Norfolk: Historic Southern Port

NORFOLK

HISTORIC SOUTHERN PORT

by THOMAS J. WERTENBAKER

SECOND EDITION   *Edited by* MARVIN W. SCHLEGEL

Durham, North Carolina DUKE UNIVERSITY PRESS

Preface

If we are to understand the history of any city, not only must we trace its origin and its development, but we must explain the causes which brought about its origin, and affected favorably or adversely its development. The history of Norfolk is much more than a series of anecdotes of interesting events and interesting people; it is an important chapter in the story of the rise of the American nation. Norfolk's part in the early tobacco trade, in the West India trade, in the Revolutionary War, in the creation of the Constitution, in the difficulties with England and France during the Napoleonic wars, in the War of 1812, in the era of internal improvements, in the Civil War, and in the World War is too important to be neglected.

American investigators have been slow to recognize the fact that national history is founded on local history, and so have left local history largely to the antiquarian and the genealogist. There are hundreds of volumes devoted to the history of this city or that county, which are moulding unnoticed on the library shelves, because they are devoted exclusively to unimportant details of local life. Although historians are becoming conscious of their neglect in this matter, the local history which shows the relationship of the community with state and national history is still comparatively rare.

In this volume the emphasis is placed on the first two centuries of Norfolk's history. Although the period from 1880 to 1930 has been treated in outline, no attempt has been made to give in detail the political, social, and industrial development. The lack of historical perspective, the difficulty of securing private letters and documents, and the impropriety of writing critically of living persons, make contemporary history exceedingly difficult. So the concluding chapters have been inserted more as a sequel to the main body of the story, than as an integral part of the history itself.

The author extends his thanks to Mr. Robert B. Tunstall, who has sponsored the work from the first, and rendered invaluable assistance; to Mr. Louis I. Jaffé and Mr. John B. Jenkins, Jr., who, together with

Mr. Tunstall, have read the manuscript throughout and aided with helpful criticisms and suggestions; to Mr. John D. Gordan, who made available the scrapbook of Miss Virginia Gordan, together with other source material; to Colonel William Couper, of Lexington, Va., who entrusted to me a set of transcripts of the letters of his great-grandfather, William Couper, of Norfolk; to Miss Mary D. Pretlow, who made available all the source material of the Norfolk Public Library; and to Miss Josephine Johnson, who contributed interesting data concerning the cultural activities of Norfolk.

THOMAS J. WERTENBAKER

Princeton, N. J.
March 24, 1931

Editor's Note

When illness unfortunately interrupted Professor Wertenbaker in the task of revising and expanding the first edition of this work, the editor agreed to try to complete the book as Professor Wertenbaker had intended. The editor has written parts of the last two chapters and has rewritten several pages in the earlier chapters in the light of new information that has appeared in the thirty years since the first edition was published. Except for occasional minor editorial alterations, the rest of the book remains as Professor Wertenbaker wrote it.

Had his health permitted, Professor Wertenbaker would have expressed here his appreciation to his daughter-in-law, Mrs. Thomas J. Wertenbaker, Jr., who furnished valuable secretarial assistance while he was working on this edition; to the Virginia State Library, which made available its microfilm of the *Virginian-Pilot* for use in the Firestone Library at Princeton; and doubtless to many others, whose names are unknown to the editor. The editor himself is grateful to Sandra Clements, who helped to prepare the manuscript for the press, and to those who read the book and offered useful comments and suggestions, including Rogers Dey Whichard, of the Norfolk Division of the College of William and Mary, Virginia H. Pinkerton, of the Norfolk Public Library, City Attorney Leonard H. Davis, and especially City Manager Thomas F. Maxwell, who co-operated at every stage of this project. Colonel E. Griffith Dodson made available his remarkable memory of the Norfolk of his youth to clear up some confused points and has also faithfully read the proofs of this edition. These all share in whatever credit this new edition may deserve, but the editor, along with the author, is responsible for whatever faults may be found with it.

MARVIN W. SCHLEGEL

Farmville, Virginia
November 10, 1960

Contents

ONE. *Colonial Days and Colonial Ways*   3

TWO. *Down to the Sea in Ships*   27

THREE. *The Maelstrom of Revolution*   48

FOUR. *The Phoenix of the Elizabeth*   74

FIVE. *Coercion—Peaceful and Otherwise*   95

SIX. *The Town and Its People*   116

SEVEN. *Strangled Commerce*   145

EIGHT. *The Fall Line Blockade*   166

NINE. *Pestilence and War*   188

TEN. *The Mailed Fist*   207

ELEVEN. *The Black Cloud*   232

TWELVE. *The New Order*   247

THIRTEEN. *A Half-Century of Growth*   271

FOURTEEN. *Mars Moulds a Great City*   300

FIFTEEN. *Peaceful Expansion*   318

SIXTEEN. *Depression and Recovery*   328

SEVENTEEN. *The Second World War*   344

EIGHTEEN. *Thinking Big*   362

NINETEEN. *Not By Bread Alone*   377

Illustrations   *following page*   214

Index   395

Norfolk: Historic Southern Port

Colonial Days and Colonial Ways

Colonial Virginia was almost entirely a rural province. From the days of the Virginia Company, when John Rolfe, celebrated as the husband of Pocahontas, discovered a satisfactory method of curing the native tobacco, the cultivation of that plant absorbed the attention of the people. From Old Point to Henrico, and from Nansemond to the Potomac, the country was dotted with fields green with the fragrant Sweetscented and Orinoco. The planters shipped their crops to Great Britain, where a part was consumed, and the rest distributed over the continent of Europe. In return they received manufactured goods— clothing, household utensils, furniture, guns, farm implements. This traffic would have necessitated one or more ocean ports, had not the many great rivers, deep creeks, and inlets made it possible for the seagoing vessels of the day to penetrate to all parts of the settled area. Every important planter had his own wharf, from which he shipped his tobacco and received his annual consignment of European goods. "No country is better watered," wrote the Reverend Hugh Jones, in 1722, "for the conveniency of which most houses are built near some landing place; so that anything may be delivered to a gentleman there from London, Bristol, etc., with [very little] trouble and cost."[1] There was no need for ports then, until the expansion of the settlements beyond deep water brought into existence the Fall Line towns.

This system, so convenient for the planter, was viewed with disfavor by the British government. Early in the seventeenth century, Governor Francis Wyatt was instructed "to draw tradesmen and handi-

---

[1] Hugh Jones, *The Present State of Virginia* (New York, reprint by Sabine, 1865), p. 34.

craftmen into towns." In 1662 the Assembly, at the command of
Charles II, passed an act, for the erection of a town at "James City,"
where all the tobacco of the three nearest counties was to be brought
for storing and export.[2] But the attempt to create a town for which
there was no need met with the failure it deserved, and the houses
were "not made habitable, but fell down before they were finished."[3]

Nonetheless, Charles persisted. In June, 1680, Governor Culpeper
announced to the Assembly that His Majesty had commanded him to
urge a measure for creating towns in Virginia. No other nation has
ever begun a colony without them, he added, and no colony has ever
thrived until they developed. Therefore, the King "is resolved as soon
as storehouses and conveniencies can be provided, to prohibit ships
trading here to load or unload but at certain fixed places."[4] Accordingly an act was passed requiring feoffees in each county to purchase
fifty acres of land for a town. For Lower Norfolk the site selected was
"on Nicholas Wise his land on the Eastern Branch on Elizabeth River
at the entrance of the branch."[5] The price was fixed by the Assembly
at ten thousand pounds of tobacco and cask. It was provided that the
town be divided into lots of one-half acre each, to be granted to such
persons as would build a dwelling or warehouse and pay the nominal
sum of one hundred pounds of tobacco.[6]

The Lower Norfolk County Court was prompt in carrying out the
provisions of this law. On August 18, 1680, it ordered the county surveyor, John Ferebee, to locate the prescribed fifty acres on October 7.[7]
The site surveyed by Ferebee was in modern terms approximately
the area lying between City Hall Avenue on the north and Water
Street on the south, bounded on the west by the Elizabeth River and
on the east by the Norfolk and Western Railroad tracks. Land-fills have
so altered the boundaries of the area that its original shape is no
longer discernible. Still, if one can imagine the Back Creek extending
from the river along the west end of City Hall Avenue as far inland
as Cumberland Street, and Newton's Creek stretching north from the
Eastern Branch at the east end of Main Street and sending one long

  [2] W. W. Hening, *Virginia Statutes at Large* (Philadelphia, 1823), II, 172.
  [3] *Virginia Magazine of History and Biography*, II, 387.
  [4] *Ibid.*, XVI, 364.
  [5] Hening, *Statutes at Large*, II, 472.
  [6] *Ibid.*, p. 474.
  [7] *Lower Norfolk County Records*, Order Book, cited in Rogers Dey Whichard,
  The History of Lower Tidewater Virginia (New York: Lewis Historical Publishing
  Company, 1959, 3 vols.) I, 328. This painstaking work, the most recent study of
  Norfolk's history, has furnished the basis for a number of revisions in the new edition of this volume.

arm over the east end of City Hall Avenue to Fenchurch Street, one can gain some conception of this narrow peninsula of woodland and old fields, lying on the northern bank of the Eastern Branch and connected to the land farther north only by a narrow isthmus.

A year after the initial survey Ferebee laid out the streets and divided the land into fifty-one lots.[8] He ran the Main Street the length of the peninsula in the east-west direction, bending it—just as it still bent in 1960—to conform to the shoreline as it then existed in order to make lots of reasonably equal size on each side of the street. Running south from the Main Street was a "street that leadeth down to the waterside" (today Commercial Place), while a "street that leadeth into the woods" (now Church Street) was laid out on the neck of land to the north. The only other street in the original plan was the Back Street, which ran north over present East Street and then turned east on what is now Bermuda Street.

In spite of the fact that the act establishing the town was vetoed by the king in 1681, the county court went ahead with its plans. Lieutenant Colonel Anthony Lawson and Captain William Robinson, appointed feoffees by the court, purchased the tract from Nicholas Wise on August 16, 1682, and proceeded to grant lots. At least one of the grantees, a sailor named Peter Smith, fulfilled the necessary provisions by constructing a house upon his land, since he received formal title to three lots on October 17, 1683, and the record states that he was then living on this land. The prospects of the town apparently were not sufficiently inviting to persuade the other grantees to build, as the next recorded grant did not come until August 17, 1687, when William Porten, the county clerk, acquired title to six lots.[9]

The town's growth began in 1691 when the legislature separated Lower Norfolk County into Norfolk and Princess Anne counties and directed that a new courthouse should be erected at Norfolk town. At that time, according to an act of the Assembly, there were "several dwelling houses and warehouses already built" there. Work on the courthouse was begun in the summer of 1691, and the structure was completed by 1694, along with the necessary public stocks and, presumably, a prison. Norfolk's first bridge was built in 1691 by Captain William Knott, the ferryman, across an arm of Newton's Creek lying on "the street that leadeth into the woods," by now promoted by the

---

[8] See the map drafted by Whichard, I, 327.

[9] *Lower Norfolk County Records*, Book 4, p. 153; *Norfolk County Records*, Book 5, p. 35, cited in Whichard, *The History of Lower Tidewater Virginia*, I, 331.

advance of civilization to "the street that leadeth out of town" (today
the intersection of Church and Charlotte streets) .[10]

These improvements caused the infant town to grow rapidly during
the 1690's. A patient search of the early records has revealed the
names of more than thirty lot-owners before 1700. Among them were
Captain William Knott, a blacksmith named Bartholomew Clarke, Dr.
Thomas Tabor, who was a merchant as well as a physician, Malachi
Thruston, Fergus Thompson, Samuel Sizemore, John Redwood, George
Newton, Francis Simpson, Thomas Walke, William Heslett, Peter
Blake, Thomas Butt, Lewis Conner, John and Matthew Godfrey,
Samuel Boush, Mary and Thomas Hodges, Israel Voss, Thomas Nash,
Edward Moseley, Captain John Dibbs, and Cornelius Tully. By the
end of the century the parish was building its first church in the pres-
ent churchyard, and Captain Samuel Boush had a silver chalice made
in London for the communion service (now preserved in the Norfolk Museum) .[11]

As the town continued to increase in population, the rest of the un-
granted lots were taken up, the last one, a narrow strip on the south
side of eastern Main Street, going to Samuel Boush, son of the chalice
donor, in 1729. Boush had already taken steps to provide room for
future expansion by laying out in lots his land on the west side of what
would soon be called Church Street; Norfolk's first suburban development was opened in April, 1728.[12] In the same year Boush, along with
Samuel Smith and Nathaniel Newton, took the first step to provide
formal education in the town by becoming school trustees with authority to build a schoolhouse on the school lot across the street from
the church and to hire a schoolmaster.[13]

By 1740 a visitor to Norfolk would have seen, as he sailed up the
river, a town of perhaps one thousand people. Along the waterfront
was a line of low-lying warehouses, behind them a mass of trees, from
which emerged here and there a gable-end, or a chimney. Upon landing he would have noted the peculiar structure of the wharves. "They
lay down long pine logs," William Byrd tells us, "that reach from the
shore to the edge of the channel. These are bound fast together by
crosspieces notched into them. . . . A wharf built thus will stand several years, in spite of the worm, which bites there very much."[14] Main

[10] *Ibid.*, I, 335-337.
[11] *Ibid.*, I, 337-340.
[12] *Ibid.*, I, 343, 353.
[13] *Ibid.*, I, 350.
[14] William Byrd, *History of the Dividing Line* (Richmond, 1866. All references to
this title are from this edition) , pp. 19-20.

Street our visitor would have found a muddy thoroughfare, lined with shops, residences, taverns, warehouses, and workshops. Here he would have seen a smithy, here a barber shop, here a shoe shop, here a cooperage. The houses were chiefly of brick,[15] were of one, or perhaps two, stories, and had chimneys at each end. The front door opened upon a hallway, flanked on one side by the withdrawing room, and on the other by the dining room. Above were several chambers.[16] The furniture was meager, but charming in design—a pair of mahogany or walnut dining tables, a bureau with a desk top, a dozen chairs with leather seats, beds, chests, a mirror, a clock.[17] In the rear was the garden, invariably enclosed with palings, while in the earlier days orchards were not uncommon. As in other parts of Virginia, the kitchen occupied a separate building, so that the food had to be brought through the yard to the dining room.[18] Around the dwellings of the well-to-do were often grouped other outbuildings—smokehouse, hen house, and stable.[19]

The stranger would have been interested in the new market house, at the north end of what is now Commercial Place. This was a frame structure, thirty feet long and fifteen wide. On either side the roof, which was overset six feet to give shelter to the vendors, was supported by four sturdy posts. Here the country people came with their poultry, eggs, butter, and vegetables; here the housewife haggled for a few pounds of beef or a peck or two of turnip-tops.[20] Other points of interest were the old Norfolk county courthouse, on the north side of Main Street,[21] the schoolhouse, and the new borough church, then but a year old.

The act of 1680 under which Norfolk was founded, made no provision for a municipal government. The residents of the Wise peninsula were under the jurisdiction of the county court. There was no mayor, no town council, no town court. If the people wished to establish a night watch, or light the streets, or put in a town pump, it was to the county justices that they had to appeal. An attempt was made to give Norfolk a government of its own in 1705, when an act of the General Assembly provided for the incorporation of towns which

---

[15] *Virginia Magazine of History and Biography*, XXIII, 407-414; *Norfolk County Deed Book*, H, p. 201.
[16] *Norfolk Herald*, Jan. 7, 1835.
[17] *Ibid.; Norfolk County Deed Book*, F, p. 103.
[18] *Norfolk County Deed Book*, H, p. 201; No. 12, p. 130.
[19] *Ibid.*, H, p. 201.
[20] *Norfolk Council Orders*, 1736-1798, p. 2b.
[21] The borough courthouse was erected later. In 1754 the council appointed "a committee to apply to Edward Travis to know his terms for his land . . . to build the said Court House on." *Ibid.*, p. 30b.

reached a population of thirty families. Although Norfolk could have complied with these terms, the act was suspended by the crown in 1710 before the town had established a separate government.[22]

At the end of the first third of the century, however, Norfolk had grown so large that a separate authority to manage its affairs was necessary. So the inhabitants petitioned the King, asking for letters patent to incorporate the town and the suburbs to Town Bridge into a borough. The place is commodious for trade and navigation, they pointed out, and "of late years" has been "very greatly increased in the number of inhabitants and buildings," so that many persons "have seated themselves upon the adjoining land." His Majesty issued his letters patent for the Charter on September 15, 1736. It authorized the establishing of a local government, "consisting of a mayor, one person learned in the law styled and bearing the office of recorder of the said borough, eight aldermen, and sixteen other persons to be common-councilmen."[23] Power was granted for the appointment of constables, surveyors, and other officers, for regulating trade, supervising buildings and streets, erecting prisons, and inflicting penalties. The town was to be represented in the colonial Assembly by one burgess, elected by freeholders, persons owning personal property to the amount of £50, or other housekeepers who had served five years at a trade. Provision was also made for the establishment of a court of hustings and a court of record, and for the holding of fairs.[24]

Governor Gooch appointed Samuel Boush, a prosperous merchant and landowner, as the first mayor. The recorder was Sir John Randolph, perhaps the most distinguished person then residing in Virginia. When he visited Norfolk to take office, the people seized the opportunity to celebrate the inauguration of their new government. "The gentlemen of the said town and neighborhood showed him all imaginable respect, by displaying the colors, and firing guns of the vessels lying there, and entertained him at their houses in the most elegant manner for several days, amply signalizing their great respect on this joyful occasion."[25]

The new borough also honored another official, the surveyor general of customs, Robert Dinwiddie, by making him an honorary citizen, and in gratitude Dinwiddie in 1741 gave the town a seal. Twelve years later, when Dinwiddie had returned to Virginia as lieutenant-

[22] Hening, *Virginia Statutes at Large,* III, 404-419.
[23] *Ibid.,* IV, 541.
[24] *Ibid.*
[25] *Virginia Gazette,* Nov. 26, 1736.

governor, he again showed his affection for the town by ordering the
London silversmith, Fuller White, to make the borough a mace, which
was presented to the council on April 1, 1754. This mace, still proudly
preserved by the city, is the only surviving bit of municipal regalia
from the colonial period.[26]

One of the problems facing the new municipal government was the
condition of the streets. A visitor to Norfolk at the end of the eighteenth century tells us that the streets were narrow, irregular, unpaved,
dirty, and poorly drained.[27] It is certain that they were not better in
1736. It is easy to picture the carts from the near-by farms, jolting over
the ruts of Church Street, and the merchants and artisans picking their
way around the mud puddles of Main. In July, 1749, the council made
Mr. Ebenezer Stevens surveyor of streets, and instructed him to "begin
to repair the same from the Town Bridge." He received permission
to "hire as many negroes as he shall think proper," and provision was
made to pay for the work by means of a tax on "every master or
mistress of a family" in the borough.[28] How unsatisfactory this work
was may be judged from the appointment of a committee to consider
"where dirt may be had to repair the streets."[29] That the borough
"fathers" were not unmindful of sanitary regulations is shown by a
"bye-law to prevent filth and so forth being hove into the streets."[30]
Nor was early Norfolk without its traffic problems. In 1755 ordinances
were passed "to prevent mischiefs from unruly horses, and oxen in
carts and wagons, and to prevent the running and training of horses
in the streets."[31] If any servant or slave rode a horse in town "faster
than a foot pace," his master was to be fined 2s. 6d.[32]

The first Norfolk police force was established in 1738, the council
passing a resolution "that a watch be kept in this town, by six or eight
watchmen," to serve at a salary of £40 each.[33] This system was so great
a drain on the town finances, however, that it was soon abandoned,
and the citizens were forced to take turns in going the rounds at
night. The presence of large numbers of sailors and Negroes was responsible for many of the "sundry robberies, insults, and disturbances,"

26 Whichard, *History of Lower Tidewater Virginia*, I, 377, 380. Benjamin Franklin
was also made an honorary citizen when he visited Norfolk in 1756 (*ibid.*, I, 380-
383).
27 Isaac Weld, *Travels in North America* (London, 1807), I, 172.
28 *Norfolk Council Orders*, 1736-1798, pp. 21b, 22.
29 *Ibid.*, p. 21b. Getting dirt has always been a difficult problem in Norfolk.
30 *Ibid.*, p. 49.
31 *Ibid.*, p. 30b.
32 *Ibid.*, p. 10b.
33 *Ibid.* p. 7a.

and made some kind of police protection necessary. Four persons kept watch at a time, going on duty at eight, and continuing until five the next morning. In case of "riot or the watch being assaulted," they were to fire three guns, one after the other, upon which every good citizen was to jump out of bed, and seizing his gun, rush to their assistance.[34] This service proved so onerous that at least one citizen, a certain John Pedrick, refused to do his part. But a fine of five shillings brought him to reason, and he was soon patrolling the streets, with gun in one hand and lantern in the other.[35] From time to time the council tried to re-establish the system of salaried police, but with no permanent success,[36] and so late as April, 1775, the citizens were still taking turns at the watch.[37]

The frequent assembling of Negroes "at unreasonable hours at night, and on the Lord's day" was a source of some alarm. So, in 1719, the county court instructed one Daniel Philips "to inspect into such meetings," and after arresting any Negro abroad after 9 P.M. without a certificate, to administer to him twenty-one lashes at the whipping post.[38] In 1741 the town council took steps to prevent the sale of intoxicating liquors to Negroes, for when drunk they were apt to be insolent and incorrigible.[39] Much of this trouble arose no doubt from the hiring of slaves for work at the wharves. When ships were loading or unloading, these men were kept busy rolling on barrels of tobacco or pork, or heaving off boxes of European goods or casks of rum and sugar. But at other times, they were prone to get into mischief. And for serious misconduct the penalty was apt to be severe. In 1717 a slave named Jack was lodged in jail for stealing some cloth from his master, and when he escaped was recaptured and put on trial for his life. He pleaded benefit of clergy; but as it was established that he could not read,[40] he was condemned to be hanged. The most frequent punishment for an offending slave was a severe lashing. The county court recorded one case in which a Negro received thirty-five lashes on the bare back, well laid on, for stealing a hoe.[41]

Yet the slave was not the only one to feel the severity of the colonial law. Even the most respected white citizen might incur a fine by ab-

[34] *Ibid.*, pp. 13b, 14.
[35] *Ibid.*, p. 18b.
[36] *Ibid.*, p. 52b.
[37] *Ibid.*, p. 69b.
[38] *Norfolk County Deed Book*, No. 10, p. 12.
[39] *Norfolk Council Orders*, 1736-1798, p. 10b.
[40] *Norfolk County Deed Book*, No. 9, p. 90.
[41] *Ibid.*, p. 122.

senting himself from church;[42] the good wife who gossiped too much might have to atone on the ducking stool. The first ducking stool in the town seems to have been erected in 1716, "at the upper end of the town, at the end of Major Samuel Boush's wharf, good and substantial."[43] "This machine was a chair fixed on the end of a long shaft, projected over the water from the town end of the county wharf," we learn from the reminiscences of an old man in 1835. "The offender was lashed to the chair. On a given signal the shaft was tipped and she was soused, until a promise of better behavior caused a halt."[44] In those days swearing was a costly matter, for a fine of five shillings was fixed for each oath. When James Spaulding ripped out ten oaths, he was fined fifty shillings. This man, a most undesirable character, was convicted of "beating, battering, cursing, swearing and drunkenness."[45] James Toomoth and his wife Mary constituted a pair of ne'er-do-wells, for the man was fined "for being a common drunkard," and Mary "for swearing five oaths and being drunk."

For many years there was no town jail, offenders being confined in the county jail. This building, an irregular structure about forty-five by thirty feet, stood beside the old county courthouse, on the north side of Main Street at the head of Market Square.[46] In 1747 the Council decided to erect a borough prison, situated "upon the public ground," probably the present Nebraska Street. However, the project had to be postponed until the Assembly granted permission to the town to levy a tax to defray the cost of construction,[47] and it was only in 1753 that work was actually begun. The building was "32 feet long, 16 feet wide, and eight feet pitch in the clear," with "three rooms, and a brick stack of chimneys."[48]

The people suffered much from the lack of good water. From the days of William Byrd to those of La Rochefoucauld, it was a common complaint of visitors that the water was brackish and unpalatable. When the first lots were laid out, the common source of water was the public spring, located at a point 110 feet north of Main, and 185 west of Church Street, and here the Negro maids must have congregated daily with their buckets to dip out the family supply.[49] For wash-

[42] *Ibid.*, p. 103.
[43] *Ibid.*, p. 161.
[44] *Norfolk Beacon*, Jan. 7, 1835.
[45] *Norfolk County Deed Book*, No. 9, p. 213.
[46] See map of Capt. Thomas Talbot's property, made in 1765.
[47] Hening, *Statutes at Large*, VI, 264-265.
[48] *Norfolk Council Orders*, 1736-1737, p. 25b.
[49] *Norfolk County Deed Book*, 1695-1703, pp. 15, 16.

ing clothes, everyone was forced to resort to the water of the river, "the place appointed for the public laving" being in the eastern end of the town.[50] How long this condition lasted it is impossible to say. No doubt some of the more prosperous citizens sunk wells in their yards at a very early date; but there seems to have been no system of public pumps until more than half a century after the founding of the town. In 1751 the council ordered the clerk of the borough to advertise on the door of the church and of the courthouse that bids would be received for four wells. They were to be twelve feet deep, five feet in diameter, to be lined with brick, and covered with two-inch plank. The pumps were to be of pine, with spouts, caps, and iron handles. One was placed near the market house, one near Captain Tucker's store, one near Captain Tatum's, and one on the schoolhouse land.[51] From time to time these wells were repaired and equipped with new and better pumps. In 1765 a well ten feet in diameter was dug on Charlotte Street, near Town Bridge, and another of the same size on the school land.[52] The people of Norfolk had the free use of these wells, but masters of ships who took on a supply of water had to pay for it.

There was never any difficulty in securing water in Norfolk in case of fire, for the people had only to form a bucket brigade, stretching from the burning house to the river, and the supply was inexhaustible. We have few records of fires in colonial Norfolk, and apparently there was no counterpart of the disastrous series of conflagrations which marked the years from 1780 to 1825. Yet one of the first acts of the council, after the inauguration of the borough government, was to order a fine of five shillings for any person "whose chimney shall blaise out." They also placed a prohibitive tax of five shillings a month on all wooden chimneys.[53] Just when the first fire engine was purchased is uncertain, but that more than one were in use in 1753 is indicated by the payment of £8 16s. to "John Jones for cleaning and repairing the water engines."[54] Three years later a shed was added to the borough prison "for the reception of the fire engines."[55] Apparently these machines soon became inadequate or out of date, for in 1763 the council ordered of Messrs. Ennes & Hope, of London, "one fire engine com-

[50] *Ibid.*, No. 6.
[51] *Norfolk Council Orders*, 1736-1798, p. 23b.
[52] *Ibid.*, p. 53.
[53] *Ibid.*, p. 3.
[54] *Ibid.*, p. 26.
[55] *Ibid.*, p. 35b.

plete of the value of about £60." An additional £40 was spent for "buckets and other utensils."[56]

Norfolk, because of its position as a seaport, was scourged by recurring epidemics. Yellow fever, so fatal during the nineteenth century, seems to have been an infrequent visitor, but smallpox was a constant source of terror. From time to time the council tried to establish a quarantine, but with doubtful success.[57] In 1744, when certain sailors from a West Indian vessel infected with the disease had taken lodgings in town, the councilmen ordered them to move at once, either back to their ship, or to some isolated house in the suburbs.[58] Two years later the unwelcome news spread that another vessel had come in with smallpox. The council at once set aside the glebe, then occupied by the Reverend Charles Smith, "as an infirmary or reception house" and engaged nurses and other attendants. "And," added the council, "all masters of ships, sloops, and other craft are not at their peril to land any infected person within this borough."[59]

The practice of inoculating persons with smallpox of a mild character, in order to render them immune to the disease in its more virulent forms, was introduced into New England early in the eighteenth century. It was only in 1768, however, that the Norfolk physicians began to experiment with it. Their first efforts gave rise to a violent controversy, some persons applauding their efforts, others claiming that they were merely spreading the disease to those who otherwise would escape.[60] The dispute spread to other communities, and waxed so hot that the colonial Assembly was forced to take action. In 1769 it passed an act prohibiting inoculation save in special cases, and under strict supervision. "Whereas the wanton introduction of the small pox into this colony by innoculation, when the same was not necessary, hath, of late years, proved a nuisance to several neighborhoods, by disturbing the peace and quietness of many of his Majesty's subjects, and exposing their lives to the infection of that mortal distemper," the importation of "small pox, or any variolous or infectious matter of the said distemper" is forbidden.[61]

One of the first practicing physicians of Norfolk was William Miller, who resided on the south side of Main Street east of Church.[62] That

[56] *Ibid.*, p. 47.
[57] *Ibid.*, pp. 12, 12b.
[58] *Ibid.*
[59] *Ibid.*, p. 17b.
[60] *Virginia Gazette*, March 5, 1772.
[61] Hening, *Statutes at Large*, VIII, 371, 372.
[62] *Norfolk County Deed Book*, No. 8, p. 41; No. 9, p. 289.

the life of the colonial doctor was not easy is indicated by a suit brought by Miller in 1715, against Mr. Anthony Walke "for £6 10s., for curing a negro's leg," and for medicines used during the illness of Walke's child. The defendant declared that "he never agreed to pay £5 for curing the negro's leg, and that to his judgment and appearance, the said negro's leg was never cured nor made whole." In the end the justices cut the doctor's bill to £1 10s., and ordered Walke to pay him that amount "for visits, physick, and attendance."[63] Other physicians, practicing in or near Norfolk in the colonial period, were "William Hunter, chyrurgeon, of Princess Anne";[64] William Happer, who was a member of the town council in 1742;[65] Calvin Campbell, who died in 1774;[66] George Ramsey, Alexander Gordon, and D. W. McClurg.

As in other parts of the colonies, social distinctions in Norfolk were sharply drawn. Merchants, men of independent means, the clergy, and other professional men constituted the first class; ship carpenters, coopers, turners, and other skilled artisans made up a highly respected second class; day laborers and indentured workers were grouped in a third class; while free Negroes and slaves formed the fourth.[67] Many of the merchants were men of ability and wealth. The original settlers, of course, came from England or the British West Indies, and the merchants of early Norfolk bear distinctly English names, such as Boush, Tucker, Taylor, Smith, and Newton. But in later years, just prior to the Revolution, many Scotchmen moved in, attracted by the advantages for trade. Between these two factions not only was there keen business rivalry, but a political division as well. On election days the Scotch party wore badges of orange, the English of "true blue." Each established headquarters at Market Square, where punch and grog were ladled out free by the workers. All bets were decided at the tavern over a bowl of hot punch and jelly.[68]

The prosperous Norfolk merchant enjoyed all the luxuries that the age afforded. His home was commodious; his table set with choice food; from England he imported clothes of the latest fashion, from Spain and Madeira the finest wines; and his slaves relieved his family of the drudgery of household work. We gain an insight into the do-

[63] *Ibid.*, No. 9, p. 119.
[64] *Ibid.*, p. 214.
[65] *Norfolk Council Orders, 1736-1798*, p. 6b.
[66] *Virginia Gazette*, Aug. 4, 1774.
[67] *Norfolk Herald*, Jan. 7, 1835.
[68] *Ibid.*

mestic economy of these men from the inventory of Robert Tucker, drawn up in 1723. His residence consisted of an entry, hall, parlor, and three chambers. There was also a kitchen apart from the main house, with a chamber above. In the hall were twelve leather chairs, three tables, a couch, a clock, a mirror, a case of drawers, four large maps, twenty-nine pictures, fire tongs, shovel, bellows, and fender. In the chambers were beds, cane chairs, chests of drawers, tables, trunks, pictures, tongs, shovels. The kitchen, the real workshop of this old home, contained two pairs of snuffers and stands, a copper chocolate pot, a coffee pot, one brass mortar and pestle, a warming pan, three spits, two dripping pans, two "aquam vittae morters," two skimmers, two ladles, two gridirons, a fender, four iron boxes, two tables, four iron pots, seven pairs of pothooks, four racks, four brass kettles, two iron hooks, one pair of tongs and fire shovel, one stew pan, and one pair of iron dogs. The pewter in the kitchen consisted of twenty-four dishes, three dozen plates, thirteen soup plates, six basins, one porringer, one bed pan, one cheese dish, two plate warmers, three chafing dishes, one teakettle and stand, one saucepan, two skillets, and a candlestick. Mr. Tucker had fifty-seven pieces of plate, presumably of silver, weighing more than twenty-three pounds; his cash on hand reached the surprising figure of £6664, Virginia currency; his Negroes numbered twenty-three; his vessels consisted of one brigantine, three sloops, and three flats.[69]

One of the most prosperous landowners of Norfolk in the days prior to the Revolution was Captain Thomas Talbot. This gentleman opened a street running north and south from Main to Back Creek through his property near the county courthouse. Although this street was but twenty-six feet wide, it led to a bridge over Back Creek, and became one of the most important thoroughfares in town. Here Captain Talbot erected a number of dwellings, which he leased to some of the leading citizens.[70] From the Talbot holdings we gain a very clear picture of Norfolk on the eve of its destruction in 1776. There was a brick store next to the county jail, on the northwest corner of Main and Talbot streets, thirty-eight feet by twenty-six feet, with three rooms below and three above. The windows of the store and of the cellar were fitted with iron bars. Some distance back of this structure was a warehouse, forty-five feet by twenty feet. Near by was another brick

[69] *Norfolk County Deed Book*, Vol. F, p. 103.
[70] W. S. Forrest, *Sketches of Norfolk* (Philadelphia, 1853), pp. 66, 67; Hening, *Statutes at Large*, VIII, 454.

building, sixty-one feet by twenty-five feet, with a room at one end
used as a store, two other rooms on the ground floor, and three rooms
above. The cellar contained three rooms, while a separate building
twenty feet by sixteen was used as a kitchen. Another brick structure
fifty feet by thirty feet served as a residence for two families. It had
"three rooms below and three above stairs at each end compleat, with
kitchen, cow-house, smokehouse for each." Near-by was a commodious
house with two rooms and a passage below, two rooms on the second
floor, and two in the garret. On the first floor were six 18-light and
four 12-light windows, on the second eight 12-light windows. In the
basement were the kitchen and two other rooms. In addition there
were other buildings—a wooden dwelling, thirty-seven feet by twenty-
five, two double houses of brick, together with stables, gardens, etc.
The entire group was valued at £3,308.[71]

Ranking next to the merchants in wealth and influence was the
large group of mariners. It was inevitable that in a seaport, where
ships were constantly arriving and leaving for foreign parts, many
young men would feel the lure of the seafaring life. Not all who
entered this profession were of humble parentage, for now and then a
Calvert, a Tucker, a Maxwell, or a Hutchings took service on a West
India merchantman. Among those who received compensation from
the state for the destruction of their property in the fires of 1776 were
thirty-five persons listed as mariners, some of them having extensive
holdings. James Maxwell owned five houses, valued at £757; Christopher Calvert, eleven houses at £1,102; Wright Wescott, five houses
on Catharine Street at £988; Paul Proby, ten houses on Bermuda
Street at £882; James Dawson, ten houses at £894; and Thomas Price,
six houses on Main Street at £638.[72] Some of the very first settlers in
Norfolk were men of the sea. Captain William Knott, "marriner,"
owned two lots, one on the south side of Main in the west end of
town, where he built his home, and another opposite on the north
side of the street. He seems to have been a well-to-do and influential
citizen.[73]

More numerous than the group of masters and sea captains were the
common sailors. So early as 1728, William Byrd tells us, the town was
provided with "sailors enough to manage their navigation."[74] Some
were married and had humble homes on the back streets; others were

[71] William H. Stewart, *History of Norfolk County* (Chicago, 1902), pp. 55, 56.
[72] *Ibid.,* pp. 363-367.
[73] *Norfolk County Deed Book,* 1685-1695, p. 187.
[74] Byrd, *History of the Dividing Line,* pp. 19, 20.

single, and when on shore, lived at one of the less pretentious ordinaries. In 1807, when the Cape Cod skipper, Elijah Cobb, was in need of men for his vessel, he went the rounds of the "sailors' boarding houses," signed up a crew, and paid "the advance to their landlords."[75] La Rochefoucauld, who visited Norfolk in 1796, says that the place housed many sea captains and sailors, so that Virginia could man her own vessels, and in this respect was not dependent upon the Northern states as were Georgia and the Carolinas.[76]

The fact that so many skilled sailors made Norfolk their headquarters did not escape the attention of the famous press gangs of the Royal Navy. In 1767 Captain Jeremiah Morgan, of the sloop-of-war *Hornet,* being short of men, decided to recruit them by force in Norfolk. So he rowed up to the county wharf in an armed tender one night at eleven o'clock, and landed thirty seamen. After refreshing themselves with "a cheerful glass" at a near-by tavern, the party marched off "to that part of town where seamen resorted to." Here they aroused the keepers of the various lodginghouses, and with oaths and threats, forced them to open the doors. A few of the sleepy tars resisted when they were pulled out of bed, but they were promptly subdued by a rap on the head, dragged downstairs and hustled through the streets to the tender. In the meanwhile the night watch had given the alarm and the people came tumbling out, partly clothed, to see what the disturbance was about. A crowd, headed by Paul Loyall, formerly mayor of Norfolk, seeing the press gang with their victims, charged boldly in among them. Morgan was so infuriated at this interference that he lunged at Loyall with his sword, and ordered his men to fire. But the citizens crowded so closely upon the sailors that they could not use their arms, and in the end not only did they lose their prisoners, but several of their own number were dragged off to jail.[77]

Rural Virginia was almost devoid of an independent artisan class. It is true that many skilled workers came to the colony, but they found it difficult to maintain themselves by their trades. So the carpenter dropped his saw, the shoemaker his adz, the bricklayer his trowel, to take up the hoe or the plow. If some few stuck to their trades, they demanded extravagant rates, and few employed them but out of pure necessity.[78] The planters frequently had to train their indentured workers and slaves as artisans, and every large estate had its carpenter,

[75] Elijah Cobb, *A Cape Cod Skipper* (New Haven, 1925), p. 64.
[76] La Rochefoucauld, *Voyages dans les États-Unis* (Paris, 1799), IV, 271.
[77] *Virginia Gazette,* Oct. 1, 1767.
[78] *Virginia Magazine of History and Biography,* IV, 267.

its cooper, its blacksmith, its shoemaker, its tanner.[79] But in Norfolk conditions were different. The artisan class was large, independent, prosperous, and the Norfolk ship carpenter or tanner had a place in the community hardly less important than that of his fellow worker of Hingham or Barnstable. Among the house owners of Norfolk in 1776 were seventeen carpenters, six ship carpenters, four bricklayers, four tanners, four blacksmiths, three blockmakers, three bakers, three silversmiths, three joiners, two sailmakers, two shoemakers, a watchmaker, a coppersmith, a cooper, a wheelwright, a tallow-chandler, a saddler, and a hatter.[80] Wages were exceptionally high. The four shillings and one pint of rum paid each ship carpenter for a day's work in refitting the ship *Phaeton* seems insignificant today, but in 1759 it provided a very respectable living. Many a Virginia clergyman wished that his income was as large.[81] The artisan group in Norfolk was recruited by the usual method of apprenticing youths to established tradesmen. In 1714 Joseph Mercer was bound to Thomas Mercer, who agreed to teach him "the trade and mystery of weaver," and undertook to instruct him in reading and writing.[82] When one Francis Brown abused his apprentice, Alexander Ross, the court transferred the latter to Thomas Nash, Jr., who contracted to bring him up to the trade of cooper.[83]

Conspicuous in the life of colonial Norfolk were the many ordinaries, or taverns. Here the weary trader just in from North Carolina sought bed and food, here the workman came at noon for a small beer, here the sparks of the town danced or gamed under the inspiration of a bowl of punch, here the idle congregated to hear the latest news of the war in Canada or the closing of Boston harbor. Among the first tavern keepers were Mrs. Ann Coverley, Peter Malbone, John Loftland, Thomas Cretcher, John Gay, Richard Josslin, Grace Powell, and Thomas Walker. The life of these good people was by no means easy, for competition was severe, prices low, and the complaints of patrons frequent. In 1717 all the innkeepers were brought before the county court, charged with using false measures. Fortunately they were able to submit their measures to the justices, who decided that they were all correct and true.[84] But poor Mrs. Coverley had to answer

[79] Jones, *The Present State of Virginia*, p. 36.
[80] Stewart, *History of Norfolk County*, pp. 363-367.
[81] Grenlees and Hardie, *Ledger*, p. 52a, Office of Corporation Court of Norfolk.
[82] *Norfolk County Deed Book*, No. 9, p. 118.
[83] *Ibid.*, p. 149.
[84] *Ibid.*, pp. 189-194.

the additional charge of "not being provided with stablidge and pasturage" for guests. There was little opportunity for the innkeeper to overcharge his patrons, for all prices were strictly regulated by the court. Rum retailed at six shillings a gallon, "punch if made good" at 16*d.* a quart, cider at 12*d.* a gallon, small beer at 7½*d.* a gallon, Madeira at 22½*d.* a quart, milk punch at 7½*d.* a gallon, claret at 3*s.* 3½*d.* a quart. For "dyat" the guest paid 3*d.* 3 farthings a meal, for "housing and foderadge for 24 hours 6*d.*," with 6*d.* a gallon extra for corn and oats for his horse.[85]

On one occasion a drinking party at Richard Josslin's tavern had so tragic an ending that all concerned were hauled into court. Samuel Rogers, Nathaniel Newton, James Hustings, and Henry Jenkins were having a gay time over a bowl of sangaree, when a certain William Finiken entered. "Come in, Mr. Finiken," they called to him, "you are as welcome as a prince." As the newcomer was noted as a dancer, they sent for a violin, and while one of the others played, he danced several jigs, pausing frequently, no doubt, for visits to the punch bowl. Then Finiken and Rogers began a game of cards called All-fours, in which Rogers won several bowls of sangaree. After this they began a friendly tussle, falling down and rolling over on the heavily sanded floor. After a pause they began this mock fighting again, and Finiken was thrown violently backward on the floor. The others lifted him to a bed, cut his neckcloth so that he could breathe freely, and after finding that his pulse was normal, left him to sleep off the effects of the sangaree. The next morning he was dead.[86]

The event of the year in Norfolk was the fair, held in Market Square. Here the merchants displayed their best wares; here the country people brought in their choicest cattle, corn, wheat, fruit, and poultry; here the court of pie-poudre, established under the charter, held its sessions. The fair was marked always by various kinds of contests. First came pole climbing. A well-greased pole was set up in the center of the square, with a gold-laced hat on top, and he whose skill in climbing was great enough to enable him to reach it, could claim the prize as his own. Usually, after others had failed, some nimble sailor boy would clamber up with ease. Next, three or four young girls would race for a fine Holland chemise. Following this event, pigs with greased tails were released in the crowd, with the announcement that they would belong to any who could catch them by the tail and

[85] *Ibid.*, p. 114.
[86] *Ibid.*, p. 163.

hold on. The "scuffling, jostling, and upsetting" which followed were received with shouts of glee. The sack race also caused great merriment. Sometimes there would be bull-baiting, accompanied by a general scamper to the roofs of houses bordering on the square.[87]

The presence of many young naval officers, who visited the town on merchantmen and warships, added much to the gaiety of social life. "My father was very hospitable and used to entertain all the strangers of any note that came among us," says one Norfolk lady in her reminiscences, "and especially the captains and officers of the British navy." One fifty-gun ship came in, with "thirty-two midshipmen on board, mostly boys and lads of good families, and several of them sprigs of nobility. They used to come to my father's house at all hours, and frequently dined with us. Sometimes, too, they would go into the kitchen to get a little something to stay their appetites. Of course I had many beaux who flattered me and danced with me, and one or two, who loved me and would have married me if I would have said yes. My father was fond of good living, and kept a famous cook—poor old Quashabee—who made the best soups, sauces, gravies, and all such things in the world. . . . [Father] was particularly fond of arrack punch, and always kept his silver tankard by him, holding about three pints, which he would empty two or three times a day till the doctors began to be afraid that he would fall into a lethargy and limited him to a single one."[88]

We gain an even more vivid picture of social life in Norfolk from a description of Governor Dunmore's visit to the town, in the days before the Revolution. "It so happened then . . . that my Lord and Lady Dunmore, and their family, came to pay a visit to Norfolk, and our people turned out to receive them in style. Indeed you never saw such a fuss as we made. For then, you know, we were all royalists, all the King's subjects, (tho' we were beginning to feel a little mannish about our rights) and we thought we couldn't do too much to honor our guests. So among other thing, we made 'em a grand ball at the old Masons Hall, and all the gentry of our town were there of course. And besides we had sent off an express to Princess Anne for Colonel Mosley, who was reckoned the finest gentleman we had, to come to town with his famous wig and shining buckles, to dance the minuet with my Lady, for our poor mayor, Captain Abyvon, was afraid to venture upon such a thing. And then we had all the British navy officers,

[87] *Norfolk Herald*, Jan. 7, 1835.
[88] *Lower Norfolk County Antiquary*, I, 97.

Captain Montague, and the rest, with their heads powdered, as white as they could be. What was best of all, all our pretty girls, far and near, came out to grace the scene. . . . So, by and by, the fiddles struck up, and there went my Lady Dunmore in the minuet, sailing about the room in her great, fine hoop-petticoat (her new fashioned air balloon as I called it) and Colonel Mosley after her, wig and all. Bless her heart, how cleverly she managed her hoop,—now this way, now that—everybody was delighted.

"Then came the reels, and here the Norfolk lads and lassies turned in with all their hearts and heels. This was my cue, and I led out my sweetheart, Nancy Wimble, in my best style, resolved to show all the sprigs of nobility what we Buckskins could do. In fact I believe I cut some wonderful capers sure enough—for I heard the young British dogs tittering one side. . . . As for Nancy, I am sure she might have danced before the Queen. It is true, she hadn't a hoop then; but she didn't want one to set her off. A young Cockney, a marine officer, who was there in his red coat, got quite smit with her . . . and talked with her about London, the King, and all such nonsense, and danced with her every time. . . . I soon found that she thought him worth two of me. . . . Then she took to reading novels, and got a new hoop petticoat to make her a lady, and began to study what she should say when she came to stand before the King."[89]

Although such distinguished guests came seldom to this little seaport town, the monotony of daily life was occasionally broken by grand celebrations in honor of the coronation of a new king or of some notable British victory. On July 23, 1746, Norfolk celebrated the defeat of the Young Pretender at Culloden. A procession wound through the streets headed by three drummers, a piper, three violinists, six men with rods and sashes, and a nurse carrying a warming pan from which peeped the head of a child, symbolizing the alleged illegitimate circumstances of the Old Pretender's birth. Next came a cart with a figure representing the Stuart claimant seated in a chair. Behind marched six men with drawn cutlasses, followed by a long line of people from the town and surrounding country. Finally the procession came to a halt, and the effigy was hanged amid the firing of salutes and the drinking of toasts. That night the town was illuminated, and the celebration was brought to an end with a brilliant ball.[90]

The presence in town of foreign sailors, a not infrequent occurrence,

[89] *Ibid.*, V, 32-35.
[90] Forrest, *Sketches of Norfolk*, p. 65.

sometimes led to excitement of a very different kind. In November, 1762, a British transport, on its way to Cádiz, with a part of the captured garrison of Havana, put in for repairs. Don Pedro Bermudez, a naval officer, with his family and attendants, together with one hundred and nineteen Spanish soldiers and sailors were disembarked. It so happened that the British vessel *Arundel* was in port, and some of her crew got into an altercation with the foreigners in the streets of Portsmouth. The Spaniards, who had no arms, fled to their lodginghouse, but the English fired in the windows, killing one man and wounding several others, and then set fire to the building. They also broke into the residence where Don Pedro was staying, and subjected him to a severe beating. Captain Wainwaring of the *Arundel* finally dispersed his enraged sailors, and, with the appearance of the Norfolk militia, restored quiet.[91]

These occasional scenes of violence did not mean that the religious life of the community was being neglected. In Norfolk, as in the rest of colonial Virginia, the Church of England was established by law. When the town was laid out, it remained part of Elizabeth River parish, which covered the same area as Norfolk County. By 1700 the parish church, like the courthouse, had been moved to the town, where it was built on the lot set aside for it at the time of the initial survey on the west side of what soon became known as Church Street.[92] Because of the loss of the vestry records prior to 1749 nothing is known of this church except that it was made of brick.

About the time that Norfolk was incorporated as a borough, the vestry seems to have decided that a new building was needed, and the church now known as St. Paul's was erected in another part of the churchyard lot in 1739. The date fortunately is preserved because the builder worked it into the wall of the south transept, where it can still be seen. Underneath the date are the initials, "S. B.," presumably for the first Samuel Boush, donor of the original chalice for the old church. Tradition has it that he donated the land, but this is improbable, since the parish already owned the churchyard. It is more likely that he promised the bricks for the church, as there is evidence that he owned a brickyard.[93]

Although the vestry had the power to levy taxes, it had difficulty in collecting enough money to maintain the church, as is apparent from

[91] Charles Stuart to Governor Fauquier, Nov. 23, 1762. Transcript in Library of Congress.
[92] Whichard, *History of Lower Tidewater Virginia*, I, 340.
[93] *Ibid.*, I, 384-385.

the surviving records. All through the 1750's the vestry hoped to build a wall around the churchyard but failed to obtain enough money, partly because the funds had to be devoted to repairing the chapel at Great Bridge and to rebuilding the poorhouse, which had to be kept up by the vestry. A greater disfigurement to the churchyard than the lack of a wall was the condition of the original church, which for years had been falling into neglected ruin. In 1750 the vestry attempted to convert the old building into a schoolhouse by offering "the Bricks and Timbers of the old church" to James Pasteur, parish clerk and schoolmaster, on the condition that he use them to build a house on the school lot on the other side of the street. This plan came to nothing, and ten years later the vestry gave Joseph Mitchell "the Bricks &c of the Old Church on condition that he clears the churchyard of all the Rubish. . . ."[94] It is to be hoped that Mitchell finally cleared away the ruins of the old church twenty years after it had been abandoned. We do not know, since the surviving records of the colonial vestry end in 1761.

The names of many of the ministers who served the Norfolk church have been recovered from other sources, but the list is necessarily fragmentary. The first minister to serve the church in town was probably the Reverend William Rudd, who was in the Elizabeth River parish in 1702. He was followed by Roger Kelsall, who died in 1709. The following year Governor Alexander Spotswood assigned James McMoran to the parish, and he served until his death four years later. James Falconer is the only known minister during the next ten years, and his stay was brief, but there must have been other ministers, as Robert Tucker gave a communion service to the church in 1722, and the service would have been useless without an ordained minister in the parish. In 1724 a clergyman with a Spanish name, John Garcia, arrived to stay for three years. When William Byrd visited Norfolk in 1728, he found John Marsden conducting the service and reported that the sermon was good; unfortunately, Marsden was not, for he departed suddenly, leaving a large sum in bad debts behind him. Marsden was succeeded by Moses Robertson, who was followed by Charles Smith about 1743. Smith remained in Norfolk until 1761, when the parts of the county south and east of the Elizabeth River were split off into separate parishes and Smith became rector of the Portsmouth parish. Alexander Rhonnald and Thomas Davis served as ministers of the Norfolk church between 1761 and the Revolution. The division

[94] *Ibid.*, I, 388-389.

of the parish required the sale of the glebe land, which had been farmed for the benefit of the minister, and, instead of buying a new glebe, the Norfolk vestry acquired four town lots to help support the rector.[95]

The earlier ministers probably also served as schoolmasters, since it was the custom in the eighteenth century for the minister to conduct an informal school for the parish children. As soon as the parish could afford it, the vestry generally hired a parish clerk to take over this duty of the minister, along with other ministerial duties such as keeping the records and digging the graves in the churchyard. The earliest known clerk-schoolmaster was James Pasteur, who held the post in 1750 and is said to have begun teaching in Norfolk as early as 1739.[96]

Since the parish school was limited to the elementary "three R's," the people of Norfolk attempted to set up a more advanced Grammar School, where boys could learn Latin and Greek as a preparation for college. In 1752 the General Assembly authorized the county court and the borough council jointly to hire a schoolmaster and establish a Grammar School on the still vacant schoolhouse lot. James Pasteur may have held this post, but the first recorded master of the Grammar School was Richard Collinson, who was examined on January 1, 1756, by the president and masters of the College of William and Mary, as required by law, and "thought capable of teaching the Grammar School at Norfolk." Inevitable differences of opinion between the county court and the borough council over the appointment of schoolmasters and other problems led to a new act in 1762, vesting sole control of the Grammar School in the borough council. The law incidentally mentioned that a schoolhouse had at last been built on the schoolhouse lot, thus fixing the date of the first school building as before 1762, most likely in 1761.[97]

The Grammar School, of course, was intended only for boys, and even the parish elementary school was apparently exclusively masculine. Girls, however, were able to obtain an education suitable to their abilities at one of the private schools in the town. One of these Norfolk girls, Mrs. Maxwell, recalled in her later years: "I was put to school to a poor dame by the name of Mrs. Drudge, and, to be sure, she did drudge to teach me my letters—spelling and reading after a fashion. . . . She taught me, good soul, to read the Bible and the

[95] *Ibid.*, I, 347-349, 385, 390-391.
[96] *Ibid.*, I, 393.
[97] *Ibid.*, I, 393-395.

stories in it pleased me greatly. . . . After I had learned out here, I was sent to a Mrs. Johnson. . . . She taught me needlework, and marking on a sampler. After this as I was shooting up, my father . . . wished to send me to a fashionable boarding school that there was then in Williamsburg. . . . Shortly after Donald Campbell imported a school master from Scotland, by the name of Buchan, who opened a select school, and I was sent to him to learn the higher branches of English, French, or Spanish."[98] Perhaps Mr. Campbell was related to the Mrs. Susanna Campbell who inserted an advertisement in the *Virginia Gazette* of August 4, 1774. "Mrs. Campbell begs leave to inform the ladies, that she has taken a house near the church, and intends opening a boarding and day school for young ladies . . . where those who will please to favor her with the care of their children, may depend upon the strictest attention."[99]

Such was Norfolk during the colonial period. The town—a busy seaport in an agricultural colony—was a thing apart from the rest of Virginia. Its people were Virginians, it is true, yet they had in many ways more in common with Boston or Philadelphia than with the planters of the James or the York. Although they rivaled the landed aristocracy in wealth, built substantial houses fitted with handsome furniture and costly plate, surrounded themselves with slaves, adhered to the Anglican Church, and acquired a certain degree of breadth and culture, there were essential differences. They were first of all practical, keen businessmen, lacking the taste for political life, the urge for study, and the philosophical view, which the plantation system fostered in their neighbors. Norfolk produced no Washington, no Jefferson, no Madison.

When William Byrd visited the place in 1728, he felt himself in such strange surroundings that in his *Dividing Line* he describes it with the same interest he would have shown in a town of Spain or Turkey. And had George Washington stopped there in 1775, his impressions would have been similar. The life of the town would have seemed strange and unfamiliar—the shipping in the river, the crowded warehouses, the wharves piled high with boxes and barrels, the throngs in the streets, the foreign goods in the shops. The fact that Norfolk was a mercantile town in an agricultural province made her position somewhat perilous. She had no great clash of interests with the ruling planter aristocracy in the colonial period, but such a clash might come

---

[98] *Lower Norfolk County Antiquary,* II, 24, 25.
[99] *Ibid.,* V, 72.

at any moment, and then, outvoted ten to one, she would be helpless. It was this separateness of interest which was largely responsible for the destruction of the town in 1776, and which many decades later produced state legislation so hostile that she seriously considered annexation to North Carolina.

CHAPTER TWO

Down to the Sea
in Ships

The founders of Norfolk selected a site admirably suited for trade. To the north lay Chesapeake Bay, stretching two hundred miles through eastern Virginia and Maryland to the borders of Pennsylvania. Within a few miles were the mouths of the James and the York, while the Potomac could be reached with a good breeze in less than a day. It seemed certain that the products of the region drained by these great inland waterways would pour into Norfolk, there to be reshipped to foreign parts. Yet Norfolk did not come into being as the port of the Chesapeake Bay country. Long after it had become a thriving town the tobacco ships, whether from St. Mary's, the York, or the James, sailed out past Cape Charles or Cape Henry, without so much as a glance in her direction. Since every plantation had its own wharf, where ocean-going vessels could tie up, a port of reshipment was not needed. So the English merchantmen went from river to river, from creek to creek, disposing of their cargoes of European goods, and taking on the hogsheads of Sweetscented and Orinoco. Not until the third or fourth decade of the eighteenth century, when the increasing size of ships made it difficult to ascend and descend the winding rivers, was a large part of the commerce of eastern Virginia concentrated at Norfolk.

The trade of Elizabeth River itself was fairly extensive, however, even in the seventeenth century, and to this the village fell heir. In colonial days the agricultural output of Norfolk and Princess Anne counties was not large. Tobacco, the basis of wealth in other parts of the colony, could not be produced to perfection in the sandy soil

which covers so much of this region, and the day of truck gardening
was far in the future. Here and there patches of the familiar green
leaves would be seen, side by side with fields of wheat and Indian
corn, but the plantations yielded at best but a moderate living. So
late as 1796, so Rochefoucauld tells us, the shores and river banks
were still covered with pine forests.[1]

But these very woods provided the chief source of income. A century
before La Rochefoucauld visited Norfolk, Edward Randolph reported
to the British government that pitch and tar were produced in considerable quantities on the branches of the Elizabeth River.[2] The industry was carried on by poor men who built their kilns unassisted by
servants or slaves, and considered a few dozen barrels a year an excellent output. The tar-burner first laid down a circular floor of clay.
Upon this he piled pine logs, covered them with a coat of earth and
ignited them through a small opening left for that purpose. This
was then closed and the fire left to smoulder. As the tar trickled down
upon the clay floor, it was drained off into barrels by an inclined
wooden pipe. If the burner decided to convert his tar into pitch, he
boiled it in large kettles, or burned it in holes made in the clay. To
secure a supply of turpentine he was put to considerably less trouble.
Going from pine to pine, he made a series of slashes, beginning as
high as he could reach and continuing to a point near the ground, so
connected as to drain off the turpentine to a bucket at the bottom.[3]

The tar-burner usually established himself upon a navigable stream
or inlet, within easy reach of Norfolk. When he had accumulated a
fair supply, he rolled his barrels on board a flat-bottomed boat or a
shallop, hoisted sail, and set off to market.[4] Before sundown his tar, or
pitch, or turpentine was reposing on one of the Norfolk wharves, and
he was busily reloading with calico, nails, an axe, a saw, a kettle, stockings, shoes, or other needed articles from the merchant's store. Perhaps
he would return with goods worth twice as much as his little cargo,

[1] *Voyages dans les États-Unis*, IV, 254.
[2] Prince Society, *Publications* (Boston, 1865-1911), XVI, 478.
[3] J. F. D. Smyth, *A Tour of the United States*, II (Dublin, 1784), 95-97. Smyth's
account was written in 1784, but there is every reason to believe that the processes
he describes were identical with those employed a century earlier. In 1742 a law was
passed to prevent frauds in this industry. "The burners and sellers of tar, pitch, and
turpentine were guilty of mixing them with sand, shavings, brick bats and such
trash."
[4] It is probable that Norfolk merchants often provided the vessels in which the
tar, pitch, and turpentine were brought to their wharves. With few exceptions the
inventories of all the larger dealers show one or more small boats (*Norfolk County
Deed Book*, H, pp. 28-31, 95, 96, 155-163).

for the Norfolk merchants were liberal in granting credit. Not infrequently he brought home a goodly sized cask of West Indian rum; in which case the merchant might have to sue for his money, for when the rum flowed freely, the tar-kiln was apt to go out and the turpentine trees go untended.[5]

If the tar-burner had on his property cypress and oak trees, he might add to his income by cutting plank and shingles. For this some capital was necessary, for he had to have horses and cart wheels for moving the timber, one or more Negroes to handle it, and axes, whipsaws, and "cutting mills" for sawing it into boards.[6] But when once the work was done, he was sure of a good return. One-inch oak plank brought nearly six shillings the hundred foot,[7] and good cypress or juniper shingles nine shillings a thousand.[8]

The proximity of the Great Dismal Swamp made the timber supply almost inexhaustible. This wilderness, lying south of Norfolk, stretched from the south branch of the Elizabeth River to the Pasquotank, in North Carolina. Here bears, wolves, wildcats, raccoons, and foxes lived under the great trees, protected from the huntsman by the marshy nature of the ground and the impenetrable undergrowth. If once a runaway slave reached the swamp, he was fairly safe from pursuit, for few masters would follow him through the half-hidden paths, where a misstep might mean death.[9] The country people for many years took timber from its borders without molestation. William Byrd, when he visited the swamp to run the dividing line between Virginia and North Carolina, remarked upon their boldness. "They get boards, shingles, and other lumber out of it in great abundance," he wrote, making "bold with the King's lands thereabouts without the least ceremony."[10]

The great swamp was used also as a free feeding ground for cattle and hogs.[11] One would secure from the county court an official mark or

[5] Mr. Matthew Godfrey was among those having extensive dealings with neighboring tar-burners. In 1716 and 1717 we find him suing successively William Maund for five barrels of tar, Walter Carling for seven barrels, and Owen Jones for nine barrels (*Norfolk County Deed Book*, No. 9, pp. 159, 168, 172, from rear).

[6] The inventory of Mrs. Ann Tatum, in 1744, showed one pair of cart wheels and chain, several whipsaws, one cutting mill, three wedges, and several thousand feet of plank (*Norfolk County Deed Book*, H, p. 116).

[7] *Ibid.*

[8] Grenlees and Hardie, *Ledger*, p. 11.

[9] Johann D. Schoepf, *Travels in the Confederation* (Philadelphia, 1911), pp. 99, 100.

[10] Byrd, *History of the Dividing Line*, pp. 19-20.

[11] *Ibid.*

brand, place it upon the stock, and turn them loose to feed.[12] At the proper seasons one would slaughter his cows and hogs, provided they could be found in the wilderness of trees and bushes, salt the meat, and pack it in barrels for market. Frequently one man would carry on simultaneously the trades of tar-burner, stock raiser, and wood cutter.[13] Partly because of this diversification of interest, partly because the proximity of the Dismal Swamp made it difficult to keep slaves, the herds were always narrowly limited in number.[14]

But had Norfolk been the mart for the adjacent counties only, it would have remained always a village. It owed its first real growth to the geography of eastern North Carolina. The settlers who moved into the marshy region south of the Virginia line found themselves upon a land-locked sea. Albemarle and Pamlico Sounds, each stretching far into the interior, the shores broken by innumerable bays and river mouths, are admirably suited for inland trade. But from Princess Anne to Cape Lookout they could be entered from the Atlantic at a few inlets only, and these were often clogged by shifting sand bars. Roanoke inlet was the best for Roanoke Sound, but even it was impassable for all save a "very few vessels and of small burden."[15] From Edenton, at the mouth of the Chowan River, vessels had to make the long detour to Ocracoke inlet.[16] So the North Carolinians, in seeking a market for their goods, were forced to take them overland to Norfolk, or to load them on light sailing vessels and bring them around by way of Cape Henry. In this way began the close commercial relations between the town and North Carolina, which, continuing to the present day, have contributed so much to its development.

In the infancy of the colony the ocean route from Carolina to Vir-

[12] In 1716 Mr. Lemuel Langley obtained an official mark for his stock, which was to be cut on the ears (*Norfolk County Deed Book*, No. 9, p. 152).

[13] There are cases in which Norfolk merchants sued one of these woodsmen for tar, shingles or plank, and salted meat, which had been contracted for but not delivered. In 1717 Walter Curling was ordered by the court to pay Matthew Godfrey forty-eight pounds of pork, seven barrels of tar, and 2,800 cypress shingles (*Ibid.*, p. 168, from rear).

[14] The inventory of John Corfrew, in 1746, showed 21 cattle, 23 sheep, and 188 hogs; that of Mrs. Elizabeth Holstead, 38 cattle, 96 hogs, and 26 sheep; that of Mrs. Ann Tatum, 11 hogs, 19 cattle, and 26 sheep (*Norfolk County Deed Book*, H, pp. 116, 196, 199).

[15] *Colonial Records of North Carolina*, IV, 169. Edward Moseley (on his *New and Correct Map of North Carolina*, published in 1733) states that Roanoke inlet had 10 feet at low tide. Currituck inlet, Hatteras inlet, and New inlet, he declares to be fit only for small sloops or shallops.

[16] "You have at Ocracock Bar 12 fathoms at low water in the range of the beacons." (Moseley, *New and Correct Map of North Carolina*.) In 1759 the schooner *Dolphin*, on its way to Virginia with pork and corn, stuck on the bar several times in coming through one of these inlets (Grenlees and Hardie, *Ledger*, p. 60).

ginia was used almost exclusively, for the roads were then impassable. Often they were little more than trails, difficult to find, cut by creeks and rivers, and clogged with mud.[17] The settlers built their homes on the water's edge, so that large vessels could tie up at their private wharves. Those who lived but a mile or two back often found it impossible to get their products down to the public landings when rain had made the "wayes too deep."[18] If the settler's land was situated up some shallow creek, he would bring his barrels of pork and tar in canoes or piraguas, down under the overhanging trees, to transfer them to vessels sturdy enough to make the dangerous voyage around to Norfolk. The sloop which took on its cargo in the Perquimans River, or at the mouth of the Chowan, if it got safely down Albemarle Sound and turned Powell's Point, might run aground on one of the islands of Currituck Sound, or stick on the sand bars in passing through Currituck inlet. Once out in the waters of the Atlantic, it must scurry along at full speed, over the thirty-five miles to Cape Henry, for fear a sudden squall would bring disaster. At that point the skipper could breathe more easily, for the remainder of the voyage to Hampton Roads and up the Elizabeth was comparatively safe.

As he approached the cluster of dwellings and storehouses which marked the early town, he headed for the wharf of the merchant to whom his cargo was consigned. If his goods had yet to be disposed of, he anchored in the river, and rowed ashore to bargain with prospective purchasers. This procedure was not likely to last long, for the demand for Carolina wares was always good. Before the day was done, the schooner would be tied up at the wharf, while sweating slaves rolled the goods ashore and into the merchant's warehouse. Some of the barrels were filled with salted pork or beef, some with Indian corn, some with tar or pitch; here were packages of beans and peas, here butter and cheese, here a bundle of hides, here boxes of beeswax and myrtle wax.[19] If the skipper, before leaving Carolina, had touched at some remote landing, far from the eyes of spying customs collectors, he probably had taken on a few hundred pounds of tobacco, without paying the duty of one penny a pound demanded of the intercolonial trade.

After the crew had regaled themselves with rum or small beer at Mrs. Coverley's ordinary, had wandered through the shops of Main

---

[17] *Colonial Records of North Carolina* (Raleigh, 1884), I, 616, 708, 715.
[18] *North Carolina Historical Review*, III, 25.
[19] *Colonial Records of North Carolina*, III, pp. xv-xviii, 621.

Street, and perhaps gotten into a brawl with the English sailors down at the county wharf, they began the work of taking on the return cargo. First came a dozen casks of Jamaica rum, then two or three hogsheads of sugar or molasses; next the men brought aboard great packages of European goods—coarse linens and woolens, hatchets, nails, scissors, hoes, axes, files, kettles, skillets, bedding, pewter, hats, shoes, clothing, guns and powder.[20] If space were left, a few slaves, newly imported from Guinea, might be taken on for sale to the Albemarle farmers.[21] At last, when all was ready, the hatches were battened down, the ropes cast loose, sails hoisted, and the return voyage begun.

In the early years of the eighteenth century this budding trade was threatened by a nest of pirates, led by Captain Teach, commonly known as Blackbeard. This rascal gathered a desperate crew, armed several sloops, and, making his headquarters near Ocracoke inlet, preyed upon incoming and outgoing vessels, or even darted out into the Atlantic to capture an occasional West Indian.[22] This was a serious matter for Norfolk, for the pirates soon created such terror in the Albemarle country that only the boldest skippers dared venture out.

The North Carolina traders appealed to Governor Spotswood, of Virginia, for protection, pointing out that their own government was too weak to grapple with Teach's band. It so happened that two British war vessels, the *Pearle* and the *Lyme,* sent, no doubt, to convoy the Chesapeake tobacco fleet to Great Britain, were lying in Virginia waters. Since they drew too much water to follow Teach into the shallows of Albemarle and Pamlico, the governor drafted fifty-five of the seamen, placed them on board two armed sloops, hired pilots, and sent them off for the Carolina coast. As they approached Ocracoke inlet, they saw Blackbeard's flag waving over a sloop armed with eight guns. Realizing that his end was at hand, the pirate "took up a bowl of liquor," "drank damnation to everyone that should give or ask quarter," and let loose a broadside. Although twenty of the King's men had fallen, the sloops came alongside, and a desperate hand-to-hand fight ensued, which ended only when all the desperadoes had been killed or disabled. Teach had stationed a Negro near the powder magazine with orders to blow up the sloop if the enemy captured it, but a prisoner, left in the hold the night before, overcame him before he

[20] *Ibid.,* VI, 968.
[21] *Ibid.,* IV, 61.
[22] On one occasion Teach brought in a ship with a cargo of sugar and cocoa. Landing the goods at a remote inlet, he applied the torch to the vessel (Public Record Office, London, CO5-1318, No. 4).

could apply the torch. Teach himself was killed, with nine of his men, while nine others, all severely wounded, were taken.[23] When the news of this engagement spread throughout the Albemarle and Pamlico region, the praises of Spotswood resounded in every home. But nowhere was the rejoicing greater than at Norfolk, for the breaking up of the pirate nest at Ocracoke meant the reappearance of Carolina sloops in Elizabeth River, and Carolina goods in the local warehouses.

In the meanwhile, with improved roads a brisk land trade had sprung up between North Carolina and Virginia. There were two main highways leading from northeastern Carolina to Norfolk, one on each side of the Dismal Swamp. Beginning at Edenton, the first went due north through the Chowan precinct, skirted the swamp on the west, and reached the Nansemond near the site of Suffolk.[24] From that point to Norfolk the road had to make a sweeping detour, passing around the head of the Western Branch, touching the northern edge of Dismal Swamp, passing over the upper reaches of the Southern Branch at Great Bridge, then turning northeast to Kemps, thence around the Eastern Branch and Broad Creek by way of Newton's Creek, to enter Norfolk from the north on Church Street. For persons on horseback, or on foot, a much shorter route was available. After leaving the Nansemond River they could turn off to the left, and following the road to Sayer's Point, at the mouth of the Western Branch, ferry over to Norfolk. Another route ran from the headwaters of the Western Branch to Crawford's Point, on the site of Portsmouth, thence by ferry to the county wharf near the market. Major Samuel Boush was running both ferries in 1715, receiving three thousand pounds of tobacco annually for his services.[25] The Assembly fixed the fee, whether for passengers or horses, at 6d.[26] Isaac Weld, who visited Norfolk in 1795, states that to cross the Virginia ferries was "a most irksome piece of business." "There is not one in six where the boats are good and well manned, and it is necessary to employ great circumspection in order to guard against accidents. . . . I heard of numberless instances of horses being drowned, killed, and having their legs broken, by getting in and out of boats."[27]

The second route from North Carolina, like the first, began at Edenton. From that point it ran northeast to cross the Perquimans

[23] *Ibid.*
[24] Moseley, *New and Correct Map of North Carolina.*
[25] *Norfolk County Deed Book,* No. 9, p. 108, from rear.
[26] Hening, *Statutes at Large,* VI, 14.
[27] Weld, *Travels through North America,* I, 169.

River at Vewby's ferry, thence through Pasquotank precinct, and over the Pasquotank River at Sawyer's ferry, touched the northern part of Currituck precinct, and then proceeded north to Great Bridge,[28] where it joined the road from the west side of the swamp. In the early days the North West River, because of the swampy nature of the adjacent ground, proved a serious obstacle. But in 1719 the inhabitants of Currituck at their own expense threw a bridge over the stream, at "Samuel Ballance's old landing."[29] The Norfolk county authorities were careful to keep these arteries of trade in good repair, appointing surveyors for the various districts,[30] inspecting bridges, and fining citizens who neglected to work their allotted days on the "King's road."[31]

The scene at Great Bridge, where the routes from both sides of the Dismal Swamp converged, must have been an interesting one.[32] Here there were two long causeways across the marshy ground on either side of the Southern Branch, connected by a wooden bridge over the stream itself. On the southern causeway where were clustered warehouses and a wharf or two, one could see two-wheeled carts from the Dismal Swamp, or the Poscaty region, or even from Currituck, unloading their barrels of tar, turpentine or pitch, or their bundles of shingles, or hogsheads of tobacco.[33] Beside the wharves a number of small vessels took on their cargoes, or prepared for the trip up the crooked Southern Branch to town. From the bridge itself came the clatter of hundreds of hoofs as the Carolina herdsmen drove across their cattle, or sheep, or hogs, on the way to the Norfolk slaughterhouses. Some were from the Currituck, others from Chowan, still others, no doubt, from the Roanoke River, eighty miles away. It was computed by Governor Barrington in 1733 that fifty thousand fat hogs, almost the whole number of fatted oxen in Albemarle county, and many horses, cows and calves, were driven into Virginia annually.[34] That most of these found their way to Norfolk is certain, as it was the only town in eastern Virginia worthy of the name.[35] When the herds reached Norfolk, they were driven to the slaughterhouses, probably on the outskirts of the town, where they were butchered.[36] The Carolinians com-

[28] Moseley, *New and Correct Map of North Carolina.*
[29] *Norfolk County Deed Book,* No. 10, p. 78a, from rear.
[30] *Ibid.,* No. 9, p. 156.
[31] *Ibid.,* p. 125.
[32] Byrd, *History of the Dividing Line,* p. 19.
[33] Jarvis Manuscript, Library of Congress, pp. 14-18.
[34] *Colonial Records of North Carolina,* III, 621.
[35] Suffolk was laid out as a town only in 1742, and Portsmouth ten years later. Hening, *Statutes at Large,* V, 199; VI, 265.
[36] *Norfolk Council Orders,* 1736-98, p. 216.

plained loudly of the lowness of prices. "He receives pay only for the meat after it is slaughtered," it was said. "For the hide, tallow, etc., the butcher pays him nothing. The same is the case with hogs. They are taken to Virginia, slaughtered, salted up, and exported and sold as Virginia pork."[37] The complaints of the North Carolina tobacco growers were also bitter. Our tobacco is generally taken to Norfolk, wrote Bishop Spangenberg, in 1752, where "it is examined by the inspectors . . . all that is merchantable is selected—the remainder is burnt. The Virginia merchants . . . pay the Carolina farmers what they please for their tobacco."[38]

So it was in very bad humor that the Carolinian, whether cattle-raiser or tobacco grower, made his purchases for the return journey. We may imagine him, picking his way through the mud of Main Street to visit the shops, or bidding for slaves at the market on the wharves. If he has left his cart at Great Bridge, he loads his purchases, whether Negroes or European manufactured goods, upon a hired boat, and starts off up the Southern Branch. If he has come on horseback, driving stock from Chowan or Perquimans, he reduces the distance by taking the ferry to Sayer's Point.

In 1733 Governor Barrington estimated Virginia's imports from Carolina, including hogs, cattle, pork, tar, pitch, tobacco, deerskins, beaver furs, hides, tallow, wax, feathers, beef, butter and cheese, at £50,000.[39] This trade not only supplied Norfolk merchants with goods for exportation and opened a market for their imports, but it gave life to many local employments. The Carolinians filled the ordinaries,[40] kept the butchers busy, and patronized the local shopkeepers. It was they whom the coopers had to thank for the steady demand for barrels,[41] the skinwrights for their hides,[42] the candlemakers for their tallow.[43]

The Carolina goods did not remain long on the Norfolk wharves, for a ready market was at hand. The mouth of the Chesapeake was considerably closer to the West Indies than was New England, and far closer than Great Britain. The Norfolk schooners could go all the way to Barbados, or Nevis, or Antigua and back, while a sugar ship was making the long passage to Glasgow or Bristol. Since, too, the islands

[37] *Colonial Records of North Carolina*, V, 1.
[38] *Ibid.*
[39] *Ibid.*, III, 621.
[40] *Norfolk County Deed Book*, No. 9, p. 114, from rear.
[41] *Ibid.*, No. 12, p. 329.
[42] *Ibid.*, p. 320.
[43] Public Record Office, London, Gooch to Board of Trade, 1742.

needed Norfolk wares, and the Norfolk merchants found it easy to dispose of the West Indian sugar, molasses, and rum, an interchange was inevitable. So early as 1697 Governor Andros reported that the Virginians were exporting to Barbados pork, beef, corn, staves, and a little tobacco.[44] However, in those early days of her history Norfolk had to compete with the New Englanders for the carrying trade from Virginia to the West Indies. The enterprising Yankees swarmed in the Virginia rivers and creeks, bartering off West Indian goods for corn, beans, bacon, and even live hogs.[45] In 1740 the *Orataro,* from Rhode Island, sailed for Virginia from Barbados, with a cargo of rum, molasses, and brown sugar, which she sought to exchange for wheat, corn, beeswax, leather, pork, beef, and staves.[46]

The Northerners were unpopular in Virginia not only because of their close bargaining, but because of their trading with the slaves for stolen goods.[47] This, together with the advantages of direct commerce to the West Indies in Virginia-built vessels, gradually made their visits less frequent,[48] and in 1739 we find William Byrd warning the Virginia merchants to do nothing to bring the Yankees "again amongst us."[49] That they did come back from time to time is vouched for by Governor Gooch, who reported to the British government in 1741 that Virginia exported to New England, "chiefly in their own vessels, which come to trade here, some pork, beef, corn, tallow, and some hides, pitch, cheese, wooden ware, and a few European goods."[50]

As the New England trade declined, that of Norfolk increased. The commerce of the Norfolk merchants "is chiefly to the West Indies," wrote William Byrd in 1728, "whither they export abundance of beef, pork, flour, and lumber. The worst of it is, they contribute much towards debauching the country by importing abundance of rum."[51] In 1742 Virginia exported to the West Indies beef and pork worth £24,-000 and corn worth £5,000, together with considerable quantities of

[44] Public Record Office, London, CO5-1359, p. 40.
[45] John J. Babson, *History of the Town of Gloucester* (Gloucester, Mass., 1860), p. 384.
[46] W. B. Weeden, *Economic and Social History of New England* (Boston, 1890), II, 906.
[47] Babson, *History of the Town of Gloucester,* p. 384.
[48] *Ibid.*
[49] *Virginia Magazine of History and Biography,* XXXVI, 359.
[50] Public Record Office, London, Gooch to Board of Trade, Aug. 6, 1741.
[51] Byrd, *History of the Dividing Line,* pp. 19-20. "A great number of vessels are fitted out there," it was stated in the *London Magazine* of July, 1746, "to trade to the northward and the West Indies."

bread, flour, hogshead and barrel staves, peas, shingles and candles,[52] taking in return "rum, sugar, molasses, money, some salt, indigo, pimento, ginger, coffee, and cocoa."[53]

The Norfolk skipper who ventured out on the Atlantic in his schooner or brigantine or ship,[54] perhaps of 150 tons, perhaps no more than 30,[55] took his life in his hands. After the Negro workmen had brought the cargo on board and the sailors had made loose from the wharf, the vessel slipped down the river with the tide. If there was a favorable breeze in Hampton Roads, she turned her prow toward the Capes, and in a few hours was out in the Atlantic. Here she tacked to the south, and with good fortune arrived four or five weeks later at St. Christopher, or Antigua, or Nevis, or Barbados. Once safely in port, the skipper set about disposing of his goods. If they had been assigned to one or more West Indian merchants, he had nothing to do but unload; but if the Norfolk exporter trusted him to find a purchaser, his difficulties would be far greater. If the New Englanders had come in ahead of him to flood the market with their provisions, he might find it necessary to hoist sail, to try his luck in another island.

Not infrequently West Indian merchants wrote to the Norfolk exporters telling the state of the market in the islands, and giving advice as to shipments. In April, 1764, Ferguson Murdock suggested to Niel Jamieson as an ideal cargo 1000 bushels of wheat, 1000 bushels of corn, 100 barrels of flour, six to eight barrels of beeswax, 40 to 45 barrels of pork, besides rice, white oak staves, pine boards, and tar.[56] In September, 1769, one of Jamieson's masters reported from Antigua that, having heard of a hurricane in San Domingo, he had visited that island with his cargo of bread, pork, flour, and corn. But upon his arrival he found that an immense quantity of provisions had come from the neighboring islands, driving prices down. Thereupon he went to Grenada, where he again met disappointment, and in the end was compelled to land his goods, and sell them himself at retail.

Usually, however, Virginia goods could be disposed of at a good

[52] "The town of Norfolk and James river have almost wholly engrossed the West Indian and grain trade," wrote Governor Fauquier in 1764. Public Record Office, London, Fauquier to the Board of Trade, Jan. 30, 1764.

[53] *Ibid.*, Gooch to the Board of Trade, 1742.

[54] Grenlees and Hardie, *Ledger*, Office of Clerk of Corporation Court of Norfolk.

[55] The schooner *Ranger*, of 40 tons, with a crew of six men, the snow *Duchess of Douglas*, sixteen men, and the brigantine *Prince of Wales*, of 120 tons burden, were active in the trade between Norfolk and the West Indies (*ibid.*).

[56] Papers of Niel Jamieson (Library of Congress), p. 701.

profit. The sugar planters needed corn, pork, bread, and peas for their slaves; lumber for building; staves, butts, and hoops for their hogsheads; pitch, tar, and turpentine for their ships.[57] If, at times, the skipper had to sell at a loss, he trusted that his return voyage would bring better luck. The Norfolk merchants gave him careful directions as to his purchases in the islands, adding at times to the usual order of rum, sugar, and molasses, instructions to take on a few boxes of limes, coffee, citron, or cocoa. Or, if the tobacco planters of the Potomac or the James were making money, he had to be on the lookout for a consignment of slaves.[58] The skippers were not overfond of the slave trade, for many of the Africans died at sea, and others were unruly. One, on a voyage from Jamaica to Norfolk with a cargo of slaves in 1761, discovered that the Negroes had been breaking into the hogsheads of rum and sugar, and also making way with the store of provisions. Fearing starvation, he had several of the captives whipped. When this had no effect, he made "an example of one of the said slaves, who was a most notorious offender, by having him hanged at the yard's end in the sight of the said slaves."[59]

In times of war the Norfolk merchants suffered severely from the depredations of privateers. The British government, when danger threatened, usually sent out a frigate or two to convoy the Chesapeake tobacco fleet and the West Indian sugar fleet across the Atlantic. But the vessels plying between the islands and the colonies on the continent had to trust to their own vigilance. During the Seven Years' War, masters often accompanied the convoy from Antigua or Nevis far out to sea, and then, turning northwest, headed for the Chesapeake. In this way they avoided the Cuban and Dominican waters, where the French and Spanish privateers were most numerous.[60]

On the return voyage, however, being unprotected, many were taken. The Norfolk owners often armed their schooners, but this did not make them a match for the privateers. It was in September, 1757, that the schooner *Catherine,* bound for Antigua with corn, pork, and lumber, sighted a sloop bearing down on her. Although she spread all

[57] The sloop *Two Friends,* bound for Antigua from Virginia in 1758, carried 100 barrels of corn, 48 barrels of pork, one hogshead of tallow, and 9,000 shingles. The sloop was valued at £530, Virginia currency, the cargo at £133. The brigantine *Jenny,* bound also for Antigua, had a cargo of 52 barrels of pork, 12 barrels of tallow, 13 casks of bread, 1,722 bushels of corn, 736 staves, and 25,000 shingles (Grenlees and Hardie, *Ledger,* pp. 11, 11a, 33).
[58] "Is there a cargo or two of slaves expected into Norfolk?" wrote one Hector Ross to Niel Jamieson, in 1766. "Some of us here would like a parcel if cheap."
[59] Grenlees and Hardie, *Ledger,* p. 109a.
[60] *Ibid.,* pp. 86, 109a, 124.

sail, the sloop crept up, and at last was close enough to open fire. The *Catherine* resisted bravely for an hour and a half, but eventually struck her colors, and was taken to Guadeloupe as a prize of war.[61] Among the vessels captured on their way from Virginia to the West Indies were the sloop *Nancy;* the sloop *Polly;* the brigantine *Jenny;* the sloop *Two Friends;* the schooner *Dinwiddie,* owned by Zachariah Hutchings, of Norfolk; the sloop *Bacca;* the schooner *Peggy;* the snow *Dutchess of Douglas;* the schooner *Ranger,* owned by John Thompson, of Virginia; the sloops *Molly, Sally, Pineapple, Kingbird,* and *Susanna;* and the schooners *Betty, Champ,* and *Dane.*[62]

The sloop *Fanny,* of 100 tons, which sailed for Barbados in 1758, was peculiarly unfortunate. Encountering a French frigate, she was overtaken and captured. After prolonged bargaining, John Anthony, the master, agreed to pay a ransom of £200, and was permitted to proceed. But Barbados was still a long way off, and the route was strewn with dangers. Once more the *Fanny* was captured, this time by a privateer, who brought her in as a prize to Guadeloupe. Anthony escaped "by stilth in the night," to report the double loss to Charles Thomas, the Norfolk owner of the sloop, but the crew long suffered in the Guadeloupe prison.[63]

The treatment of captured American sailors by the French and Spaniards was often harsh. When the Virginia sloop *Friendship,* bound for St. Christopher, was taken three leagues off the island of St. Martin's, the men were put in a long boat, and told to row ashore.[64] The crew of another captured vessel, after remaining for months in prison at Cape François, were sent to Denan Castle, in France. "Quite stripped of our clothing," they wrote, "short of provisions," disheartened by "bad usage and confinement," they despaired of getting home.[65]

The suffering was not all on one side, however, for the colonists themselves sometimes fitted out privateers to prey upon the enemy's commerce. In 1739 Governor Gooch announced in the *Virginia Gazette* that he was prepared to issue writs of marque and reprisal on the Spaniard. Upon which the editor remarked that the Virginia merchants who had so long complained of their losses now had an opportunity for revenge. "No doubt," he added, "there are men of spirit in Vir-

[61] *Ibid.* pp. 6, 6a.
[62] *Ibid.*
[63] *Ibid.,* p. 40a.
[64] *Ibid.,* p. 26a.
[65] *Ibid.,* p. 73.

ginia who will do so."[66] During the Seven Years' War a merchant named Sprowle was among those who sent out privateers from Norfolk.[67] That others followed his example is shown by the statement that at the outbreak of the Revolution Norfolk was unarmed save for "some cannon belonging to some gentlemen who had fitted out privateers in the last war."[68]

The perils of the West India trade were by no means confined to the activities of the privateers, for the skippers had to reckon also with the Atlantic storms. It was in 1760 that the schooner *Lancastershire Witch*, of Norfolk, on her way home from Jamaica, struck on the Coloradoes rocks, thirty-five leagues from Havana, and went to pieces. The crew brought off nineteen hogsheads of rum and some coffee and ginger, which they placed aboard the ship *Kingston*, bound for Philadelphia. Unfortunately a gale overtook this vessel, carried one mast overboard, beat in some of the hatches, and threatened to send her to the bottom. Some days later on sighting a ship on its way to South Carolina from Quebec, both crew and refugees went on board her, leaving the *Kingston* a derelict. But their deliverers, being short of water and provisions, were compelled to send them ashore in a long boat thirty-five leagues off the coast of North Carolina, where the exhausted company landed shortly afterward on Shallote island, near Cape Fear.[69]

The Norfolk merchants seem to have traded extensively with the French West Indies during the first third of the century. Whereas the British sugar islands were too small to absorb the exports from the English continental colonies, the French islands found that Canada could not supply all their needs. In other words, both the British and French colonies were overbalanced, the first on the continental side, the other on the side of the West Indies. Thus by international trade alone could an equilibrium be established. Consequently cheap sugar and molasses at Guadeloupe, or Martinique, or San Domingo, and the excellent market there for provisions and lumber, made an interchange with Virginia inevitable. The British government at first sanctioned the trade, with the understanding that it must not continue in case of war with France. But it was in war times that profits were greatest,

---

[66] *Virginia Gazette*, Aug. 31, 1739, photostat copy, Library of Congress.
[67] *Journals of the House of Burgesses*, 1758-1761, p. 296.
[68] Peter Force, *American Archives*, Fourth Series (Washington, 1837-1853), III, p. 1191.
[69] Grenlees and Hardie, *Ledger*, p. 76a.

and the colonial merchants did not hesitate t[
their vessels with corn, pork, and beef, and s[
for Jamaica, they often headed for the neutr[
and Curaçao, where they exchanged their carg[
molasses.[70] In January, 1710, the Board of T[
Virginians were supplying the French in this [
ernor Spotswood to put an end to the illega[

The planters of the British West Indies obj[
the French islands, whether in times of war or peace, and united in a
petition to Parliament to put an end to it. The continental colonies,
on the other hand, represented that to deprive them of this market
would bring ruin to their merchants, without in any way benefiting
the British sugar planters, and for months the Board of Trade was
bombarded with petitions and counterpetitions. Virginia's interest
was great enough to draw a formal protest from Governor Gooch, and
a "representation from the Council."[72] However, the West Indians
had their way, for in 1733 Parliament passed the so-called Molasses
Act, placing prohibitive duties on molasses and sugar brought into the
British colonies from the foreign islands.[73]

The act seems to have been universally disregarded. Jamaica became
a clearinghouse between the continental colonies and the French islands, vessels leaving Kingston with papers indicating a full cargo,
when in fact their holds contained nothing but empty hogsheads.
They then headed for San Domingo, filled up with sugar and molasses,
and set out for New England or the Chesapeake.[74] Governor Gooch, the
easy-going Governor of Virginia, denied all knowledge of this traffic,[75]
but it seems certain that the Norfolk merchants participated in it. The
very year that Gooch made his report, a ship came in at Ocracoke inlet
from Guernsey, laden with French wines, brandy, and woolens, all prohibited under the Navigation Acts; they were transferred to a colonial
vessel and taken to Virginia by way of Pamlico and Albemarle
Sounds.[76]

In the infancy of Norfolk, few of the merchants owned ocean-

[70] Frank W. Pitman, *The Development of the British West Indies* (New Haven,
1917), pp. 189-195.
[71] Public Record Office, London, CO5-1363, pp. 39-43.
[72] *Ibid.*, CO5-4, pp. 204-207.
[73] Pitman, *British West Indies*, pp. 242-270.
[74] Pitman, *British West Indies*, p. 278.
[75] Public Record Office, London, Gooch to Board of Trade, May 24, 1734.
[76] *Colonial Records of North Carolina*, IV, 169-170.

s. The materials for shipbuilding were at hand—tar, pitch, ne, rosin—but labor was dear, and seafaring men few.[77] Of enty sloops and brigantines which William Byrd saw at the Norlk wharves in 1728, it is probable that not five were built or owned in the colony.[78] Two years later there were but sixteen sloops, six brigantines, and one ship belonging to all Virginia. In the next decade, however, shipbuilding made appreciable advances, and Governor Gooch could state, in 1739, that sloops were often built in Virginia, to be disposed of in the West Indies.[79] The inventory of John Tucker, in 1736, shows that this Norfolk merchant owned three sloops, one of them, 40 feet long, valued at £230.[80] Captain Nathaniel Tatum, of Norfolk, owned the ship *Caesar*, worth £625, and the sloop *Indian Creek*, worth £25.[81]

Yet in 1742 four ships, six or seven brigantines, two or three snows, seven or eight schooners, and five or six sloops, constituted the entire Virginia merchant marine.[82] In the next two decades, the expansion of trade so stimulated shipbuilding that in 1764 Virginians owned 102 seagoing vessels, totaling 6,168 tons, and manned by 827 sailors.[83] It is certain that shipbuilding was engaged in actively in or near Norfolk from an early date. So early as 1736 the sloop *Industry*, "lately built at Norfolk," was taking on tobacco on the James for London. Some of the first to take up lots in the town were ship carpenters,[84] while the numbers in this trade steadily increased. In 1761 the firm of John Glasford & Co., of Glasgow, contracted with Smith Sparrows for a ship built at Norfolk,[85] 60 feet long, 22 feet wide, 10 feet in the lower hold, and 4 feet between decks. The charge was 50 shillings the ton.[86]

Upon the arrival of the fleet from Great Britain, especially after bad weather, the Norfolk ship carpenters were kept busy refitting damaged vessels. When a ship limped up the Elizabeth, her cargo was unloaded, her sails and rigging stored in some near-by loft, and her crew lodged at the various ordinaries. She was then conducted to shallow water and careened by the aid of fall and blocks. Next a lighter, with

[77] Public Record Office, London, CO5-1359, pp. 40-41.
[78] Byrd, *History of the Dividing Line*, pp. 19, 20.
[79] Public Record Office, London, Gooch to Board of Trade, July 13, 1739.
[80] *Norfolk County Deed Book*, H, pp. 32-59.
[81] *Ibid.*, pp. 28-31.
[82] Public Record Office, London, Gooch to Board of Trade, 1742.
[83] *Ibid.*, Fauquier to Board of Trade, January 30, 1764.
[84] *Norfolk County Deed Book*, No. 12, pp. 233, 274, and No. 9, pp. 204-5.
[85] Papers of Niel Jamieson, p. 43.
[86] *Ibid.*, p. 295.

its steaming kettles of pitch or tar, was run up beside her bottom, so that the Negro workers could caulk up every leaky seam. After this the various groups of artisans had their turn, for glaziers were needed to replace the broken glass, iron-workers to fit in new bolts, coopers to repair damaged hogsheads, sailmakers to patch the torn canvas, carpenters to make new hatches or replace masts or spars which had gone overboard.[87] It was a sad time for the owner and the master, but for the Norfolk workmen it meant full employment at high wages. When the good ship *George,* of Glasgow, came up the river in 1762 with a leaky hold,[88] she had to remain for 43 days. In addition to the cost of oakum, pitch, tar, and nails, her master paid £8 for wharfage, £12 for storage for the cargo, £2.12 for a lighter, £17. 16. 3 for Negro hire, £12 for rum with which to refresh the workmen, £12 for bread, £11 for a ship carpenter, and £9. 8. 6½ for cooperage.[89]

In the meanwhile, the increasing size of the English tobacco ships, together with the gradual diversification of Virginia and Maryland agriculture, were making Norfolk the entrepôt for the entire Chesapeake region. It was a matter of no great difficulty for a vessel of sixty or seventy tons to move from plantation to plantation up the rivers and creeks, but for a ship of 250 tons it was a tedious and dangerous operation. Moreover, the British owners objected to taking on their cargoes piecemeal. It was more economical to have the tobacco brought down the rivers to a point near the coast, where the vessels could load in one operation, and start on their return voyage to England or Scotland with the least possible delay. Norfolk was ideally situated for this trade, so the merchants thought, because of its ample harbor and its proximity to the ocean. It is true that many of the planters on the upper James considered the distance too great, and some on the Potomac hesitated to trust their frail shallops to the mercy of the Chesapeake, so that many tobacco ships went for their cargoes directly into the York, or the Rappahannock, or the James, without stopping at the little port on the Elizabeth. But others, in increasing numbers, found it profitable as well as convenient, to make Norfolk their final destination.

---

[87] "The inhabitants consist of merchants, ship carpenters, and other useful artisans," declared William Byrd in 1728. *History of the Dividing Line,* pp. 19-20.

[88] Grenlees and Hardie, *Ledger,* p. 174a.

[89] *Ibid.,* Loose sheet (see pp. 19-22). Among the well-to-do artisans living in Norfolk in 1775 were John Gardner, Joyce Edwards, Samuel Danby, Willis Bramble, Josiah Deane, and Christopher Busten, ship carpenters; James Gay and Talbot Thompson, sailmakers; Samuel Blows, George Jamieson, and John Williamson, blacksmiths (Stewart, *History of Norfolk County,* pp. 363-367).

During the middle decades of the eighteenth century many Virginia farmers began to devote a part of their acreage to wheat and corn, and the market for wheat and corn was in the West Indies, not Great Britain. To find vessels loading for Antigua or Jamaica they had to come to Norfolk.[90] So it became a common occurrence to see shallops or even sloops, laden with barrels of flour, wheat and corn, winding down the rivers to the bay and across Hampton Roads to the Elizabeth. And when this traffic was well established, it was not long before it began to embrace tobacco. The Norfolk merchants had factors on all the great rivers, who bargained with the farmers for their produce, and at times it was not possible for them to secure a full boatload of corn or wheat. They had to roll on a few hogsheads of tobacco to make the trip to Norfolk worthwhile. Tobacco began to pile up on the wharves there, English ships came in to take it off, and a trade with Great Britain developed, which for decades rivaled that to the West Indies.

Among the Norfolk merchants who traded extensively with Virginia and Maryland points, was Niel Jamieson. Connected with the firm of John Glasford & Co., of Glasgow, he possessed all the business insight and thrift for which Scotchmen are noted. One of his agents described him as the "most perfect master of trade in the bay."[91] From Cabin Point, in Surry County, Jamieson secured large quantities of corn, wheat, peas, pork, and tobacco, through his factor, Adam Fleming;[92] from Maryland he got wheat, iron, and tobacco;[93] from Petersburg flour and corn;[94] from Falmouth, on the Rappahannock, tobacco, butter, and beeswax;[95] from Alexandria flour and herring;[96] from Richmond, wheat;[97] from Fredericksburg, corn and pig iron. To Suffolk, which now enjoyed a trade with the Chowan region, he sent regularly for pitch, tar, and turpentine.[98] In short, his sloops could be seen in

---

[90] In 1739 William Byrd wrote to a Norfolk merchant warning him against purchasing Maryland wheat and neglecting that of the Virginia growers. If you leave our wheat on our hands, he said, we will have to sell it to the New Englanders, in exchange for the "West India commodities," which now we receive from you (*Virginia Magazine of History and Biography*, XXXVI, 395).

[91] Papers of Niel Jamieson, p. 2407.

[92] *Ibid.*, pp. 2475, 2875.

[93] *Ibid.*, pp. 2959, 3379.

[94] *Ibid.*, p. 964.

[95] *Ibid.*, p. 2866.

[96] *Ibid.*, pp. 2144, 2938.

[97] *Ibid.*, pp. 2142, 2184.

[98] "Turpentine of late comes down very slow," one of Jamieson's Suffolk factors wrote in 1766. "The people are busy with their crops."

every river and almost every creek of tidewater Virginia and Maryland.

Jamieson's warehouses in Norfolk and Gosport presented a busy scene. Side by side with barrels of flour and hogsheads of tobacco were casks of Jamaica rum and Antigua molasses; boxes of manufactured goods from England or Scotland; wine from Lisbon or Cádiz, or Madeira; salt from Turks Island; barrels of coffee, pimento, chocolate, spices, cocoa nuts, from various parts of the world. At his wharves were sloops or brigantines making ready to leave for the West Indies, or perhaps a two-hundred-ton ship just in from London or Glasgow. Seated on one side one might see a dozen or more slaves just in from the Guinea coast, watching with wondering eyes, while their more civilized fellow Africans worked busily loading or unloading the cargoes.

When the sloops went back to Cabin Point, or Osborne's warehouse, or Falmouth, they took with them a wide variety of European goods— Irish linens, canvas, Holland thread, broadcloth, shalloon, fustian, druggets, silk crepe, worsted hose, pillows, handkerchiefs, buttons, gloves, pins; guns, powder, and shot; hoes, scissors, fishhooks, scales, axes, feather beds, grindstones, hour glasses, chafing dishes, spinning wheels, spoons, knives, forks; pewter plates, basins, porringers, and candlesticks; tables, chairs, cupboards, chests.[99] Piled in with these goods were often West Indian rum and molasses, Madeira wine, and a few barrels of salt. It was not unusual for British masters to put in at Norfolk, and there hire shallops and sloops to go up the rivers for a cargo of tobacco. After these little craft had flitted from store to store, or from plantation to plantation, they returned to the Elizabeth and tied up to the ship, where the crew hoisted the hogsheads on board.[100]

The trade with Great Britain was, of course, the foundation of the economic life of Virginia. In 1742 exports to the mother country comprised £180,000 in tobacco; £4500 in pig-iron; £2670 in pitch, tar, and turpentine; £2000 in skins.[101] An increasingly large share of this trade left from Norfolk. "The seat of trade is altered," wrote Governor Fauquier, in January, 1764, "the northern part of the colony employing fewer vessels than heretofore, the southern many more."[102] At a very early date the stores of the Norfolk merchants were filled with European goods, which unquestionably came directly to them

[99] *Norfolk County Deed Book,* No. 9. Inventory of Matthew Godfrey, pp. 639-641.
[100] Grenlees and Hardie, *Ledger,* p. 77a.
[101] Public Record Office, London, Gooch to Board of Trade.
[102] *Ibid.,* Fauquier to Board of Trade, Jan. 30, 1764.

in British ships.[103] We know that the ship *Moseley* was trading from Norfolk to Great Britain in 1736,[104] the *Thomas and Sarah,* in 1758,[105] the ship *Peggy,* in 1766,[106] and the ship *Loyal Hunter* in 1762, and that in 1770 the firm of Balfour and Barraud, of Norfolk, advertised themselves as importers from London, Bristol, and Glasgow. The Virginia and Norfolk *Intelligencer,* for February 16, 1775, lists the ships *Elizabeth,* from Bristol, the *Betsy,* from London, and the *Hodge,* from Liverpool, as having just entered.

We gain an insight into the commerce of Norfolk from the vessels in her harbor and in Hampton Roads, on December 30, 1775. In addition to Dunmore's fleet were the sloop *Christian,* of Norfolk, bound for Glasgow with wheat and staves; the sloop *Agatha,* from Grenada to Norfolk with forty-five hogsheads of rum; the brig *Cornet,* from Glasgow to Norfolk with dry goods; the schooner *Peggy,* from St. Vincent's to Norfolk with rum and sugar; the sloops *Molly* and *Swallow,* from Turks Island for Norfolk with salt.[107]

The Norfolk merchants were alert, enterprising, close-bargaining businessmen. "The two cardinal virtues that make a place thrive, industry and frugality, are seen here in perfection," wrote William Byrd in 1728.[108] No doubt the spirit of thrift was a part of Norfolk's Scotch inheritance, for many of her leading merchants came from Glasgow. John Joyce, who visited the place in 1785, went so far as to state that before the Revolution the inhabitants "were almost all Scotch."[109] Some came over as agents for Glasgow firms, and after accumulating a little capital, opened business on their own account. They might start by shipping a few barrels of pork or corn to the West Indies, or bringing in a cask or two of rum. If things went well they would broaden their operations, until eventually they could boast of their own warehouse and wharf on the Elizabeth, their own stores on the James or the York, their own sloops for carriage in the rivers and the bay, perhaps their own brigantine or ship for the voyages to Jamaica or Antigua. Others migrated from Scotland as clerks,

103 *Norfolk County Deed Book,* No. 9. Inventory of Matthew Godfrey, 1717, pp. 639-641.
104 *Virginia Gazette,* Jan. 21, 1736.
105 Grenlees and Hardie, *Ledger,* p. 19.
106 *Virginia Gazette,* Jan. 6, 1766.
107 *American Archives,* Fourth Series, IV, 577.
108 Among the early merchants were Samuel Smith, George Mason, Robert Tucker, Lewis Conner, Peter Malbone, Lawrence Smith, Thomas Nelson, Samuel Boush, John Phripp, Nathaniel Tatum, John Hutchings, Anthony Walke, Mason Calvert, and John Taylor.
109 *Virginia Magazine of History and Biography,* XXIII, 407-414.

with letters of introduction to the Norfolk firms, hoping to learn the details of the American trade in the offices along the water front. These too, in many cases, because of ability and industry, became well-to-do merchants.

The inventories of the Norfolk merchants, even in the first part of the eighteenth century, show how extensive were their operations. When John Tucker died in 1736 his warehouses contained European goods to the value of £469. 4. 0½, including woolens, sheeting, silks, ticking; thread, tape, ribbons, laces; razors, lancets, combs, buckles; Bibles, primers, horn books, writing paper; rugs and blankets; dishes, basins, and plates of pewter; hatchets, chisels, hammers, locks, saws; hour-glasses, kettles and compasses of brass. His three sloops and one shallop were appraised at £445. His stock of Madeira wine totalled £690, his rum £851. 14. 1, his sugar £223. 15. 4¾. He had European goods yet unpacked worth £239. 19. 10; wares at "Mr. Mason's store" worth £2014. 18. 11¼; he owned six slaves worth £147. 10; 88 ounces and 13 pennyweight of gold wedges worth £310. 5. 6; and cash to the amount of £2443. 12. 1½.[110]

The close of the colonial period found Norfolk prosperous, progressive, full of hope. In less than a century the town had grown from an insignificant village to the most important place in Virginia. Its population, at most a few hundred in 1700, was estimated at six thousand in 1775.[111] At first merely the port of southeastern Virginia and northeastern Carolina, it became in time the chief point of shipment for all tidewater Virginia. Its spacious harbor was crowded with vessels, its streets with busy purchasers, its wharves and warehouses with all kinds of wares; its citizens were never without employment, in its shipyards were always the frames of sloops, schooners, or ships. Its citizens had every right to look forward to a future of continued growth and prosperity, which would make it the queen of the Chesapeake, the chief port of Maryland, Virginia, and North Carolina. They could not foresee that in a few years the town of which they were so proud would be but a heap of smouldering ruins, its people scattered, its leading merchants disgraced, its commerce prostrated.

[110] *Norfolk County Deed Book,* H, pp. 32-59.
[111] Johann D. Schoepf, *Travels in the Confederation,* pp. 98-100.

CHAPTER THREE

The Maelstrom of Revolution

The accession of George III to the throne marked the culmination of a conflict which had long been in progress between the British government and the colonies. Ever since the meeting of the first representative assembly, at Jamestown, in 1619, the colonists had exercised almost complete control over internal taxation. This proved an effective weapon. In imitation of the House of Commons, who thwarted the king at every turn by threatening to cut off his revenues, the colonial assemblies mastered his representatives in America by holding tight to the purse-strings. In internal affairs the colonies had become practically self-governing republics before the middle of the eighteenth century.

When, then, the failure to reapportion representation in Great Britain thrust into power a group of reactionaries, a clash with America was inevitable. To George III, to his prime minister, George Grenville, to the entire Tory faction, the authority exercised by the assemblies seemed to threaten, not only British control in the colonies, but the foundations of conservatism in England itself. So they set to work to strengthen the hands of the governors. The obvious, if rather dangerous, way to do this, was to supply them with funds for the payment of their salaries and for the expenses of their governments by taxing the colonies by act of Parliament.

The changed temper of the British government was not at first apparent to the Americans. When Grenville forced through the so-called Sugar Act, they did not take alarm. "England has always controlled our commerce," they said, "this is just one more troublesome regulation. Perhaps like the Molasses Act, it will not be strictly enforced." But Grenville intended that it should be enforced. Revenue vessels were sent over to guard the coasts, and customs officers were ordered to proceed against offenders. Since the old duty of 6*d*. a gallon on molasses, if actually collected, would put a complete stop to the trade to the French West Indies, the new duty was fixed at 3*d*. a gallon. The colonists suddenly awoke to the unpleasant realization that a new era had dawned in British imperial control.

Norfolk was deeply stirred. When several vessels were seized by Edward H. Moseley, surveyor of Elizabeth River,[1] public rage vented itself against one of the informers. This unfortunate man, a certain Captain William Smith, was taken by a number of leading citizens, tied to the tail of a cart, and marched off to the county wharf. Here, after treating him to a coat of tar and feathers, they sent him on the ducking stool, and pelted him with rotten eggs and stones, the mayor himself, the sedate Maximilian Calvert, taking a leading part in the proceedings. They next marched him through "every street in the town," with two drums beating, returning finally to the market house. There, "all the principal gentlemen of the town being present," they deliberated his fate, and ended by throwing him "headlong over the wharf." Had not a passing boat pulled him out of the water, more dead than alive, he would have been drowned.[2] Thus in the early years of the quarrel with the British government, Norfolk was enlisted with a whole heart in the colonial cause. Grenville had touched the life blood of the town when he interfered with the West Indian trade.

Norfolk was in bad humor, then, when news arrived of the passage of the Stamp Act. On March 29, 1766, about thirty of the leading citizens met in one of the taverns to discuss this obnoxious measure, repairing in the evening to the residence of Mayor Calvert, where "they brought daylight on." It was decided to summon the Sons of Liberty, and two days later the patriots crowded into the courthouse to draw up resolutions of protest. "We will by all lawful ways . . . defend ourselves in the full enjoyment of, and preserve inviolate to posterity, those inestimable privileges of all free-born British subjects of being taxed only by representatives of their own choosing. . . . If we quietly submit to the execution of the said stamp act, all our claims to civil liberty will be lost, and we and our posterity become absolute slaves."[3]

[1] *Tyler's Quarterly*, III, 293.
[2] *William and Mary Quarterly*, XXI, 167.
[3] *Virginia Gazette*, April 4, 1766; *William and Mary Quarterly*, XXI, 49.

The resentment was changed to rejoicing and intense patriotism, when, six weeks later, the ship *Peggy*, from Glasgow, glided into the Elizabeth with the tidings that the Stamp Act had been repealed. May 22, 1766, was set aside as a day of thanksgiving. At dawn the people were awakened by the ringing of bells and the discharge of cannon. The courthouse and the borough church were gay with colors, while the ships in the river were beautifully decorated. On the courthouse was a painting, depicting King George, with the imperial diadem over his head, before him prostrate America introduced by Pitt, offering her tribute of duty and gratitude; on one side were Manufacture, Agriculture, and Commerce, raising their drooping heads; on the other Slavery and Oppression with downcast faces. After a sermon by Mr. Davis, and more salutes from the ships, the leading citizens sat down to a dinner, where King George, the Prince of Wales, the Queen and the royal family, were successively toasted. The company then drank to Pitt, "the man who rejoiced on hearing the sound of British liberty echoed back from the forests of America." With the coming of evening the town was illuminated, and bonfires were kindled, while the common people washed down vows of eternal loyalty to the King with copious drinks of West Indian rum.[4]

But rejoicing turned to anger the next year, when it was learned that Parliament, under the leadership of Charles Townshend, had imposed new taxes on the colonies. This was followed by a long series of coercive measures—the suspension of the New York Assembly, the sending of troops to Boston, the Tea Act, the Boston Port Bill, the overriding of the Massachusetts charter—and in Norfolk, as elsewhere, the spirit of resistance grew intense. A Committee of Public Safety was organized to keep alive the spirit of liberty by corresponding with patriots in other communities.[5] Upon hearing of the closing of Boston Harbor, this body set aside June 1, 1774, as a day of fasting and prayer. To the Boston committee they wrote, "Our bosoms glow with tender regard for you, and we will support you to the limit of our ability." On June 27, the Norfolk citizens, in a meeting at the courthouse, denounced the blocking up of the harbor as a "most tyrannick exercise of unlawful power." The acts for altering the

---

[4] *Virginia Gazette,* June 6, 1766.

[5] The committee was composed of Matthew Phripp, chairman, William Davies, secretary, John Boush, Thomas Claiborne, John Hutchings, Joseph Hutchings, James Holt, Samuel Inglis, Niel Jamieson, John Lawrence, Thomas Newton, Jr., Thomas Ritson, Robert Taylor, and John Taylor (Stewart, *History of Norfolk County,* p. 35).

Massachusetts constitution and for suppressing riots, they characterized as violent infractions of the solemn chartered rights of the colonies and melancholy proofs of the despotic spirit of the times.[6]

Late in August, 1774, Norfolk was shocked by the news that nine
chests of tea, consigned to some leading merchants of the town, had
just arrived on the brigantine *Mary and Jane.* At a meeting in the
courthouse, it was unanimously resolved that the tea must be sent
back, and a special committee was appointed to urge compliance
upon the importers. When the merchants assented readily they received a vote of thanks, and Norfolk's "tea-party" ended peaceably.[7]
In March, 1775, the committee condemned John Brown, a Norfolk
merchant, as an enemy of American liberty, for bringing in a number
of slaves from Jamaica on the brig *Fanny,* in violation of the Continental Association.[8] A few weeks later Captain Sampson, of the snow
Elizabeth, of Bristol, incurred the anger of the committee. Sampson
had secured their permission to store a load of salt brought in contrary to the Association, pending repairs to his vessel; but when ready
to depart, instead of taking on the salt again, he had begun loading
with lumber. "We trust the merchants, planters, and skippers of vessels
will make him feel their indignation, by breaking off all kinds of dealings with him," said the committee.[9] Walter Chambre, of Whitehaven,
was also denounced for shipping goods to Norfolk in opposition to
the non-importation agreement,[10] while the local firm of Eilbeck, Ross
& Co. was ordered to send the ship *Molly* back to England without
breaking cargo.[11]

It was inevitable, however, that as the boycott became more stringent, discontent and even violent opposition should manifest itself
among some of the importers. The Norfolk merchants who traded
with Glasgow or Liverpool faced ruin if they could not land British
goods. "Why should the entire brunt of the attempt to coerce the
government fall upon us?" they asked. "It is well enough for the
planters to talk about boycotting the English manufacturers, for they
can make out with the goods they have on hand. But for the trader
it means going out of business." "Everything is managed by committee," one grumbler wrote in January, 1775, "settling and pricing

[6] *American Archives,* Fourth Series, I, 370, 371, 518.
[7] *Ibid.,* p. 727.
[8] Stewart, *History of Norfolk County,* p. 352.
[9] *American Archives,* Fourth Series, I, 174.
[10] *Ibid.,* III, 431.
[11] *Ibid.,* II, 897.

goods, imprinting books, forcing some to sign scandalous concessions, and by such bullying conduct they expect to bring the Government to their own terms."[12]

The Scotch merchants had no deep and lasting sympathy with the Revolutionary cause. Many had been swept along with the current during the protests against the Stamp Act or the Townshend measures; but when it came to interfering with commerce, or to taking up arms against the mother country, they quickly drew back. There were few among them, Colonel Robert Howe pointed out, "who from local attachments, could feel any strong prepossession in favor of America, or its cause, suspicious friends therefore at best. . . . By habit attached to traffic, by interest induced to pursue it," they could but be hostile to the Continental Association.[13] In December, 1775, one of the officers under Dunmore wrote that the Norfolk Scotch "to a man are well-affected to the [British] government."[14]

There were others, too, who looked upon the Revolution as a "cursed dispute," certain to bring ruin to their business and their families. In July, 1775, the Norfolk committee itself wrote to the Virginia Convention, protesting against the restriction placed upon the exportation of provisions. The merchants "have made large contracts for the articles so prohibited," they pointed out, "and have now on hand considerable quantities of those perishable commodities. . . . They have had no opportunity to regulate their trade agreeably to this unexpected resolve, but are suddenly prohibited from commerce in the midst of their engagements." They asked for delay "to give time for vessels that are now loading to take in their cargoes," and to permit the merchant as best he could "to blunt the edge of this sudden calamity."[15]

The Norfolk merchant had to consider that in case of war British privateers would prey upon his West Indian commerce, British frigates would block up the entrance to Chesapeake Bay, British fleets might even enter Elizabeth River to knock his house about his head. There was little ammunition on hand, the supply of arms was inadequate, and the few old cannon in Norfolk which had served on privateers of other times were not mounted, the old fort, on the site of Town Point, had crumbled away. "What could be expected from a

---

[12] *Virginia Magazine of History and Biography*, III, 157.
[13] *Richmond College Historical Papers*, I, 152-153.
[14] *American Archives*, Fourth Series, IV, 350.
[15] *Virginia Magazine of History and Biography*, XIV, 51.

people whose whole property was at stake in their houses, and whose lives were beset on all sides?"[16]

Yet the borough government did not begin to waver until British guns were actually leveled at their warehouses and their homes. In 1775 Lord Dunmore broke off communications with the Virginia Assembly, and, fleeing to the British fleet, made use of it in an attempt to force the people back to their allegiance. In July he was in the Southern Branch with the *Otter* and several other warships. A clash with the Norfolk Committee of Public Safety followed. When a certain Alexander Main was pointed out to Dunmore by John Shaw as one who wore a hunting-shirt, which was the accepted uniform of the minutemen, Milord imprisoned him on board the *Otter*. The next time Shaw set foot in Norfolk he was roughly handled by a mob.[17] Dunmore was still fuming over this incident when Andrew Sprowle, a prominent Portsmouth merchant, received a summons to attend the Committee of Public Safety, to answer the charge of having "harbored his Majesty's troop in his store at Gosport."

This aroused the governor to action. A few days later Mayor Paul Loyall received a letter from Captain John McCartney, commander of the *Mercury*. If those who supply the King's ships with provisions are to be held up as enemies of American liberty, he wrote, they are the more entitled to my protection. "I shall, the first opportunity, place his Majesty's ship under my command, abreast the town . . . and if it becomes necessary, use the most coercive measures in my power."[18] The answer of the mayor and aldermen was worthy of American freemen. "This corporation . . . notwithstanding their exposed and defenseless situation, which cannot be remedied, unbiased by fear, unappalled at the threats of unlawful power, will never desert the righteous cause of their country, plunged as it is into dreadful and unexpected calamities."[19]

These were brave words, but it became every day more evident that the Norfolk patriots were helpless. Dunmore's forces were strengthened by the arrival of additional war vessels; the Scotch element in town was co-operating with him; many of the country people were openly loyal, declaring, "Dem it, they will be for the old King George."[20] For some time the printer, John Holt, continued to urge

[16] *Ibid.*, III, 7.
[17] *American Archives*, Fourth Series, III, 66, 92.
[18] *Ibid.*, p. 92.
[19] *Norfolk Council Orders*, 1736-1798, pp. 71, 716.
[20] *Virginia Magazine of History and Biography*, III, 154.

the people not to give up their liberties without a struggle, but on September 30, 1775, he was effectually silenced. A party of seventeen British rowed up to the county wharf, landed, and marched to the printing office. While a crowd of several hundred looked on, they carried off the types and other "printing implements," and arrested two of the workmen. On their way back to their boat, the drums beat to summon the citizens to arms. Yet few answered, and the British, after giving three huzzas, in which a crowd of Negroes joined, embarked with their two prisoners. So long as the guns of the warships pointed out over the town, Norfolk had to be submissive.[21]

Lord Dunmore and Virginia were now at the point of open warfare. The famous minutemen of the upper counties were concentrating at Williamsburg, preparatory to marching on Norfolk. The Revolutionists of Norfolk and Princess Anne, under the leadership of Matthew Phripp, Colonel Lawson, and others, assembled in arms and posted themselves at Kemp's Landing and other strategic points. Many of the staunchest patriots in Norfolk had already left to join the militia,[22] and a general exodus of all save those well affected to the British now took place. For days Church Street and the road to Great Bridge were crowded with fugitives, many of them driving carts filled with household goods.[23]

Dunmore began active operations against the local companies on October 12, when Captain Leslie ascended the Southern Branch and carried off or destroyed nineteen cannon concealed in a wood.[24] Five days later the governor, with a party of grenadiers, sailors, and marines, sailed up the Eastern Branch to Newton, where he landed and marched on Kemps. The militia took to their heels, and the British, after breaking open the stores and taking off some small arms, returned unmolested to their ships.[25] On the night of October 19 thirty-nine men landed at Norfolk and marched out into the country, where they took twenty cannon. By November 1 the British had captured no less than seventy-seven pieces of ordnance, and could boast that they had rendered all Norfolk county defenseless.[26]

---

[21] *American Archives,* Fourth Series, III, 847, 923; *Virginia Magazine of History and Biography,* III, 160; *Richmond College Historical Papers,* I, 197.
[22] The fact that Dunmore's men met with no resistance in raiding Holt's press is explained by the absence from town of almost all save "Tories and negroes." (*American Archives,* Fourth Series, III, 1137.)
[23] *Ibid.,* III, 923; *Richmond College Historical Papers,* I, 100.
[24] *American Archives,* Fourth Series, III, 1716.
[25] *Richmond College Historical Papers,* I, 98.
[26] *American Archives,* Fourth Series, III, 1716.

On November 7 Dunmore issued a proclamation declaring martial law, summoning the people to his standard, and offering freedom to all slaves belonging to rebels, who would take up arms for the King.[27] This aroused the ire of all Virginia. Even in times of peace the people were haunted by the fear that the blacks might rise and murder them in their beds; for the governor to put arms in their hands was an unpardonable sin.

In the meanwhile news reached Dunmore that the local militia were assembling again in various places to guard the road over which the approaching State troops must pass on their way to Norfolk. These forces he decided to attack at once. With a reinforcement of sixty men from St. Augustine, he was able to muster two hundred soldiers and marines and a few Norfolk Tories for a descent on Great Bridge. Finding no militia at this place and learning that a force under Colonel Lawson was stationed at Kemps, he marched overland to that village. Here he won an easy victory, for the militia, after firing one volley, fled from the field, their leaders "whipping up their horses as they streamed through Kemps." Several were killed, two were drowned in their flight, and fourteen were taken. Upon entering the village, Dunmore set up his standard, and summoned the people to take the oath of allegiance. To escape this humiliation many fled to the sand dunes of Cape Henry, but some came in, took the oath, and pinned upon their breasts the strip of red cloth accepted as the badge of loyalty to the Crown.[28]

The British and Tories were guilty of many outrages. We have been compelled to abandon "our aged parents, and wives, and children and families," wrote the Norfolk and Princess Anne patriots, "leaving them to the mercy of invidious neighbors, the lawless, plundering soldiery, and the more savage slave. Our plantations have been ravaged, our wives and children stripped to nakedness, and our very bed chambers invaded at midnight by ruffians with drawn daggers and bayonets. Our houses have not only been robbed of plate, specie, etc., but reduced to ashes."[29] One lady tells how she found an "ugly looking negro man" in the house, "dressed up in a full suit of British regimentals, and armed with a gun." "Have you got any dirty shirts here? (this is the name by which our soldiers are known.) I want

---

[27] *Colonial Records of North Carolina*, X, 308, 309.

[28] *American Archives*, Fourth Series, III, 1717; *Lower Norfolk County Antiquary*, II, 132-133; *Richmond College Historical Papers*, I, 100-103; *Virginia Magazine of History and Biography*, XIV, 387.

[29] *Virginia Magazine of History and Biography*, XVII, 176, 177.

your dirty shirts. . . . Then he went up stairs to look for them, he said, but no doubt to see what he could steal." The lady laid her complaint directly before Lord Dunmore. "Why, madam," said he, "this is a provoking piece of insolence indeed, but there is no keeping these black rascals within bounds. . . . We must expect such things whilst this horrid rebellion lasts."[30]

On November 16, Dunmore, in high good humor at his easy success, marched into Norfolk, where he lost no time in raising the standard. The Scotch merchants and their clerks, many Negroes, and some others who feared the confiscation of their property, took the oath, and pinned on the badge.[31] Of those who did so, however, many secretly resolved that they would go over to the patriot cause the moment Dunmore's troops were gone. "I would rather have seen you dead than with this red badge," one good wife told her husband. "Phast!" he replied, "Do you think it has changed my mind? If I can save my property by this step, ought I not in common prudence to wear it, for your sake and the children?"[32] Milord next enlisted the Scotchmen into a regiment which he called the "Queen's Own Loyal Virginians,"[33] and the runaway slaves into the "Etheopean Corps."[34] He then laid out a plan of fortifications for the town, and began the construction of earthworks.[35]

In this Dunmore made a mistake. Norfolk's real strength against attack by land lay in the long, circuitous route by which alone it could be approached. Had the British devoted all their energies to erecting works at Bachelor's Mill on the edge of the swamp and at Great Bridge, it is probable that the Virginia troops would never have gotten within sight of the town. At the last moment this fact dawned on Dunmore, and he set some of his men at work hastily fortifying Great Bridge. This was a place of great natural strength. The Southern Branch flowed here between marshes, extending one hundred and fifty yards or more on either side. From the northern side a long causeway crossed the marsh to an island of firm earth, where a wooden bridge forty yards in length had been thrown over the stream to a similar island on the other bank. This island, in turn, was connected with the village of Great Bridge by another long causeway over the

[30] *Lower Norfolk County Antiquary*, II, 133, 134.
[31] *American Archives*, Fourth Series, IV, 343; *Virginia Magazine of History and Biography*, XIV, 387.
[32] *Lower Norfolk County Antiquary*, II, 136.
[33] *American Archives*, Fifth Series, II, 159-161.
[34] *Ibid.*
[35] *Richmond College Historical Papers*, I, 137.

marsh on the southern side. On the south island were a number of warehouses, where goods were taken on and off the river boats.[36] The British now threw up a stockade fort on the north island, and planted guns to command the bridge.[37]

In the meanwhile, the Virginia troops under Colonel William Woodford had left Williamsburg, crossed the James, and were now swinging through Suffolk. They were good fighters and deadly shots, while their ardent patriotism fired them with anger against Dunmore.[38] Many wore hunting shirts with a tomahawk or scalping knife stuck in the belt,[39] which made the British suppose they would fight after the manner of Indians. They came muttering threats against Norfolk. "The town is a nest of Tories," they said, "who are aiding Dunmore to subdue the colony, either by provisioning his ships, or actually taking up arms against their fellow countrymen. It would serve them right should we burn their houses over their heads."[40] Woe to the Tory who fell into their hands, for it was with difficulty that the officers prevented their men from hanging them as traitors. Woodford took the milder and more logical course of handcuffing them to their black comrades, and so marching them through the country to Williamsburg, there to be tried by the Convention.[41]

Upon their arrival at Great Bridge, the Virginians threw up breastworks across the southern end of the causeway, which they manned lightly, posting the main force in the village behind. There they remained inactive for several days, awaiting reinforcements from North Carolina under Colonel Robert Howe. Whether Woodford could have forced his way over the Southern Branch, even with this accession to his force, is doubtful. To charge across the causeway and bridge against the British works would have been most costly; to flank the position on the right was impossible because of the swampy nature of the soil; on the left the river was guarded by the British sloops. Fortunately, the enemy solved the problem for him by themselves taking the initiative. A slave of Major Marshall's who deserted to the British, apparently at his master's command, informed Dunmore that the Virginians numbered no more than three hundred.

---

[36] B. J. Lossing, *Field Book of the Revolution* (New York, 1851-1852), II, 327, 328; Jarvis Manuscript, pp. 17, 18.
[37] *Richmond College Historical Papers*, I, 106.
[38] *Ibid.*, I, 101.
[39] *Virginia Magazine of History and Biography*, III, 159.
[40] *Richmond College Historical Papers*, I, 99; *American Archives*, Fourth Series, IV, 343; Smyth, *A Tour of the United States*, I, 10.
[41] *Richmond College Historical Papers*, I, 122.

Thereupon the Governor, remembering how the local militia had fled at Kemps, and thinking the shirtmen of the same caliber, decided to attack.[42]

So he sent to Great Bridge all his available regulars, sixty Tories, and some sailors from the war vessels,[43] and this force, added to the thirty whites and ninety Negroes already there, brought the garrison to several hundred men.[44] On the morning of December 9 the Americans heard the reveille in the British fort, followed by the discharge of cannon and musketry, and saw the regulars emerging, followed by the Tories and Negroes. The foremost ranks carried planks, which they laid down over the broken bridge to permit the troops and two pieces of cannon to cross to the south island. Here, after burning a few houses and piles of shingles, they opened fire on the American breastwork. The regulars under the command of the gallant Captain Fordyce then advanced over the south causeway. The Americans, crouching behind their breastworks, waited calmly as the dreaded redcoats drew near. "Reserve your fire until they are within fifty yards," ordered Lieutenant Travis. Then, at the proper moment, he gave the signal, and the shirtmen, aiming as coolly as though at target practice, let go with deadly effect. Down went many of the brave fellows upon the causeway, some dead, others desperately wounded, while the back ranks began to falter. Fordyce waved them on, however, reminding "them of their ancient glory." But as he approached the breastwork he too fell, covered with wounds, and his men retreated hastily back to the island.

Here they were rallied by Captain Leslie. The Negroes and Tories had not advanced beyond the island, and the two field pieces continued to play upon the Virginians. But now Colonel Woodford brought up reinforcements, opened a heavy fire from various points, and forced a retreat across the bridge. So enraged were the regulars at their defeat that Captain Leslie had to entreat and even threaten them before they would retire. There was no time for dragging the two cannon back over the bridge, so they were spiked and abandoned. As the fire slackened, several of the Virginians clambered over their breastwork to succor the wounded men on the causeway. The poor fellows, when they saw the shirtmen approach, cried out in terror,

[42] Jarvis Manuscript, p. 13; *Richmond College Historical Papers*, I, 117, 119; *American Archives*, Fourth Series, IV, 292.

[43] *American Archives*, Fourth Series, IV, 540.

[44] *Richmond College Historical Papers*, I, 112.

for Dunmore had reported that they would scalp the wounded.[45] "For God's sake do not murder us," they said. "Put your arm around my neck, and I will show you what I intend to do," the Virginian replied. In this way they assisted the prisoners to the lines, where their wounds could be dressed. Seeing this act of bravery, Captain Leslie stepped out in front of the fort, in plain view of both parties, and bowed his thanks.[46]

The victory was decisive. With the regulars cut to pieces and the Tories and Negroes demoralized, it was no longer possible to hold the fort; so on the evening of the battle the British retreated. Some hours later they streamed into Norfolk, the wounded men crying out for water as the wagons in which they were lying jolted over the rough streets.[47] In the town all was confusion and panic. As for Dunmore, when he learned of the defeat of his troops he raved like a madman, actually threatening to hang the boy who brought the news.[48] There was no thought of defending the half-finished breastworks, and the regulars, followed by the Ethiopian Corps, marched down to the wharves and rowed out to their ships. The Tories, expecting no mercy from the shirtmen, put their movable property on board their own schooners and swung out under the protection of the warships. Whole families had to hurry away, taking their household effects and casting perhaps lingering glances at the homes they were never to see again. Many a dainty lady, who had been accustomed to every luxury, now found herself crowded into some dark hold, intended only for hogsheads of tobacco or barrels of rum or molasses.[49]

The triumphant Virginians, reinforced by a part of the expected Carolina force, were not long in discovering that the road to Norfolk was open. The advance guard, under Colonel Stephens, reached Kempsville on the night of December 11, and two days later Colonel Howe, with his Carolinians, entered Norfolk. Woodford followed from the Great Bridge, arriving on the night of the fourteenth with "up-

[45] "They look like a band of assassins," one correspondent writes, "and it is my opinion if they fight at all it will be that way." *Virginia Magazine of History and Biography*, III, 159.
[46] Jarvis Manuscript, pp. 10-24; Stewart, *History of Norfolk County*, pp. 40-41; *American Archives*, Fourth Series, IV, 540; *Richmond College Historical Papers*, I, 115-121.
[47] *Lower Norfolk County Antiquary*, II, 138.
[48] *Richmond College Historical Papers*, I, 121.
[49] "All the principal Tories, with their families and effects, have retired on board the ships-of-war, and other vessels in the harbor, of which there is a very large fleet." *Ibid.*, I, 121, 129, 130; see also *American Archives*, Fourth Series, IV, 14.

wards of 1000 men."[50] The few remaining inhabitants of the town sent
a petition to the two commanders, declaring that they had "at all
times wished for liberty," and craving protection for their "small
substance."[51] Woodford and Howe replied that they had no intention
of injuring them "either in their persons or their property, unless
they should attempt to resist."[52] The resentment of the two commanders against the town was obvious, however, and they gave free
vent to their indignation when several of their men were wounded
in the streets. "Some of our people say they received the fire from
houses," Woodford wrote the Virginia Convention. "You may be
assured the town of Norfolk deserves no favor."[53]

A few days later Howe pointed out to the Convention that Norfolk, because of its unique position, would be a menace to the Americans throughout the war. The enemy will certainly seize the place,
"which could so conveniently barrack almost any number of troops,
is so well calculated for defense, situated between two colonies, so that
the same troops could execute their purposes upon both, and from
which their shipping could convey their men to any part of this
colony." The neighboring counties would supply them with provisions. Norfolk harbor, "near the mouth of the James River, within
five or six leagues of the Capes, commanding the navigation of two
colonies, makes it perhaps the most noble place for arms for them the
world ever produced." On the other hand, "it cannot be the least
benefit to you, unless you command the navigation, without which it
would only serve to sacrifice whatever troops you might happen to
station there, who would be hemmed in on the one side by the
shipping, and on the other by their army. . . . Upon the whole, I
think Norfolk cannot be maintained with any troops you can place
there. . . . In short, though this is a situation extremely desirable to
your adversaries who have shipping, it will ever remain in the kind of
war we are waging a place disadvantageous and dangerous to you.
This, I can assure you, is the sense of every officer in the line."[54]

While the two commanders were thus hinting broadly for permission to apply the torch to Norfolk, the folly of Dunmore gave them
an unexpected opportunity. The situation on board the fleet was
becoming intolerable. Men, women, and children on the crowded

[50] *Richmond College Historical Papers*, I, 126.
[51] *Ibid.*, p. 123.
[52] *Ibid.*, p. 129.
[53] *Ibid.*, pp. 127, 128.
[54] *Ibid.*, pp. 138, 139, 148.

vessels were suffering for food and water; many were ill, and several died. Petitions began to reach Howe and Woodford for permission for the refugees to come ashore. They replied that all women and children who landed would be protected, provided they gave no information to the enemy, and that the men would receive a fair trial "by their country for taking up arms against it."[55] Thereupon, Dunmore, remembering how easily he had cowed the merchants by threatening destruction to their homes, tried the same tactics on the two commanders. Having been joined by the *Liverpool*, a frigate of twenty-eight guns, the fleet moved up to a position opposite the town. Milord then assumed an imperious tone. Was it the intention of the troops to attack his men, he asked, if they came ashore to get food and water? If so, he would not answer for the consequences. Later, when some of the backwoods riflemen, firing from the cover of houses and wharves, began to pick off his soldiers whenever they put their heads above decks, he sent another warning. This must stop, he said, or he would knock the town about their ears.[56]

Now began a general exodus. Wagons, carriages, and carts were backed up to the fine residences on Main, or Church, or Talbot streets and filled with household goods. While the mistress stood by to direct the work, Negro men and women went back and forth bringing out beds, chairs, tables, linen, clothing, pewter dishes, silver, heaps of clothing, bread, salt meat, and other provisions. When all was ready, there would be a chirrup to the horses, and off they went, the ladies and children riding in front with the driver, the slaves following on foot. In the business districts shopkeepers and merchants made desperate efforts to hire conveyances—a wagon, a dray, a cart, anything to take their wares out of town. Even in the narrow lanes, the resorts of laborers and sailors, the owners and landlords were bringing out their furniture, and pressing carts and wheelbarrows into service. As the strange, tragic procession moved along the streets and over the Princess Anne road, there was no complaining, and now and then someone would strike up a song to keep the spirits up. The fugitives went wherever shelter offered, some to Portsmouth, some to various parts of Princess Anne and Norfolk counties, some to Suffolk, others to Nansemond county, some even to North Carolina.[57]

[55] *Ibid.*, p. 145.
[56] Smyth, *A Tour of the United States*, I, 10; *American Archives*, Fourth Series, IV, 540. Colonel Howe assured the British that his sentinels had received orders not to fire on the boats. "If they exceeded this order, we would punish them ourselves." *North Carolina Colonial Records*, X, 372.
[57] Norfolk *Argus*, Jan. 1, 1856.

On the afternoon of January 1, 1776, the British fleet, consisting of the *Liverpool,* the *Otter,* the *Kingfisher,* and the *Dunmore,* drew up before the town, from Town Point to the upper wharf. At 3:15, persons on shore heard the rattle of drums on board and immediately afterward the warships opened with every gun. The Americans answered as best they could from the buildings on the water front, but the fire from the ships was so hot that they had to retire.[58] Thereupon, several boatloads of British rowed up to the wharves and, stepping ashore, set fire to the warehouses and other buildings next to the water. This they did, so Dunmore afterwards protested, not with a view to destroying the town, but to deprive the shirtmen of their cover. But the Americans seized upon the occasion as an excuse for laying Norfolk in ashes. The soldiers, probably acting without orders, went from house to house applying the torch,[59] and as the British watched from their ships, flames arose, at first one point and then another, until the whole town was burning.[60]

With the roar of the cannon, the crashing of the balls, and the crackling of the flames, it was a truly terrifying time for those inhabitants still remaining. Women and children rushed through the streets, seeking safety in flight, some hugging a few precious belongings. Several were killed.[61] The troops added to the confusion by plundering shops and residences, determined "to make hay while the sun shone." As cask after cask of rum was rolled out of the warehouses and opened, some became drunk. Gangs would approach a house, beat down the door, drag out whatever they fancied, and then set the place on fire.[62] The bombardment continued without interruption throughout the afternoon and far into the night, and Dunmore, finding that the fire had swept away so many houses that the balls now had a free sweep into the heart of the town, was emboldened to land attacking parties. One group actually brought several field pieces which they planted in the streets, but the American fire was so deadly that they were forced to beat a hasty retreat.[63] The town burnt fiercely all that night, lighting up the country for miles around,[64] and the next day the plundering was resumed. It was only on January 3, when

[58] *Lower Norfolk County Antiquary,* II, 80.
[59] *American Archives,* Fourth Series, IV, 540.
[60] Smyth, *A Tour of the United States,* I, 10.
[61] *Richmond College Historical Papers,* I, 149.
[62] H. J. Eckenrode, *The Revolution in Virginia* (New York, 1916), pp. 86, 87.
[63] *Richmond College Historical Papers,* I, 149; *American Archives,* Fourth Series, IV, 539.
[64] *American Archives,* Fourth Series, I, p. 540.

nearly nine hundred houses, or more than two-thirds of Norfolk, was in ashes,[65] that Howe and Woodford restrained their men.[66]

The plight of the people was heart-rending. Many took refuge in the houses still standing in the suburbs, others trudged wearily over the roads to seek shelter in the adjacent counties. The troops gave what assistance they could, lending their wagons and driving the women and children out of the danger zone. "How they will be removed further," wrote Woodford, "it is not in our power to say."[67] But their situation, however pitiable, was preferable to that of the wretched Tories on board the fleet. Dunmore did what was possible for the prominent merchants. The families of John Hunter and Andrew Sprowle occupied the brigantine *Hammond,* Jonathan Eilbeck's family the sloop *Peace and Plenty,* the Robert Speddin and John Goodrich families seven little sloops, Niel Jamieson was on his brigantine *Fincastle,* John Brown with his family on two schooners. But the tradespeople and Negroes were crowded into small craft, intended as carriers of merchandise in the rivers and the bay.[68] Not only were food and water scarce, but smallpox broke out, taking a terrible toll, especially among the blacks. These unhappy creatures rued the day they had left their masters, for every landing place of the British was marked by their graves,[69] while their bodies by the score were dumped into the waters of Hampton Roads. "We have daily carcasses driving up on the surf," wrote a correspondent from Hampton.[70]

Woodford and Howe received orders from the Virginia Convention to do all in their power to make Dunmore's position untenable. The fleet had been supplied in large part from a distillery, several mills and some bakehouses on the right bank of the Elizabeth, and from the buildings and wells at Gosport.[71] While Norfolk was still burning, a detachment marched off at night and set fire to the distillery.[72] A few days later they returned, and after giving notice to the residents of that vicinity to move, destroyed the wells and the remaining property of the distillery company.[73] The British made desperate efforts to

[65] *Virginia Magazine of History and Biography,* XXIII, 408-414.
[66] Eckenrode, *The Revolution in Virginia,* pp. 86, 87.
[67] *Richmond College Historical Papers,* I, 151.
[68] *American Archives,* Fifth Series, I, 151, 152.
[69] *Richmond College Historical Papers,* I, 162.
[70] *Randolph Macon Historical Papers,* I, 114.
[71] *Ibid.,* p. 27; *Richmond College Historical Papers,* I, 145, 150.
[72] *American Archives,* Fourth Series, IV, 540.
[73] *Richmond College Historical Papers,* I, 150.

protect the buildings, opening on the Americans from the war vessels, and sending ashore an attacking party, but in vain.[74] Another detachment of shirtmen crossed to Gosport, where they fired the warehouses and pumps and attempted to burn a windmill.[75] Howe and Woodford also scattered small detachments along both banks of the river from Tanner's Creek to Craney Island to drive off landing parties.

In the meanwhile the two commanders were making preparations to evacuate Norfolk. Their mission had been fulfilled; many of their men were asking permission to resign, others were ill. But it was not their intention to leave anything for the possession of the British, and early in February, 1776, by the command of the Virginia Convention, they burned down what was left of the town, 416 houses in all, valued at about £50,000.[76] Then, after demolishing Dunmore's entrenchments, they marched out, taking the remnants of the wretched inhabitants with them. They left behind complete desolation, charred timbers, blackened foundations, ashes. Gone were the courthouse, the market, the warehouses, the shops, the handsome residences. Where a few months before singing bands of slaves had loaded and unloaded vessels fresh from Glasgow or the West Indies, where merchants had bargained for molasses or sugar or tobacco, where the country people had gathered to sell their produce, where children had laughed and played, was now only silence. Caught between the upper and the lower stones of the Revolution, Norfolk had paid the supreme penalty.

The burning of Norfolk started a controversy which has continued to the present day. In March, 1776, the Earl of Richmond rose in Parliament to condemn the "barbaric rage" with which the British were conducting the war. What excuse is there for "our naval commanders," he asked, who reduced the loyal town of Norfolk to ashes? Thereupon, the Earl of Sandwich explained that the "Norfolk people set fire to the town; that is, the fire from the men-of-war set fire to part of it, and the inhabitants burnt the rest."[77] The matter should have been put to rest by the report of a commission of investigation, appointed by the Virginia government in 1777.[78] They found that of 1331 houses destroyed in and near Norfolk, 32 had been burnt by

[74] *Ibid.*, p. 152.
[75] *Ibid.*, pp. 145, 152; *Randolph Macon Historical Papers*, I, 27.
[76] *Ibid.*; *Virginia Magazine of History and Biography*, XXIII, 414.
[77] *American Archives*, Fourth Series, VI, 294, 299.
[78] The Commissioners were Richard Kello, James Prentis, Daniel Fisher, and Robert Andrews.

Dunmore on November 30, 1775; 19 by Dunmore the day of the bombardment; 863 by the troops of the State before January 15, 1776, and 416 by the order of the Convention in February.[79] Yet two decades later Rochefoucauld smiled incredulously when informed that the patriots themselves had burned the town. "You recall that the Jacobins of France said that the aristocrats burned their own chateaux," he said. "Party heat gives rise to the greatest absurdities. Men are the same everywhere."[80] Modern English historians of established reputations, who would do well to examine the facts more closely, still place the blame for Norfolk's destruction at Dunmore's door.[81]

Major General Charles Lee, who was appointed commander of the American forces in the Southern Department, now assumed the direction of the operations on the Elizabeth River. Detachments were maintained at Great Bridge, Kemps, Ferry Point, on Tanner's Creek, at Newton, and elsewhere.[82] But they could not prevent Dunmore from landing under the cover of his war vessels, at Tucker's Mill, west of Portsmouth, and establishing a camp there. The British made an entrenchment and a ditch eight feet deep, extending a quarter of a mile in length, from one cove to another, which gave them about four acres of land. Here they drilled their few remaining regulars, the Norfolk Tories, and several hundred blacks. The *Liverpool* and *Otter* were stationed close to the shore to protect this improvised fort, while the *Dunmore* remained on the other side of the river near the ruins of the distillery.[83] Although the British and their unhappy wards were comparatively safe from attack here, their position became increasingly uncomfortable. The sinking of several wells afforded a plentiful supply of water, it is true, but provisions were scarce, and the fever still raged among the blacks.[84]

In fact, Dunmore could not have remained here a week, had not the Tories on both sides of the river constantly rowed out to the fleet under cover of darkness, with bread, wheat, and corn. After trying in vain to put an end to this traffic by guarding the shores, the Committee of Safety decided upon the drastic expedient of moving the entire population. On April 10, 1776, they ordered that "all the inhabitants

[79] *Virginia Magazine of History and Biography*, XXIII, 414.
[80] La Rochefoucauld, *Voyage dans Les États-Unis*, IV, 225.
[81] W. E. H. Lecky, *The American Revolution* (New York, 1908), p. 236.
[82] New York Historical Society, *Collections*, 1871, p. 462.
[83] *Ibid.*, pp. 365, 385.
[84] *Richmond College Historical Papers*, I, 162.

of Norfolk and Princess Anne counties, at present residing between
the enemy and our posts at Great Bridge and Kemp's Landing, and
in a direct line from Kemp's Landing to the ocean, be immediately
removed to some interior parts of this colony."[85] This order caused
consternation. To force five thousand souls to abandon their homes
and their fields, and move many miles over a wretched road in quest
of shelter among strangers, would cause endless suffering.[86] Yet the
order would probably have been enforced, had not the flight of the
British rendered it unnecessary.

In the meanwhile General Lee was leaving no stone unturned to
tighten the lines around the Elizabeth and cut off parties communicating with the fleet. A certain Mr. Hopkins, seized as he was
returning from the vessels, was conducted to his own residence, and
made to look on while the troops rifled it of furniture and set it on
fire.[87] The Americans now occupied Portsmouth, not only because it
afforded quarters for the troops, but because it was an excellent
position from which to watch the British at Tucker's Mill. Explaining
to the Convention that "even the women and children had learned
the art of spies," Lee ordered the entire population to leave. He then
confiscated the movable goods of the most prominent Tories—Andrew Sprowle, Niel Jamieson, John Goodrich, and Robert Speddin,—
and applied the torch to their residences and stores.[88] One attempt
was made to set fire to the merchant vessels clustered in the river
near the ruins of Norfolk, but the unexpected arrival of the *Dunmore*
forced the boats to scamper for shore before they had succeeded in
their purpose.[89]

One morning in May, the lookouts in Portsmouth observed that the
British were preparing to leave. As they watched, men, women, and
children embarked, anchors were hauled up, sails spread, and prows
pointed down the river. The fleet made an interesting spectacle—the
war vessels, their guns ready for action; brigantines; schooners; and
sloops, nearly a hundred in all, their decks crowded with troops,
Negroes, and Tories.[90] A few days later the fleet came to anchor at
Gwynn's Island, off the coast of Mathews County. There Dunmore
established a camp, erecting breastworks, mounting cannon, and

[85] New York Historical Society, *Collections*, 1871, p. 407.
[86] *Virginia Magazine of History and Biography*, XV, 154.
[87] *Richmond College Historical Papers*, I, 155, 156.
[88] *Ibid.*, p. 155; New York Historical Society, *Collections*, 1871, pp. 457, 458.
[89] New York Historical Society, *Collections*, 1871, p. 459.
[90] *Richmond College Historical Papers*, I, 161.

stationing several small armed vessels in the channel between the island and the mainland. The *Dunmore, Otter, Roebuck,* and other warships were anchored in close in order to protect the camp, while the wretched band of fugitives came ashore, hoping that at last they would be safe from the relentless Virginians.[91]

But Dunmore had blundered again. General Andrew Lewis, hero of the Battle of Point Pleasant, brought up troops and erected batteries on the mainland opposite the island. On July 8, 1776, he opened upon the camp, fortifications, and shipping with two 18-pounders and several smaller guns. The first shot, fired by Lewis himself, passed through the *Dunmore.* Then a nine-pounder entered her quarter, smashed the china, splintered a large timber, and wounded Lord Dunmore himself. "Good God, that ever I should come to this!" shouted his lordship. By this time the entire fleet, in the greatest confusion, began to slip their cables and move out into the bay. On shore the cry was raised, "The shirtmen are coming!" and away everyone scampered to get on board the vessels. Some of the sick were placed in carts and conveyed to the point of embarkation; others were left to their fate. When some brush huts were accidentally set on fire, those who were too ill to crawl out were burned to death. The next day, when the Americans took possession, they found a scene of horror. Bodies were strewn about "without a shovelful of earth upon them; others gasping for life; some had crawled to the water's edge, who could only make known their distress by beckoning. . . . In short, such a scene of misery, distress, and cruelty," they had never seen before. The Norfolk Tories were paying a terrible penalty for their adherence to the royal cause.[92]

Dunmore lingered near Gwynn's Island for a day or two, taking care to keep out of range of Lewis's 18-pounders, and then left for the Potomac in search of recruits and provisions.[93] After remaining there three weeks, in which time two hundred more deaths occurred, he burnt thirty or forty of his vessels, and dividing the rest into two divisions, sailed down the bay and out through the Capes. The squadrons then separated, one heading north and the other south.[94] On August 15 Dunmore, with twenty-five sail, entered New York harbor.[95] As for the refugees, many never saw Norfolk again. "Some go imme-

91 New York Historical Society, *Collections,* 1872, pp. 44, 52.
92 *American Archives,* Fifth Series, I, 150, 151, 431, 432.
93 *Ibid.*
94 *Ibid.,* p. 862.
95 *Ibid.,* p. 949.

diately to Great Britain," Dunmore announced on July 31, "others to
the West Indies, and others to St. Augustine."[96] Some, we know, accompanied him to New York, where they established themselves as merchants and shippers.[97] All their warehouses, stores, and residences in
Virginia had been destroyed, while their building lots in Norfolk or
Portsmouth were confiscated.[98] Some, however, who owned one or
more merchant vessels, were able to bring them off with their cargoes;
others had property in Europe or the West Indies,[99] which they were
able to capitalize for a new start in business. The larger number were
never able to restore their fortunes and would have sunk into poverty
had it not been for assistance rendered by the British government.[100]

The lot of the Norfolk people who remained in Virginia was
hardly less deplorable than that of those who left with Dunmore.
Hundreds who before the war had enjoyed every comfort were reduced to want.[101] It is true that all who could prove their allegiance
to the Revolution received some compensation for the destruction of
their property in the two fires, but the sums were quite inadequate.[102]
It was the interruption of trade and the consequent loss of employment which in the end proved most disastrous. The people took refuge wherever shelter was to be found. Some lived miserably in huts
in the woods;[103] some rented houses in Princess Anne and Norfolk
counties, some moved many miles into the interior. Everywhere they
were charged excessive rents,[104] and those who had relatives or
friends to offer shelter in the hour of need were fortunate indeed.

"I shall not attempt to describe what we have suffered within these
last three years," wrote one brave woman. "[We all] live together on
dear deceased Mr. Aitchinson's plantation. It is a small house for two
families that have been used to be better accommodated, but we are
very thankful for such an asylum. Many of the poor inhabitants of
Norfolk are greatly distressed for any house at all. We spin our own
clothes, milk, sew, raise poultry. . . . Everything has got to such
prices here that we buy nothing that we can do without. Our girls are

---

[96] *Richmond College Historical Papers*, I, 196.
[97] New York Historical Society, *Collections*, 1901, p. 122.
[98] Stewart, *History of Norfolk County*, pp. 56, 57.
[99] *American Archives*, Fifth Series, I, 152.
[100] Dunmore seems to have taken away with him a thousand refugees from eastern Virginia and Maryland (*ibid.*, p. 432).
[101] *American Archives*, Fourth Series, VI, 1540; *Virginia Magazine of History and Biography*, XXIII, 408.
[102] Stewart, *History of Norfolk County*, pp. 363-367.
[103] *Virginia Magazine of History and Biography*, XXIII, 407-414.
[104] *American Archives*, Fourth Series, VI, 686.

all dressed in their own spinning, even little Molly. Ann assists and your Jenny is as notable at the country work as if she had been brought up to it. . . . I am sorry our present circumstances prevents them from improving themselves by reading, writing, keeping polite society, etc."[105]

Despite the ruin which befell Norfolk, despite the Tory sympathies of many of her leading merchants, despite the dispersal of her people, the town did its share toward winning the Revolution. Virginia had to have a navy to protect the Chesapeake and her great navigable rivers, and for the work of creating and directing a navy the people of Norfolk were pre-eminently fitted. There was need not only for naval officers and for sailors, but for ship carpenters, caulkers, sailmakers, ropemakers. Upon the first Naval Board were two Norfolk men— Thomas Newton and John Hutchings.[106] James Maxwell was chief superintendent of the state navy yard in Charles City County.[107] "Mr. Maxwell had thought of buying a farm and setting us down on it," wrote his wife, "when he received a letter from Gen. Washington, I think, or some one, inviting him to come and take charge of the Navy Yard. . . . He determined, at once, to accept the invitation and join the standard of the country, which, I was both proud and pleased to have him do."[108] Christopher Calvert was given charge of the construction of vessels.[109] Other Norfolk men who served in the navy were George Muter, Wright Wescott, Nicholas Wonycott, and John Harris. The little Virginia war vessels could offer no resistance to a real invasion of Virginia waters; but they did excellent work in protecting trade, keeping the Tories quiet, facilitating the movement of troops, transporting arms and ammunition, and guarding the channels of communication.[110]

It was under their wings that the trade of Norfolk began its first stirrings after the great fire. In November, 1779, when Miss Jenny Stewart visited "that once agreeable place," she found it still desolate. "Nobody could conceive that did not see it how much it is altered," she said. "It shocks me exceedingly." But even then there were "a

---

[105] *Virginia Magazine of History and Biography*, III, 214.
[106] *The Researcher*, I, 15.
[107] *Ibid.*, p. 69.
[108] *Lower Norfolk County Antiquary*, II, 138. This shows that some of the Norfolk men who pinned on the red badge of loyalism under compulsion afterwards served their country well.
[109] *The Researcher*, I, 70.
[110] *Ibid.*, pp. 9-16, 62-76, 129-136, 197-203; *Virginia Magazine of History and Biography*, XVII, 364.

great many small huts built up in it," occupied by former residents who could not "be happy anywhere else."[111] So early as the winter of 1778-1779 some of the prominent families were planning to rebuild their homes,[112] a clear indication that commerce was not entirely dead. We know that goods from the French West Indies and even from France itself continued to find their way to Virginia during the Revolution, despite the activities of British frigates and Tory privateers. In May, 1779, there were two large French ships in Elizabeth River, while at the wharves of Portsmouth, Gosport, Suffolk, and Norfolk were scores of vessels of various sizes, unloading French goods, or taking on tobacco, tar, pitch, turpentine, and pork.[113] Fleets of Virginia vessels left for Nantes with tobacco, which was exchanged for salt, blankets, woolens, sail duck, medicines, linens, arms, powder, and other articles needed by the people and government of the state.[114]

The Virginians sought to protect this growing commerce by the erection of a fort on the Elizabeth, just west of Portsmouth. They made a parapet fourteen feet high and fifteen feet thick facing the river, brought up heavy guns, and accumulated stores of ammunition and provisions. But they made the mistake of manning this post too lightly, and when, in May, 1779, Sir George Collier entered the river with a large fleet, the garrison could offer no resistance. Sir George landed a force west of the fort, with the purpose of making a joint attack by water and land, and the Americans, in fear of being cut off, retreated during the night, leaving Portsmouth, Gosport, and all the shipping a prey to the enemy. It was a rich prize. "The quantity of naval stores, of all kinds, found in their arsenals was astonishing," reported Sir George. "Many vessels were taken on the stocks . . . one of 36 guns, one of 18, three of 16, and three of 14, besides many merchantmen." The whole number taken, burnt, and destroyed, while the King's ships were in the river amounted to 137 vessels.[115] After burning Suffolk and committing numerous other outrages, the British hoisted sail and headed out of the Capes. Their unannounced visit had cost Virginia £1,000,000, and had struck a blow at her commerce from which she was years in recovering.[116]

[111] *Virginia Magazine of History and Biography*, III, 215.
[112] *Ibid.*, p. 214.
[113] *Virginia Historical Register*, IV, 188, 189.
[114] *Virginia Magazine of History and Biography*, XVII, 364; *Official Letters of Governors of Virginia*, I, 146, and II, 92.
[115] *Virginia Historical Register*, IV, 187, 188.
[116] *Ibid.*, pp. 188-195.

In the meanwhile, fighting had been going on in Princess Anne and Norfolk counties between patriots and Tories. Many families were hopelessly divided. "Long and what were thought valuable friendships are now entirely dissolved," wrote one observer, "and persons that thought themselves a few years ago the best of friends, are now the most inveterate enemies. Even the very near and dear ties between father and son are in many instances quite done away."[117] After the departure of Dunmore, this enmity broke forth in a long series of murders, robberies, and burnings. Bands of ragged Tories, making their headquarters in the swamps of Princess Anne, would descend upon a plantation, strip it of provisions, burn the buildings and drive off the livestock. The most notorious of these bandits was Josiah Phillips, leader of a force of fifty men, who for several years spread terror far and wide.[118] In May, 1778, the legislature outlawed Phillips, and before the year was out, he was captured, tried in the civil court, and hanged.[119]

But there were other Tory leaders to take his place. "The county of Princess Anne has neither civil or military law in it," wrote Thomas Newton, Jr., in September, 1781. "Murder is committed and no notice is taken of it. . . . A few desperate fellows go about on the sea coasts and large swamps, and do mischiefs in the night."[120] It was proposed to erect a redoubt at Cape Henry to "overawe those ragamuffins" until troops could arrive from the upcountry.[121] Yet so late as August, 1782, the swamps were still harboring many refugees, who, however, seemed anxious to come in under an offer of immunity. Colonel Newton suggested that it would be wise to issue a general pardon, excepting from it "Levi Sikes and Robert Stewart, the great offenders."[122]

The hopes of the refugees were aroused from time to time by the arrival of the British in Elizabeth River. In October, 1780, a fleet from New York arrived at Portsmouth and landed an army under General Leslie. Fortunately they were bent on gaining touch with Cornwallis in the Carolinas rather than conquering Virginia, so that after a short stay they sailed for Charleston. They took with them some Norfolk and Princess Anne Tories; but the slaves who had flocked in at the

[117] *Virginia Magazine of History and Biography*, III, 215.
[118] *Official Letters of Governors of Virginia*, I, 282, 283.
[119] *Richmond College Historical Papers*, I, 199, 200.
[120] *Calendar of Virginia State Papers*, II, 450, 451.
[121] *Ibid.*, II, 671.
[122] *Ibid.*, III, 252.

news of their arrival, they were compelled to leave behind.[123] Even more unwelcome than Leslie was Benedict Arnold, who entered the Capes in December, 1780, and after a brief excursion up the James, established himself at Portsmouth. The traitor came, not like his predecessors for a brief stay only, but with the purpose of devastating and perhaps conquering Virginia. He set to work to fortify the town, throwing up works from Gosport Creek to "a creek which empties itself below Portsmouth," and mounting heavy cannon. The *Charon,* he posted off Craney Island, while the other warships were drawn up from Tucker's Mill to Gosport.[124] Arnold made his headquarters in the home of Patrick Robinson, on the northwest corner of High and Middle streets,[125] setting aside the old sugarhouse on Crawford Street, near the Gosport bridge, for a prison and a barracks for his troops.[126] Immediately slaves began to come in. By this time, however, the British had learned that the blacks were more of an encumbrance than a help, being useless as soldiers, costly to maintain, and serving only to spread disease among the troops.[127] Yet Arnold could not refuse to accept them, and many remained with the army until after the surrender at Yorktown. General Washington hoped to trap the traitor by sending a French fleet to cut his communications by sea, while troops closed in upon him by land. But the French were tardy in carrying out their part of the program, so that when they approached the Capes, they found Admiral Arbuthnot waiting for them. After an indecisive engagement the French withdrew to Newport, and the offensive broke down.[128]

As the stay of Arnold in Virginia lengthened and as other forces joined him, first under General Phillips, and then under Lord Cornwallis, the Tories of Princess Anne and Norfolk counties assumed a bolder attitude. They began to enlist in considerable numbers, while some of the exiles came back to take possession of their confiscated estates.[129] The conquest of Virginia they thought certain. But their confidence was sadly shaken again when the British marched out of Portsmouth to establish their camp at Yorktown. Unwilling to face their outraged countrymen, they gathered up what belongings they could carry, and to the number of several hundred followed in the

[123] *Official Letters of Governors of Virginia*, II, 222, 234, 321.
[124] *Calendar of Virginia State Papers*, I, 557.
[125] Burnt before 1859.
[126] Jarvis Papers, p. 36.
[127] *Calendar of Virginia State Papers*, I, 557.
[128] Lossing, *Field Book of the Revolution*, II, 334.
[129] *Calendar of Virginia State Papers*, I, 476.

wake of the troops.[130] Once more they were forced to endure the pangs of hunger and fear as Washington, Rochambeau, and De Grasse closed in upon the British. When it became obvious that Cornwallis would have to surrender, some stole away at night and, crossing the bay, sought their old refuge in the Princess Anne swamps. Many crowded into the sloop-of-war *Bonetta,* which was permitted to sail unsearched, and so escaped to New York. Others fell into the hands of Washington's victorious army, and later were tried for taking up arms against their native land.[131]

No community in America suffered more in the Revolution than Norfolk. With its buildings laid in ashes, its people scattered far and wide, many of them in dire poverty, its slave population in part carried off, its prosperous trade ruined, the vessels which had once crowded its harbor captured or destroyed, many thought that the place would never again raise its head. Even though the tobacco trade to England were resumed, even though the British should be generous enough to open their West Indian ports to American goods, it would not profit Norfolk, they said. Portsmouth would be the future port of Virginia, and the once proud town across the river would remain an unimportant village. Whether their predictions were to prove correct, whether Norfolk's ruin was to be permanent, or whether independence was eventually to bring increased prosperity and growth, time alone could show.

---

130 *Virginia Magazine of History and Biography,* III, 215.
131 *Richmond College Historical Papers,* I, 201-203.

CHAPTER FOUR

The Phoenix of the Elizabeth

The rebuilding of Norfolk continued under the British and Tories. During the occupation of the Elizabeth River in 1780 and 1781, some of the exiles came back and, believing that the Revolutionists would never regain possession of Norfolk, settled down on their old estates, and began building. In September, 1783, the State of Virginia confiscated two dwellings, seven storehouses, and other smaller structures belonging to Niel Jamieson. A few weeks later it took over a two-story brick house and kitchen near Main Street, the property of Jonathan Eilbeck.[1] In January, 1785, two dwellings on Church Street and another at Town Bridge, taken from William Chisholm, were sold by act of Assembly.[2] In addition to these structures, which stood out here and there amid the "heap of ruins and desolation," the Americans found "two houses built on the public by the enemy" when they re-entered the town in 1781.[3]

With this as a nucleus, Norfolk slowly emerged from its ashes. The mayor and aldermen met in March, 1782, to start the wheels of government. The consent of the Assembly was gained for a new borough plan in which Main Street was widened and Church Street altered.[4] In restoring their homes, property owners were permitted to run their steps five feet into the street, while an additional five feet was set aside

[1] *Norfolk Borough Register,* 1783-1790, Corporation Court, pp. 4a, 14.
[2] *Ibid.,* p. 65a.
[3] *Norfolk Council Orders,* 1736-1798, p. 76. *The Norfolk Directory* for 1806 states that "at the close of the year 1783 there were not twelve houses rebuilt."
[4] *Norfolk Council Orders,* 1782, October. The George Nicholson map of 1802 shows two buildings projecting into the street at Main and Church. They doubtless were erected by the Tories in 1781, before the streets were laid out under the new plan.

for a footway, which they must "post" and pave.[5] The borough government next rebuilt the market, purchased fire engines, reopened wells, erected bridges, and constructed a town hall and prison.[6]

Immediately after the war, a number of Scotch and English merchants migrated to Virginia, some as representatives of British firms, others to enter business for themselves. Believing that Portsmouth would displace Norfolk as the chief seaport of Virginia, most of them planned to settle in that town. But since the Portsmouth people, still resentful against the British, refused to receive them,[7] they went to Norfolk, where they were welcomed. These newcomers, because of their mercantile connections as well as their personal ability, played a vital rôle in restoring the town's prosperity.[8]

As for the Norfolk patriots, many were still living in the backwoods in extreme poverty. These unfortunates, themselves lacking the means to restore Norfolk's ruined stores and warehouses, often refused to sell their lots to those who could. Therefore many merchants had to rent ground upon which to build at very high rates, some paying no less than one hundred guineas a year for a lot large enough for a storehouse only. Since leases could be had for no more than seven years, the tenant built a mere shack, "anything that would answer the business," knowing that in a short time he would have to relinquish his right to it.[9] Consequently, Norfolk was rebuilt chiefly of small, poorly constructed, wooden houses.[10] Only after several decades, when whole streets of frame buildings had been swept away by fire, did the town regain the aspect of the old substantial Norfolk of pre-Revolutionary days.[11]

With the conclusion of peace in 1783, ships from London, Liver-

[5] *Ibid.,* p. 80.

[6] *Ibid.,* pp. 80, 81, 85b, 87, 91.

[7] One account says they "formed a mob and drove them off." (Norfolk *Herald,* Aug. 10, 1802.) La Rochefoucauld declares, "Les habitans exaltés contra les Anglais, ont refusé d'y recevoir aucun négociant de cette nation." (*Voyage dans les États-Unis,* IV, 255.)

[8] The Scottish mercantile houses did not, of course, send back as their representatives the men who had incurred such enmity because of their Tory principles during the Revolution. It was stated that there were not above forty Scotchmen of ante-bellum days living in Norfolk in 1785. *Virginia Magazine of History and Biography,* XXIII, 407-414. Among the Scotch names listed in the *Directory* of 1806 are Nathan MacGill, Alexander McClure, John Mackenzie, John MacGowan, George McIntosh, Duncan McDonald, John McNeil, James Menzies, and David McAllister.

[9] *Virginia Magazine of History and Biography,* XXIII, 407-414.

[10] La Rochefoucauld, *Voyage dans les États-Unis,* IV, 257.

[11] One observer stated that the houses were few and far between and of humble dimensions, while the merchants, from lack of storerooms, often had to leave their goods in the open air under watch. (Norfolk *Herald,* July 11, 1828; H. B. Grigsby, *Governor Tazewell* [Norfolk, 1860], p. 27.)

pool, and Glasgow once more began to enter the Capes, laden with European manufactured goods. Most of them headed for the James, the Rappahannock, or the Potomac, but some came to the Elizabeth and discharged their cargoes at the wharves of Norfolk.[12] Here they took on tobacco, brought down from Richmond, Petersburg, and other river ports, and set out on the return journey. Before a year had passed the interchange of goods between the Chesapeake Bay and Great Britain was in full swing. "Our trade was never more completely monopolized by Great Britain . . . than it is at this moment," wrote James Madison in June, 1785. "Our merchants are almost all connected with that country, and that only, and we have neither ships nor seamen of our own."[13]

With remarkable rapidity Norfolk resumed its old place as the chief export town for this overseas trade. "It is the only port of the southern part of this great State," wrote La Rochefoucauld in 1795, "for boats of 100 or 120 tons only can go up to Petersburg and Richmond. The products of the back country which come to those places by land, are usually sent by barges to Norfolk, whence they are exported. Thus, this port practically monopolizes the commerce of all Virginia from the Rappahannock, and that of North Carolina well beyond the Roanoke."[14]

Yet Norfolk's former prosperity had been based chiefly upon the West Indian trade, and future growth would be slow unless the British government opened her islands to the products and the ships of the United States. At first hope ran high. William Pitt, in March, 1783, introduced a bill in the Commons permitting the free importation of American goods in American ships into the British West Indies. But this liberal policy, so sharply at variance with the British colonial system, met immediate opposition. England must stimulate shipbuilding at home, not in America, it was argued; otherwise the time might come when the Admiralty would have to send to the United States whenever they wanted a new frigate. Pitt's bill was blocked. On July 2, 1783, an order in council was published restricting the trade between the United States and the British colonies to a limited number of articles to be carried exclusively in British vessels.[15]

---

[12] *Norfolk Borough Register*, 1783-1790, pp. 30a, 32a, 43a, 46a.
[13] Gaillard Hunt, *Letters and Writings of James Madison* (Philadelphia, 1865), I, 91.
[14] *Voyage dans les États-Unis*, IV, 258.
[15] F. Lee Benns, *The American Struggle for the British West India Carrying Trade, 1815-1830* (*Indiana University Studies*, X, Bloomington, 1923), pp. 8, 9, 10.

At first this seems to have aroused no serious apprehension in Norfolk. The lumber, provisions, and naval stores of Virginia could still find a market in the British West Indies, the sugar and molasses of Antigua and Jamaica could still be had in exchange. That this trade was to be carried on exclusively in British bottoms would prevent the revival of shipbuilding on the Elizabeth, it was true, but this could be endured so long as the trade itself was restored.

But the merchants were not long in finding their mistake. The entire British West Indian trade was monopolized by foreign firms. The Norfolk trader who wished to send a bill of goods to the islands had to bargain with the English shipowners, who might charge him what they would, or if he wished to ship a cargo on his own account, refuse to give him space at any price. "What makes the British monopoly the more mortifying is the abuse they make of it," said Madison. Many Virginia planters and merchants "have received accounts of sales this season, which carry the most visible and shameful frauds in every article."[16] As for the shipbuilders, the ropemakers, the block makers, the ship carpenters, the caulkers, who had looked to peace for a return of prosperous days, they all suffered from idleness and low wages. There was no call for American vessels, and very little occasion for repairing and reconditioning. The foreign ships which came into the Capes "were for the most part well fitted, and wanted little or nothing, except when they met with some damage on the voyage." So the Norfolk mechanics "had scarcely employment to afford a scanty subsistence for themselves and their families."[17]

It was useless to appeal to the feeble Congress, which, under the Articles of Confederation, did not have the power to regulate foreign commerce, to retaliate for the discrimination against American shipping. The Virginia merchants had to turn to their own state legislature for relief, and at the session of 1785 their complaints poured in.[18]

The Assembly itself was at a loss what to do. Should they assent to the regulation of foreign commerce by Congress, or should they attempt to play a free hand? The Federalists argued that England could be forced to make concessions only by the united action of all the states, and for this a grant of power to Congress was necessary. It would be idle for Virginia to place a heavy duty on West Indian rum or sugar brought in by British ships if Maryland refused to follow

[16] Hunt, *Letters and Writings of James Madison,* II, 151.
[17] Norfolk *Gazette and Public Ledger,* Oct. 30, 1804.
[18] Hunt, *Letters and Writings of James Madison,* I, 200; Hugh B. Grigsby, *Virginia Federal Convention* (Richmond, 1855), II, 127.

suit. And if Maryland and Virginia agreed to have a like duty, would not England ignore their action, so long as she could supply her islands from Massachusetts or New York? After a long debate the Assembly voted by a large majority that "the power over trade ought to be vested in Congress, under certain qualifications." But it was not so easy to secure agreement on just what these "qualifications" should be. Madison, who led the battle for a liberal grant of power, was opposed by Meriwether Smith, Carter Braxton, and Benjamin Harrison. When the Federalists introduced a bill to authorize Congress to retaliate upon foreign nations and to impose a 5 per cent duty on imports to raise funds for the state quotas, these men protested vigorously. The time had not yet come, they said, for Virginia to surrender her customs to the Federal government. The power to tax was the essence of liberty and must be controlled solely by the people of Virginia through their representatives in the Assembly. In committee the bill was so weakened by amendments that the Federalists turned from it in disgust.[19]

In the meanwhile, a petition came in from Petersburg, complaining that the restrictions of the European powers were ruining the commerce of Virginia, and urging immediate relief. Something must be done, they declared, to foster shipbuilding and to open the trade routes to Virginia-built ships, owned by Virginia merchants.[20] A similar petition from the Norfolk merchants had been presented at the previous session, and it was deemed necessary to mollify the shipping interests. If relief was not to be had by Federal action, Virginia must bring the British lion to terms. Accordingly Braxton introduced a bill to prevent the importation of goods from the British West Indies in British bottoms, and another granting a drawback on goods imported in Virginia vessels.[21] These measures pleased nobody. Few imagined that they would cause England to alter her navigation acts, while the effect upon the Virginia trade would be ruinous. In the end they were dropped by the Antifederalist majority, and in their place a bill was passed placing a tonnage of five shillings on entering vessels of countries having no commercial treaty with the United States.[22]

It was obvious, however, that this could benefit the shipping and mercantile interests little, so long as American vessels were excluded from the British West Indies, and the session was about to close with

[19] Grigsby, *Virginia Federal Convention*, II, 140-145.
[20] *Ibid.*, II, 143.
[21] *Ibid.*, II, 145; Hunt, *Letters and Writings of James Madison*, I, 200.
[22] Hunt, *Letters and Writings of James Madison*, I, 222.

Norfolk, Petersburg, and Alexandria bitterly dissatisfied. At this moment, when the Antifederalists were looking around for some means of mollifying these towns, Madison suggested an interstate convention to consider means for regulating American commerce. John Tyler had made this motion before, only to have it ignored. Now, however, on the last day of the session, it was rushed through with but two dissenting voices. It was this resolution which led to the Annapolis Convention, and out of the Annapolis Convention grew the Constitutional Convention at Philadelphia. Thus the demand of the Virginia merchants for retaliation against England's trade restrictions played an important and wholly unexpected part in the creation of the new Federal Union.[23]

When once the movement had been launched, the people of Norfolk gave it their hearty support, looking to the proposed constitution as their only salvation. All through the summer of 1787, while the convention was in session, they waited impatiently for the report. When at last the Constitution was placed before them, and they saw that it meant the creation of a real nation with a government strong enough to battle for American rights the world over, hope grew strong in the "ancient borough." Crowds gathered in the Borough Tavern and the old coffee house opposite Town Hall to read the numbers of the *Federalist* as they appeared, and each point in favor of the new union was loudly applauded.[24] At the celebration of Washington's birthday, toasts were drunk to the United States, to the members of the Federal Convention, to the Rhode Island minority, to the author of the *Federalist*, and to the commerce and manufactures of America.[25] George Mason's objections to the Constitution, when published in the *Norfolk and Portsmouth Journal*, were immediately answered in an article running through three numbers of that paper,[26] while an Antifederalist "Address to the People of Virginia," brought forth vigorous protests from "Virginian" and "Alexander M. Sarcasm."[27] In April the borough elected as its representative in the Virginia ratifying convention General Thomas Mathews, a staunch Federalist.[28]

Although Mathews was Speaker of the House of Delegates and a

[23] T. J. Wertenbaker, *The American People, A History* (New York, 1928), pp. 111-113.
[24] *Norfolk and Portsmouth Journal*, Jan. 30, 1788.
[25] *Ibid.*, Feb. 13, 1788, Library of Congress.
[26] *Ibid.*, Feb. 20, 1788.
[27] *Ibid.*, March 12, 1788.
[28] *Ibid.*, April 23, 1788; Grigsby, *Virginia Federal Convention*, I, 306.

man of great influence in the state, he was not the spokesman for the mercantile group in the convention. That honor fell to Francis Corbin, of Middlesex. When Patrick Henry, in one of his bitter attacks on the new constitution, stated that the state was prospering under the Articles of Confederation, Corbin took him sharply to task: "Let him visit the sea coast," he said, "go to the ports and inlets. In those ports, sir, where we had every reason to see the fleets of all nations, he will behold but a few trifling little boats—he will everywhere see commerce languish—the disconsolate merchant, with his arms folded, ruminating in despair, on the wretched ruin of his fortune, and deploring the impossibility of retrieving it. The West Indies are blocked up against us."[29] It is not difficult to imagine the applause with which this statement was greeted by the delegates from the shipping centers. When the final vote was taken, the southeastern counties cast a solid vote for ratification. James Webb and James Taylor for Norfolk County, Thomas Mathews for Norfolk borough, Anthony Walke and Thomas Walke for Princess Anne, Willis Riddick and Solomon Shepherd for Nansemond, James Johnson for Isle of Wight, Miles King and Worlick Westwood for Elizabeth City, John Blair and George Wythe for York, John Stringer and Littleton Eyre for Northampton, all voted in the affirmative.[30]

The news that Virginia had joined the new Union reached Norfolk late on Friday, June 27. It was announced by the firing of cannon at the fort and on the ships; with darkness, the borough was illuminated, while excited people thronged the streets to discuss the good tidings.[31] The next week the town celebrated jointly the Fourth of July and the ratification of the Constitution. A long procession formed at 11 A.M., and marched through the principal streets out to Town Point. In the lead was a band, followed by the various tradesmen of the town and county, holding aloft standards with mottoes emblematic of their crafts—butchers, fishermen, bakers, brewers and distillers, printers, merchants, grocers, pilots, ship carpenters, ropemakers, blacksmiths. Then came the good ship *Constitution,* commanded by Captain Maxwell and drawn by ten horses. Behind marched more tradesmen, seamen, carpenters, bricklayers, glaziers, cabinetmakers, coopers, hatters, shoemakers, saddlers, peruke makers, goldsmiths, candlers, draymen, physicians, lawyers. The tailors at-

[29] Jonathan Elliot, *Debates on the Constitution* (Philadelphia, 1836-45), III, 123, 124.
[30] *Ibid.*, pp. 589-590.
[31] *Norfolk and Portsmouth Journal,* July 2, 1788.

tracted especial interest, for with them were two boys representing Adam and Eve, "whose uncommon garb of fig leaves" drew attention to the advances made in the art of making clothes. Next in order were the schoolmasters, with their scholars carrying their books, then the sergeant with the famous mace presented by Governor Dinwiddie in 1754,[32] and last of all the mayor, aldermen and councilmen. At Town Point a repast had been set in the open, and here the people regaled themselves while the caterer, Mr. Smith of the Borough Tavern under the assumed character of old Will Boniface, flitted from table to table. Speeches, toasts, and songs followed, after which a bonfire of ten barrels of pitch was set off.[33]

In the heat of the struggle for the Constitution, it seems not to have occurred to the Federalists that even the new government might be powerless to force Great Britain to open her colonies to American shippers. All was now confidence and expectation. Hardly had Congress assembled when an act was passed placing discriminating tonnage duties on foreign-built and foreign-owned ships.[34] Next Gouverneur Morris was sent to London to take up with the British government the matter of a commercial treaty, opening their islands to our products carried in our own vessels. But the British showed no inclination to yield merely because the states had created a real union. The ministry decided to wait for the United States to make the first move, and Morris had to report that he could accomplish nothing. Apparently this left the American government the alternative of acquiescing in the existing situation, or of retaliation. The former course was not to be thought of, for petitions were pouring in from the seaport towns demanding relief; while the latter would be costly and probably ineffective. In this quandary Washington, at the suggestion of Hamilton, decided to try again for a treaty of commerce, and so sent over our ablest diplomat, John Jay. The British now proved more amenable, and Jay sent back a treaty technically consistent with his instructions and in some respects highly advantageous. But Article XII, which related to the West India trade, was unsatisfactory. True, it opened the island ports to American vessels, but only of seventy tons, and it pledged the United States to export no molasses, sugar, coffee, cocoa, or cotton, either from the United States or from the islands.[35] While the treaty was under consideration

[32] *Norfolk Council Orders*, 1736-1798, p. 27b.
[33] *Ibid.*, July 9, 1788.
[34] Benns, *American Struggle for the British West India Carrying Trade*, p. 13.
[35] *Ibid.*, pp. 17, 18.

in the Senate in secret session and the mercantile centers were awaiting anxiously to know its provisions, Stephen T. Mason sent an abstract to a Philadelphia paper. A tremendous outburst of disappointment and of anger against Jay followed. "Why should we be restricted to vessels of 70 tons," men asked each other, "while the British use their largest ships? Why are we excluded from the West Indian carrying trade? Why shall we not export cotton of our own growth? Why does the treaty not require recompense for the carrying off of our slaves in 1783, contrary to the treaty of that year?" At Norfolk the excitement ran high. Early in August a crowd from the town and county pushed into the courthouse, where they passed resolutions denouncing the treaty as injurious to American interests and obviously intended to promote British influence.[36] The hubbub throughout the country continued until the Senate struck out the clause relating to the West Indian trade, and in this mutilated form ratified the treaty. This left the status of affairs relative to the islands just as it was before the opening of negotiations.

To make matters worse, there was a steady falling off in the tobacco trade. The exports of hogsheads from Norfolk in 1793 was 15,000, and in 1795 only 9,968.[37] This rapid decline is accounted for in part by the European war, but it also resulted from the gradual exhaustion of the Virginia soil. In colonial days, when land was cheap and labor dear, the planters had found it necessary to exploit their soil without regard to the future, and tobacco was planted year after year on one plot without rotation of crops or the use of fertilizers, until it had become worn out. All tidewater Virginia was full of "old fields" reverting to timber.[38] By 1796 the larger part of the tobacco crop came from the upper counties, while the total was growing less and less important in the agricultural output of the state.

Alarmed at this situation, many of the more enterprising planters began to increase their wheat acreage. Wheat grew readily in Virginia, it was not exhausting to the soil, and it commanded a steady market. Among the extensive wheat growers was George Washington, who found time amid the cares of the presidency to instruct his overseer in the setting out of the crop and the grinding of the grain. Some of the growers had their own mills, and shipped flour directly from the plantation wharves; others sent the wheat to the mills of Richmond, Petersburg, or Alexandria.

[36] Norfolk *Herald*, Aug. 12, 1795.
[37] La Rochefoucauld, *Voyages dans les États-Unis*, IV, 266.
[38] T. J. Wertenbaker, *Planters of Colonial Virginia* (Princeton, 1922), p. 105.

The Virginia millers were unable to turn out so fine a variety of flour as their competitors in New York and Pennsylvania, and could not command so high a price in the foreign market. As a result the planters began to send a large part of the wheat crop each year to be milled in Philadelphia, the Brandywine, or New York.[39] Norfolk became the chief point of transhipment for this northern trade, since the coastal packets seldom ventured up the rivers to the Fall Line. The method of loading is shown by the voyage of the *Lady Walterstoff*, of Philadelphia, in 1790. This vessel came in the Capes and sailed up the James to City Point, where the Richmond firm of Stephen and Moses Austin sent down two thousand bushels of wheat. She then came to Norfolk to receive the rest of the cargo from the York River. One after another the river boats sailed into the Elizabeth, made fast to the *Lady Walterstoff*, and transferred their wheat and corn. After a stay of several weeks the brig weighed anchor and set sail for Philadelphia.[40]

Norfolk's northern trade was greatly stimulated by the rise of the Fall Line towns, for the merchants of these places rarely dealt directly with Europe or the West Indies. The more produce which came down the upper James to Richmond or down the Appomattox to Petersburg, the greater would be the amount to be shipped from Norfolk's wharves. There were a few agents for English firms at Richmond, but most of the traders carried on merely a commission business. "It is from the merchants of Richmond and Petersburg that those of Norfolk usually purchase the grain, flour, and tobacco, which they themselves export," wrote La Rochefoucauld.[41] And Richmond was growing rapidly. The James, extending above the falls far back into the interior, poured into her warehouses the products of a dozen counties. Despite its shallow waters, this river for many years was the greatest commercial highway of the state, since the cost of bringing down bulky commodities over the mud roads was prohibitive. The tobacco growers of Albemarle or Fluvanna or Amherst would lash two canoes together, place on board a hogshead of tobacco weighing one thousand pounds, and steer down the stream to Westham.[42] From this point they had to take it by land seven miles to Richmond, or, if it was to be transhipped to Norfolk, down to Shockoes.[43] Later a canal

[39] La Rochefoucauld, *Voyages dans les États-Unis*, IV, 264.
[40] *Norfolk Borough Register*, 1783-1790, p. 244a.
[41] *Voyages dans les États-Unis*, IV, 302.
[42] Smyth, *Tour in the United States*, I, 32.
[43] *Ibid.*

was dug around the falls, so that river boats and canoes could descend, through three locks, to a basin at Richmond. This left a portage of one mile only for goods going further down the river. The proposal to extend the canal to Rocketts was blocked by Richmond merchants to prevent the products of the back country from going directly to Norfolk without stopping at their warehouses.[44]

In addition to its growing northern trade and to the European trade, Norfolk was enjoying a fair interchange of goods to the West Indies. British restrictions could not keep her vessels out of the French islands, and many left each year for Martinique or Guadeloupe with lumber, livestock, and some salted provisions. "The restrictions in the Danish and Dutch colonies were habitually avoided. With the Spanish colonies the trade was forced."[45] Moreover, trade to the British colonies in British bottoms continued on a large scale, for Jamaica, Antigua, Nevis, and Barbados could not dispense with American provisions, lumber, and naval stores. The columns of the Norfolk newspapers in the years from 1785 to 1800 are full of notices of the departure of vessels for the Indies, and of advertisements of sugar, molasses, and rum for sale in the warehouses on the waterfront.[46] In 1791 the exports of Norfolk and Portsmouth reached $1,028,789.00. The port sent out that year 35,071 barrels of flour, 341,984 bushels of wheat, 29,376 tons of naval stores, besides large quantities of lumber, provisions, and tobacco.[47] The duties from imposts and tonnage for the same year mounted to $209,519.84.[48]

Still, recovery might have been slow had it not been for the outbreak of war in Europe in 1792, following the excesses of the French Revolution. British shipping now was so greatly in demand in other parts of the world that her navigation acts could not be enforced in the West Indies. One after another the governors of the various islands, fearing starvation for the people, issued proclamations, permitting the importation of flour, grain, bread, lumber, and other American products in American bottoms of all sizes. Since the French islands also needed American goods and American carriers, the West India trade mounted by leaps and bounds. In the years from 1792 to 1801, exports from the United States to the British islands rose from

[44] La Rochefoucauld, *Voyages dans les États-Unis*, IV, 303-305.
[45] *American Commercial Beacon*, Aug. 28, 1821.
[46] Norfolk *Journal*, Dec. 31, 1788; *Virginia Chronicle*, June 29, July 6, Sept. 21, Nov. 23, 1793; *Norfolk and Portsmouth Chronicle*, Sept. 26, Oct. 10, 1789; July 10, 1790, etc.
[47] La Rochefoucauld, *Voyages dans les États-Unis*, IV, 260-266.
[48] *Virginia Magazine of History and Biography*, VIII, 289.

$2,144,638 to $9,699,722.[49] Nor was this all. A large part of the carrying trade to Europe fell into American hands. From San Domingo, Jamaica, Martinique, Guadeloupe, and Antigua, our ships sailed for the United States, there to take on new clearance papers and turn eastward to Europe. In 1789 the tonnage of American-owned vessels engaged in foreign trade was 127,000; in 1801 it was 849,000.[50]

Norfolk participated fully in this startling revival. Her Indian corn, lumber, tobacco, and naval stores were cheaper than those of the North, and superior in quality to those of South Carolina and Georgia. She could supply all the demands of the islands save that for rice and yellow pine. Clearances for foreign ports from Norfolk and Portsmouth rose to 307 in 1798, to 405 in 1799, and to 448 in 1801.[51] On one day alone of January, 1803, there were in the Elizabeth River forty-two ships, thirty-one brigs, fifty-six schooners and forty sloops.[52] The number of vessels from foreign ports to enter at Norfolk rose from 356 in 1800, to 368 in 1801, to 453 in 1802, and to 484 in 1803.[53] In 1804 and 1805 the number entering declined, but the total tonnage from foreign countries continued to mount. Exports rose from a little over a million dollars in 1792, to two millions in 1795, to four and a third millions in 1804,[54] and, in the years from 1804 to 1807, from five to seven millions annually.[55] Tonnage owned by Norfolk citizens, negligible in 1785, was 15,567 in 1796, and 31,292 in 1805.[56] In 1806 her merchants owned 120 vessels, aggregating 23,207 tons, used exclusively in the foreign trade, some of them stately ships of from 350 to 450 tons.[57] "Six years ago there were not ten large vessels belonging to Norfolk," wrote La Rochefoucauld in 1796; "to-day there are fifty, to say nothing of fifty more smaller ones, engaged chiefly in the West India trade."[58]

The shipbuilding industry, so lately entirely prostrated, now enjoyed an unexampled expansion. Old shipyards sprang into life, Gosport was crowded with partly finished hulls, while every slip along the banks of the Elizabeth and its tributaries resounded to the hammer

[49] Benns, *American Struggle for British West India Carrying Trade*, pp. 19, 20.
[50] Wertenbaker, *The American People, A History*, pp. 180, 181.
[51] Norfolk *Herald*, Oct. 26, 1835.
[52] *Ibid.*, Jan. 13, 1803.
[53] *The Norfolk Directory*, 1806, p. 59.
[54] La Rochefoucauld, *Voyages dans les États-Unis*, IV, 260; Forrest, *Sketches of Norfolk*, p. 102.
[55] Norfolk *Beacon*, Dec. 13, 1834; *The Norfolk Directory*, 1806, p. 59.
[56] Norfolk *Beacon*, Dec. 13, 1834.
[57] Norfolk *Herald*, Oct. 26, 1835.
[58] *Voyages dans les États-Unis*, IV, 265.

and the saw.[59] "In those days we were so prosperous," wrote one old citizen afterward, "that no carpenter could get a wharf to build a ship on. They were built along shore and up the creeks. . . . The whole harbor was continually full of shipping and there were an immense number of ship carpenters and sea captains."[60] Even then it was impossible to supply the demand for new ships. "There was no haggling about prices; the only question was, 'How soon can the work be done?' "[61] From eighty to ninety vessels of all sizes were built at Norfolk annually, most of them for the Philadelphia market.[62] The capacity of some of the shipyards is indicated by the launching from the establishment of John Foster, at Portsmouth, of a 380-ton ship, the *Dumfries,* intended for the London trade.[63]

The cost of construction for the hull of a vessel of 120 tons or more was $24.00 a ton; for completed ships, ready to put to sea, from $47 to $50. The pay of ship carpenters, which was very high for the times, being from two to three dollars a day,[64] attracted laborers for many miles around. Every man who had ever built a shallop or a row boat represented himself as a skilled ship carpenter, and few were turned away. "The rapid growth of Norfolk has drawn hither an immense concourse of people, poor as well as rich," stated the *Herald* of February 7, 1795. Despite the fact that building had gone on rapidly and that the number of houses by 1796 had risen to eight and nine hundred, it was very difficult to secure lodgings.[65] In 1800 the population was 6,926, of whom 3,850 were whites and 3,076 blacks.[66] "Your harbor, capacious as it is, was filled with ships from foreign parts," wrote a visitor to Norfolk. "The coasting trade, which distributed your imports, employed hundreds of vessels, whose streamers, mingling on a gala day with the flags of the foreign ships, presented a cheering spectacle. . . . It was difficult . . . to cross in a ferry boat from Norfolk to Portsmouth, on account of the great number of vessels in the harbor. Your warehouses were full of foreign and domestic products. Besides your stated population, there was always a body of transient people, . . . demanding houseroom and board."[67]

[59] *Ibid.*
[60] Jarvis Manuscript, p. 51.
[61] Forrest, *Sketches of Norfolk,* p. 107.
[62] La Rochefoucauld, *Voyages dans les États-Unis,* IV, 270.
[63] Norfolk *Gazette and Public Ledger,* Oct. 30, 1804.
[64] *Ibid.*
[65] Forrest, *Sketches of Norfolk,* p. 102. La Rochefoucauld places the number between seven and eight hundred (*Voyages dans les États-Unis,* IV, 256) .
[66] *Second Census of the United States* (Washington, 1801) . There were 2,312 white males, 1,538 white females, 352 free Negroes and 2,724 slaves.
[67] Forrest, *Sketches of Norfolk,* p. 115.

The columns of the Norfolk *Herald* picture the life of the town at this period. From the issue of January 5, 1805, we find that the ship *William and Mary* and the brigs *Martha Johnson* and *Sophia* had just arrived from Jamaica, the schooner *Adeona* from Antigua, that other vessels from Guadeloupe, Port Republic, and Kingston were lying at Hampton Roads. The American ship *Alexander* was advertising for a cargo of six hundred hogsheads of tobacco, the schooner *Brothers* for passengers for Edenton, N. C., the British ship *Phoenix* for tobacco for Liverpool. George McIntosh had for sale a consignment of cloth, hardware, cutlery, and nails, just in from Liverpool on the *Sukey and Juno;* Donaldson, Thorburn & Co. two hundred crates of queen's ware, glass, and copperas; James B. Timberlake & Co. rum from Jamaica, Antigua, and New England, wines from Madeira and Sicily, sugar, tea, green coffee, spices, glass, Spanish cigars and cheese; James Taylor and Thomas Armistead had Teneriffe wine and old port; Martin Fiske rum, brandy, whiskey, mackerel, mould candles, chocolate, pepper, sugar, and paper; Lewis E. Durant & Co. ship chandlery, iron, brass, and tinware in from London on the *Alexander;* R. Bowden & Co. thirty thousand pounds of green coffee; Phinehan Dana thirteen bales of India cotton; N. Macgill one hundred and eighty barrels of beef and ten pipes of gin.

If one were inclined to venture his money in a voyage to Europe or the Indies, he could purchase the brig *Drake,* of 108 tons; the *Fair American,* a ship of 317 tons; the ship *George,* of 232 tons; the brig *Maria,* of 130 tons; the British ship *Prince of Wales,* of 456 tons, "pierced for 20 guns" and having three decks; the ship *Carpenter,* of 235 tons; or a dozen other ships or brigs. From the same paper we learn that Tildsley Graham operated a bakery at Town Point, that Hillary Lambert conducted a shoe-repairing business at Calvert's wharf, that Thomas Lester of Rothery's Lane was a tinplate worker and coppersmith; that Francis Lynch sold bonnets, calico, and playing cards at No. 20 Market Square; that William Wright was a "silk and muslin dyer, lately from Europe." Madden and Whitehurst, tailors and habit-makers, of 115 Main Street, assured "those who honor them with their commands, that no exertion of theirs shall be wanting to give satisfaction, of which they are confident from their long experience and practice. They are well acquainted with the latest fashions, and as for despatch, none of their profession in this borough can, they flatter themselves, surpass them."[68]

Norfolk was a cosmopolitan spot in the last two decades of the

[68] Norfolk *Herald,* Jan. 5, 1802. Norfolk Public Library.

eighteenth century. On its busy wharves and crowded streets one could brush elbows with merchants from Glasgow, or Liverpool, or Kingston, or Philadelphia; with North Carolina shippers, just in from Albemarle Sound with a cargo of lumber, tar, and turpentine; with traders from Richmond and Petersburg; perhaps with sailors from some French brigantine lying in the river awaiting a consignment of tobacco. The town numbered among its prominent merchants not only native Virginians and recent Scotch immigrants, but Englishmen, Irish, and French West Indians. There were a few Dutch, Spanish, and Portuguese. "Our Norfolk born people, and the people from the neighboring counties, formed the base—a pretty broad base, but only a base."[69]

In July, 1793, there came into Hampton Roads a fleet of one hundred and thirty-seven square rigged vessels, under the escort of two ships of the line, three frigates, and three smaller warships, all carrying the flag of France. Their decks were crowded with men, women, and children, many of them ill. They were French refugees, driven from their homes in San Domingo by an uprising of the slaves.[70] Some of the ships came up the Elizabeth and landed hundreds of these unhappy people at Norfolk. Most of them were in complete destitution, many families formerly wealthy now depending on charity. The borough government took steps to provide for them until they could find employment, or could move on to the interior.[71] At the same time subscriptions from private sources poured in, not only from Norfolk, but from almost every town in Virginia, while the state legislature voted a considerable sum.[72] This kind reception, the alliance between France and the United States, and the fact that in Virginia they could make use of the few slaves they had brought with them, were deciding factors in the decision of many to remain.[73] Isaac Weld states that there were between two and three thousand in Norfolk at one time, but that afterwards most of them dispersed to other parts of the country. Those who remained opened little shops, in an effort to restore their fortunes. Among the Frenchmen who conducted dry goods stores in 1806 were M. Blanchard, and Louis Santegan on Church Street, and Gabriel Leleivie, Mary Lemasurier, and Peter Vizenneau on Main Street. The Norfolk *Journal* of De-

[69] Grigsby, *Governor Tazewell*, p. 23.
[70] *Virginia Chronicle*, July 13, 1793.
[71] *Norfolk Council Orders*, 1736-98, pp. 165, 165b.
[72] La Rochefoucauld, *Voyages dans les États-Unis*, IV, 277.
[73] *Ibid.*

cember 7, 1873, states that many of the stores on the west side of Market Square were kept by Frenchmen. The officers of the French Lodge of Wisdom included Jean Pierre Laperouse, Jean Baptiste Campamagy, Pierre Chabaner, Gabriel Bernard, François Blanchet, Gaspard Ducamp, Louis Lepage, and Louis Durand.[74] At least one of the exiles prospered, for we are told that "Monsieur Delisle, a Frenchman from the West Indies," went extensively into the brickmaking business, and established himself on Church Street, near Princess Anne Road.[75]

The mixed nature of the population accentuated the violence of party spirit at Norfolk. Everywhere in the United States the people were divided into the partisans of France and of England; at Norfolk, where Scotchmen and Englishmen every day elbowed French republicans, matters often came to the verge of blows. On one occasion, when some French sailors on shore-leave got into a controversy with a party of British tars, "the whole people were up and ready to join them on one side or the other in open contest," and peace was restored only by the calling out of the militia.[76] La Rochefoucauld declares that the friends of France were the prevailing party. In proof of this he states that when a French convoy was leaving the Capes for the north, all the pilot boats at Norfolk were mysteriously scuttled as the result of a rumor that one of them was to be used to warn the English at Halifax.[77]

When the news of the French victory at Valmy reached Norfolk in January, 1793, the guns at the fort were fired, while a large group of republicans at the Borough Tavern celebrated with songs and toasts. The company drank to the Republic of France, to Citizens Dumouriez and Custine, to the National Convention, and to the Rights of Man.[78] In February of the next year the French were hosts to the patriots of "Norfolk Borough," and, while the French ships in the river kept up an incessant fire, a long procession moved through the principal street. A dinner followed, marked by the usual huzzas, toasts, and French and American songs.[79] Still another celebration took place in 1795, on the anniversary of the signing of the Franco-American treaty of alliance in 1778.[80]

[74] *Norfolk Directory for 1806-7*, p. 75.
[75] Forrest, *Sketches of Norfolk*, p. 103.
[76] Weld, *Travels in North America*, p. 176.
[77] La Rochefoucauld, *Voyages dans les États-Unis*, IV, 278.
[78] *Virginia Chronicle*, Jan. 26, 1793.
[79] *Ibid.*, Feb. 22, 1794.
[80] *Ibid.*, Feb. 7, 1795.

On the other hand, the Federalists formed themselves into the Society of Constitutional and Governmental Support, with Alexander Gordon as president, and Duncan McPherson as vice-president, to "contradict the Jacobin clubs."[81] This group grew stronger as news of the excesses of the Convention filtered in, and as the realization grew that Norfolk's prosperity was contingent upon peace with England. They were never able to swing the full weight of public sentiment, however, until news reached the town of the outrageous X. Y. Z. affair. Then, when it became known that the French Directory had insulted the United States by refusing to treat with her envoys until they had handed over a *douceur* or bribe, anger rose to white heat. The Norfolk Frenchmen were troubled and downcast, their friends mute. A great gathering of citizens gave President Adams a unanimous vote of confidence. "We are friendly to France," they said, "but we reject with indignation her demands. We are determined not to purchase peace at the price of national character and individual security."[82]

The borough took on a warlike appearance. A meeting in the Town Hall on June 28 opened a subscription to raise money for purchasing or building a warship to be lent to the United States government.[83] A group of young men, from sixteen to twenty-four years of age, wrote to President Adams, offering their services to fight for the nation.[84] Those citizens who were exempt from military duty formed themselves into a volunteer company to show "no lack of patriotism in this alarming crisis."[85] On July 4 the Fifty-fourth Regiment, made up of Norfolk militia, paraded before General Thomas Mathews and several Federal officers.[86] The excitement increased when merchantmen came scurrying into the Capes with the news that French privateers had begun preying on American commerce. In July the *Triumphant* took the brig *Elizabeth* on her way from Grenada to Norfolk, and later made a prize of the *Abigail*, which was headed for Havana. The schooner *Ranger* was boarded by the privateer *Sanspareil*, but escaped with the loss of some bread, beef, and the skipper's watch and wearing apparel.[87] Not until the ap-

81 Norfolk *Herald*, March 4, 1795.
82 *Ibid.*, May 10, 1798.
83 *Ibid.*, June 30, 1798.
84 *Ibid.*, June 23, 1798.
85 *Ibid.*, July 7, 1798.
86 *Ibid.* The chief officers of the regiment were Colonel Graves, Major Westweed, Captains Reynolds, Smith, Nestle, Nivison, and Myers.
87 *Ibid.*, July 19; Nov. 24, 1798.

pointment of Adams' new commission to renew negotiations with France did the excitement subside; but even then the old enthusiasm for France, born of French assistance to the United States and sympathy for the early principles of the French Revolution, did not return.

Such was Norfolk at the close of the eighteenth century—crowded, busy, turbulent, full of life and hope. With expanding business, with fortunes being made rapidly, with the population doubling, with shipbuilding enjoying an unprecedented boom, with people flocking in from all parts of Virginia and North Carolina, with the Chesapeake Bay and Albemarle Sound tributary to her commerce, she looked forward to the day when she would rival Boston and Philadelphia. This was the time when "one might walk from Norfolk to Portsmouth on the decks of the vessels at anchor in the harbor," wrote one enthusiast, "when the rich products of the Indies were piled on our wharves, and stored in our warehouses, when our merchants bought cargoes of cotton, corn, and tobacco, and shipped on private account, when Richmond and Petersburg were tributary to Norfolk and their merchants flocked periodically hither to purchase their supplies, when the business of Norfolk was comparatively larger than that of New York, and really larger than that of Baltimore."[88]

Main Street was a busy thoroughfare, lined with shops and houses from one end to the other, and "thronged with a heterogeneous mass of human beings."[89] Among the conspicuous buildings were the Custom House at the head of Washington Street; the post office and the Exchange Coffee House side by side; the *Public Ledger* office, the courthouse and archives office on the north side of the street; the market house in Market Square; the new Borough Tavern a few doors west of the corner of Church Street; and the old Borough Tavern farther east. In the west end of Main were the residences and offices of a number of prominent persons, No. 6 being the law office of Littleton W. Tazewell; No. 12 the residence of John Nivison, borough recorder; No. 4 the house of John Cooper, editor of the *Public Ledger;* No. 32 the law office of William Lindsay; No. 13 that of Robert B. Taylor. Further east were several boardinghouses, followed by a group of dry goods stores, with here and there a barber shop, a confectionary, a grocery store, a shoemaker's shop, a cut-nail manufactury, a chemist's store, a tailor shop, a watchmaker's shop, a

---

[88] Forrest, *Sketches of Norfolk*, pp. 116-117.
[89] *Ibid.*, p. 107.

bookstore, or even a residence. East of the intersection with Church
the street was devoted almost entirely to residences. Here dwelt
Dr. James Taylor; the sea captain Miles King; Colonel John Hamilton, British vice-consul; Mrs. West, proprietor of the theater; and
Edward Archer, member of the town council.[90]

Church Street, "still the only avenue by which the town could be
entered by vehicles," was a "noisy, brisk thoroughfare," built up with
stores and tenements. The southern end was filled with dry goods
stores, shoe-shops, and grocery stores, but from No. 50 northward were
dwellings occupied by the middle classes—tailors, cabinetmakers, sea
captains, blacksmiths, plasterers, butchers. St. Paul's, with its burying
ground, was on the west side, while opposite was the Academy and
the new Episcopal church. Although both Main and Church were
unpaved, and were muddy in winter and dusty in summer, they were
always crowded with "horses, carriages, phaetons, chairs, carts, and
drays," not to mention the swarms of pedestrians. Water Street had
been laid out all the way from Parker Street to the site of the Union
depot, but from Reed Street to Merchant Street it was still under
water. The completed section was lined on the south with wharves,[91]
around which centered the activities attendant upon commerce. Here
were the warehouses of the merchants, the wholesale grocery companies, ship chandlers, blacksmiths, block and pump makers, ship
joiners, coopers, sailmakers, ship carpenters.

Back Creek still separated the old town from the new section to the
northwest, but bridges at Catharine and Granby streets made com-
munication possible. It was proposed at this time to fill in both the
Back Creek and Newton's Creek, leaving canals deep enough for large
boats to ascend to Catharine Street on the west and on the east up to
Fenchurch, but the matter was left to the future.[92] In the section
north of Back Creek were a number of residential streets, of which
Freemason was the most important. Here was the home of Moses
Myers, here the residences of H. Richard Lee, Jonathan Eilbeck,
W. A. Armistead, and J. Charles Catlett. "The houses had no con-
veniences," H. B. Grigsby tells us, "except here and there a closet.

[90] *The Norfolk Directory,* 1806.
[91] Among these were the wharves of Pennock, Warren, Woodside, Rothery, Marsden, Maxwell, Campbell, Newton, Moor and Meburne, Loyall, John Calvert, C. Calvert, and Lee.
[92] Nicholson, Map of Norfolk, of October 22, 1802; Forrest, *Sketches of Norfolk,*
pp. 116-117.

They were, however, substantially built, and were neatly finished within. They invariably had . . . the smokehouse in which every housekeeper cured his meat; and there was the dairy. . . . The people had cows, but there was no running water, and there was no ice. Long years passed before ice was introduced. The equinoctial storms sadly worried our fathers. From the imperfect filling in of the streets and wharves the tides rose high; and then . . . Norfolk was another Venice. The canoe was our gondola, and 'yo heave ho' were our echoes of Tasso."[93]

In this period before the Revolution, the merchant class was the wealthiest and most influential in the town. Moses Myers, William Pennock, John Southgate, John Mackenzie, Alexander Maclure, Robert Maitland, and many others carried on an extensive trade, largely in their own ships. These men possessed handsome residences and surrounded themselves with every comfort the age afforded. The beautiful residence of Moses Myers is still standing, a monument to the charm of the buildings of that day. The professional men—lawyers, doctors, ministers, town officials—constituted another highly respected group, while the fifty or more sea captains who made Norfolk their home were a class to themselves.

Far more numerous, of course, were the artisans—carpenters, bricklayers, plasterers, bakers, shoemakers, brewers, coopers, cigarmakers, chairmakers, cabinetmakers, blacksmiths, dyers, turners, joiners, saddlers, hatters, whitesmiths, painters, glaziers, goldsmiths, watchmakers, gunsmiths, brass founders, cutlers, tanners, printers, wheelwrights; and workers connected with building and repairing ships—ship carpenters, ship joiners, ship chandlers, riggers, sailmakers, block and pump makers. There was a considerable group of free Negroes, most of them working for wages as day laborers, but a few establishing themselves as little tradesmen or artisans. Thus a free black named Armistead Lewis kept a livery stable on Wolfe Street, Isaac Anderson was a carpenter, Leonora Byers had a shop on Main Street, Betty Cross was a midwife, George Johnson was a shoemaker, Thomas Knight a barber. As for the hundreds of sailors who at all times could be seen walking the streets, wandering around the Wigwam on Briggs' Point, or swarming on the wharves, those who were unmarried took up their residence at the sailors' boardinghouses. Of these there were thirty-five or more, most of them located on Little

93 Grigsby, *Governor Tazewell*, p. 25.

Water Street, Woodside's Lane, and Water Street on both sides of its intersection with Commerce Street.[94]

The rapid rise of Norfolk from ruin in 1783 to prosperity and riches in 1800 attracted wide attention. It was freely predicted that the town would become one of the greatest commercial cities of the Union. Few stopped to consider that the present flourishing condition was the result chiefly of the opening of the West Indies to American merchantmen, that this in turn was purely the result of the European war, and that with the return of peace and the enforcement of the British colonial trade laws would come stagnation and hard times. The day was not distant when Norfolk was to learn that a prosperity which is at the mercy of foreign commercial restrictions is apt to be fleeting.[95]

[94] *The Norfolk Directory*, 1806.

[95] "The trade of our fathers in 1802 was an unnatural trade," wrote Hugh Blair Grigsby. "It was a fungus that sprung from the diseased condition of foreign powers. It was not the result of developed productive wealth, but the accident of the war between the two greatest commercial nations of the globe, which gave us the carrying trade. It was born of other people's troubles, and destined to die when those troubles were appeased." (Grigsby, *Governor Tazewell*, p. 27.)

CHAPTER FIVE

Coercion—Peaceful and Otherwise

From the opening of the European war in 1792, the West Indian trade and the American carrying trade to Europe was seriously hampered by the belligerents. Although the French and Spaniards were glad to have the ships of Boston, New York, or Norfolk supply their islands with provisions and lumber and carry off molasses and rum, now that the British frigates had made the sea so unsafe for their own shipping, they were on the alert to break up any trade between the United States and the British West Indies. Their cruisers and privateers roved in Caribbean waters ready to pounce upon any vessel headed for Jamaica, or Antigua, or Nevis. So early as January, 1795, the *Happy Return,* belonging to John Calvert of Norfolk, was captured by the French schooner *Resolution* and sent as a prize to Charleston.[1] Following the X. Y. Z. affair French seizures became so frequent as to bring ruin to many American shippers. "Our merchants have been plundered of many millions," complained the Norfolk *Herald,* in January, 1801. "In this town claims against the French are . . . in all about $2,000,000." A year later the principal sufferers organized to petition Congress for relief, and to correspond with victims elsewhere.[2]

The treaty of September, 1800, with Napoleon did not end the French depredations. In December, 1802, when the schooner *Maria,* of Norfolk, was at anchor at Tobago, a boatload of sailors from the French frigate *La Badine* boarded her and took her out to sea.[3] In

---

1 Norfolk *Herald,* Feb. 28, 1795.
2 *Ibid.,* Jan. 28, 1802.
3 *Ibid.,* Jan. 29, 1803.

April, 1804, the Norfolk schooner *Sarah,* on her way from San Domingo to Norfolk with a cargo of coffee, was taken by a French
privateer and sent as a prize to Cuba.[4] Especially thrilling was the
case of the ship *Eliza.* This vessel, the property of Conway and
Fortescue Whittle, was returning with rum from Jamaica when she
was captured by a Frenchman. Captain Evans and his crew were put
on shore on the Isle of Pines, where they remained three weeks, suffering from exposure and hunger. By working night and day they
succeeded in constructing a raft, which bore them over to the Cuban
shore. Here they spied the *Eliza* at anchor, manned by Frenchmen,
but no longer under the protection of the privateer. Thereupon they
"sallied out," apparently on their raft, clambered on board, and
made themselves masters of the ship. The French sailors were set
ashore, the cargo removed to a safe spot, and the vessel burnt to
prevent its recapture.[5]

As the bitterness of the European struggle increased, conditions in
the West Indies grew worse. It was calculated that from January 1
to July 1, 1805, one out of every four vessels plying between the
United States and Jamaica was captured by French or Spanish privateers.[6] In May of the same year a vessel of ten guns, at times flying the
French flag, at others the Spanish, stationed herself outside the
Capes, robbing every merchantman she encountered.[7] From the renewal of war in 1803 to August, 1805, French and Spanish privateers
took no less than thirteen Norfolk vessels, including two ships, three
brigs, seven schooners, and one sloop. The total value was $196,000,
of which $120,000 was covered by insurance.[8] The Norfolk *Gazette*
pleaded with the government to provide cruisers to convoy American
vessels to the West Indies, but with little effect. Not until the merchants began arming their ships and sailing in fleets did they secure a
measure of safety. In the fall of 1805, when two ships of twenty guns
and several schooners of from four to eight guns encountered a
French privateer on their way from Port-au-Prince to the United
States, they had little difficulty in driving her off.[9]

But it was not always possible for the ships to go in groups, and

---

[4] Norfolk *Gazette and Public Ledger,* Sept. 18, 1804.
[5] *Ibid.,* Sept. 18, 1804 and April 10, 1805.
[6] *Ibid.,* Aug. 5, 1805.
[7] *Ibid.,* May 24, 1805.
[8] *Ibid.,* Aug. 5, 1805.
[9] *Ibid.,* Oct. 11, 1805.

news of captures was constantly filtering into Norfolk. In September, 1807, the town was aroused by the intelligence that the brig *Sumner* had been taken, and its crew subjected to ill treatment. The *Sumner* was on its way to Norfolk from Jamaica when she was brought to by the *Revenge*, a French privateer manned by a motley crew of French, Spaniards, and Italians. The brig was conducted to Philipia bay, in Cuba, where the captain and crew were robbed of all their possessions, and, half-naked, were transferred to another prize, the *Catherine-Eliza* of New York. This little vessel, overcrowded, with a very short allowance of food and water, was fortunate to reach New York in safety. The *Sumner*, with its own cargo as well as that of the *Catherine-Eliza*, was taken to a port on the Spanish Main, where it was condemned.[10]

Serious as were the depredations of the French privateers, they were overshadowed by those of the British. The government at London was determined to use its naval supremacy to isolate the French West Indies and deprive them of colonial imports, and, having driven most of the French merchantmen from the sea, would not permit American vessels to take their place. So they placed food and provisions on the contraband list and, declaring a "paper blockade" of the French islands, sent over their frigates to enforce it. Before the war was a year old, the Norfolk merchants were complaining of the "arrogance and insolence" of British captains and the British courts. At a meeting of Norfolk and Portsmouth citizens, on March 14, 1794, a memorial to Congress was drawn up. They had beheld the depredations upon American commerce with indignation, they declared, and would not be silent when the honor and interest of the whole country was involved. The seizing of American vessels, their detention in British ports, their condemnation by British courts could be stopped only by the Federal government. "We in Norfolk and Portsmouth would be exposed to ruin in case of war, but we will support war, if it is necessary to secure our rights."[11] In fact, many in Norfolk thought war preferable to the existing situation. "If we were at war with England," they said, "our vessels would leave armed and our privateers would retaliate. But now we have nothing to get but blows." In November the merchants of Norfolk and Portsmouth again petitioned Congress asking that compensation for the seizures

10 *Ibid.*, Sept. 2, 1807.
11 Norfolk *Chronicle*, April 5, 1794.

by the British be insisted upon. The majority of those who signed were "not victims of these piracies," but were directed by sympathy for their fellow citizens.[12]

Yet the seizures continued year after year, many accompanied by unnecessary insults and abuse. On October 1, 1805, the brig *Ann Elizabeth*, on her way from Malaga to Norfolk, was brought to by an armed British brig of fourteen or sixteen guns. Ten or twelve men came on board, armed with pistols and cutlasses, and proceeded to rifle the crew's belongings. "They broke open my trunks," stated Captain Williams, "took away my wearing apparel, $200 in cash, my watch, hat, shoes, hammock, and sheets, did not leave me one shirt . . . , all my navigation books; also my mate's clothes and $20, also . . . destroyed my papers and accounts. They beat the mate and people most dreadfully." Finding the brig's papers regular, they told them to proceed. As the *Ann Elizabeth* slowly drew away in the light breeze, the British let loose a full broadside, with round and grape, cutting the rigging and sails, and splintering the hull in many places.[13]

The bitterness caused by such incidents was heightened by the constant impressment of American sailors. With the enormous expansion of American trade and the growth of American shipbuilding, it became a serious problem to find sailors. The shipyards could turn out a brig in twelve months, but it took years to make a real jack-tar. The Norfolk skippers could not take on a farm hand or a wood chopper and expect him to know the difference between the main mast and the jib boom. So they, like owners in the northern states, began signing up British sailors, whenever they could induce them to desert. Nor was this difficult. Life on board the British war vessels and merchant ships was desperately hard, with unwholesome food, rigid discipline, low wages, and brutal punishments. When a British vessel came into an American port it was usual for one or more sailors to jump overboard and swim ashore, there to take out naturalization papers, assume new names, and sign up on some American vessel at twice or three times their former wages. Albert Gallatin stated that of the four thousand seamen required to man the seventy thousand tons of new shipping turned out each year, half were British, presumably deserters.[14]

[12] *Ibid.*, Nov. 20, 1794.
[13] Norfolk *Gazette and Public Ledger*, Oct. 23, 1805.
[14] Wertenbaker, *The American People, A History*, pp. 181, 182.

Great Britain was not inclined to submit to this kind of thing. If her ships were undermanned, her commerce must lag, her sea power would decline, and she would be unable to resist the giant blows of Napoleon. So the British frigates took to stopping American vessels on the seas, lining up the crew on deck, and taking off all the British tars on board, with perhaps an American or two thrown in. In April, 1795, a British sloop-of-war stopped the ship *Harriot,* as she was about to enter the Capes, and sending an officer on board to inspect her papers and crew, took off three men, two of them Americans. They were on the point of impressing the mate, also, but were finally persuaded to leave him.[15] Quite similar was the case of the *Charles Carter.* This ship sailed from Norfolk, on July 23, 1803. When six leagues off Cape Henry, she fell in with the British frigate *Boston,* which took off four of the crew, all of them Americans who had recently shipped in Norfolk. The *Boston* then proceeded to Hampton Roads. Here one of the impressed sailors, Augustus Topham, rather than remain on what the Americans called a "floating hell," braved the danger of drowning by swimming ashore.[16]

Public sentiment in Norfolk, while resenting these injuries, was strongly in favor of removing all excuse for their perpetration. The entire crew of a foreign merchant ship in any Virginia port might desert, and the master be powerless to force them back. If he appealed to the magistrates, it would avail nothing, for the law provided a severe penalty for them should they attempt to interfere. In 1804 the Norfolk representative in the House of Delegates sponsored an act to discourage desertion from merchant vessels.[17] "We believe that the people are not inclined to go to war in order that our flag shall protect British deserters," wrote one Norfolk editor. "As advocates for a national navy we do not wish to see foreign seamen employed in our merchant ships, because those form a nursery for seamen for our navy. . . . The foreigners are not to be relied upon when we fight their own country."[18] Nonetheless, the people of the borough continued to press for action on the part of Congress for the protection of their rights. A crowded meeting in the Town Hall in February, 1806, passed a series of resolutions, declaring that "Great Britain has shown her hostile temper towards the United States, by impressing our citizens into her service, and compelling them to fight her battles, and

---

15 Norfolk *Herald,* April 22, 1795.
16 *Ibid.,* Aug. 4, 1803.
17 Norfolk *Gazette and Public Ledger,* Jan. 30, 1805.
18 *Ibid.,* Aug. 12, 1807.

to contribute to the capture and plunder of their own countrymen, by her various abuses of the law of blockade, by the new principle which she hath prescribed as a part of the law of nations, and by which she effectually blockades the whole of every nation with which she is at war."[19]

In June, 1807, the people of Norfolk were thrown into a passion of humiliation and anger by the attack of the British frigate *Leopard* upon the *Chesapeake,* ten miles off Cape Henry. The American cruiser was just leaving for the Mediterranean, with a crew short-handed and untrained, her decks littered, her powder flasks and loggerheads stored. When the *Leopard* drew up beside her and Captain Humphrey announced that he intended to come on board to search for British deserters, she was in no condition to resist. Commodore Barron, who was in command, made desperate efforts to clear the decks, but before this could be accomplished the British frigate poured in her whole broadside. The Americans held out for fifteen minutes, and only after three had been killed, eighteen wounded, and the vessel riddled, did they lower their colors. The British then came on board, picked out four alleged deserters, three of them Americans, and left the luckless *Chesapeake* to limp back to Hampton Roads.[20]

As news of this outrage filtered into Norfolk, the people, dumfounded and incredulous, swarmed out in rowboats to every vessel which came in from the Capes, to question the crews or passengers. When, at last, they saw approaching a boat conveying eleven wounded men, all doubts were dispelled, and Norfolk gave itself up to thoughts of revenge. "Greatly as we have always deprecated war," wrote the editor of the *Gazette,* "conscious as we are that our country will experience infinite distress, we look upon it as degrading beneath contempt if we are to submit to such an insult."[21] At a meeting in Town Hall the crowd found it impossible to jam into the building and so adjourned to the "large church." Resolutions were passed expressing indignation and horror at the attack upon the *Chesapeake,* and promising support to the government in securing satisfaction. They were determined to refuse all intercourse with the British ships of war, either by providing them with pilots or by selling them supplies or water. A subscription was opened for the wounded and for the families of the killed.[22]

[19] *Ibid.,* Feb. 14, 1806.
[20] Wertenbaker, *The American People, A History,* pp. 183-185.
[21] Norfolk *Gazette and Public Ledger,* June 24, 1807.
[22] *Ibid.*

On June 27, Robert MacDonald, one of the injured sailors, died of his wounds. His funeral the next day became the occasion for the expression of the public humiliation. As the body was brought across the river from the hospital to the county wharf, attended by a procession of boats, the American shipping kept their colors at half-mast, while minute guns were fired by the artillery on shore. No less than four thousand citizens were waiting at Market Square, and while the coffin was being landed, formed themselves in a long procession. In the lead were the Junior Volunteers, the minister, the committee, the surgeons of the hospital; then came the coffin, attended by pallbearers selected from masters of vessels in the river; next in order were the captains, mates, and seamen; then the band, with drums muffled; next the United States officers, the volunteer companies, the borough officers, and last a long line of citizens in columns of fours. The procession marched up Catharine Street to Freemason Street, thence to Christ Church, where Mr. Davis delivered the funeral sermon.[23]

In the meanwhile, active preparations were under way to fortify Norfolk. In a crowded meeting at the Exchange Coffee House, the young men formed themselves into a volunteer company; slaves by the score worked feverishly to put Fort Norfolk in repair; powder was collected and stored; Commodore Stephen Decatur directed the sailors in the work of rigging and arming the dismantled government gunboats. Then the State militia began arriving, the Richmond Light Infantry Blues, the Republican Blues, a company from Petersburg. If there was to be war, Norfolk was going to put up a strenuous fight.[24]

For a few days it seemed that hostilities might start at once. Commodore John E. Douglas, commander of the British fleet in Hampton Roads, because of the refusal of the citizens to have intercourse with his ships, thought that an attempt would be made to prevent communication between him and the British consul in Norfolk. On July 3 he sent a menacing letter to Mayor Richard E. Lee. "I am determined," he wrote, "if this infringement is not immediately annulled, to prohibit every vessel bound either in or out of Norfolk, to proceed to their destination, until I know the pleasure of my government. . . . You must be perfectly aware that the British flag never has, nor will be insulted with impunity." Mayor Lee's reply, written on July 4, was both spirited and biting. "The day on which this answer is written, ought of itself to prove to the subjects of your sovereign, that the American people are not to be intimidated by menace. . . . Seduced

23 *Ibid.*, June 29, 1807.
24 *Ibid.*, July 1, 3, 13, 1807.

by the false show of security, they may be sometimes surprised and slaughtered, while unprepared to resist a supposed friend; that delusive security is now however passed forever. The late occurrence has taught us to confide our safety no longer to anything but our own force. We do not seek hostility, nor shall we avoid it. We are prepared for the worst you may attempt. . . . We therefore leave it with you either to engage in war, or to remain on terms of peace." To make it clear that there would be no interruption of communication with the British consul, the mayor added, "Your letters directed to the British consul at this place have been forwarded to him."[25]

This reply was delivered to Commodore Douglas by L. W. Tazewell on July 6. He was received courteously in Douglas' own cabin on the *Bellona,* where the captains of the squadron were assembled. Silently the letter was passed around the circle, while the faces of the officers showed that they grasped the seriousness of the situation. Finally Douglas spoke. His letter had been misunderstood, he said. He had no orders to start hostilities with the United States, and nothing was more remote from his intentions. What he had written could not properly be construed as insulting and menacing. And so the immediate crisis passed. But it left the people of Norfolk still smarting. "We would ask who was it that first departed from the usual course?" asked the *Gazette.* "If the *Chesapeake* had deserters from the British navy, why not leave that affair to the two governments? The fact, as it appears to us, is that Commodore Douglas is disposed to leave the governments to act only when the force he commands cannot operate."[26]

The storm of indignation which gripped the nation at the news of the attack on the *Chesapeake* did not persuade President Jefferson that war was necessary. Jefferson was a man of peace. So he contented himself with a proclamation requiring armed British vessels to leave American waters and prohibiting intercourse with them, and then sought reparations through the usual diplomatic channels. This course seemed tame to the Norfolk people, who had seen the crippled *Chesapeake* return to Hampton Roads, and the wounded sailors brought to the hospital; but as passions cooled, they became reconciled to it. "Nothing could have been more judicious," said one editor. The proclamation "will no doubt induce a powerful movement in the people of England, who . . . will insist on the government's rendering us justice. . . . If the British government should sanction the conduct

25 *Ibid.,* July 6, 1807.
26 *Ibid.*

of Admiral Berkeley, or refuse to punish him, war must be the conse-quence."[27] Norfolk was to have five more years of peace, such as it was, before the British cannon were actually pounding at her gates.

But the *Chesapeake-Leopard* affair had given ample warning of what lay ahead. Impressments and seizures continued; Americans were still robbed and insulted on the high seas; something must be done to protect our rights and to prepare for war. Although the experience of Norfolk in the Revolution made her sensitive to the condition of the river defenses, the War Department could not be induced to keep them in repair. In 1802 Secretary of War Henry Dearborn visited Norfolk and gave orders for the dismounting of Fort Norfolk, and the creation of a new fort at Ferry Point in what is now Berkley. This bit of stupidity stirred the Norfolk *Herald* to sarcastic comment. A fort situated here, above both towns, it said, "is an invincible protection to the little place called Kemps, ten miles up the Eastern Branch, and to Great Bridge, twelve miles up the Southern Branch, to both of which places a lighter for wood can go with tolerable safety on the flood tide." So the people learned to rely on their own efforts to keep Fort Norfolk and Fort Nelson in condition, and at the first alarm of war hastened out, pick and shovel in hand, to work on the crumbling ramparts.

Jefferson's plan of putting the American frigates in dry dock and entrusting the defense of our rivers and harbors to a fleet of little gun-boats, came in for unending derision. "We understand Gun-boat No. 1 was by the late storm safely moored in the middle of a corn-field," stated the *Gazette*.[28] "The gunboats were planned by Mr. Jefferson himself, upon principles altogether new, but, withal, perfectly philo-sophical. From the dissection of a gnat to the construction of a man-of-war, our beloved chief is equally useful."[29] When a French privateer seized the schooner *Anna-Maria*, in January, 1805, in sight of the Cape Henry lighthouse, the editor asked, "What has become of our gun-boats, those redoubtable defenders of our trade? Why do they not come forward and protect our trade, which is insulted in our very harbors?"[30] Seven years later, when the American frigates were showing their mettle in single combat with the English, the *Gazette* returned to the subject. "What will be said of that wretched system of gun-boats, on which millions have been expended, that ought to have been spent on an efficient navy?"

27 *Ibid.*, August 3, 1807.
28 *Ibid.*, Sept. 20, 1804.
29 *Ibid.*, Nov. 1, 1804.
30 *Ibid.*, Jan. 18, 1805.

The only safe policy, thought the people of Norfolk, was to build as many frigates and ships-of-the-line as the finances of the nation would permit. With a number of swift-sailing cruisers to convoy the American merchantmen, seizures and impressments would be less frequent; with a respectable navy to reckon with in case of war, the European countries would not be so free with their insults. "We have always held one opinion, that to avoid war, we must show that we are not afraid of it or its consequences," said the *Gazette.* This paper suggested the construction of seven ships-of-the-line, eight frigates, three sloops of war, and four bomb ketches, to carry in all nine hundred and eight guns, and to cost $2,655,000. But President Jefferson was obdurate. We are not justified, he said, in running into debt to prepare for some future war we know not when. So, far from adopting a program of naval construction, he would not keep in condition the few frigates already built. "Foreign nations must form a high opinion of our energy and activity," it was complained, "when they observe the whole attention of the Navy Department directed to one frigate, and that she can be got to sea in something less than six months."[31]

Jefferson, however, put his trust in something else than frigates. While Great Britain was trying to weaken France with her Orders in Council, while Napoleon was retaliating with his arbitrary decrees, while Americans found it difficult to engage in foreign commerce of any kind without seizure and confiscation, the President remained confident. He could bring the war-maddened powers to reason, he believed, by his policy of peaceful coercion. Calling his cabinet about him, he took a loose sheet of paper and wrote out a message to Congress, recommending an embargo on foreign trade. When Britain realized that the American market was closed to her manufactures, he thought, that her imports from the United States were cut off, that her West India islands were suffering for provisions, she would be forced to do us justice. The shipping centers protested, but the embargo bill was rushed through both Houses, and on December 22, 1807, Jefferson affixed his signature. The embargo forbade the departure of any ships for foreign ports, while coasting vessels were required to give bond to put in only at ports of the United States. With a stroke of the pen Jefferson threw thousands of sailors out of employment, paralyzed the shipping business, and cut off imports and exports totaling $246,-000,000.

In Norfolk there was a general scamper to load the vessels in port

31 *Ibid.,* Jan. 26, 1807.

and get away before the embargo took effect. An interesting case is that of the Cape Cod skipper, Elijah Cobb, whose vessel was tied up at Norfolk when the news arrived. Cobb had to store one hundred tons of ballast, secure a crew, take on three thousand barrels of flour, stow away provisions, water, and fuel, secure clearance papers, and get the ship to sea, all between Friday afternoon and Sunday morning. So he set two gangs of stevedores to work, one discharging ballast at the main hatch, and the other taking on flour forward and abaft. At noon on Saturday he asked for his papers. "Why Cobb," said the collector, "what is the use of clearing the ship, you cannot get away. Even if you get your ship below, I shall have boats out that will stop you." Nonetheless, as Cobb insisted, he drew up the papers. In the meanwhile the skipper had gone the rounds of the sailors' boarding houses, engaged his crew, and paid their landlords for back board. At 8 A.M. on Sunday morning, two hours before the embargo came in force, he weighed anchor and dropped down the river with the tide. Unluckily the wind died out, and it was 11 o'clock before he drew into the Roads. An hour later, Cobb spied a boat approaching "with sail and oars," and realized that the collector was making good his promise to intercept him. "Well," he said to his mate, "we are gone." But at the same moment he saw a fresh breeze coming from the south, and ordered all the light sails out. When the boat was so close that the features of the men could be seen, the sails bellied out and the ship pulled away. Cobb headed for Cádiz, where he sold his flour at the enormous price of $20.00 a barrel.[32]

The embargo proved disastrous to Norfolk. Her warehouses were locked, her wharves empty, the ships in port moved away to fresh water to avoid the worms, property values declined, many merchants faced ruin, her shipyards were idle, her artisans out of work, hundreds of sailors walked the streets or packed their bags to leave for foreign countries, the gangs of Negro stevedores loafed in the back alleys, the taverns and boarding houses were without guests. The more substantial citizens sat around in their homes or offices, with overcast faces, discussing the folly of the administration. If the embargo were intended to distress Great Britain, it would certainly fail of its purpose. The British had long complained of the desertion of their seamen; well, the embargo was driving them back again. Already hundreds had left Norfolk. As for the West Indies, they were getting some supplies from Canada, some from Europe. Moreover, they were beginning to

[32] Elijah Cobb, *A Cape Cod Skipper*, p. 64.

raise their own food, and so were making themselves forever independent of the United States. Certainly, also, Great Britain could have no serious objection to a measure which forced her chief competitor out of the carrying trade. It was well enough for the planters to accuse Norfolk of selfishness in opposing the embargo, but the planters did not have to lose their all. True, tobacco had fallen from $6.00 a hundred pounds to $3.50, and flour was selling for only $4.50 a barrel, but the farmer could keep his produce in his barn and wait for better times. But the trader's entire income was cut off, the value of his estate had sunk by half, if he had pressing obligations he fell into the sheriff's hands.

"Will it not appear wonderful that persons who have contended for commercial rights, suddenly abandon all commerce," complained the *Gazette,* "who lately rejected any accommodation with Great Britain unless the rights of our seamen were effectually protected, should suddenly adopt a line of policy, that must force these seamen into the service of that or some other country, or leave them to starve?" How can one contemplate calmly a total cessation of commerce? "Better, far better would it have been for the nation to have incurred a debt of $100,000,000 or more, for military and naval preparations, than to pursue a policy which leads to national bankruptcy, and to the destruction of all public spirit."[33]

We get a glimpse of how far-reaching were the effects of the embargo from the complaints of a Nansemond tar-burner. This man had on hand two hundred barrels of tar, one hundred barrels of turpentine, and twenty thousand staves. The stopping of exports had ruined the sale for these products, so that he could get hardly seventy-five cents a barrel for the tar and turpentine, while the staves were worth nothing. A neighbor who owned a raft, formerly employed in carrying produce from Suffolk to Norfolk, by which he supported his family, was now literally starving. At Washington they may call this "preserving our resources, but so long as the present measure lasts, we cannot see that we have any resources to preserve."[34]

Amid this universal suffering, it was the seamen who fared worst. These poor fellows were like fish out of water. They could not secure even odd jobs to tide them over the period of idleness, because unemployment was almost universal. Many an honest tar, his little earnings exhausted, his wife and children hungry, his furniture, clothes,

[33] Norfolk *Gazette and Public Ledger,* April 25, 1808.
[34] *Ibid.,* March 16, 1808.

and tools sold, took to drink to forget his misery. "We might as well shut up shop," declared William Couper, "for there is nothing but dullness and complaining. . . . Working people's wages here is almost reduced to nothing on account of nothing to be done."[35] To make matters worse, the Federal government dismantled a number of gunboats at Norfolk, throwing one hundred and seventy more sailors out of work. The mayor called a meeting of citizens in March to devise measures of relief, but it was impossible for "a community bowed down by their own sufferings" to contribute largely to charity.[36] In December, 1808, there were three hundred persons in the borough supported by public bounty, and perhaps as many more by private charity. The number of those whose pride kept them from asking aid cannot be estimated.

With the approach of autumn, the complaints of the Norfolk citizens grew louder. "Twelve months continuation of the present measures, and the area which is covered by the town of Norfolk will be worth more as a field for cultivation, than . . . with its numerous and costly buildings [as a port]. . . . To the next election alone can we look for safety."[37] The merchants feared that even when the embargo was lifted, they would not regain their markets. Spain, Portugal, and other European countries were getting supplies from the East, the West Indies, and from Canada. A letter from Jamaica tended to confirm the worst fears. "We consider the embargo helpful to Jamaica," it said. "We are raising our own provisions, splitting our hogshead staves and headings, while we get out puncheons from Quebec. Every day we feel ourselves more independent of you and laugh at the policy of your government." An Antigua planter wrote in similar vein. "I shall raise enough provisions to supply my estate for one year from January 1 next, so that I shall want only a little corn for my horses and mules, instead of buying three thousand bushels a year, and all my brother planters are as well off."[38]

There were occasional violations of the embargo by Norfolk men. Taking on a cargo of flour, they would secure clearance papers for New York or Boston, and then head for the West Indies. This brought a swarm of Federal officers down on the town to pry into the merchants' business, look over their books, and examine their cargoes. They had

35 Letters of William Couper, March 15, 1809. (Transcript copies in possession of Colonel William Couper, of Lexington, Va.)
36 Norfolk *Gazette and Public Ledger*, March 14, July 29, 1808.
37 *Ibid.*, Sept. 2, 1808.
38 *Ibid.*, Nov. 16, Dec. 14, 1808.

directions to detain any coaster whose cargo was "unusual," and in their zeal greatly hampered the legitimate northern trade. "Richmond flour is generally consumed in every considerable seaport in the United States," the merchants complained, "for the northern bakers prefer it to their own. And so far from the shipments this year being unusually large, less than twenty-eight thousand barrels have left Richmond in the past four months. This is less than half the amount for the same months last year. Surely the President will not deprive us of this little remnant of our trade, merely on the suspicion that one or two ships have slipped away to Jamaica?"[39]

Early in March came the joyful news that the embargo act had been repealed, and Norfolk burst into activity. True, non-intercourse with Great Britain and France was continued, but even the most inexperienced trader knew that there were ways of circumventing this restriction. He could take on flour, beef, tobacco, or lumber, secure clearance papers for some Spanish port, and upon his arrival there sell his cargo to Frenchmen or Britishers, who, in turn, would take it to France or England or one of their colonies. So the Norfolk wharves once more were alive with merchants, clerks, sailors, and stevedores, the Elizabeth was dotted with sails. "Commerce has again spread her swelling wings to favorable gales," it was said. In less than a week after the reopening of trade, eight vessels had left for St. Jago de Cuba, and four for St. Bartholomew's, the two ports selected as entrepôts of the new trade, while others had headed for Cádiz, Sweden, Buenos Aires, Havana, or Algeciras. It seemed that Norfolk would soon be more prosperous than ever.

But early in May many of the first shippers were returning disappointed. They had found St. Jago glutted with produce, prices had fallen, the cost of transhipment for bulky goods such as tobacco and flour had been heavy. So trade lagged once more, conversation in the coffee houses turned again to criticisms of the administration. In the days before the embargo, all of the trade to the British colonies had been carried on in American bottoms, they said, and 80 per cent of that to Great Britain. Now the American produce went only so far as St. Jago, Amelia Island, or St. Bartholomew's in our ships, while English vessels secured the carriage from these points to Great Britain. On one day alone, there were seventy-five British ships at Amelia. Obvi-

---

[39] The extent of the coasting trade may be judged by the marine lists of the Norfolk papers. The *Gazette* for Oct. 31, 1808, listed only one schooner bound for Richmond, one for Boston, and a brig for New Orleans.

ously non-intercourse was a failure, for instead of stopping trade between the United States and Great Britain, it merely aided British shippers at the expense of Americans.[40]

To make matters worse, seizures by both British and French continued. In June, 1809, the sloop *Venus* was boarded off the Isle of Pines by a privateer, supposed to be French, and robbed of provisions, stores, a boat, a quadrant, clothes, and some sugar.[41] In the spring of 1810, the Norfolk ships *Susan* and *Eliza* were detained in France, while their captains were thrown in prison, and the crews treated with great cruelty. "We were marched through the town tied together like felons," wrote one of the men, "and for five days fed on bread and water only."[42] Later news arrived that three more Norfolk vessels had been detained by the French, the *Fame* at Calais, and the *Planter* and the *Vigilant* at Amsterdam. "If our vessels go to any port of Europe except Great Britain," complained the merchants, "they are seized by Napoleon. If they go to Great Britain, they are seized by the United States when they come home. Between the Emperor and Mr. Madison, our merchants, shipwrights, and all concerned in commerce may soon cease their avocations."[43] The bitterness against France expressed itself in an act of violence against the privateer *Ravanche de Cerf*, at anchor in the Elizabeth. On the night of April 15, 1811, when the crew was on shore two boats filled with armed men came alongside, overpowered two youths left as a guard, and placing a tub of combustibles in the hold, set it on fire. The ship burned to the water's edge.[44]

Norfolk was opposed to the War of 1812. Her merchants were ready to do their part in upholding the honor of the nation, but they considered it folly to lock horns with the greatest naval power of the world, when our own navy was insignificant. "How can we fight without frigates and ships-of-the-line?" they asked. "Will Mr. Jefferson's gunboats protect our commerce? Can they prevent the enemy from blockading our ports? Can they even defend our rivers and harbors?" But when war was actually declared, Norfolk prepared to make the most of a bad situation by putting her defenses in readiness and by sending out a bevy of privateers. Late in the summer of 1812 the armed schooner *Mars*, of Norfolk, captured the British brig *Leonidas*, of ten guns, and sent her, a prize, into Savannah. This was a rich haul, as her

[40] Norfolk *Gazette and Public Ledger*, June 5, 1810.
[41] *Ibid.*, June 26, 1809.
[42] *Ibid.*, March 30, 1810.
[43] *Ibid.*, Feb. 25, 1811.
[44] *Ibid.*, April 17, 1811.

cargo of sugar and coffee was worth fifty thousand dollars, and the brig itself twenty thousand dollars.[45] Nor was trade, even with Great Britain and her colonies, entirely interrupted. The British government made Bermuda a place of deposit for her islands, permitting American products to land there from neutral ships. Later the West India governors were empowered to open their ports even to United States vessels in case of dire need.[46] The Norfolk papers in October, 1812, were full of notices advertising English fall goods for sale.[47] It was said also that the British let the American vessels pass, in order to provision her armies in the Peninsula. "Our valuable coasting trade . . . has as yet been subject to but slight interruptions," stated the *Gazette*. All in all, Norfolk suffered little during the first eight months after the declaration of war.

But matters took a different turn in February, 1813, when a British squadron came in the Capes and blockaded Chesapeake Bay. Before them fled the United States frigate *Constellation,* crowding on all sail to reach the protecting guns of Fort Norfolk. In her haste she missed the channel and ran aground in the river, but swarms of citizens came down in boats, and lightened her until she floated.[48] She remained at Norfolk throughout the war, aiding greatly in its defense with her officers, crew, guns, and small boats. Many incoming merchantmen, less fortunate than the *Constellation,* were taken as they entered the Capes. An attempt was made also to break up the traffic down the James River to Norfolk. Two frigates, anchoring off Newport News, sent out an armed tender, which took a ship, two brigs, and three schooners, while a bevy of barges pursued a number of lighter vessels into shallow water and captured or drove them ashore.[49] On one occasion several of these barges were driven by the wind so far into the Roads that they could not get back to the fleet. One surrendered to the *Constellation,* while others were pursued up James River and captured by boats filled with militia.[50]

At the moment when news reached Richmond that a powerful British squadron was within the Capes, a large part of the Virginia militia, under General Joel Leftwich, was absent upon an expedition to the northwest.[51] Other detachments were called to the colors, however,

[45] *Ibid.,* Sept. 4, 1812.
[46] Benns, *American Struggle for the British West India Carrying Trade,* p. 27.
[47] Norfolk *Gazette and Public Ledger,* Oct. 19, 1812.
[48] Jarvis Manuscript; Norfolk *Gazette and Public Ledger,* June 1, 1816.
[49] Norfolk *Gazette and Public Ledger,* March 17, 20, 24, 1813.
[50] *Ibid.,* April 14, 1813.
[51] *Ibid.,* Dec. 12, 1812; March 13, 1813.

and rushed to Norfolk. The first to arrive was a Richmond company, followed by the Henrico Rifles, the Albemarle cavalry under Captain Carr, the Petersburg Blues, and a small body of regulars.[52] These, together with the militia and volunteer companies of Norfolk, and the sailors from the *Constellation* and the merchant ships in port, made a very respectable force. The command was given to General Robert B. Taylor, an officer of energy and ability. Taylor found the men enthusiastic but lacking in discipline, and poorly drilled and equipped. His first task was to whip them into an effective military machine. In many of the companies the officers were related to some of the privates, and on the road it was not unusual for one in the ranks to call out to the captain, "Uncle Tom, don't march so fast," or "Halt a little, Cousin Bill, till I tie my shoe." General Taylor, therefore, broke up the companies, and distributed the men in new units, without regard to the locality. He then organized the companies into regiments, and began the arduous work of drilling and maneuvering.[53] Breastworks were thrown up at strategic points—on Lamberts Point, at the bridge over Tanner's Creek, and at the junction of Church Street and Princess Anne Road. The British could expect a warm reception if they landed a force on the south shore of Hampton Roads and attempted to make their way over the creeks and inlets which separated it from Norfolk. To attack with any hope of success, they must approach by water, up the Elizabeth. But the river too was well guarded by Fort Norfolk, on the right bank below Smith's Creek, and Fort Nelson on the site of the Naval Hospital. As they were equipped with twenty heavy pieces of artillery, each manned by experienced gunners, it would be a hazardous matter for frigates or ships-of-the-line to run past them.

But General Taylor was determined that the British vessels should never get up so high as these forts. Several miles down the river, near the left bank, is Craney Island, at that time connected with the shore by a narrow foot bridge. On the west side of the island he threw up redoubts, and on the east erected a fort. Upon these he placed two 24-pounders, one 18-pounder, and four 6-pounders, manned by 150 seamen from the *Constellation,* four hundred militiamen, one company of riflemen, two companies of light artillery, and thirty men from Fort Norfolk.[54] In the river channel, stretching in a wide arc from Craney Island to Lamberts Point, were twenty gunboats, carrying one or

[52] *Ibid.,* Feb. 12; April 17, 1813.
[53] Jarvis Manuscript; Norfolk *Gazette and Public Ledger,* June 2, 1813.
[54] Norfolk *Argus,* June 22, 1855; Jarvis Manuscript, pp. 132, 133.

more 18-pounders, and commanded by experienced shipmasters.[55] An advancing British squadron would be exposed in front to the fire of this mosquito fleet, and raked on their right from the batteries on the island.[56]

In June a number of warships and transports, filled with marines and soldiers, joined the British fleet, and preparations were made for an attack on Norfolk. On June 21 the watchers on Craney Island saw the entire squadron move across Hampton Roads and anchor off the mouth of Nansemond River—four great ships-of-the-line, with their frowning sides pierced by three tiers of guns; seven frigates, their graceful lines suggestive of alertness and speed; three sloops-of-war; two transport ships; and numerous smaller craft. On deck the red uniforms of the infantry could be seen plainly, and it was no longer to be doubted that a landing in force was in preparation.[57]

That night the Americans waited at their post until daylight. They were then permitted to rest. But when the British boats were seen to make for shore filled with redcoats and marines, the call to arms was again sounded, as it was now obvious that the enemy intended to advance on Craney Island along the river bank. The Americans made their preparation with coolness, shifting some of the guns to the west side of the island and drawing up the militia behind them. The sailors from the *Constellation* stood at the heavy guns at the breastwork, waiting for the signal to fire. At this moment some of the men, noticing that the colors were nowhere displayed, hunted up a pole and hoisted the Stars and Stripes. In the meanwhile the British had been lost to view in a pine forest on the plantation of Captain George Wise, but when several rockets, sent up as signals to the fleet, revealed their position, the batteries opened upon them. The gunners, using grape and canister, fired with great rapidity and precision. The British had not expected so hot a reception. As men began to drop, the line faltered, and then fell back. This part of the attack had failed ingloriously.

In the meanwhile, two long columns of barges, crowded with marines and sailors, approached the island from the west. In the lead was Ad-

[55] Among these were John Nants, Richard I. Cos, David Hall, George Davis, Joseph Middleton, Briscoe I. Doxey, Joseph Melvin, and William Lee. Jarvis Manuscript, pp. 132, 133.

[56] *Ibid.*

[57] The force available for the attack consisted of one thousand regimentals, one thousand seamen, the Royal Marine Brigade of sixteen hundred men, four hundred marines, and three hundred Frenchmen taken in the Peninsula, in all 4,300 men (Norfolk *Gazette and Public Ledger*, June 23, 1813).

miral Warren's beautiful barge, the *Centipede,* a brass 3-pounder mounted in the bow. The American gunners, cool and confident from their victory over the land force, waited for them to get within range. At last Captain Emerson shouted, "Now my brave boys, are you ready? Fire!" The first discharge of grape and canister threw the head of the British column into confusion. Several boats were sunk, leaving their men to struggle in the water, others were grounded. Still the flotilla advanced, the barges behind pressing on as those in front went down. But no courage could face that merciless fire. At last a round shot passed through the *Centipede* diagonally, cutting off one man's legs, and wounding several others. As the barge sank, orders were issued to retreat, and the British oarsmen turned and pulled for their fleet. So ended the attempt to capture Norfolk, Portsmouth, the *Constellation,* and the shipyard at Gosport. The victory of Craney Island shows how unnecessary was the disgrace which befell the nation a year later when Washington was taken and the Capitol burned.[58]

The British fleet, though repulsed in its attack on Norfolk, by no means relinquished its grip on the trade of Virginia and Maryland. Stationing itself in Lynnhaven Bay, it kept a close guard over the entrance to the Chesapeake. At times their barges entered the Roads, or rowed a short distance up the James to intercept the traffic on that river.[59] Occasionally a merchantman would elude the blockading ships, either by her swiftness or because her pilot was acquainted with channels through which they were afraid to pursue.[60] Of twenty-nine vessels among those which made the attempt to get out, one was captured in Chesapeake Bay, one taken at sea, and twenty-seven escaped. In addition, five Norfolk privateers got to sea during the time of the blockade.[61]

Moreover, the British, in their anxiety to watch the main entrance to Norfolk, left the back door wide open. The produce of all southeast Virginia began to pour into Albemarle Sound, whence it went out to foreign countries or further south to Wilmington or Charleston. Of thirty-seven vessels insured by one company for voyages between North Carolina ports and the West Indies, thirty arrived safely, six were captured, and one lost at sea; of eleven vessels sailing to or from Europe, three were captured, and two lost at sea; of twenty-one

[58] Jarvis Manuscript; Benson J. Lossing, *Pictorial Field-Book of the War of 1812* (New York, 1868), pp. 677-680; Norfolk *Gazette and Public Ledger,* June 23, 1813; Norfolk *Argus,* June 22, 1855.
[59] Norfolk *Gazette and Public Ledger,* November 27, 1813.
[60] *Ibid.*
[61] Norfolk *Herald,* June 5, 1818.

coasters, nineteen arrived safely, one was captured, and another taken and recaptured.[62] The enemy were aware of this trade, but they found it most difficult to blockade the coasts of North Carolina. If their frigates should be caught by an eastern gale between Cape Lookout and Cape Hatteras, they could not clear the land on either tack; while in the calmest sea the Frying-pan shoals, and Cape Roman shoals made it hazardous for large vessels to approach the coast.[63]

So the flour and tobacco of Richmond and Petersburg came down the James to Norfolk, whence it was shipped to Kempsville in light boats, and then overland about ten miles to North Landing. Here it was transferred to sloops, which passed through Currituck and Pamlico Sound to Beaufort. From this point larger vessels were constantly leaving for Europe, the West Indies, or Charleston. In the summer of 1813 about one hundred voyages were made from the ports of Pamlico and Albemarle to Wilmington without one capture, while between Wilmington and Charleston there were only three captures. The insurance on goods going from Norfolk to Charleston was between 15 and 20 per cent.[64] In June, 1814, all Norfolk was thrilled by the passage of a vessel of twenty tons, laden with bacon, brandy, and other goods, through the Dismal Swamp canal from Scotland Neck, on the Roanoke River. The opening of this waterway, which connected the Southern Branch with the North River, greatly facilitated communication with the North Carolina sounds.[65]

Unfortunately, at this moment all hope of foreign trade was lost because of the embargo of December, 1813. This act caught a number of Norfolk vessels in port at Charleston, and forced them to discharge and store their cargoes. The Norfolk merchants were still complaining of this, when news came that even the trade from Petersburg and Richmond to Norfolk in flour, wheat, meal, and corn had been prohibited. The government was determined that no provisions should fall into the hands of the enemy through the capture of river boats crossing from the James to the Elizabeth. This restriction seemed "arbitrary and useless" to the Norfolk traders, especially "since rice and spirits were still permitted to pass from Norfolk up the James, and whiskey, beef, pork, and butter from Baltimore to Norfolk."[66]

The New Year of 1815 found the people bitter and despondent. The

[62] Norfolk *Gazette and Public Ledger,* June 21, 1815.
[63] *Ibid.,* Jan. 15, 1814.
[64] *Ibid.*
[65] *Ibid.,* June 11, 1814.
[66] *Ibid.,* Feb. 2, March 14, 1814.

British blockade and the Federal restrictions together had paralyzed business. "Some years ago," writes one observer, "walking through Wide-Water street, I was much incommoded by rum puncheons, sugar hogsheads, bales of goods, flour and tobacco hogsheads. I heard the bawling of negroes as they hoisted these goods in and out of vessels, I got the odor of tar and turpentine, I was in constant danger of breaking my shins on the skids of passing drays. Recently I again went through Water Street, Market Square, and Main Street. No rum puncheons, no bales of goods, no sugar and tobacco hogsheads, no bawling negroes, no drays passing. Instead of plodding merchants, and busy clerks, I see only some military officers, ten or twelve idle youths, a few recruits, and a group of negroes. From the near-by dram shops come the fumes of egg-nog and cigars, and the sound of fiddles and tamborines." The war and the restrictions it brought to her trade had reduced Norfolk to a shadow of her former self.[67]

At this moment, when all seemed dark, the town received the news of Jackson's great victory at New Orleans. It seemed "almost incredible" that the undisciplined Westerners should have crushed Pakenham's veterans, fresh from their triumphs in the Peninsula. The killing of two thousand Britishers with a loss of only twenty-one Americans seemed to Norfolk a just revenge for her own wrongs at the hands of the British—the *Chesapeake* affair, impressments and seizures, the Orders in Council, the blockade of their harbor. But pride and satisfaction gave way to unbounded joy, when immediately after came the announcement that peace had been concluded—honorable peace with not an inch of territory ceded, not one of our rights surrendered. Once more the wharves became alive with industry, once more ships began to come in from distant points; once more Norfolk vessels cleared for Liverpool, London, Boston, New York, New Bedford. The *Constellation* hoisted sails, and amid the grateful cheers of the people, fell down the river on her way to New York. Peace, the long hoped-for peace, was here at last. It remained to be seen whether it would restore the prosperity of the borough, whether her "sails would whiten every sea," or whether with the end of the conflict in Europe would come new restrictions to commerce and hard times for her merchants, sailors, and artisans.

[67] *Ibid.*, Jan. 4, 1815.

CHAPTER SIX

The Town and Its People

In this day of rapid changes, of tenseness and activity, it may be imagined that life in Norfolk a century and a quarter ago was hopelessly monotonous. To the people of that day it did not seem so. In place of moving pictures there were strolling entertainers and theatrical companies; as a substitute for football they had bandy, for baseball the races, for automobile rides, picnics at Lake Drummond. There were parties, school entertainments, and balls; there were the annual fair, the only too frequent excitement of fires, the Fourth of July parade, and the never-to-be-forgotten occasion when some distinguished guest came to town—General Lafayette, or Louis Napoleon, or Colonel Robert Y. Hayne, or Henry Clay, or Stephen A. Douglas.

Even in the eighteenth century Norfolk was visited from time to time by wandering performers, the predecessors of the modern circus. Some were tumblers and gymnasts, others ventriloquists, still others jugglers; some brought menageries. Among these early troupes was that of Mr. Godwin, who entertained with "lectures, paintings, transparencies, songs, catches and glees."[1] More thrilling was the performance of Robertson and Sully, in the Long Room of Riffand's Garden. After Robertson had given an imitation of birds, he and his partner threw back-somersaults from three tables and a chair piled one on the other. This was followed by an "astonishing leap" by Robertson over twelve men with fixed bayonets, and by music on the "much admired Egg Hornpipes." Robertson closed the performance with the "Antipodean Whirligig," in which he "whirled on his head at the rate of 250 a minute, without the assistance of his hands."[2] This pair found a

[1] Norfolk *Journal,* Nov. 12, 1788.
[2] Norfolk *Herald,* Jan. 23, Feb. 2, 1802.

worthy successor in Mr. Rannie, "so well known for his ventriloquel powers in Europe, etc." Rannie informed Norfolk that his performance stood almost alone, "as we have no accounts of any ventriloquist but three since the days of Adam or the Woman of Endor."[3] Seven years later the people flocked to Matone's Garden to see a pair of Bengal tigers. The management announced that "these curious animals, lately imported from Surat, are the first that reached any part of the continent."[4] By 1836 the circus had made its appearance at Norfolk, a troupe giving a performance on a lot at the corner of Hill and Talbot streets. This was followed by an animal show containing an elephant, a lion, a tiger, a zebra, two leopards, a gazelle, a coypu, two hyenas, and numerous monkeys and South American birds.[5]

Of a very different character was the lecture of Edgar Allen Poe on "The Poetic Principle," in September, 1849. "Chaste and classic in its style of composition, smooth and graceful in its delivery, it had the happiest effect upon the fashionable audience. . . . His recitations were exquisite and elicited the warmest admiration. For about an hour every one present seemed charmed and delighted with the rich intellectual entertainment."[6] Four years later a large audience at Mechanics Hall listened to the great violinist, Ole Bull, accompanied by the "musical wonder" Adelina Patti, then only eight years old.[7] Perhaps it was the large German group in Norfolk who were responsible for the development of music in the town. So early as 1818 James H. Swindell, the organist of Christ Church, organized and trained a chorus of men and women. In May they gave a concert of sacred music, chiefly from Handel, before one thousand people, "the largest assemblage of beauty and fashion ever seen in Norfolk."[8] In later years a number of young men, forming what they called the Philharmonic Association, continued the musical tradition.[9]

The Norfolk people were devoted theatergoers. In colonial days a wooden pottery, in the rear of a lot on Main Street near King's Lane, was converted into a theater. After the Revolution, so early as 1790, the people were flocking to see *The Irish Widow*, or the *School of Scandal*,[10] but there was no regular playhouse until 1793, when a

3 *Ibid.*, Feb. 17, 1803.
4 Norfolk *Gazette and Public Ledger*, Jan. 12, 1810.
5 Norfolk *Beacon*, July 16, 1836.
6 Norfolk *Argus*, Sept. 17, 1849.
7 H. W. Burton, *History of Norfolk* (Norfolk, 1877) , p. 14.
8 Norfolk *Herald*, March 23, May 22, 1818.
9 Forrest, *Sketches of Norfolk*, pp. 238, 239.
10 Norfolk *Chronicle*, May 8, 1790.

wooden warehouse on Calvert's Lane was used for that purpose. In 1795 a new brick theater was erected on the east side of Fenchurch Street, between Main and Bermuda,[11] where for many years professional troupes and local amateurs had their performances.[12] "Last week our theatre opened," said the *Herald* in February, 1802, "with a new comedy, 'The Contrast,' advertised as the virgin essay of an American genius. If the author's future lucubrations are not the contrast to his first endeavors, we hope his productions will not be baptized in Norfolk. Great negligence of scenery was observed; even the curtain was left to Jonathan (Mr. Sully) who had not weight sufficient to influence its descent."[13] Despite an occasional failure of this kind, the theater was popular. "We do not recollect to have witnessed a greater display of ladies in any small theatre," said the *Herald* of March 24, 1803, "and it is to be lamented they could not be more agreeably accommodated. Some ladies were annoyed, being surrounded by well-dressed noted damsels from Water Street, Bank Street, Lee's wharf, etc." Such persons and the sailors who accompanied them ought to be relegated to the galleries, thought the editor, so that decent people would not be offended by their "Bank street dialect."

In November, 1821, Norfolk was excited by the arrival of Junius Brutus Booth, then a young man of twenty-five. The people were surprised to find him a mere lad, who wandered around town in "an old straw hat and linen roundabout," gazing at everything he saw.[14] His rendition of Richard III delighted his audience, the tent scene, which was called "a finished piece of action," coming in for especial applause.[15] With the passing of years Norfolk lost much of its interest in the stage. The theater fell into disrepair, and in April, 1833, it was sold to the Methodists, who used it as a house of worship until 1845, when it was destroyed by fire.[16]

A few years later a Mr. George Jones started a movement which resulted in the erection of the Avon Theater, on the new public square, just east of the site of the present City Hall.[17] This building which seated from eleven hundred to twelve hundred persons, was classic in design, the interior handsomely decorated. The drop curtain was an object of admiration, with its painting of Pericles and Phidias, look-

[11] Norfolk *Herald*, June 19, 1839.
[12] Norfolk *Beacon*, Oct. 23, 1839; Forrest, *Sketches of Norfolk*, p. 253 n.
[13] Norfolk *Herald*, Feb. 16, 1802.
[14] Forrest, *Sketches of Norfolk*, p. 160.
[15] Norfolk *Beacon*, Nov. 12, 1821.
[16] Norfolk *Herald*, April 17, 1833.
[17] Forrest, *Sketches of Norfolk*, p. 212; Norfolk *Beacon*, Oct. 23, 1839.

ing out from Mars Hill upon the Acropolis. The theater faced west, and the beautiful portico with its Doric columns, its pilasters, and its bust of Shakespeare, could easily be seen across the Granby Street bridge from vessels coming up the river.[18] It was formally opened on October 17, 1839, with a presentation of Knowles's *Hunchback*.[19] Unfortunately the theater was destroyed by fire in February, 1850.[20] The Avon was not rebuilt, but in 1856 a new theater, later known as the Opera House, was opened by Henry C. Jarrett.[21] Here appeared, in the days before the Civil War, some of the ablest actors and actresses of the day—James E. Murdoch in several of Shakespeare's plays, Mary Devlin in *London Assurance,* D. W. Waller in *Hamlet,* Joseph Jefferson, and Maggie Mitchell.[22]

Although Norfolk did not produce a literary school of national distinction during the period before the Civil War, her citizens published verse and prose in considerable volume. Forrest says that even the merchants found time for writing. "Often while attending to the peculiar duties of his vocation, the man of business, who has the mind for the more exalted pursuits of literature, forms his plans, arranges his thoughts, and then embraces the first opportunity to retire a while from his merchandize, his books, his customers, and his dollars and cents, to commit them to paper. These casual and hasty attempts sometimes possess real merit." The productions of the Norfolk writers appeared in the local papers, or in the *Southern Literary Messenger,* or perhaps were published separately as books of verse.

One of the ablest writers of this period was Hugh Blair Grigsby (1806-1881), editor, biographer, scholar, and poet. Grigsby as a boy studied under tutors and later entered Yale. From early youth he showed a predilection for biography, in his eighteenth year writing a series of sketches of prominent Virginians. In 1827 he published the *Letters of a South Carolinian,* while in 1890, nine years after his death, the Virginia Historical Society published his work on the *Virginia Federal Convention of 1788.* Both are made up largely of biographical sketches. Grigsby's editorial writing was clear, forceful, and logical, while he ranked high as an orator. His verse, although not large in volume, has considerable merit. Among the best of his poems are "Hymn," "I Cannot Die," and "Lines to My Daughter." Grigsby col-

[18] Norfolk *Beacon,* Oct. 23, 1839.
[19] *Ibid.,* Oct. 16, 1839.
[20] Forrest, *Sketches of Norfolk,* p. 252.
[21] Burton, *History of Norfolk,* p. 25.
[22] *Ibid.,* pp. 25, 26, 29, 31, 24, 27.

lected a library of six thousand volumes, many of them formerly belonging to John Randolph, of Roanoke.[22a]

Among the Norfolk poets of this period was William Maxwell, whose *Walcott* and *Columbian Bards* attracted attention in New England and abroad. William Roscoe ranked Maxwell among the best of the minor American poets. Thomas Blanchard, "a ripe scholar, a fine classic writer, and a gifted poet," was widely known for his ode "To the Memory of George Washington," written in 1800. Richard Halstead, signing himself "Quilp," published a volume of verse in 1846. Another Norfolk poet, who contributed to some of the leading literary journals of the day, was Abram F. Leonard. His "Song of the Emigrants," and "Ode to Solitude" are not without merit. Byron Walthall, whose early death ended a career of great literary promise, was the author of "The Stag Hunter." Other Norfolk writers of poetry were R. James Keeling, William Wallace Davis, and S. S. Dawes.[22b]

Perhaps Norfolk's most famous poet was Abram Joseph Ryan, universally known as Father Ryan. He was born at Norfolk in 1839. Entering the priesthood of the Roman Catholic church, he became a chaplain in the Confederate army. After the war he moved to Augusta, Georgia, where he founded and edited *The Banner of the South*. In 1880 he published *Poems, Patriotic, Religious and Miscellaneous,* among them the "Conquered Banner," "The Sword of Robert E. Lee," "The Lost Cause," etc. Father Ryan is the outstanding poet of the Confederacy, and his works were read in almost every household in the South.

In the ante-bellum days Norfolk produced one distinguished sculptor —Alexander Galt. This young man had a distinct spark of genius. At fifteen he was drawing excellent pencil portraits, and a few years later went to Florence to study under the best Italian teachers. While there his bust "Virginia" and his "Psyche" were exhibited and attracted very favorable comment. Upon his return to the United States, he visited several Southern states, filling important orders, and everywhere showing a ripening talent. In 1856 he was again in Florence, where he executed his statue of Thomas Jefferson, for the library of the University of Virginia.[22c] Galt enlisted in the Confederate army and died of smallpox, in Richmond, on January 19, 1863. Many of his best

[22a] A. A. Brock, *Virginia Federal Convention of 1788* (Richmond, 1890), pp. v-xxi.
[22b] Forrest, *Sketches of Norfolk*, pp. 346-372.
[22c] When the Rotunda of the University burned, a group of students took this statue from the pedestal, wrapped it in mattresses and brought it down the winding stairs to safety.

works were destroyed in the fire which accompanied the evacuation of Richmond in 1865.

Ever popular with the Norfolk people was the race track. In the early years of the nineteenth century the races were held at Thorowgood's Farm, in Princess Anne.[23] Here gathered a motley crowd— gaily dressed ladies with their escorts, farmers, merchants, clerks, sailors, urchins, everyone who could get away from work. On one occasion when the harbor was full of shipping waiting for loading or unloading, it was suggested that the races be prohibited, lest clerks, sailors and stevedores forget their duties to view this all-absorbing sport.[24] The races of 1802 lasted four days, the first being devoted to four-mile heats for a purse of $400, the second to two-mile heats for sweepstakes, the third to three-mile heats, and the fourth to ladies' and gentlemen's elegant saddle and bridle races.[25] There was good sport throughout, but some of the jockeys were criticized for appearing in old and dirty jackets.[26]

But the races were soon over, and then the young had to turn to cards, billiards, cricket,[27] or bandy. The last named game was often played in the streets or in vacant lots, much to the disgust of passers-by. "The national, manly, and innocent game of bandy ought not to be suppressed by the officers of the police in the borough," said a sarcastic article in the *Herald*. "The loss of an eye now and then by the force of a ball helps the [medical] faculty a little, as the sickly season is over; and the panes of glass that are broken put a few dollars in the pockets of the glazier. All trades must live and the practice of bandy, it is hoped, will be tolerated."[28]

If one were too old for cricket or bandy, he could seek amusement at the Vauxhall Gardens and baths, or Rosainville's Bower, or Lindsay's Retreat, or the Museum of Nature, or the Wigwam Gardens. The Wigwam, on Briggs' Point, was kept open all summer. It was "adorned with a variety of trees and flowers," arranged to represent stars, the American eagle, an elephant, a camel, lambs, Egyptian pyramids, etc. "Refreshments of the best kind, good wines, and liquors, with complaisant and attractive waiters," together with "the pleasantness of the situation," were expected to lure all who wished to "unbend the

[23] Norfolk *Herald*, Aug. 28, 1802.
[24] Norfolk *Gazette and Public Ledger,* Nov. 25, 1805.
[25] Norfolk *Herald*, Oct. 2, 1802.
[26] *Ibid.,* Nov. 9, 1802.
[27] *Ibid.,* Nov. 13, 1818.
[28] *Ibid.,* Dec. 2, 1802.

wrinkled brow of care." The admission price, of one shilling and sixpence, commanded also "some value at the bar."[29]

Dancing was universal, and no young lady considered her education complete unless she knew the minuet, or could follow the intricate figures of the cotillion. Among the early masters was a certain Mr. Thuillier, who had a school for dancing and music in 1788. Two years later Joseph Martin opened a dancing academy in the Old Coffee House, opposite the Town Hall. He taught the most "approved methods of modern dances, together with the new figures, lately introduced into the polite world, with their proper steps and attitudes."[30] Private dances were everyday occurrences, while Washington's birthday, or other great occasions, were frequently marked by formal balls.[31]

October 22, 1824, was the never-to-be-forgotten day on which Lafayette visited Norfolk. The old general arrived on the *Petersburg* and was rowed to the county wharf in a handsome barge. With him were his son, Secretary of War Calhoun, General Taylor, General Cocke, George Newton, and others. As he mounted the wharf steps, a thrilling scene presented itself. On one side of Market Square were four companies of infantry, on the other a line of civic societies, between them, at Main Street, a beautiful arch, decorated with flowers and evergreens and bearing the words, "Welcome Lafayette." The sidewalks, every window, many near-by roofs, and the shipping were crowded with people eager to do homage to the nation's guest. After an address of welcome by Mayor John E. Holt, the general proceeded to the "elegant apartments prepared for him at Mrs. Hansford's boarding house." That night the town was illuminated, Main Street being a "continuous blaze of light." Many houses showed transparencies, with mottoes and words of welcome, while the shore front was lit up by forty-two bonfires. On Saturday afternoon there was a banquet at the Exchange with plates for three hundred, and on Sunday the general paid a visit to Fort Monroe.

There had been some misgivings concerning the grand ball, for there was no floor in town capable of accommodating more than one hundred and twenty-five couples. At last some one thought of the new custom house, on Water Street, then in course of construction.[32] A large

---

[29] *Ibid.*, June 22, 1802.
[30] Norfolk *Chronicle*, April 24, 1790.
[31] Norfolk *Journal*, Feb. 13, 1788.
[32] The present custom house was completed in October, 1858. In 1800 the office was located in a large building at the west end of Main Street. After that it was moved from place to place until the construction of the government building of 1824 on Water east of Market Square.

force was set to work planing the rough floor and concealing brick walls and rafters with flags and decorations, so that on Monday night all was ready. Upon entering the door one passed down a hall through bowers of myrtle and ivy, and ascended richly carpeted steps. Here the "brilliancy of the ball room burst upon the sight with an over-powering effect." Overhead was a thickly woven artificial ceiling of myrtle, ivy, and cedar boughs, apparently growing out of eight trees arising from the floor. From this green canopy were suspended in-numerable lamps in rows and circles, like "gems of various hues." In the windows were illuminated transparencies, depicting "landscapes, cascades, etc." At one end of the room was a sofa, reserved for the gen-eral, decorated with banners and overhung with evergreens and roses.

By eight o'clock Secretary Calhoun arrived, after which the room rapidly filled. The handsomely gowned women and military and naval officers in their dress uniforms added to the brilliancy of the scene. While waiting for the general many couples promenaded around the room to the music of the violins. At last, at nine, Lafayette came in, and was led to his seat. Thereupon the orchestra struck up, and danc-ing began. After the first cotillion the general was conducted around the room and introduced to the ladies. At 10:30 the company sat down to supper, and at 11:30 Lafayette left to take the boat for Richmond.[33]

Prior to 1850 the Fourth of July was invariably celebrated with processions, oratory, and feasting. The observance of the day in 1831 was typical. Long before the procession started, the line of march was crowded with spectators, who looked on from the sidewalks, porticos, doorways, and windows. The militia led the way—the Independent Volunteers, the Light Artillery Blues, the Junior Volunteers. Next came the tailors, bearing a banner depicting Adam and Eve, with the motto: "Naked and ye clothed me." The blacksmiths, riding on a mounted platform drawn by two fine horses, worked busily with forge, bellows, and anvil, and after completing various simple articles, dis-tributed them to the crowd. The carpenters also plied their trade in a moving workshop. The next car, with the stone-cutters, masons, bricklayers, and plasterers, represented the brick and stone foundation of a building and men at work slaking lime and laying brick. Other cars followed depicting in like manner the work of tanners, curriers and morocco dressers; cordwainers; painters; hatters; coppersmiths, brass-founders, and tin-plate workers; gunsmiths, watchmakers and

[33] Norfolk *Beacon*, Oct. 25, 27, 29, 1824.

silversmiths; ropemakers, shipwrights; and teachers with their pupils. The procession halted before the residence of Dr. N. C. Whitehead, at the corner of Catharine and Freemason streets, while all who could find seats crowded into Christ Church to hear Hugh Blair Grigsby deliver the oration.[34] Nineteen years later, when the South was finding itself outvoted in Congress and its status as a minority section fixed permanently by the famous compromise of that year, the Fourth of July passed almost without notice. "It is a question whether the South have at this day any independence to boast of," said the *Argus,* with a touch of sadness.[35]

In the Norfolk of ante-bellum days, there were many able men, some of them known throughout the Union—the distinguished merchants Moses Myers,[36] William Pennock, Phineas Dana, and John Newell, Jr.; William Plume, the Irish immigrant who grew rich from the manufacture of rope;[37] Hugh Blair Grigsby, editor and historian; General Robert B. Taylor, soldier and jurist; Commodore James Barron; William Wirt, attorney-general under Monroe; Governor Littleton W. Tazewell; and Thomas Newton, who represented Norfolk in Congress for thirty years.[38]

A visitor in 1828 describes Tazewell as a man of "middle size, and thin visaged; his countenance is grave, but intelligent, and his manners evince a highly cultured man."[39] "Whoever regards his tall, spare form, and the unusual, yet dignified, motion of his limbs, his expressive countenance, his elevated forehead partially shaded by light grayish hair, curling negligently down his neck, his eye brows arched, . . . his cheeks furrowed . . . his lips remarkably thin and well-formed," instinctively marks him as a man of unusual powers.[40] Commodore Barron was "of middling height, and robust make. His face is round and full, and his countenance open, benevolent, and pleasing. His air and manners are altogether affable and gentlemanly."[41] "In his family circle he was cherished with unspeakable fondness and affection; and this whole community, in which he was for so large a

---

[34] Norfolk *Herald,* July 6, 1831; Forrest, *Sketches of Norfolk,* pp. 177, 178.
[35] Norfolk *Argus,* July 6, 1850.
[36] The beautiful residence of Moses Myers, on Freemason Street, is still standing, a monument to the architectural taste of the times.
[37] Norfolk *Gazette and Public Ledger,* Feb. 23, 1807.
[38] Forrest, *Sketches of Norfolk,* p. 55.
[39] Anne Royall, *The Black Book* (Washington, 1828) , p. 254.
[40] Forrest, *Sketches of Norfolk,* p. 384.
[41] Royall, *The Black Book,* p. 258.

portion of his life beloved and esteemed, will ever honor and revere his memory."[42]

Barron was a principal in an unfortunate duel. Commodore Decatur, famed for his exploits in Tripoli, having made some slurring remarks concerning Barron's conduct in the *Chesapeake-Leopard* affair, the latter sent him a challenge. The duel was fought with pistols at Bladensburg, Maryland. When all was ready, Commodore Bainbridge began to count, and at the word "two" both fired. Barron was wounded in the hip. Decatur stood for a moment erect, and then fell. "I am mortally wounded," he said. "At least, I believe so, and I wish I had fallen in defence of my country." He died the same evening in great agony.[43]

Like other seaport towns, Norfolk had its share of grogshops and gambling houses, its brawls and murders. In the alleys leading from Water Street to Main were many "filthy, tobacco-impregnated barrooms," and "licentious dance cellars," where sailors drank and squabbled. On one occasion, in 1803, bands of drunken sailors rioted in the streets, creating great excitement and injuring a number of people with stones. One unfortunate had his head nearly severed from his body by a stroke with a shingle.[44] "From the almost continual rioting in the streets, sometimes for nights together, . . . it might be doubted whether we have any police, or legal authority whatever, to protect the peace of the borough," complained the *Gazette* in February, 1805. At times the denizens of the tippling houses came forth, not to fight, but to make night hideous with song. "Saturday night about twenty friends of mirth, fellows of fun, took it into their heads to let the inhabitants know they were alive," said the *Herald,* "and with something they conceived was music, but which no ear could relish and no beast dance to, amused themselves and kept awake every child, and of course every nurse within the sound of their humdrum concert."[45] Sometimes young men, drunk and armed, would resort to the theater, or public gardens, where they were a nuisance and a danger.[46]

There was no organized crime in Norfolk, similar to that in many of our modern cities, but drinking and gambling not infrequently led to stabbings or shootings. In 1806 two brothers named Davis kept a

[42] Forrest, *Sketches of Norfolk,* p. 275.
[43] *Ibid.,* pp. 274, 275.
[44] Norfolk *Herald,* July 19, 1803.
[45] *Ibid.,* Oct. 2, 1802.
[46] *Ibid.,* April 16, 1802.

faro table on the third floor of a house in Water Street. One night an Italian named Colmini, having broken the bank, was accused of cheating by the Davises and one of the other players. When they tried to seize him Colmini fled down the narrow, dark stairway and hid at the landing. As the three men in pursuit passed him, he gave each in turn a vicious stab with a stiletto, and then made good his escape. All of his victims died.[47]

Fifteen years later Norfolk was stirred by the brutal murder of a Frenchman named Peter Lagaudette, by two Spaniards, Manuel García and José Castillano. A young man named Cherry, happening to enter a frame building in the fields between Church and Cumberland streets south of Bute, was horrified to find the mutilated remains of a man. The torso was on the floor, the head, hands and feet badly burned were in the fireplace, the arms and legs in a tub. In a few minutes the whole town was aroused. It was learned that the two Spaniards, a villainous-looking pair, had occupied the house with Lagaudette, and a general alarm was sent out for them. They were arrested at Lamberts Point. It is supposed that the three men had quarreled over the division of booty attained by a robbery, and that the two Spaniards, having murdered Lagaudette, dissevered the body and attempted to dispose of the fragments piecemeal. They were tried for murder, found guilty, and executed. The hanging took place in a field near Portsmouth, in the presence of a crowd of between three thousand and four thousand persons.[48]

Norfolk has always had a large proportion of Negroes. In 1820 in a total population of 8,608 there were 3,261 slaves and 599 free blacks; in 1830 with a total of 9,816 there were 3,757 slaves and 928 free blacks; in 1840 of 10,920 persons, 3,709 were slaves and 1,026 free blacks; in 1850 the total was 14,320, the slaves 4,295 and the free Negroes 957. The blacks served as cooks, waiters, chambermaids, nurses, washerwomen, coachmen, porters, and stevedores. The unusually large proportion of free Negroes is explained by the fact that when plantation slaves were manumitted, they usually moved to town. There were some complaints of unruliness on the part of the blacks, but usually they were guilty of nothing more serious than gathering on vacant lots in Loyall's Lane or Calvert's Lane to play dice or five corns, or to skylark, or to pitch pennies.[49] The plot of 1802 was

[47] Norfolk *Gazette and Public Ledger*, Nov. 24, 1806.
[48] Library of Congress, Miscellaneous Papers, No. 724.
[49] Norfolk *Herald*, May 19, 1819.

an exception. A group of Negroes conspired to rise on Easter of that year, set fire to the town, and make good their escape. One of their number made a confession, naming the guilty men. Every available white man was immediately called to arms, and for weeks, in April and May, the militia remained on duty night and day.[50] The two leaders, Jeremiah and Ned, were tried, convicted, and condemned to death. They were conveyed to the place of execution in a cart, and Jeremiah was turned off in the presence of a great crowd. When it became Ned's turn and he stood trembling under the gallows, he received a reprieve and was conducted back to prison.[51]

The people of Norfolk were not blind to the evils of slavery. Thoughtful men complained of the inefficiency of Negro labor and the diversion of European immigration from the South. When Mrs. Anne Royall visited the town in 1828, she thought the insolence of the blacks insufferable. "This is the case in most of the towns of Virginia, and gives the lie to the reports charging them with cruelty to their slaves. But this slavery, nevertheless, is a great curse, as it takes all they make to feed and clothe them; they are, on every account, prejudicial to the country."[52] Considerations such as these no doubt were influential in the forming of the Norfolk Colonization Society,[53] to aid in sending Negroes to Africa. In January, 1821, fifty Negroes sailed from Norfolk for Africa on the *Nautilus*, with clothing, furniture, tools, etc. With the vessel were a number of native Africans, apparently just rescued from slave dealers and on their way home. At the sight of these uncivilized creatures mingling with their American cousins, "all hearts were touched, and many eyes were filled with tears. After the service numbers came forward and joined the Society, while others gave contributions. Several poor blacks gave their little mites to their brethren who were going out."[54]

For many years after the Revolution, Norfolk was an unsightly town, built largely of wood, the narrow streets and lanes leading into Main from north and south crowded with ramshackle tenements. The lack of adequate drainage, the proximity of marshes and stagnant pools, and the presence of decaying matter thrown into the river at the docks combined to create unpleasant odors. The streets were unpaved and poorly lighted; Market Square was almost a quagmire;

[50] Letters of William Couper, Aug. 19, 1802.
[51] Norfolk *Herald*, May 11, 13, 29, 1802.
[52] Royall, *The Black Book*, p. 255.
[53] Norfolk *Herald*, Jan. 1, 1821.
[54] *Ibid.*, Jan. 17, 1821.

Water Street was "knee deep in mire from the Custom House east."[55]
"It is one of the ugliest, most irregular, dirtiest towns that I have ever
seen," said La Rochefoucauld in 1796. "The houses are low and mean,
almost all of wood, . . . not twenty being of brick. The streets are
unpaved; the town is surrounded by a marsh."[56] A few years later Tom
Moore visited Norfolk and carried away an even more unfavorable impression. "At the time we arrived, the yellow fever had not disappeared,
and every odor that assailed us in the streets, accounted very strongly
for its visitation." The best that can be said is that the place "abounds
in dogs, in negroes, and in democrats."[57] "The streets are surely a little
too crooked for beauty . . . and are in some places intolerably dirty,
that is, where they haven't yet been paved," wrote a visitor about
1815. "The principal ones, however, are kept clean, and handsomely
lighted. The houses too, for the most part, even on Main Street, are
built in a very slovenly style, tho' I see with pleasure, some signs of
better taste in the new ones which are shooting up. The public buildings are but few, and not over-elegant. The court house is rather a
shabby affair, altogether unworthy of such a place."[58]

This unprepossessing Norfolk was practically swept away in a series
of conflagrations. The first of these occurred in 1799, when many
buildings on the east side of Market Square between Main and Union
were destroyed.[59] On February 22, 1804, a second fire swept over the
district south of Main Street, from Market Square to Town Point,
destroying over three hundred warehouses, stores, and dwellings. The
loss of goods of every description was so great that some merchants
were never able to restore their fortunes. One old man, seeing that
it was impossible to save his property, rushed into the flames and was
burned to death.[60] "On Wednesday, being the 22nd of February a fire
broke out in a gentleman's store in the lower part of the town about
11 o'clock at night," wrote William Couper, "where it burned down
and laid to ashes not less than 260 houses in the space of six or seven
hours, and the houses being chiefly built with wood, all the exertions that could be made were in vain. . . . I received no bodily hurt
as many a one did, some that were burned to ashes, some that were
killed by the blowing up of houses with powder to save the rest from

[55] Norfolk *Beacon*, Aug. 29, 1854.
[56] La Rochefoucauld, *Voyages dans les États-Unis*, IV, 256, 257.
[57] Norfolk *Gazette and Public Ledger*, Sept. 12, 1806.
[58] *Letters from Virginia* (Baltimore, 1816), p. 18.
[59] Burton, *History of Norfolk*, p. 5.
[60] Norfolk *Beacon*, May 3, 1836; Forrest, *Sketches of Norfolk*, p. 112; Stewart,
History of Norfolk County, p. 358.

catching fire, some that were hurt that is supposed will never recover. With the ships getting on fire, drifting about in the harbor, kindling one another, indeed it was a most awful sight to see, the columns of smoke, the bursting out of the flames, the cries of those that were on the streets saving their little properties, exposed to a most terrible, drifty and snowing night."[61]

A fire in 1805 destroyed ten or twelve houses on Water Street,[62] another in 1813 burnt twenty-five more, all of wood;[63] still others in 1814 cost nineteen more.[64] The last of these fires started in the old shingled Market House, whence it spread to the wooden buildings on the east side of Market Square. In a short time all had been consumed and the flames were sweeping on over the lanes between Union and Water streets. The fire engines were late to arrive, there were few buckets, and the conflagration was checked only by blowing up houses in its path.[65]

In April, 1819, occurred another destructive conflagration. One hundred houses were consumed, including many stores and dwellings, and thirty-four families were rendered homeless. This fire extended along the north side of Main Street, and up Talbot Street, Mitchell's Lane, and Willock's Lane.[66] A few months later the crowded tenements of Bank Street, where Negroes and poor whites herded together, were swept away, despite the efforts of a new fire company and of soldiers from Fort Norfolk.[67] In 1827 a fire destroyed Christ Church, together with sixty other buildings, most of them of wood;[68] while six years later twenty old houses on the south side of Main Street were carried away.[69]

As the wooden houses were destroyed, substantial brick buildings took their place. "Strangers were astonished at the improvement in our streets and buildings in the past eight or ten years," said the *Herald* in 1818. "Where miserable hovels . . . showed their contemptible fronts, stately and elegant piles have sprung up." "I expected to have seen an old, dirty-looking, gloomy, clownish town," said Mrs. Anne Royall, in 1828. "On the contrary . . . the houses are

61 Letters of William Couper, April 27, 1804.
62 Norfolk *Gazette and Public Ledger,* Nov. 22, 1805.
63 *Ibid.,* March 8, 1813.
64 *Ibid.,* March 28, 30, 1814.
65 *Ibid.*
66 Norfolk *Herald,* April 9, 12, 1819.
67 *Ibid.,* Sept. 24, 1819.
68 *Ibid.,* March 9, 1827; Burton, *History of Norfolk,* p. 7.
69 Norfolk *Herald,* Nov. 4, 1833.

large and elegant, and many of them surrounded with beautiful trees.
. . . The town is not only neat, it is beautiful. The streets are well
paved, lighted, and the neatest kept in any town in the Union, except
Providence. I will not except Philadelphia."[70] Joseph Martin, writing
in 1836, tells us that "many buildings with stone fronts, and in improved style, have been erected within a few years."[71] Freemason
Street became the fashionable part of town, and its handsome houses
and flower gardens attracted the attention of every visitor to Norfolk.
"Blooming roses of various hues, flowering vines, evergreens, and rare
flowers" attested to the taste and care of the owners.[72] "Arriving at the
corner of Freemason Street," wrote a correspondent to the *Beacon* in
1853, "we marched along viewing our magnificent churches, our noble
palaces of the wealthy, and admiring the extreme cleanliness that prevailed, together with the taste displayed in all the private gardens.
This street is undoubtedly the most magnificent in the city." Granby
Street he found somewhat behind the times. "We expressed some surprise to ourselves that the various owners of the fine, large, old-time,
well-built houses on this street do not improve their outward appearance."[73] "Entire new and beautiful streets have taken the place of
old marshy lanes and alleys," said another writer. "New and capacious
buildings have gone up, where, some years ago, were nothing but
old shanties and ruins. . . . In fact the place wears a new aspect, and
seems to have been thoroughly renovated."[74]

The borough authorities, from the days when Norfolk began to rise
from its ashes, were not inattentive to the streets. So early as 1786 the
council was receiving estimates for a "sink or drain, through the Main
street, from the Church street to the river."[75] But the people were
poor, the borough income small, and little could be done. An order
was issued to prevent the throwing of refuse and dead animals in the
streets, but even this was not always obeyed.[76] Later the town was divided into districts with an overseer of streets in each, whose duty it
was to fill in mud holes, repair bridges, make drains, and keep the
streets in good condition.[77] One district embraced all Main Street,
another Church Street, a third Fenchurch and Bermuda streets, a

[70] Royall, *The Black Book*, p. 254.
[71] Joseph Martin, *Gazetteer of Virginia* (Charlottesville, 1836), p. 247.
[72] Norfolk *Argus*, May 5, 1854.
[73] Norfolk *Beacon*, Aug. 1, 1853.
[74] Forrest, *Sketches of Norfolk*, p. 407.
[75] *Norfolk Council Orders*, 1736-98, p. 100b.
[76] Norfolk *Chronicle*, Aug. 7, 1794.
[77] *Norfolk Council Orders*, 1736-98, pp. 262b, 166b.

fourth Freemason and Cumberland, the fifth Catharine Street, including Farmer's Lane, the sixth Market Square, Holt, Maxwell, Concord,
Granby, and Boush.[78] Stone for streets could be purchased cheaply at
any wharf, for tons were brought over from Europe as ballast.[79] In
1802 the principal streets were graded and the gutters paved, "with
proper descents for carrying off water."[80]

Still the complaints of rubbish, dirt, and stagnant water continued.
In 1807 the legislature empowered the borough to pave the streets,
and shortly afterward the old mud-choked thoroughfares became a
thing of the past. "All the principal streets are paved," wrote a visitor
in 1818. Where a few years ago one "in crossing the street stuck ankle
deep in the mud, he now finds a smooth and solid pavement."[81] Joseph
Martin, too, spoke of the paving of the streets and the excellent system
of draining.[82] "The streets are well paved and tolerably clean," said a
visitor in 1834, "besides being very decently lighted up at night."[83]
Main Street and other business thoroughfares were the first to receive
attention, but in time Bermuda and other residential streets had their
turn. "Church street, formerly a bog in winter and dusty in summer,
is now a handsomely paved street from the lower termination near the
Court House to the Town Bridge," stated the *Herald* in 1835. This
street was lined with stores at the southern end, with many fine residences further north. "It is one of the most delightful promenades in
Norfolk," said the *Beacon*. In 1836 Fenchurch Street was extended
northward over marsh land toward the creek, and handsomely paved.
At this time Norfolk had more miles of paved streets than any other
city in the South.[84] In the meanwhile, the work of filling in Water
Street was resumed, so that by 1839 it could be used as far as Hunter's
shipyard. Later it was completed to its eastern terminus at Main Street
and paved throughout.

An unattractive feature of early Norfolk was the marshy ground
along the shores of Back Creek, between the old town and the new
residential district centering around Freemason and Granby streets.
At high tide the water came up to the present intersection of Metcalf
and Plume at one point, to Market and Court at another, and actually
touched Freemason just west of Granby. "The creek is a foul blotch

78 *Ibid.*, p. 208b.
79 *Ibid.*, p. 166b.
80 Norfolk *Herald*, Jan. 8, 1803.
81 *Ibid.*, May 1, 1818.
82 Martin, *Gazetteer of Virginia*, p. 248.
83 Norfolk *Beacon*, Jan. 7, 1834.
84 *Ibid.*, May 3, 1836.

on our fair town," said a writer in the *Herald* in June, 1827. "Whenever the tide ebbs, it is left dry and covered at the edges with slime. It can be seen clearly from the thoroughfare where Bank Street joins Catharine. Why not shut out the water at the Granby Street bridge? This would permit the mud to harden, and trees and grass to grow." This suggestion aroused great interest. All were agreed that the marsh should be eliminated, but some thought it wise to leave a canal to connect with Cove Street, others preferred a public square, still others a promenade with shade trees.[85] The final vote was in favor of the public square, with a space at one end reserved for a new city hall.[86] It was not until 1839, however, that the work of filling in was actually accomplished, and then only for the area east of Bank and Catharine streets.[87] The more extensive marsh ground west of Bank remained until many years after the Civil War.[88]

On August 23, 1847, the cornerstone was laid for the new City Hall. This building, which still stands, imposing and beautiful amid the business structures of the modern city, faced west, overlooking Back Creek and the harbor beyond. It is eighty feet by sixty, with a portico, supported by six Tuscan columns. A cupola, thirty-two feet in diameter, and rising one hundred and ten feet above the street, dominates the structure, and in former days made it a conspicuous object for miles around. Granite steps lead to the portico, and the front wall is faced with granite. The building contained court rooms, mayor's office, sheriff's office, council chambers, and jury room, while beneath the first floor was a cistern, with a capacity of forty-five gallons. The entire cost was about fifty thousand dollars.[89]

A few years later a new Custom House was erected on Main Street, at Granby. Its handsome portico, with the long flight of steps leading up from the street, its granite walls, its six columns with their Corinthian capitals, added a touch of dignity and beauty to this part of the city.[90] Other new structures dating from this period were the prison, on the site of the Avon Theater; the Norfolk Academy at Catharine and Charlotte streets; the great naval hospital at Portsmouth; the National Hotel at Main and Church streets; the Atlantic Hotel, which was opened in 1859;[91] the Presbyterian Church; Mechanics Hall, on

[85] *Ibid.*, June 22, 1827; March 26, 1830.
[86] *Ibid.*, Jan. 7, 1834.
[87] Forrest, *Sketches of Norfolk*, p. 211.
[88] Robert W. Lamb, *Our Twin Cities* (Norfolk, 1888) , p. 54.
[89] Forrest, *Sketches of Norfolk*, p. 255.
[90] The building is still standing.
[91] Burton, *History of Norfolk*, p. 36.

the south side of Main Street, a few doors east of Market Square;[92] and the Cumberland Street Methodist Church.

In the early days the streets of Norfolk were unlighted, and the pedestrian had to take his lantern with him or depend upon such friendly rays as came from the near-by houses. In 1811, however, the legislature of Virginia passed an act empowering the borough to set up lamp posts.[93] Even then the streets remained dark and gloomy, for the oil lamps gave but a faint gleam, and were often neglected by the attendants. "Why is there no light in the lamps?" complained one man in February, 1823. "Have the citizens refused to pay the lamp tax?" "Is there no oil?[94] Last night while walking in the street, I stumbled over a pile of bricks and measured my length in the gutter."[95] Relief came in 1849, when the Norfolk Gas Light Company, composed of enterprising citizens, established its plant on Briggs' Point, at the corner of Mariner and Walker streets. The laying down of pipes continued in the summer of 1849, and on October 1, in the presence of a crowd of spectators, the lights were lit in several buildings.[96] Freemason Street seems to have been the first equipped with gas lights. "It is a pleasure to walk at night on this street, now brilliantly lighted," wrote a correspondent to the *Argus* in March, 1850. "These beautiful lights should be diffused over the entire city."[97] This was done as speedily as possible. "When the storm howls . . . it is pleasant to look out upon the city below, all mantled with a silvery light. Here and there, on this side and that, as far as the eye can reach, the friendly lamps are seen, like so many faithful sentinels at their posts."[98] The company made the mistake of using rosin for the manufacture of its gas, with the result that their building was burnt down twice in the same year. This warning was sufficient, and thereafter rosin was discarded in favor of coal.[99]

It was many years later that Norfolk acquired modern water works. Far into the nineteenth century the town wells, placed at convenient points in the streets, provided almost the sole supply of water. But the unavoidable pollution, together with the brackish taste, made it un-

[92] Forrest, *Sketches of Norfolk*, p. 251.
[93] *Ibid.*, p. 119.
[94] In 1825 the lamp tax amounted to $577.80, and the cost of maintaining the lights was $461.25 (Norfolk *Beacon*, Jan. 13, 1826).
[95] Norfolk *Herald*, Feb. 12, 1823.
[96] Forrest, *Sketches of Norfolk*, p. 245.
[97] Norfolk *Argus*, March 14, 1850.
[98] Forrest, *Sketches of Norfolk*, p. 246.
[99] Burton, *History of Norfolk*, pp. 215, 216.

desirable for drinking purposes. So, in the summer of 1800, when a certain Johnny Rouke, who owned a large well of pure water at his home on Briggs' Point, began peddling water around town, he was heartily welcomed. The sight of his "tea-wagon" standing before some residence, while the colored maid filled the drinking bucket, became familiar to all. Later the "tea-water" was sold in the streets by old Negro men at a half cent a gallon.[100]

The first person in Norfolk to equip his residence with a cistern is said to have been Caleb Bonsal, the bookseller.[101] But others followed his example until in 1853 it was stated that "much the larger portion of the regular supply" was obtained in this way. The cisterns were of brick, below the surface of the earth, and were fed by pipes connected with the house gutter.[102] This system, too, was far from satisfactory, and there gradually arose a demand for a modern water works system. "Why drink rain water, flavored with the dirt and dust of the roof," it was asked, "when Lake Drummond or Deep Creek can so eaily be tapped?" But this suggestion at once stirred the opposition of the conservatives. It was merely a plan of speculators to line their pockets; it would double taxes; Lake Drummond was too far away. And who wanted to drink juniper water, strong enough to stain one's clothing or one's face, water full of alligators and snakes? In the midst of this controversy came rumblings of the Civil War, and so Norfolk had to wait for another twelve years before the actual construction of a system of water works was begun.[103]

The people of Norfolk in the early days were recompensed for the poor quality of their water by an abundance of good and wholesome food. The market was always stocked with meat, fowl, fish, and vegetables. "The market of Norfolk is a subject of much astonishment to a person from the North," said Mrs. Royall. "This was the 25th of April; of course I was surprised to find ripe strawberries, peas, potatoes, green beans, cucumbers, and all sorts of vegetables in the greatest perfection and abundance; but their meat of every sort is very indifferent. They, however, have fine fish, fowl, and game."[104] At Christmas time, especially, the country people flocked in with their carts, driving little horses the size of a two-year-old cow, and bringing geese, ducks, chick-

[100] Norfolk *Herald*, Aug. 2, 1826.
[101] Forrest, *Sketches of Norfolk*, p. 217.
[102] *Ibid.*, p. 216.
[103] Norfolk *Argus*, Aug. 27, Sept. 2, 1858; Cary W. Jones, *Norfolk as a Business Centre* (Norfolk, 1881), p. 57; Lamb, *Our Twin Cities*, p. 38.
[104] Royall, *The Black Book*, p. 255.

ens, opossums, raccoons, rabbits, squirrels, eggs, vegetables, mutton, lamb, etc. On Christmas eve, 1819, it was computed that there were 311 carts in town, besides scores of boats from Princess Anne and elsewhere, bringing in all no less than six thousand turkeys.[105] If one went the round of the stalls, he would be sure to hear something like the following: " 'Friend, how d'ye sell port? Eight dollars. Mr. Shuster, how does beef go to-day? Ten cents. Boy, how much do you ask for chickens? Two and three pence, and half a dollar, master. Madam, what's the price of your geese? Three and nine pence, sir. Old gentleman, how much do you ask for turkies? Nine shillings."[106] To the farmer who moved into Norfolk to partake of the prosperity of the days when the West Indian trade was in full swing, the prices of food seemed excessive. One complained bitterly that he had a simple meal for his family, consisting of a hog's jowl, greens, two fowls, butter, bread, and toddy, and the cost came to no less than $2.62½.[107] William Wirt, who came to Norfolk in 1804, also felt high prices a serious grievance. "Indian meal, through the winter is nine shillings per bushel," he wrote, "flour, eleven and twelve dollars per barrel, a leg of mutton, three dollars, butter three shillings per pound, eggs two shillings, and three pence per dozen, and so on."[108] Half a century later prices were far more reasonable. A visitor at the market in 1853 found there 178 carts supplied with all kinds of food—eggs at ten cents a dozen, chickens at thirty-seven and a half cents per pair, apples, tomatoes, fish, potatoes, collards, beef, pork, lamb, veal, geese, figs, corn, grapes, quinces, pears, "snap-beans," peaches, and cantaloupes.[109]

The religious life of Norfolk was also much transformed in the post-Revolutionary decades. The most significant change was made by the Revolution itself, which resulted in the overthrow of the Established Church and the creation of complete religious freedom. The parish vestry ceased to be a government agency, surrendered its charitable duties to the newly created overseers of the poor, and lost the right to tax; deprived of its customary revenues, the Protestant Episcopal Church, as the reorganized church was called, declined everywhere in Virginia and almost died. In Norfolk the newly organized vestry had to face the problem of rebuilding the old borough church, whose fire-blackened walls alone had survived the burning of Norfolk in

---

[105] Norfolk *Herald*, Dec. 29, 1819.
[106] Norfolk *Gazette and Public Ledger*, Jan. 4, 1815.
[107] Norfolk *Herald*, March 4, 1818.
[108] Burton, *History of Norfolk*, p. 6.
[109] Norfolk *Argus*, Aug. 15, 1853.

January, 1776. For this purpose the General Assembly in October, 1785, authorized the vestry to raise £700 by lottery.[110] The lottery apparently was successful, since the vestry the following year elected Walker Maury minister of the parish. Maury was at the same time appointed master of the revived school by the borough council, which had just appropriated £300 for a new building on the old school lot.[111] When Maury died of yellow fever two years later, he was succeeded in both positions by the Reverend Alexander Whitehead.[112]

At this point a bitter quarrel split the old church. Two rival vestries were elected by the opposing groups; in 1789 one summoned William Bland to be minister of the parish, and the other invited James Whitehead, possibly a relative of Alexander Whitehead, who continued to serve as schoolmaster until 1792. Although the Whitehead faction was recognized by the Virginia Convention of the Episcopal Church as the legal group and Bland was refused a seat in the Convention, Whitehead's supporters eventually withdrew all claim to the old borough church and on June 24, 1800, laid the cornerstone of a new church at the north end of the schoolhouse lot. This building, later known as Christ Church, was destroyed by fire in 1827 and was replaced by a new structure on a new lot, at the corner of Freemason and Cumberland streets, where it still stands. Meanwhile, the Bland congregation disintegrated after his death in 1803, and the old borough church was not used again for Episcopal worship until 1832, when a revived congregation had it reconsecrated as St. Paul's Church, the name it has borne ever since.[113]

Many former Episcopalians probably joined the newly organized Methodist Episcopal Church, which appeared in Norfolk in 1793. Methodism had been preached there before the Revolution, when it was still a movement inside the Church of England, but it now returned as an independent church. The first Methodist bishop, Francis Asbury, bought a lot on Fenchurch Street, just below the school lot, and, according to tradition, Methodist services were held in a barnlike building there for seven years. In 1800 the Methodists acquired another lot on Cumberland Street, where they still maintain a church.[114]

The first Catholic church was erected about the same time as the

110 Whichard, *History of Lower Tidewater Virginia*, I, 442.
111 *Norfolk Council Orders*, 1736-1798, pp. 99, 104.
112 Whichard, *History of Lower Tidewater Virginia*, I, 442.
113 *Ibid.*, I, 442-444.
114 *Ibid.*, I, 446.

first Methodist building. The Catholic Church had not been tolerated in colonial Virginia, and there were no known Catholics in Norfolk before the Revolution. The first Catholics arrived in 1791 as refugees from the French Revolution, and their number was increased two years later by other Frenchmen fleeing from the slave insurrection in Santo Domingo. In 1794 these exiles purchased a lot at the corner of Chapel and Holt streets, the one now occupied by St. Mary's, and built there a wooden chapel. This was replaced in 1842 by a more substantial structure, which is used today as a parish hall.[115]

The next denomination to appear in Norfolk was the Presbyterian. Before the Revolution the town had contained many Scotch merchants, who would have been of the Presbyterian faith, but they seem to have been content with the services at the borough church. Although many of these returned after the war, it was not until 1800 that a Presbyterian church was formally organized. By 1802 the new congregation had built a church on the northwest corner of what is now Bank and Charlotte streets and put a bell on its roof, a distinction so unusual in Norfolk in that day that it soon came to be known as the "Bell Church." The building still stands, much altered in appearance, but it is no longer used by the Presbyterians.[116]

The last of the major denominations to arrive was the Baptists, who at first had a biracial congregation. The Norfolk Baptists began as a branch of the Portsmouth Baptist Church and did not form a separate organization of their own until 1805. They worshiped in the then-vacant borough church until 1816, when they erected a building of their own on Cumberland Street. Shortly afterwards the two races separated, the Negroes assuming the name of the First Baptist Church. The First Baptist Church in 1830 acquired a lot on Bute Street and built a church there. Ten years later part of the congregation seceded and moved into the old Presbyterian church on Bank Street.[117]

In addition to its many churches, Norfolk was fortunate in having one of the finest academies in the South. Soon after the Revolution, when most of the town was still in ashes, when taxes were high, and the people impoverished, the council appointed a committee to "contract for the rebuilding of the free school."[118] Accordingly in 1786, £300 was appropriated, as has been mentioned, and a building, sixty feet by twenty-two feet and two stories high, was erected on the school

[115] *Ibid.*, I, 446-447.
[116] *Ibid.*, I, 445-446.
[117] *Ibid.*, I, 447-449.
[118] *Norfolk Council Orders,* 1736-1798, p. 97b.

land on Church Street.[119] A set of rules and regulations drawn up by a committee of aldermen was adopted by the borough council in March, 1787, when the school was for the first time named Norfolk Academy. The subjects to be taught were reading, writing, arithmetic, book-keeping, English grammar, geography, Latin, Greek, French, and the use of the globes. There was to be a committee of aldermen to examine the school twice a year and to sit with the master in cases of serious misconduct on the part of pupils. Expulsion might be resorted to for lying, swearing, obscenity, quarreling, or fighting. The children of those days had to be early risers, for in summer school was in session from six to eight and nine to twelve in the morning, and from two to five in the afternoon. In winter the early session was omitted. There were to be two vacations, four weeks at Whitsuntide and a month at Christmas. Each member of the first class was to wear a broad black band thrown over the right shoulder and under the left arm, while a student in one of the other classes wore a blue ribbon in the button-hole of his coat.[120]

In 1796, when La Rochefoucauld visited Norfolk, he found the school flourishing. "There is a very good school for boys there," he said, "the tuition being $40 a year for each pupil."[121] The headmaster at that time was James Whitehead, minister of one of the Episco-palian factions, who had been appointed to the post when the other Whitehead resigned in 1792. In 1796 he was involved in a dispute with the borough council, which attempted to exercise its right to dismiss him. When the schoolmaster stubbornly refused to accept his dismissal, however, the council surrendered and left him in his position.[122] The headmaster usually had two assistants; at least he did in 1802 when a Mr. Maguire was teaching Latin and a Mr. Beraule was the French instructor.[123]

The academy was removed from borough control and made an independent corporation in 1804, when the General Assembly named a board of trustees, consisting of Littleton W. Tazewell, Thomas Newton, Jr., Richard H. Lee, Arthur Lee, and other distinguished citizens.[124] This board at once took legal possession of the frame school-

---

[119] *Ibid.*, p. 99.
[120] *Ibid.*, pp. 106, 107b.
[121] La Rochefoucauld, *Voyages dans les États-Unis*, IV, 271.
[122] Whichard, *History of Lower Tidewater Virginia*, I, 438.
[123] Norfolk *Herald*, Oct. 2, 1802.
[124] *Ibid.*, Feb. 5, 1836; Samuel R. Borum, *Norfolk, Port and City* (Norfolk, 1893), p. 28.

house and the lot on Church Street; it also replaced James Whitehead with a new headmaster.[125] Hoping to move the school to a more convenient location, the trustees on August 29, 1806, purchased from the overseers of the poor the old glebe land on the south side of Charlotte Street.[126] It was a full third of a century, however, before the new academy was built, the school continuing to use the old building until it became so ramshackle that it was totally unfit for further service.

At the public examination held on September 19, 1816, "more than 100 scholars" were tested "in the several branches of English and classical education." At that time the headmaster was a Mr. Edmonds.[127] In November, 1814, Dr. Augustine Slaughter, after making provision in his will for emancipating his slaves, established a fund of three thousand dollars for scholarships at the academy. These were to be used for training poor boys in reading, writing, and navigation. After receiving an adequate schooling, each boy was to be apprenticed to a shipmaster. It is stated that Mr. Philip R. Thompson, of Culpeper County, one of Dr. Slaughter's heirs, secured a lawyer to examine the will and found that a technical defect rendered it null. It was expected that he would demand the entire three thousand dollars, but instead he directed the lawyer to draw up a new instrument to carry out the original intent of the donor, to which he affixed his signature. In 1853 there were ten boys at the academy profiting by the generosity of these two men.[128]

In the years from 1830 to 1836 the academy suffered a decline and the trustees were concerned to find that Norfolk boys were turning elsewhere for instruction. The school building was "merely rented to some teacher who kept a school on his own private account." The revenues were inadequate, consisting of $200 for the rent of the Academy, $56 from the rent of other buildings, $132 interest on $2,200 owed by the Presbyterian church, and $30 dividends on $550 in stock of the Farmers' Bank—in all $418. So it was proposed to sell the Church Street property and with the proceeds build a handsome schoolhouse on the Charlotte Street lot.[129] All Norfolk became interested, and by 1840 "public and private munificence" had made it possible to erect one of the finest school buildings in the country.

The cornerstone was laid on May 25, 1840, with impressive cere-

[125] Whichard, *History of Lower Tidewater Virginia*, I, 439.
[126] Norfolk *Beacon*, Feb. 5, 1836.
[127] *Lower Norfolk County Antiquary*, V, 145.
[128] Forrest, *Sketches of Norfolk*, pp. 143, 144.
[129] Norfolk *Herald*, Feb. 5, 1836.

monies.[130] The procession formed at French's Hotel,[131] and moved through Main, Fenchurch, Holt, Church, Main once more, and Catharine, to "Academy Square." The line, extending nearly a mile, was led by a band, followed by the mayor, the sergeant with the Borough mace, the recorder, the council, trustees of the Academy, clergymen, foreign consuls, military and naval officers, civic societies, hundreds of schoolchildren, the naval apprentices from the *Delaware,* and citizens and strangers. "As the long line passed down Main street, to the sound of music, with the mystic symbols of the different institutions borne along and with banners all flying, the windows in the lofty houses on either side crowded with the fair," the scene was enough to stir the soul. After prayer by Bishop Philander Chase, of Illinois, and an address by Colonel William Garnet, various objects—coins, newspapers, documents, etc.—were deposited in the cornerstone, and the stone itself lowered into place.[132]

The building is ninety-one feet long by forty-seven, and is modeled after the temple of Theseus at Athens. There are two porticos with six Doric columns each, on the east and west ends. The architect was Thomas U. Walter, of Philadelphia, noted for his work on the national Capitol at Washington. In its new building the school took on a new lease of life. The first choice for principal seems to have been unfortunate, however. John P. Scott, an Irishman by birth, was a classical scholar and a man of high character, but he lacked the patience essential to a successful teacher. It is stated that when the weather was hot and the boys were disorderly, he would seize the chief offenders and hustle them out of the nearest window. His administration was short-lived.[133]

"In this institution are taught, as thoroughly and extensively as in any college, all branches necessary to the attainment of an English, mathematical and classical education," said the *Argus,* in 1848. "There being two departments, pupils of any age over eight years may be admitted. . . . Besides the ordinary branches taught at colleges generally, this institution presents the additional advantage of a military education. . . . The managers of the institution avoid as much as possible corporal punishment. . . . In the junior department pupils study the lower branches of English, and the first principles of algebra

[130] Norfolk *Beacon,* May 25, 1840.
[131] Afterward the National. The building was demolished in 1959 as part of the downtown redevelopment program.
[132] *Lower Norfolk County Antiquary,* IV, 150-163; Norfolk *Beacon,* May 27, 1840.
[133] *Lower Norfolk County Antiquary,* IV, 38.

and commence Latin. They are then transferred to the Senior department." At this time the faculty consisted of John D. Strange, Mathematics and Military Science; Richard B. Tschudi, Ancient Languages; George W. Sheffield, English; and Hilarus Magnin, Modern Languages.[134]

Important in the life of early Norfolk was the local newspaper. The advent of the Revolution found one sheet in the borough, *The Virginia Gazette or Norfolk Intelligencer,* edited by James Holt. The few musty copies of this journal, now reposing in the Library of Congress, make interesting reading. The news is chiefly national and foreign, picked up from the crews of passengers of incoming vessels, or copied from other papers. Events at Norfolk, unless of unusual importance, were omitted, perhaps on the theory that they were known to all the readers of the *Gazette* long before they could be put into print. But the lists of vessels entering or clearing, the notices of runaway slaves, the advertisements of houses or of ships for sale, give a vivid glimpse of what was going on in Norfolk at the end of the colonial period. Holt's paper came to a sudden end in September, 1775, when Lord Dunmore seized his presses and set them up on his fleet.[135]

After the Revolution, when Norfolk was rising from its ashes, *The Norfolk and Portsmouth Journal* made its appearance,[136] followed in 1788 by the *Norfolk and Portsmouth Chronicle,* a weekly edited by J. McLean and A. McLean;[137] and in 1793 by *The Virginia Chronicle and Norfolk and Portsmouth General Advertiser. The Herald and Norfolk and Portsmouth Advertiser,* a little biweekly, eighteen inches by twenty-four inches, was first issued on August 13, 1794. It later became a daily, and under the able guidance of Thomas G. Broughton, was for decades the standard paper of southeastern Virginia and northeastern Carolina. *The Norfolk Gazette and Public Ledger,* founded in 1804, by William Davis, was an anti-Jeffersonian paper, ridiculing the policy of peaceful coercion and opposing the War of 1812.[138] In April, 1815, *The American Beacon* made its appearance. This paper, at first neutral in politics and later Whig, was long ably edited by William Cunningham.[139]

[134] *Ibid.,* IV, 30-32; Forrest, *Sketches of Norfolk,* p. 213.
[135] See p. 54.
[136] The copies in the Library of Congress date back to September, 1787.
[137] Forrest, *Sketches of Norfolk,* pp. 99, 100. A number of copies are preserved in the Library of Congress.
[138] It was still issued in 1816.
[139] In 1834, Hugh B. Grigsby was owner and publisher.

Still another paper, *The Southern Argus,* appeared in January, 1848. It was Democratic in politics, and after urging Virginia on to secession in 1860 and 1861, collapsed in the storm which it helped to brew.[140] The *Norfolk Day Book,* established in 1857, was suppressed during the war by the Federal authorities, and *The New Régime,* the mouthpiece of General Benjamin F. Butler, issued in 1864 and 1865, took its place.[141]

The descriptions of Norfolk by visitors or historians give us a vivid picture of the town in the days before the Civil War. "Passing one or two neat country boxes on your left, you come to Fort Norfolk, a strong fortification with a brick wall, in the shape of a half-moon," wrote a visitor in the second decade of the century. "Fort Nelson is little above on the other shore, and makes quite a pleasing show with its green banks and white houses in the rear. You are now up, and the town sits to you in all her charms, to paint her if you choose. It is on your left in the landscape, and appears to be almost divided into two parts, by the water running and shining between. Bridges are thrown over to unite these divisions, and the lower one, or the Point, as they call it, shows a number of neat, white houses, almost lost in trees. On your right the harbor opens before you in a beautiful basin, nearly a mile wide. The Marine Hospital, on Washington Point, at the head of it, comes out to meet you in front. Portsmouth, a neat rural village, sits in smiling silence on the other side; and still further up, Gosport with her navy-yard, ships and bridge, finishes the prospect."[142] "It was late in the evening, or night rather, when we landed at Norfolk," wrote Mrs. Anne Royall, in 1828. "The captain sending a man, both as a guide and porter, to conduct me to Mrs. . . . who kept a boarding house. I was pleased to find the family up, and met an obliging old lady in my landlady, and some genteel company, which at once interested me in favor of Norfolk. . . . The streets are not regular, but they are lively, and display much fashion, politeness, and business. . . . The town contains three banks, a court house, a jail, an academy, three insurance offices, an orphans' asylum, an atheneum containing 6,000 volumes of well chosen books, and seven churches."[143]

"Approaching Norfolk," said another visitor in 1834, "you sail

[140] The student of Norfolk history must turn to the Library of Congress for the Norfolk newspapers prior to 1802. From that year until 1861 he will find most of the files in the Norfolk Public Library.

[141] A set of *The New Régime* is to be found in the Princeton University Library.

[142] *Letters from Virginia,* pp. 17, 18.

[143] Royall, *The Black Book,* pp. 253, 254.

up bold Elizabeth River, passing Craney Island on your right, where you see the remains of military works, and two or three country boxes on your left. You reach Fort Norfolk, now dismantled, on the same side. The new Naval Hospital is on the opposite shore, and forms a splendid vision with its Doric colonnade in front. Before you is the town, divided, as you see, into two parts, but united again by yonder stone bridge.[144] And there, a little to the left of it, is the house of our ex-senator, Mr. Tazewell, with its white portico and green lawn in front, making a very agreeable point in the picture. The right, or business part of the town, is well built up with brick houses, and appears to be a thriving mart. Passing on you enter the harbor itself, which opens into a beautiful basin, about three-fourths of a mile wide, and something longer; and full, you see, of ships and brigs and innumerable smaller vessels, all along the wharves."[145]

At the wharf is a swarm of Negroes, all shouting, "Shall I take your baggage, Marsa?" "There are no hacks, and you have to walk to your hotel, while the negro lugs your bags behind."[146] "The streets I find, are not quite as straight, nor the houses, in general, exactly as well built as I would have wished to see them. The public buildings, too, with two or three exceptions, are quite unworthy. . . . The Court House particularly, is a shabby affair, and ought to be demolished . . . and the three banks are only dwelling houses converted into offices of discount and deposit. The new Episcopal church, however, has some pretensions to architectural style, and is, on the whole a handsome edifice. . . . The people here are sociable, lively, and agreeable, the ladies especially being charming."[147]

A few years later Norfolk presented a different appearance. "Many beautiful public buildings, elegant family residences, large and splendid stores, well-paved streets, and a thriving and healthful population of about 16,000" mark the recent improvements, stated the historian Forrest.[148] If we view the city from some central eminence, a picture of great beauty and interest presents itself. To the northeast we "have a fine view of the Academy building, and its proportionate dimensions, standing in the center of its handsome square. East by south, and only a few rods distant, Christ Church shoots up its spire towards the sky. Southeast by east, stands old St. Paul's, amid the slumbering

144 Granby Street Bridge.
145 Norfolk *Beacon,* Jan. 7, 1834.
146 *Ibid.,* Aug. 23, 1839.
147 *Ibid.,* Jan. 7, 1824.
148 Forrest, *Sketches of Norfolk,* p. 309.

dead. . . . [Beyond] is the Eastern Branch of the Elizabeth, as it glides under the draw-bridge. [Nearer] stands St. Patrick's Church, . . . and the towering cupola of the Presbyterian Church, and the neat front of the Cumberland Street Baptist Church. Southeast by south, the Cumberland Street Methodist Church presents its bold and massive proportions. Due south, and over the water, at Washington Point, stands the Marine Hospital, a tidy and airy structure, half hid amid trees, and surrounded by evergreens and shrubbery. [In the foreground are] the Mechanics' Hall, with its showy front and architectural peculiarities, and other handsome buildings. . . . [To the south is] the City Hall, which the beholder sees with admiration,— its massive columns, lofty dome, solid walls, and fine proportions. . . . [Across the water is Portsmouth] and the Naval Hospital, an elegantly constructed pile of masonry, a grand ornament to the harbor. . . . [To the west] Elizabeth River spreads out its deep, broad bosom, floating in their majesty and pride, some of the most formidable war-steamers, many smaller vessels, and numbers of boats, with their white sails inviting the breezes; and then on, five miles in the distance, lies Craney Island. . . . [To the north are] several African churches, Plume & Company's Rope and Oakum Works, the Gas Works, Cotton Factory, the Almshouse, Cedar Grove and Elmwood cemeteries, steam saw-mill, farm-houses, cottages and lawns, with a thick growth of pine, oak, and maple in the background." Such was Norfolk in 1852, three years before it was blighted by the great yellow fever epidemic, and nine before the scarcely less terrible scourge of civil war.

CHAPTER SEVEN

Strangled Commerce

With the Peace of Ghent the British government closed her West Indies to American vessels. The island authorities were permitted to suspend the order for six months more, but the time was later reduced to four months. St. George and Hamilton, in Bermuda, were opened to our ships, it is true, but the duties here were heavy and the character of the cargoes restricted. And, since Bermuda was much nearer to the United States than to the West Indies, thus assuring the British carriers the lion's share of the freight, the Americans considered this a dubious favor. When, on July 3, 1815, Great Britain concluded a commercial treaty with the United States, opening the ports of each country to the vessels of the other, she made an exception of her West Indies. "We cannot reverse our two-century-old colonial policy," the British negotiators said. "It is enough that we will admit your produce, we will not permit shipment in American bottoms." In vain the Americans protested that this violated the spirit of true reciprocity, that the interchange of goods ought to be carried on jointly by British and American shippers, and that if the United States retaliated by excluding British vessels, the West Indians would starve. The English stood their ground, and waited to see what President Madison and Congress would do about it.[1]

The new arrangement proved most injurious to American shipping. The British started a triangular trade, from which we were excluded and with which we could not compete. England had few articles to send to her islands; so her ships now loaded for the United States and took on new cargoes there for the West Indies, whence they returned home with sugar and molasses. In the direct trade between the United States and Great Britain the eastward voyage with

[1] Benns, *American Struggle for the British West India Carrying Trade*, pp. 29-32.

the bulky American products always required far more cargo space than the return trip with the manufactured goods of Europe. The new triangular route now made it possible for the British to charge nominal freight rates from England to the United States, getting their profit from the other two legs of their voyage. As a result, many American merchantmen had to come home from England in ballast, with the profits from their eastward trip eaten up by the failure to secure a return cargo. Before many months shipbuilding fell off, artisans were thrown out of work, seamen began to seek employment under foreign flags, many vessels were "dismantled at the wharves, and literally rotting in the docks."[2]

Yet few complaints were heard from Norfolk. The only way to secure reciprocity was to retaliate with prohibitive duties or with non-intercourse, and Norfolk had had its fill of both. She knew from experience that it was not easy to coerce the British lion. Moreover, the merchants were doing fairly well as it was, for British vessels swarmed in the Elizabeth River. Norfolk was the only port in which an assorted cargo could be had for the West India trade—flour, grain, meal, naval stores—so it was selected by many British traders in preference to Philadelphia, New York, or the New England ports. The Norfolk merchants, although their own vessels were often idle, made a good commission on every cargo which left for Jamaica or Antigua, and on every cask of sugar or molasses which came back. One house alone exported to the British West Indies an average of $260,000 annually in 1816, 1817, and 1818. It was estimated that produce worth two million dollars went out each year to these islands during the period the trade was open, some of the British ships making seven or eight round trips. Although peace did not restore the decaying shipyards of the Elizabeth nor give employment to shipwrights, sea captains, and seamen, it did bring a degree of prosperity to the town and its people.[3]

So while the Northern seaports were urging retaliation against Great Britain, Norfolk was content to let well enough alone. "There is an uncommon bustle in our port at present," stated the Norfolk *Herald,* in April, 1818, "vessels daily arriving and departing for the West Indies. Rum, molasses and sugar are cheap, flour and provisions up to the clouds, the demand for lumber cannot be met. We hope

---

[2] *Ibid.,* pp. 34-36.
[3] Norfolk *Beacon,* Aug. 28, 1821; Norfolk *Herald,* Oct. 2, 1818; Forrest, *Sketches of Norfolk,* p. 156.

Congress will not interfere and close our ports to the British." Yet
that is just what Congress did. An act was passed forbidding trade in
British vessels between the ports of the United States and those
British colonies which were closed to American vessels. The law
was to be in force September 30, 1818.[4] For weeks the Elizabeth was
crowded with vessels trying to unload and take on their cargoes before the interdiction came in force. The schooner *Favorite*, from
Barbados, arrived early on the morning of September 29, and by
nine o'clock was discharging her cargo of sugar and rum. In eleven
hours she had cleared her hold, filled up again with flour, bread, and
staves, and battened down her hatches. The next morning she loaded
her deck with shingles, stowed her longboat, and cleared before ten
o'clock. Many others were less fortunate. Some were ready for sea at
the last moment but could not get out; some that had escaped in time
were driven back by a severe northeast gale. "It is with deep regret
that we see them go," said the *Herald*. "Since the peace they have
been regular customers here, . . . bringing valuable cargoes, paying
heavy duties, and taking away lumber, naval stores and flour."[5]

Despite the distress which followed the exclusion act, the people of
Norfolk waited patiently to see what impression it made on the
government at London. Apparently the effect was wholesome. When
Richard Rush, the American minister, began negotiations for the
renewal of the commercial treaty of 1815, Lord Castlereagh offered
equality of trade in the West Indies. British and American vessels
were to be treated alike both as to articles of import and export,
ports of entry, and duties in tonnage and cargoes. But now the Americans overreached themselves. Fearing that duties on American goods
coming directly from the United States would be so much heavier
than on those going by way of Great Britain or Canada that their
shippers would not be able to hold their own, they demanded that
the customs be uniform. This the British refused to consider, and the
treaty of 1815 was renewed without opening the West India trade.

The Northern shippers were not deeply concerned, but Norfolk
complained bitterly. "It will be perceived that the treaty is perfectly
silent upon the subject of the West India trade, the great desideratum
with the Southern States," said one paper. "This is a heavy disappointment. . . . We feel the loss of this trade here perhaps more
than it is felt in any part of the Union; but all hopes of retrieving it

---

[4] Benns, *American Struggle for the British West India Carrying Trade,* pp. 52, 53.
[5] Norfolk *Herald*, Oct. 2, 1818.

are now permanently extinguished. . . . We have neither loaves nor fishes to comfort us."[6]

The trade to the British West Indies, crippled though it was, did not cease entirely. Great Britain, alarmed lest the islanders starve, opened St. John's, Halifax, and Bermuda to American vessels, and our goods poured into these ports, whence they were transhipped to the West Indies in British bottoms. This new course of commerce deprived Norfolk of the advantage of position, for her Northern rivals were as close to Bermuda as she, and much closer to Halifax. In 1820 only sixty-four vessels, aggregating six thousand tons, with exports valued at $181,500, left the port for these two places.[7] This was less by eighty thousand dollars than the average shipments of one Norfolk firm prior to the Act of 1818.[8]

A bad matter was made worse, when Congress, in 1820, decided to end trade with the British West Indies, even by the circuitous route. Great Britain could be forced to yield, it was thought, only when every leak had been stopped and her colonies brought to the verge of ruin. So it was enacted that after September 30, 1820, no British vessels coming from any North American colony should enter a port of the United States, and goods from such a colony would not be received if transhipped at some intermediate point. Although this severe measure had the approval of Representative Newton, of the Norfolk district, it was condemned by the Norfolk merchants. "There is not the remotest chance that our restrictions will force Great Britain to change her colonial system," they said. "Is Congress trying to teach the West Indies to become independent of us? We have succeeded only in injuring ourselves. How amazing it is that representatives from the lower counties of Virginia and North Carolina are supporting a measure so ruinous to those sections! If Congress had not interfered it is probable that by this time a full half of the trade to the British West Indies would have been centered in Norfolk."[9] A visitor to the town in November, 1821, found the people, not only in Norfolk, "but in all the country round about," unanimous in their demand for the removal of the restrictions; the merchants because their warehouses were empty; the farmers because they could not dispose of their foodstuffs; sailors, caulkers, ropemakers, coopers, and riggers,

---

[6] Benns, *American Struggle for the British West India Carrying Trade,* pp. 55-60.
[7] Norfolk *Beacon,* Aug. 28, 1821.
[8] *Ibid.*
[9] *Ibid.*

because they were unemployed; newspaper owners because their advertising columns were empty.[10]

In December the mayor, recorder, aldermen, and councilmen passed resolutions voicing the general discontent. The acts prohibiting British ships "from bringing the productions of the British colonies to our ports, and taking away the agricultural productions of our state and other staples," were denounced as "highly injurious to Norfolk and this district."[11] A few days later the citizens crowded into the Town Hall to add their voice to that of the borough government. After an address by William Maxwell, the meeting passed resolutions declaring the navigation acts pernicious to Norfolk, destructive of its commerce, and injurious to all classes of citizens. Congressman Newton was instructed to work for their repeal, while a committee was appointed to correspond with the people of Richmond, Petersburg, and Fredericksburg.[12]

But Congress would not yield. The Northern ports poured in memorials urging them not to surrender our shipping interests to our rivals, it was known that the West Indies were suffering severely, and word came from England that Parliament was preparing to admit American vessels. Even Colonel Newton, despite the appeal of his constituents, remained "inflexibly firm" in support of the American restrictions. Before the session came to an end, an act was passed authorizing the President to open our ports to British vessels from the West Indies, in case Great Britain removed her prohibition upon our vessels.[13] This measure awakened no enthusiasm in Norfolk. "We know that the sugar plantations have petitioned for relief," said the *Herald,* "but we fear the British government will do just as much for their relief as Congress has for ours—nothing."[14]

Nonetheless, in July, Parliament did pass an act permitting the importation to certain ports of the West Indies of provisions, lumber, naval stores, tobacco, etc., from the United States in American vessels, provided this country would remove her restrictions. This looked like a complete victory for the United States, and President Monroe, on August 24, 1824, issued a proclamation opening American ports to British vessels from the North American colonies. But the duties, which were much higher on British than on American ships, he left

---

[10] *Ibid.,* Nov. 8, 1821.
[11] *Ibid.,* Dec. 18, 1821.
[12] *Ibid.,* Dec. 18 and 22, 1821.
[13] Benns, *American Struggle for the British West India Carrying Trade,* pp. 80, 81.
[14] Norfolk *Herald,* March 20, 1822.

unchanged. This, thought the Norfolk *Herald*, hardly seemed like real reciprocity. So, too, thought British foreign minister Canning. While he was still complaining to Secretary Adams on this point, Congress passed an act directing the President not to yield until Great Britain agreed to lay no higher duties in her colonies on goods from the United States than from Canada, or even from England itself. This was too much. The British retaliated with an order in council imposing a discriminating tonnage duty on American vessels entering her colonies, and a discriminating duty of 10 per cent on their cargoes.[15]

The situation caused a heated controversy in Norfolk. The *Beacon* supported Colonel Newton and the Federal government; the *Herald* was sharp in its criticisms. Our muddling representatives have worked us into an untenable position, said the latter, which delays a settlement indefinitely. In the meanwhile our merchants are ruined, our memorials treated with contempt, and the people of the islands are learning to become independent of us. On the other hand, the *Beacon* placed the blame on England. "She thinks the ocean is her birthright," it said, "and expects us to submit to unequal duties in the West Indies in order to drive most of the trade to Canada. It is not to our interest to build up strong British colonies on either side of us, for in time of peace they would lure our seamen from us and in time of war would be a serious menance to our safety. If she expects us to feed her islands, we must be on an equal footing with vessels from St. Johns and Halifax. Let us remain firm. The West Indians are already mortgaging their estates; while some are migrating to foreign islands. In the end Great Britain must yield."[16]

Nor was the existing arrangement entirely without its advantages. The West Indian trade, which had fallen off sharply in 1820, 1821, and 1822, now began to revive. Whereas the exports to the islands from Norfolk in those three years averaged less than $100,000, in the years from 1823 to 1825 the average was $216,000. Of this amount $168,000 represents goods carried in American bottoms. In the first nine months of 1826 exports in American ships were $176,000, in British ships $43,174.[17] In the face of the discriminating tonnage and customs duties, of high export duties, and of onerous port charges, this was all that could be expected. Yet, as compared to the golden days prior to the embargo it seemed trifling, and Norfolk

---

[15] Benns, *American Struggle for the British West India Carrying Trade,* pp. 87-99.
[16] Norfolk *Beacon,* Oct. 7, 1823.
[17] Norfolk *Herald,* Oct. 11, 1826.

hoped against hope that Great Britain eventually would yield. But the English now made an unexpected move. Believing that the government at Washington was taking advantage of the dependence of the West Indies upon American food and lumber to seize the lion's share of the carrying trade, they suddenly threw open their island ports to all the world. Perhaps the new Latin-American republics could supply their needs, and so break the chains which bound them to the United States. Our vessels were to be admitted, but only on condition that we abolish our discriminating duties and place Great Britain on the footing of the most favored nation. This we hesitated to do, and while we were hesitating, an order in council was issued prohibiting all trade in American vessels with the British West Indies.[18] Renewed negotiations through Albert Gallatin failed to budge the British, so President Adams, under authority of the Act of May 1, 1823, once more closed our ports to British vessels from any British colony in the western hemisphere.[19]

The proclamation, which went into operation at once, caught many Norfolk merchants unprepared. They had made purchases in the Indies, to be brought home in British vessels, and though some were on their way when the proclamation was issued, they were refused admission at Hampton Roads. "In the whole of our restrictive measures, we know of none that has borne so hard upon our merchants as this," complained the *Herald*.[20] Intercourse with the British islands continued, of course, through indirect channels. Goods were shipped to the French, Swedish, and Danish West Indies, where British vessels took them to Jamaica, or Antigua, or Nevis. But Norfolk's share of this trade was small. Her commerce at a low ebb, "a fearfully large proportion of her population idle, or employed at half time," the surrounding country impoverished, with grass growing in her streets, Norfolk was described as "a pensive and desponding city."[21]

A permanent settlement of the dispute over the West India carrying trade came in 1830. Andrew Jackson had promised in 1828, in case he were elected president, to open the British colonies to American vessels, and he kept his word. Instructing Louis McLean, his minister at St. James's, to reopen negotiations, he brought the British to terms by alternate concessions and threats. In the final settlement,

[18] Benns, *American Struggle for the British West India Carrying Trade*, pp. 104-119.
[19] *Ibid.*, pp. 143-145.
[20] Norfolk *Herald*, April 2, 1827.
[21] *Ibid.*, June 25, 1827; Feb. 15, July 9, 1828.

England retained the right to discriminate in favor of Halifax and St. John's, but agreed to admit American vessels to her West Indies on equal terms with British vessels from American ports. The diplomatic battle, which had been waged so fiercely for fifteen years, was over.

History furnishes no clearer example of the injury which may be done by economic war. The efforts of Great Britain, and to a lesser extent of the United States, to gain the lion's share of the carrying trade reacted disastrously upon both. The unending series of laws, orders in council, and proclamations, kept the merchants in a state of uncertainty, and only too often entailed heavy losses. In former days many Norfolk firms had had close ties with the traders of Antigua, or Jamaica, established by years of mutually profitable dealings. It was impossible to maintain these ties when one year the trade was direct to the British Indies, the next through Bermuda, the next by way of Halifax or St. John's. Many Norfolk traders had been ruined, and now were in no position to take advantage of the permanent settlement. Moreover, necessity had forced upon the West Indies a certain degree of economic independence, and they were no longer compelled to come to the American ports for provisions and lumber. In 1831 only seventy-nine vessels, forty-three of them British and thirty-six American, cleared from Norfolk for the British West Indies.[22] A sad decline this from the days when the town ranked fourth or fifth in the tonnage of American ports, and the Elizabeth was crowded with vessels loading for Antigua, Nevis, and Jamaica. The *Herald* might well ask whether it had not been a mistake for Norfolk to found its prosperity upon a trade so dependent upon the "fluctuating caprice of a foreign power."

Despite all, it is probable that Norfolk would have regained much of the West India trade after the agreement of 1830 had it not been for the protective tariff. The fostering of the production of sugar and molasses in Louisiana by heavy duties put a damper upon the intercourse with the Antilles. When the tariff bill of 1820 was introduced in Congress, it met with a violent protest from the Norfolk *Herald*. "If it is designed with any view to relieve the manufacturing interests, there is no excuse for it. In the name of common sense, is not every section of our country crying out under the afflictive pressure of the times, as well as the manufacturers?"[23] In 1824, when a

[22] *Ibid.*, March 23, 1832.
[23] *Ibid.*, April 26, 1820.

new and more radical tariff was proposed, the citizens met in the Town Hall to protest. Declaring that the measure would be ruinous to the commerce and the agriculture of the South, of the state, and Norfolk in particular, they appointed a committee to draw up a memorial, addressed to Congressman Newton, directing him to do all in his power to oppose the new duties.[24] As successive acts built the tariff wall higher and higher, the Norfolk merchants renewed the attack. On September 9, 1831, another meeting was held in the court-house, with Giles B. Cooke chairman, and Alexander Tunstall secretary. The tariff was called unequal, unnecessary, and oppressive; injurious to agriculture, commerce, and other interests; and aimed directly at the prosperity of the South.[25]

But these protests were in vain. Under the protecting wing of high duties, the sugar production of Louisiana doubled and tripled, until it supplied the larger part of the home market. Once or so in a decade, when the Southern crop was a failure, the West Indian vessels reappeared in the Elizabeth, but normally the sugar and molasses imports were small indeed. In 1844 the entire amount brought into the United States, over the tariff wall of 71 per cent, was valued at $2,467,290.[26] No wonder a visitor to Norfolk in 1835 was struck by "the stillness and inactivity that pervaded her wharves, streets, in fact the whole town. . . . Poor Norfolk! how are thou fallen; how different from the early days. . . . Then all was bustle, activity and life. I remember looking through the cabin window of my state room on board the packet . . . upon the huge vessels . . . in rows at her wharves, while my ears were greeted with the new (to me), though pleasing song of the laborers, as they lustily shouted their hoisting chorus, in almost deafening peals, from a hundred different wharves and vessels. . . . Now all appeared still—still as the grave."[27]

While the merchants were still repining over the West India trade, they suddenly awakened to the fact that New York was taking from them a large part of their century-old commerce with Great Britain. The opening of the Erie canal was making that city the central mart of all America, and other cities of the Atlantic seaboard, which at one time aspired to be her rivals, now humbly paid tribute to her commercial supremacy. Packet lines to Charleston, Norfolk, and Baltimore poured the produce of the South upon her wharves, whence it

[24] *Ibid.*, March 1, 1824.
[25] *Ibid.*, Sept. 12, 1831.
[26] *Niles' National Register*, LXVIII, 329.
[27] Norfolk *Herald*, Nov. 16, 1835.

was shipped to all parts of the world. To an even larger extent she became the distributing center for European goods, her merchants importing in vast quantities and reshipping to other ports on the seaboard.

Norfolk viewed this development with alarm. Our town, "with all its advantages for foreign and domestic trade, has become nothing but a thoroughfare between the north and south," it was said. "Instead of being what its geographical position entitles it to be—the great southern seaport—it is reduced to the humiliating condition of waiting on the pampered aristocracy of New York. In other days Norfolk was a large exporting and importing port, but now, since the concentration of capital in the North, she has become a hewer of wood and drawer of water to the lordly merchants of the northern city. New York imports for the whole South, and we, the consumers, not only pay the duty, but the commissions of her merchants, the freight, and insurance on the transhipment coastwise. Without foreign commerce Norfolk must dwindle to a village, and Virginia sink to the lowest scale in the Union, while New York, vampire-like, is sucking her blood to the last drop."[28]

"Norfolk ought to have 100,000 people," wrote a correspondent, signing himself a Friend of the Old Dominion. "Thirty years ago our population was nearly as large as it is now, and for one ship they had a dozen. All branches of business flourished then as much as they languish now, when there is a general approach to bankruptcy. We were better off as a colony. The present system takes away our foreign trade, and I have little hope for the preservation of our liberties, when one city is to swallow up all the commerce of the country. I am utterly opposed to the present course of trade, and will go as far as any to break it up, 'peacefully if we can, forcibly if we must'."[29]

In the letters and articles which deluged the newspapers, figures were marshaled to show Virginia's commercial decline. In 1791 the exports of the state had been three million dollars or one-sixth of all from the United States; in 1816, eight million dollars or one-tenth of the whole; while in 1833 they had sunk to $4,500,000 or one-twentieth of the whole. In 1806 Norfolk and Portsmouth merchants had owned one hundred and twenty vessels, aggregating 23,207 tons, engaged in foreign commerce; in 1835 Virginia as a whole could not boast of thirty. As for imports, they had fallen to almost nothing. In the days

[28] Norfolk *Beacon*, March 13, 1834.
[29] *Ibid.*

before the embargo from five to seven millions in foreign goods had entered Virginia ports; in 1833 the total was $670,000. "This is a decline," said the *Beacon,* "which in rapidity and amount, has no parallel in the history of commerce." No wonder Virginia is becoming impoverished, when her people pay in commissions to the cities of other states $8,000,000, or one-fourth of her entire surplus production. If this sum were kept at home, it would arrest the torrent of emigration to the West, restore the mercantile credit of the state, build up her waste places, and bring back in bottoms of her own the fruits of every clime.

Some of the Norfolk merchants looked up the commercial statistics for New York and compared them with those of Virginia. This made interesting reading. In 1791 the imports of New York and of Virginia were nearly equal; in 1821 those of New York were $23,000,000, of Virginia $1,078,000; in 1832 the figures were $57,000,000 and $550,000 respectively. "Why," it was asked, "should the Old Dominion buy directly from abroad less than one-hundredth as much as New York? Why is it that in Norfolk there is now to be seen not a single square-rigged vessel? Why were Virginia's imports in 1769 eleven times greater than in 1837?"[30] The custom house figures for 1837 showed that the exports of Virginia amounted to $11,254,539, of which only $5,265,461 went directly from her ports abroad. At the same time her direct foreign imports were $816,887, and her imports from other states $10,427,652. The foreign imports reshipped to Virginia from Northern ports were estimated at $4,448,574.[31] Virginia's foreign trade, formerly almost entirely direct, was now for exports nine-tenths direct and one-tenth circuitous, for imports one-seventh direct and six-sevenths circuitous.

So vital did this matter seem to the state and the South, that on November 14, 1838, a commercial convention met in Norfolk to consider measures of relief. The delegates, who came chiefly from the business centers of Virginia and North Carolina, assembled in the Methodist church on Cumberland Street. It was known that Colonel Robert Y. Hayne, of South Carolina, famous for his debate with Webster, would be among the speakers, and the building was crowded beyond its real capacity. "The brightness of the lamps showed off every object with the clearness of day"—the dignified figure of Governor Tyler in the chairman's seat, the gay gowns of the la-

[30] *Ibid.,* Sept. 21, 1838.
[31] *Ibid.,* Oct. 22, 1838.

dies who thronged the galleries, the earnest, determined faces of the delegates, the speaker himself, fluent and logical as ever. After the addresses various resolutions were passed: recommending steps to remove all state taxes on goods directly imported, to increase banking capital, and to develop roads and canals; urging the citizens to pledge themselves to buy only from those merchants who themselves bought abroad. At a brilliant dinner Colonel Hayne summed up the spirit of the convention in the following toast: "To our brothers of the North, . . . it is our duty and our interest to cherish the most intimate commercial relations with our Northern brethren—not, however, as dependents, but on terms of reciprocal advantage."[32]

The Virginians blamed the decline of their European trade upon their lack of capital. When purchases were made abroad, the importer had to pay cash to the manufacturer, and, upon the arrival of his goods, sell on long time. This required large reserves of capital, which the Norfolk merchants, because of their many reverses, did not have. They were forced to become mere agents, or purchasers at second hand, from the Northern importers. Nor was this all. The New Yorkers established packet lines to Europe, with vessels whose speed and size gave them an advantage over all rivals. They could afford to lower freight rates, especially upon imports, to a point where it was impossible for the Southern shippers to compete. Their attempts to absorb also the export trade were less successful, because of the bulky character of the Southern products. It was a costly business to send a cargo of tobacco, or flour, or cotton to New York, there to be transferred to the trans-Atlantic liners. So ships continued to leave Norfolk for London and Liverpool, but, having taken on their return cargo, they sailed for New York. There they unloaded, and returned to Norfolk, sometimes with a small consignment of goods, sometimes in ballast.[33]

An important factor in this development was the increase of immigration from Europe. In the seventeenth century, when thousands of indentured servants came to Virginia, the master of every tobacco ship, after he had stowed away his boxes of manufactured goods, had room for from ten to twenty persons. But the nineteenth century immigrants avoided the South, where they would be thrown into competition with slave labor, and settled in the great commercial and

---

[32] *Ibid.*, Nov. 14, 16, 17, 1838.
[33] *Ibid.*, March 4, 1834; Dec. 29, 1838.

manufacturing centers of the North. In 1820 only 8,385 entered the country, but the numbers rose rapidly, to 27,382 in 1828, to 60,482 in 1832, and 79,340 in 1838. Many a ship which formerly left Europe directly for Norfolk now headed for New York in order to carry its share of the immigrant horde. Better the short trip from New York to Norfolk in ballast, than the long trip from Liverpool or Glasgow to Norfolk with a hold two-thirds empty.

The character of Norfolk's trade at this period is made clear by a reference to the list of entries of vessels for a part of March, 1839. Five came in from New York, three from other Northern ports, fourteen from places in Virginia and Maryland, three from other Southern states, four from the West Indies, and none from Europe.[34] Of the forty-one vessels entering the Elizabeth from Northern ports in the early weeks of 1839, fourteen came in ballast, ten brought "merchandize," five potatoes, three hay, two ice, one "produce," one plaster, one oil and candles, one lime and potatoes, one hay and apples, and two fish and potatoes.

There would have been some consolation for Norfolk had the loss of her European trade been accompanied by a corresponding growth of the coastal trade. But the development of the steamboat threatened to deprive Norfolk even of the American trade she had long enjoyed. The people of the town had greeted with enthusiasm the first steam-driven vessel to enter her port, not foreseeing that for decades this type of ship would prove a menace to her prosperity. "We have at length had the satisfaction of seeing in our harbor one of those valuable improvements in internal navigation, a steamboat," said the *Gazette and Public Ledger* on May 24, 1815. "The elegant steamboat *Washington*, Captain O'Neale, is now here. She is intended to run between Washington city and Powtomac creek." When, a year later, the steamboat *Powhatan* arrived from New York, to begin a biweekly schedule between Norfolk and Richmond, the press hailed the event as the beginning of a new era.[35] "A Norfolk merchant may leave here one day," they said, "buy a cargo in Richmond, and be back the next day." It would be equally easy for the Richmond merchant to come down the river to charter a ship to take off his produce.[36] In truth, so long as the steamboats were used only for inland navigation,

[34] *Ibid.* (Consult all numbers for March, 1839.)
[35] *Ibid.*, May 28, 1816.
[36] *Ibid.*, July 30, 1816.

they served to strengthen Norfolk's position as the chief port of tide-water Virginia, to which the merchants of the Fall Line towns brought their goods for transhipment to ocean-going vessels.

But when the New York packets began running under steam power, the effect upon Norfolk proved unfortunate. Since their compara-tively light draft made it possible for them to ascend the James and the Potomac, they could trade directly with Richmond, Petersburg, and Alexandria, and so eliminate the necessity of transhipment at Norfolk. In former days ocean-going vessels, then entirely dependent upon the winds for locomotion, preferred to stop at Norfolk, in order to avoid the tedious ascent of the crooked Virginia rivers. But to the steamboat, curves offered no serious obstacle.

"The introduction of steam made seacoast towns no longer neces-sary to commerce," pointed out the Norfolk *Post* many years after-ward, "and, for the time being, the old town was left gradually to fall to ruin and decay on the small business and traffic of the immediate neighborhood. . . . Steamers that can take goods direct to the point of destination on the rivers and bays, and receive their return cargoes at the same points, possess a great advantage over the old sailing vessels, which were compelled to discharge their cargoes . . . at the large harbors on the seacoast. This is the true cause of the gradual decadence of cities on the seacoast like Norfolk, which, unlike New York, New Orleans, Boston, and other great centers of trade, had not become fully established as commercial marts before the era of railroads and steamboats."[37] So, while Norfolk languished, the Fall Line towns prospered on the Northern trade. In 1855 no less than sixty packets entered the Richmond basin from New York, forty from Baltimore, and twenty-nine from Boston.[38] Clearly Norfolk had to regain her foreign trade, or see the commerce even of Chesa-peake waters pass her by as well.

At this juncture the opening of the Dismal Swamp canal brought a ray of hope. The people had waited impatiently for the long-delayed completion of this work upon the larger scale. "Wait until the corn, fish, tobacco, pork, and lumber of eastern Carolina begin pouring in through the canal," they said, "and prosperity will once more be ours." The advantages of a canal to connect the waters of the Eliza-beth River with those of Albemarle Sound were obvious even in

[37] Norfolk *Post*, Sept. 27, 1865.
[38] W. F. Dunaway, *History of the James River and Kanawha Co.* (New York, 1922) , p. 165.

colonial days. To bring the produce of Bertie or Halifax down the rivers, transfer them to larger vessels, and then make the voyage out to the ocean and around to Norfolk was a costly and dangerous undertaking. So, in 1787 a company was formed, under a joint charter of Virginia and North Carolina, to dig a canal from Deep Creek, a tributary of the Southern Branch, to Pasquotank River.[39] Because of the slowness of subscribers in paying for their shares, the actual work of digging began several years later.[40]

At the outset two serious mistakes were made. The channel was too narrow and shallow, and no competent engineer was employed. With gangs of Negroes at work on either end, the route had not been correctly surveyed, the company did not know how many locks would be necessary or how much dirt must be removed, and so could form no accurate estimate of the cost. La Rochefoucauld inspected the work in 1796 and found the channel completed for five miles at the Virginia end, and six at the Pasquotank end. Although digging had then been going on for three years, the most difficult part of the work remained to be done.[41] As it turned out, the company had underestimated the cost, for the locks proved expensive, and it was found necessary to dig a feeding canal from Lake Drummond, in the heart of the swamp. When the funds ran out and the company had exhausted its credit with the banks, the work came to a standstill. The best the company could do was to connect the two sections of the canal by means of a road. Boats took the Carolina produce to the end of the south section, whence it was carried by wagons to the northern section, there to be transferred to the waiting Norfolk boats. In this way a large traffic was carried on in the years prior to the War of 1812, tolls in one year alone amounting to six thousand dollars, or 7 per cent on the capital invested.[42] At intervals, as funds came in, digging was resumed, and in 1808 had progressed to a point where it was estimated that five hundred men could complete it in three months.[43] "Why not employ the sailors thrown out of work by the embargo," it was suggested, "and enjoy without further delay the full benefits of the great project?" But the company either would not or could not follow this advice, and the nibbling process continued. As one writer expressed it, the canal went on as slowly as though "the age of

[39] Forrest, *Sketches of Norfolk*, p. 97.
[40] *Virginia Chronicle*, Jan. 5, 1793.
[41] La Rochefoucauld, *Voyages dans les États-Unis*, IV, 258, 259.
[42] Norfolk *Gazette and Public Ledger*, April 14, 1808.
[43] *Ibid.*

Methuselah, and not that of the Psalmist, were the prescribed period of human life."[44]

The British blockade of Chesapeake Bay in the War of 1812 and the resulting urgent demand for an inland waterway to Albemarle Sound seem to have provided the needed impetus, and at last, in June, 1814, boats began coming through the canal. The first to reach Norfolk came from Scotland Neck, on the Roanoke River, with bacon and brandy. The boat was of twenty tons burden, and at one place in the canal the master was obliged to lighten the cargo.[45] Immediately the North Carolina produce began to come through in large quantities. One person alone paid tolls, from December 8, 1815, to June 1, 1816, on 394,000 staves, 478,000 shingles, 2,233 barrels of corn, 10,000 pounds of bacon, 370 barrels of tar, 6 barrels of pitch, 371 barrels of fish, 27 barrels of oil, 59 casks of flax seed, 2 casks of beeswax, and 16 kegs of lard, in all worth $32,000, or enough to load four ships of three hundred tons.[46]

However, the traffic, born of the necessities of war, served only to show the inadequacies of the canal. Vessels which were large enough to navigate safely the waters of Albemarle and Pamlico sounds were too large to get through the new waterway. The depth and width of the canal must be increased at once, the number of locks reduced, or trade would resume its old channels. The company, having had proof of the volume of traffic which might be expected, appealed to the state legislature for support. In all they secured three loans, two for $50,000 each and one for $37,500. They also received permission to increase the number of shares, and soon after sold a large block to the United States government.[47] Yet it was only in the winter of 1828, thirty-six years after the first shovelful of dirt was removed, that the canal, completed on the larger scale, was ready for traffic.[48] The people of Norfolk, when they thought of the rapidity with which the Erie canal had been pushed through, had reason to rue the delays in digging their own waterway. Nonetheless, they were proud of the work. The canal was twenty-two and a half miles long, had an average width of forty feet, and accommodated vessels drawing 5½ feet.[49] There were five massive stone locks, two at the north end rising

[44] Norfolk *Beacon*, May 3, 1836.
[45] Norfolk *Gazette and Public Ledger*, June 11, 1814. See above, p. 114.
[46] *Ibid.*, June 1, 1816.
[47] Norfolk *Beacon*, March 17, April 10, 1826.
[48] Norfolk *Herald*, June 13, 1828.
[49] *Ibid.*, April 2, 1838.

thirteen feet, another ten miles south rising 3½ feet; the Culpeper lock six miles further on, falling 3½ feet, and finally the lock at the south end, falling thirteen feet. At Deep Creek, fifteen feet above sea-level, was a basin a half mile long. The entire work cost eight hundred thousand dollars.[50]

Expectations of a rich trade through the canal were heightened by recent improvements in the navigation of the Roanoke River. This stream, with its tributaries, the Dan and the Staunton, drained a country whose soil, unlike that of eastern Virginia, had not been exhausted by tobacco. Heretofore, the falls above Weldon had prevented boats above from passing down stream into Albemarle Sound, but there was now a canal around these obstructions. Thus the Dismal Swamp canal opened not only the trade of the sounds with their tributary rivers, the Black Water, Nottoway, Meherrin, and Chowan, but that of the upper Roanoke as well; and it was expected that the tobacco, cotton, flour, hemp, and flax of Warren, Mecklenburg, Halifax, and Charlotte counties would pour in upon Norfolk.[51] But in June, 1828, the *Herald* reminded the Norfolk people that the new system of waterways would prove of no benefit unless the proper vessels were provided. The light river boats were expected to deposit their cargoes at Weldon, where steam towboats and barges must be ready to take on the goods for the long journey to Norfolk. Accordingly the Virginia and North Carolina Transportation Company was organized, and some months later a steamer, the *Petersburg,* and eight barges were ready for work.[52]

The canal was opened December 31, 1828, and the long-expected stream of traffic began. The people of Norfolk watched anxiously as some of the larger vessels sailed past to Richmond, or to Baltimore, but they soon found that the bulk of the goods came directly to their wharves. From June 15 to June 29, 1829, eighteen lighters with shingles and staves, twelve rafts of timber and spars, one sloop, and three schooners came through bound for Norfolk. The traffic south from Norfolk in the same period consisted of two schooners for Weldon, two sloops and one schooner for Currituck, three schooners for Beaufort, two sloops and one schooner for Elizabeth City, five schooners and two sloops for Edenton.[53] This was merely the beginning. In 1829 the northbound trade comprised 770 hogshead of tobacco,

[50] *Ibid.,* Nov. 11, 1829; Martin, *Gazetteer of Virginia,* pp. 243, 244.
[51] Norfolk *Herald,* June 16, 1828.
[52] *Ibid.,* June 13, 1828; July 16, 1830.
[53] *Ibid.,* July 16, 1830.

1,964 bales of cotton, 2,937 barrels of flour, 2,507 barrels of fish, 30,000 bushels of corn, 1,170,000 staves, 14,296,000 shingles, and 2,037 barrels of turpentine.[54] The cotton trade was especially interesting to the Norfolk people, and when the steamboat *Petersburg* came in, towing the barges *Dan* and *Roanoke,* piled high with bales, crowds came down to the wharf to view them.

As the months passed, the Norfolk papers noted exultantly that the traffic through the canal was increasing rapidly. The cost of shipping tobacco, flour, or cotton in wagons over the dirt roads of Virginia from the upper Roanoke to Richmond or Petersburg was so heavy that Norfolk had visions of monopolizing the trade of the entire Roanoke Valley. The freight charges from Danville to Norfolk on a hogshead of tobacco were $8.50; to Richmond by way of Lynchburg and the James River, $24.50.[55] Yet it was not the trade of the upper Roanoke, but of the lower river and of Albemarle Sound which crowded the canal. So great was the increase that tolls grew from $11,658, in 1829 to $18,437 in 1830 and to $27,030 in 1831. In the year ending April 30, 1833, tolls were $34,059.[56] In the same twelve months the northward traffic rose to $1,713,796. Of this sum forest products, mast timber, planks, scantling, stoves, shingles, posts, fence-rails, firewood, and naval stores accounted for $724,918; cotton for $478,842; tobacco for $205,793; flour for $57,792; corn for $136,021; and wheat, flax seed, and sweet potatoes for $34,667; fish for $47,908; provisions for $20,304; and wine, molasses, and sugar for $7,500. The southbound vessels carried merchandise, salt, coffee, molasses, sugar, flour, pork, liquors, and other products valued at $780,088, making a grand total for both ways of $2,493,884.[57]

The breaking down of the south lock interrupted traffic in 1835, but the next year it was resumed in greater volume than ever.[58] In October, 1836, sixty-seven schooners, three sloops, sixteen lighters, and twenty-one rafts passed through to Norfolk, nine schooners and sloops to Baltimore, and two schooners to the District of Columbia; while sixty-four schooners, three sloops, and seventeen lighters returned from Norfolk, two sailing vessels from Richmond, seven from Baltimore, three from the District of Columbia, and one from New York.[59] In October, 1837, northward traffic consisted of eighty-seven

[54] *Ibid.,* March 19, 1832.
[55] *Ibid.,* May 18, 1829.
[56] *Ibid.,* March 19, 1832; May 22, 1833.
[57] *Ibid.,* May 22, 1833.
[58] *Ibid.,* Sept. 21, 1835.
[59] *Ibid.,* Dec. 6, 1836.

schooners, seven sloops, sixteen lighters, and twenty-one rafts, and southward traffic of ninety-five schooners, five sloops, and seventeen lighters.[60] At a time when Norfolk was bemoaning the shrinkage of her foreign trade, this canal commerce was all-important. Without it business would have been dead.

From time to time there were criticisms of the canal company. "Nine-tenths of the trade of Norfolk comes from Albemarle Sound," it was said, "yet the chief artery through which it must flow is sluggish. The shoals and logs in the canal are so bad that boats often have to lighten their cargoes, the locks and bridges are antiquated, in places the channel is too narrow for vessels to pass each other, the water is often low, the approaches at each end are crooked and obstructed by stumps."[61] North Carolina threatened to make itself independent of the canal by deepening the outlets from her sounds; the Norfolk merchants to cut a new canal to connect the waters of the Southern Branch with those of Currituck Sound. Yet decade after decade the stream of commerce continued, until the company had met all its obligations and was paying a regular dividend of 6 per cent. For the year ending September 30, 1852, tolls were $45,119, the northbound trade alone including 4,947 bales of cotton, 24,395 barrels of fish, and 837,748 bushels of corn.[62] Four years later the amount of corn carried had risen to 1,300,000 bushels.[63]

Had the Carolina products been reshipped directly to Europe or the West Indies, as in former days, the canal would have made Norfolk once more an important commercial center. But the larger part was loaded on coasters and sent to New York, Boston, Philadelphia, or Baltimore. To those who remembered the golden days before the embargo, when the port was crowded with ships from foreign lands, this seemed at best an humble and unprofitable business. "Norfolk has the best harbor in the United States," they declared. "She should gather into her lap the products of the back country within a radius of 500 miles, and ship them out to every part of the globe, in packet lines controlled by her own merchants. But before she can fulfil this destiny, she must have great avenues of commerce reaching out into the west, enterprising merchants of the stamp of Moses Myers and William Pennock, and capital to back them. Otherwise Norfolk will remain a mere stopping place in the north and south traffic. The

60 *Ibid.*, Nov. 24, 1837.
61 Norfolk *Beacon*, May 12, 1845; *Daily Southern Argus*, Jan. 22, Jan. 25, 1849.
62 *Daily Southern Argus*, Nov. 29, 1852.
63 *Ibid.*, Feb. 9, 1857.

canal is invaluable, it has staved off ruin, but it will take more than a ditch through to Albemarle Sound to make Norfolk a second New York."

It was fortunate, in these hard times, that the Federal government selected Gosport as the site of one of its navy yards. The outlay of money for docks, workshops, storehouses, and warships not only provided a market for timber, rope, ironware, and sails, but it gave employment to scores of carpenters, stone masons, bricklayers, shipwrights, and sailors. The construction of one great warship alone, such as the ship-of-the-line *Delaware,* meant the expenditure of many thousands of dollars. The launching of the *Delaware,* in October, 1820, was acclaimed as an evidence not only of America's determination never again to leave her commerce without protection on the ocean, but of the mechanical skill of the Southern shipwrights. A throng of twenty thousand people assembled. The river was dotted with boats of all descriptions, among them the steamships *Virginia, Richmond, Petersburg,* and *Sea-Horse,* and the famous frigate *Guerrière,* her masts gay with streamers. Color was lent to the crowd on shore by the presence of the famous Richmond Light Infantry Blues. As the ship glided into the water, a shout arose, accompanied by the blare of bands and the roar of cannon.[64]

Ten years later, the *Delaware,* then completed, graced another event of great significance for Norfolk—the opening of the stone dry dock at the Navy Yard. This work, the first of its kind in America, required six years for its completion and cost nearly a million dollars. The chamber was 253 feet long, 85½ feet wide and accommodated our largest vessels. On June 17, 1833, when the gates swung open and the sailors, tugging away at the capstan, drew the *Delaware* slowly in, thousands of people looked on from stands erected on either side. It was a scene long to be remembered—the gaily dressed ladies, the handsome uniforms of the naval officers, the warship, with her towering masts, her three rows of gun-ports, the Indian figurehead, and the Stars and Stripes flapping behind; in the background the Southern Branch with its wooded shore. At last the ship came to rest. The gates were closed, and the pumping began. The day of careening vessels at the Navy Yard was past.[65]

Among the vessels built at the Navy Yard were the frigate *St. Lawrence,* the sloop *John Adams,* the surveying brig *Pioneer,* the

[64] Norfolk *Herald,* Oct. 23, 1820.
[65] Stewart, *History of Norfolk County,* pp. 433-437.

sloop *Yorktown*, the steamer *Union*, the brig *Perry*, the sloop *James-town*, the store-ship *Southampton*, and the steam-frigates *Powhatan*, *Roanoke*, and *Colorado*.[66] At the same time extensive shipbuilding operations were carried on by private concerns. Among their more noteworthy feats were the construction of the ship *General Washington*, of 420 tons, by Porter and Dyson, launched in 1815;[67] the packet *Newburn*, by John P. Colley, and the steamship *North Carolina*, by Ryan and Gayle, both launched in 1829;[68] the ships *Madison*, of 470 tons, and *Washington*, of 530 tons, launched from the yards of Isaac Talbot, the former in 1828 and the latter in 1833.[69] In 1853 Page and Allen, of Portsmouth, had under construction a clipper of 1500 tons, at that time the largest vessel ever laid down south of New York.[70]

From time to time in the period between the War of 1812 and the Civil War, we catch glimpses of the industrial life of Norfolk. Joseph Martin, in his *Gazetteer of Virginia*, published in 1836, tells us that the place boasted of three banks—the United States Bank, the Virginia Bank, and the Farmers' Bank of Virginia—ten hotels, three steam mills, three tanyards, two ropewalks, in addition to the various "mechanical pursuits." Ten steamboats plied from Norfolk to Baltimore, Richmond, and other places. In 1853 there were seven banks, five hotels, five daily papers, an insurance company, a gas company, three shipbuilding concerns, an iron foundry, cordage and oakum works, besides carriage, furniture, and cotton plants. The capital invested in manufactures was about $570,000.[71] The population was 14,320.[72]

For a place possessed of one of the best harbors in the world, within an hour or two of the ocean, and flanked by a network of inland waterways, the situation was disappointing indeed. Completely outdistanced by New York, Boston, Philadelphia, and Baltimore, the people of the "old borough" ruminated sadly over her unfortunate history, and inquired among themselves for the proper measures to secure the prosperity and commercial greatness which by right was theirs.

[66] *Ibid.*, pp. 429-442.
[67] Norfolk *Gazette and Public Ledger*, Oct. 21, 1815.
[68] Norfolk *Herald*, June 3, Dec. 2, 1829.
[69] *Ibid.*, Nov., 29, 1833.
[70] Forrest, *Sketches of Norfolk*, p. 345 n.
[71] *Ibid.*, pp. 344-345.
[72] *Ibid.*, p. 270.

CHAPTER EIGHT

The Fall Line Blockade

In the United States the period of canal building was quickly followed by that of railroad construction. The Erie canal, which was opened in 1826, worked wonders for New York. DeWitt Clinton had declared that it would make the city "the granary of the world, the emporium of commerce, the seat of manufactures, the focus of great moneyed operations," and the fulfilment of this prophecy began at once. The products of the West came through the canal and down the Hudson, the wharves of Manhattan were piled with bags and barrels, packet lines were organized to carry them to foreign lands, the population of the city doubled, tripled, quadrupled. Philadelphia, Boston, Baltimore, became alarmed. If New York drained the entire western country, they would be eclipsed. Anxiously they looked for some means of communication with the trans-Allegheny region, which would permit them to share in the great prize.

Baltimore was the first to hit upon the railway. Having behind it no long navigable river, out of touch with the Chesapeake and Ohio canal, it grasped eagerly at the new carrier. So, three years after the opening of the Erie canal, the cornerstone of the Baltimore and Ohio railway was laid. "We are commencing a new era in our history," said John B. Morris, one of the directors. "It is but a few years since the introduction of steamboats effected powerful changes. Of a similar and equally important effect will be the Baltimore and Ohio Railroad. While the one will have stemmed the torrent of the Mississippi, the other will have surmounted and reduced the heights of the Allegheny." The foresight of Baltimore gave her a long start over Norfolk, her natural rival in the race for the western trade.

Norfolk first thought of the railway, not as a means of crossing the mountains, but as a supplement to river transportation. She had seen Richmond outdistance her because of the James River trade; she now sought to draw to her wharves the products of another fertile river valley. The failure of the Dismal Swamp canal to attract the upper Roanoke trade had caused keen disappointment. The necessity of transferring goods at Weldon, together with the dangers and delays of the trip down the lower Roanoke, through Albemarle Sound, up the Pasquotank, and through the canal, had discredited this route. The bulk of their produce still went overland to the James or the Appomattox, and so to Richmond or Petersburg.

In August, 1829, came the disconcerting news that Petersburg was planning a railway to the upper Roanoke, a general town meeting having requested that the President of the United States detail an engineer to examine and report on the route.[1] Later a company was organized, the town subscribed $130,000, aid was asked from the state and Federal governments, and the actual work of construction began. The rails ran south through Dinwiddie, Sussex, and Greensville counties, to a point on the Roanoke just below the falls. Twelve months later forty miles of track had been completed, and in 1836 the road was in full swing. "They now have three engines upon the road," says Martin's *Gazetteer*, "a part of which have been at work upward of nine months, and make their trips with as much regularity as could have been expected from horse power."[2]

Norfolk was stirred into action. "It is absurd for Petersburg to aspire to be a great port," said the Norfolk papers. "Why, most of her people never saw a ship. At the same time we must not lose sight of the fact that they may draw off the Roanoke trade from our canal, if this railway goes through. The question is this: Will Norfolk, within hail of the sea, or Petersburg, on the tiny Appomattox, become the market of North Carolina and the Roanoke Valley? We must bestir ourselves and lay down a railway of our own to the Roanoke, if we hope to retain our share of this trade."[3] Accordingly the Portsmouth-Weldon railway was projected, to run seventy-six miles through Norfolk, Nansemond, Southampton, and Northampton counties to the Roanoke near the terminus of the projected Petersburg line. The people of Norfolk—merchants, storekeepers, mechanics—subscribed liberally, the borough took one hundred thousand dollars in stock,

[1] *Niles' Weekly Register*, Sept. 5, 1829.
[2] Martin, *Gazetteer of Virginia*, pp. 162, 163.
[3] Norfolk *Herald*, Feb. 27, 1833.

Portsmouth added fifty thousand dollars and the work of construction was begun.

But when the company went to the state legislature with a request for financial aid, the Petersburg interest was able to block it in the Senate through a tie vote of fourteen to fourteen.[4] This caused great indignation in Norfolk. "Thus we stand, the goose to be plucked for the benefit of our more favored neighbors," said the *Herald*. "The legislature have demanded from our canal company the money lent them, at interest, some years ago; whether convenient to them or ruinous to the work, it matters not. The money is wanted to build up other towns. But when we ask a small portion to aid us in a work essential to our interest, the door of the treasury is slammed in our face. . . . That the Petersburg interest should have been arrayed against us . . . is only what might have been expected, . . . but the opposition of the Richmond interest can be stimulated by nothing but a deep-rooted jealousy. Well, go on gentlemen, you have for a time succeeded . . . but you have not put us down. With our own resources we will complete the railway."[5]

This was the opening of a wordy battle between the Norfolk and Petersburg papers. The Petersburg *Intelligencer* reminded the *Herald* that the legislature had already done its share in aiding Norfolk by the purchase of the canal bonds. Petersburg, it pointed out, was a far better market than Norfolk. Even after the digging of the canal, the greater part of the Roanoke produce had come to the Appomattox in wagons. "The truth is," it added sagely, "Norfolk is too far out toward the sea, cut off from the fertile regions of the interior by swamps and sterile plains. The produce of the back country will always change hands at more convenient market towns, near the head of navigation." To this the *Herald* replied in sarcastic vein. "So it is not desirable to have shipping ports near the sea," it said. "In view of this severe handicap, we wonder why New York has grown so great. Perhaps the *Intelligencer* will enlighten us on this point." But the Petersburg editor was not to be floored. True New York was near the ocean, but were not Philadelphia, Baltimore, London, and Paris, like Petersburg, all up rivers? Let Norfolk explain that if it could. "This is very good again," came back the *Herald*. "But is there no difference between the Patapsco, the Delaware, the Thames, and the Seine, and your poor little, muddy Appomattox? Is it nothing that

---

[4] *Ibid.,* March 1, 1833.
[5] *Ibid.*

gallant ships can go to all those places, but cannot go to Petersburg?"

In 1834 the Portsmouth-Weldon railway again applied for aid from the legislature, and, despite the renewed opposition of the Fall Line towns, was successful. The vote in the Senate was sixteen to fifteen. When on Sunday, January 19, the steamship *Patrick Henry* arrived with the glad tidings, she was greeted with cheers from the crowds who lined the wharves on both sides of the river. Church bells rang out, guns were fired, bonfires blazed in the principal streets, every house was illuminated, rockets shot up over the river. The news was conveyed to Suffolk by field-pieces placed at intervals along the railway, which were fired in succession. Prosperity seemed at hand. Now that the success of the railway was assured, the tobacco, flour, cotton, and grain of the Roanoke would come to Norfolk, the merchants would once more be busy, the wharves piled high, the river full of vessels.

Work proceeded rapidly. A brick shop, 118 feet by 30 feet, was erected at Portsmouth, and equipped with lathes and other machinery for manufacturing and repairing locomotives and cars.[6] The rails were of heart pine, nine inches by five, the upper side plated with two-inch iron bars, fastened to ties with white oak wedges. Although it was decided to use steam power for locomotion, the ties were notched in the center to admit a path for horses in case of emergency. Whenever trains were to run into sidings, at depots and water stations, a turntable, worked by a hand lever, was made use of. This device was preferable to iron switches, so it was thought, since the latter were apt to throw the locomotive off the track.[7] The management at first was puzzled as to whether their cars should be equipped with wooden wheels, cast iron wheels, or wheels with cast iron spokes and wrought iron rims and flanges. After long deliberation the last named type was adopted.

In August, 1833, the tracks had progressed four miles from the west end of High Street. Four months later "three beautiful cars" arrived, two from Baltimore, and one, having three compartments large enough for thirty people, from Hoboken.[8] At last, in July, 1834, the line was completed to Suffolk, and the president and directors made the trip in one of the new cars, drawn by horses. And now produce began to come in. Jesse Lankford, of Southampton, arrived

[6] Virginia Board of Public Works, *Reports* (Seventeenth, Eighteenth, and Nineteenth), 473.
[7] *Ibid.*, p. 470.
[8] Norfolk *Herald*, Dec. 16, 1833.

at Portsmouth over the railway with ten thousand pounds of bacon and lard, and ten barrels of vinegar.[9] This was an earnest, so it was said, of what was to follow. By August 17 a regular schedule for horse cars had been established to Suffolk, with carriages in attendance at Ferry wharf to convey passengers to the High Street depot.

Excitement reached its height in September, with the arrival of the first locomotive. This tiny engine, weighing about five tons, was christened *John Barrett,* in honor of the first white man to ascend the Roanoke River above the great falls.[10] On its first trip to Suffolk it drew an excursion train, with the president, the directors, prominent citizens of Norfolk, a brass band, and the Portsmouth Grays. The passengers held their breath as the train rushed along at fifteen miles an hour and laughed to see horses and cows snort with terror and rush to the woods. They could hardly credit their eyes when they arrived at Suffolk in one hour and twenty minutes. On the return journey "night came upon us, and the chimney of the locomotive, with its stream of sparks lighting up the gloom of the swamp, was a source of general admiration."[11] In July, 1835, the line had been completed to Nottoway, forty-two miles from Portsmouth. Trains, drawn by another locomotive, the *General Cabell,* made the trip in three hours. The route lay through a desolate country, with "no hamlets, no villas, no churches, no towns, nothing to relieve the monotony of the sylvan scene except a few small farm-steads . . . and here and there a barren field or half-grown crop of old-field hickory."[12] By December Margarettsville, across the Carolina border, had been reached,[13] in August, 1836, the terminus was Garysville, a few miles from the Roanoke,[14] and in June, 1837, the entire line was completed, the bridge over the river built, and trains running to Weldon.[15]

Now came disappointment. Railroad building was still in the experimental stage, and it was soon discovered that the management had made several serious blunders. Experience showed that the company could not economically manufacture its own rolling stock, and the outlay on machine shops was practically wasted. Two new locomotives proved too heavy for the wooden rails, and after a few months of use, wrecked large sections of track. Before the end of

9 Norfolk *Beacon,* Aug. 9, 1834.
10 Virginia Board of Public Works, *Report* (Twentieth).
11 Norfolk *Beacon,* Oct. 6, 1834.
12 Norfolk *Herald,* July 29, 1835.
13 *Ibid.,* Dec. 7, 1835.
14 Norfolk *Beacon,* Aug. 4, 1836.
15 Norfolk *Herald,* June 9, 1837.

1837 it was reported that all along the line many rails were crushed and that between Portsmouth and Suffolk especially, the road was entirely broken down and almost impassable. Here and there the iron plates had become loose, leaving the ends projecting several inches above the timbers. In December, 1837, a train of three passenger cars, carrying twenty-five or thirty people, and nine freight cars laden with cotton, ran into one of these "snake-heads." The locomotive left the track, upsetting the tender, wrecking the coaches, and injuring seventeen people.[16] Nor was this the only accident on the road. Earlier in 1837 two trains had collided, splintering a number of cars, killing three persons, and injuring many others.[17]

Staggering under these accumulated misfortunes, the company elected a new president,[18] employed a new engineer, and set about the work of reconstruction. The damaged rails were replaced and edged with new iron, many rotten ties were discarded, the heavy locomotives were exchanged for lighter ones. An "agent" was placed on the top of the baggage car on each train as a lookout, ready to apply the brakes in case of need, and to signal the engineer by means of a rope attached to the bell.[19] These improvements were accompanied by increased facilities for traffic. In Portsmouth the rails were extended to the water's edge, a ferry connection was established with Norfolk, and new and better cars were purchased.[20]

But, when, despite all, the bulk of the traffic continued to go to Petersburg, the people of Norfolk became discouraged. "The railroad which cost us so much, and from which we expected such great things, is now completed," they said. "Why does not the tobacco, flour, cotton, bacon, lard, and corn come through?" The Petersburg road, it seems, had outmaneuvered its rival by intercepting the traffic of the upper Roanoke by means of a branch from Hicksford, on its main line, to Gaston on the river above the falls. There was no reason why the farmers should take their produce over the falls, or through the dilapidated locks to Weldon, when they could transfer them to the Petersburg trains higher up the river.[21]

But hope was revived by the construction of a railway from Weldon to Wilmington, to which Norfolk citizens subscribed liberally,

[16] *Ibid.*, Dec. 13, 1837.
[17] *Ibid.*, Aug. 7, Sept. 29, 1837.
[18] Colonel Andrew Joiner.
[19] Virginia Board of Public Works, *Report* (Twenty-third).
[20] Norfolk *Herald*, Sept. 1, 1838.
[21] Norfolk *Beacon*, Jan. 25, Feb. 1, 1839.

opening a new north and south connection all the way from Baltimore to Wilmington. Passengers could leave Baltimore on the fine
Chesapeake Bay steamers, transfer at Norfolk to the Portsmouth line
for Weldon and then take the train for Wilmington. The Petersburg
company, cut off from this trade by the fact that its terminus at
Blakely was on the north bank of the Roanoke, attempted to purchase a half-interest in the bridge at Weldon. Protracted negotiations
followed, in an effort to agree on the price, the Petersburg trains
using the bridge in the meanwhile. In the end the Petersburg company declined to purchase, and when the bridge was closed to them,
made connection with the Wilmington line by sending their passengers by wagon and boat to Halifax. This proved a serious inconvenience. Passengers complained that after leaving the train at Blakely,
they had "to walk down a most miserable dirty way, in mud knee
deep," then descend the river in an open boat, and finally to jolt over
a bad road in a wagon to Halifax, where they waited twenty-four
hours for the train.[22] To offset this disadvantage, the Petersburg company made an agreement with the Richmond and Fredericksburg to
lower the fares from Washington to the Roanoke River. "They have
come down to a fraction of their former rates," stated the *Beacon,*
and threaten to "run for nothing and give a bottle of wine," should
their rivals meet the reduction. Nonetheless, the Portsmouth connection did announce a new through rate of $7.00 from Baltimore to
Weldon.[23]

Yet disaster lay ahead. The bridge over the Roanoke had been exceedingly costly, and over thirty thousand dollars was still due the
various contractors. Rochelle and Smith, the largest of these creditors,
made repeated efforts to collect, and, failing in this, sold their claims
to Captain Francis E. Rives, a representative of the Petersburg line.
This practically delivered the Portsmouth railway into the hands of
its rival, and Captain Rives at once took steps to seize the company's
property in North Carolina in default of payment. One night he
brought forty Negroes to a point on the railway south of Margarette-
ville, ripped off the iron and displaced the ties at intervals for a distance of two miles. When news of this vandalism reached Portsmouth
thirty or forty citizens rushed by train to the scene and set to work to
repair the damage. They found that Rives had continued the work
of destruction while they were on the way, tearing up the floor of the

[22] *Ibid.,* April 28, 1841.
[23] *Ibid.,* Sept. 29, 1840.

bridge over the Petersburg line, and cutting the timbers of a trestle nearby. In the end Rives was arrested, the damage repaired, and train service renewed. But in the legal battle which followed, the railway was the loser, the Supreme Court of North Carolina deciding that Rives had a legal title to the seventeen miles of the road in that state, and that he had a right to stop traffic if he so desired. This he did at the earliest notice. "We have not one word to say against the decision of the court," remarked the *Herald;* "it shows us, however, that the law is a paradox in some cases; for while guarding individual rights, it may subserve the most reprobate purposes."[24]

The end was now close at hand. For some months an effort was made to continue service to the North Carolina border, but in the spring of 1845 the trains had to be taken off. Norfolk's first effort to turn the new method of transportation to her benefit, had ended in failure, and disappointment and gloom pervaded the town. On September 4, 1846, the Portsmouth railway with its cars, engines, and depots was purchased by the Board of Public Works of Portsmouth for sixty-two thousand dollars and the rolling stock was stored for possible use in the future.[25]

In the meanwhile the question of a scheme of internal improvements embracing all Virginia had been engaging the public attention. The Old Dominion was sinking lower and lower in the list of states in wealth and population; thousands of her youth were leaving to seek their fortunes in the West;[26] her foreign commerce had fallen to the lowest ebb. Something must be done to restore her ancient prestige. In 1831, when the legislature met, a system of internal improvements was proposed. But now sectional jealousies arose to render these efforts futile. West was arrayed against east; the Fall Line towns against the seaports; one Fall Line town against another; canal interests against railroads. "There has been as much talk about internal improvements in the legislature as would fill many folio volumes," it was said, but the "system proposed was debated and amended to death."[27] Some of the members could not see that canals were needed, to say nothing of the absurd dream of cars drawn over rails by puffing steam engines. These "old fogies" drew the fire of a fellow representative. Virginia has too many "let-us-alone politicians," he said; "very

[24] *Niles' National Register,* April 12, 1845.
[25] Norfolk *Beacon,* Sept. 5, 1846.
[26] "Upwards of 30 or 40 of our most promising young men will, in the short period of one month, bid adieu to our good old borough." *Ibid.,* 1835.
[27] *Niles' Weekly Register,* March 26, 1831, p. 58.

pious too—as much so as the Council of Castile, who said that if God
had intended a certain river to be navigable, he would himself have
made it so. They would not fight against God, No! No!"[28] "Hogsheads of tobacco will yet be rolled to market," was the sarcastic comment of one paper, "and if it had been the practice in Virginia to
make horses draw the plough by their tails, what a world of words
should we have had before any change could be made in that respect!"[29]

In 1832 the ultra-conservatives were so far overcome that the legislature took a step of far-reaching importance—it passed an act incorporating the James River and Kanawha Company, and subscribed
a hundred thousand dollars of its stock.[30] This company was charged
with the task of connecting Richmond with the Ohio, either by canals
or railways, or by both. Unfortunately the corporation, influenced
chiefly by Joseph C. Cabell, elected to continue the James River
canal to a point not lower than Lynchburg, to make the Kanawha
navigable, and to connect the two waterways with a railway.[31] The
results of this blunder were far-reaching indeed. It cost Virginia
hundreds of millions of dollars, it cut her off from the Ohio valley
trade, it made the economic union of east and west impracticable,
and played an important part in the eventual disruption of the state.
Perhaps it was not to be expected that the legislature and the company should see at this early date, when the period of experimentation was not yet over, the possibilities of railroad transportation. The
weight of tradition was on the side of canals. George Washington had
dreamed of a canal over the mountains to the Ohio; was it wise to
abandon his plans? Was it not the Erie canal which had made New
York so wealthy and powerful? They did not stop to consider that in
their own scheme profits would be eaten up by constant tranship-
ments—from the Kanawha to the railway, from the railway to the
canal, from the canal to the lower James. They did not dream that
eventually railways would prove so efficient that even the great Erie
canal could not compete with them. Without serious misgivings they
based Virginia's bid for economic unity and for trade with the Ohio
region upon canal construction.

A few years later, when the blunder was obvious to all, it was too
late to effect a change. Those who had invested their money in the

28 *Ibid.*
29 *Ibid.*
30 Dunaway, *History of the James River and Kanawha Co.,* pp. 97, 98.
31 *Ibid.,* pp. 119-121.

James River Company formed a solid phalanx against every proposal to parallel their route with a railway. So late as 1846, when a bill was introduced for a railway from Richmond to the Ohio, in which the state was to invest $4,800,000, the canal interest gathered enough votes to kill it.[32]

Had Virginia been able to grasp fully the significance of the new era of transportation, had she placed her dependence upon railways and laid out a wise and comprehensive scheme of construction, how different would have been her history! Instead of squandering millions on unwise projects, her outlay would have been returned many times over in increased commerce and manufactures; instead of rushing on to disunion, she would have bound her western counties with the bands of economic interest. It is easy today to see what should have been done. Starting with Norfolk, the state's only great ocean port, a railway should have been built west to Petersburg, Richmond, Charlottesville, Staunton, Charleston, and the Ohio River. There should have been no delay for minor undertakings, no side lines, until the one central trunk railway had been put into operation. Then the north and south lines could have been added; from Washington to Richmond, from Danville to Lynchburg to Charlottesville, from Winchester to Staunton, from Abingdon to Staunton, from Wheeling and Parkersburg to Charleston.

Had this been done the products of all Virginia—the tobacco and cotton of Pittsylvania and Halifax, the fruit of the Shenandoah, the grain of Mason and Cabell, would have poured through this system down to Norfolk. Here it would have gone out to the ports of the world in vessels of Virginia's own making, in exchange for direct imports. Norfolk would have rivaled Baltimore and Philadelphia; migration from Virginia to the West would have been checked; prosperity, wealth, growth would have returned to the Old Dominion.

But this was not to be. The Fall Line towns would not consent to the connecting of Norfolk with the back country. Having developed under the old system of river navigation, they were determined to maintain their ascendency by legislative action. If trainloads of goods came through from the west to Norfolk without so much as stopping at Richmond or Petersburg, would not Richmond and Petersburg sink to mere villages? They would see to it that whatever lines were built, whether railways or canals, should stop at the Fall Line, so as to perpetuate the present conditions. Norfolk must be isolated, out of

[32] *Niles' National Register,* Jan. 10, 24, 1846.

touch with the country beyond Petersburg, Richmond, Fredericks-burg, and Alexandria. True, large liners could not ascend the James or the Appomattox, but smaller vessels could continue to take the produce of the state to New York, there to be transhipped. A great port in Virginia was a desirable thing, no doubt, but not if it could be had only at the cost of ruining the river towns. And since the "central interest" was powerful enough to swing the legislature, in this matter they had their way.

"We were among the first to enter upon a system of improvement with a view to develop our great and varied resources," said the Norfolk *Argus* some years later, "but our efforts were misdirected and our means so misapplied that we were among the last to accomplish any great practical result. . . . The mistake was in locating the termini of the railways at the head of our rivers instead of at a sea-port. . . . Other states and nations have pursued a course the reverse of ours, and hence their success. They commenced near the sea and projected their lines of railway into the interior. . . . Look at New York, Pennsylvania, Maryland, North Carolina, Georgia, and Ala-bama, who followed this wise policy, and see the happy fruits. . . . Virginia owns a noble seaport . . . but this she long neglected, and until lately absolutely ignored. . . . Near $30,000,000 have been lavished on inland cities, with no great and general result . . . be-cause the seaport was cut off from all connection with the producing sections of the State. . . . The idea of converging our improvements on the glorious Appomattox or the upper James at the falls, 150 miles from the ocean, is a farce. . . . The seat of power is along the central line, and aspirants from all other quarters of the State pander to that interest."[33]

One of the most important results of this unwise policy was the di-version of traffic from Virginia to the seaport of another state. The Baltimore and Ohio was slowly, but steadily, advancing towards the Ohio. In 1836 the line entered Harpers Ferry, and connecting there with the Winchester and Potomac, began drawing off the produce of the Shenandoah to the Baltimore market. This was bad enough, but when a request followed to extend the Baltimore and Ohio up the valley and thence to the Ohio by way of the Kanawha, Richmond was alarmed. "Baltimore is spreading her arm around us," pointed out the Richmond *Times,* "and is not only endeavoring to secure the trade of the west by obtaining an avenue through our territory, which

[33] Norfolk *Argus,* March 14, 1856; July 9, 1858.

she flatters herself she will be able to secure through our sectional jealousies and our want of enterprise, but is taking from us even the trade which we have hitherto enjoyed. A large portion of the trade of the Valley of Virginia, which formerly came to Richmond, now goes to Baltimore upon the macadamized road down the valley."[34] Not only did the legislature reject the request, but in the session of 1844-45 refused to accede to petitions from the western part of the state, asking that the Baltimore and Ohio be permitted to extend its line to the Ohio at Parkersburg. They would concede nothing except the privilege of skirting the upper Potomac to Wheeling, thus leaving practically all western Virginia free for the day when the James River and Kanawha would reach out to the Ohio.[35]

The people of the west were bitterly angered at this decision. A convention, with delegates from thirteen counties, met at Clarksburg to protest to the legislature. They had looked to the proposed extension into their territory as a means to market their grain and their coal, they said, so that a vast country, now almost a wilderness, would become populous and wealthy. They had been taxed heavily for canals and railways in other parts of the state; to discriminate against their region was unjust and tyrannical. "We deny that any line of improvement is entitled to exclusive privileges to the injury of others, or that the northwest must be deprived of an outlet to its natural market, because it might abridge the trade of the James River and Kanawha Company. We are determined that our claims shall not be treated as though we were a mere colonial dependency, and in future will vote against all appropriations for railways and canals in other parts of the State until our rights have been recognized."[36]

Apparently this threat broke the opposition. In February, 1851, the state incorporated the Northwestern Virginia Railway, to run from Parkersburg to a point on the Baltimore and Ohio near Clarksburg. Almost at once the new line came under the direct control of the Baltimore and Ohio. Work was begun in 1852, pushed on vigorously in the face of great physical difficulties, and completed in 1857. Thus it was that Baltimore assumed the position to which Norfolk rightly aspired, as the seaport, not only of the Shenandoah valley, but of northwestern Virginia. A fourth of a century had passed since the

[34] *Niles' National Register,* June 21, 1845, p. 255.
[35] Dunaway, *History of the James River and Kanawha Co.,* pp. 189-190; Edward Hungerford, *The Baltimore & Ohio Railroad* (New York, 1928), pp. 148-200.
[36] *Niles' National Register,* June 21, 1845.

legislature at Richmond committed the state to the James River line of improvement, ample time certainly in which to carry out the most comprehensive scheme. Yet the west still remained isolated from central and eastern Virginia, for the canal ran only to Buchanan, about forty miles west of Lynchburg, and the Virginia Central terminated at the foot of the Alleghenies.

The act incorporating the James River and Kanawha Company stipulated that its lower termination at Richmond should be connected with tidewater, "so as to enable the boats . . . to descend the river or return."[37] If the people of Norfolk entertained a hope that this meant that they were to share at once in the benefits of the canal, they were doomed to disappointment. Sixteen years passed and nothing was done. As the *Argus* complained, the canal had one end stopped by a mountain and the other rested on a hill—cut off from tidewater except by a costly transit in drays and wagons. In 1847 the legislature instructed the company to make the connection,[38] and in 1851 the work was well under way.[39] Despite many delays, calling forth sarcastic comment from the Norfolk papers, this really formidable undertaking was completed in 1854. It consisted of a series of locks and basins extending from the canal for one mile to a ship dock, and a ship canal from the dock to the river at Rocketts. The whole cost was $851,312.[40] Even now Norfolk benefited but slightly, for the products of the upper river were transferred at the dock directly to packets bound for New York, Boston, and Baltimore. Until Norfolk regained its foreign trade, or until coasting vessels became too large to navigate the James River to Rocketts, Richmond would remain the chief point of transhipment.[41]

Blocked from all connection with the canals and railways of Virginia, Norfolk once more looked to North Carolina as her only salvation. The railroad to Weldon must be rebuilt and linked with the new line now under construction from Raleigh to Gaston. Who knew but that Norfolk would become the chief port of northern and western Carolina, just as Baltimore was the chief port of northern and western Virginia. There were actually some suggestions of annexation. "I am for hitching teams with the old North State," said a correspondent in the *Argus,* "for it has long been my notion that Vir-

[37] Dunaway, *History of the James River and Kanawha Co.,* pp. 98, 99.
[38] Norfolk *Beacon,* March 22, 1847.
[39] Norfolk *Argus,* March 21, 1851.
[40] Dunaway, *History of the James River and Kanawha Co.,* p. 164.
[41] *Ibid.,* p. 165.

ginia cares little for Norfolk. We cannot be worse off, and we may be better. Huzza for North Carolina and annexation."[42] The editor of the *Argus* commented on this seriously. Pointing out that Norfolk was the natural outlet for a large part of North Carolina, he suggested that the town apply to the Virginia legislature for permission to secede. This petition they would base upon the ill-treatment and neglect of the Old Dominion, the good treatment expected of North Carolina, and finally, on the fact that nature evidently intended it should be so.[43] Although this threat, for so it obviously was, seems to have been ignored, the restoration of the old Portsmouth-Weldon railway soon was an accomplished fact. Hershaw and Company, a Boston firm, bought the property, new charters were secured from Virginia and North Carolina, and reconstruction began under the name of Seaboard and Roanoke Railway.

At this juncture the entire situation was changed by a bitter quarrel between the old enemies of the Portsmouth line. Formerly two separate groupings had competed for the north and south traffic—the Richmond, Fredericksburg and Potomac, the Richmond and Petersburg, and the Petersburg and Roanoke on the one hand, and the Baltimore Steam Packet Company to Norfolk, and the Portsmouth and Weldon on the other. In each case through tickets at low rates were issued. After the collapse of the Portsmouth line, passengers from the Baltimore steamers for the south ran up the James in river boats to City Point, where they transferred to the Petersburg and Roanoke. This company, now the southern link of both competing routes, refused to renew its agreement with the Richmond and Petersburg and the R. F. & P., and assumed a neutral position. "If our Company combined with the railroads north of us," stated President H. D. Bird, "and thus threw our influence against the Bay company, the inevitable result would be to excite that company against us, and drive them to use their influence in favor of reviving the Portsmouth railway."[44]

The result was by no means what Mr. Bird expected. In September, 1846, the Richmond and Petersburg railway, with the co-operation of the R. F. & P., organized a subsidiary company to run steamships from Walthall, on the James River, to Norfolk. This, it was thought, would force the Bay line boats off the river and break up their

[42] Norfolk *Argus*, April, 1849.
[43] *Ibid.*, May 10, 1849.
[44] Virginia Board of Public Works, *Report* (Thirty-third), p. 676.

through system from Baltimore. This move was followed by the purchase of a controlling interest in the Baltimore Steam Packet Company, by the stockholders of the R. F. & P. The Baltimore Steam Packet Company as a corporation then purchased a controlling interest in the Seaboard & Roanoke, and the two systems, formerly such bitter rivals, fell under one control. The effect upon Norfolk was unfortunate. It now became the policy of the combination to divert traffic over the R. F. & P., while the close union of the Seaboard and the Bay line made it to the interest of both to encourage the long haul rather than local traffic. So far as circumstances permitted, they made Portsmouth no more than a place of transfer for goods from North Carolina to Baltimore. So late as February, 1871, the *Journal* charged that the Seaboard was an incubus to Norfolk, whose chief object was to enrich other cities at her expense.[45] This was no doubt an exaggeration, for the railway played an important rôle in the development of Norfolk, but the benefits would have been far greater had the line been controlled by Norfolk men, shaping its policies in conformity to the interests of the city.

However, the people rejoiced as the work of construction was rushed to completion. The old wooden rails which had caused so much trouble were replaced with the latest T rails, imported from Wales.[46] Progress was facilitated by the fact that the old roadbed could be utilized, and by November, 1851, trains were running from Portsmouth to Weldon. Very different were both locomotives and cars from those used on the Portsmouth and Weldon, and when the town councils of Norfolk and Portsmouth traveled over the line as guests of the company, they were amazed at the smoothness and speed with which the train moved.[47] The farmers along the route now began flocking into town with their bacon, cotton, peas, and corn. One, from Halifax county, had not seen Norfolk since the collapse of the old line. "In those days the trains made eight miles an hour, and we all were in danger of our lives from the 'snake heads' in the track," he said. "Now one can go 30 miles an hour in the parlor-like cars, in perfect safety."[48]

At Weldon the Seaboard connected again with the Wilmington railway, and through north and south passenger traffic was renewed. But it was upon the west that Norfolk had her eyes. A railway from

[45] Norfolk *Journal,* Feb. 4, 16, 1871.
[46] Norfolk *Argus,* June 9, Dec. 7, 1849.
[47] *Ibid.,* Nov. 27, 1851.
[48] *Ibid.,* Nov. 29, 1851.

Raleigh to Gaston was nearing completion, and Gaston was but twelve miles from the Seaboard terminus at Weldon. So the Gaston-Weldon Company was formed to bridge the gap. It proved a difficult bit of engineering to cut through the rocks on the south bank of the Roanoke, but the work was completed in 1853, and in August of that year the first train passed amid the cheers of the workmen.[49] A few days later two trains arrived at Portsmouth from Raleigh, crowded with North Carolinians, bent on celebrating the completion of the link. Among the guests were former President Tyler and Governor Reid of North Carolina, and there was much feasting and toasting and words of friendship between North Carolina and Virginia.[50] In the meanwhile, work was progressing upon the Roanoke Valley Railway, from Ridgeway, on the Raleigh and Gaston, to Clarksville, on the upper Roanoke River. This branch line was expected to drain not only Granville County in North Carolina and Mecklenburg County in Virginia, but the valleys of the Staunton and the Dan as well.

The Seaboard proved successful from the first. Long freight trains were constantly pulling into the Portsmouth station, laden with staves, lumber, tobacco, flour, naval stores, and cotton. "Well may the editor of the Petersburg *Intelligencer* be alarmed at the diversion of travel, and at our superior facilities for trade and business," boasted the *Beacon*. "We would advise him to keep cool, and if that be impossible, at his domicile at this time, he had best come to the seaboard, bathe in its briny waters, and cast off all visions of an inland seaport on the banks of the mighty Appomattox."[51] Norfolk seemed to awaken as from a long sleep under the influence of the new trade.[52] On one day alone seven carloads of staves came in for Reid and Soulter, two hundred and sixty-four barrels of rosin and one car of flour for Josiah Wills, three cars of staves and nine barrels of turpentine for K. Biggs, ten bales of cotton for William Reid, eighteen barrels of turpentine for J. B. Odum.[53] In the year ending January 31, 1855, the receipts of the Seaboard were $201,893.61; the next year, including the months of the yellow fever epidemic, they were $173,-723.58,[54] for the following year $203,666.08,[55] for the year ending

[49] Norfolk *Beacon*, April 19, 1853.
[50] *Ibid.*, April 22, 1853.
[51] *Ibid.*, June 27, 1853.
[52] Norfolk *Argus*, Oct. 22, 1853.
[53] *Ibid.*, April 28, 1854.
[54] *Ibid.*, May 29, 1856.
[55] *Ibid.*, April 17, 1857.

January 30, 1860, $240,546.50.[56] At first goods from North Carolina were piled up on the streets of Portsmouth, hauled in drays to the water's edge, and brought to Norfolk in small boats. Later a railway ferry boat was constructed on which the loaded cars were taken across the river so that they would be unloaded on the Norfolk side.[57] Cars were hauled in and out of the boat at any state of the tide by a pony engine placed under the deck.[58]

Although this was like food to a starving man, the railway situation as a whole remained essentially unfavorable to Norfolk. Her one line had to compete with the Petersburg and Roanoke for the Carolina trade, while the Richmond and Danville was reaching its arm out to the upper Roanoke to divert the traffic of that region to the James. The Southside Railway, which, with the Virginia and Tennessee, drained southwest Virginia, had its terminus at Petersburg. All central Virginia was tributary to Richmond, parts of the Valley and all northwestern Virginia to Baltimore, and Norfolk was completely cut off from the railway system of the state to which it belonged.

In 1851 the city made a determined effort to secure a railway to Petersburg. This would link her with the Southside Railway, which connected with the Virginia and Tennessee at Lynchburg, which, in turn, was linked up at Bristol with the railway system of Tennessee. As talk of the new line grew more definite, the Norfolk merchants began to dream of long through freight trains, bringing to their wharves the grain of the Cumberland Valley and the cotton of the Mississippi. The charter for the Norfolk and Petersburg railway was secured with comparative ease, but it was another matter to get the legislature to give financial support.[59] The Petersburg interest opposed violently, because they wished their own town to remain the terminus of the group of railways; the Richmond interest because traffic from the southwest might be drawn off at Lynchburg from their canal. Although in February, 1852, the Committee on Internal Improvements of the House of Delegates recommended appropriations of about three millions to aid various state lines, including $1,705,000 for the James River and Kanawha Canal, the appeals of the Norfolk and Petersburg were ignored.[60] "In all this great program," said the *Argus* bitterly, "which is destined, probably, to cover the land

---

[56] *Ibid.*, March 26, 1860.
[57] *Ibid.*, April 26, 1854.
[58] Burton, *The History of Norfolk*, p. 10.
[59] Lamb, *Our Twin Cities*, p. 26.
[60] Norfolk *Argus*, Feb. 13, 1852.

with wonders and its inhabitants with rags, the only seaport town in the State is not once mentioned, nor a single dollar appropriated from the common treasury towards the advancement of her prosperity. . . . We do not hesitate to express the hope that our representatives in that body will return home, and our people take prompt and decided steps to release themselves from bondage by annexing the city, come what may, to North Carolina. . . . To this the alternative will be to submit to galling, degrading, and hopeless oppression, or to take refuge in revolution."[61] Fortunately a few days later the committee supplemented its report with the suggestion that the state subscribe $480,000 to the stock of the Norfolk and Petersburg, and excitement in Norfolk died down.[62] The Norfolk councils then subscribed $200,000, on condition that there be "a satisfactory connection with the Southside Railway at or near its terminus in Petersburg."[63]

The road had already been partly surveyed, and the work was now pushed forward under the able direction of William Mahone.[64] Beginning in Norfolk at the east end of Main Street, the tracks made a wide circle over the Eastern and Southern branches, and cut through the Dismal Swamp to Suffolk, whence they swung northwest in almost a straight line to Petersburg. Mahone did the railroad and Norfolk a great service by insisting that the roadbed, the bridges, the rails, and the rolling stock be of the latest and most substantial type, that the grades be easy, the ditching deep, the curves few.[65] Much had been learned about railway construction since the days of the Portsmouth and Weldon, and the new line profited fully from the mistakes of the old. In July, 1858, trains were running, and a few weeks later all Norfolk was thrilled by the arrival of several carloads of fruit and flour from Lynchburg.[66] The transferring of goods from freight cars to the wharves was made easy by the laying down of track along Water Street from the station to Town Point.[67]

In the meanwhile Norfolk, for the moment forgetting her many defeats at the hands of the central interests, asked for permission to extend the Norfolk and Petersburg to Charlottesville. This would

[61] *Ibid.*, Feb. 11, 1852.
[62] *Ibid.*, Feb. 19, 1852; May 14, 1857.
[63] Burton, *The History of Norfolk*, p. 13.
[64] *Ibid.*, p. 15.
[65] Norfolk *Beacon*, April 5, 1855.
[66] Norfolk *Argus*, July 1, 1858.
[67] The track still remained in 1961 and standing freight cars often blocked the street, rendering vehicular traffic difficult.

give a connection with the Virginia Central, and divert western traffic from Richmond to Norfolk. The bill met a stone wall in the Senate and the project had to be abandoned. Once more all Norfolk shook with indignation. "I know not whether North Carolina will receive us, but it may be worth while to make the experiment," said the *Argus*. "Since grave Senators have publicly declared that . . . we are of no use to the State, our neighbors may perchance think our port not worthy of acceptance. The Old North State has appropriated nearly as much to works looking to Norfolk as Virginia herself, our principal trade is with her farmers, and a large number of our best citizens are natives of her soil. The United States ceded Alexandria to Virginia, why not Virginia cede Norfolk to North Carolina?"[68] Richmond had four railways, the editor pointed out, terminating near her limits. "No one connects with the other, and never will. She may well be called the railway rat-trap of the State. The policy deserves no other name. It is conceived in folly, hedged in by jealousy and selfishness."[69]

A few days later an indignation meeting was held in Ashland Hall, presided over by Mr. Charles Reid. It was resolved that "the Senate of Virginia in refusing to Norfolk the privilege of connecting with the works which are now constructing on State account on the Central line (including the tunnel[70] and the Covington road) towards the construction of which Norfolk and the eastern counties are heavily taxed, . . . have perpetrated an act of tyranny worthy of the dark ages of mail-clad despotism. . . . Since we are to be taxed without participation, since such tribute is demanded of us as we cannot honorably pay, we ask that the ruling power of the land make us outcasts rather than slaves, by ceding us to North Carolina. We regard our representation in the Senate and the House of Delegates as mere mockery, and we therefore request that our Senator and Delegate will vacate their seats."[71]

The Norfolk and Petersburg had not had time to build up a paying traffic before the advent of the Civil War. The tonnage carried in 1860 was only 7,502, as compared with 32,660 by the Seaboard. Yet the southwestern connection had been secured, and time alone was needed for this line, with the Southside, and the Virginia and Ten-

---

[68] Norfolk *Argus*, March 13, 1856.
[69] *Ibid.*, March 14, 1856.
[70] This was the great tunnel through the Blue Ridge at Rock Fish Gap. It was a work of great expense, and constituted a vital link in the east and west traffic.
[71] Norfolk *Argus*, March 18, 1856.

nessee, to form a great artery of trade. The Norfolk and Western, into which these lines were eventually merged, was one day to accomplish wonders for the development of the city.

Still another important line of communication was opened for Norfolk in 1859, with the completion of the Albemarle and Chesapeake canal. This project had been in contemplation for years. The Dismal Swamp canal was too small for steamers, and the farmers of northeastern Carolina were loud in their complaints. When at last the Carolina government began to consider plans for making a deep cut to the ocean through the sand bar at Nag's Head, so that large vessels could have access to both Albemarle and Pamlico sounds, Norfolk became alarmed. So early as 1840 the noted engineer, Colonel Crozet, had surveyed a canal route from the Eastern Branch, near Kempsville, to the head of North River. Later, this route was abandoned for one from Great Bridge across the swamp to North River into Currituck Sound, thence through another canal into Doctor's Creek and Albemarle Sound.[72] Both cuts were to be fifty feet at the top, thirty feet at the bottom, and seven feet deep. There was to be but one lock, the largest in the United States, two hundred and twenty feet by forty feet wide, through which vessels of six hundred tons could pass. After the company had been incorporated and the stock subscribed the work of digging went on rapidly. Great advances had been made in engineering since the days when swarms of Negroes armed with spades had dug out the channel of the old canal. Now steam engines did most of the work. It was a popular recreation for the people of Norfolk to go down to Great Bridge to watch the machines pulling up stumps and digging up mud and depositing it on the bank, with loud "coughings and gruntings."[73] The *Enterprise* from Wilmington, Delaware, had the honor of being the first boat to pass through. On January 9, 1859, the company's steamer *Calypso*, taking her in tow, entered the great lock and passed on south to Albemarle Sound.[74] The new canal opened a ready means of communication with the cotton lands of the Pamlico, the Neuse, and the Tar, and added greatly to the volume of trade. In 1867-68 over sixteen thousand bales came through. In 1878-80 the number had risen to 77,608.[75] The Albemarle and Chesapeake canal played an important rôle in

[72] Forrest, *Sketches of Norfolk*, p. 261.
[73] Norfolk *Argus*, April 20, 1857.
[74] Burton, *History of Norfolk*, p. 31.
[75] Jones, *Norfolk as a Business Centre*, p. 35.

strengthening Norfolk's position as the chief port for northeastern Carolina.

In the long and elusive quest for prosperity, Norfolk at last seemed to be on the road to success. With one railway giving direct communication with central North Carolina, with another linking the city with southern Virginia and Tennessee, with a fine canal opening afresh the great Carolina sounds, it was thought that trade must increase rapidly. True, the city was still largely cut off from central and western Virginia, but the people were disposed to overlook this fact, now that the prospect was so bright for becoming an entrepôt for the cotton, flour, corn, and lumber of the South. Little did they dream that disaster lay immediately ahead; that their harbor would soon be blockaded, their streets filled with hostile troops, the South of which they expected so much, devastated and exhausted.

The period of internal improvements was for many states and cities marked by glorious success, by expanding trade, growing wealth, increasing population. For Virginia, and especially for Norfolk, it was a time of wasted opportunities and bitter disappointment. The proud Old Dominion, once the undisputed leader in the Union, saw one state after another pass her in all that makes for influence and power. And there were many to say that the fault was her own; that when other states were acting promptly and planning wisely to profit from railway communication, she was distracted with petty jealousies and local interests, and held back by shortsighted old fogies. Norfolk, of course, laid the blame upon Richmond. Richmond, because of the suffrage law, controlled the elections of at least twelve counties, and so exercised an overwhelming influence in the legislature. Looked up to as the metropolis, the great social and commercial center of the state, her men of wealth connected by relationship or interest with the leaders of other sections, she partitioned out the honors of the government to those who would aid in her aggrandizement. "Such corrupt logrolling was hardly ever seen in any other legislature in the United States, the whole system enduring to the advancement of Richmond, and a few other favored points. Even the Panhandle could obtain privileges to which no citizen of Norfolk would dare aspire."[76]

Whether or not these charges be true, it is certain that Virginia's policy of internal improvements was shortsighted, wasteful, expensive, ineffectual. And the penalty was swift and terrible. In the Civil

[76] Norfolk *Journal*, Feb. 18, 1867.

War Virginia needed warships to break the blockade and protect her commerce, but the discrimination against her one natural port made the creation of a navy most difficult; she needed the support of all sections of the state, but the isolation of the western counties left them no alternative save separation; she needed a network of modern railways to move and supply her troops, but her mileage was comparatively low, her lines improperly located; she needed all her sons to fight her battles, but tens of thousands of young Virginians had gone west to seek new opportunities and build new homes.

CHAPTER NINE

Pestilence and War

Like other seaports, Norfolk in former days was constantly exposed to epidemics of smallpox and yellow fever. Whenever a vessel came in from the West Indies, from Cádiz, or even from England, there was the possibility that it might spread wholesale death. Little was known of the causes of these epidemics, so that preventive measures were misdirected. It was thought that they resulted from damp cellars, or from the proximity of marshes, or from insanitary and crowded conditions of living, or from the presence of pigpens in town, or from the pumping of bilge water near the wharves. In cases of smallpox the quarantining of patients did much to protect the community, but nothing save the approach of cold weather could stem the sweep of yellow fever.

From time to time the borough government, or the medical fraternity, made efforts to secure a general inoculation for smallpox. In 1795, when a seaman from the schooner *Antelope* started an epidemic, the council set aside a sum of money for this purpose.[1] But there was so much danger attached to inoculating, even with the mildest form of real smallpox, that the public resisted strenuously. It was only in 1802, four years after Edward Jenner made his first test with cowpox, that smallpox vaccine was brought to Norfolk from Europe. On March 2 Doctors Balfour and Ward inserted a notice in the *Herald* "informing the public that they have now under inoculation several persons with the true kine-pox, the matter certainly genuine." Still the people hesitated. "What was cowpox but smallpox under a different name?" it was asked. "Who could say how fatal it might be! True the doctors claimed that the matter had been tested, but doctors were often mistaken." Many persons refused to be inocu-

[1] *Norfolk Council Orders*, 1736-1798, pp. 173b, 175, 175b.

lated, and some even objected to having this "artificial disease" spread in the community. Nonetheless, in the spring of 1802, inoculation proceeded, with excellent results. "We have succeeded after so many unsuccessful trials, in introducing into this town the mild antidote to smallpox," stated the doctors. "So many attempts had been made before, without success, that even medical men declared they did not believe the disease (cowpox) could be brought here. It will no doubt take some time to remove the obstinate prejudice of the public; but like all great truths, it ultimately must prevail, and surmount every obstacle ignorance can oppose. Eighteen have had the disease (cowpox) in its mildest form, and numbers are under inoculation."[2]

But while medical science was conquering one of Norfolk's greatest enemies, the other continued its occasional visits to the town, spreading always terror, suffering, and death. In 1795 yellow fever broke out in the crowded tenements in the narrow lanes near the river, and before it was checked by the frosts of October, had carried off no less than five hundred people.[3] At that time this district was swarming with strangers—mechanics, attracted by the high wages current in Norfolk; sailors, seeking a berth in a tobacco ship or a West India trader; small merchants from the rivers and creeks of tidewater Virginia; North Carolinians, in port with a cargo of farm produce. These visitors proved easy victims to the scourge. Some fled at the first warning of danger, only to die miserably on the way or after reaching their homes; others were struck down before they could move. The borough authorities were helpless. The number of doctors was inadequate, it was difficult to secure nurses, impossible to isolate the patients, and whole families were wiped out, who, with proper care and food, might have been saved.[4] The doctors, groping for the causes of the epidemic, stated that "the air was evidently impregnated with putrid effluvia, arising from decayed substances of every sort, brought down upon the creeks and rivers—together with filth thrown from the shipping and docks."[5] If they had only known the truth, what future terror and suffering Norfolk would have been spared! But more than a century was to elapse before a modest army surgeon, born in Virginia, not forty miles from Norfolk, made the discovery which prepared the way for the conquest of this terrible scourge.[6]

[2] Norfolk *Herald*, April 13, 1802.
[3] La Rochefoucauld, *Voyages dans les États-Unis*, IV, 257.
[4] *Letter of Doctors Taylor and Hansford*. Miscellaneous Pamphlets, No. 685, Library of Congress.
[5] *Ibid.*
[6] Walter Reed. He was born in Gloucester County.

In 1802 yellow fever again visited Norfolk, claiming its victims by the hundreds. "We had the yellow fever raging very much among us this season," wrote William Couper, a recent arrival from Scotland, "where it cut off many one every day. . . . But I have reason to thank my preserver for preserving me in the midst of 20 or 30 or 40 that died every day, for the matter of seven or eight weeks, and the country were no better. But all is well again, and hardly any complaints to be heard."[7]

For two decades Norfolk remained comparatively free from yellow fever. Then, on July 20, 1821, a vessel from Point Peter, Guadeloupe, arrived with a cargo of rum, sugar, and molasses, and tied up in the slip between Southgate's wharf and Warren's wharf. With her, apparently, came yellow fever. On August 1, a Mr. Price, clerk of the adjacent warehouse, became ill, and shortly after a Negro cook in a near-by house contracted the disease. Both men died. Other cases followed rapidly, and once more Norfolk knew the terror of a yellow fever epidemic. The disease crept up Woodside's Lane, a narrow alley crowded with persons of low character, many of them weakened by "intemperance and debauchery," whence it spread to Little Water, now Upton Street. In a few weeks it had extended over the entire area south of Main Street from Market Square to Town Point. Fortunately, the epidemic seemed to be held within these bounds by some invisible quarantine, and it was stated "that persons living in that district had just to remove to the north of Main Street, and they were as safe from the fever as they would have been a thousand miles off."[8] As in 1795, there was a wholesale exodus at the first approach of the epidemic, and this undoubtedly saved hundreds of lives. Unfortunately, some of the fugitives were imprudent enough to return early in October, before the first frost, and of these some contracted the disease and died. In all there were about one hundred and sixty deaths. An unusual feature of the epidemic was the fact that the Negroes, who were thought to be almost immune, suffered as heavily as the whites. Of the whites who died, the larger part were recent Irish immigrants and Northern visitors.[9]

The borough authorities were greatly puzzled by this epidemic. It had been stated repeatedly that yellow fever resulted from filth and refuse; yet in 1821 Norfolk was far cleaner, far better drained, than in

[7] Letters of William Couper, October 11, 1802.

[8] George D. Armstrong, *History of Yellow Fever in Norfolk* (Philadelphia, 1856), p. 23.

[9] Report of Dr. Robert Archer, Norfolk *Herald*, March 1, 1822.

former years. "Our police have been improved," it was pointed out, "most of our streets and alleys, particularly in that district, have been paved." The health officer traced the origin of the epidemic to the dock near Woodside's Lane, but when he gave his theory as to how the disease was carried from the merchantman to near-by residents, he was wide of the mark. It was observed, he said, that the crew pumped out on the dock a stream of bilge water, so offensive that the doors and windows in the houses near-by had to be closed. It was this foul air, he believed, that infected Price and other early victims.[10]

The next spring Norfolk bestirred itself to prevent a return of the terrible visitor. Shallow, stagnant slips were filled up, unsanitary houses pulled down, the street drains kept open. The quarantine against infected ports was strictly enforced, although many thought that "the theory of importation of the disease was a chimera."[11] Fortunately, there was no recurrence of the fever. Four years later, however, it became known late in September that yellow fever had made its appearance in Norfolk, as on former occasions, in the district south of Main. In two days almost every family on Main Street from the Virginia Bank to Town Point had fled. This prompt action, together with the short time left before frost, made the mortality comparatively light. Yet twenty-seven persons had succumbed by September 30.[12] As to how many more perished before the end of October, the Norfolk papers are silent.

After this, twenty-nine years passed in which Norfolk was practically free of yellow fever. An entire generation had grown up since the epidemics of 1821 and 1826 caused such widespread terror, and only a few old persons could remember the harvest of death in 1795. People began to think that the paving and draining of the streets and the widespread use of cisterns for drinking water had rendered the town immune to yellow fever. Then, on June 7, 1855, the steamer *Ben Franklin,* bound from St. Thomas to New York, put into Hampton Roads in distress, with yellow fever on board. It was imperative that the steamer be repaired, and upon giving assurances that his crew were all in good health, the captain, on June 19, was permitted to take her to Page and Allen's shipyard, at Gosport. A few days later a laborer employed in "breaking up her hold," contracted yellow fever, and, on July 8, died. The steamer was at once put in quaran-

---

10 *Ibid.*
11 Norfolk *Herald,* July 22, 1822.
12 *Ibid.,* Sept. 22, Oct. 2, 1826.

tine, but Pandora's box had been opened, and the furies let loose over Portsmouth and Norfolk.

The first cases occurred in a row of buildings near the Navy Yard, "small, sadly out of repair, overcrowded with inhabitants, and filthy in the extreme." The authorities built a fence around this district, apparently after all of the residents had been removed, and for a time it was fondly hoped that this would localize the disease. A tremor of apprehension went over Portsmouth, then, when it became known a few days later that cases had been reported in various parts of the town. In Norfolk the people were still hopeful. The Elizabeth was broad and deep; would it not interpose an impassable barrier to the progress of the epidemic? Unfortunately the Norfolk authorities had permitted a number of poor families from Gosport, presumably persons forced to leave the "infected houses," to move to Barry's Row, a tenement district south of Main Street, and on July 30, yellow fever made its appearance there. Thereupon, the Board of Health had all the families, "well and sick," removed, and boarded up the streets in the vicinity. The patients were taken to an improvised hospital at Oak Grove, but so fixed was the idea that the disease was spread, not from person to person, but by contact with infected houses or decaying matter, that the well, it seems, were permitted to go at large. When it was reported a few days later that certain poor families were moving into Barry's Row in defiance of the Board of Health, someone set fire to the buildings, and, while eight thousand persons looked on, they burned to the ground.

As new cases began to appear in various parts of the city, terror seized the people. Every head of a family had to decide whether to leave his business engagements and flee, or to remain, facing the danger of death for himself, his wife, and children. Thousands chose the former alternative, and every train which left Portsmouth, every steamer for Baltimore or Richmond, were crowded with fugitives. Then came the announcement that other cities had declared a quarantine against the stricken towns—first New York, then Suffolk, Richmond, Petersburg, Weldon, Hampton, Washington, Baltimore. The question now was where to go. Must all remain "to grapple with the pestilence, no matter how deadly it might become?" Fortunately, Mathews County and the Eastern Shore threw open their doors. Henry A. Wise, governor-elect of Virginia, not only took some of the fugitives in his residence, but equipped his outhouses so as to accommodate as many of the poor as possible. By August 11, it was estimated, one-half of the people of Norfolk had left. The ministers, doctors, undertakers and nurses, however, almost without exception, remained. "The physician and the Christian pastor are, by their profession, called to minister to the sick, the dying, and the afflicted," wrote the Reverend George D. Armstrong, "and certainly, a time of pestilence, when their services are most needed, is no time for them to flee."[13]

August 14 was set aside as a day of humiliation and prayer, but the fever continued to spread. The district south of Main Street was almost entirely deserted, the post office being removed to the Academy building, and the merchants transacting business from their residences. But the disease passed north of Main, appearing first in one district, then in another, until almost every part of the town was infected. The doctors and nurses were entirely insufficient in numbers and persons began to die for want of care. One family, who kept a boardinghouse, became so terrified that they fled from town, leaving a lodger, an Irishman, named Stapleton, ill in an upper room. When the poor man found himself deserted, he staggered downstairs and up the street to Dr. Constable's office. There his strength gave out, and he fell dead on the door-stoop.[14] Fortunately noble persons came from other cities—physicians, nurses, and druggists—to risk their lives in the cause of humanity. The first to arrive was Miss Annie M. Andrews, of Syracuse, New York, who offered her services to Mayor Hunter Woodis as a nurse. Others came from Richmond, New York, Philadelphia, Baltimore, Savannah, Charleston, and even far off Mobile and New Orleans. Many of these men and women met the martyr's death, no less than thirteen from Philadelphia alone succumbing to the pestilence they came to combat.[15]

Before the end of August the city had become a great hospital. Many patients had been taken to the buildings at Lamberts Point, and others to the City Hotel, but neither sufficed to hold the multitude of sick. Dr. Armstrong gives a heart-rending account of the scenes he encountered in his pastoral rounds. In one house, from which a widowed mother and two of her children had just been buried, three other children were ill; in another were two families, all stricken with the fever; at the home of Mr. S. the eldest daughter had had the "black vomit," and was upon the point of death; at a near-by home a captain

---

[13] *Ibid.,* Jan. 31, 1856; Armstrong, *History of Yellow Fever in Norfolk,* pp. 28, 29, 37, 38, 39, 40, 41.
[14] Armstrong, *History of Yellow Fever in Norfolk,* pp. 44, 45.
[15] Burton, *History of Norfolk,* pp. 22, 23, 31; W. S. Forrest, *Great Pestilence in Virginia* (New York and Philadelphia, 1856), p. 53.

of the marines, his wife, her sister, and one child were dead. "We have burials, but no funerals now," he wrote, on September 6. "It is the mother we are to bury; and the daughter is now so extremely ill that we dare not let her know that her mother lies dead in the very next room. . . . Enough are present to carry the coffin to the hearse; and . . . we drive off . . . at a rapid pace. The principal grave-digger opens the cemetery gate; but instead of simply pointing us to the grave . . . he asks us in very much the style of the challenge given by a sentry on guard, 'who's this?' . . . Arrived at the lot belonging to the family, we find no grave dug there as yet. . . . The hearse cannot wait; the carriages cannot wait; all we can do is to deposit the coffin where the grave is to be dug, and, offering a short prayer, there leave it."

The deaths now mounted to seventy, eighty, or even a hundred a day. On one of his visits to the cemetery, Dr. Armstrong asked how many graves had been ordered for the day. The reply was forty-three. Passing on to the potter's field he saw large numbers of coffins and rough boxes, "piled up like cord wood" as high as a man could reach, while close by laborers were at work on a pit in which to bury them. In addition there were a number of interments in the Catholic cemetery. Since this was before five in the evening, and since for days past the burials had continued until nine or ten at night, it seemed certain that more than a hundred were buried that day. At one time the supply of coffins gave out, and the bodies had to be interred in boxes, in one instance four to a box. Others were tied up in the blankets in which they died, and carried out to the potter's field, in furniture-wagons, carts, or drays, there to be buried layer upon layer in pits.[16]

Not only the streets of Norfolk, but the harbor as well, reflected the desolation of the city. "As we look out along the water-front we see that wharves and warehouses, with the names of occupants painted in large letters upon their fronts, all appear as usual, saving that their doors and windows are closed, and there is no living thing to be seen about them. The names painted there will, many of them, if they are to give true directions, soon have to be blotted out, and graven, instead, upon the sign-stones in the 'city of the dead.' But look along the wharves, where at every season of the year there are many vessels lying, and in the winter and early spring they often line the wharf-heads five or six deep. There is now not one single vessel to be seen afloat, from the draw-bridge to Town Point. There are the two slender masts of a

16 Forrest, *Great Pestilence in Virginia*, pp. 94-97.

fishing-smack sunken in the county dock; and here, in this shipyard, there is a vessel drawn up as if for repairs; but there is no shipwright at work upon her. . . . The only boat which enters our harbor now is the little steamer, *J. E. Coffee,* run to meet the boats from Baltimore and Richmond in Hampton Roads. By her our mails are carried, and all our commerce done. Yesterday she came in with her whole deck piled with empty coffins; and coffins for the dead are one main article of import now. . . . Poor desolate Norfolk! The coming of a ship into her harbor today would cause almost as much surprise . . . as the coming of the first ship . . . to the Indians, who then dwelt here. The sun shines as brightly, and the sea-breeze seems as balmy, as at other times; and yet this, one of the finest harbors on the Atlantic seaboard, the unseen pestilence has made to be shunned by the mariner more than if it were full of quicksands and sunken rocks."[17]

All through that terrible September and until late in October the fever raged. In Bermuda Street every house had its sick or its dead, while the district north of Back Creek, where dwelt the wealthy and aristocratic, was swept from one end to the other. "It was then that some were appalled and chilled with fright, while others were apparently callous, careless and reckless, and went about the work of boxing and removing the dead, with but little appearance of fear or agitation." It was felt by all that it was too late to flee, that "the venom had entered the blood," and they could resist it as well in Norfolk as elsewhere.

"The city was wrapped in gloom. All the stores, and the dwellings of the absentees, were closed; few were seen passing in the streets on foot, and these on some errand of mercy or necessity. . . . Most of the inhabitants present were either confined at home by sickness, or in attendance on the sick. . . . And though there was the perpetual din of carriages, continually passing, from early dawn till a late hour of the night—the physicians' carriages, the hacks conveying nurses and members of the Howard Association, and the hearses, and the ever-moving 'sick-wagon'—rattling and rumbling to and fro in every direction—there was no sign of wholesome animation."[18]

Finally, when the coming of frost put an end to the pestilence, Norfolk lay suffering, stunned, still unable to grasp the full meaning of the fearful calamity. Of those who remained through those terrible ninety days, "every man, woman, and child, almost without exception,

17 *Ibid.,* pp. 101-104.
18 *Ibid.,* p. 87.

had been stricken with the fell fever, and about 2,000 had been buried." Two-thirds of the whites, and one-third of the whites and blacks together had succumbed to the disease.[19]

Among the dead were some of Norfolk's leading citizens: Mayor Hunter Woodis; John G. H. Hatton, president of the Select Council; Alexander Feret, of the Exchange Bank; William D. Roberts, delegate-elect to the legislature; Bray B. Walters, proprietor of the National Hotel; Josiah Wills, merchant and banker; former Mayor W. D. Delany; Alexander Galt, postmaster; William Reid, ship broker; Caleb Bonsal, miller; John D. Gordan, banker. The mortality among physicians was very severe, including ten local doctors[20] and twenty-six out of forty-five who came from other places. Of the eight ministers who were in town during the epidemic, all became ill and four died.[21]

On November 11 Dr. Armstrong, who had contracted the fever but recovered, held services for the first time since the pestilence. "In all the congregation . . . I noticed but three families that were not clad in mourning. And in every part of the house there were vacant seats which, as the eye rested on them, called up to memory the forms of those accustomed to occupy them. . . . In one part of the church sat the orphans, now gathered under the protecting care of the Howard Association. There they sat, some sixty in number, ranging from fourteen to two and three years in age, all made parentless by the terrible pestilence. Some of them when found, were in the house alone with the dead body of their remaining parent; and they, poor little things, so young that they did not know their own names. . . . Through the assistance sent us from abroad, in connection with what we can do at home, I hope we . . . can provide comfortably for them all."[22]

Dr. Armstrong, in seeking to solve the mystery of the rapid spread of the yellow fever in the city, made some exceedingly interesting observations. He dared to express the opinion that the disease was not contagious. "I was for more than six weeks almost constantly during the day among the sick, the dying, and the dead; . . . yet I did not take the fever until as an epidemic it reached the part of the city in which I lived. . . . Those who resided in the adjoining country, and came into the city during the day only, in no instance that I have heard of took the fever. . . . So with the country-people who attended

[19] Burton, *History of Norfolk,* p. 23.
[20] R. W. Sylvester, T. F. Constable, G. I. Halson, R. J. Sylvester, F. L. Higgins, J. A. Briggs, Thomas Nash, G. L. Upshur, R. B. Tunstall, and Henry Selden.
[21] Burton, *History of Norfolk,* pp. 23, 24.
[22] Armstrong, *History of Yellow Fever in Norfolk,* pp. 158, 159.

our markets; and there were some who attended throughout the season. Not one of them, that I have heard of, died of the fever. . . . The disease . . . spread rapidly in the direction of the prevailing winds, and but slowly in a direction across the track of those winds. . . . If we map down the whole region over which the yellow fever prevailed and then draw a line in the direction of the prevailing winds, this line will be found to measure not much short of five miles; while a line drawn at right angles to this will not, at the widest point, measure more than one and a half miles. . . . Besides this, the liability to take the disease was found to be far greater by night than by day." Had Dr. Armstrong drawn the proper conclusions from these remarkable observations, had it occurred to him that they pointed directly to the mosquito as the agent of transmission, he might have put the medical fraternity upon the right track a half century before the days of Reed. But his only inference was that "to pen up the inhabitants upon the infected ground is to aggravate the disease a thousand fold," and that they should be permitted, even encouraged, to flee wherever they would.[23]

While Norfolk was still staggering from this terrific blow, it was hurled headlong into the maelstrom of the Civil War. Although the people of the town resented so deeply the control of the state legislature by the central group, although they had little in common with the planter aristocracy of the wheat and tobacco sections, in the long-drawn-out struggle for national supremacy between North and South, their hearts were entirely with their own section. While admitting the economic and social evils of slavery, they resented the attacks of the abolitionists, and defended the treatment of the Negroes. On July 31, 1835, the aldermen of the borough instructed the mayor to request the postmaster to withhold delivery of the *Emancipator* and other similar papers addressed to free Negroes or slaves. This they deemed necessary to prevent disobedience and dissatisfaction among the blacks.[24] A few weeks later a meeting of citizens at the courthouse, presided over by Mayor Miles King, passed resolutions denouncing the abolition movement, demanding that Congress refrain from interfering with the slave trade, and calling for action by the states to protect slavery and to close the doors to abolition literature.[25]

The general sentiment of the town may be gathered from the dis-

23 *Ibid.*, pp. 182-192.
24 *Lower Norfolk County Antiquary*, II, 11.
25 Norfolk *Herald*, Aug. 17, 1835.

cussion of slavery by W. S. Forrest, in his *Sketches of Norfolk,* published in 1853. "Our colored people, the slaves particularly, are generally happy and contented. They are entirely free from those cares and troubles which necessarily grow out of the responsibilities and duties of life, that devolve on those upon whom they depend for support. . . . Very many of them seem as free as any beings on the face of the earth; having, generally, liberal, kind and indulgent owners, who allow them many privileges and who look anxiously to their welfare, providing for them comfortable lodging-rooms, sufficient clothing, and a full quantity of wholesome food. . . . Many of the slaves in this part of Virginia live an exceedingly easy life. They labor, it is true, in many cases well and faithfully; but they sleep soundly, eat heartily, sing cheerfully. . . . They are allowed, without constraint, to attend church several times on the Sabbath, and often on other days of the week." As to *Uncle Tom's Cabin,* the people of Norfolk regarded it as the work of a well-meaning but deluded woman, an entirely false picture of slavery and life in general in the South.[26]

Yet they were puzzled at the growing differences between the two great sections, and not a little concerned at the rapidity with which the South was being outdistanced in wealth and population. While King Cotton was fixing the plantation system and slavery more firmly on the South, the Northern states were turning to manufactures. From Boston to the Ohio factory towns had sprung up, and many a spot, formerly given over to corn or wheat, now resounded to the clash of machinery. The country became a dual nation, with two sections of contrasting economic systems, and so of conflicting interests. Since both were under the same Federal government, it was inevitable that there should be a struggle for the control of Congress and the presidency.

In Norfolk, as in other parts of the South, alarm and despondency grew as the North gradually threw its wall of free territory around slavery and used its overwhelming majority in Congress to pass laws harmful to the Southern system. There were some who deplored Virginia's dependence upon agriculture, and urged the shifting of capital and labor into industries. So early as 1827 the Norfolk *Herald,* pointing out that "a fearfully large proportion" of the population was either idle or working part time, suggested the establishment of cotton mills. They "would set the idle to work, draw out hidden wealth, and revive our drooping trade. If the agricultural States of Pennsylvania, Delaware, and Maryland are prospering through manufactures,

[26] Forrest, *Sketches of Norfolk,* pp. 426-428.

why not Virginia and North Carolina? We *can* employ slave labor, but
we have also an abundant free population which needs employment.
At least let us make an effort before resigning ourselves to poverty and
ruin."[27] Despite this appeal Norfolk, like the rest of the South, did not
succeed in building up a system of manufactures. It remained what it
had always been, a port for the agricultural South, shipping out the
tobacco, cotton, and corn of Virginia and North Carolina.

In politics the town was predominantly Whig.[28] For many years there
was a long succession of Norfolk Whigs in the state legislature, and
that party's candidates for the presidency usually carried the borough.
In 1840, when William Henry Harrison was elected, Norfolk celebrated with parades, speeches, and illuminations.[29] Again, in 1848, the
town was wild with joy at the news of the election of General Zachary
Taylor. On November 28 the Whigs held "a grand uproarious, jolly
celebration, marked by a great display of fireworks—in which both
old and young joined—sky-rockets, flying pigeons, Roman candles, pin-
wheels, spit-devils, and fire-crackers." At seven in the evening the procession started amid cheers for "Old Zach." In the lead were a number
of boys bearing torches; then came a band blaring away at "Old Dan
Tucker," and "Old Zach is Coming," followed by a group bearing flags
and portraits of Taylor and Fillmore. Next in order was a wagon
filled with "fat old Whigs," the Hampton Rough and Ready Club,
the Princess Anne Club, the Portsmouth Club, another band, and
finally the Norfolk Rough and Ready Club. As the procession proceeded from street to street, it was greeted with cheers from the throngs
on the sidewalks, and with the waving of handkerchiefs by the ladies
on the balconies and porches. Later that night there was a supper
at Ashland Hall, while throughout the town bonfires flamed, torches
flickered, and cannon thundered.[30]

During the administration of Pierce, the Know-Nothing party gained
hundreds of adherents in Norfolk, and for a time had complete control of the city government. Although the number of immigrants in
the town was small compared with the hordes swarming each year
into the Northern cities, they had aroused no little antipathy. The
Irish were unpopular because they were Roman Catholics; the Germans because of their competition with the native artisans. But, if we
may believe the *Argus,* the Know-Nothing government in Norfolk not

[27] Norfolk *Herald,* Oct. 29, 1827.
[28] Forrest, *Sketches of Norfolk,* p. 394.
[29] Burton, *History of Norfolk,* p. 9.
[30] Norfolk *Beacon,* Nov. 30, 1848.

only tyrannized over Catholics and foreigners but Protestant Americans as well. They opposed and thwarted Mayor Woodis at every turn, displaced able men from the city services and "struck at men in the dark."[31] In 1854 Know-Nothingism had become a burning issue in the town. When the Democrats nominated Henry A. Wise for the governorship, a number of Norfolk citizens asked him if he were a member of the Know-Nothing organization. "No," he replied, "the present state of affairs is not such as to justify the formation, by the people, of any secret political society. . . . In every character, in every relation, in every sense, with all my head, and all my heart, and all my might I protest against this secret organization of native Americans and Protestants to proscribe Roman Catholics and naturalized citizens." With the election of Wise the Know-Nothing movement subsided in Virginia, most of its adherents returning to the Whig party.[32]

On March 21, 1856, the Whigs held a large and enthusiastic meeting in Ashland Hall, where they promised their ardent support to Fillmore and Donelson. The Norfolk _Herald_, on September 20, "hoisted at the head of its editorial columns the Old Line Whig flag," and urged all to vote for Fillmore. For weeks the people could think of nothing, talk of nothing save the approaching election, and Whig or Democratic rallies followed each other in rapid succession. Finally, when election day had passed and it became known that James Buchanan had been elected president, it was the turn of the Democrats to rejoice. On November 26 they held a noisy torchlight procession, while the Whigs looked on in silence.[33]

And now Norfolk watched with growing resentment and alarm, as the march of events hastened the country on to the maelstrom of disunion and civil war—the continued troubles in Kansas, the Dred Scott decision, the Lincoln-Douglas debates, the John Brown raid, the rift in the Democratic party. During the session of the Democratic convention at Charleston, men gathered in groups in the hotel lobbies or on the streets to discuss the latest developments. Excitement reached fever heat when it was known that the Northern Democrats had insisted upon inserting the so-called Freeport Heresy in the party platform,[34] and that the delegates from some of the Southern states had withdrawn from the convention. With a divided Democratic party

[31] Norfolk _Argus_, Feb. 29, 1856.
[32] Burton, _History of Norfolk_, pp. 18, 19.
[33] _Ibid._, pp. 26, 27.
[34] The Freeport Heresy was an attempt to reconcile Squatter Sovereignty with the Dred Scott decision.

and with no more than a remnant of the old Whig party remaining in the field, the triumph of the Republicans was a live possibility. And for the Republicans, the avowed enemies of the Southern economic and social system, to be in control of the government seemed to most Southerners the worst of disasters. "We will not be governed by our enemies," they said; "we will not be reduced to the condition of a conquered people."

Foreboding and gloom increased when the Democrats reassembled at Baltimore, and, after additional Southern states had withdrawn, nominated Stephen A. Douglas for the presidency. The parties were now split along sectional lines, and it seemed certain that the next president would be a Northern man, elected almost entirely by Northern votes. The nomination of John C. Breckenridge by the Southern Democrats, and John Bell by the so-called Constitutional Union party, composed chiefly of Whigs, did not alter the situation, for the chance of success for either was slight. On August 25 Douglas paid Norfolk a visit. He was received with great respect, a committee meeting him at the wharf in Portsmouth, to conduct him across the river to his rooms at the National Hotel. In the evening, when he spoke from the portico of the City Hall, five thousand people, not only from Norfolk and Portsmouth, but from Old Point, Hampton, and the country for miles around, packed every corner of the public square. Douglas pleaded earnestly for Squatter Sovereignty, trying as usual, to reconcile this, his favorite doctrine, with the Dred Scott decision. The crowd listened attentively, but without enthusiasm.[35]

For weeks, now, excitement remained at a high pitch. On all sides could be seen the party standards, some advocating Breckenridge and Lane, some Douglas and Johnson, some Bell and Everett. On September 3 William L. Goggin came to Norfolk to speak in the interest of Bell, and was greeted with the booming of cannon and the cheers of the Whigs.[36] Two weeks later a joint debate between champions of Douglas, Bell, and Breckenridge was held before a large audience in Ashland Hall. Here passions ran so high that fisticuffs occurred between a Bell elector and a Breckenridge elector.[37] A few days before the election Henry A. Wise spoke in the Opera House, packed to its

[35] Norfolk *Argus*, Aug. 27, 1860. "I drove to Norfolk," says John S. Wise in *The End of an Era*, "and seeing a great crowd assembled, paused and heard part of a speech by Stephan A. Douglas. I was greatly impressed by his tremendous voice, every tone of which reached me more than a block away." J. S. Wise, *The End of an Era* (Boston, 1899), p. 156.

[36] Burton, *History of Norfolk*, p. 40.

[37] *Ibid.*, p. 40.

utmost capacity, in favor of "the Constitution, the Union, and the true National Democracy."[38] The vote in Norfolk followed traditional lines, for Bell received a clear majority over the other three candidates, with 986 votes, to 438 for Breckenridge, 232 for Douglas and none for Lincoln. In Portsmouth Bell polled 676 votes, Breckenridge 558, Douglas 210 and Lincoln 4.[39]

In the country as a whole the result was quite different, Lincoln securing 180 electoral votes to 72 for Breckenridge, 39 for Bell, and 12 for Douglas. The fact that Lincoln had triumphed was known in Norfolk the next day, the *Argus* carrying an article headed "Triumph of the Black Republicans." "Aaron's rod had swallowed up all the rest," it said. "The returns which came pouring in upon us yesterday, confirmed our fears by showing, in the roundest figures, that fanaticism and hostility to the social conditions of the South, have received a sectional sanction to take possession of the administrative powers of the Federal Government. The program of aggression is fully marked out; and the demon of discord may now stalk on 'with pomp and circumstance' 'conquering and to conquer' so far as any hope of protection of our rights by the Federal arm remain to us. If we wish to preserve our liberty, we must look to ourselves, and not to those who scarcely deign to call themselves our fellow countrymen. Thanks to the blood of our forefathers, there is spirit yet left in the South, and the few coming months may prove themselves big with deliverance from the yoke of what is fast growing to be an intolerable bondage."[40]

Two days later this article was followed by another, openly suggesting secession. "Sooner or later the ties which now link together the North and South must be sundered. How closely the inevitable effect will follow the cause, may be a matter of speculation, but it can only be a matter of time. When those shall govern the confederacy who pronounce Southern life utter 'barbarism,' and denounce as 'the sum of all villanies' a practice on which our whole section sustains itself, the South must secede if secession be practicable."[41] But such utterances were premature. A majority of the people of Norfolk were not yet ready to sever the bond of union which had existed for over seventy years, and which they still regarded with pride. The traditions of friendship with the North were strong—those memories of the Revolution, of the War of 1812, and of the still more recent sympathy

---

[38] Norfolk *Argus*, Nov. 2, 1860.
[39] *Ibid.*, Nov. 7, 1860.
[40] *Ibid.*, Nov. 8, 1860.
[41] *Ibid.*, Nov. 10, 1860.

and aid which Norfolk herself had received during the yellow fever epidemic. One correspondent to the *Herald* actually advised Virginia to throw in her lot with the North rather than the cotton states. "Their slave property, both by the duty and policy of the free States, would be secured, until it could be gotten rid of by gradual sales. There would be, on the part of the free States, a cordial and sincere co-operation in this scheme."

This suggestion found little favor, however, and the spirit of resistance, fanned by news of happenings in the cotton states, made rapid progress. In December a large group of Norfolk men formed an association to resist any hostile aggression upon Southern rights by the Federal government. "In order to present a united front to the bigotry and fanaticism which possess those who war against our institutions and social conditions," they declared, "we ignore all former political ties. . . . In consideration of the impending crisis, caused by the threatening attitude and triumph of a sectional party, who are pledged to deadly hostility against our institutions, our section, and our dearest interests, we form a society, the Southern Rights Association, and Minute Men of Norfolk, Virginia. We pledge ourselves to sustain the equality of Virginia in the Union, or failing in that, to unite under her authority, with any or all of our sister States . . . to resist the aggressive and fanatic power of the North, even (as a last resort) to secession from such an odious Union as now exists."[42]

A few days later the entire town was thrown into intense excitement by the news that South Carolina had passed her ordinance of secession. Many of the older men considered this act rash and premature, and earnestly advised Virginia against following suit. The *Herald* was strongly Unionist in sentiment. Why should we "dance crazily out of the Union to the fiddling of South Carolina?" it asked. On the other hand, the *Argus* greeted the news with enthusiasm. "Right nobly have the proud and brave sons of South Carolina met the emergency! At one stroke they have severed the chains which bound them to a tyrannous North, and they now stand before the world an independent people! . . . Other States will follow. . . . A new confederacy will be formed, one of equal rights and honest execution, and American will become what destiny has writ of her—the cynosure of mankind."[43] On December 21, the Norfolk Minute Men sent their greetings to the South Carolina Convention: "With the

[42] *Ibid.,* Dec. 15, 1860.
[43] *Ibid.,* December 22, 1860.

glorious Palmetto flag thrown to the breeze, and flying over our heads, we have just fired fifteen guns in honor of the first step taken by your gallant State, emblematic, we hope, of coming events. All honor and glory to 'the game cock' of the South.''[44]

As one Southern state after another went out of the Union, the excitement in Norfolk grew. On January 4, the people observed the "fast and prayer day" proclaimed by President Buchanan;[45] on the fifth, hundreds of men thronged into Ashland Hall, to take steps for the organization of the military forces of the city. All the speakers emphasized Norfolk's attachment to the Union, but demanded guarantees for the safety and honor of the state. Should the Federal government continue to trample on Southern rights, Norfolk must do her part in defending them, by force of arms if necessary.[46] In the meanwhile all eyes were turned on Richmond, where the legislature was debating the question of calling a state convention. In the street, at the dinner table, everywhere, men asked each other, "What is the news from the Capitol?" At length it became known that the bill for the convention had passed by large majorities, and Norfolk made ready for the election of her delegate.

On January 24 the secession group met in Ashland Hall to nominate their candidate and, after several fiery addresses, named James R. Hubard.[47] The Union Conservatives nominated General George Blow. For the next few days the town was filled with the contentions of the two groups, every street corner being turned into a debating club, in which the merits of Secession or of Unionism were loudly proclaimed. The election itself, which was held February 4, resulted in a victory for the Union men. General Blow receiving 992 to 442 for Mr. Hubard. In fact the Unionists swept all Virginia, and entered the convention with an overwhelming majority. Apparently the new Confederacy, which was even then forming at Montgomery, would have to fight its battles without the aid of the Old Dominion.[48]

Yet the Norfolk secessionists did not despair. When word came of the election and inauguration of Jefferson Davis, sentiment began to swing their way. Now that an organized union of Southern states existed, ready and anxious to welcome her, to break with the old Union

[44] *Ibid.*
[45] Burton, *History of Norfolk,* p. 42.
[46] *Ibid.*
[47] *Ibid.,* pp. 42, 43.
[48] James C. McGregor, *The Disruption of Virginia* (New York, 1922), p. 110.

seemed less like a leap in the dark. Some of the more ardent young men began leaving for Charleston to join the Confederate army.[49]

Such was the situation when Abraham Lincoln was inaugurated. In his address the President announced his intention of maintaining the Union, if necessary, by force. "I shall take care," he said, "as the Constitution itself expressly enjoins upon me, that the laws of the Union be faithfully executed in all the States." This declaration produced a profound impression in Norfolk. The *Day Book,* an anti-secessionist paper, was bitter in its denunciation. "Lincoln, the wild, political despot of the West, whose head has been crazed by the doctrines and isms of Horace Greely, has proclaimed to those who had patience to hope better things of him, that they must hope no longer. His inaugural has gone forth to the world—carrying with it the declaration of coercion, fully and explicitly announced. It has told the millions of inhabitants of this country, who hoped for peace from his lips, that they shall have no peace. He proclaims to the South war! war! war!"[50] Even the *Herald* warned the people that the address had extinguished the last hope of a peaceful settlement.[51]

The Union delegates at Richmond were now in a quandary. With the press of all eastern and central Virginia unanimous that the state could not continue in the old Union should it begin war on the Confederacy, and with Lincoln's assurance that he intended to use the army and navy for that purpose, the secessionists pressed the fight with renewed hope. They were seconded by a volley of resolutions from meetings in many cities and towns, all demanding immediate withdrawal from the Union.[52] In Norfolk a huge assemblage of people in Mechanics Hall, after listening to many fiery addresses, adopted a resolution instructing General Blow to cast his vote for secession.[53] Already some impatient soul had unfurled the Confederate flag, with its seven stars encircling the letters "Va.," from the roof of a house on Wolfe Street,[54] and now a party of young men sailed down to Craney

---

[49] Burton, *History of Norfolk,* p. 43.

[50] *Ibid.,* pp. 43, 44.

[51] Norfolk *Herald,* March 6, 1860.

[52] McGregor, *The Disruption of Virginia,* p. 143.

[53] Burton, *History of Norfolk,* p. 44. Mechanics Hall was built in 1850 on the south side of Main Street a few doors east of Market Square (now Commercial Place) (Forrest, *Sketches of Norfolk,* p. 251). This apparently was the building at 159 Main Street, listed in the 1886 directory as Heptasophian Hall. It was on the site later occupied by the Gaiety Theater (earlier called the Majestic) until it was demolished in 1960. Letter of Col. E. Griffith Dodson to the editor, March 20, 1961.

[54] Burton, *History of Norfolk,* p. 44.

Island and hoisted the colors over the old blockhouse there.[55] The city was expecting and ready for secession and war.

Events moved rapidly to the climax. On April 12 a dispatch was received from Charleston telling of the bombardment of Fort Sumter. Then came the news of the surrender, followed by President Lincoln's call for seventy-five thousand volunteers. "Business was almost suspended. The people assembled upon the streets, discussing the situation, breathlessly awaiting the decision of the convention at Richmond, and listening to popular harangues. The local militia, anticipating the result, assembled, and paraded the streets with bands and Southern flags."[56] When news arrived that the convention, amid scenes of excitement bordering on hysteria, had passed an ordinance of secession by eighty-five votes to fifty-five,[57] "it was greeted with great cheering, the firing of guns, and every demonstration of excited enthusiasm."[58] Virginia had remained loyal to the Union until Mr. Lincoln forced upon her the option of fighting for or against the new Confederacy. Acquiescing heartily in the decision of the convention, Norfolk now began active preparations for the struggle.

[55] *Ibid.*
[56] Wise, *The End of an Era*, p. 160.
[57] McGregor, *The Disruption of Virginia*, p. 176.
[58] Wise, *The End of an Era*, p. 160. Many of the officers at the Navy Yard at once resigned to take service under the Confederacy. A prominent exception was David Farragut, who turned his back on his old associates and his wife's family, to remain faithful to the Federal government (Albert Mordell, *Farragut at the Crossroads*, Annapolis, 1931).

CHAPTER TEN

The Mailed Fist

Saturday, April 20, 1861, was a day of intense excitement in Norfolk. One rumor had it that the frigate *Cumberland* was about to bombard the city, another that the Navy Yard was to be destroyed, still another that all the vessels there were to be scuttled. The Norfolk and Portsmouth militia were under arms, and during the day the Richmond Grays and six companies from Petersburg, arrived by railway.[1] General William B. Taliaferro would have done well, perhaps, to employ these troops for an immediate attack upon the Navy Yard. Here were the *Merrimac*, the old *Pennsylvania*, the *Columbus*, the *Delaware*, the *New York*, and other vessels which would have been invaluable as a nucleus to the Confederate navy; here were vast stores of guns, small arms, rope, sails, and naval stores of all kinds; here machine shops, foundries, and docks. But General Taliaferro lacked the guns to contend with the warships, or marines to carry them by boarding. It would have required only a few minutes to capture the Navy Yard, he thought, but to hold it under the guns of the ships was another matter.[2] While he was debating this point, a Federal officer came from the yard under a flag of truce. He was conducted to the Atlantic Hotel, where in the presence of the Confederate commanders he gave assurance that none of the vessels would be removed, and that not a shot would be fired.[3] This confirmed General Taliaferro in his determination to withhold his hand.

The conference was no sooner over, however, than Commodore Charles S. McCauley, in command at the Navy Yard, gave orders

---

[1] B. J. Lossing *Pictorial History of the Civil War* (Philadelphia, 1866-68), I, 395.
[2] Stewart, *History of Norfolk County*, pp. 69, 70.
[3] Lossing, *Pictorial History of the Civil War*, I, 395; Virginia Gordan Scrap Book (an unpublished collection of clippings from newspapers during the Civil War, in possession of Mr. John D. Gordan, of Norfolk).

for the scuttling of all the Federal vessels save the *Cumberland*. Hardly had this been done when the *Pawnee,* bearing Rear-Admiral Paulding and several hundred men, came steaming up the Southern Branch. Paulding had orders to take off every ship afloat there, and was deeply chagrined when he found the *Merrimac* and others slowly settling to the bottom. So he made preparations to destroy the Navy Yard and to draw off the men. All that afternoon and evening the Federals worked, knocking the trunnions off cannons, breaking machinery, placing combustibles in buildings and vessels preparatory to firing them. One man spent his time rolling cannon balls into the river. At last, at two in the morning, the soldiers, marines, sailors, and workmen were taken on board the *Pawnee* and the *Cumberland*. At 3:20 A.M., when these vessels moved out into the river, a rocket was sent up from the *Pawnee,* as a signal for the firing of the Navy Yard.[4] In a few moments the flames shot up from building after building, while the great ship-of-the-line *Pennsylvania,* the *Merrimac,* and other vessels became floating furnaces. "The scene was grand and terrific beyond description. The roar of the conflagration was loud enough to be heard at three or four miles distance, and to this were added occasional discharges from the heavy guns of the old *Pennsylvania.*"[5]

No sooner had the Federals gone than the Virginia troops rushed in to grapple with the flames. Despite their efforts, when morning came the ship houses, some workshops, the old marine barracks, and several other buildings were in ashes; the *New York,* on the stocks, was totally consumed; the *Pennsylvania, Dolphin,* and *Columbia* were burned to the water's edge; the *Merrimac* and *Germantown* partly burnt and sunk; the *Plymouth, Columbus,* and *Delaware* scuttled. Yet many valuable buildings escaped, and the dry dock was uninjured. It is stated that the master's mate, who had orders to blow up the dry dock, lighted the fuse, but instead of igniting the powder train with it, threw it in the water. This he did in order to prevent loss of life to women and children from stones hurled into the city by the powder mine.[6] Hundreds of fine cannon were found ready for duty.[7] The importance of this capture for the Confederacy can hardly be overestimated. Could the Southern naval constructors secure seasoned timbers and proper engines, eventually they might send out from the Elizabeth warships

[4] Lossing, *Pictorial History of the Civil War,* I, 395-397.
[5] Virginia Gordan Scrap Book; Edward L. Pierce, *Addresses and Papers* (Boston, 1896) , pp. 8-10; J. W. H. Porter, *A Record* (Portsmouth, Va., 1892) , pp. 12-16.
[6] Porter, *A Record,* pp. 15-16.
[7] *Ibid.,* p. 22.

capable of contesting with the Federal navy. They might break up the blockade, open the channels of trade, and secure for the Confederacy the all-important European goods. They might guard the sounds, bays, and rivers, closing them to the Northern warships and transports, and rendering invaluable aid to the Confederate armies. In other words, Norfolk was the sole hope of a Confederate navy, and a navy was almost the sole hope of victory and independence.

General Taliaferro took immediate steps to fortify Norfolk and Portsmouth. Earthworks were erected on Hospital Point, a battery set up at Fort Norfolk, the works on Craney Island repaired, and a battery placed on Sewells Point.[8] It was at the last named place that the first encounter with the Federal navy took place. On May 19, 1861, when the Confederates were just mounting their guns, a shot from the steamer *Monticello* landed in their midst. "Never was a battery worse prepared. The guns were not in order, not a sight had been placed on them, . . . consequently the firing was at random and very few shots were effective." The *Monticello* was joined by an armed tug, and the two vessels continued the cannonade until the close of day. The next morning the *Monticello* opened again, but during the night the Confederates had completed their preparations, and their fire was now so hot that after an hour and a half she retired to Old Point.[9] The fortification of the Elizabeth now went forward rapidly. Twenty-nine guns were set up at Sewells Point, fifteen at Fort Norfolk, sixteen at Fort Nelson, eleven at Pinner's Point, ten at Lamberts Point, five on Tanner's Creek, five on Boush's Bluff, and forty-five in various entrenchments.[10]

Those were exciting days for Norfolk. Troops were constantly arriving over the Seaboard and the Petersburg railways, and marching off to the encampments around the two towns.[11] As they swung through the streets, under the flags of North Carolina, of Georgia, or of Virginia, people lined the sidewalks or crowded the windows, waving handkerchiefs and cheering. Nothing was too good for the visiting troops. The ladies sat up at night to mend their clothes and darn their socks, while in the day they visited the camps with fruit and other delicacies. There were frequent field ceremonies, in which this regiment received a Confederate flag, or that colonel a spirited horse. One week the soldiers gave a concert in the Opera House for the sick

[8] Stewart, *History of Norfolk County*, p. 70.
[9] *Ibid.*, pp. 74, 75; Burton, *History of Norfolk*, pp. 47-50.
[10] Stewart, *History of Norfolk County*, pp. 75, 76; Porter, *A Record*, p. 23.
[11] Richmond *Dispatch*, May 10, 1861.

in camp, the next a group of little girls held a fair, the next the ladies of the Catholic church gave a benefit for the families of the city volunteers. When word came that Governor Letcher had appointed as commander of the Virginia forces General Robert E. Lee, there was much surprise among soldiers and townspeople. "Who is he? Where did he come from?" everyone asked. Few dreamed that their new leader was destined to become one of the greatest military leaders of all time. There was less surprise and more satisfaction when General Benjamin Huger, of South Carolina, arrived to take command of the Norfolk district.[12]

Brawls and barroom fights were not uncommon in Norfolk in the first weeks of the war, but with the arrival of General Huger they were suppressed with a stern hand. "There were no important cases in Mayor Lamb's court this morning," wrote a correspondent to the Richmond *Dispatch* on August 17, 1861. "The watchmen of the night reported no arrests or cases of disorder." A powerful Federal fleet, assembled in Hampton Roads, maintained a complete blockade of the Elizabeth, and so stopped all direct trade with foreign countries and with other Virginia ports. For a time vessels continued to pass through the canals to North Carolina, but this trade, too, eventually was blocked. Prices for foodstuffs began to rise, flour selling at $8.50 a barrel, coffee at fifty cents a pound, sugar at fifteen cents, potatoes at one dollar a bushel. Fish were plentiful, and, together with corn bread, formed the mainstay of every table. There was no unemployment, for the men who had not joined the army or navy were needed in the small manufacturing plants which had been started to supply goods formerly imported.[13]

In the midst of the general confidence and enthusiasm, came news of a disaster, so unexpected and so far-reaching as to shroud the city in gloom. It was on January 11, 1862, that a fleet of over a hundred gunboats, tugs, and transports, bearing sixteen thousand Federal troops, sailed from Hampton Roads out into the Atlantic. This expedition, under General Ambrose E. Burnside and Flag-Officer Louis M. Goldsborough, was directed against Pamlico and Albemarle sounds. These leaders found the Confederates unprepared. The government at Richmond would have been wise had it established at the outset of the war, at each of the inlets through the North Carolina bars, impregnable forts, backed by every available gunboat. It was of vital importance to

[12] Burton, *History of Norfolk*, pp. 46-67.
[13] *Ibid.*, p. 61.

keep the Federals out of these inland seas. Here was a doorway for European commerce which the Federal blockading fleet would have found it difficult to close, for the storms off Cape Hatteras were frequent, and there were no near-by harbors. On the other hand, a Union force in Albemarle Sound would be a constant menace to Norfolk and the Navy Yard, and so to the infant Confederate navy, for a short march up the Chowan would place them athwart the Seaboard Railway, the chief artery of communication with the South. But Fort Hatteras and Fort Clark, at the Hatteras inlet, had been captured by a Federal fleet in August, 1861, and the way into Pamlico Sound was now open to Burnside's expedition.[14]

However, the way to Albemarle Sound was still blocked by Confederate fortifications at Roanoke Island. Situated between the two great sounds with a narrow channel on each side, this place, which was a bulwark for all northeastern Carolina, could easily have been made impregnable. But the Confederates had contented themselves with placing batteries, mounting forty guns in all, on either side of the island, sinking vessels in the main channel, sending up a flotilla of pigmy gunboats, and reinforcing the garrison until it numbered several thousand men. General Henry A. Wise, realizing that his force was inadequate, implored the government at Richmond to send him a part of the sixteen thousand men at Norfolk. Roanoke Island is the key to Norfolk, he said. It unlocks two sounds, eight rivers, four canals, two railways, and the region from which the city draws four-fifths of its supplies. It should be defended at the expense of twenty thousand men, and many millions of dollars.[15] But his warning availed nothing, and he was left alone to fight Burnside's overwhelming force.

On February 7 the Federal gunboats moved up the west channel and began an engagement with the batteries. The Union guns were of heavier caliber and far more numerous, so that after a short encounter, the redoubts began to crumble, the flagstaff was shot away, and one battery after the other put out of action. Thereupon the Federal troops landed, and the next morning, moved forward to the attack. The little Confederate army fought desperately, several times repulsing the enemy, but they were outnumbered three to one, and at last began to waver. At this moment a determined charge by the New York Zouaves broke their line and swept it back toward the shore.

---

[14] Lossing, *Pictorial History of the Civil War*, II, 168, 169.
[15] Lossing, *Pictorial History of the Civil War*, pp. 173, 174.

Here, since there were not enough boats to convey the men over to Nag's Head on the bar, most of them had to surrender. A few escaped and made their way up the bar to Norfolk.[16]

The Southern press criticized the administration bitterly for this disaster. "We all knew of the fitting out of the Burnside expedition, of its presence off the Carolina coast, of its intention of attacking Roanoke Island; we all knew that the force on the island was inadequate to its defence," said the Norfolk *Day Book*. "Yet that handful of brave and devoted men were suffered to remain there insufficiently reinforced, . . . to be 'butchered to make a Northern holiday.' . . . If the vulnerable points on our extended coast are to be defended at all, let them be defended effectively. . . . We ought to have had in the sound twenty gunboats or more. . . . Ten months have elapsed since the Navy Yard here came providentially into our possession—and fifty such gunboats might have been easily constructed there. . . . But there has not one single such been here constructed. . . . Let it never be lost sight of for a moment at a time, that this point, this Navy Yard, is one of incalculable importance to the Southern Confederacy."[17]

Although there was much truth in this criticism, it is not true that the Navy Yard had been put to no important use. In fact Secretary Stephen R. Mallory had been moving heaven and earth to turn out warships capable of holding their own with the Federal frigates, by converting one or more of the scuttled vessels in the Southern Branch into ironclad steamers. Since the *Plymouth* and the *Germantown* were sailing vessels, it was decided to make the experiment with what was left of the *Merrimac*. In November 1861, the New York *Tribune* published a letter from one Henry Davis, a Northerner just returned from Norfolk. "The *Merrimac* has been transformed into a great battering ram, with a steel nose, for running down vessels," he wrote. "All her internal works are completed, but her plating is only partially effected as yet. . . . Her engines are four feet below the water line, and her sides slope inward. She is to be covered overhead with a bomb-proof network of railroad iron. . . . Her armament is to be of the heaviest and best rifled cannon known, and there is no doubt, if she has a

[16] *Ibid.*, pp. 170-176; Richmond *Dispatch*, Feb. 13, 1862; Norfolk *Day Book*, Feb. 12, 1862.

[17] Norfolk *Day Book*, Feb. 12, 1862. It is stated by J. W. H. Porter in *A Record*, that Naval Constructor John L. Porter, in June, 1861, urged upon Secretary of the Navy Mallory the importance of importing from England steam engines and armor plate for gunboats before the Southern ports were blockaded. Mallory turned a deaf ear, and awakened to the importance of the matter only when it was too late.

chance, she will do an immense amount of damage to our fleet." This strange monster, which could no longer be recognized as the graceful *Merrimac*, the Confederates christened the *Virginia*. The transformation was accomplished under the supervision of William P. Williamson, John L. Porter, and John M. Brooke, all formerly officers in the United States Navy.

In the meanwhile, President Lincoln, Secretary Stanton, and General McClellan were preparing to hurl the great Army of the Potomac against Virginia in an effort to capture Richmond. Two routes presented themselves: by water to Fort Monroe and up the York River; or by land through Manassas and Fredericksburg. The former was selected, and warships and transports assembled at Washington. But before the expedition could move, the absolute mastery of Chesapeake Bay had to be assured, and early in March this mastery was challenged by the *Virginia*. It was at eleven on the morning of the eighth that the ironclad left the Navy Yard, accompanied by the little river boats *Beaufort* and *Raleigh,* and passed slowly down the Elizabeth, amid the prayers of the throngs on shore and the salutes of the Confederate batteries. A few minutes later the lookouts on the Federal warships were startled to see the strange vessel pass Sewells Point and head west for Newport News. To them she looked like "a submerged house, with the roof only above water," set off by the Confederate flag and a smokestack.[18]

At the mouth of the James River, riding at anchor, were the *Cumberland,* of twenty-two guns, and the *Congress,* of fifty guns, so little expectant of danger that their boats were swinging at the lower booms and washed clothes were hanging in the rigging. As the *Virginia* bore down upon these vessels, inactivity gave place to stir and bustle, as the crews prepared for the battle. "My hearties," said the captain of the *Congress,* "you see before you the great Southern bugaboo, got up to fright us out of our wits. Stand to your guns, and let me assure you that one good broadside from our gallant frigate, and she is ours." With a tremendous roar the *Congress* opened. But when the balls glanced off harmlessly from the ironclad superstructure, all on board the frigate realized that their vessel was doomed. In the meanwhile, two Confederate steamers, the *Patrick Henry* and the *Jamestown,* had come down the James River to enter the battle. On the other hand,

[18] Virginius Newton, *Merrimac or Virginia* (Richmond, 1907), pp. 10-11; Virginia Gordan Scrap Book; John M. Brooke, "The Merrimac, or Virginia, her Real Projector," *Southern Historical Society Papers,* XIX, 1.

the Federal batteries at Newport News began firing upon the Southern warships, in a vain effort to save the two frigates. Slowly the grim *Virginia* approached the *Cumberland*. Reserving her fire until within close range she opened with her bow rifle with telling effect. Then, without stopping, she rammed the frigate, "striking her about midships, and literally laying open her side." Reversing her engines, the *Virginia* drew off, leaving her ram in the wound it had made. The *Cumberland* at once began to sink, her crew cheering and firing to the last.[19]

The *Virginia* now turned around and headed for the *Congress*. The latter had slipped her cable, and was making for shoal waters under the protection of the land batteries when she grounded. With head inshore, and unable to use all her guns, she was raked by the great ironclad and the James River gunboats. A shot from the *Virginia's* bow gun crashed through one of the ports, overturning two cannon, and killing sixteen men. As the ship was now littered with dead and dying men and was afire in three separate places, after an hour's gallant resistance, she struck her colors. When the crew of the *Beaufort* boarded the *Congress* to take off the wounded, a terrible scene met their eyes. "Confusion, death, and pitiable suffering reigned supreme, and the horrors of war quenched the passion and enmity of months." Unfortunately as the Confederates were about to move the prisoners, Federal infantry on shore fired with deadly effect, forcing the *Beaufort* to draw off. Thereupon the *Virginia* opened again on the luckless *Congress*. In the meanwhile, the *Minnesota, Roanoke,* and *St. Lawrence,* which had been lying off Old Point Comfort while trying to come to the assistance of the two helpless frigates, all went aground. The *Minnesota* stuck so fast that all efforts to get her afloat proved futile, and she would have proved an easy victim for the *Virginia,* had not the lowering tide forced that vessel to withdraw to deep anchorage off Sewells Point. That night several boatloads of Confederates rowed out to the *Congress* and set her on fire.[20]

As the news of this battle was flashed over the country, something akin to panic seized the North. "The blockade . . . could not last long before this mighty and invulnerable engine of destruction," it was said. "New York, Boston, and Washington would soon be threatened. . . . As the sun went down that night over Hampton Roads,

[19] Newton, *Merrimac or Virginia;* Virginia Gordan Scrap Book.
[20] Virginia Gordan Scrap Book; E. V. White, *The First Iron-Clad Naval Engagement* (New York, 1906) .

Illustrations

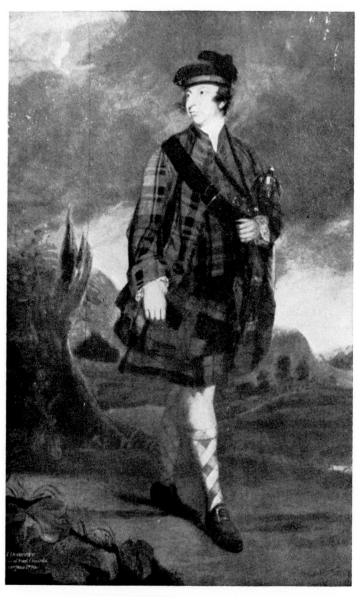

Plate I. Lord Dunmore. The last royal governor of Virginia. His occupation of Norfolk led to the city's destruction during the Revolution. From the Virginia Historical Society copy of the portrait by Sir Joshua Reynolds.

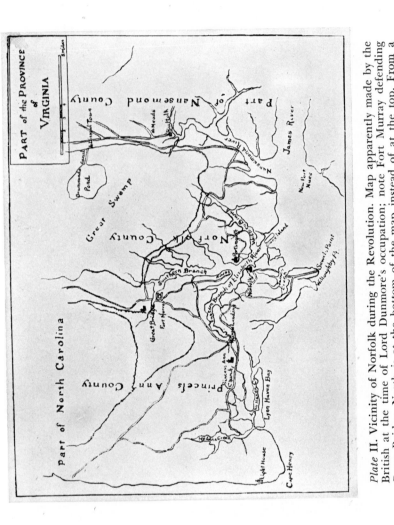

Plate II. Vicinity of Norfolk during the Revolution. Map apparently made by the British at the time of Lord Dunmore's occupation; note Fort Murray defending Great Bridge. North is at the bottom of the map instead of at the top. From a tracing of the original in the Library of Congress.

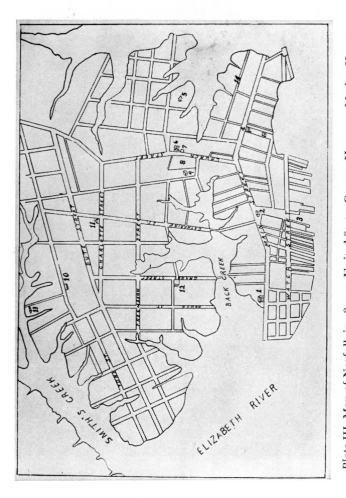

Plate III. Map of Norfolk in 1802. 1, United States Custom House; 2, Market House; 3, County Dock; 4, Town Hall; 5, Catholic Church; 6, Christ Episcopal Church; 7, Norfolk Academy; 8, Old Borough Church (now St. Paul's Church) and Graveyard; 9, Methodist Church; 10, Work House; 11, Presbyterian Church; 12, United States Bank; 13, The Magazine; 14, Bermuda Street. Traced from the George Nicholson map of 1802, so far as known the earliest complete map of Norfolk extant.

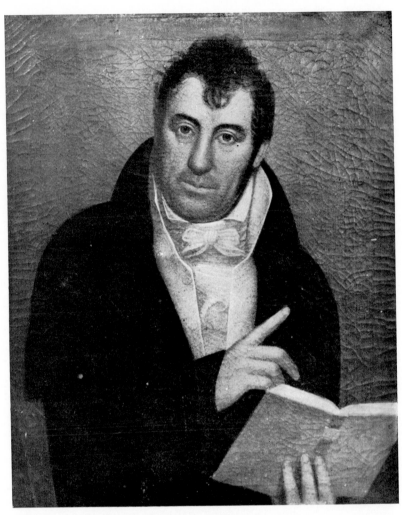

Plate IV. General Robert B. Taylor, commander of the American forces in the battle of Craney Island.

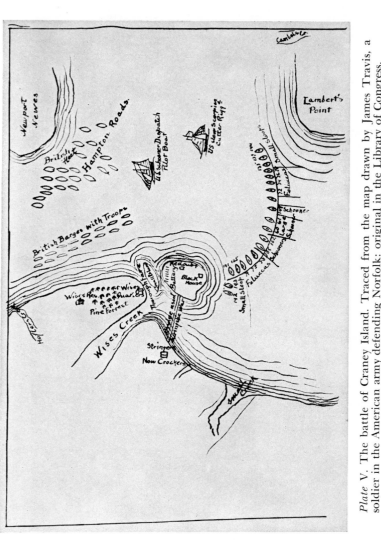

Plate V. The battle of Craney Island. Traced from the map drawn by James Travis, a soldier in the American army defending Norfolk: original in the Library of Congress.

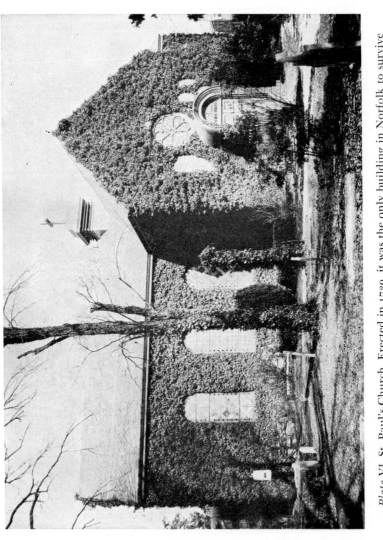

Plate VI. St. Paul's Church. Erected in 1739, it was the only building in Norfolk to survive the Revolution.

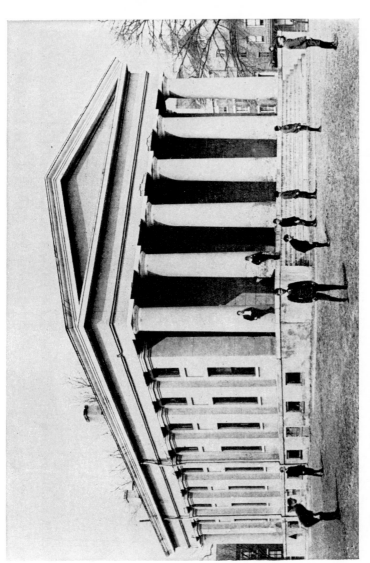

Plate VII. Norfolk Academy. Modeled on the temple of Theseus in Athens, the building was constructed in 1840.

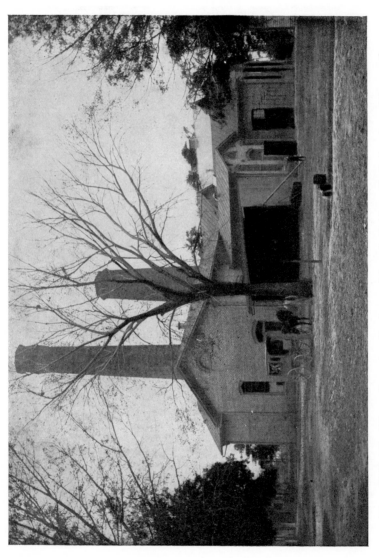

Plate VIII. The Water Pumping Station at Moore's Bridges. Built in 1873, this was the beginning of the city water system.

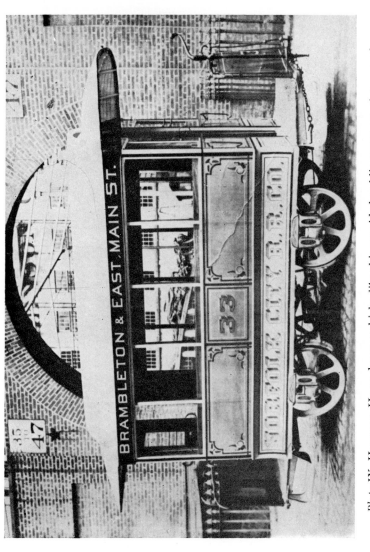

Plate IX. Horsecar. Horse-drawn vehicles like this provided public transportation over the city streets until the arrival of the electric trolley car in 1894.

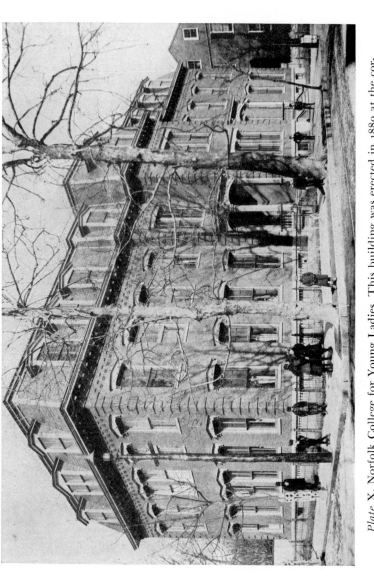

Plate X. Norfolk College for Young Ladies. This building was erected in 1880 at the corner of Granby Street and College Place.

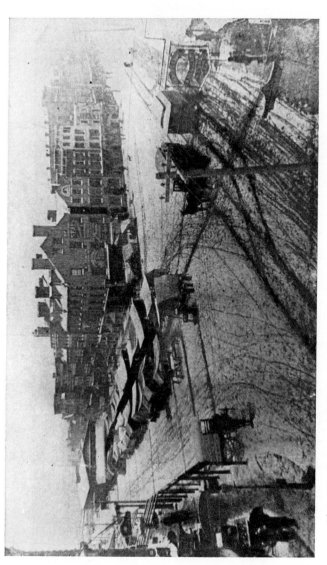

Plate XI. Commercial Place Looking towards the Ferry. This view, taken in 1888, shows the market stalls. One of the Main Street horsecars is directly behind the telephone pole.

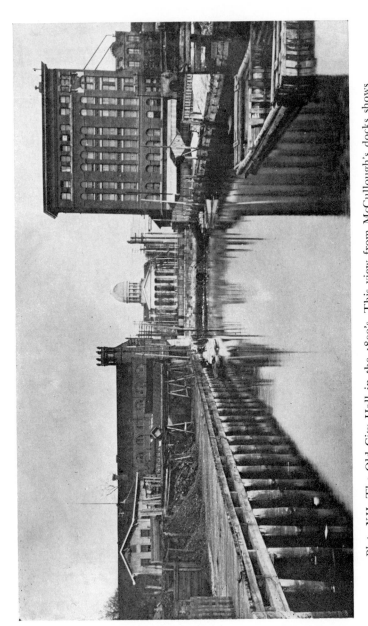

Plate XII. The Old City Hall in the 1890's. This view from McCullough's docks shows City Hall Avenue after it was filled in 1884, ending on Granby Street. To the left is the Armory, to the right the Haddington and Taylor buildings.

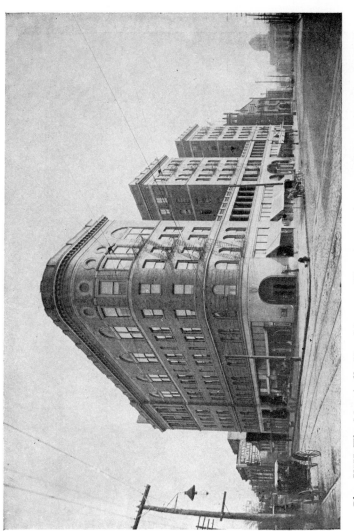

Plate XIII. The Monticello Hotel in 1902. The view on the opposite page was transformed by the erection of this hotel. Note the Armory and the old City Hall on the right; to the left is one of the family homes still surviving in 1902, and beyond it is the Granby Family Theatre.

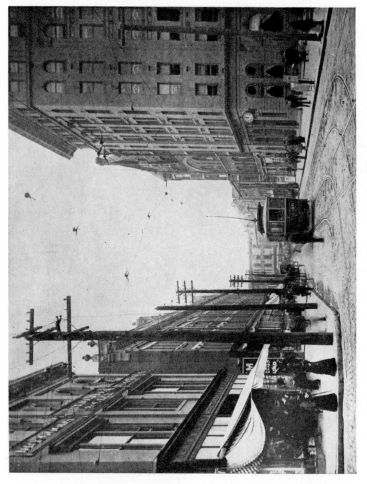

Plate XIV. Main Street looking east from Granby. This 1902 view shows one of the new trolley cars, introduced in 1894.

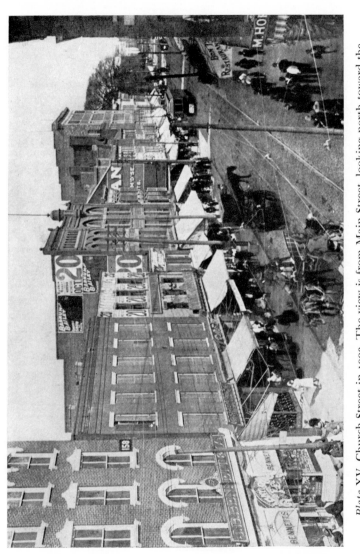

Plate XV. Church Street in 1902. The view is from Main Street, looking north toward the churchyard of St. Paul's.

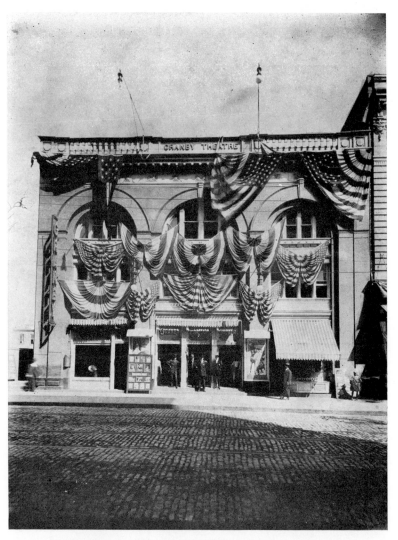

Plate XVI. The Granby Family Theatre. The theater is decorated with flags in honor of the opening of the Jamestown Exposition, April 24, 1907. Note at the right the edge of a new building erected between the theater and the Monticello after the picture of the hotel was taken in 1902.

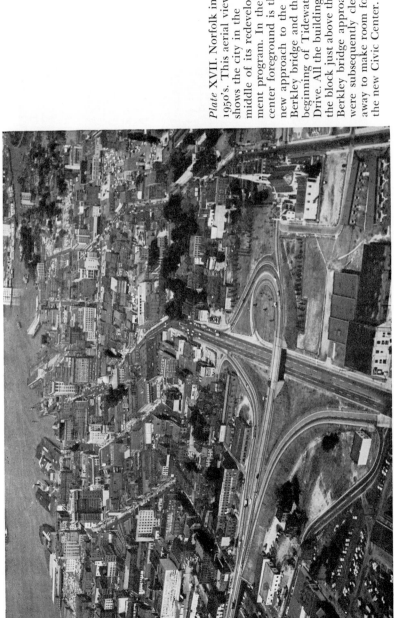

Plate XVII. Norfolk in the 1950's. This aerial view shows the city in the middle of its redevelopment program. In the center foreground is the new approach to the new Berkley bridge and the beginning of Tidewater Drive. All the buildings in the block just above the Berkley bridge approach were subsequently cleared away to make room for the new Civic Center.

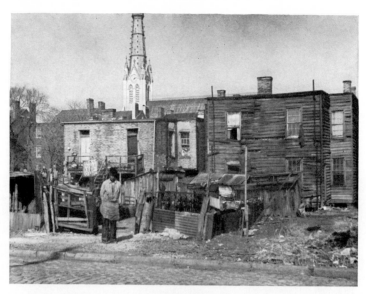

Plate XVIII. The Norfolk Redevelopment Program: Public
Housing. Above are several of the houses torn down in the
slum clearance program; below is a view of one of the housing projects that replaced the slum.

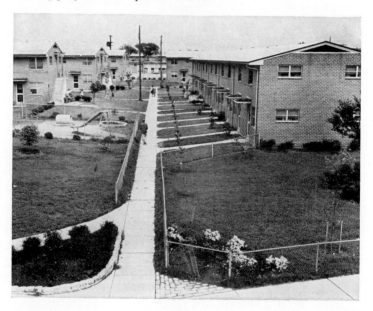

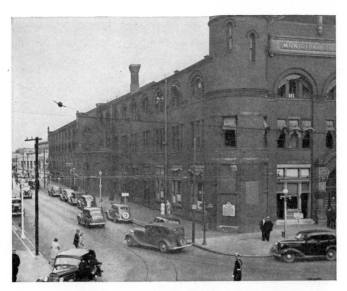

Plate XIX. The Norfolk Redevelopment Program: Private Investment. Above is the old Armory, converted into the Municipal Building, as it looked in 1936, with the city market behind it; below is the Rennert building, with its Maritime Tower, which replaced it at the end of the 1950's.

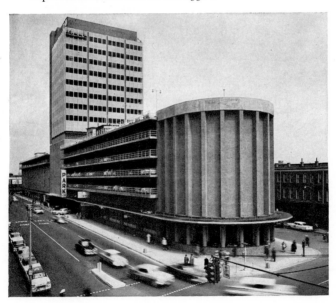

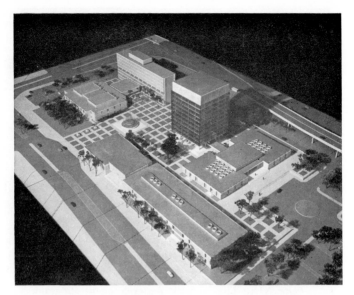

Plate XX. Norfolk of the 1960's. Above is a model of
the completed Civic Center; the Public Safety Building at the top was opened in 1961, with the other
structures scheduled to be finished by 1964. Below is
an artist's drawing of the new public library building
as it would look when completed.

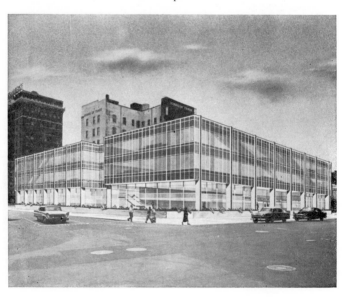

every Union heart in the fleet and in the fortress throbbed with despair." "Oh! what a night that was!" said an eyewitness at Old Point.
"The heavens were aflame with the burning *Congress.* The hotel was
crowded with fugitives. . . . There was nothing to dispute the empire
of the seas with the *Merrimac,* and had a land attack been made by
Magruder then, God only knows what our fate would have been!" Yet
this alarm was in large measure groundless. The *Virginia* could not
lift the blockade and attack New York, because she was not a seagoing vessel and would have foundered the moment she got outside
of the Capes; she could not go to Baltimore or Washington, because
she drew too much water. She was suited only for fighting in Hampton
Roads and adjacent waters, and even there the enemy, in order to
elude her, had only to avoid the deepest channels. This should have
been obvious to all after the next day's battle.

At 8:30 on the morning of March 9 the *Virginia,* with the *Patrick
Henry* and the *Jamestown,* opened fire on the *Minnesota,* which was
still fast aground. Before they could disable her, however, "the Ericsson Battery, now called the *Monitor,* was discovered off Newport
News," bearing down upon them. This strange craft had arrived late
the evening before, and was now ready to try conclusions with the
dreaded Southern fighter. As she approached, the *Patrick Henry* and
the *Jamestown* now retired, for they could not face her heavy guns, and
a battle royal followed between the two ironclads. Shot after shot
was hurled against the slanting sides of the *Virginia,* broadside after
broadside pelted the iron turret of the *Monitor.* In her efforts to keep
her sides presented to her more agile antagonist, the *Virginia* ran
aground. For fifteen minutes she remained immovable, while the
Monitor circled at will, searching for weak spots in her armor. At
last she broke away, and the battle continued on more even terms.
Once the *Virginia* rammed the *Monitor,* but without her iron beak
could do her no serious damage. At last, after six hours of incessant
fighting, the *Monitor* retired to the shallow water, known as the Middle Ground, where the *Virginia* could not follow. "The pilots declared
that we could get no nearer the *Minnesota,*" Flag-Officer Buchanan
reported afterwards, "and believing her to be entirely disabled,
and the *Monitor* having run into shoal water, which prevented our
doing her any further injury, we ceased firing at twelve, and proceeded to Norfolk." He was anxious, also, to repair the damages
to the *Virginia,* for her stem was twisted, her armor damaged, the
smokestack riddled, the muzzles of two guns shot away, and she was

leaking badly.[21] That night the *Minnesota* was gotten afloat and towed below Old Point.[22]

The first battle between ironclads is frequently misunderstood. The *Monitor* did not save Washington and New York, because they were never in danger from the *Virginia*. She did not even win the mastery of Hampton Roads, for the *Virginia* later moved out freely in those waters, and was unmolested. More important, she did not clear the way for McClellan's invasion of the Peninsula. Late in April, when General Joseph E. Johnston appealed to Flag-Officer Josiah Tatnall to bring the *Virginia* around to the mouth of the York, the latter considered the project impracticable. "Even though we should succeed in running past Fort Monroe and the warships there," he said, "we could not get at the transports, because their light draught would make it easy for them to retire to shallow water out of our range."[23] In other words, it was not the *Monitor,* but the limitations of the *Virginia* itself, which put such narrow restrictions on her activities. From the outset the *Virginia* could be expected merely to defend the mouth of the James, Nansemond, and Elizabeth rivers, and this she continued to do until the day of her destruction.[24]

That day was now at hand. McClellan had landed one hundred thousand men on the Peninsula and was pushing on toward Richmond. With the York open, exposing the left flank and rear of the Confederate army to attack, General Joseph E. Johnston had no alternative save to retire. This in turn placed the Federals in possession of the left bank of the James, and thus menaced the right bank and the Petersburg Railway. Since Burnside was operating in the Albemarle region, within striking distance of the Seaboard, Norfolk had become untenable. "If they get possession of the country west of this place, through which the railroads pass, as well as the waters on the other three sides, any escape from here is very doubtful," wrote General Huger on April 29.[25] With this view General Lee concurred. "His [the enemy's] possession of James River will render the evacuation of Norfolk in time necessary," he wrote on April 30.[26] Since, moreover, Huger's division was urgently needed by Johnston at Richmond, the order to

[21] Stewart, *History of Norfolk County,* p. 84.
[22] F. T. Miller, *Photographic History of the Civil War* (New York, 1911) , VI, 154-182; White, *The First Iron-Clad Naval Engagement;* Virginia Gordan Scrap Book.
[23] *War of the Rebellion: A Compilation of the Official Records of the Union and Confederate Armies.* Series I, Vol. XI (Washington, 1889) , pp. 477, 478.
[24] Newton, *Merrimac or Virginia,* p. 23.
[25] *War of the Rebellion,* Series I, Vol. XI, p. 475.
[26] *Ibid.,* p. 476.

evacuate the city was issued, and on May 2, Secretary of War Randolph went to Norfolk to prepare for the removal of ammunition, provisions, heavy guns, and rolling stock.

The rumor that Norfolk, the Navy Yard, and the *Virginia* were to be abandoned, caused consternation, not only in Norfolk, but throughout Virginia. "There has been some vague talk lately of a possible evacuation of Norfolk, destruction of the Navy Yard, etc.," said one of the Richmond papers on May 7, "but it would seem incredible that the government harbored such an idea. . . . We would lose the finest navy yard in the whole country, and a ship, which, besides performing so great a part in the maintenance of Norfolk, etc., protects James River and Magruder's right flank from the enemy's gun boats." Moreover, if Norfolk is lost, will not Burnside immediately move on Weldon, and so cut off communications between Richmond and the South? Despite these protests the removal of men and stores continued rapidly, and, by the evening of May 9, was practically completed.

Early on the morning on May 10, General John E. Wool, accompanied by President Lincoln, Secretary Stanton, and Secretary Chase, landed a large body of troops at Ocean View, and marched on Norfolk. Upon arriving at Tanner's Creek, they found the bridge in flames, and so were forced to make a detour around the head of the creek to the Princess Anne road. At four in the afternoon they reached the Confederate earthworks, but finding them deserted and the guns spiked, they continued until they were within sight of the spires of Norfolk peering through the trees. Here they were halted by Mayor Lamb and several councilmen, with a flag of truce. The mayor stated that the Confederates had evacuated Norfolk, that there would be no opposition, and requested protection for citizens and property. Thereupon the men bivouacked on the field, while General Wool, Secretary Chase, and General Viele, with an escort, entered the town and proceeded to the City Hall. Here the mayor addressed a crowd of citizens. He regretted the abandonment of the city, and, had the decision rested with him, would have defended it to the last. But since the step had been taken, he begged them to acquiesce and abstain from violence and disorder. A call for three cheers for President Davis received an enthusiastic response, and after giving three groans for Lincoln, "with less heartiness," the people dispersed.[27]

While the Union forces were occupying Norfolk, the Confederates

[27] *War of the Rebellion*, V, 40-46; XII, 677-679; Virginia Gordan Scrap Book.

had been engaged in destroying the Navy Yard and the shipping in the river. The dry dock was mined and seriously damaged, machinery was broken up, buildings burned, and valuable stores of tobacco thrown in the river. One party rowed out to the fleet, and set fire to the *William Selden,* the *Cayuga,* and *Harmony,* the *Plymouth,* the *Pilot Boy,* and other craft. Two of the burning vessels floated over toward Norfolk, but before they could do any damage firemen succeeded in towing them out from the docks. The work of destruction continued far into the night. From the Norfolk side "the incendiaries could be seen moving about in the darkness, with their pitch-pine flambeaux, like so many diabolical visitants. The scene strongly reminded the spectator of the panorama of the burning of Moscow, and with the immense flame that it threw forth made the scene one of terrible grandeur." The next day found the Navy Yard in ruins, "scarcely anything left but black walls and tall chimneys."[28]

In the meanwhile, anxiety and uncertainty prevailed on board the *Virginia,* off Sewells Point. When Flag-Officer Tatnall learned that Norfolk and the Elizabeth River batteries had been abandoned, he determined to run the vessel up the James. He had been assured by his pilots that by lightening the ironclad until she drew only eighteen feet, she could ascend to within forty miles of Richmond. So, calling all hands on deck, he explained the situation, adding that he hoped to surprise the Federal fleet in the James, and aid in the defense of Richmond. The men replied with three cheers, and went heartily to their task. But late that night, after the unarmored sides of the vessel had been brought above the water line, rendering her unfit for action, the pilots announced that it would be impossible to float her over the Jamestown Flats. Such a thing could have been done with a strong eastern wind, they said, but not now, when there had been westerly winds for two days. Tatnall was in a serious dilemma. He could not go forth to a desperate battle with the Federal fleet and batteries in the vessel's present condition. "I had no time to lose," he wrote afterwards. "The ship was not in condition for battle, even with an enemy of equal force, and their force was overwhelming. I therefore determined, with the concurrence of the first and flag lieutenants, to save the crew for future service, . . . and to destroy the ship, to prevent her falling into the hands of the enemy." So the *Virginia,* in which such fond hopes had been reposed, was grounded near Craney

[28] Virginia Gordan Scrap Book; *Photographic History of the Civil War,* VI, 73, 75, 155.

Island, tar, oil, fat, and grease spread over the decks and set on fire.[29] When she had been burning fiercely for an hour and a half, a terrific explosion tore her to pieces. "The air was thick with large and small pieces of timber. Huge sections of red-hot iron plate were torn off, and whirled through the air like so much paper. The shore and water for miles around were covered with pieces of the wreck, in every conceivable shape and size. The noise made by the explosion was terrific, shaking everything, even the very ground. . . . The fated vessel sank immediately after the explosion, not a vestige of her remaining above water."[30]

The days which followed were full of anxiety, hardship, and humiliation for the people of Norfolk. While the enemy camped at their front doors, while Negro troops paraded through their streets, while business was almost dead, and actual famine to be apprehended, they waited anxiously for news from the dear ones fighting under Lee and Johnston. From the first, however, good order prevailed. "It being Sunday, of course all places of business were closed, and the city presented a quiet aspect," said a Northern reporter the day after the Federal occupation. "The wharves were crowded with blacks, male and female, and a goodly number of working people, with their wives and children, were strolling about. Soldiers were stationed on the wharves, and picketed through the city, whilst the flag of the Union floated in triumph from the cupola of the Custom House. The houses through the city were generally closed, especially most of those of the wealthier classes."[31] A few weeks later another visitor spoke of Norfolk as "a city of the dead, almost all the stores being closed, grass growing in the streets, and few residents to be seen." Food was scarce, but country people still came in with strawberries, vegetables, chickens, and eggs.[32] The Atlantic Hotel was open and doing a thriving business; the proprietors rejoicing at the sight of gold and silver coins.

Although the officers and soldiers were usually orderly and cases of rudeness rare, friction with the civilians began from the first. One lady, who had threatened a soldier for trespassing upon her premises, was marched off to headquarters under guard; country people who came in to summon physicians were detained until they took the oath of allegiance to the United States; the Norfolk *Day Book* was sup-

29 *War of the Rebellion*, V, 46, 47.
30 Virginia Gordan Scrap Book.
31 Baltimore *American*, May 13, 1862.
32 Virginia Gordan Scrap Book.

pressed, and a sheet called the Norfolk *Union* issued in its place.[33] Feeling at all times ran high. The Federals looked upon the citizens as rebels, the citizens despised the Yankee invaders. "No person of any respectability holds any intercourse whatever with the Yankees," it was asserted. "They will not even look at them, and our contempt for them cuts. . . . They tried in every way to overcome this hatred, but finding it impossible, at length have given up the attempt."[34] General Wool, soon after taking possession of the city, inquired of the councils whether they considered themselves "as of the United States, of the Confederacy, as neutrals, or as a conquered people?" At first the councils evaded the question, but when pressed, stated that they considered the city as conquered territory. "The surrender of the city was giving it up to superior force. . . . Force implies the . . . overpowering of the people; to overpower the people is to conquer them, and to conquer them is but to subject them to the rule of the conqueror. Thus the status of Norfolk is plain." General Wool then urged the city officials to take the oath of allegiance, but they would not. Thereupon civil government was suppressed and military rule substituted.[35]

Norfolk's cup of bitterness was full when the Federal authorities began recruiting the slaves, organizing them into regiments, and using them for garrison duty and for expeditions into the surrounding country. To see Negro soldiers drilling in the streets was bad enough, but to have them arrest some old-school Southerner, or ransack his house, or stand guard over him in prison, was almost too much to be endured. On January 1, 1863, the Norfolk Negroes held a parade in honor of the Emancipation Proclamation. The procession was led by a line of hacks filled with colored women, some in white, others in Union colors. Next came an old butcher wagon drawn by two half-starved horses, in which Negro women trampled and tore Southern flags, while behind was a column of black marchers, about five hundred strong, directed by marshals mounted on Federal horses and decorated with blue sashes looped up with red and white. The procession moved down Main Street, where it was joined by another division, and the two proceeded to the residence of General Viele, the

---

[33] From the old *Herald* Office.

[34] Virginia Gordan Scrap Book. A Delaware soldier testifies to the hostility of the Norfolk ladies. "They are proof against the charms of brass buttons. They care nothing for sash or sword. You may get yourself up exquisitely and they wont deign you a look, except through the blinds." (*Delaware State Journal and Statesman,* June 17, 1862.)

[35] *The New Régime,* March 11, 1864.

military governor. The general came out, accompanied by Mrs. Viele, and addressed the crowd briefly. Thereupon the Negroes marched out to the fair grounds, and thence to the cemetery, where they buried Jefferson Davis in effigy.[36]

The resentment aroused by such scenes was accountable for a tragic incident. On the afternoon of June 17, 1863, a company of Negroes, under the command of a white officer named Sanborn, was marching down Main Street. Among the spectators was Dr. David M. Wright, a prominent physician, beloved because of his heroic work during the epidemic of 1855. Dr. Wright could not conceal his disgust, and approaching Lieutenant Sanborn, with clenched hands, exclaimed: "Oh! you coward!" Thereupon, Sanborn halted, and turning to Wright said: "You are under arrest." Maddened at the thought of having the Negro soldiers seize him and imprison him in the Custom House, Wright drew his pistol and fired twice at the officer. Sanborn staggered into Foster and Moore's store, where he died. Dr. Wright was tried before a special military commission and found guilty of murder. Although not approving of his rash act, the people of Norfolk considered the doctor, in a sense, a martyr to the Southern cause, and while he was awaiting execution, deluged him with delicacies.

On one occasion he nearly escaped. His eldest daughter, Penelope, changed clothes with him in his cell, and not until he was hastening away was the ruse detected. President Lincoln approved of the findings of the court, and he was sentenced to be hanged. The execution took place at the fair grounds in the middle of the race track, on October 23, 1863. The Federal troops were posted in a square around the gallows, while thousands of spectators looked on from housetops, or stood on tiptoe in buggies, carts, and wagons. Among them, however, "few old citizens could be recognized," for the better classes stayed at home.[37]

Norfolk continued under military rule for thirteen months, in which time municipal affairs went from bad to worse. The public buildings fell into disrepair, the street lamps were broken, the fire equipment was stolen, the bridges became unsafe. In June, 1863, civil law was resumed, under the authority of Governor F. H. Peirpoint. When Virginia seceded in 1861, the people of the western part of the state, declaring this action of no effect, organized a government to replace

[36] Virginia Gordan Scrap Book.
[37] *Ibid.* While Dr. Wright was being conducted to the scaffold, the sound of wailing could be heard from various houses along the route. The doctor had made many friends by his work during the epidemic. During those terrible days in 1855 he contracted yellow fever, but was spared by fate for an even worse death.

the one at Richmond. They elected Peirpoint governor, chose a legislature, congressmen and senators, and received recognition from President Lincoln as the legal government of Virginia. Later, when West Virginia was formed, Peirpoint made Alexandria his capital, and at once took measures to restore civil rule in the small part of Virginia under Federal control. In Norfolk the attempt was farcical. General Viele and Peirpoint permitted none save Union men to vote, and of these there were not more than one hundred.[38] The mayor, councilmen, and justices were, of course, hostile to the Confederacy, and many of them were Northerners. Eventually, some Southern sympathizers took the oath of allegiance, for no ministers, physicians, lawyers, merchants, and clerks in the stores, were permitted to pursue their vocations without it. They did so with the understanding that they were merely accepting amnesty, and not manifesting any change of heart.[39] "He [General Wool] tells them that unless they take the oath of allegiance, they shall have nothing to eat. . . . There is positive suffering among the women and children of Norfolk. . . . To every cry of distress, to every appeal for the observance of the ordinary humanities, to every demand for the usages of civilized war, this old man . . . has but one answer: 'Take the oath of allegiance or starve!' "[40]

It cannot be said that General Viele was popular in Norfolk, but the people looked back upon his rule as benevolent indeed after they fell into the hands of General Benjamin F. Butler. This officer, notorious because of his severity at New Orleans, regarded the Peirpoint government with contempt, and ruled Norfolk almost as though no such thing existed. The provost marshal and the provost court took over the functions of the civil courts, and arbitrary orders were issued to levy taxes on business, open schools, inspect banks, and issue licenses to traders. In June, 1864, by the vote of the Union men in Norfolk, all of them in Butler's power, he overthrew even the pretense of civil government, and restored the military régime.[41] Peirpoint was so enraged that he complained to the Secretary of War, and later to President Lincoln. Butler, he said, had not only been guilty of an unwarranted assumption of power, he had not only ignored the government of Virginia which the President himself had

[38] *The New Régime*, Aug. 23, 1864, Princeton University Library.
[39] Virginia Gordan Scrap Book; *Governor Peirpoint to the President* (Washington, 1864) , p. 9.
[40] Richmond *Enquirer*, June 4, 1862.
[41] *The New Régime*, Aug. 23, 1864.

recognized, but his régime had been marked by tyranny and injustice.[42]

"In November [1863] General Butler was appointed to the command of the eastern district of Virginia and North Carolina," wrote Peirpoint. "I sighed when I heard it—I remembered New Orleans. There was short rejoicing at Norfolk among the ultra Union men, but in a short time the wail of woe came up. . . . Among the first orders . . . was one threatening punishment to any person who used any disrespectful language to any officer or soldier in the Union army. Next was an order directing all permits granted by his predecessors be returned to him. Then came an order charging one per cent on all goods shipped into his military district, to go to the support of the provost marshal's fund. All vessels clearing from his district pay from five to fifteen dollars. . . . Oyster men were taxed from fifty cents to one dollar per month for the privilege of taking oysters."[43]

If we may believe the governor, the Butler régime was as corrupt as it was oppressive. No man could do business without a permit from the military authorities, and permits were distributed to those who offered the highest bribe. "One man in Norfolk, who has been there two or three years, has a permit, and says he got it in such a disgraceful way that he is ashamed to tell how he got it. . . . The liquor business now stands thus in Norfolk: a few men from Boston and Lowell, Mass., have the exclusive monopoly of importing it into the city. . . . You pay twenty-five cents per drink, two dollars for a bottle holding three half-pints of common whiskey, and three dollars for a bottle of good. The restaurant keepers pay these Boston men three dollars per gallon for whiskey that costs in Baltimore from 95 cents to $1.05."[44]

Butler's conduct in relation to the Norfolk gas works was typical. He "seized the whole concern, and put them into operation himself, although the president of the company assured him that he would . . . supply all the gas needed. Yet General Butler sent to Lowell for a man and fixtures to repair at a cost of $10,000. . . . I suppose the profits go into the provost marshal's fund. He sells the gas at nearly double the price paid in Washington. . . . A large amount of the stockholders are widows, old maids, and orphans—all their subsistence is taken from them. . . . Their slaves are all gone, and in the language

[42] *Private and Official Correspondence of General Benjamin F. Butler* (Norwood, Mass., 1917) , III, 282-285, 321-324, 450-460; IV, 304-310, 431-434; *Governor Peirpoint to the President*, pp. 11-49.
[43] *Governor Peirpoint to the President*, p. 9.
[44] *Ibid.*, p. 23.

of Dr. Cook, one of their number, they are only respectable vaga-
bonds, and must, many of them who were once wealthy, soon become
objects of charity."[45] "He refused to allow the company to bring
coal to the city because the president and directors refused to take the
oath of allegiance. He then declared gas to be a military necessity,
seized the works, and put his friends from Lowell, Mass., in possession."[46]

On March 7, 1864, an order was issued that every fourth dog in
the Norfolk district be killed. This created consternation until it was
learned that any owner could save his dog by paying two dollars for a
license. "I met a soldier with a line around a little dog's neck," wrote
Governor Peirpoint, "he was between a spaniel and the poodle—
white wool—but dirty; his chin was close to the ground, his eyes upturned meekly, and wagging his tail gently as he went along." A Negro
standing on the sidewalk remarked as he passed, "Little doggie, if you
don't get two dollars, Marse Butler will take de wag out of your tail."[47]
Perhaps the most heartless act of Butler was the seizure of the funds
of the Howard Association, used to support children who had lost
their parents in the yellow fever epidemic of 1855. "There are some
twelve or fifteen of the orphans which are still a charge upon them
[the Association]. Last year they had a small surplus of interest which
they devoted to the poor. . . . General Butler, with the same propriety
and more, might seize the assets of Girard College, or that of any
professorship in Harvard."[48]

"Ever since the Union troops occupied the city of Norfolk and
Portsmouth," the governor continued, "the military have had possession of the ferry and boats between the two cities, using them for its
own profit and benefit. . . . The receipts of the ferry before the war
amounted to from $15,000 to $18,000 per annum." All this money, together with confiscated property, fines, the 1 per cent tax, the tax on
oysters and dogs, clearances of vessels, etc., went to the provost marshal's fund. "It is estimated by those who have pretty good opportunity of knowing, that there has been collected since General Butler
went to Old Point last fall, from two to three hundred thousand dollars into this fund. . . . It is strange to me that such a system should
have grown up whereby military commanders collect tens and hun-

---

45 *Ibid.,* p. 24.
46 Burton, *History of Norfolk,* p. 216.
47 *Governor Peirpoint to the President,* p. 28.
48 *Ibid.,* p. 29.

dreds of thousands of dollars into this post or provost marshal's fund, which is held by men who give no bonds."[49]

Late in 1863 Butler sent General E. A. Wild, with two Negro regiments, on an expedition through Princess Anne, and northeastern Carolina, which practiced such severities that for years the people of those sections looked back upon them with horror. A Union man, a friend of Peirpoint, told the governor that for weeks afterwards, "he could stand on the portico of his house and trace the track of the raid for ten miles by the turkey buzzards, feeding on the carrion made by destruction of animal life. Union men and widows shared the same fate; all they had was taken or destroyed. . . . While near where Captain Coffee lives, General Wild came to the house owned by a man by the name of White, who was a captain in the Confederate service. General Wild arrested Mrs. White, the wife, as a hostage. . . . She was in a delicate situation. Her daughter, a young girl of about nineteen years of age, stepped forward and said, 'General, you cannot take my mother, take me.' He took the daughter and set fire to the house, and burnt everything in it, with all the knickknacks of an expectant mother." While on their way to Norfolk the troops happened to meet a regiment of New Yorkers, who were so outraged at the sight of a white girl marching along the road under custody of Negroes that they were on the point of rescuing her by force. But Miss White herself interposed, stating that she had not been dishonored, and so was led off "to be imprisoned in the second story of Wild's headquarters at Norfolk."[50] A few days later General Butler reported: "General Wild took the most stringent measures, burning the property of some of the officers of guerilla parties, seizing the wives and families of others as hostages for some of his negroes that were captured, and appears to have done his work with great thoroughness, but perhaps with too much stringency."[51]

We have seen that some of the Federal officers at Norfolk had smoothed the way for Southern men and women to take the oath of allegiance by explaining that it meant no more than passive obedience to the United States government. Butler took a different view of the matter. "The oath of allegiance means fealty, pledge of faith to love, affection and reverence for the government," he explained. So, ignoring the fact that love and reverence are not instilled by oppression

[49] *Ibid.*, pp. 47, 48.
[50] *Ibid.*, pp. 36, 37.
[51] *Correspondence of General Benjamin F. Butler*, III, 269.

and cruelty, he withheld his licenses from all whom he suspected of sympathy for the South. Business fell almost entirely into the hands of Northern men.[52] The Norfolk and Portsmouth schools were closed, and a school for Negro children, conducted by Northern teachers, was opened in their place.[53] "I am glad to learn from your letter that your school has been closed since Christmas," Butler wrote to a teacher in Accomac, "and with my consent until you change your sentiments, and are a loyal woman in heart, it never shall be opened."[54]

One day Butler sent for Dr. George D. Armstrong, one of the heroes of the yellow fever epidemic of 1855, and questioned him concerning the spirit with which he took the oath of allegiance. "I regard Norfolk as for the present a conquered city," he answered. "I wished, in accordance with the scriptural injunctions, to obey the powers that be, and I believed the United States to be the powers that be. I took the oath with the intention of keeping it so far as my actions were concerned. My feelings, of course, I cannot control. My words and actions I can." Thereupon Butler subjected him to a quizzing to draw out what his feelings were. "You said you looked upon the hanging of John Brown as just and right because he interfered with the peace of the country. . . . Would you look upon the hanging of the prominent rebel, Jefferson Davis, for instance, as just and right?" "I would not, sir," was the answer. "Are your sympathies with the Union or Confederate cause?" "With the Confederates." "You took the oath, sir, for the purpose of having the United States protect you while you should by your conduct and your life aid and comfort the rebels. . . . (To an aide) Make an order that this man be committed to the guard house, in close confinement, there to remain until he can be consigned to Fort Hatteras."[55] Later he wrote Secretary of War Stanton: "I do not consider that I am bound to feed and house a rebel at the expense of the United States without an equivalent. Therefore I directed that he should be put to labor."[56] While Dr. Armstrong was thus working for his food and lodging, his pulpit was filled by the Reverend C. L. Woodworth, chaplain of the Twenty-seventh Massachusetts Infantry.[57]

On February 11, 1864, an order was issued placing all houses of

[52] *Ibid.*, III, 452.
[53] *Ibid.*, III, 459.
[54] Virginia Gordan Scrap Book.
[55] *The New Régime*, Feb. 24, 1864.
[56] *Correspondence of General Benjamin F. Butler*, III, 56, 57.
[57] Virginia Gordan Scrap Book.

public worship in Norfolk and Portsmouth under the control of the provost marshals. These officers were directed to see that the pulpits were "properly filled, by displacing when necessary, the present incumbents, and substituting men of known loyalty." They were to see that "the churches are open freely to all officers and soldiers, white and colored, . . . and that no insult or indignity be offered to them, either by word, look, or gesture, on the part of the congregation."[58] Two weeks later General Wild ordered the arrest of the Reverend S. H. Wingfield, of Portsmouth, for manifesting disapproval of the reading of the prayer for the President of the United States. The provost marshal was directed to turn the minister "over to Colonel Sawtelle to work for three months cleaning the streets of Norfolk and Portsmouth, thus employing his time for the benefit of that government he has abused, and in a small way atone for his disloyalty and treason."[59]

Butler's detectives were spread over the city to report all who showed hostility to his régime or sympathy for the Confederacy. His officers, scorning "arrest warrants, search warrants, etc., did what they pleased, entered where they chose, and carried off anything they coveted."[60] "Spies are as thick as flies in a sugar bowl," wrote one lady.[61] When Governor Peirpoint visited the city in March, 1864, he "met men, who six months ago, stood erect and talked like freemen. . . . But now the hand of oppression is upon them, they look dejected, and disheartened. When they spoke to one of their troubles, it was far from the presence of anyone, and then in an undertone. When they came into my room to talk with me, they would look around the room to assure themselves that there was no spy concealed, and see that the doors were closely shut."[62] It is not hard to understand the spirit of desperation which gripped the people. "I would be willing to be hanged for the sake of seeing dear old Norfolk free," wrote one Norfolk lady. "I hope never to see another city given up. I would rather see my home laid in ashes than live as we are now living. What is wealth compared with freedom? . . . My hand trembles and my blood boils with rage when I think of the scenes I saw yesterday at headquarters."[63]

[58] *Ibid.*
[59] *Ibid.* On March 1, the remainder of Mr. Wingfield's sentence was commuted to confinement at Fort Monroe.
[60] Norfolk *Journal,* Aug. 4, 1868.
[61] *The New Régime,* May 23, 1864.
[62] *Governor Peirpoint to the President,* p. 49.
[63] Virginia Gordan Scrap Book.

We catch a glimpse of the suffering of some of the old families of Norfolk from a letter written by Mrs. Munroe Winthrope, in April, 1864. "I have made $7.00 lately," she states, "and I wanted to buy about seventy things with it. But alas! it would not be persuaded but to supply two wants, that is, to repair my watch that has been silent for three years, and to purchase a few pairs of stockings. . . . I have bought two new dresses for each of us, but one of them is not paid for yet. Now we are in need of shoes. There is a great deal of suffering among our people who have no income and have exhausted their money. . . . Many are privately selling furniture. Those who have been in affluence are reduced to the utmost. . . . The smallpox is very bad and very fatal. At the pest house white persons and negroes often occupy the same bed, which has increased the aversion to the place."[64]

Still more vivid is the picture of Norfolk during the last year of the war from the pen of a visitor. "The city looks gloomy," he says, "the people for the most part sullen. . . . Of the houses, one-fourth appear to be unoccupied, having been deserted by their inhabitants. . . . A part of these have been seized by the government for storage purposes; of some, the newly arrived mechanics from the north have taken possession; in others the freedmen and their families have squatted. No repairs are perceptible on any hand. Those which were burned or have since crumbled to ruin, are suffered to remain so. In spite of the cold blasts of winter, there is still a lamentable lack of glass in the windows. Sadness and gloom, if not despair, have settled upon both people and houses. Broken glass, crumbling walls, opening roofs, creaking doors, and general dilapidation follow disappointed hopes. . . . I left Norfolk as sad as the large company of women, both white and black, standing in front of the commissary's office to receive rations for the support of their families, as sad as the hundreds of ladies I had met draped in the weeds of mourning, as sad as the winds which howl through the deserted habitations of the hundreds of secessionists."[65]

When the Norfolk soldier, whether marching into Maryland and Pennsylvania, or bivouacking in the field, or facing the enemy, got word of the sufferings of the loved ones at home, it steeled him to meet the hardships and dangers of his life. Perhaps, as he swept on to victory at Chancellorsville, or hurled back the Union troops at Cold

[64] *The New Régime*, April 26, 1864.
[65] *Ibid.*, May 23, 1864.

Harbor, or at Spotsylvania, visions rose before him of wife and children, insulted and abused by Wild or Butler and their Negroes. No troops in the Confederate army had a finer record than those from Norfolk. Individuals were scattered in the regiments and batteries of various states—South Carolina, North Carolina, Alabama—but the larger number went into the service of Virginia with old Norfolk companies, or with new organizations formed to defend the city in 1861. The Norfolk Junior Volunteers became Company H of the 12th Virginia infantry; the Independent Grays and the Woodis Rifles entered the Sixth Virginia, as Company H and Company C respectively, together with three new Norfolk companies, which became Companies A, D, and G. Both regiments entered Mahone's brigade. The Norfolk Light Artillery Blues, under Captain C. R. Grandy, had an especially distinguished career, fighting nobly at Seven Pines, Oak Grove, Second Manassas, Sharpsburg, Fredericksburg, Chancellorsville, Gettysburg, the Wilderness, Spotsylvania, and Petersburg. The Huger Battery, the United Artillery, and the Atlantic Artillery also fully upheld Norfolk's honor.

The Sixth Virginia, comprising in addition to the five Norfolk companies, two companies from Princess Anne, one from Portsmouth, one from Manchester, and one from Chesterfield, had a distinguished career. Colonel William Mahone was in command until with his promotion to brigadier general he made place for Thomas J. Corprew. In April, 1862, Colonel Corprew in turn was succeeded by Colonel George T. Rogers. The regiment remained near Norfolk until February, 1862, when it was ordered to Currituck Bridge, to protect the Albemarle and Chesapeake canal and to cover the retreat of General Wise from Roanoke Island. Wise brought it back to Great Bridge, where it remained until the evacuation of Norfolk. On May 10, 1862, the troops filed into town over the drawbridge, bade a hasty goodbye to wives and children, and entrained for Petersburg.[66] The regiment was then posted along the James River, to assist the batteries to block the passage of the Federal gunboats, and so was not with the rest of Mahone's brigade at the battle of Seven Pines.[67]

During the retirement of McClellan's army from the Chickahominy to the James, the Sixth fought continuously. On one occasion, on the Charles City road, when the first battalion was sent forward to engage the enemy, the second battalion mistook them for Federals and

---

[66] Companies G, H, and I joined the regiment at Petersburg.

[67] Porter, *A Record*, pp. 279-280.

fired upon them from behind. In this unfortunate affair twenty-eight men were killed or wounded. The Sixth was heavily engaged at the battle of Oak Grove, on June 25, and again on July 1, at Malvern Hill. At Second Manassas it took part in the famous charge of Mahone's brigade, which aided so materially in hurling Pope's army back upon Washington.[68]

Perhaps the most gallant action of the Sixth was at Crampton Gap. Lee had crossed the Potomac early in September, 1862, dispatching Jackson to capture Harpers Ferry and open communications with the Shenandoah Valley. Unfortunately, an intercepted dispatch revealed his plans to McClellan, who thereupon moved westward to the South Mountains in Maryland, with overwhelming forces, to place himself between the two Confederate commanders. The peril was very great, for should the meager forces in the mountain gaps give way, the retreat of Lee's men would be cut off. General Cobb, in command at Crampton's Gap, received orders to hold on, "even if he lost his last man in doing it." So the brigade, now but eight hundred strong, resisted hour after hour the assaults of Franklin's entire corps. The enemy were repeatedly repulsed, relates Captain James H. Toomer, of Portsmouth, "leaving the ground blue with their dead and wounded. After three hours hard fighting we were flanked on both our right and left, and order was given for the regiment to fall back. . . . Pulling ourselves up by laying hold of branches of trees and climbing from ledge to ledge, with the music of Minie balls continually in our ears, we succeeded in getting safely over the mountain. When the brigade reformed in Pleasant Valley, only four in our company and 17 in the regiment answered to their names." The sacrifice of the Sixth was not in vain, however, for its gallantry had not only made possible the capture of Harpers Ferry, with twelve thousand five hundred men, but the juncture of Lee and Jackson at Sharpsburg.[69]

The regiment, after being reorganized and recruited, continued to fight throughout the war. Over and over Lee called upon it, now to storm a battery, now to repel an attack, now to relieve some shattered detachment, and always the men responded gallantly—at Chancellorsville, in the Wilderness, at Spotsylvania, Cold Harbor, North Anna River, Hanover Court House, Turkey Ridge, Second Frazier's Farm, Wilcox's Farm. At the Crater only eighty-five members of the regiment were in camp when the Federal mine was set off under the

[68] *Ibid.*, pp. 281, 282.
[69] *Ibid.*, 283-286.

Confederate works. These men fell in with the rest of the brigade, and, hastening to the breach, were in the thick of the engagement. At the roll call after the battle, it was found that only ten had escaped, thirteen being killed, fifty wounded, and twelve missing.

Such were the men who returned to Norfolk in the spring of 1865, bearing the parole of General Grant. They were received by their families and friends with reverence and affection. Even the Northern men who had moved to Norfolk honored them for their bravery and treated them with respect. Not so Butler's provost marshal. By his order they were arrested on the street, dragged before him, and there "in the presence of gaping, motley crowds of negroes and whites," he cut the buttons from their uniforms.[70] The people of Norfolk accepted the outcome of the war in good faith, were ready to come back into the Union as loyal citizens, were willing, even happy to be rid of the curse of slavery,[71] but the bitterness occasioned by the unnecessary cruelties of the three years of Federal occupation has hardly yet died out. The name of Butler will ever be infamous in Norfolk.

[70] Stewart, *History of Norfolk County,* p. 100.
[71] Norfolk *Journal,* Jan. 4, 1867.

CHAPTER ELEVEN

The Black Cloud

The people of Virginia, in the days immediately after Appomattox, gave little thought to the political future of the state. They were too deeply concerned with procuring food for their families, repairing their homes, laying out crops, and plowing their fields. But there were some who wondered whether Virginia would remain long under the military rule, or whether the President and Congress would permit Peirpoint to establish civil government. In either case, it seemed unlikely that the mass of the people would have any part in the conduct of affairs, for the new constitution, adopted by the Alexandria convention of 1864, had limited the suffrage to Union men. However, after President Johnson had recognized Peirpoint, his legislature passed an enabling act, permitting former Confederates to vote. In Norfolk the civil courts resumed their jurisdiction, the police, the fire companies, the ferries, the town finances were restored to the municipality, and an election was held in which Thomas Tabb was chosen mayor. Butlerism and the mailed fist seemed things of the past. With an honest governor at Richmond, with no immediate fear of Negro suffrage, it seemed that the people could ignore politics amid the vital task of restoring the prosperity of the state. They were not long in discovering their error.

The legislature made the mistake of passing a stringent vagrancy law, intended to put an end to idleness and petty larceny among the Negroes. This, together with the desire of the Republican national leaders to gain permanent control in Virginia, was largely responsible for the refusal of Congress to recognize the state government or seat their senators and congressmen. Thaddeus Stevens, in his demands that the suffrage be accorded the blacks and taken away from "disloyal" whites, found a ready echo from a group of Virginia Radicals. These men, headed by the carpetbagger John C. Underwood, met in convention at Alexandria and petitioned Congress to overthrow the Peirpoint government. They watched eagerly the battle between Johnson and the Radicals in Congress, in the hope that the President's defeat would make them masters of Virginia. In the meanwhile they tried to win over the Negroes, by assuring them that their only hope of justice lay in the success of the extreme group of Republicans, both in Congress and in the state.

At this time Norfolk had an abnormally large black population, since during the war hundreds of slaves had fled there to the protection of the Union troops. A Federal officer in January, 1866, reported that "in the neighborhood of Norfolk, Fortress Monroe, and Yorktown, about 70,000 negroes have been collected during the war."[1] Under the tutelage of Northern officers, Northern businessmen, and Northern teachers, the freedmen had learned to demand equality with the whites. In 1864 they had celebrated the abolition of slavery in Virginia by the Peirpoint convention,[2] and now, on January 1, 1866, they observed the anniversary of Lincoln's Emancipation Proclamation. A long procession, directed by mounted marshals and decorated with tricolored scarfs, formed on Bute Street and marched through the town. In the lead was the band and two companies of the Twentieth New York infantry, followed by various Negro organizations—the Sons of Houn, Humble Sons of God, Zion's Sons, Hebrew Union, Independent Society—with a long line of Negro citizens in the rear.[3]

Although the Northern troops remaining in Norfolk acted officially as the protectors of the blacks, hostility developed between individual soldiers and the freedmen. The Northerners, while according the Negro a degree of social equality, were more intolerant than the Southerners of his characteristic weaknesses. Whenever a bluecoat off duty wandered down to Little Water Street or other parts of the town where the Negroes were concentrated, there was apt to be trouble, perhaps bloodshed. On June 22, 1865, a number of soldiers, armed with pistols, rocks, and bricks, swarmed through this district, terrifying the blacks, and raiding several of their disreputable dance halls.[4] The Negroes vowed revenge. The next day scores repaired to near-by woods, where they cut hundreds of bludgeons, several feet long and heavy enough to fell an ox. That night, as they moved down Main Street to the guard house, muttering threats against all "white trash," they en-

[1] J. P. McConnell, *Negroes in Virginia, 1865-1867* (Pulaski, Va., 1910), pp. 48, 49.
[2] Virginia Gordan Scrap Book; *The New Régime*, March 13, 1864.
[3] Norfolk *Post*, Jan. 2, 1866.
[4] *Ibid.*, June 29, 1865.

countered a lone soldier and set upon him. Although the man seized one of the bludgeons and knocked down his nearest assailant, he would have fared badly had not a group of his fellow soldiers come to the rescue. The soldiers charged, scattered the blacks, and took six or seven prisoners.

Later in the evening a group of Negroes fired on some soldiers at the circus grounds, wounding one in the leg. Thereupon, his comrades formed a mob and set out for Roanoke Square, felling every Negro who came in their path. After an unsuccessful attempt to break into the dance hall, they scattered a few blacks on Union Street and retired to their barracks. The police were not numerous enough to cope with riots of this kind, so that Mayor Tabb called upon General Mann to preserve order with his troops. With armed sentinels posted throughout the town, something like order was now restored.[5] But several months later, when the Thirtieth regiment of Negro troops passed through Norfolk on their way to Baltimore, a pitched battle with members of the Twentieth New York was narrowly averted.[6]

These riots were represented in the Northern press as unprovoked attacks on the Negroes by Norfolk whites. The better classes in Norfolk felt this injustice keenly, for they had no animosity toward the blacks and were anxious to maintain peaceful relations. In the riots many had offered shelter to individuals when pursued by the mobs of soldiers. Yet the demoralization of the times, the tendency of the freedmen to turn liberty into license, and the fear of carpetbag control in government, made a clash of the races possible at all times. On April 16, 1866, the Negroes celebrated the passage of the Civil Rights Bill. A procession formed in Market Square and marched through the principal streets in orderly fashion. At the corner of Bute and Dock streets a few bricks were thrown at the marchers, but there was no serious trouble until they arrived at the field where the speaking was to take place. Here somebody fired a pistol, and when the only policeman in sight attempted to make an arrest, the Negroes, many of them discharged soldiers, resisted with arms in their hands.

In some way, a young Confederate veteran, named Whitehurst, became involved in the melee and was pursued by the Negroes to his father's house near-by. Here, while standing in the doorway, firing at the mob, he accidentally shot his step-mother. The Negroes rushed in upon him, seized him, and were beating him with palings

---

[5] *Ibid.*, June 26, July 7, 1865.
[6] *Ibid.*, Dec. 18, 1865.

when two of their marshals on horseback interposed. These men were leading Whitehurst down the street between them, one holding him by the collar, the other by the hair, when he was shot down from behind. A few minutes later order was restored by the arrival of Major F. W. Stanhope with Federal troops. But the whites were now thoroughly aroused, and that night armed bands roved the streets, killing several Negroes and wounding others.[7]

Such incidents, duly misrepresented in the Northern press, served only to strengthen the hands of the Radicals in Congress. The fear of the Northern people that the fruits of the war might yet be lost, together with the antagonism aroused by the tactlessness and intemperate utterances of President Johnson, gave Stevens and his group a sweeping victory in the elections of 1866. Thus fortified, they proceeded to reconstruct the South according to their own views. The Peirpoint government was swept aside, Virginia was made into Military District Number 1, and General John M. Schofield placed in command with instructions to summon a convention to draw up a new constitution. In making out the list of voters the act required that all Negroes be admitted, and that persons who had held Federal offices prior to the war and later aided the Confederacy should be excluded. When the registration was completed, it was found that 120,101 whites and 105,832 blacks had qualified, apparently leaving the control with the former. Unfortunately, however, the Negroes were so distributed as to have a majority in most of the counties, and, upon a strictly racial division, could count on fifty-eight delegates in the convention to forty-seven for the whites. In the city of Norfolk the black voters numbered 2,049 and the whites 1,910.

It was a time of foreboding and despair in Virginia. "What is the use of struggling?" men asked each other. "Congress is determined to ruin and degrade us, and even if we rescue this convention from the carpetbaggers and negroes, will find some other way of forcing its will upon us." In Norfolk the Radicals nominated Henry M. Bowden, and a runaway slave who for some years prior to the war had practiced dentistry in Boston, named Thomas Bayne. The Conservatives named Colonel Gilbert C. Walker and Dr. W. W. Wing. Walker, a native of New York, was president of the First National Bank of Norfolk. His business ability, his interest in the welfare of the city, and his honesty of purpose, had won the confidence of all. However, from the first the Conservatives had little hope, for the carpetbaggers and

[7] *Executive Documents*, 1866-67, Vol. XI, Norfolk Riots.

scalawags, with the assistance of the Union League, had organized the blacks into a solid political phalanx. October 22, when the election was held, was a gala day for these simple souls. Long before the hour for opening the polls, they gathered in crowds at the booths, waiting to cast their ballots as their Northern friends had instructed them. Throughout the morning carriages were kept busy bringing in the blacks from distant parts of the city, and by two o'clock almost the entire Radical vote had been polled. On the other hand, many whites refused to vote, and Bowden and Bayne were elected by substantial majorities. How distinct the Radical alignment was, is shown by the fact that only nine whites voted for Bayne, and only six blacks for Wing.[8] As went Norfolk, so went Virginia. Of the one hundred and five delegates for the convention, thirty-five were Conservatives, sixty-five were Radicals, and five were doubtful. The Radicals counted twenty-five Negroes, fourteen native Virginians, thirteen New Yorkers, and thirteen more from other Northern states or from foreign countries.[9]

Such was the body, which on December 3, 1867, assembled in the Capitol at Richmond, where for decades the representatives of the old aristocracy had debated the affairs of Virginia. As the work of drawing up the constitution proceeded, the Negroes, under the leadership of Bayne, more than once threatened to desert their white allies. Bayne was disgruntled over the refusal of the convention to place white and black children in the same schools. Finally one of the leading white radicals turned upon him sharply. "He makes no recognition of any white man," he said, "but wants a party . . . to be composed entirely of colored men, in order, as I suppose, as he thinks, that he might be the leader and head of them."[10] But the former slave frankly avowed his desire to place the Negro in control of the state. "The colored race, Mr. President, have always been leaders in all de great revolutions of history, and they do say that it was de black man who drove Jeff Davis out of Richmond," he declared. "Certain it is that a negro-so-called led (now he didn't follow, mind that) the attack on de British troops on State Street, in Boston, and this was de commencement of de Revolutionary war, and if this black man had not led de whites on to victory, I spects there wouldn't have been no Revolutionary war at all, and you would still be groaning under the British

[8] Burton, *History of Norfolk*, p. 114.
[9] Richard L. Morton, *The Negro in Virginia Politics* (Charlottesville, 1919), p. 50.
[10] *Debates of the Constitutional Convention of Virginia, 1867* (Richmond, 1868), p. 545.

yoke."[11] Enlivened by touches of this kind, the convention proceeded with its work, and in April, 1868, reported a constitution enfranchising the Negroes and disqualifying the vast majority of white men from holding office and many from voting. General Schofield, with his usual sound sense, pleaded for moderation, but he succeeded only in bringing down upon him the denunciations of the Radicals. Bayne yelled out that he "wa'nt gwine to be timidated by no general, and dat it would be a pretty ting to go home and say dat de convention was skeered of de General."[12]

While the convention was still in session, civil government was partly overthrown and many offices filled by military appointees. In April, 1868, Mayor John R. Ludlow, John Williams, city register, R. Q. Drummond, city collector, and others, having refused to take the ironclad oath, were removed from office.[13] The few who could take the oath, Northern men, most of them, were held over. The military authorities then appointed Francis DeCordy, mayor; A. D. Campbell, city treasurer; O. M. Dorman, judge of the corporation court; and W. T. Harrison, president of the common council. These men were not mere political adventurers, seeking personal gain and plunder. Most of them, though not native Virginians, had made Norfolk their permanent home, held real estate there, and were deeply interested in her advancement.[14] This was fortunate indeed, for there was urgent need of energy, foresight, and wisdom. The city treasury was empty, a debt of nearly two million dollars hung over the people, taxes were high, the police were inefficient, there was no water works. Although, in the two years they were in power, it was impossible for the military appointees to rectify all these evils, they gave the city an efficient administration and earned the gratitude of the people.[15]

But the rule of Northern businessmen was quite a different thing from the domination of Negroes, carpetbaggers, and scalawags, threatened by the new constitution. The people of Norfolk made it clear that men who came among them to invest capital and start legitimate enterprises were welcome. "It is the paper-collared, half-shirted, mean, low carpet-bagger, who is lured to us only to get offices here, which his worthlessness at home forbade his even aiming at there, who cheats and humbugs the poor negro out of his money and his vote . . . it is to

[11] Norfolk *Journal*, Jan. 13, 1868.
[12] *Ibid.*, April 20, 1868.
[13] *Ibid.*, June 2, 1868; Burton, *History of Norfolk*.
[14] Norfolk *Journal*, June 26, 1868.
[15] Burton, *History of Norfolk*, p. 131; Lamb, *Our Twin Cities*, p. 35.

this class of Northern men to whom we object and are hostile."[16] Yet this was the class who would rule, should the constitution be adopted. So the white men began to organize what they called the Conservative party to save the state. Forgotten were the old quarrels of Democrats and Whigs, to some extent even the quarrels of Union men and Confederates; it was now a question of white rule or black.

So early as December 11, 1867, a convention met in Richmond to organize the Conservative forces. Walker was selected as one of Norfolk's delegates, but he refused to serve on the grounds that the movement was premature.[17] But as the farcical work of the convention proceeded and it became obvious that the carpetbaggers and Negroes were seeking, not political equality, but complete supremacy in the state, Walker turned from them in disgust. He could but agree with the Norfolk *Journal* when it stated the issue as follows: "The simple question before the people is this—are we to have our State officers and our judiciary filled by intelligent white men of character, or are we to have all our officials, from the Governor to the coroner, composed of negroes and their radical friends, our Legislature of the same, our judges radical pettifoggers, our magistrates negroes, and our children forced into mixed schools, or denied the privileges of education?"[18]

"Organize! organize! organize at once!" urged the *Journal*. "Let the people appoint committees in every ward in our cities, in every precinct in our counties. There never was such an issue presented to Virginia as the present."[19] On the evening of April 28 a great throng assembled before the City Hall to listen to Colonel J. W. Hinton and other Conservatives. The mass of upturned faces, the glare of bonfires, the deafening applause, showed that the whites of Norfolk were aroused to the need of united action to save the state.[20] The next day Hinton, John Goode, and others went up to Great Bridge, where they spoke to a gathering in Berea Church. After describing the new constitution, Hinton called out, "Will you ratify it?" "Never! never!" the crowd roared back. "I thought so," said the speaker.[21]

The Conservatives nominated Colonel R. E. Withers for governor to oppose the carpetbagger H. H. Wells. On July 3, 1868, Withers

[16] Norfolk *Journal*, Sept. 2, 1868.
[17] *Ibid.*, Dec. 5, 1867.
[18] *Ibid.*, March 10, 1868.
[19] *Ibid.*, April 18, 1868.
[20] *Ibid.*, April 29, 1868.
[21] *Ibid.*, April 30, 1868.

visited Norfolk. A stand had been erected in front of the courthouse, for a vast crowd was expected, but a pouring rain drove the assemblage in doors. Here all who could secure seats or standing room listened indignantly while the speaker dwelt on the iniquity of the constitution. In conclusion he advised them to cast their votes against ratification, stating that it was better to remain forever under military government then to fall into the power of carpetbaggers and scalawags.[22]

As for the Negroes, it was for them a time of hardship and suffering, but of glorious anticipation. Refusing steady work, many wandered about the streets, picking up chance jobs, sawing wood, putting away coal; the women and children in rags, gathering sticks and junk. "Idle, shiftless, wretched, and nearly naked," they found their consolation in listening to harangues, holding secret political meetings, and joining in parades. Of these there was an abundance. The struggle between the Negro leaders and the scalawags and carpetbaggers, begun on the floor of the convention, was continued with great bitterness in Norfolk. Opposed to the noisy Bayne were Lucius H. Chandler and the obnoxious carpetbagger James H. Platt. Chandler, a native of Maine, had come to Norfolk in 1850, where he attained success as a lawyer and politician. At the outbreak of the war he had thrown in his lot with the Union, receiving as his reward an appointment as United States district attorney. His loyalty, his reputation for honesty, and his close Southern affiliations made him the outstanding candidate for Congress in the Second District in 1865, and he was elected with the support of Democrats and Republicans alike. Now, however, with the people divided into Radicals and Conservatives, he alienated his white friends by throwing in his lot with the carpetbaggers and Negroes.[23]

Late in April, 1868, certain Radical leaders held a convention at Suffolk to propose a candidate for Congress. Bayne appeared in company with a group of his black supporters, but the whites excluded him. They then proceeded to nominate Chandler, while the irate Bayne, ranting on the outside, denounced their action as irregular and of no effect.[24] A few days later the Negro dentist spoke from the City Hall steps to an enthusiastic gathering of blacks, declaring that they had been tricked and must refuse to vote for Chandler.[25] In the mean-

[22] *Ibid.*, July 4, 1868.
[23] Norfolk *Landmark*, April 18, 1876.
[24] Norfolk *Journal*, April 29, 1868.
[25] *Ibid.*, May 1, 1868.

while, the Platt men were also working against Chandler. When the state radical convention met at Petersburg, with from fifteen hundred to two thousand delegates, most of them Negroes, it soon became obvious that Platt held the whip hand. The Suffolk delegates reported the action of their meeting, but the convention voted down Chandler's name with howls of derision, and then proceeded to nominate Platt.[26]

Platt was no more acceptable to the Norfolk Negroes than Chandler, for they were almost entirely under the influence of Bayne, and Bayne wanted the nomination himself. Every attempt of the Radical organization to force them into line failed. Since Chandler, too, refused to abide by the decision of the convention, night after night City Hall green resounded to the speeches of the three factions. On the evening of May 19 a pitched battle between the Chandler and Bayne men was narrowly averted. A crowd of Negroes had jammed into the court room expecting to hear Bayne speak, and were inclined to make a disturbance when they found Chandler in possession of the floor in the midst of a long-winded address. The Chandler men, on their part, resented the interruptions and the calls for Bayne, so that Mayor DeCordy found it necessary to threaten to arrest the first man who offered violence. In the end he awarded the floor to Bayne, and the dentist launched forth on one of his characteristic jumbles of religion, politics, and Negro rights, while Chandler had to finish his address on the outside.[27]

The opposing forces met in wordy combat again, during the Negro celebration of the Fourth of July, 1868. An excursion train arrived from Petersburg, bringing Platt "with all the scalawags, carpetbaggers, negroes, and cur dogs he could rake up." This motley crowd, joining the Norfolk Negroes, repaired to the City Hall green to listen to the speakers. Chandler began with a bitter address, abusing the whites of Norfolk, who had ostracized him since his defection to the Radicals, and advocating equality of the races and mixed schools. J. Parker Jordan spoke next, and then Platt. But feeling ran so high between the factions that Bayne, with most of the Negroes, drew off from the crowd, and marching out to Linsey's Gardens, held a meeting of his own.[28] A few days later, when Bayne was about to take a steamer at City Point for Norfolk, he was violently assaulted by a group of

---

[26] *Ibid.*, May 4, 1868.
[27] *Ibid.*, May 20, 1868.
[28] *Ibid.*, July 7, 1868.

Negroes, probably at the instigation of Platt, knocked down a long flight of stairs leading to the wharf, and severely injured. When he arrived in Norfolk the next morning, battered and bruised, he was escorted to City Hall Square, where his friends took turns in thundering against the Chandler and Platt ruffians.[29] Two days later the Platt faction had another inning, when a Negro named Givens spoke at the City Hall, roundly denouncing Bayne and his two white lieutenants, Sykes and Smith.[30]

By this time the blacks had become highly excited, and political gatherings were almost daily occurrences. Black orators, some of them former slaves, and unable to read and write, stood on the City Hall portico, giving vent to high-sounding, meaningless phrases.[31] In the midst of this hubbub, when the blacks were being victimized by unscrupulous leaders, they received one bit of sound advice from a real friend. Early in August, General O. O. Howard, head of the Freedmen's Bureau, visited Norfolk, and spoke first at the Bute Street Methodist Church, then at the old Baptist Church, and finally at the Baptist Church at Catharine and Charlotte streets. He told the Negroes that they must get to work, save money, educate their children, and keep their houses clean.[32] But they were not ready for such advice. They were looking forward to political supremacy in the state, perhaps to the distribution of the property of the whites, and disillusionment was not yet at hand.

In the meanwhile, General Schofield had advised Congress, in submitting the new constitution, to permit the people to vote separately on the clauses which disfranchised so many whites. This would give the state an opportunity to restore civil government, saddled with Negro suffrage, it is true, but with the white vote almost intact. A committee of nine prominent Virginians, who visited Washington to interview the President and the leaders in Congress, agreed to this arrangement as the best the state could expect,[33] while Gilbert C. Walker and other influential Northerners residing in Virginia urged it upon President Grant. Accordingly, having been so authorized by Congress, Grant named July 6, 1869, as the date for the election, and ordered those sections relating to the test oath and disfranchise-

[29] *Ibid.*, July 10, 1868.
[30] *Ibid.*, July 13, 1868.
[31] *Ibid.*, July 25, 1868.
[32] *Ibid.*, Aug. 6, 1868.
[33] Alexander H. H. Stuart, *Popular Movement in Virginia in 1869* (Richmond, 1888), pp. 28-58.

ment to be voted on separately. The giving of the vote to the Negroes was bitterly resented, but the people had to accept this phase of the constitution in order to save the remainder of their political fortunes. The moderate Republicans had already nominated Walker to oppose H. H. Wells, the Radical candidate for governor, and Colonel Withers withdrew in his favor.[34]

A short but exciting contest followed. On May 12, Walker was welcomed in Norfolk, where he was acclaimed Virginia's only hope. Although the whites expected to carry the state as a whole, and perhaps win in the Second District, it was obvious that the vote in Norfolk would be very close. General Canby, who was now in command in Virginia, by a revision of the lists had so reduced the white majority in the city that a handful of carpetbaggers and scalawags might turn the scale. On the other hand, the Radicals were weakened by their factional disputes. Not only were Bayne and Platt still in the field, but in Norfolk alone there were two Negro candidates for the state Senate, and three for the House of Delegates. The Conservative candidate for the state Senate was Colonel W. H. Taylor; the two candidates for the House, A. S. Segar and W. H. Burroughs.

Each party strained every nerve to enlist its full strength. On June 24, the last day for the registration of voters, the *Journal* made an earnest appeal to the whites. "To-day, if the true men of the city will register, all will be saved. . . . To-day, the best and dearest interests of every freeman in Norfolk hangs upon the discharge of duty, which his duty to his wife, children, home, friends, and country, points out as the only path of safety. To-day you aid in freeing your State from the vile influence of hired, itinerant demagogues, or you bind Virginia with manacles. . . . We are requested to say whether we prefer to live henceforth as free men or in subjection to an inferior and ignorant race, under the guidance of corrupt and degraded leaders."

Despite the intense excitement, practically no violence attended the election in Norfolk, for all the saloons were closed and policemen guarded the polls. The Negroes had the first inning, swarming around the booths in the early hours, before going to work, and voting in a solid phalanx. Later in the morning the whites began to arrive in an ever-increasing stream so that by twelve o'clock the Conservatives led by 220 votes. But the battle was not yet over. With the sounding of the noon-day whistle black voters poured in from the warehouses and

[34] Morton, *The Negro in Virginia Politics*, pp. 66-73.

wharves in such numbers that at nightfall it was impossible to tell which side had won.[35] It was only the next day that it became certain that in the local voting the Radicals had been generally successful. Not only did Wells carry the city by 2,094 votes to 2,014 for Walker, but Crane defeated Segar for congressman-at-large. On the other hand, Goodwin, the Conservative candidate for Congress for the Second District, came off an easy victor, while the Radicals split their vote between Bayne and Platt.[36]

The successes of the Radicals in the city were forgotten upon receipt of the news that in the state as a whole the whites had won a great victory. Although the constitution had been adopted almost unanimously, the objectionable clauses had been voted down; Walker had defeated Wells by 119,535 to 101,204; and the Conservatives had won forty-three seats in the Senate to thirteen for the Radicals, and ninety-six in the House of Delegates to forty-two for the Radicals. Only twenty-seven Negroes were elected to the Legislature, six in the Senate and twenty-one in the House.[37] Norfolk Conservatives celebrated. On the evening of July 7 a great crowd assembled on Main Street before the *Journal* office to listen to A. S. Segar and other Conservative leaders. The mass of upturned faces, the glare of the bonfires lighting up the street from Granby to Church, the deafening applause which greeted the speakers, testified to the intensity of feeling. Later the crowd fell in behind Weisdorf's band and marched down the street to the Atlantic Hotel, where they called for the governor-elect. When Walker appeared on the Granby Street balcony, a fine figure of a man, six feet in height, the picture of health and vigor, he was greeted with deafening cheers. He congratulated Virginia upon her deliverance from "vampires and harpies," and promised an honest, capable administration. As he concluded, amid immense applause, the band struck up "Dixie," and the crowd surged back to the *Journal* office, there to listen to still more addresses.[38]

The Norfolk papers were profuse in their praise of the Northern men for their part in the victory. "Almost every man of Northern birth who settled here since the war has aided in the glorious work of redemption," said the *Journal*. "All honor to them. . . . We wish for more such men, not tens, but hundreds."[39] But now, as the people

[35] Norfolk *Journal*, July 7, 1869.
[36] *Ibid.*, July 19, 1869.
[37] Morton, *The Negro in Virginia Politics*, p. 77.
[38] Norfolk *Journal*, July 8, 1869.
[39] *Ibid.*

settled down to the regular routine of life, the realization came that they had yet to win control of the city government. Another bitter struggle lay ahead. The new Constitution required each city of five thousand or more to hold elections on the fourth Thursday of May for mayor, judge, clerk, sergeant, commonwealth's attorney, treasurer, and other officers. Since in the recent election the Radicals had carried the city, the whites had good reason to regard the future with apprehension. Fortunately, about two hundred white men were enfranchised at this time by the removal of disabilities, and this reversed the small Negro majority in the city; but the margin was small at best.[40]

Ten months of comparative quiet ensued, while Norfolk remained under the able direction of Mayor DeCordy. Then, on April 22, 1870, the *Journal* sounded the tocsin by urging the Conservatives to register. "If you fail in this duty," it warned, "our city will surely fall under the control of the Radical gang."[41] The people, once more thoroughly aroused, responded with such good will that the registration books showed a white majority of 171.[42] This was encouraging, but it by no means made a white victory certain, for with the carpetbag and scalawag vote subtracted from the white column and added to the list of black voters, no one could predict the result. Once more the white Radicals, lured on by the hope of lucrative city jobs, set to work to organize the blacks; once more the City Hall resounded to the oratory of Bayne and Dilworth and Jordan.

Typical of these gatherings was that of May 14, 1870, when the hustings court room was jammed with the Negroes and their friends. The meeting was proceeding quietly as J. Parker Jordan was dilating on the needs of Negro education, when someone called out: "How many Negroes did you ever sell?" An uproar followed, and there would undoubtedly have been a free-for-all fight, had not Mayor De-Cordy jumped upon a chair and roared out a command for silence. "The first man who disturbs this meeting, black or white, I will send to jail," he said. This brought forth cheers, and the speeches continued.[43]

The "black and tan" party nominated Peter Dilworth for mayor, while the Conservatives named John B. Whitehead.[44] As election day

40 *Ibid.*, Aug. 16, 1869.
41 *Ibid.*, April 26, 1870.
42 *Ibid.*, May 11, 1870.
43 *Ibid.*, May 16, 1870.
44 *Ibid.*, May 14, 18, 1870.

approached the *Journal* continued to harp upon the momentous issues involved. A black victory means the "subordination of property, intelligence, and industry to pauperism, ignorance, and sloth. It means the debasement of Christian civilization and of Anglo-Saxon enterprise beneath the heels of Fetish Superstition and African unthrift. It means negro magistrates on your bench, negro policemen on your streets, negro legislators in your councils . . . negro commissioners in your schools."[45] On the evening of May 23, the whites held a monster demonstration, in which over two thousand men paraded the streets, shouting for Whitehead, and bearing aloft transparencies with significant mottoes. "White schools for white children," read one, "Scalawags for office, negroes to vote," said another, while a third showed the Radicals hugging the Negro before election and kicking him afterwards. A band from Richmond led the parade, which wound in and out of the streets, amid the glare of fireworks and the cheers of the crowd.[46]

The election was marred by one serious incident. When two Negroes approached the polls to vote the Conservative ticket, they were attacked by a group of their fellow blacks. The whites rushed to their rescue, and in the riot which ensued one Negro was shot in the hip while trying to slash a white man with a razor. With this exception the voting proceeded in an orderly manner. The outcome was a decisive victory for the Conservatives, Whitehead defeating Dilworth, Thomas W. Pierce being elected city clerk, Thomas T. Cropper commonwealth's attorney, Joseph M. Freeman treasurer. The Radicals had to content themselves with the commissioner of revenue, the inspector of streets, the clerk of the market, the keeper of the almshouse, and five whites and four blacks in the city councils. Mayor Whitehead took his seat at noon on July 1, 1870, and Reconstruction, so far as Norfolk was concerned, was practically a thing of the past.

The bitter memory of the struggle remained for many years, however, affecting party alignments and even personal relations, for the people of Norfolk were not quick to forgive those who had deserted the white man's cause in the hour of need. It was this, perhaps, which was responsible for a tragedy which shocked the community in the spring of 1876. On the morning of April 6 Lucius H. Chandler disappeared from his home, leaving no hint as to his whereabouts. Although his family gave the alarm promptly and a careful search was

45 *Ibid.*, May 20, 1870.
46 *Ibid.*, May 24, 1870.

made, ten days passed and still no trace of the missing politician could be found. At five o'clock on the morning of April 17, a Negro named Tyler left his home to take oysters in the river. Unfastening his boat from the pile to which it had been tied, he got in, took the oars, and pushed off. At this moment the body of a man moved from under the boat, and floated toward shore. In alarm Tyler rowed ashore and calling a white man to his assistance, removed the body from the water. It was Chandler. That the unhappy man had committed suicide was made evident by the discovery in his pockets of five heavy cobblestones.[47] Such was the end of the man who once had possessed the universal esteem of the people of Norfolk, but who had committed the unpardonable sin of aligning himself with the blacks at a time when white supremacy hung in the balance.

[47] Norfolk *Landmark*, April 18, 1876.

CHAPTER TWELVE

The New Order

Like all other Southern cities, at the conclusion of the Civil War Norfolk was prostrate. She had escaped the complete destruction which had been her lot in the Revolution, but her commerce was at a low ebb, her tributary railways broken, her finances deranged, her streets out of repair, her citizens impoverished. To her sons who came trudging home from the war, she seemed desolate indeed. "But for the occasional appearance of an idle white vagabond, sauntering along the wharf, gazing wistfully into the water," said one observer, "we should have imagined ourselves wandering amid the ruins of a lost city."[1]

Recovery was rapid, however. The broken railways were repaired, the river and bay steamers resumed their regular schedules, and, with the final assurance that the whites would remain in control of the state and the city, capital began to emerge from its hiding places. Northern men who made Norfolk their home during or immediately after the war aided materially in the revival of business. Some possessed wealth, others had valuable business connections in the North, still others aided solely by their enterprise and acumen. All who devoted themselves to business and kept aloof from Radical politics received a hearty welcome. The municipal government fell into the hands of honest, able men, and progress became the order of the day.

So early as 1865 a movement was started for a new water supply. To the more enterprising citizens existing conditions were intolerable. "How can we attract manufacturers," they asked, "if we have not the water essential for their needs? How can we ask capitalists to settle among us, and partake of contaminated water from our cisterns and wells? How can we insure public health by means of a sewerage

[1] Norfolk *Journal,* Dec. 6, 1866.

system, unless we have water in abundance?" The Norfolk *Post* declared that "half the cisterns and nearly all the pumps ran dry during the summer," and people have to borrow water even for cooking purposes.[2] "Just imagine, ye advocates of pumps and cisterns, the contents of such inconvenient receptacles." We ourselves saw taken from the old well on the corner of Main and Nebraska streets, "four copies of the old *Index,* any quantity of tin-pots and kettles, several infantile genus canine, one old tabby, and boots and shoes accordingly."[3]

None the less, the "Old Fogies," closing their ranks, fired broadside after broadside in the papers. "These people have water on the brain," declared "Common Sense," "but, I, for one, can't see the point. We have a very good supply of water and every time it rains, it is freshened and the supply renewed."[4] Another scribe, signing himself Madison, wished to know "what is the use of talking of a luxury which is to cost $1,000,000 to a people that haven't got the money?"[5]

The controversy waxed doubly hot when Mayor Tabb announced that he would place the matter before the voters on October 12, 1865.[6] If one ventured on Main Street, he found the people discussing water, if he entered Beardsley's to enjoy a game of billiards or partake of a bowl of oyster soup, water was the all-absorbing topic. At Tuttle's soda fountain, in the parlor of the Atlantic, the saloon of the National, at Sangster's, the post office, the Custom House, in the photographic saloons, in Freemason and Granby streets, at Town Point, water was the unceasing topic of conversation. The night before the election the advocates of good water formed a procession, led by the band of the Thirtieth Illinois Regiment playing "The Juniper Quickstep." Behind came the fire companies with torches, followed by decorated wagons and citizens bearing transparencies with such inscriptions as: "Sacred to the memory of the town pump," "Juniper will be our greatest blessing," "Vote for the new drink—water," "Mix Juniper with your whiskey to prevent chills."[7] The next day the "Old Fogies" were overwhelmingly defeated, and the government was empowered, by 451 votes to 149, to borrow five hundred thousand dollars to erect the water works.[8]

Unfortunately the city's credit was low, and so difficult did it prove

2 Norfolk *Post,* June 23, 1865.
3 *Ibid.,* Aug. 19, 1865.
4 *Ibid.,* June 29, 1865.
5 *Ibid.,* July 1, 1865.
6 *Ibid.,* Sept. 22, 1865.
7 *Ibid.,* Oct. 12, 1865.
8 *Ibid.,* Oct. 13, 1865.

to float bonds that the matter had to be postponed. But a severe drought in the summer of 1869, with the attendant shortage of drinking water, brought matters once more to a crisis. With the cisterns going dry, with well water brackish and unwholesome, with many depending upon barrels left out to catch an occasional shower, the cry for immediate action became insistent. "For five years we have been talking, writing, and voting," said the *Journal*. "The time has come when we must have water." And now began a lively controversy as to the proper source of supply. The old suggestion that water be pumped from Lake Drummond brought forth renewed protests. Juniper water was not fit to drink, it was so strong it would eat through iron in a few month's time, it would stain clothes, it could not be used in factories. When a letter appeared in one of the papers dilating on the advantages of Doyle's Lake, at Ocean View, the writer was overwhelmed with ridicule. "This little pond has no outlet," it was pointed out, "and does not contain enough water for a week's supply. It is to be doubted if the pond were filled with lager, it would supply our German fellow citizens with the beverage for one week."[9]

In November, 1869, three engineers[10] made an examination of a number of small lakes northeast of the city, in Princess Anne County, and reported favorably. The nearest available body of water was Broad Creek, at Moore's Bridges, they said. The stream at this point was brackish from the ebb and flow of tide water, but by building a dam across the creek, a sufficient supply of pure water could be had. However, since the new basin would have to be dredged and dyked and ditches cut in the near-by marshes to bring in the water, they considered the two Bradford lakes, near the shore beyond Little Creek, as the best source. Here the water basin was already made, the water excellent, the supply adequate for present and future needs.[11]

William J. McAlpine, who made a thorough study of the situation and reported in February, 1871, came to an entirely different conclusion. Believing that the Princess Anne lakes and creeks would prove inadequate for a growing city, he thought that the water should be brought from Lake Drummond or from the Nansemond River. The belief that the juniper water from the lake was so highly charged

9 Norfolk *Journal*, Oct. 5, 1869.
10 Virginius Freeman, H. W. Williamson, and John F. Dezendorf.
11 Merchants and Miners' Exchange, *Report*, 1869, pp. 78-83.

with tannin as to corrode iron, he denied vigorously. "The lock-gates of the feeder were taken off a year since," he said, "after having been in the water directly from Lake Drummond for twenty-three years. The wrought iron clamps, spikes, etc., were found to be so little oxidized that they were all used in the new gates." With a supply of pure water sufficient for a city of a million people, the greater cost of the Lake Drummond plan should not influence the councils to reject it. "The streams at Moore's Bridges and the lakes beyond will furnish a supply for a population of 50,000," he said, "and when the city increases beyond this demand, all of the expenditure . . . will be lost."[12]

After a careful consideration of McAlpine's report, the councils decided to draw their water, neither from Moore's Bridges nor Lake Drummond, but from Deep Creek, a tributary of the Southern Branch. The contract was let to William H. Allen and Co., and the work of laying down pipes begun.[13] This, however, was a palpable infringement upon the rights of the Dismal Swamp Canal, and when that body protested,[14] the city turned to the Moore's Bridges plan.[15] A few months later the work had been completed, and the water began to course along the conduit and throughout the city. But now that the people had water at their very doors, they were slow to avail themselves of it, many continuing for twenty years or more to depend upon cisterns. In January, 1874, only 185 connections had been made,[15a] while so late as 1893 the Chamber of Commerce reported that some rain-water cisterns were still in use, although "almost entirely out of date."[16] However, for the time being the vexed water question had been settled.

But now another vital need intruded itself on the public attention. Norfolk was a city devoid of hills; so, after heavy rains the water, instead of running off, stood in pools in the streets or in vacant lots. With the completion of the water works, and the draining into the gutters of the waste from hundreds of spigots, this nuisance became intolerable, and the cry for a system of sewerage and street drainage

[12] W. J. McAlpine, *A Supply of Water,* reprinted in *Norfolk's Water Supply* (Norfolk, 1904), pp. 33, 36, 58, 59.
[13] Norfolk *Journal,* Jan. 10, 1872.
[14] *Ibid.,* Feb. 8, 1872.
[15] *Ibid.,* Aug. 6, 1872.
[16] Lamb, *Our Twin Cities,* p. 40; Borum, *Norfolk, Port and City,* p. 24. On Jan. 1, 1875, there were 535 connections, a year later 771, and on Jan. 1, 1877, the number was 955. From time to time the supply was increased by tapping lakes adjacent to Moore's Bridges—Lake Lawson, Lake Smith, and Lake Bradford.

grew insistent. "If existing conditions continue," it was said, "we ourselves will be to blame if the city is swept by pestilence." Matters
came to a head in 1878 with the news that Memphis was in the grip
of an epidemic of yellow fever. Norfolk did not wish another visitation of that dread disease, so a noted civil engineer was employed and
a system of drains and sewers was adopted.[17] There were to be twenty-
eight miles of iron, stone, and terra cotta pipes, connected with a great
cesspool from which sewerage was pumped into the harbor.[18] But the
work progressed very slowly, and in 1887 it was stated that the system
was "still incomplete, many of our important thoroughfares being in
a state of sad upheaval, giving full opportunity for our people to
enjoy the winter's mud."[19]

No feature of the new drainage system was more welcome than the
elimination of the last remnants of Back Creek, between Bank and
Granby streets. For some years after the Civil War the imposing City
Hall looked out to the west over what the *Journal* called a "great,
pestiferous, noisome, odorous, odious, and unsightly marsh."[20] On the
east the marsh extended from Plume Street almost up to Freemason,
but further west it was so narrow that Granby Street crossed it on an
old stone bridge.[21] It had been suggested repeatedly that this area
should be filled in to enlarge City Hall Square. Not only would
this remove a menace to health, but it would fill the long-felt need of
a park. Year after year passed, however, and nothing was done.
Finally, in 1881, an enterprising citizen, A. A. McCullough, "took
hold of the matter on his own responsibility and account, and transformed the old cesspool into a busy mart of real healthy business
life."[22] In this way sixty acres were added to the city, which were soon
covered with stores, warehouses, and residences, but the opportunity
for a park in the heart of the old section of town was lost.

Mr. McCullough, in redeeming the land on either side, had made
no effort to eliminate the old ditch from Bank to Granby, to which
Back Creek was confined. With the adoption of a sewerage system this
eyesore was removed. In 1884 the canal was replaced by a four foot
underground iron culvert, the space filled in with shells,[23] and a wide

---

17 Norfolk *Journal*, Feb. 18, 1882.
18 Borum, *Norfolk, Port and City* (1893) , pp. 25, 26.
19 Lamb, *Our Twin Cities*, p. 59.
20 Norfolk *Journal*, July 21, 1871.
21 *Ibid.*, July 29, 1869; Oct. 20, 1872.
22 Lamb, *Our Twin Cities*, p. 54.
23 It may well be said that the people of Norfolk have been raised on oysters, and
the city itself on the shells.

boulevard constructed from the City Hall to Granby. The old Granby Street Bridge was removed, the street there graded, and the marshes to the west filled in to the edge of the canal.[24] Today as motor coaches and automobiles rumble over the wide surface of City Hall Avenue, few indeed realize that the site was once occupied by a creek deep enough for navigation, that where now stand tall office buildings, busy slaves once loaded or unloaded produce at their masters' wharves.

During and immediately after the Civil War the streets of Norfolk fell into disrepair. The condition of Main Street was described as wretched, while Water Street, from Jackson to the Lorillard Steamship wharf, was a quagmire.[25] In 1887, when the city finances were much improved, the work of repairing was begun.[26] In Main Street, save at the eastern end, the old cobblestones were removed, and Belgian blocks substituted.[27] In the course of time this work was pushed in other parts of the city, until, in 1896, of Norfolk's thirty-two miles of streets, eighteen were permanently paved with stone. It was far from a pleasant experience to jostle over the cobbles of the business section, and the fashionable denizens of Freemason doubtless preferred shopping on foot to venturing over them in their carriages. But for the country people who brought their produce to market, the stones were far preferable to mud.[28] That the parking problem was not born with the automobile is shown by the frequent complaints against the farmers for blocking traffic on Main Street, their carts often extending all the way from Granby Street to Church. After 1870, when the councils forbade this practice, the farmers for a time "parked" on Union Street, but the police were lax in enforcing the law, and the line of carts eventually reappeared on Main.[29]

The spirit of improvement next demanded electric street lights. It was a long cry from the day when Norfolk marveled at the first twinkling gas jets, for gas lights were now out of date. In February, 1883, the mayor placed the matter before the councils, and before the close of the year a number of arc lights were in operation. Many of the old gas lamp posts long remained like sentinels of a by-gone day, but their picturesque lamps were dark. By 1888 the Electric Light Company of Virginia was providing one hundred and ninety-two pub-

[24] Lamb, *Our Twin Cities*, p. 64; Norfolk *Journal*, April 8, 1884.
[25] Norfolk *Journal*, Dec. 10, 1873.
[26] *Ibid.*, January 4, 1877.
[27] Lamb, *Our Twin Cities*, p. 78.
[28] Borum, *Norfolk, Port and City*, p. 25.
[29] Norfolk *Journal*, Sept. 15, 1872.

lic arc lights and the old City Gas Light Company one hundred. The time when brawling sailors or drunken Negroes could break a head in the darkness of Norfolk's many narrow lanes was gone forever.

The return of peace found Norfolk still trusting to volunteer fire companies for protection against conflagrations, the Aid Fire Company, the United Fire Company, the Hope Hose Company, and the Hook and Ladder Company. There was one "steam" engine, the *General B. F. Butler*. But the organization was imperfect and the equipment antiquated, and when Chief Folger tested the engine, in August, 1865, with water pumped from Roanoke dock, several sections of hose burst.[30] Later the *General B. F. Butler* was removed to Fort Monroe, and its place taken by a new and better engine.[31] Still fires continued, and the dread of a widespread conflagration hung always over the city.

The completion of the water works afforded a protection from fire, in itself worth the money spent on this project. Unfortunately, it was in July, 1872, while the workmen were still laying pipes, that a severe conflagration swept the fire-trap section of Main Street, from Market Square to Union, destroying property valued at $250,000.[32] It was with a deep sense of relief, then, that the crowd looked on at a fire in February, 1874, while the firemen poured in a stream of water from one of the new mains. As the hissing steam arose and the flames died down, a great shout went up, in recognition of the fact that an important victory had been won over one of Norfolk's most deadly enemies.[33] In 1876 the Fire Corps consisted of Chief Thomas Kevill, an assistant, and three companies, each with a steam engine, a fireman, and a driver, and a number of extra men. Kevill received $60 a month, the firemen $20, drivers $70, and extra men $10 each.[34] Twenty years later the corps comprised fifty-one men, all receiving a regular salary, while the equipment embraced "five steamers, two of them new; two hook and ladder trucks, five hose carriages, thirteen horses, and a chemical engine."[35]

When the Federal authorities withdrew the provost guard from the streets of Norfolk in 1865, the little police force proved entirely incapable of maintaining order. With the Negroes demoralized, with soldiers on leave thronging the streets at night, with the usual groups

[30] Norfolk *Post*, Aug. 15, 1865.
[31] *Ibid.*, Jan. 31, 1866.
[32] Lamb, *Our Twin Cities*, p. 38.
[33] Norfolk *Landmark*, Feb. 17, 1874.
[34] Burton, *History of Norfolk*, p. 219.
[35] Borum, *Norfolk, Port and City*, p. 27.

of sailors seeking excitement, there should have been thirty-five or forty men constantly on duty. Instead there were six. "Thirty years ago one captain and two policemen were enough," pointed out the *Post*. "At that time a man could stand in the center of the city and throw a stone to its corporate limits, if it did not strike the water. Now the limits join Springfield," and a large force is necessary.[36] Throughout 1865, conditions grew worse. Crowds of idle boys thronged Main Street by day, sailors, vagrants, and Negro women at night; certain parts of the town were infested with notorious dance-houses, collisions between soldiers and Negroes were frequent; hold-ups and burglaries became nightly occurrences.

On the evening of July 4, a young man named William Martin was attacked by George King, a Negro of giant proportions. While a crowd of blacks stood by crying "Kill him! Murder him!" King slashed Martin's neck with a razor, and the white man was saved only by the timely arrival of a policeman. On the same night an officer was scuffling with a drunken sailor, when two other tars came to the aid of their comrade. Thereupon Little Water Street poured forth a horde of blacks, anxious to get into the melee, and it was only with the arrival of the guard that something like order was restored.[37]

In January, 1866, the *Post* complained that thugs and garroters had instituted a reign of terror on the streets. Among the victims were Joseph G. Fiveash, knocked down and robbed by white ruffians on Freemason Street at Catharine; Charles E. James waylaid on Granby, near Main; George Griffen, attacked by thugs on Catharine Street.[38] On February 4 George Brown was attacked on Holt Street, but felling one assailant and shaking off another, he made good his escape.[39] The same night burglars entered the house of R. G. Broughton, Jr., at 155 Bute Street. "The police ought to know every man in Norfolk," complained one editor, "and should be able to spot garroters and house-breakers, as fast as they arrive." But the robberies continued until times were more settled and improved finances made it possible to increase the police.

In 1877 there was a force of forty-two men under the leadership of Chief C. C. Benson. By this time holdups were less common, but trouble was still frequent with disorderly sailors who came ashore to visit the "havens," concert halls, saloons, and variety halls. At any

[36] Norfolk *Post*, Oct. 4, 1865.
[37] *Ibid.*, July 6, 1865.
[38] *Ibid.*, Jan. 22, 1866.
[39] *Ibid.*, Feb. 5, 1866.

moment the noise of quarreling from the gaming houses, or of open battle from some dark alley, might give warning that Jack was making trouble. And though the Negroes were more orderly than in the first months of their freedom, individual offenses were still frequent. On the other hand, there was no organized crime in Norfolk. In 1887 the police force, under Chief Joseph A. Pollard, numbered fifty-four, all uniformed and equipped like the police of New York City, while in 1896 the number had mounted to sixty-five.[40]

Norfolk was one of the first cities in the South to inaugurate a system of public schools. The legislature passed an act authorizing public schools in Norfolk as early as 1850, but it was only in 1857 that the system was actually put into operation with Thomas C. Tabb as superintendent. Four years later came the Civil War. The ensuing demoralization, the depletion of the city treasury, General Butler's dismissal of all teachers refusing to take the oath of allegiance, and the proposal to associate white and black children in the same schools tended to discredit public education. Gradually, however, with the return of prosperity and the passing of the fear of Negro control, the people began to regard it with more favor. In 1874, when W. W. Lamb was superintendent, there were four schools for whites, with sixteen teachers, and 526 pupils; and two Negro schools with eight teachers and 359 pupils.[41] But adequate buildings were still lacking, and often the school rooms were crowded. In 1878 the school committee assigned to each room four pupils in excess of the number of seats, explaining that four was the average number of absences.

In the next few years substantial progress was made, however, and in 1893 the city could boast of ten school buildings, five of them new, with thirty-eight teachers. The first high school was opened in 1894. Superintendent K. C. Murray, grasping the urgent need for more advanced work, won over the city to this step in the face of violent opposition. The Hemenway School, at Park and Lovitt avenues, was purchased, a staff of five teachers engaged, and on September 15, 1894, classes were begun. In 1899 there were twelve public school houses in Norfolk, with a total of sixty-five rooms; fifty-four white and eleven Negro teachers; and a total of 3,343 pupils.[42]

In the meanwhile, the old Norfolk Academy had been experiencing many vicissitudes. During the Civil War it had been taken over by the

40 Burton, *History of Norfolk*, pp. 221, 222; S. R. Borum, *Norfolk and Its Environs* (Norfolk, 1896) , p. 27; *Norfolk and Portsmouth* (1888) , p. 32.
41 Norfolk *Landmark*, Jan. 27, 1874.
42 Stewart, *History of Norfolk County*, p. 182.

Federal troops and used for a hospital. When the Norfolk *Post* in September, 1865, urged that the property be returned to its owners, as the need for a preparatory school was urgent,[43] the government complied willingly. The building was renovated, equipment hastily supplied, and teachers engaged, and in October the academy was re-opened with the Reverend R. Gatewood as principal.[44] In 1877 the city council attempted to take over the property for use as a public high school, claiming that the land upon which the academy stood had been donated to the trustees for public education, and that the school owed certain sums to the city. This effort met with failure, however, and the academy, continuing as a private school, entered upon a new period of growth and usefulness. In 1882 Robert W. Tunstall, a graduate of the University of Virginia, was elected principal, and under this able organizer and teacher the curriculum was recast, well-trained teachers were engaged, and adequate equipment was added. In 1893 the attendance was 136.[45]

In November, 1865, the first number of the Norfolk *Virginian* was issued. This paper, which fell in 1867 under the management of Michael Glennen, exerted a widespread influence in eastern Virginia. Mr. Glennen was one of the first Southern editors to plead for reconciliation with the North after the Civil War, and was largely responsible for the participation of the Federal government in the Yorktown centennial and for the first parade in which Confederate veterans and United States troops marched side by side. On March 31, 1898, the *Virginian* was merged with the *Daily Pilot,* and has continued as the *Virginian-Pilot,* one of the best edited papers in the South. The *Public Ledger,* an afternoon paper, appeared first on August 3, 1876, and was later merged with the *Dispatch* into the *Ledger-Dispatch,* a large and up-to-date paper. The *Journal* was first issued in 1866, and after a short but useful career was merged with the *Landmark.* This paper, under the able editorship of Captain James Barron Hope, known as "Virginia's poet laureate," long played an important rôle in the life of Norfolk.

The typical Norfolk residence of the period from 1865 to 1885, although lacking the charm of the Moses Myers house and other early homes, had the merit of extreme simplicity. It was built usually of brick, and abutted directly upon the street. There was always the

---

[43] Norfolk *Post*, Sept. 8, 1865.
[44] *Ibid.,* Oct. 9, 1865.
[45] Borum, *Norfolk, Port and City,* p. 28.

little portico, with its two columns, its flat roof, its railing, its long flight of steps leading down to the street; two basement rooms, used for dining room and kitchen; two rooms above; two in the second story with halls and stairs on one side. There were no window screens, no central heating plant, no bathroom, no gas pipes, no electric wires, no telephones. However, these modern conveniences were widely adopted in the last decade of the century, together with the highly ornate architecture and furniture of the mid-Victorian period.

The residential streets in 1865 must have presented a quiet and not unpleasing spectacle. "The houses, though ancient, are beautiful, picturesque, and the abodes of wealth and refinement. The streets are lined with huge trees, planted more than 100 years ago," while the gardens are "filled with the rarest, most fragrant, and many colored flowers."[46] Twenty years later the appearance of the older streets was much the same. The old houses, the broad sidewalks, the hitching posts, the long lines of shade trees, the blooming gardens, the pedestrians in the quaint dress of the day, perhaps an open carriage drawn by two fine horses, combined to give an impression of quiet dignity and charm.

A visitor to Norfolk in 1887 was struck by the beauty of some of the older residences. "The side-walks are skirted with trees, the front yards . . . are ample and gladden the eye with their green carpets; the buildings are all of brick and are large and roomy. . . . Wide stone steps lead up to the hospitable-looking doorways. All, with one exception, have porticos which show that the Virginian of old not only studied the classics, but also made his knowledge useful, for the first has Ionic columns, the second Doric, and the third Ionic." On the opposite side of the street was another charming old residence. "A handsome porch with Corinthian columns is the leading feature of this building, and two quaint and curious-looking brick erections at each limit of the front grounds give it quite a feudal appearance."[47]

Main Street, twenty years after the war, presented a varied and interesting scene. The buildings were uniformly of brick, three stories high, with shops on the first floor, and offices or storerooms above. On the north side was an endless row of canvas awnings, protecting from the sun the wares piled up for display on the sidewalk. In front of many stores were wooden images—an Indian gripping a bundle of cigars, or a man in long coat and high hat carrying a suitcase. Most

[46] Norfolk *Post*, Aug. 14, 1865.
[47] George I. Nowitzky, *Norfolk* (Norfolk, 1888), pp. 58, 59.

of the signs were affixed to the front walls of the buildings, but many jutted out over the sidewalks. Over the rough cobblestones jostled an endless procession of country carts laden with meat, vegetables, fish, oysters, or chickens; low-slung wagons, drawn by mules, and piled high with boxes and bales; or now and then a horsecar, clanging vigorously for the right of way down the middle of the street. "The street is utilized for the display of the best office, commercial and hotel buildings in the city," says a visitor in 1887.[48]

Strolling down Main Street from west to east, one would have been struck first by the new addition to the Atlantic Hotel, stretching 250 feet from Randolph to Granby. The Atlantic, which had its main entrance on Granby, was built in the French chateau style, with large, airy windows, pilasters on its front, and a row of flags waving from its mansard roof.[49] Opposite it, on the corner of Main and Fayette, was the Hare Building, its gold-lettered signs gleaming in the upper windows. Beyond it was the new Dodson Building with its marble front, the home of the cotton exchange and the Citizens' Bank of Norfolk. A little farther east the old Custom House, "a noble link with the ante-bellum days," faced up Granby Street. Next to this building was the St. James Hotel (then called the Virginia), built in 1879, a plain structure, devoid of beauty. "Hugging the St. James, in what appears a most Christian-like manner," was the Y. M. C. A., "the most showy edifice in the city." Across from the Custom House, on the eastern corner of Granby and Main, was the Ames and Stevens furniture building. Proceeding farther east along Main Street, one would notice on the north side the Lowenburg stores, the Academy of Music, and three of Norfolk's most important banks, the Bank of Commerce, the Norfolk National, and the Marine. The time-honored Purcell House, on the southeast corner of Church and Main, marked the end of the commercial district. From here east the business houses gave way to substantial residences, until the street terminated at the Norfolk and Western railroad station.[50]

Market Square at this time was described as "the busiest and most

[48] *Ibid.*, p. 25.
[49] Lamb, *Our Twin Cities*, pp. 73, 78. The original Atlantic Hotel was located at the corner of Main and Atlantic (then Gray) streets; it was destroyed by fire on Jan. 8, 1867. The new Atlantic Hotel was then built on Granby at Main and reopened Oct. 8, 1867. R. S. Dodson, who took over the hotel in 1871, added the wing on Main Street ten years later. The new Atlantic was in its turn destroyed by fire on Jan. 31, 1902. Burton, *History of Norfolk*, pp. 106, 112, 140; letters of Col. E. Griffith Dodson to the editor, Jan. 18, March 20, 24, 1961.
[50] Lamb, *Our Twin Cities*, pp. 78-80; Nowitzky, *Norfolk*, pp. 25-34; letter of Col. E. Griffith Dodson to the editor, March 20, 1961.

crowded place of the same area in Virginia or the Carolinas, for not only does most of the population of Norfolk and suburbs do their marketing and shopping here, but the two ferries" at one end, and the streetcar line at the other, pour in a continuous stream of human freight. "The huckster-stands and market wagons filled with the choicest of vegetables from the great truck-farms of Virginia and North Carolina; the fish-stands; . . . game from the marshes of Currituck Sound, Chesapeake Bay and the great Dismal, is a sight worth seeing. . . . In the fruit line we have everything from an egg to an apple, fresh fish, alive and kicking, plums, blackberries, whortleberries, raspberries, cherries, etc. . . . It is pleasant to walk through this great center of attraction about five o'clock in the morning, to view the luscious fruits, and listen to the haggling of exacting hucksters and butchers with economical housewives. . . . Much human nature can be seen in a market house."[51]

On Saturday nights the scene was made picturesque by "hundreds of smoking, glaring torches." Then it was that the wandering merchants stood up in their wagons to harangue the crowd. Some dilated on the virtues of the soap which would "even remove the stains from the character of a New York 'boodle alderman'; or medicine that will cure every disease from corns to consumption; or microscopes with which a man can look through a foot plank; or cement that will mend anything from the main shaft of an ocean steamer to a broken heart."[52]

Church Street in the eighties had "a blending of everything in the shape of habitations upon its long and crooked length . . . churches, synagogues, hospitals, grave yards; dry goods, boot and shoe, furniture, and grocery stores; meat markets, stables, liquor houses, bars, undertaking establishments, human hair stores, junk stores, alligator-tooth jewelry establishments." Here one encountered the Odd Fellows' Hall; beautiful old St. Paul's Church, dense masses of ivy clinging to its walls; the Central Presbyterian Church; St. Vincent de Paul Hospital, and finally Lesner's Garden. This popular resort is described as "a zoölogical garden, and also a flower garden," where visitors could wander among the trees, fountains, ponds, flowers, and shady bowers, or gaze in wonder at the line of cages filled with wild animals.[53]

As for the water front it was as busy and picturesque as ever.

[51] Norfolk *Post,* June 22, 1865.
[52] Nowitzky, *Norfolk,* p. 92.
[53] *Ibid.,* pp. 34-42.

"As I crossed over from Portsmouth on the ferry boat, the city of Norfolk stood before me," wrote a traveler in 1887, "her buildings so densely massed that I could scarcely trace a single street. . . . . Her substantial looking wharves, fringed with the tall masts of stately ships and the smoke-stacks of a fleet of steamers; further back the solid walls of the warehouses and stores that line her water-front; and above them all a grand display of spires, towers, pinnacles and domes." Upon landing the visitor marveled at the vast variety of goods piled up on the wharves and in the warehouses—huge blocks of stone from Tennessee, marble from Italy, oranges from Florida, rice from South Carolina, iron ore from southwest Virginia, steam engines from New York, plate glass from Paris, lime from London, tons of coffee from Brazil, tea from China, fish from the Chowan River, cotton from Alabama.[54] Everywhere were busy merchants and clerks, and scores of perspiring Negroes engaged in loading and unloading the steamers and sailing vessels.

"Here is life with a dash of foreign and strange in it all along shore," says another observer, "with a spice of brine and pungence of bilge and oakum and tar. . . . Ships and barks and barkentines, brigs and brigantines, and schooners and sloops; steamships and steamboats, towboats and toy launches, yachts, pilot-boats, racing-shell, cat-boats, and 'bug-eye' canoes, rafts even, enormous Naval cruisers, and little revenue cutters, clippers and old tubs, 'lime juices' and ocean tramps . . . discharging, loading, under tow and in dock. . . . There are lights to guide shipping on every point; buoys marking the channel; fog-bells and sirens, stentor throated and tempest tuned. Wharves—cotton wharves, with compress yards and warehouses and platforms behind; coasters' wharves, . . . stave wharves like India Dock; coal wharves, truck landings, oyster and fish landings; ferry slips; wood wharves; lumber wharves; shipyard and ship railways, and floating docks."[55]

Norfolk, despite its rapid growth after the war, occupied but a fraction of the area included in the present limits. In 1872 the town was squeezed in between Smith's Creek on the north and Newton's Creek to the east. Brambleton had but a few scattered houses, Atlantic City was a separate village, while a trip down Church Street to Huntersville brought one out into the open country. One branch of Smith's Creek extended out to Elmwood Cemetery, the other past the site of

[54] *Ibid.*, pp. 12, 51, 52.
[55] Borum, *Norfolk, Port and City*, p. 21.

Stockley Gardens, while between were farms and woodland. Newton's Creek was a broad body of water stretching from the A. M. & O. station to Princess Anne Road, and from Bermuda Street to Park Avenue, crossed by Noe's Bridge and Lovitt's New Bridge.[56]

On July 1, 1887, Brambleton was annexed to Norfolk. This suburb was formerly owned by George Bramble, his farm extending from the creek to Mississippi Inlet. In 1856 he sold fifty acres to the Norfolk and Petersburg railway, retaining 145 acres for his own use. Part of this land he put under cultivation, but much remained a wilderness of scrub oaks and chinquapin bushes. In 1870 E. H. C. Lovitt, as executor for Bramble, sold part of the land, and soon thereafter the Queen Street causeway (later to become Brambleton Avenue) was constructed, streets laid off, and lots placed on sale. In 1872 the Campostella bridge and the Holt Street bridge were built, while two years later Park Avenue was opened to Princess Anne Road. For the first time in the history of Norfolk, the town could be entered from the east by any save the old Church Street route. After this Brambleton grew rapidly. "Bath houses were built on Campostella bridge; boat and tub races were organized, and a band played in summer evenings in the grove at the end of the Holt Street bridge." In 1886 there were 840 families in the new community, with three churches, a public library, and lodges for several fraternal orders. In later years Newton's Creek was in large measure filled in, chiefly with millions of oyster shells, and Brambleton lost even the appearance of isolation.[57]

Another flourishing suburb was Atlantic City, near the site of old Fort Norfolk. This was a thriving little community, "with its variety of industries and many small stores."[58] In 1872 Atlantic City was connected with the city by two bridges, one to York Street, and the other to Botetourt Street. Here was the Norfolk Knitting and Cotton Manufacturing Company, several outposts of the lumber trade, and a number of concerns engaged in the oyster business.[59] In February, 1890, Atlantic City, together with a large tract of adjacent territory, was annexed to Norfolk.[60]

For many years after the Civil War Norfolk theatergoers continued to patronize the old Opera House, in Odd Fellows' Hall, on Church

[56] Norfolk *Journal*, Oct. 20, 1872.
[57] Lamb, *Our Twin Cities*, pp. 53, 114-116.
[58] Nowitzky, *Norfolk*, p. 43.
[59] Lamb, *Our Twin Cities*, pp. 52, 89, 90.
[60] Stewart, *History of Norfolk County*, p. 331.

Street. The building was "in the mediaeval English style, which rejoices in a grand display of great windows and pinnacles."[61] In this period, as in earlier days, the people always patronized liberally even mediocre performances. In June, 1865, when members of the crew of the British warship *Styx* presented *Black-Eyed Susan,* the heavy masculine heroine, who showed little regard for her *h*'s, came in for generous applause.[62] Several weeks later Kate Fisher appeared in the *French Spy,*[63] followed by *The American Cousin, The Taming of the Shrew, Waiting for the Verdict, Jack Cade,* and *Youthful Days of Richelieu.*

Jean Hosmer proved quite a favorite, her portrait of Lucretia Borgia attracting the "elite of Old Point" and other neighboring places. The part "was powerfully rendered, and the audience was chilled with horror."[64] Strolling opera companies occasionally visited Norfolk, but whether from lack of ability or from the failure of the audience to appreciate their efforts, often received a cold reception. "A few broken-down, voiceless, and expressionless operators, an orchestra but little superior to three blind fiddlers and a Scotch bagpipeman, a chorus of invalids in the last stages of consumption, . . . this is a tax upon the patience," said one critic. The rendition of *Norma* was bad; that of *Faust* worse. "Such demoniac howlings and screechings were never heard outside of Pluto's dreary kingdom, and we can only compare the entire performance to a midsummer night when all the cats and dogs" are loose.[65]

In October, 1867, when the theater was under the management of Sardo and Company, the tragedian Eddy delighted the "play-goers in the great character of Damon."[66] Three years later the room was crowded to see Laura Keene in *She Stoops to Conquer.*[67] This was followed by a performance by a burlesque and opera bouffe company, and later by Fox and Denier in *Three Blind Mice.*[68] In April, 1872, Edwin Booth appeared as Iago several evenings in succession before large audiences.[69] Eight months later Fannie Janauschek "created

[61] Nowitzky, *Norfolk,* pp. 36, 37.
[62] Norfolk *Post,* June 22, 1865.
[63] *Ibid.,* July 11, 1865.
[64] *Ibid.,* Nov. 4, 1865.
[65] *Ibid.,* March 24, 1865.
[66] Burton, *History of Norfolk,* p. 144.
[67] Norfolk *Journal,* Oct. 5, 1870.
[68] *Ibid.,* November 5, 1870; December 14, 1870.
[69] Burton, *History of Norfolk,* p. 143.

quite a sensation among the theater-goers" as "Mary Stuart in Schiller's beautiful representation of the hapless queen."[70] In December, 1873, Norfolk greeted Joseph Jefferson enthusiastically in his famous role of Rip Van Winkle.[71]

In January, 1876, "the charming little Lotta," a favorite in Norfolk, played the part of Musette, in the *Secret of Guilde Court,* while on February 7 and 8, the Kellogg Opera Troupe presented *Fra Diavolo* and *Faust.* Ten days later Maggie Mitchell, remembered by many in Norfolk for her appearances before the Civil War, won new admirers for her acting in *The Pearl of Savoy.*[72] But the greatest treat of all was the performance of Lillian Adelaide Neilson, as Juliet, in January, 1877. The Grand Duke Alexis, the Grand Duke Constantine, Rear Admiral Boutakoff, and other distinguished Russians who were visiting Norfolk graced the occasion with their presence. "Every seat in the house was occupied, and extra chairs were placed in all available places—even then standing room was in demand, and the walkway in the rear of the dress circle was literally packed. The auditorium was very handsomely decorated with the flags of all nations—the front of the gallery being festooned with small foreign flags, and the private boxes tastefully draped with large American and Russian flags. . . . The distinguished guests were the cynosure of all eyes, when the curtain was down. . . . In the character of the pure and constant Juliet, Miss Neilson fully sustained the reputation she had so justly won as the ideal of the immortal poet's beautiful conception."[73]

In 1880 the old Opera House, the scene of so many notable gatherings, was eclipsed by the erection of the Academy of Music, on Main Street. The exterior of the new building was unattractive, the lower floor being occupied by shops, but a surprise awaited those who walked through the long vestibule to the auditorium. "The two circles are rich in relief work; but the crowning glories are the proscenium and the ceiling. The first is a scholarly blending of emblems appertaining to music and drama in semi-relief," set off by two angels sitting half-poised on the cornice of the top boxes. "The ceiling is rich in magnificent frescoes and large medallions, with the busts of dramatic authors and musical composers." The stage was

[70] *Ibid.,* p. 148.
[71] *Ibid.,* p. 154.
[72] *Ibid.,* p. 165.
[73] Norfolk *Virginian,* Jan. 23, 1877; Norfolk *Landmark,* Jan. 23, 1877.

forty-five by sixty feet, and the auditorium seated sixteen hundred people.[74]

In 1899 the Norfolk Conservatory of Music, one of the first of its kind in the South, opened its doors under the management of Anton F. Koerner. A year later the Conservatory's symphony orchestra, composed partly of professionals, partly of amateurs, gave its first concert in the Y. M. C. A. hall. It was only in 1920, however, that a permanent civic symphony orchestra was organized.

The cultural activities of Norfolk during this period and in subsequent years derived their inspiration largely from the lives of two remarkable women—Irene Leache and Anna Cogswell Wood. In 1873 these ladies established the Leache-Wood School, which was later housed in a two-story, vine-covered building on Freemason Street. The girls who attended this seminary took away not only a knowledge of Latin, mathematics, and English, but a lasting love for the beauties of art, music, and literature. After the death of Miss Leache, Miss Wood began a memorial art collection, which for many years was housed in the Norfolk Public Library. In 1905 the Leache-Wood Alumnae Association took over the care of this collection. Eleven years later the latter organization changed its name to the Irene Leache Art Association, which was expanded in 1917 into the Norfolk Society of Arts.

The Norfolk women, like their sisters in other parts of the world, accepted without complaint the changing vogues in dress—the tunic of 1868; the loose sleeves, the bustle, the wide skirts and flowing train of 1873; the close-fitting skirt and tightly laced corset of 1877. The men looked on, uncomplaining save in the case of the "crown" bonnets of 1865, the "barber pole" stockings of 1875, and the Dolly Varden costume of 1872. Then they protested mildly. "An excitement of more moment than the Fenian demonstration, the Mexican Emperor, the national debt, Negro suffrage, or the restoration of the South . . . is the sudden change in fashions," said the editor of the *Post* in 1865. "We are to have crowns now, instead of the neat little crownless and modest republican bonnets and jaunty hats of the past year. This revolution will cost the country more than the debt. Our present styles of bonnets are very becoming, and we desire no change. The rents are too high and business too dull."[75]

A few years later "the ridiculous Dolly Varden lunacy captured the

---

[74] Nowitzky, *Norfolk*, p. 31; Borum, *Norfolk, Port and City*, pp. 10, 33.
[75] Norfolk *Post*, Sept. 25, 1865.

ladies of Norfolk, and swept off its victims by the hundred. It was revealed in linen, cotton, silk and woolen goods, the dark ground of which was illuminated with figures of leaves, vines and flowers, such as roses, hollyhocks, sunflowers, etc. of all the beautiful hues of the rainbow." "It gives to lovely woman the appearance of a perambulating conservatory," thought Burton. "But the Dolly Varden must run its course, and we must make up our minds to encounter it in parlor and kitchen as well as at church and on the streets."[76]

The Norfolk men suffered greatly from the universal curse of receptions, or "socials" as they were then called; and on occasions ventured to put their complaints into print. "You have to stand duty in a crowd, with kid gloves on your hands and weariness in your heart," one wrote. "Your shoes pinch, but you cannot sit down. Your companion bores you, but you must listen and smile. If you try to move about, you tread on thirteen hideous dress trains, that drag themselves like half-dead boa-constrictors at the heels of their fair possessors. You eat cake and drink coffee, though you know it will give you a headache in the morning."[77]

No doubt this long-suffering male was more in his element in some of the baseball games, or in the rowing matches, or perhaps on the race tracks. So early as October, 1865, the Juniper baseball club was practicing on a field near the cemetery. "The feats of dexterity displayed by the fielders in catching the ball on the fly, rather astonished some of the spectators who had never witnessed the game before."[78] On November 24, the Junipers played the Unions, of the Thirty-ninth Illinois Regiment, and were defeated 44 to 30.[79] Two weeks later they redeemed themselves by overwhelming another Norfolk club, the Creightons, 94 to 25. "On the part of the Junipers, Panchon, the pitcher, showed decided tact and experience in giving the ball to the bat, guarding against any possibility of ground balls, which is quite a big item in a match game," reported the *Post*. "Moore at short stop was all over, but was too excitable in the interests of others, and lost sight of his own position. . . . The basers and fielders did very well, but need practice."[80] In 1867 the Creightons played a home and home series with the Petersburg Independents. The odd game was played on neutral ground in Suffolk, the Creightons winning 43 to

76 Burton, *History of Norfolk*, pp. 142, 143.
77 Norfolk *Journal*, Nov. 15, 1870.
78 Norfolk *Post*, Oct. 26, 1865.
79 *Ibid.*, Nov. 25, 1865.
80 *Ibid.*, December 9, 1865.

9.[81] The Norfolk boys met their Waterloo in August, 1868, however, when they fell before the Maryland Club, of Baltimore, by the score of 87 to 10.[82]

After this the energies of athletic youths turned to the equally exciting sport of rowing. The Undine and the Chesapeake Boat clubs were organized in Norfolk, and the Seaboard Club in Portsmouth, so that long ship's boats, pulled by six lusty youngsters, became a familiar sight on the Elizabeth. In August, 1871, the Undines tried their prowess against the Potomac Club of Georgetown, but were defeated.[83] This race was overshadowed in interest by the match between the two Norfolk clubs on May 7, 1872. The entire city was on tiptoe. The wharves on both sides of the river, the warehouses, the bridges were crowded, and the decks of the monitor *Canonicus* swarmed with people. On the United States tug *Standish* a brass band played, while the course was lined with rowboats, tugs, sloops, and yachts. The Undine crew consisted of William Webber, J. C. Lynch, James O'Rourke, J. C. Carroll, James McMenamin, John A. Hebrew, and E. B. Le Page; the Chesapeakes, of William C. Dickson, L. W. Tazewell, J. C. Baker, W. C. Hardy, George McIntosh, Fred Hardy, and P. T. Moore. The course covered three and an eighth miles. At 4:36 P.M. the boats got away, with the Undines in the lead. But the superior training of the Chesapeakes soon told, for they crept up on their opponents, passed them, and won by a good margin, in the excellent time of nineteen minutes and twenty seconds.[84]

In May, 1873, an exciting race took place between the Chesapeakes and the Seaboards, of Portsmouth. The Norfolk crew was unchanged save that Moore had given way to William Waller, McIntosh to William A. Graves, Jr., and W. C. Hardy to F. B. Dornin. The Portsmouth boat, named the *Ripple,* seems to have been superior to that of the Chesapeakes, and won handily in eighteen minutes and forty-five seconds. But Norfolk forgot this setback, when the Chesapeakes, three weeks later, won from the Anacostian Club of Washington, in a race of four-oared shells on the Potomac. The victorious crew were welcomed on their return to Norfolk with a banquet at the Atlantic Hotel, featured by an address by Colonel J. W. Hinton.[85] The interest in rowing gradually waned, despite the organiza-

[81] Burton, *History of Norfolk*, p. 110.
[82] *Ibid.*, p. 125.
[83] *Ibid.*, p. 140.
[84] Norfolk *Journal*, May 8, 1872.
[85] Burton, *History of Norfolk*, pp. 149, 150, 151; Lamb, *Our Twin Cities*, p. 38.

tion of the Norfolk Boat Club with a large membership, and the erection of a club house.[86]

While some of the young men were thus distinguishing themselves as oarsmen, others were winning favor in the lists. In the tournament held at the old Fair Grounds in 1870, S. S. Gresham, Jr., entered as the Knight of the Sable Plume, J. M. Hardy as Fra Diavolo, Henry L. Turner as Norfolk, Asa Biggs as the Old North State, L. C. Salusbury as Golden Spur, W. H. Gresham as Sir William Delaraine, C. H. Quarles as True Heart, W. A. Boykin as Ivanhoe, F. M. Halstead as the Lost Cause. The roads to the Fair Grounds were crowded, and the cars, each drawn by six horses, jammed to suffocation. Although the sun shone in the eyes of the knights, they displayed great skill in managing their horses and in spearing the ring. The Knight of the Sable Plume won first honors, with Fra Diavolo second. The next evening, at an elaborate ball in the Atlantic Hotel, Miss Maggie Sterling, of New York, was crowned Queen of Love and Beauty, Miss Jennie Taylor, Miss Lula Blow, and Miss Mollie Webb being Maids of Honor.[87]

Not to be outdone by their brothers, in June, 1879, the ladies of Norfolk organized a six-day walking match at the Opera House. Hour after hour, day after day, the fair contestants, unmindful of weary, aching feet, trudged round the main floor of the orchestra. On the sixth day the race had narrowed to Laura T. Douglass, Estelle Fillmore, Jennie Thorne, and Minnie Horton. As the day wore on so many spectators crowded on the stage that it seemed a "sea of eager and expectant faces." At last, when it was known that Miss Douglass had won, "a storm of applause" broke forth. In the six days the winner had walked 310 miles and three laps.[88]

Horse racing, the sport of colonial and ante-bellum days, was by no means eclipsed by the introduction of baseball and rowing. Year after year the Norfolk Turf Association arranged races in the Trotting Park at the end of Colley Avenue, or Fort Norfolk Road as it was formerly called, which were watched by eager crowds.[89] It was in November, 1873, that the Norfolk mare Nellie was matched against a New York trotter named Huntress, for a purse of $1,500, at the Campostella track in the new Fair Grounds, south of the Eastern Branch. Hundreds came from Norfolk, some in carriages over the

[86] Borum, *Norfolk, Port and City,* p. 32.
[87] Norfolk *Journal,* Oct. 5 and 6, 1870; Burton, *History of Norfolk,* pp. 137, 138.
[88] Norfolk *Journal,* June 8, 1879.
[89] *Ibid.,* July 6, Oct. 20, 1872.

draw-bridge or the toll-bridge, some came on foot, others crowded into a special train on the N. & P. railway, which ran directly to the grounds. Enthusiasm was unbounded when Nellie won three out of five heats, her best time for the mile being two minutes and thirty-two seconds.[90]

Hunting, too, was popular. The whole Tidewater region abounded in water fowl, canvasback, mallard, teal, and other ducks; geese, swans, partridges, pigeons, pheasants, wild turkeys, and even deer. Several gunning clubs were in existence, with headquarters on the Currituck Sound, at Two Penny Point, and elsewhere. The Norfolk Fox Hunting club held frequent meets, a favorite ground being near Indian Pole Bridge.[91]

The circus, of course, was always popular. "Everybody goes to the circus," declared the *Post* in June, 1865, when Nixon's show visited Norfolk. "The fondness for horses and athletic exercises, the mad antics and clever jokes of the clown, the daring feats of the bold riders, the graceful attitudes of the lady who rides the dashing white horse, the fearful acts of the two brothers—they're always brothers—delight all classes. The canvas is crowded every night, a goodly portion of the audience being black."[92] The tent was erected on a vacant lot on the corner of Main and Granby streets, opposite the Custom House. Seven years later the entire community was thrilled at the daring of "Professor" Donaldson, in ascending from the Fair Grounds in a balloon. To the horror of the crowd the balloon burst while in mid-air, but the cloth seems to have flattened out into a kind of parachute, so that the Professor's descent was retarded, and he fell into a clump of trees with no serious injuries.[93]

From time to time the quiet life of Norfolk was broken by some great event which stirred deep emotions or aroused curiosity and excitement. In April, 1870, General Robert E. Lee visited the city. As his train pulled into the Seaboard station, the Portsmouth veterans greeted him with a salute from a gun borrowed from the fire company. The general's carriage, from the station to the ferry, passed through masses of people, while the Rebel yell rang out over and over again. On board the ferry itself, the general retired to his cabin to avoid his admirers, but as he stepped ashore in Norfolk, all had a chance to show their respect. Here the United Fire Company awaited

[90] Burton, *History of Norfolk*, p. 154.
[91] Norfolk *Journal*, Jan. 27, 1877.
[92] Norfolk *Post*, June 22, 1865.
[93] Norfolk *Journal*, Jan. 9 and 16, 1872.

him, together with a crowd which packed Market Square and pressed forward eagerly, amid the glare of Roman candles and the boom of cannon, to catch a sight of "Marse Bob."[94] Six months later the city once more paid homage to the great leader, but this time at the sad tidings of his death. Public buildings, stores, residences were everywhere draped in mourning, business was temporarily suspended, bells tolled. Norfolk had accepted the verdict of the war, was loyal to the restored Union, but her affection for the hero of the Lost Cause was constant.[95]

On the morning of January 13, 1877, the Russian frigate *Swetlana* arrived in the Elizabeth, with Grand Duke Alexis, Grand Duke Constantine, Rear Admiral Boutakoff, Prince Obolinski, and other notables, for a visit of two months. This event caused a flutter among the Norfolk ladies, who awaited eagerly an opportunity to meet the distinguished foreigners. When it was announced that the Norfolk German Club would give a dance on January 25 in honor of Grand Duke Alexis, there were hasty refittings of gowns of silk or tarlatan. "The ballroom floor and spectators' seats were thronged with the elite, beauty, and fashion of our ancient borough, and the scene presented was of unusual splendor and brilliancy. The hall was decorated with Russian and American flags, and the music was splendid. Beautiful belles, graceful and courtly gentlemen, and stately matrons were present to mingle in the social festivities of the evening. . . . At 9 o'clock the band played, and the German was begun. . . . At 10 o'clock the Grand Duke and his staff entered the room, and were formally introduced by Captain B. P. Loyall to many ladies and gentlemen. After a few minutes of pleasant conversation, *les Lanciers* claimed the attention of the dancers, and partners took their places." Mrs. James Y. Leigh danced with Grand Duke Alexis, and Miss Hattie Parks with Prince Obolinski.[96] On February 8 there was a grand naval ball at the Navy Yard in honor of the Russians, while a few days later the Grand Dukes gave a *matinee dansante* on board the *Swetlana*.[97]

The period from 1865 to 1890 in Norfolk was marked by profound changes. Many of the oldest families had suffered terribly from the war, some having been reduced to poverty, others having left many of their members upon the battlefield. The military funerals, of almost

[94] Burton, *History of Norfolk*, p. 133.
[95] Norfolk *Journal*, Oct. 13, 1870.
[96] Norfolk *Virginian*, Jan. 26, 1877.
[97] Burton, *History of Norfolk*, pp. 183, 194.

weekly occurrence in 1865, when the bodies of Norfolk's soldiers were brought home, typified the end of the old social order. Norfolk still revered the ante-bellum tradition; charm, courtesy, and hospitality still marked her social intercourse, but she could not escape the moulding influence of a new era. New railway lines were opened, new steamship connections made, manufactures sprang into life, Northern businessmen came with new ideas, the young men of Norfolk imbibed the spirit of progress. The advent of electric lights, street-cars, water works, sewerage, clean streets, an efficient police force, better schools; the elimination of marsh lands, the erection of substantial business houses, the extension of the city limits were but symptoms of the changed spirit of the time. The Norfolk of other days, the Norfolk of General Robert B. Taylor, Governor Tazewell, Hunter Woodis, and Hugh Blair Grigsby, was making way for the commercial and industrial city of the future.

CHAPTER THIRTEEN

A Half-Century of Growth

The conclusion of the Civil War found Norfolk practically cut off from the interior. Vessels were still coming through the Albemarle and Chesapeake canal, and traffic on the James was immediately restored, but months elapsed before the Norfolk and Petersburg, and Seaboard and Roanoke railroads could be put into operation. For miles the tracks had been torn up and bridges destroyed. It was only in the fall of 1865 that trains began to move over the Seaboard, and in April, 1866, that connection with the south was restored by the completion of the new bridge over the Roanoke at Weldon. The Norfolk and Petersburg was opened for traffic in February, 1866.

This long expected event was marked by an excursion from Richmond to Norfolk, graced by the presence of Governor Peirpoint and many senators and delegates. Cigars and liquor were passed around in the special guest coach, and one could hardly see across the car. "Loud talking is heard, and songs, facetious remarks, and anecdotes, laughter, mock speeches, and a disposition to romp. Looking out, a low, flat country, with here and there a clump of trees, seen through a veil of smoke, and a stream of whirling, delirious sparks. . . . We are going very rapidly, but the track is new, and we go smoothly. . . . Trees, swamps, the Elizabeth River, the Dismal Swamp, the canal go by, and we are at Norfolk. Here we are met and escorted to Pepper's, where a supper awaits us. In an anteroom are bowls of fluid. . . . Legislators close round in firm circles, and after a preliminary pull," they listen to an address of welcome by Mayor Tabb. Governor Peirpoint replies, pledging the state's support to measures aiding in the development of Norfolk. He is followed by Colonel J. P. Baldwin,

Gilbert C. Walker, and others. "After this, things got sort of lively all around the board." "Gentlemen," said one legislator, "Norfolk is by nature a great commercial 'mporium. . . . S'got a magnificen harbor. We are going t' make it blossom like a rose. I mean to say be full of ships, 'n things, masts, an' sails, an' Jib-booms, an' ship ahoy."[1]

The resumption of railway traffic had a magical effect upon Norfolk. The city awakened as from a troubled sleep, and activity was resumed with a vim unknown since the days before the Embargo. "Everywhere there is bustle and noise, and the pleasing sound of labor," said an observer, in December, 1866.[2] "Turn where we might, we saw huge piles of cotton. . . . The wharves everywhere groaned beneath the weight of the products of the great North State—tar, turpentine, rosin, staves, shingles, lumber. Hundreds of merry-faced laborers were busy discharging or loading the many vessels that lined the wharves, or moved freight to and fro."[3]

On February 24, 1866, two carloads of cotton from Georgia which arrived over the Norfolk and Petersburg awakened the city to the fact that at last connection had been established with the Far South. Cars could be loaded at Memphis, and passing over the Memphis and Charleston to Chattanooga, thence over the East Tennessee and Georgia to Bristol, over the Virginia and Tennessee to Lynchburg, the Southside to Petersburg, and thence over the Norfolk and Petersburg, discharge their loads in the warehouses on the banks of the Elizabeth. Before the lapse of a year this group of railways was pouring into Norfolk various agricultural products—cotton, corn, flour, fruit, peanuts, potatoes, tobacco, and wheat—together with millions of feet of lumber.

However, the linking of Norfolk with the cotton states would have proved of little ultimate benefit had it not been for the consolidation of the three lines from Norfolk to Bristol. This move, one of the first of its kind in the South, was sponsored by General William Mahone. Had the proposal been made prior to the Civil War, the Richmond interest could probably have blocked it, for it was certain to divert traffic from the James River and Kanawha canal and from the Richmond and Danville Railway, but Richmond no longer wielded the power of old. First winning the support of Governor Walker, Mahone secured the passage of a bill to merge the Norfolk and Petersburg,

[1] Norfolk *Post*, Feb. 19 and 20, 1866.
[2] Norfolk *Journal*, Dec. 6, 1866.
[3] *Ibid.*

the Southside, and the Virginia and Tennessee into the Atlantic, Mississippi and Ohio Railway; to provide for its extension to meet the railroad system of Kentucky; and to authorize a loan of fifteen million dollars for repairs and new equipment.[4]

The new system, which stretched 408 miles across southern Virginia, was in a strategic position to intercept traffic to Richmond, not only from Lynchburg and the Valley of Virginia, but from West Virginia. No wonder the Richmond press dubbed Mahone the "Railroad Ishmael."[5] For Norfolk, however, the merger was most beneficial. The lumber, wheat, and tobacco of southern Virginia, and the cotton of the Far South poured into her lap in increasing volume, and the old isolation of ante-bellum days was forgotten in the optimism of dawning prosperity.

There was one moment of great anxiety. With the financial panic of 1873, the road became financially embarrassed and could not meet the interest on its mortgage bonds. In March, 1876, the bondholders applied for a receivership,[6] and three months later the receiver took control. With returning prosperity receipts mounted steadily, so that in time every obligation could have been met, but it was deemed expedient to end the receivership by selling the road. Norfolk awaited in breathless suspense. Should unfriendly interests acquire this line and divert its traffic to Richmond or Baltimore, the effect would be ruinous. Fortunately, the purchaser, Clarence H. Clarke, of Philadelphia, made Norfolk the key to a much expanded system.[7] Changing the misleading name of Atlantic, Mississippi and Ohio, to Norfolk and Western, he launched a progressive program, making contracts for joint traffic with the Virginia and Georgia, and the East Tennessee, and reducing through passenger and freight rates.[8]

Even more important was the extension of the line into the vast coal fields of southwest Virginia and of West Virginia. The New River Railway, controlled by the Norfolk and Western, was pushed westward, until, in 1883, it reached the Pocahontas region. On this side and that, wherever coal was discovered, branch lines were run up the narrow valleys beneath the mountain ranges. This was the

---

[4] C. C. Pearson, *The Readjuster Movement in Virginia* (New Haven, 1897), pp. 27, 28; Jones, *Norfolk as a Business Centre*, pp. 21-26; Norfolk *Journal*, Nov. 15, 1870.
[5] Pearson, *The Readjuster Movement in Virginia*, p. 70.
[6] Norfolk *Journal*, March 16, 1876.
[7] The purchase was made on Feb. 10, 1881, and the owners took possession of the road on May 3, 1881 (Norfolk *Journal*, Jan. 12, 1882).
[8] *Ibid.*

beginning of a movement which was to make Norfolk one of the greatest coal ports of the world. But the management was not yet satisfied. Extending its line northwest along the boundary of West Virginia and Kentucky to the Ohio River, and thence to Columbus, it tapped the Middle West, and opened to Norfolk the possibility of becoming also a great grain port.[9]

In the meanwhile, the Seaboard and Roanoke was also doing its share to build up Norfolk. In the ten months preceding April 1, 1867, this line brought in 52,000 bales of cotton, 760,000 pounds of dried fruit, 17,000 barrels of naval stores, 670,000 staves, and 2,500,000 feet of lumber.[10] It was chiefly by the Seaboard and Roanoke that Norfolk maintained its position as the most important port for North Carolina. Goods in large volume flowed over the North Carolina railway from Charlotte and Salisbury to Raleigh, then over the Raleigh and Gaston to the Seaboard, and thence to Norfolk. This caused many protests from the Carolinians. "Why," they said, "should our produce aid in building up a port in another State, when we have suitable harbors of our own? The traffic which now goes to Norfolk should be diverted to Beaufort, by means of the Atlantic and North Carolina." But the old difficulties of shallow water, sand bars, and dangerous capes operated now as in former generations to force Carolina freight to go to Norfolk. Of 39,285 tons of goods passed on by the North Carolina railway to other roads in 1869, no less than 31,767 tons found their way to the Elizabeth, 4,950 tons to Wilmington, and only 2,568 tons to Beaufort.[11]

Though Norfolk easily maintained her superiority over the Carolina ports, she had good reason to fear the competition of Baltimore and other great Northern cities. She was in constant fear that her connections to the west and south would be interrupted by the formation of north and south railway mergers. From the mass of little lines in North Carolina, it was inevitable that trunk railways would eventually be created. Whether the new combinations would radiate from Norfolk, or from Washington and the North, was of supreme importance. The north and south trend is shown by a statement of President W. A. Smith, of the North Carolina railway. "Our true

---

[9] Poor's *Manual of Railroads* (New York, 1887, 1894).

[10] Norfolk *Journal*, Feb. 13, 1867.

[11] C. K. Brown, *State Movement in Railroad Development* (Chapel Hill, 1928), pp. 156-160.

policy is to work with the shortest, quickest, and the cheapest lines north and south," he reported to his stockholders in 1869.[12]

That the Carolina eventually became linked with the Richmond and Danville, and not with the Seaboard, is due in part to the Civil War. In 1861 there was one serious gap in the railway lines from Richmond to the Far South, that between Danville and Greensboro. So the Confederate Congress, acting upon the advice of President Davis, chartered the Piedmont railway, which at once became a subsidiary of the Richmond and Danville. After the war the latter company, with its southern terminus in Greenville, suddenly envisaged a far-reaching system in Georgia and other parts of the South. And for this system the tracks of the North Carolina, between Greenville and Charlotte, were a necessary link. In 1871, despite the bitter opposition from many Carolinians, the entire North Carolina railway was leased to the Richmond and Danville, and the dream of a trunk line from Norfolk to western Carolina for the time being vanished.[13] On the other hand, the Seaboard, taking a leaf from the book of its rivals, gradually built up a north and south system of its own. Gaining control of the Raleigh and Gaston, the Raleigh and Augusta, and the Wilmington and Shelby, by 1884 it was draining into its warehouses at Portsmouth the products of all central and southern North Carolina.[14]

Norfolk's two railways, with the Albemarle and Chesapeake canal, succeeded in making the place one of the nation's greatest cotton ports. "Cotton is pouring in," stated the Norfolk *Journal,* in January, 1867. "As formerly we were the greatest corn port on the Atlantic, so we may soon be the greatest cotton port." In 1858 Norfolk received only 6,174 bales of cotton, eleven years later the number was 137,-339,[15] while in the year ending March 1, 1874, it was no less than 437,031 bales.[16] For the time being, it was receiving more cotton than either Charleston or Savannah, and was surpassed only by New Orleans and Galveston.[17]

At first the agreements for through freight rates between both railways and connecting steamship lines caused much complaint. "The

[12] Brown, *State Movement in Railroad Development,* p. 162.
[13] *Ibid.,* pp. 165-173.
[14] Poor's *Manual of Railroads,* 1884, p. 406.
[15] Norfolk *Landmark,* Feb. 12, 1874; Merchants and Mechanics Exchange, *Report,* 1869, p. 31.
[16] Norfolk *Landmark,* March 11, 1874.
[17] *Ibid.,* March 17, 1874.

Atlantic, Mississippi and Ohio carries cotton to New York at the same rate it does to Norfolk," stated the *Journal*. "Out of the 70,000 bales (brought here last year) every one remained at Norfolk except 68,500 which were dumped into steamers and carried north."[18] But this state of affairs was short-lived. In 1874 a cotton exchange was organized, with offices in the warehouse of Reynolds Brothers, on Water Street. Later the exchange moved to the Dodson Building on Main Street, the handsome marble front of which had once stood in Baltimore and had been brought to Norfolk by boat in its entirety.[19] In addition the establishment of two compress houses made possible foreign shipments directly from Norfolk's wharves. "My attention was attracted by the grim-looking tower of the Virginia Compress," states a visitor to Norfolk in 1888, "which showed plainly what it was intended for, not only by the white clouds of escaping steam and deafening noise that accompanied them, but also by the many bales of cotton that would find their way into its somber-looking interior large and clumsy, and leave reduced to less than half their former size, in order to take up less space in a ship's hold."[20]

In short, cotton, almost unknown at Norfolk before 1855, restored the city's foreign trade, and with it the long-dreamed-of prosperity. In 1866 the number of bales sent directly from the Elizabeth River to Europe was only 733, in 1873 it had mounted to 8,282, in 1874 to 47,342, in 1875 to 87,753, in 1876 to 106,421.[21] In the year ending August 31, 1888, the number of bales sent to Great Britain alone was 230,983.[22] At that time more than half the cotton received at Norfolk and Portsmouth was shipped abroad.[23] Norfolk's exports in 1866 totaled $411,397,[24] in 1874 they had risen to $1,831,036, in 1875 to $5,243,986,[25] in 1876 to $7,825,112,[26] in the year ending August 31, 1885 to no less than $14,279,835.[27] Once more the Elizabeth took on the character of old, with great ocean liners at anchor or tied up at the wharves. Here is the Allen liner *Hibernian,* loading for Liverpool; here the steamer *Strasburg,* of 2,662 tons, bound for Reval;

---

[18] Norfolk *Journal*, March 23, 1871.
[19] The building was erected in 1885 by R. S. Dodson, owner of the Atlantic Hotel. Letter of Col. E. Griffith Dodson (his grandson) to the editor, Jan. 13, 1961.
[20] Nowitzky, *Norfolk,* p. 24.
[21] Norfolk *Landmark*, Jan. 7, 1877.
[22] *Ibid.,* Sept. 2, 1888.
[23] *Ibid.,* Oct. 8, 1885.
[24] *Ibid.,* March 11, 1874.
[25] *Ibid.,* Dec. 11, 1875.
[26] *Ibid.,* Jan. 7, 1877.
[27] *Ibid.,* Sept. 4, 1885.

here the great ship *Gregory*, there a bevy of barks, brigs and schooners. In 1883 no less than 121 vessels, aggregating 97,955 tons, left the Elizabeth for foreign ports,—59 for Liverpool, 15 for Demerara, 11 for Jamaica, 7 for Reval, 4 to Barbados, 3 to Barcelona, 3 to Belfast, 3 to Trinidad, and one or two to other widely scattered ports.[28]

It was in the decade from 1870 to 1880 that the port of Norfolk once and for all outdistanced the Virginia Fall Line cities. As ocean liners grew larger and larger, it became increasingly difficult for them to ascend the James or the Appomattox. If one wished to ship cotton or wheat from Richmond or Petersburg for foreign ports, it had to be done in vessels of light draft, and vessels of light draft were finding it difficult to compete with the new and larger type of steamer. So it was to Norfolk that the southern cotton was brought, while the exports of her ancient rivals gradually sank. In 1874 Richmond exports had totalled $3,483,626, while those of Norfolk were but $1,831,036; the next year the figures for Norfolk had risen to $5,243,986, while those for Richmond had declined to $2,944,642.[29] It was in vain that the Richmond *Enquirer* protested that Norfolk's trade was chiefly in small vessels, which could easily come up the James to Rocketts. The *Landmark* retorted that the ship *Gregory* of 27$\frac{7}{12}$ feet draft, and the frigate *Colorado* of 24$\frac{3}{12}$ feet had recently visited Norfolk, whereas at Rocketts there was but 14 feet of water.[30] The Fall Line cities had either to become manufacturing and financial centers, or look forward to gradual decay.

It was now no longer a matter of whether Norfolk could induce the Virginia and Carolina railways to come to the Elizabeth, or to Hampton Roads, but of whether they could find the means of doing so. So early as 1868 the Chesapeake and Ohio, the railway on which Richmond had relied to open the commerce of the Ohio region, was planning to extend its tracks to deep water. A company pamphlet of that year shows three alternate termini, at Norfolk, West Point, and Newport News. Norfolk made a determined effort to bring the line to the Elizabeth, sending a committee composed of Charles Sharp, George W. Johnson, and James McCarrick, to interview President Huntington. They received no encouragement. Huntington had already selected Newport News, not only because the distance from

[28] *Ibid.*, Jan. 1, 1884.
[29] *Ibid.*, Dec. 11, 1875.
[30] *Ibid.*

Richmond was shorter than to Norfolk, but because there was no
rival line on the peninsula between the James and the York.[31]

In the meanwhile, another new railway had been laid down, which
strengthened Norfolk's hold upon the trade of eastern North Carolina—the Elizabeth City and Norfolk, later called the Norfolk and
Southern. This line was chartered in 1870, but the delays of financing
and construction postponed the opening until January 1, 1881.[32]
During the same year the line was extended to Edenton. In 1891 it
was sold under foreclosure, repurchased by the stockholders, and
consolidated with the Albemarle and Pantego; fifteen years later it
was extended westward to Charlotte by a combination with four
other railways.[33] The Norfolk and Southern to some extent superseded the two canals as the artery of commerce from the North
Carolina sounds to Norfolk, and great quantities of cotton, lumber,
naval stores, corn, peanuts, and early vegetables flowed in to its
terminus at Berkley.

And now the Atlantic Coast Line and the Richmond and Danville
began to cast longing eyes at the Elizabeth River, for neither had a
satisfactory deep water outlet. They could not extend their lines to
this point, however, because of an agreement not to build in the
territory of the Seaboard. But in case a new line, under a separate
management, was laid down to the Elizabeth, they considered themselves free to use its tracks. So, in 1886, when Mayor Barton Myers, of
Norfolk, sought an interview with William P. Clyde and John H.
Inman, they suggested that he organize a company for a railway from
Pinner's Point to Tarboro. This Mr. Myers did, buying the charter
of the Western Branch Belt Railroad, and laying down tracks to
Suffolk. He next purchased the narrow-gauge railway of the Tunis
and Serpell Lumber Co., and made it a standard-gauge road, without
changing the charter or personnel. The next step was to organize the
Chowan and Southern Railway, with tracks entering Tarboro. In
1889 Harry Walters and John F. Newcombe, representing the Atlantic Coast Line, came to Norfolk, and received the charters of the
three connecting lines. They were then combined as the Norfolk and
Carolina railroad, and became a part of the Atlantic Coast Line
system.[34]

[31] Interstate Commerce Commission, Finance Docket 4943. Testimony of Barton
Myers.
[32] Poor's *Manual of Railroads*, 1884.
[33] *Ibid.*, 1907, p. 380.
[34] Norfolk *Landmark*, July 1, 1888; Testimony of Barton Myers, *loc. cit.*

In the meanwhile, the Southern Railway, with which the Richmond and Danville had been consolidated, backing out of the deal with Mr. Myers, had begun active preparations to make West Point, at the head of the York River, its deep water terminal. Mr. Inman was warned that the place was ill chosen, but he persisted for several years, wasting millions of dollars in the attempt. In the end he was forced to make an arrangement with the Atlantic Coast Line, whereby the Southern used its tracks to the Elizabeth.[35] But the Southern management was not satisfied to remain permanently dependent upon another company and looked around anxiously for an outlet of its own upon Virginia's great harbor. This opportunity came through the Atlantic and Danville.

So early as February, 1867, the newspapers were discussing a proposed railway from Norfolk to Danville,[36] which was to be called the Norfolk and Great Western. The plan envisaged the ultimate extension of the line to Bristol, where it was to connect with other railways leading to Nashville.[37] The people of Norfolk were asked to subscribe to this ambitious venture, and the old bait of a rapid increase in growth and wealth through the western trade was dangled before their eyes. But the city's finances had not yet been straightened out from the Civil War entanglements, and the people voted against the subscription by a narrow margin. For the time being the project dropped from view. However, in 1882, a new company was chartered under the name of Atlantic and Danville, and the next year the work of construction was begun.[38] The line was completed to Danville in 1890. But in 1891 it passed into the hands of receivers, and on April 3, 1894, was sold in the interest of the bondholders. In 1895 the company was reorganized, with capital stock totalling $5,-700,000.

In the meanwhile the Southern had secured a temporary outlet on the Elizabeth River, by purchasing trackage rights over the Wilmington and Weldon, and the Norfolk and Carolina railways from Selma, N. C., to Pinner's Point. During the year ending August, 1895, the company acquired by purchase and lease real estate in Norfolk and at Pinner's Point sufficient for the establishment of terminals for local traffic and railway connections. During the next three years many thousands of dollars were expended in improvements—in the

[35] *Ibid.*
[36] Norfolk *Journal*, Feb. 1, 1867.
[37] *Ibid.*, Jan. 25, 1869.
[38] Poor's *Manual of Railroads*, 1884.

purchase of additional real estate at Pinner's Point, in dredging, in erecting new wharves, docks, and warehouses. On January 1, 1896, Southern trains began to move from Selma to Pinner's Point, and in a few years the tonnage handled at the new terminus was nearly three times as large as that handled at West Point in 1896. The next step was the lease for fifty years of the Atlantic and Danville, on August 31, 1899. This entrenched the Southern's position by making it independent of trackage agreements with other companies, and so gave definite assurance of a satisfactory ocean outlet for its vast network of railways.[39]

Norfolk now looked back upon the ante-bellum days, when she was struggling vainly to secure railway connections with the south and west, as an unpleasant, hazy memory. With great railway systems fighting to reach her harbor, with the Fall Line towns eliminated as rival ports; with the products of Virginia, West Virginia, North Carolina, Tennessee, and the Far South pouring into her lap, she realized that the long-expected prosperity was at hand.

Yet there was one weakness in the railway system at Norfolk. The lines all centered on the Elizabeth River, some on the left bank, others on the right, in most cases without convenient connection one with the other. This necessitated delays in the movement of cars and proved a serious inconvenience to shippers. It was A. J. Cassatt, then a director of the Pennsylvania Railway, who found the remedy. Mr. Cassatt in 1883 had commenced the construction of the New York, Philadelphia, and Norfolk Railroad and the rebuilding of the old Eastern Shore and Peninsula railroads. When these lines were opened for traffic, the barges from Cape Charles City brought cars from the north to the car float bridges of the various railways on the Elizabeth. In 1898 Mr. Cassatt ended this unsatisfactory arrangement by building his own terminal, where all freight cars of his road could be assembled, and where his barges could be loaded by his own crews. To secure direct connection with the other railways, he built a belt line from this terminal south and west of Portsmouth, turning over to each railroad an eighth interest without profit. The Norfolk and Portsmouth Belt Line proved of great benefit to the community, not only in facilitating exchange of freight, but in attracting industries. A plant located on this "clearing house of transportation" had access to seven great railways,[40] as well as to overseas and coastal

---

[39] *Ibid.*
[40] Later eight.

steamers. In 1927 the Belt Line was serving 116 different industrial concerns.[41]

In the long and interesting history of Norfolk, her commerce has been dependent, at various periods, upon different articles of export. From the date of foundation until the third decade of the nineteenth century, tobacco, lumber, and naval stores were the basis of the town's commerce; from 1870 to 1885 cotton was mainly responsible for the city's growth; from 1885 to the present day coal has been the chief article of export.

So early as 1853 it was predicted that Norfolk would become the greatest coaling station in the United States. The James River and Kanawha canal, so it was thought, would lead to great shipments from the western Virginia fields to the Elizabeth, where "the whole steam-marine of the Atlantic would be supplied with fuel." With a ready means of transportation, "the best fuel in the world for steam would be supplied at Norfolk cheaper than any accessible point on the Atlantic border."[42] After the Civil War, visions of a huge coal trade continued to flit before the eyes of the Norfolk merchants, and the proposed Norfolk and Great Western had as one of its chief objects the tapping of the mining region. "Norfolk can become one of the great coal-marts of the Union," said the *Journal,* in April, 1870, "and can compete with Baltimore and Philadelphia in furnishing the whole seaboard. The English mines are going deeper, and the time will come when Virginia coal can be exported. We look to the development of the coal mines of Virginia and West Virginia, when connection is made with our city, as the commencement of a new era in the growth and commerce of Norfolk. . . . She will become the Newcastle of America. May the day come when we shall see long trains arriving many times a day, laden with every kind of coal."[43]

With the creation of the Norfolk and Western and the completion of the New River line, this hope became a reality. In 1881 and 1882 extensive preparations were made for the reception of coal trains, the company extending its freight yard, building a coal pier into the Eastern Branch, and removing the old drawbridge, so that large vessels could approach it.[44]

It was on March 17, 1883, that the first carload of coal came through from the Pocahontas fields, and was presented to the city of

---

[41] *The New Norfolk* (Norfolk, 1927) , pp. 15, 16.
[42] Forrest, *Sketches of Norfolk,* pp. 298, 299.
[43] Norfolk *Journal,* April 25, 1870.
[44] Norfolk *Landmark,* Jan. 12, 1882.

Norfolk by Vice-President Kimball, of the Norfolk and Western. "Its arrival was greeted by a salute fired by a detachment of the Blues. The car was then detached from the rest of the freight train, and gayly decorated with bunting. The Mayor and others then mounted the engine and car for an ovation tour up the tracks as far as McCullough's wharf. The novel sight attracted crowds along Water Street, and cheer after cheer greeted the 'first car.' People rushed to the track to get specimens of the coal, and sometimes they were kindly supplied with more chunks of it than they wanted. . . . As the car moved slowly along many a head that appeared at a window to catch a glimpse of the sight, caught something else. . . . The car then returned and ran up on the elevated railway to the coal chutes. . . . Engineer E. H. Reams had the honor of running the train down from Pocahontas. The locomotive that pulled the 'first fruits' so to speak, is a Mogul engine, No. 83. The car is a gondola No. 6,212, bearing on one side this inscription: 'From Pocahontas to Norfolk, For Mayor Lamb.' "[45]

It became immediately obvious that the pier on the Eastern Branch would be inadequate for the needs of the new trade. So the Norfolk and Western carried its track in a wide sweep around the city to Lamberts Point, where the water was twenty-six feet deep, and built a great pier out over the water, 894 feet long, 60 feet wide, and 48 feet high. From this point the coal deliveries were 504,153 tons in 1886, and over a million tons in 1889. In all 3,821 vessels took on coal here in these four years.[46] "At Lambert's Point, a dingy mass of piers, trestles, and buildings marks the coaling station of the Norfolk and Western," said the New York *Evening Post*. "Coal from thence is now shipped so far north as Portland, Maine, and southward to Havana."

The presence of cheap coal gave Norfolk an advantage over other Atlantic ports, which aided both the coastwise and foreign trade. The steamer which came into the Elizabeth for a cargo of cotton or grain had but to stop at Lamberts Point to fill its bunkers, while those at a rival port might have to make a wide detour for fuel.

With the opening of the twentieth century the coal trade had grown so rapidly that it induced a great capitalist to construct an entirely new railroad from the coalfields to Norfolk. It was H. H. Rogers who envisaged the Virginian Railway and provided the capital for its construction. In 1905 representatives of Mr. Rogers

---

[45] Norfolk *Virginian*, March 18, 1883.
[46] *Facts and Figures about Norfolk* (Norfolk, 1890) , pp. 8, 9.

promised the mayor and council that if they would grant a right of way around the city, he would bring the line to Norfolk, secure frontage on the right bank of the Elizabeth, and construct the terminus there. Thereupon Barton Myers and others secured an appropriation of ninety-five thousand dollars for the purchase of the right of way, and got an option upon five hundred acres at Sewells Point. They then went to New York and closed the deal with Mr. Rogers. The rights of way cost more than the ninety-five thousand dollars, so the committee paid the balance from their own pockets. In the end Mr. Rogers not only reimbursed them, but repaid the ninety-five thousand dollars to the city.[47]

The Virginian, which was built from Deepwater, West Virginia, to Sewells Point, a distance of 442 miles, was opened for business on April 1, 1909. The construction was unique. The engineers were told to connect the two terminal points, regardless of intervening towns, in the most direct and convenient way. This made it possible to construct what is practically a gravity road from west to east, so that great trains of coal cars can move down from the mountain region to Hampton Roads, with a minimum of steam power. At Sewells Point a steel pier 1,040 feet long was erected, with provision for coaling four large vessels at a time. This remarkable road entered upon extensive operations at once. In 1910 it hauled nearly a million tons, in 1913 four and a half millions, in 1916 six millions and a half.[48]

The three great coal carrying railroads—the Norfolk and Western, the Chesapeake and Ohio, and the Virginian—made Hampton Roads the greatest coal port in the world. There was a constant procession of trains from West Virginia to Lamberts Point, Sewells Point, and Newport News, where ocean liners, bay steamers, tramps, and coasting vessels awaited for cargo or bunker coal. The demand seemed limitless, for the factories, railroads, electric power stations, and gas works of the Eastern and Middle Atlantic States were constantly in search of cheap fuel. So early as 1911 the requirements of New England alone took nearly four million tons from Hampton Roads. In 1926 the port sent out no less than twenty-seven million tons.

In measure as the railways brought freight into Hampton Roads, the facilities of the steamship lines increased to carry it off. In 1869 there were but twenty coastal steamers plying regularly between Norfolk and other American ports. In addition, however, there were

---

[47] Testimony of Barton Myers, *loc. cit.*
[48] The National City Company, *The Virginian Railway* (New York, 1917).

many steam craft used in the bay, the rivers, and the two canals. The canal boats were from twenty to three hundred tons burden, many of them making regular trips from Philadelphia and Baltimore to Norfolk, and thence through to points on the North Carolina sounds. At this time the New York liners consisted of the *Isaac Bell*, the *Niagara*, the *Saratoga*, the *Albemarle*, and the *Hatteras*, all side-wheelers, and the propeller steamship *Virginia*. The Boston line had the *William Lawrence*, the *George Appold*, and the *Blackstone*, all propeller steamers, and the side-wheeler, *William Kennedy*.[49]

The export trade in the 1860's was still small, and was carried on almost entirely in sailing vessels. During the year 1868 eighty-three craft left the Elizabeth for foreign ports—four steamers, thirty-six brigs, two ships, twelve barks, twenty-nine schooners.[50] But with increasing shipments of cotton, the tonnage of vessels engaged in foreign trade rapidly mounted—from 12,530 in 1870, to 30,598 in 1873, to 65,521 in 1876, to 86,279 in 1878,[51] to 121,420 in 1882, to 789,396 in 1891. In the five years from 1891 to 1895 inclusive, over 2,500 vessels left for foreign ports, 2,100 of them steamers. Exports rose from $728,000 in 1871, to $1,255,000 in 1873, to $7,815,000 in 1876, to $9,820,000 in 1879, to $16,264,000 in 1881, and to $19,845,-000 in 1882.[52]

The pioneer in restoring Norfolk's foreign trade was William Lamb. As commander of the Confederate forces at Fort Fisher, North Carolina, Lamb in the course of his duties in assisting British blockade runners had established many friendships with the ship owners. At the close of the war these men offered to aid him in building up an export business, and in 1866 he sent out the *Ephesus*, the first steamship ever loaded in Norfolk for Europe. Although the *Ephesus* was wrecked on Sable Island and a part of her cargo of cotton lost, Lamb's export business grew steadily. He became manager of a line of Spanish steamers plying between Norfolk and Liverpool, as well as the Norfolk agent for the Baltimore-Liverpool steamers, and the Allen Line.[53] Reynolds Brothers, Ricks and Milhado, Barry Brothers, and other firms also aided in the restoration of Norfolk's transatlantic trade.

In the meanwhile the coasting trade was also making great strides.

[49] Merchant and Mechanics Exchange, *Report*, 1869, pp. 71-73.
[50] Norfolk *Journal*, Jan. 25, 1869.
[51] Norfolk *Landmark*, Aug. 6, 1879.
[52] *Facts and Figures about Norfolk*, p. 13.
[53] *Norfolk and Vicinity*, pp. 74-75.

The Old Dominion line operated a fleet of seven steamers to New York; the Merchants and Miners steamers plied between Norfolk and Baltimore, Savannah, Boston, and Providence; the Clyde liners went to Philadelphia. In 1879 the number of vessels engaged in the coastwise trade was 1,068, totaling 973,459 tons; in 1887 the number was 1,500 vessels, of 1,396,071 tons.

A surprisingly large part of the coastwise traffic was in peanuts, fruit, and vegetables. In colonial days the soil of the southeastern counties was not esteemed highly, for only in limited areas was it suited for tobacco, the one great staple. There were few wealthy planters. Even after the Revolution the forests extended for miles along the shores, and it was only in the years just preceding the Civil War that the farmers awoke to the fact that their land was unsurpassed for truck gardening and peanuts. In early days peanuts were almost unknown in Norfolk. When first introduced the farmers cultivated them in an irregular and careless manner, little dreaming that they would ultimately prove a gold mine. But during the Civil War a demand arose from Federal soldiers and other newcomers, and after the war extensive cultivation began. The output, which in 1867 was only 75,000 bushels, grew to 324,000 bushels in 1872, to 780,000 bushels in 1876, to 1,000,000 in 1879, and 2,250,000 bushels in 1888. Before the end of the century Norfolk had become the greatest peanut-growing region of the country. Before 1876 the nuts were cleaned in fan mills by the farmers, but in that year K. B. Elliott erected the first factory in Norfolk, with machinery for polishing and assorting. In 1910 Virginia and North Carolina together produced about 10,000,000 bushels, valued at $8,000,000.

It was in 1842 that two New Jersey farmers came to eastern Virginia and began intensive truck raising. They were immediately successful, receiving from $40 to $50 a barrel for cucumbers, and from $15 to $20 a barrel for peas. It was a revelation to the local farmers, who had been devoting their time to tobacco, wheat, and the other time-honored products of the region. Immediately they began to turn their attention to tomatoes, beans, potatoes, cabbage, strawberries, beets, lettuce, peas, onions, and similar crops. The value of land rose rapidly. A farm which sold for $4,000 in 1842 would bring $6,000 in 1845, and $18,500 in 1855. The first truck farms were on the Western Branch, but they spread rapidly, first throughout Norfolk County, and then into Princess Anne, Nansemond, Isle of Wight, and elsewhere. In time all tidewater Virginia and North Carolina, from

Northumberland on the Potomac, to Carteret on Pamlico Sound, became practically one vast garden. Here one might see acres of green peas, vast fields of cauliflower, farms devoted to cucumbers, whole fields of strawberries, potatoes, and cabbage plants. Everywhere were Negro workers planting, or weeding, or spraying, or harvesting.

In many cases the farmers brought their wares to market on the rivers, sounds, and canals, in small sailing vessels. "Often 150 of these little vessels enter the harbor a few hours before the sailing time of the steamers, racing at full speed, with everything set and loaded high above the decks with a profusion of boxes and barrels packed with melons, cabbages, tomatoes, and vegetables of every description. They dash straight in to get the best positions at the wharves, and often crowd up so thick that steamers and large vessels cannot make their berths. In consequence numbers of them are obliged to cast off and go swarming out into the bay, and there cruise aimlessly back and forth like a cloud of butterflies, until they are signalled to return, when they come in with a rush, jostling and crowding, the air meantime ringing and rent with the good natured jabbering and chaffing and cries of the crews."[54] The frequent sailings of the coastwise and bay steamers, together with the use of express freight cars on the Eastern Shore branch of the Pennsylvania and other railways, gave quick and ready access to all the great eastern markets. In 1893 the annual shipment of truck from Norfolk amounted to three million packages. At this time the acreage of the truck farms was forty-five thousand, the number of hands 22,500, and the value of the product seven million dollars.

Thus for Norfolk the post-Civil War period was one of prosperity, growth, optimism. With the reopening of old railways and the laying down of new lines, with the growth of coastal trade, with the revival of direct commerce with foreign ports, with the development of the cotton trade, with the opening of communication with the great coal fields of Virginia, with the transformation of eastern Virginia and North Carolina into a vast trucking garden, Norfolk awoke from the lethargy of olden days and claimed its rightful place as one of the leading ports on the Atlantic seaboard. It was in 1885 that a representative of the New York *Evening Post* "discovered Norfolk." Hitherto the attitude of the Northern press had been hostile and often unfair. One paper had derided the place as "that decrepit victim of the slave power, poor old imbecile granny Norfolk, who

[54] Borum, *Norfolk, Port and City*, p. 105.

spends her feeble breath in sighing still for the system which made her a municipal specimen of what the naturalists call arrested development."[55] Now the reporter was astonished to find the place awake, throbbing with life and hope. "It is a city of the New South," he wrote. "Already it is the third cotton port of the United States, while a beginning has been made of a coal trade, which has limitless opportunities. There are 60,000 people within a radius of three miles of the market house. On the wharves all is bustle and stir. Negro workers are moving the bales of cotton to and fro, while clerks and factors in long ulsters are sampling the product. In a nearby building a cotton compress, with the force of 6,000 tons in its iron jaws, is putting two bales into one to prepare them for shipment. Here we see negroes rolling barrels of garden truck into the New York steamers; nearby a collier and lumber schooner is taking on its cargo. The great clouds of dust which come from this building mark it as a peanut factory, where the nuts are graded and cleaned. In the harbor are steamers with red funnels, black and white funnels, steamers of all kinds, from almost every country; around them a bevy of ships, brigs, schooners, and lesser craft. If one drives out beyond the city limits, he finds himself passing between the truck gardens which cover the peninsula on which Norfolk is built. As far as the eye can reach are green things—beets, parsley, spinach, turnips, strawberries, peas, onions, potatoes, corn, lettuce, cabbage, cucumbers, watermelons."[56]

Even before the close of the Reconstruction period it was obvious that Norfolk's rapidly growing commerce would eventually double and triple the city's population. But it was not so easy to predict the effect of this expansion upon the physical character of the place, and upon the life of the people. Already streets and houses had overrun the entire region south of Smith's Creek. Would it in time become as densely settled as Main, and Bank, and Church streets? Would Freemason and Bute be lined with houses, built directly upon the street, touching elbows, with only a bit of green in the garden plot behind? Would narrow lanes be cut from street to street, and built up with crowded tenements?

No doubt this is what the people of Norfolk expected, and, no doubt this is what would have happened, had the future offered no readier means of street transportation than the past. When the aver-

55 Norfolk *Post*, Oct. 30, 1865.
56 Norfolk *Landmark*, Jan. 26, 1885.

age citizen had to walk to and from business, it was not practical for him to build his residence more than a mile from the center of town. The fields north of Smith's Creek lay invitingly before him, but unless he owned a horse and carriage, he could not take advantage of them. It was most opportune, then, that just at this moment his problem was solved by the advent of the streetcar.

It was in 1869 that the Norfolk City Railroad Company, fortified with a liberal franchise,[57] began laying down tracks over the entire length of Main Street.[58] In August of the next year the people were thrilled by the arrival of "five elegant street cars," from Wilmington, Delaware.[59] These tiny vehicles, with their narrow front and back platforms, their hard benches, and their four wheels, were drawn by horses or mules. If traffic was light, one horse only was assigned to a car, but when large crowds had to be moved, one, two, or even three more were added. There was but a single track on Main Street, with switches at Bank Street, at Peter Smith and Company's store, and elsewhere. Later rails were laid on Church Street, Granby Street, and in the residential sections. In 1893 the Norfolk City Railroad Company was operating one mile of double track, and four and a half miles of single track, with cars running on a five-minute schedule, from Market Square to Brambleton, to Huntersville, and to Atlantic City. The equipment consisted of 120 horses and forty cars, handled by a force of sixty men. The Suburban and City Railway, organized in 1887, operated three and a half miles of track, having, in 1893, fifteen cars and sixty horses.[60]

Year after year the horse-drawn cars continued to serve Norfolk, until the clang of the bell and the clatter of the horses' feet on the cobblestones had become a part of the everyday life of the city. But already their doom had been sounded. In 1887 an electric car had been put in service in Richmond, the first in the United States, and a few years later electricity was rapidly replacing horse-power on the street lines of many other cities. Public sentiment demanded that Norfolk should not lag behind. The companies had prospered under the old system, however, and were reluctant to lay out thousands of dollars in new equipment until they were certain enhanced returns would justify it. But in 1893, in return for an extension of their franchises, they decided to make the change, and at

---

[57] The franchise was granted in 1866 (Borum, *Norfolk, Port and City*, p. 26).
[58] Norfolk *Journal*, Aug. 28, 1869.
[59] *Ibid.*, Aug. 3, 1870.
[60] Borum, *Norfolk, Port and City*, p. 26.

once began electrifying their roads.[61] It was October 17, 1894, that the first trolley car went into operation in Norfolk. Although by this time the electric-driven car was no longer a marvel, its appearance on the streets created no little excitement. Before the end of the year the horse-drawn cars were entirely superseded, and many faithful horses and mules were thrown out of a job. A decade later, the streetcar system, intertwined in the map of Norfolk like a tangled web, wound in and out of the business section, and then reached out in all directions to the suburbs—to Sewells Point, Ocean View, Willoughby Spit, South Norfolk, Berkley, Portsmouth, Pinner's Point.[62] The people had become as dependent upon the unending stream of fine new electric cars, as those of New York today upon the subways.

Hard upon the laying down of streetcar tracks came the development of new suburbs. The most important of these, located across Smith's Creek near Atlantic City, was called Ghent.[63] This expanse of farm land was taken over by a real estate company, plotted off into streets and avenues, and in a remarkably short period converted into one of the most exclusive residential sections of Norfolk. The west branch of the creek, which had extended back across Princess Anne Road, was filled in to Olney Road, and the lower part, lined with a stone buttress, was rechristened the Hague. The new community was provided with paved streets, granolithic sidewalks, sewerage pipes, water mains, and gas pipes. Hundreds of silver maples and magnolia trees were planted along the thoroughfares, while several public squares were laid off on reclaimed tracts. In 1893 only a score of houses, "all of handsome and modern design," had been erected, or were in course of construction.[64] A decade later the entire suburb was built up.

The phenomenal success of the Ghent undertaking led immediately to other development schemes. Farms were bought up, wide avenues and cross streets marked off, and building operations started. A map of Norfolk published in June, 1900, shows a maze of streets all the way from the Hague to Tanner's Creek, with unplotted spaces on Lamberts Point, just south of the Norfolk and Western Railway west

[61] *Ibid.*, p. 27.

[62] *Virginian-Pilot,* June 1, 1902.

[63] It is related that Commodore Drummond, because of the fact that he brought home a copy of the treaty of Ghent in his ship *Rob Roy,* gave the name Ghent to his home across the creek from Botetourt Street, and that the new suburb was named for the old residence.

[64] *Industrial Advantages of Norfolk* (Norfolk, 1893) , pp. 24-26.

of Colley, and at one or two other places. In 1902 even these bare spots had disappeared. Houses were going up every day in sections which a few years ago had been considered far out in the country. It is not too much to say that the streetcar, especially the trolley car, tripled the area of Norfolk and gave to thousands of its people who otherwise would have been cooped up on the crowded streets of the old town the advantages of suburban life, with its lawns, its open spaces, and its quiet.

But this movement, so wholesome in most of its aspects, was viewed with no little apprehension by some of the older citizens. The old West End, which for generations had been the aristocratic section of Norfolk, now had to meet a new and vigorous rival. While the wealthy and the distinguished were moving over the creek to Ghent, the older residential sections gradually assumed an appearance of neglect and decay. The old West End had not yet been deserted by the older families, for some still lived in the charming houses handed down to them by their fathers and their grandfathers. But others followed the trolley to the newly created city "across the bridge."

As the horsecar period was succeeded by the trolley-car period, so was the latter in turn superseded by that of the automobile. In the last decade of the nineteenth century when the motor-driven vehicle was slowly being perfected, the people of Norfolk apparently were not especially interested in its progress. Many were skeptical of its ultimate success, and no one seems to have foreseen its tremendous effect upon modern civilization. In the summer of 1899 a steam Locomobile, using kerosene for fuel, appeared upon the streets of Norfolk. This little car, shaped like a buggy, with wire spokes and solid rubber tires, could make short spurts of a mile a minute with a full head of steam. It is supposed to have been the first automobile ever operated in Virginia.[65] In March, 1900, T. S. Oliver, of Swift and Company, inserted a notice in one of the daily papers stating that he would introduce the delivery automobile to the citizens of Norfolk. This vehicle, of a type already used in various cities as delivery cars, he said, "is compact, neat, attractive in appearance and readily controlled by the operator." Exhibitions would be given on the streets for a week or ten days.[66] If the sight of this vehicle, rattling and chugging up and down the streets, elicited any excitement, the papers failed to record it. During the same year Mr. F. W. McCullough purchased a

[65] Letter of John G. Wallace (in possession of the author), May 27, 1930.
[66] *Virginian-Pilot,* March 6, 1900.

Ford. How great a curiosity a car was in those days is shown by the fact that in a trip from Baltimore to Staunton, Mr. McCullough met only one other car. From Staunton he was forced to ship his Ford to Norfolk by freight, since one of the counties he wished to visit prohibited automobiles on the road.[67]

During the next few years a number of Norfolk people purchased automobiles, and established dealers began advertising new and used cars for sale. "We have secured the agency of the Columbia Electric and the Pope-Hartford gasoline automobiles," stated the White Hardware Company. "Also we have a second-hand Locomobile for sale at a very low price."[68] By the year 1910 hundreds of automobiles were in use in the city and suburbs, and at any time one might see parked on Main or Granby a dozen or more of the touring cars typical at that date. At the first airplane ascension on Lee's Parade, in November, 1910, more than one hundred cars were parked around the field.[69] The delivery of merchandise was still done almost entirely by horse-drawn vehicles, however, and Commercial Place presented the same aspect as of old, with its long line of wagons backed against the curb, or drawn up in the center of the square, the horses waiting patiently with lowered heads.[70] But so early as 1904, it had been predicted in Norfolk that "the day of the 'plug' would soon be over," and that delivery wagons and even heavier trucks would be propelled by motor.[71] The next two decades saw the fulfilment of this prophecy, and the horse-drawn vehicle became in Norfolk, as in other American cities, a comparative rarity.

The era of the automobile saw many changes in the development of Norfolk. New suburbs—Colonial Place, Lamberts Point, Park Place, Larchmont—filled in with modern residences, churches, schools, and stores, until the entire region between the Elizabeth River and Tanner's Creek became one uninterrupted city. Moreover, building extended over the creek, now rechristened Lafayette River, where many beautiful homes went up in the neighborhood of the country club. The man of means could live upon what amounted to a diminutive country estate, and yet make his daily trip to the business centers in his automobile in less than half an hour.

Yet the automobile by no means converted Norfolk entirely into a

---

[67] Letter of Mr. F. W. McCullough (in possession of the author).
[68] *Virginian-Pilot*, March 31, 1904.
[69] *Ibid.*, Nov. 2, 1910.
[70] *Norfolk* (Norfolk Industrial Commission, Norfolk, 1912), p. 23.
[71] *Virginian-Pilot*, Feb. 21, 1904.

city of homes, for the development of apartment houses kept pace with the building of suburban cottages. The compactness of the apartment, its many modern conveniences for housekeeping, and its proximity to the retail and theater district, conspired to make it attractive to many families. "Norfolk is to become a city of apartment houses," said the *Virginian-Pilot* so early as 1904, "and in this respect will rival Washington, the home of the flat-dwellers, should buildings of this character be continued at the present rate." The typical apartment house of that day was from three to five stories high, with dining hall, doctor's office, and barber shop. The apartments consisted of two or three bedrooms, dining room, living room, kitchen, pantry, and bath.[72] Soon there were scores of such buildings in the city, scattered over West Ghent and other comparatively new sections.

While the residential section of the city was shifting westward and northward, the business section was also on the move. In former days wholesale houses had centered around Water Street and Commercial Place, while the shops had been located on Main and Church streets. At the conclusion of the Civil War, when Granby Street crossed Back Creek on the old bridge, and when on the corner of Main and Granby was an open lot large enough to accommodate the tents of the visiting circus, business had not yet turned the corner. The northwest trend, however, was already drawing the retail houses up Main, and by 1880 the S. A. Stevens furniture warehouse had occupied the corner of Main and Granby. In the next few years commercial enterprises took over the street as far north as City Hall Avenue, which in 1884 replaced Back Creek east of Granby. The Taylor Building, three stories tall, erected in 1885, was soon overshadowed by its towering neighbor, the Haddington Building, on the southeast corner of Granby and City Hall Avenue, and in 1893 the Columbia Building, next to the Atlantic Hotel, provided more shops and offices.[73] Opposite the Taylor building stood the old Newton home, built almost a hundred years earlier on the shores of Back Creek, the last outpost of the old residential era south of City Hall Avenue. On the north side of Back Creek was Lawrence's oyster house, marked by a huge pile of shells, and the docks of the McCullough Lumber Company.

North of this point in 1893 Granby was still dominated by stately

---

[72] *Ibid.*, April 12, 1904.
[73] The Columbia Building was destroyed in the great fire of Jan. 31, 1902, which also destroyed its neighbor, the Atlantic Hotel. Letter of Col. E. Griffith Dodson to the editor, January 23, 1961. In 1961 the Haddington Building was destroyed by fire, and a new façade on the Taylor Building concealed its name and date.

old residences. Most impressive was the charming old Tazewell mansion, set off in spacious grounds behind a brick wall which stretched from what was to become Brooke Avenue almost to College Place. Next to it, the home of the Newton family had just become the public library, and across College Place was the Norfolk College for Young Ladies. Opposite the entrance to the Tazewell residence was the McIntosh home, with the Dickson place just below it and the Hardy house a little farther up the street. These homes, however, were soon destined to yield to the remorseless march of business northward. In 1898 the massive Monticello Hotel rose just south of the Dickson house on land which had been under the waters of Back Creek not many years before. Four years later the Tazewell mansion, then nearly a century old, was moved to make room for a block of business houses, leaving only Tazewell Street to mark its former site. By 1905 Back Creek had completely disappeared, as City Hall Avenue was extended west of Granby to provide more commercial sites.[74] In another five years the northward advance had reached the corner of Freemason, and lower Granby had become one of the most crowded, busy streets in the South.

At the same time fine structures were going up on other streets. The post office, a handsome stone building, with classic façade, on Plume Street at Atlantic, was completed in August, 1900.[75] At this time the tallest building in Norfolk was the seven-story Citizens Bank Building, on Main Street, next to the Custom House. But in December, 1904, the people were thrilled by the announcement that the city was to have a real skyscraper, a thirteen-story structure on Main, at Atlantic, to be erected by the Bank of Commerce.[76] This building, when it was completed, stood out like a lone tower, above Norfolk's skyline, to greet visitors on incoming steamers. Gradually, however, other high buildings arose to challenge its ascendency, the most conspicuous being the Royster Building, on Granby near the Monticello. Norfolk was not yet a city of skyscrapers, but the river front presented a very different picture from the days before the Civil War, when Forrest described it so accurately. The little wooden wharves had been replaced by modern piers and warehouses; in place of the groves of trees, with here and there a private residence peeping through the

[74] *Virginian-Pilot,* Nov. 30, 1907. City Hall Avenue was extended west of Granby Street before May 25, 1905. Letter of Col. E. Griffith Dodson to the editor, July 20, 1961.
[75] *Virginian-Pilot,* June, 1900.
[76] *Ibid.,* Dec. 11, 1904.

foliage, were massive hotels or department stores, or office buildings; the dome of the City Hall, which then stood out above the neighboring roofs, was almost hidden from view. One now saw tugs or ferry boats, or the bay steamer, with occasionally a great ocean liner, where once scores of schooners or brigs had been tied up.

In 1903 the cornerstone was laid for a building which, although not comparable in size to the Bank of Commerce or the Royster Building, was not less important to the people of Norfolk. It was in August, 1870, that the Norfolk Library Association was organized, with Dr. Samuel Selden as the first president. A charter was secured in February, 1872. The library was first opened to the public in a large room in the Norfolk Academy, and here it remained for many years. In 1883, however, the books and other equipment were moved to the Y. M. C. A. building on Main Street. When the agreement with the Y. M. C. A. expired in 1893, the library was once more moved, this time to the Newton house, at the corner of Granby and College Place. The next year a new corporation, the Norfolk Public Library, took over the property of the old association. In 1901, when Andrew Carnegie offered the city fifty thousand dollars for a library building and the councils appropriated five thousand dollars for maintenance, this organization set to work to secure a suitable lot. Their problem was solved in less than a year by the donation of a site on Freemason Street by the children of Dr. William Selden as a memorial to their father. Building operations began in October, 1903.

The reputation of the Hampton Roads section as an all-year resort dates back to the days of the famous old Hygeia, at Old Point. The original building was erected in 1821, the lumber being supplied by Tunis and Park, of Norfolk. It was situated near the entrance to Fort Monroe, and consisted of one large room which served the double purpose of parlor and dining hall, with four chambers on either side, and the kitchen in an outhouse in the rear.[77] Here came in the days before the Civil War "public men weary of their cares, army and navy officers on furlough or retired, and the gay daughters of Virginia."[78] In 1863 the Hygeia was razed by order of the United States government, and another building was erected farther away from the fort. In 1874 the property fell under the control of Mr. Phoebus, who developed it into one of the most famous resorts of the country. In 1880 the Hygeia was a long frame structure, with verandas

[77] *Ibid.*, Sept. 2, 1902.

[78] Edward L. Pierce, *Enfranchisement and Citizenship: Addresses and Papers* (Boston, 1896), p. 32.

for each of its three stories, running the entire length of the building. There was "ample capacity for 600 guests" who could enjoy, in addition to the bathing and the breezes of Hampton Roads, such modern improvements as "elevator, gas, and electric bell in every room," and bathrooms on every floor. In 1902 this building was torn down. Although the Hygeia is now but a memory, the fame of Old Point Comfort as a resort has been upheld by the Chamberlin Hotel. The bringing of various trunk lines to Norfolk accelerated a development already under way, which made the Hampton Roads section a popular all-year resort.

In the meanwhile, Ocean View, on Chesapeake Bay, a few miles north of Norfolk, was also attracting many visitors. This suburb was established as a private summer resort in 1854, and after the Civil War it grew steadily in popularity. "For several winters past, invalids from the North have been making Norfolk their retreat," it was stated in 1880. "Stopping over here for a rest, on their way to Florida, they have been so pleased with our genial clime as to give up the idea of going further south."[79] So a hotel was erected at Ocean View, which from the first was crowded. Many were attracted, not only by the mildness of the climate, but by the facilities for hunting, fishing, and riding. The beach served also as a playground for the people of Norfolk, and in the summer months crowds went out daily. The Ocean View Railroad Company ran trains from its station at Church and Henry streets eight times a day, the "wheezing and puffing little coffee-pot engines," covering the eight miles in twenty minutes.[80] The round-trip fare was thirty cents. With the advent of electric streetcars, the steam engines were discarded, and the road electrified. In time Ocean View grew to the proportions of a large summer resort, with numerous hotels, cottages, and pavilions. In the 1920's the old Ocean View Hotel was torn down.[81] One of the most attractive features of this resort was the tourist camp, carved out of a forest of water-oaks, bay-berries and hollies, and equipped with water, sewers, and electric lights. Ocean View, once regarded by the people of Norfolk as a remote suburb, was annexed to the city in 1923.

The development of Virginia Beach, on the Atlantic Ocean directly east of Norfolk, followed hard on that of Ocean View. In 1883 Norfolk residents, with the aid of some Northern capital, purchased a

[79] Jones, *Norfolk,* p. 37.
[80] *Ibid.,* p. 39; *Virginian-Pilot,* Aug. 23, 1901.
[81] *Virginian-Pilot,* Jan. 3, 1928.

large tract of land at this place, erected the Princess Anne Hotel, and connected it with Norfolk by a narrow-gauge steam road. The hotel was a four-story structure with a veranda along the ocean front, bedecked with the towers, bay windows, and broken roof lines of the day. A rough log wall, topped by a board walk, protected the lawn from the inroads of the sea. At the same time, privately-owned cottages were put up, while "an artificial wood and labyrinth, a switchback railway, boats on the lake, a race course, and a zoölogical garden" added to the attractions of the resort. Virginia Beach grew rapidly, until its hotels, boardinghouses, and cottages could accommodate twenty thousand people. The old narrow-gauge soon gave way to a modern electric line, run by the Norfolk Southern Railway. In the 1920's great advances were made—the erection of a splendid new hotel, the Cavalier, the construction of two miles of concrete seawall and promenade, and the development of a fine highway to Norfolk. The Princess Anne Country Club added much to the charm of Virginia Beach. The club golf course, constructed in the center of a pine forest between the ocean and Linkhorn Bay, was one of the best in the country. Five miles north of Virginia Beach is Cape Henry, famed as the spot first touched by the Jamestown settlers, in 1607. Here is the picturesque old lighthouse, the first to be erected by the United States government, and here is Fort Story guarding the entrance to the Chesapeake.

The period between the Civil War and the First World War found its culmination for Norfolk in the Jamestown Exposition of 1907. So early as 1900, a move had been made to commemorate the three-hundredth anniversary of the establishment of the first permanent English settlement in America. Many took for granted that the exposition would be held at Richmond, but a delegation of prominent citizens from the Norfolk section appeared before the Assembly, and carried the day for Hampton Roads. On March 10, 1902, a bill was passed granting a charter for an exposition company on condition that capital stock of not less than $1,000,000 be subscribed by January 1, 1904. Despite the appointment of the popular General Fitzhugh Lee as president and the great enthusiasm for the project in tidewater Virginia, considerable difficulty was experienced in raising this sum.

On December 23, 1902, the Academy of Music was filled to overflowing with an enthusiastic crowd, bent on stimulating interest in the exposition and increasing the stock subscriptions. General Lee was absent, but disappointment at this fact was forgotten in the warmth with which the crowd greeted the appearance of Governor Montague. When Mr. Montague pointed out the importance of the exposition to Virginia, and especially to Norfolk, the house rang with applause.[82] Although subscriptions began to come in more rapidly after this meeting, they still fell far short of the million-dollar mark. In fact, on December 31, 1903, with but a few hours of grace left, more than one hundred thousand dollars were needed. That evening a group of representative men gathered in the rooms of the Board of Trade, determined on heroic efforts to close the gap. Slowly but surely the remaining shares were subscribed, until at eleven o'clock only $5,400 was needed. Ten minutes later the news arrived that a meeting at Newport News had taken five thousand dollars. "Who will subscribe the remaining $400?" it was asked. "I will, on behalf of the Norfolk-Hampton Roads Company," said M. D. Lowenberg, director general of the exposition, and the great project was saved. That night the people of Norfolk greeted the New Year with especial enthusiasm, and the corridors of the Atlantic Hotel rang to cheers of the crowd and the strains of "Dixie."[83]

In the meanwhile a tract of 340 acres at Sewells Point had been purchased, and the work of construction begun. It was no light task to erect a miniature city on this isolated spot, to lay down a boulevard ten miles to Norfolk, to pipe drinking water, to build piers, to provide lights and telephone service, to make streets and pavements, to erect a group of beautiful and permanent buildings, to set out flowers and shrubs. So many unavoidable delays occurred that when the day appointed for the opening arrived, the grounds were far from complete. Nonetheless there was a grand parade, and President Roosevelt, who arrived on the *Mayflower* with a group of distinguished diplomats, made a characteristic address.

Virginia Day, marked by a great military and naval pageant, was the high water mark of the exposition. Despite threatening clouds the crowds began to assemble early, and by ten o'clock were surging through the Virginia building in an endless stream. At two all repaired to the Lee Parade. Here, when Thomas Nelson Page had read his poem *The Vision of Raleigh* and Governor Swanson had followed with the address of the day, the great parade passed in review before the governor, Admiral Evans, and General F. D. Grant. It

[82] *Ibid.*, Dec. 23, 1902.
[83] *Ibid.*, Jan. 1, 1904.

was an inspiring sight, the regulars and sailors swinging by in perfect form; the naval cadets in their white caps, blue blouses and trousers, and white leggings; the Virginia Military Institute cadets with white trousers and plumed caps; the Virginia Polytechnic Institute boys in full dress; and the Virginia and Georgia militia.[84]

Despite these activities it was only on September 14 that the exposition was actually completed and in full operation. Visitors who arrived after that date were rewarded by an interesting and beautiful spectacle. The two great government piers, shining white against the water of Hampton Roads, were united by an artistic arch to form a basin called Smith Harbor. To the south was Raleigh Square, leading up to the Court of Honor, with its sparkling fountain and its two lagoons, and beyond was the stately administration building. The central group of buildings included structures devoted to art, to machinery and transportation, to food, to medicine, to manufactures and liberal arts, to mines and metallurgy, to marine appliances. To the south of the administration building was the Lee Parade, and beyond this the military encampment. To the right and left, facing Hampton Roads were the state buildings, many being replicas of historic structures—the Old State House, for Massachusetts; Independence Hall, for Pennsylvania; the Bullock House, for Georgia; the Carrollton mansion, for Maryland. The dignified buildings, the thousands of lights, the avenues set with trees and bushes, the waving pennants, all set off by the broad expanse of Hampton Roads, presented a picture of rare beauty.

The Jamestown Exposition was harshly criticized by certain Northern journals. Some censured the delay in completing the grounds and buildings, others thought there was too much emphasis on the past and not enough on the present and future. Yet on the whole, the great undertaking had been well done. Its influence in calling attention to the progress of the tidewater section and the vast opportunities which lay before it can hardly be exaggerated. No doubt the interest of many visitors was centered in the charming statue of Pocahontas, or the Captain John Smith group, or the Peter Stuyvesant portrait; but others noted also Norfolk's splendid shipping harbor, her rich back country, her network of railways. The Jamestown Exposition was the forerunner of the greater Hampton Roads of the twentieth century.

The half century from 1865 to 1915 was vital in the history of

[84] *Ibid.,* June 13, 1907.

Norfolk. Prior to this period the town had been the victim of one malicious whim of fate after another. While other Atlantic ports, although less favorably located and possessing inferior harbors, had outdistanced her in the race for wealth and power; while New York, Boston, Philadelphia, and Baltimore counted their populations by the hundreds of thousands, Norfolk had remained an unimportant town of from ten to twenty thousand people. The burning of the town in 1776, the loss of the West India trade, the absorption by New York of her import trade, the invention of the steamboat, the blocking of all attempts to connect the town with the interior by rail, the yellow fever epidemic of 1855, and the Civil War had been successive blows too severe to be parried even by the most enterprising and alive of populations.

Now, however, these misfortunes were but unpleasant memories. With a network of splendid railways entering her doors, with numerous steamship lines ready to carry off the products which they brought in, with cotton and coal calling back to life the old foreign trade, with the city's health guarded by the advance of medical science, with her adjacent territory transformed into a garden spot, fortune at last was smiling upon the hitherto ill-fated place. Moreover, there was every reason to expect continued growth, because of the rapid development of the South. After all, Norfolk was a Southern port; if that section doubled and quadrupled its annual output, so would Norfolk's trade double and quadruple. The opening of mines, the development of intensive agriculture, the establishment of factories meant new business for the Southern railways, and greater activity on the wharves of the Elizabeth.

It is unfair to say with the Northern press that Norfolk had been the victim of the slave system. The slave-made tobacco of the Virginia plantations was long one of her main exports, the slave-made cotton of the Far South would eventually have reached her port had not emancipation intervened. But there can be no question that the freeing of the slaves was the prelude to the rise of the New South, and that the rise of the New South heralded a new era of prosperity for Norfolk. With the annual output of Virginia's manufactures totaling $675,000,000, of her crops nearly $300,000,000, with her coal mines yielding 12,000,000 tons, and her iron mines 63,000 tons, and with other Southern states keeping step, there could be no fears for the future of the South's most convenient gateway.

CHAPTER FOURTEEN

Mars Moulds a
Great City

The course of Norfolk's history has been affected profoundly by war. In the Revolution the town was destroyed; the War of 1812 paralyzed her West Indian trade and brought on commercial stagnation; the Civil War, despite the immediate misfortunes it entailed, was the beginning of a new era of prosperity; the First World War greatly increased the population and made Hampton Roads one of the nation's greatest ports. In 1914 Norfolk's exports were $9,500,000, and imports $3,125,000; in 1926 exports had risen to $137,208,000, and imports to $16,868,000. As for the metropolitan area of Norfolk, including Portsmouth, Newport News, Suffolk, and other towns around Hampton Roads, the population in 1926 was a third of a million, the foreign trade $220,000,000, and the entire water-borne commerce twenty million tons. Such rapid expansion was revolutionary. The little Norfolk of a few decades before had become a great prosperous city, with exports equal in value to those of San Francisco, and far in advance of those of Baltimore, Philadelphia, or Boston.

Like other American communities, Norfolk watched with breathless interest the commencement of hostilities in Europe in 1914. Most of the people sympathized openly with the Allies, condemning the German invasion of Belgium, rejoicing in the victory of the Marne, protesting against the submarine sinkings of neutral shipping. As for the problems of the government at Washington arising from the interference by both groups of belligerents with American trade, Norfolk gave the policies of President Wilson its full support. The proclamation of neutrality, the protests against British seizures of

American vessels, the request for the recall of the Austrian ambassador, the various notes concerning submarine sinkings, the peace proposals, all elicited approving editorial comment.[1]

At first few anticipated that the United States would be vitally concerned. True, shipments to the Allies, and to a lesser extent to Germany through neutral countries, brought about a rapid increase in the exports from Hampton Roads, shipments from Norfolk rising from $9,500,000 in 1914 to $19,000,000 in 1915, and to $36,000,000 in 1916, and those of Newport News from $5,000,000 in 1914 to $70,286,000 in 1915.[2] True, in 1916 Norfolk took fourth rank among the cotton ports, her shipment of truck amounted to five million packages, and her bank clearings increased $41,000,000 over 1915. But these changes were regarded as transitory, and few were prepared for the more startling advances of the next few years.

Norfolk applauded President Wilson's war message of April 2, 1917. "That Congress will hesitate to take the steps urged on it by President Wilson . . . is inconceivable," said the *Virginian-Pilot*.[3] "The words of the President are those of truth and soberness; positive as befitted the occasion, and solemn as in keeping with a decision as momentous as that taken by the Continental Congress when it issued the Declaration of Independence."

Immediately the city resounded to the bustle of military preparation and the tramp of soldiers. Recruiting for the Navy began the day after the declaration of war, when several hundred pretty girls, stationed at street crossings, sought to persuade young men to enlist.[4] When Admiral Sims made an especial appeal to fill the complement of the great battleship *Nevada,* mass meetings were held in various parts of the city, while bluejackets drove through the streets in a drizzling rain to sign up the applicants.[5]

By this time all Norfolk was aroused. It was imagined that Uncle Sam's chief contribution to the war would be naval, and the press and public speakers pointed out that every seaport must do its part. At a mass meeting in the Colonial Theatre, on April 15, impassioned pleas for enlistment repeatedly brought the audience to its feet.[6] Five days later a great parade wound its way through the streets. In the

---

[1] Norfolk *Ledger-Dispatch*, Feb. 13, 1917.
[2] *Year Book of Hampton Roads*, 1927, p. 23.
[3] April 4, 1917.
[4] *Virginian-Pilot*, April 7, 1917.
[5] *Ibid.*, April 9, 1917.
[6] *Ibid.*, April 16, 1917.

lead was a squad of police, then came Chief Yeoman Quigley representing Uncle Sam, next a platoon of mounted citizens, followed by a brass band, a company of seamen, the Boy Scouts holding placards urging enlistment, high school girls, two army trucks decorated with the flags of the Allies, a big fire engine, and a long line of automobiles.[7]

Enthusiasm reached its height on April 28, when a little band of French sailors took part in a parade of marines, sailors, and national guardsmen. As the Frenchmen passed the Virginia Club, a number of women standing on the balcony beneath the tricolor showered them with tulips. "For once forgetting discipline, the Frenchmen mingled their shouts with those of the crowd, many of them catching the flowers as they fell. As the marine band burst into the 'Marseillaise,' hats were lifted and the throng went wild." Fired by scenes such as these, young men enlisted in such numbers that by the first of May Norfolk led the list of cities in naval recruiting.[8]

However, the full realization of the meaning of war came only with the departure of the Norfolk detachments of the National Guard. The Light Artillery Blues, famous for their work in the Civil War, were mustered in on June 30, 1917. On the day of their departure for Fort Oglethorpe, Georgia, wives, sisters, sweethearts, and mothers gathered at the armory to say goodbye. It was a touching scene as khaki-clad youths, surrounded by admiring groups, awaited in the drill hall or in front of the building. At last came the whistle, a few last kisses or handshakes, and Norfolk's first contingent had gone.[9]

In the next few months the city was to become accustomed to such scenes. The Fourth Virginia Regiment, with a number of Norfolk companies, was called to arms, recruited, properly equipped, drilled, and made ready for inclusion in the new National Guard Army. On August 24 the troops paraded in Norfolk, through dense throngs of cheering people. Early on September 4, the day of their departure for Camp McClellan, at Anniston, Alabama, Colonial Avenue, at the point where it crosses the Norfolk and Western, was obstructed by a crowd of men, women, and children, assembled to bid their loved ones goodbye. As the trains pulled out the men waved from the windows to mothers and sweethearts, who sobbed out their distress or

[7] *Ibid.*, April 21, 1917.

[8] *Ibid.*, April 28; May 2, 1917.

[9] Arthur K. Davis, *Virginia Communities in War Time* (Richmond, 1926), p. 306; *Virginian-Pilot*, July 8, 1917.

smiled with pride. "It is not that I am sorry to see my boy go," said one mother; "these tears are tears of pride."[10]

When it became known that the United States might send thousands to the battle front, necessitating the drafting of hundreds of men from Norfolk, the people gave immediate approval. On June 5, 1917, nearly ten thousand men went to the polls and registered under the draft act,[11] and in September the first contingent to be called to the colors left for Camp Lee, near Petersburg. Norfolk was not less proud of these men than of her other soldiers, and on September 22, the city and county united in a farewell dinner to one of the departing detachments. There were patriotic addresses, in which the men were lauded as "the flower of the section's young manhood," who would stand before the German advance as immovable as the French at Verdun. The second quota of 447 men came at the end of June, 1918, and three weeks later 292 Norfolk Negroes were summoned. Altogether the city's contribution to the services, military and naval, whether members of the National Guard, volunteer recruits, or drafted men, totaled several thousand men.[12]

Norfolk also responded promptly to all calls for aid in financing the war. Each Liberty Loan quota was met and passed. A War Campaigns committee labored "to raise funds to help win the war." All Norfolk rallied behind these organizations. Four-minute men, speaking at concerts, plays, and lectures, urged the people to invest with Uncle Sam; Liberty Loan posters explained the need of the government for funds; religious and social organizations urged on the campaign; the banks lent their facilities. Norfolk oversubscribed her quota for the first loan by $1,131,900, the second by $1,759,080, the third by $1,986,700, the fourth by $2,191,850, and the Victory Loan by $858,850. In all nearly $36,000,000 was subscribed. The extent to which the people, poor as well as rich, supported the government with their savings is indicated by the fact that on the fourth loan there were 39,686 purchasers. Norfolk also passed her quota for war savings stamps, the public schools alone taking no less than $400,000.[13]

In the meanwhile the port of Hampton Roads, so long neglected by the state and the nation, was becoming a great gateway for ocean traffic. With the wharves and piers of New York inadequate to the

10 *Virginian-Pilot*, Sept. 5, 1917.
11 *Ibid.*, June 6, 1917.
12 Davis, *Virginia Communities in War Time*, pp. 310-313.
13 *Ibid.*, pp. 314-317; *Virginian-Pilot*, April 5, June 15, 1918.

sudden demand upon them, with the railways leading to the metropolis congested, it was necessary for both the government and private
shippers, to seek additional outlets. Inevitably their eyes turned to
Norfolk and Newport News. Their unsurpassed harbor, with its
eight trunk railways, its nearness to the ocean, its accessibility to the
great coal and cotton regions of the South, had obvious advantages
over other Atlantic ports. So its commerce doubled, tripled, quadrupled.

Looking out from Sewells Point, one can see "great hulls from
Norway, Sweden, and Denmark, uncamouflaged and beaten by the
seas until they are the sea's own gray," said the *Virginian-Pilot;*
"French barks and British merchantmen; ships from China and from
Russia, from Argentina, and from the West Indies. . . . The whole
beautiful expanse of Hampton Roads is today populous with merchant craft, that fly the flags of all the world. One can watch the
harbor from dawn until dark, and the number and variety and
fascination of the vessels there seems endless. From the Norfolk side
ships are to be seen taking on cargo and bunker at the great coal
piers; still others are in the stream waiting their turn, while all about
them ply the small, busy harbor craft, and an occasional big government dredge engaged in the work of making anchorages. In the distance, tramps and sailing vessels, barges and schooners, show dim
against the horizon. Then, towards Newport News, one sees the
merchant ships in great array—numbers of them anchored in long
lines, others clustered in groups about the busy docks and piers."[14]

The principal article of export was coal. There was urgent need of
fuel in war-torn Europe, and nowhere could it be had more readily
than at Hampton Roads. Long trains moved in unending streams
from the West Virginia fields, to dump their burdens into the holds
and bunkers of the vessels at the piers at Sewells Point, Lamberts
Point, and Newport News. In 1917 the exports of Norfolk and Portsmouth alone totaled 10,903,137 tons, of which 10,469,060 were coal.

The next year, when the United States was straining every nerve
to perfect her new war industries and when the railways were taxed
to the limit to carry troops and war supplies, much of the coal from
Hampton Roads was diverted to domestic ports. New England needed
fuel for her factories, and since sufficient coal could not be carried by
rail through New York, the coal-carrying steamers from Virginia
waters began turning their prows northeastward. In 1917 Norfolk's

[14] *Virginian-Pilot,* Dec. 1, 1918.

domestic shipments of coal were only 289,710 tons, in 1918 they jumped to 5,525,758.[15]

It is rare indeed for the commerce of Hampton Roads to be interrupted by cold weather, for the winters are mild and open, the harbor usually free from ice. But in the winter of 1917-1918, the water froze, shipping was paralyzed, and freight piled up on the piers and wharves. Great battleships, which were set to work to break the ice, often could make little headway. Even when a channel was cleared to the coal piers, the steamer might have to wait for its cargo, because the coal had frozen and could not be dumped until steam pipes had been run through the cars. Jack Frost was proving a valuable ally for the Kaiser.[16]

Nor did coal stand alone in Norfolk's war commerce. Norfolk and Portsmouth sent out to other American ports in 1917 half a million tons of fruits and vegetables, 76,000 tons of tobacco, 66,000 tons of petroleum products, 36,000 tons of lumber, 76,000 tons of cotton, 23,000 tons of fish, oysters and clams; receiving in return 546,000 tons of iron and steel manufactured articles, 300,000 tons of petroleum products, 136,000 tons of dry goods, 200,000 tons of fertilizer, 337,792 tons of canned goods, 85,000 tons of sugar, and miscellaneous goods to the amount of five and a half million tons.[17] To foreign ports the cities sent flour, wheat, cotton, steel billets, and tobacco. Imports, while small compared with exports, were vastly greater than in former years. The chief item was nitrate of soda, for when the blockade of Germany cut off the supply of kainite, the manufacturers of fertilizers were forced to turn to the nitrates of Chile. The War Board, not wishing to use American bottoms, forced many Norwegian, Swedish, and Danish vessels to carry on this trade, by threatening to withhold bunker coal. In 1917 no less than 363,865 tons of nitrate was brought to Norfolk, the next year 411,195 tons.[18]

Commerce was still further augmented by the activities of the Naval Overseas Transportation Service. When the United States entered the war there were but six transports in commission on the Atlantic seaboard, chiefly employed in the Panama service. When it was decided to send a great army to France and to supply it from the United States, this little nucleus had to be expanded into a fleet of ocean carriers. The interned German ships, totaling 460,000 tons, and

[15] War Department, *Port Series* (Washington, 1927), No. 15.
[16] *Virginian-Pilot*, Jan. 6; Feb. 2, 1918.
[17] War Department, *Port Series*, No. 15.
[18] *Virginian-Pilot*, Dec., 1918; War Department, *Port Series*, No. 15.

a Dutch fleet of 300,000 tons were pressed into service, and these, with other accessions, brought the total, on December 1, 1918, to 512 vessels of 3,246,000 tons.[19] A large part of the fleet operated from Hampton Roads, 288,000 troops and vast quantities of supplies going out from its wharves. Here the scene during the rush months of 1918 was a busy one indeed, when the men in khaki were transferred from their trains to the transports, and workmen loaded the supply ships with everything needed by the Army in France—uniforms, stockings, blankets, shoes, hats, canned food, sugar, meat, locomotives, motor trucks, steel rails, horses, mules, airplane parts, medical supplies, guns, rifles, ammunition.

The advantages of Norfolk for both ocean and railway[20] traffic induced the Federal government to establish there the greatest Army base in the country, with concrete warehouses, miles of track, a rifle factory, and one or more huge piers. At the time, work was in progress on a municipal terminal near Sewells Point, which was to be connected with the railways entering Norfolk by an extension of the Belt Line. The government, taking over this property, pushed on the work vigorously. Workmen were brought in from all parts of the country,[21] new mains extended the city water system to the base,[22] lumber and other materials poured in over the railways. Buildings and piers rose as if by magic. "No private terminals were ever so lavishly provided with everything in the way of modern equipment. The derricks and giant cranes could shift a crate of eggs delicately and softly, or they could swing a locomotive from the piers to the hold of a transport with the same ease." It is estimated that the base cost the government thirty million dollars.

Though Norfolk was the center of a great food-producing region, and though food and fuel were pouring through Hampton Roads, the people suffered during the war for lack of both food and coal. While the needs of the Allies were so pressing, those of this American community, a community from which shipment abroad was easy, received secondary consideration. The gas company was forced to limit its output, certain "lightless nights" were set aside, at the request of the Federal Fuel Administration, and electric signs and lights in front of theaters were prohibited. "With the dimming of lights on the white way the moon, after almost a half-century of neglect, became an

[19] Colonel Leonard P. Ayres, *The War with Germany* (Washington, 1919) , p. 39.
[20] *Ibid.*, pp. 44-47; *Virginian-Pilot*, Jan. 19, 1919.
[21] *Virginian-Pilot*, Sept. 2, 1918.
[22] *Ibid.*, Jan. 10, 1918.

important factor of the life of Norfolk," said the *Virginian-Pilot*. During the winter of 1917-1918, heatless days and a temporary suspension of industry to economize in coal caused no little suffering,[23] and on one occasion a number of people in Newport News, desperate at the prospect of sickness in their families, actually raided the coal yards.[24]

Although the food shortage was not so acute, Norfolk's situation in this respect also was unusual. The housewives, as everywhere, were urged to save food. "You are called upon to render a blow to Kaiserism by helping to keep the soldiers of America and the Allies in food," they were told. Thousands of families voluntarily reduced their consumption of wheat, butter, sugar, and meat, and so early as October, 1917, the hotels were observing the rule of meatless Tuesdays. This abstinence, aggravated by a serious shortage of sugar, bread, and milk, resulting in part from the unexpected influx of strangers to Norfolk, was not the least of the people's sacrifices.[25]

For the trucking interests of Norfolk the situation became tragic. With city dwellers converting their back yards into gardens, with thousands of schoolchildren becoming amateur farmers, with the Food Administrator calling loudly for more and more vegetables, they had a right to look forward to a great expansion of their activities. Instead, they were forced to curtail production. The government drained off so many of their laborers for work at Norfolk that they could not cultivate all their acres, and with the railways choked with troops and war supplies, it was difficult to market what they did raise. Their complaints poured in on the government. One farmer stated that he had only three men to work seven hundred acres of land, another, one man for four hundred acres. "How can we hold our laborers," they said, "when the government contractors offer them $3.50 for an eight-hour day, with 66 cents an hour for overtime? While the Food Administrator is urging production, we have hundred of acres of wheat uncut, whole farms of potatoes undug." But the government could do nothing for them, and thousands of acres of the most fertile land in the United States remained idle at the moment when food was of supreme importance.[26]

In the meanwhile the Navy Department had decided to create on Hampton Roads the greatest naval base in the United States, and was

---

23 *Ibid.*, Feb. 1, 1918.
24 *Ibid.*, Jan. 4, 1918.
25 Davis, *Virginia Communities in War Time*, pp. 318-321.
26 *Virginian-Pilot*, Jan. 29, Feb. 2, Feb. 3, Feb. 5, 1918.

considering the relative advantages of Sewells Point and a site near Yorktown. The former was finally selected. On June 28, 1917, President Wilson set aside $2,800,000 for the purchase of the land and the erection of the first storehouses and piers. A tract of about 474 acres was secured, of which 367 had been the old Jamestown Exposition grounds, while one hundred belonged to the Pine Beach development. The first step was to create a naval training camp. Work on this unit was begun on July 4, and pushed forward with such rapidity that by August 4 barracks, mess halls, and storehouses for seven thousand five hundred men had been completed, roads constructed, and three miles of railway laid down.

This was the beginning. The government designed for the base not only an enormous supply station, but an aviation station, a submarine base, and another training camp. A preliminary step was the erection of a great bulkhead, 22,150 feet long, at a cost of $3,104,281. Next came the work of dredging, to provide thirty-five foot channels to the merchandise piers, and to fill in the areas back of the bulkhead. This work, which cost $2,373,000, added over three hundred acres to the area of the base. All during the autumn of 1917, and throughout 1918, the work continued. The cry was for speed, regardless of expense. Two piers, 1,400 feet long, and 125 feet broad, were thrown out into the Elizabeth River; on the northwest point was made a submarine basin with room for thirty-one vessels; on the north a lagoon for airplanes; and further east a landing field for airplanes and dirigibles. Great buildings of concrete arose as if by magic—hangars, two six-story warehouses, a huge cold-storage warehouse and ice-plant, an aircraft storehouse, mine-storage warehouses, hospital wards, laundries, barracks, mess halls, garages, bakeries, machine shops, armories, drill halls, officers' quarters, and hundreds of other buildings.[27]

The historic old Navy Yard at Gosport also became the scene of intense activity. The yard was enlarged; fitting-out piers were constructed with cranes, trolley, tracks, capstan, and conduits; a dry dock, 1,011 feet long, 144 feet wide, and 40 feet deep, was laid down for the accommodation of the greatest battleships. The dock, which required the removal of 625,000 cubic yards of earth and the pouring of 184,000 cubic yards of concrete, has been called "the most complicated piece of mass concrete construction ever built in this coun-

[27] Navy Department, World War, *Activities of Bureau of Yards and Docks*, pp. 132-143.

try."[28] At the naval hospital, also, a program of expansion was undertaken. Eight temporary wards were built in the rear of the main hospital, and a large group of emergency buildings added on the west, including subsistence house, corps barracks, and wards. Before the close of the war the establishment had become the largest naval hospital on the Atlantic coast.[29]

The problem of securing labor proved difficult. Not only was every available workman in the vicinity of Norfolk employed, but agents scoured other parts of Virginia and the nation. Men were brought in from Minnesota, Kansas, Kentucky, and Texas. "If you see any unbelievably wide-brimmed hat," said the *Virginian-Pilot*, "there is either a Texan or a Kentuckian under it."[30] Hundreds of country girls, lured by stories of high wages and city life, came to Norfolk to seek employment as stenographers or clerks. One agent brought 294 youths from Evansville, Indiana, and then left them to shift for themselves. Private concerns entered the competition for workers, adding to the already acute shortage, and boosting wages. The effect on the laborers themselves was bad. Regular mechanics were content to work steadily, but many of the transients became insolent and shiftless, wandering from job to job, in quest of the highest wages and lightest work. Month after month the stream of laborers poured into the city, until the population swelled to twice its normal size.[31]

The housing problem became acute. Men in the services found it difficult to secure houses or apartments for their families; workmen were forced to crowd in wherever there was a vacant room; rentals shot up at an alarming rate. Accusations of profiteering became rife, and the appeals for government regulation insistent. In some cases servicemen refused to vacate at the expiration of their leases, on the grounds that they could not live on the sidewalks while engaged in activities vital to the success of the war. Finally the government decided to erect houses of its own and laid plans for three residential communities: at Glenwood, near the Naval Base; at Truxton, outside Portsmouth; and at Cradock, on Paradise Creek. The Glenwood project was eventually discontinued, and the other two were merely in the preliminary stages when the Armistice was signed.[32]

28 *Ibid.,* pp. 239, 240.
29 *Ibid.,* pp. 108-111.
30 *Virginian-Pilot,* Sept. 2, 1918.
31 Davis, *Virginia Communities in War Time,* pp. 331-335.
32 *Ibid.,* pp. 334, 335; Navy Department, *Activities of Bureau of Yards and Docks,* pp. 498-500.

Hand in hand with the huge government activities went the development of private industry. Many new plants came to Norfolk during the war; old concerns doubled their capacity. The American Chain Company, the British-American Tobacco Company, E. I. DuPont de Nemours and Company, the Linde Air Products Corporation, the Virginia Coal and Navigation Company, the Standard Oil Company were among the important concerns which opened new plants in or near the city. The Norfolk Shipbuilding and Dry Dock Company, in Brambleton, which in 1916 employed forty men, in June, 1918, employed seven hundred. The Chesapeake and Potomac Telephone Company doubled the size of its exchange and added ten thousand new telephones.[33]

These great changes, so revolutionary in character, so rapid and unexpected, strained the public and private utilities of the city to the utmost. "Within the space of a few months Norfolk has sprung into the dimensions of a great city," the *Virginian-Pilot* pointed out in January, 1918. "It has become almost overnight the center of government activities, involving the expenditure of millions, and transforming its outlying districts into hives of industry crowded with busy workers. The population has increased by leaps and bounds, transportation lines are overtaxed with shipments by land and water. The harbor is filled with vessels flying the flags of all nations awaiting their turn to discharge or take on freight. Business of all kinds has expanded beyond facilities to handle it. Public utilities are inadequate to the business imposed on them. In short Norfolk has outgrown the conditions existing when swept down upon by a tidal wave of progress, and in order to ride upon the flood of prosperity must put aside her outgrown garments and equipments."

While this transformation was in progress, Norfolk men were fighting gallantly at the front. The Fourth Virginia, upon its arrival at Camp McClellan, was absorbed into other units, most of the men going into the 116th Infantry. The Light Artillery Blues, which had been Battery B of the First Regiment, Virginia Field Artillery, became a part of the 111th Field Artillery. Both the 116th Infantry and the 111th Field Artillery were a part of the Twenty-ninth Division, known as the Blue and Gray.[34]

[33] Davis, *Virginia Communities in War Time*, pp. 322, 323; *Virginian-Pilot*, Dec. 29, 1918.

[34] *Ibid.*, pp. 306, 307; John H. Cutchins, *History of the Twenty-ninth Division* (Philadelphia, 1921), pp. 13, 14.

The men remained at Camp McClellan until June, 1918. Here, in the beautiful foothills of the Blue Ridge, they went through their preliminary training. Under the able direction of Major General Charles G. Morton, assisted by French, British, and American tutors, they were instructed in trench digging, grenade throwing, the use of the bayonet, and rifle shooting. With the approach of the summer of 1918, the division was ready to leave for France, and the Norfolk men with the 116th went to Hoboken, where they sailed on the transport *Finland* on June 15.[35]

Arriving at St. Nazaire, the regiment disembarked, and moved in box cars, each labeled "hommes—40, chevaux—8," to the camp at Champlitte. France seemed strange and interesting indeed to the Norfolk boys—"the neat little gardens, the quaint peasant women with their rosy cheeks, white caps, black frocks, and wooden shoes, and the solemn 'undertakerish' looking men in their wide brim felt hats." When the train pulled into Champlitte, "the men with all equipment slung, marched up the dark, silent, winding, cobbled streets of the small French village. . . . No tents now—the companies were split up into small groups of ten, fifteen, or twenty men, and assigned to a hay loft there, a cow stable there, or possibly, to an abandoned monastery, built in the fourteenth century."[36]

The stay at Champlitte was short. Every available division was needed at the front, and the 116th took over a quiet sector in Alsace to release more seasoned troops. Here they got their "first view of hostile aircraft" and had their first experiences with life in the trenches, with German raids, and American counter-raids. Late in September came the order to proceed to the front. "Then began a series of night hikes and one day stands." We catch a glimpse of the hardships of war from the reminiscences of one of the men. "About 1:30 in the morning it began to rain very hard. Those sleeping on the ground in the open were rather out of luck. So were the rest of us at 3:00 A.M., when orders came to pack up once more. With mud up to the shoe tops and inky blackness, and with a high wind blowing, it was no easy matter to roll our soaking blankets in the packs. But we were not amateurs, and we were soon on a ten mile hike to the town of Bruges. We arrived there at 8:00 A.M., drenched through and through. Our hike was lightened by thoughts of securing dry billets,

---

[35] Cutchins, *History of the Twenty-ninth Division,* pp. 1-62; Davis, *Virginia Communities in War Time,* p. 307.
[36] Cutchins, *History of the Twenty-ninth Division,* pp. 74-75.

but no such luck. We arrived at a worse place than that which we had left; a bleak, cold, muddy hillside."[37]

On September 26 General Pershing had launched his great Argonne-Meuse offensive. Day after day, week after week, the American divisions had been battling their way north through forests, over ravines, fortified hills, ruined cities, trenches, and machine-gun nests, until, early in October, they had made a great salient in the German lines from Samogneux along the Meuse to Brieulles, and thence west to the Argonne. The salient itself was a source of danger to the Americans. Not only did it permit the Germans to fire down upon their right flank from the heights east of the Meuse, but it exposed them to counterattack in the rear. So General Pershing planned an offensive east of the river to straighten out the line, and placed the brunt of the attack upon the Twenty-ninth.[38]

It is probable that few of the brave men who took part in the offensive of October 8 realized just what it was their commanders asked them to do. Ornes, a few miles to the east, was the point of junction for several of the great German lines of defense. From it radiated, like spokes from the hub of a wheel, the Brabanter Stellung, the Hagen Stellung, the Volker Stellung, and the Kriemhild Stellung. To advance five miles the troops would have to storm as many lines of fortifications as their comrades farther west in ten or fifteen miles. In other words, they had to break a pivotal point of the entire German system of fortifications.[39]

The 116th and 115th regiments, associated with the Eighteenth French Division under the command of General Andlauer, were placed in line from the Meuse to Marmont Farm, with the Thirty-third American Division on the left and the Twenty-sixth French on the right. On the night of the seventh, French and American engineers built four bridges over the river, while the various units toiled through the night to gain their positions. "It was nearly dark, and a misty rain was falling when the battalion set out on its 23 kilometer hike to Samogneux. It was fair going to the Meuse crossing at Vacherauville, but from there across Talou Hill to Samogneux was a hell of barbed wire, debris, shell holes, and trenches, the wreck of a battlefield, which in the pitchy blackness of the night seemed to be a frenzied mass of shattered but still living forms blocking the way." Shortly after

[37] *Ibid.*, p. 131.
[38] Shipley Thomas, *History of the A. E. F.* (New York, 1920), p. 311.
[39] Cutchins, *History of the Twenty-ninth Division*, p. 147.

midnight the head of the column arrived at Samogneux, and the various infantry and machine gun companies were conducted to their places.

At five o'clock the next morning the silence was broken by the crash of hundreds of guns; and the men, lighting their cigarettes as they went, advanced under the cover of the barrage. On they went, over the Brabanter Stellung, past Haumont, over the Malbrouck Hill, through the Bois de Brabant. After the first half hour the Germans resisted bitterly, and the Americans were repeatedly subjected to machine-gun, rifle, grenade, and *minenwerfer* fire. Yet they pushed on, unmindful of their losses, until at nightfall their line ran through the northern outskirts of the Bois de Consenvoyne, three miles from Samogneux, and the threat to Pershing's right flank had been removed.

Days of bitter fighting followed. Now the men were cleaning out the machine-gun nests at the ruins of Ormont Farm, now charging across the open ground in the face of a withering fire, now sweeping over the Ravin de Molleville, now charging into the hell of the Bois de la Grande Montagne, until, on the night of October 29, the division was relieved by the Seventy-ninth. It was a record to be proud of, the record established by the Blue and Gray division, in this, its only great battle. For three weeks they had fought unceasingly, working their way forward slowly, through a maze of German defenses, responding nobly to every call, accomplishing all that was humanly possible. As they marched to the rear, weary in soul and body, emaciated, with eyes sunken, voices husky, their clothes in tatters, they had the consciousness of duty courageously performed. The division had advanced four and a half miles, had captured 2,148 prisoners and 21 pieces of artillery, and had suffered the loss of 6,159 men.[40]

The war record of Norfolk's draft men was equally fine. Most of the men were sent to Camp Lee, at Petersburg, where they were incorporated in the 318th Infantry of the 80th Division.[41] After months of intensive training, on May 18, 1918, they left for their port of embarkation. The men thought they were destined for Newport News, but as the train passed Waverly, Wakefield, Suffolk, and other familiar stations, they realized that they were headed for "good old Norfolk." But their glimpse of home was fleeting. At seven-thirty in the morning they arrived at the west Boissevain government pier, and

---

[40] Thomas, *History of the A. E. F.,* p. 461.
[41] *Virginian-Pilot,* Sept. 5, 1917.

filed on board the transport *Red Italia*. At noon they steamed down the river and, heading north, joined a fleet of transports and supply ships, guarded by destroyers. The voyage across was uneventful until within a short distance of the French coast, when, near Belle Isle, they were attacked by submarines. The destroyers opened with so deadly a fire that one of the attackers was sent to the bottom, and the others forced to submerge. Although the U-boats renewed their attempt the next day, the entire fleet arrived safely at St. Nazaire.[42]

On June 3 the men crowded into French box cars and moved off slowly for Calais. If they thought this mode of traveling uncomfortable, they soon discovered that it was superior to hiking along a highway with a heavy pack on one's back. "After going awhile a fellow imagines some one has hung the Post Office or the Royster building on his back," wrote one of the soldiers.[43] The division assembled in the Sammer training area for instruction by the Sixteenth Irish and the Thirty-fourth English divisions.[44] At Montaign Farm, near Hesdigrieuf, they were practiced in the manual of arms and the use of machine gun, bayonet, rifle, grenade, and gas mask. The Eightieth next moved to the Third British Army sector, to take post in the secondary lines between Arras and Albert. Here certain units were attached to British divisions, and got their first taste of fire in the trenches. Four hundred casualties occurred at this point.[45]

The division was then moved across northern France to join the First American Army around the St. Mihiel salient, and was held in reserve during the offensive of September 12-15. It was then hastened off to take part in the great Argonne-Meuse advance. Taking its place in line before Bethincourt, between the Thirty-third Division on the right, and the Fourth on the left, it was in readiness for the attack on the night of September 25. "The next morning our artillery opened with the heaviest fire I ever saw," wrote one Norfolk boy. "The artillery was placed hub to hub. At 6:00 A.M. we went over the top in a light fog, advancing against the Germans seven kilometers. We took many prisoners and saw many German dead. Most of the prisoners were pleased, apparently, and imagined they would be sent to the United States."[46] The right of the division reached the

---

[42] *Ibid.*, March 19, 1919.
[43] *Ibid.*
[44] Thomas, *History of the A. E. F.*, p. 109.
[45] *Ibid.*, p. 110.
[46] *Virginian-Pilot*, March 9, 1919.

Meuse that day beyond Dannevoux, but the left was held up before the Bois de Septsarges.

"On the 27th, while mopping up, six or seven of us captured 29 Germans and two pieces of heavy artillery," wrote one of the men. "The dead and dying about were awful, and the narrow escapes a fellow has are truly unbelievable. We advanced more on the 27th and 28th, when we met strong resistance at the Meuse River."[47] Early on the twenty-eighth the Germans counterattacked from the town of Brieulles, but were checked by determined rifle and machine-gun fire. But the Eightieth, when in turn it tried to take Brieulles, was repeatedly thrown back. Since the town seemed impregnable, and since the frontage of the division was now greatly reduced by the character of the terrain, it was taken out of line and held in reserve. It had "made a brilliant success" in its first great battle.[48]

The men were not permitted to rest long. On October 3 they were back in line in front of Nantillois. On the fourth, when they went forward again, they encountered a concentrated fire from the Bois des Ogons, and could make little headway. "We went over the top four times in three days. Living in filth, thirsty, hungry, unshaved, covered with mud, blood and cooties, we never fully appreciated the danger." It was only after a terrific struggle that they swept through the Bois des Ogons. And when this had been accomplished a new obstacle presented itself in the Madeleine Farm. Several more days of heroic fighting continued, but this point could not be carried, and the division was once more withdrawn for rest and recruiting. As the weary men marched back to Le Chemin, the devastation through which they passed reminded them of Dante's *Inferno,* and upon emerging into the peaceful country beyond, they were awakened as from a nightmare by the sight of cottages and gardens, and the laughter of little children.

But the end was not yet. With the men refreshed and with ranks once more filled, the division took its place in line for the third and last phase of the Argonne-Meuse drive. This time the resistance was weaker, the advance more rapid. In one mighty push they went forward with the Seventy-seventh on their left and the Second to the right, past Imecourt, Verpel, through the difficult Bois de Four and Bois de Gerache, on to the strongly held town of Yoncq. Here, in the

47 *Ibid.*
48 Thomas, *History of the A. E. F.,* p. 251.

face of a terrible flanking fire from the hills across the Meuse, the division swept the Germans back and advanced to the Yoncq-Beaumont road. "The 80th division, commanded by General Cronkhite, left the field with conscious pride in its battle record. Three times, in each of the three phases, it had smashed its way forward in the Meuse-Argonne battle, and its fighting was in the open rolling country where the German resistance was greatest. It advanced . . . 24 miles, and captured 103 officers, 1,710 men, and 88 pieces of artillery, and lost a total of 210 officers and 5,464 men."[49]

Five days later when Norfolk's soldiers were still resting from their heroic exertions, the city of Norfolk itself was aroused by the din of shrill whistles. Instantly men, women, and children, abandoning business, housework, and school, poured into the streets. Main and Granby soon were jammed with a mob of joy-crazed people, shouting, singing, gesticulating, laughing, weeping. The din was deafening. Added to the cheering of many thousands of people was the noise of toy-drums, cow-bells, automobile horns, and whistles. Every building was decorated with the flags of the Allies, many automobiles were gay with bunting. When a detachment of bluejackets came swinging down the streets the crowd parted to make room, at the same time redoubling their cheering. Not until the small hours of the next morning did the city regain its composure and its people retire to rest. Thus did Norfolk celebrate the signing of the Armistice.[50]

A long wait followed for the return of the soldiers. It took time to bring back to the United States the vast American army in France, and it was only in May, 1919, that it became known that the Twenty-ninth Division was on its way home. On May 20 a committee on the *Gratitude* went to Newport News to welcome the 16th Infantry. Five days later the 111th Field Artillery, containing the old Light Artillery Blues, came in on the *Virginian*. Only a favored few were permitted on the dock, but hundreds of impatient mothers, fathers, wives and sweethearts waited outside. As the transport docked, "one had only a glimpse of power at first, then every inch of space above and below decks massed with living khaki. There was a deep silence, then in an instant the spell was broken. The band played the Stars and Stripes Forever, the boys were waving and shouting." Asked if they were glad to get home, the soldiers merely breathed in one mighty chorus 'Ah!' "[51]

[49] *Ibid.*, p. 350.
[50] *Virginian-Pilot*, Nov. 12, 1918.
[51] *Ibid.*, May 26, 1919.

June 22 to June 28 was set aside as "Home-Coming Week." A committee of prominent citizens prepared an elaborate program, marked by church services, song festivals, parades, athletic sports, a water carnival, a picnic and barbecue, the demobilization of flag service, receptions, a ball, the conferring of medals upon servicemen. A triumphal arch was erected at Granby Street and City Hall Avenue, while the whole city was a mass of flags. Everywhere were booths, run by fraternal societies, where food, drinks, and cigarettes were handed out to all in uniform. The men who had gone through the inferno of the Meuse heights, of the Bois des Ogons, and Madeleine Farm, were made to feel that Norfolk was not unmindful of their bravery and their sacrifices.[52]

[52] Davis, *Virginia Communities in War Time*, pp. 349-350.

CHAPTER FIFTEEN

Peaceful Expansion

The tremendous activities of the war period convinced the people of Norfolk that a change in the city government was necessary. With the population increasing by leaps and bounds, with the water problem acute, with the schools, police, transportation, housing inadequate, there was need for prompt and vigorous action on the part of the councils. But the councils, from their very nature, found it difficult to act either promptly or vigorously. The board of aldermen served as a check on the council, the council as a check on the aldermen, and the mayor as a check on both. Unless a change was made at once, it seemed that the city must be strangled by its own rapid growth.

So the commission-manager form of government was proposed, and November 20, 1917, set as the date for the people to decide. Under the new plan the voters were to elect a Council of five members, who, in turn, selected a city manager to act as the chief executive in all business matters. To assist him the city manager appointed, subject to the approval of the Council, the heads of the departments of Public Welfare, Public Works, Public Safety, Law, and Finance. In this way it was hoped to bring vigor, efficiency, and progressiveness into the government without depriving the people of their ultimate control.

But the conservative group had no idea of submitting without a battle. "The city-manager will be an autocrat," they said. "The ring in its palmiest days would look like a society for the prevention of cruelty to children, compared to this new form of government," said one. "The old time boss would look like a tissue-paper sport, compared with the City Manager."[1] So intense were the "Old Fogies" that some began speaking on the street corners, and it became a common

[1] *Virginian-Pilot,* Nov. 15, 1917.

occurrence to find at Granby and City Hall Avenue, or Main and Church, large crowds gathered around listening to their arguments.[2] On the evening of November 14 both the advocates and the opponents of the change held meetings, the former in the Maury High School, and the latter in Eagles' Hall, on Church Street.[3] "I favor the new charter," said one speaker, "because it has a tendency to promote efficiency and economy in the government of the city. There is too much lost motion in the machinery of our municipal organization."[4]

That the people of Norfolk concurred in this view is indicated by the overwhelming majority accorded the charter, 3,403 votes being cast for, and only 1,222 against it. According to the *Virginian-Pilot*, the success of the movement was largely due to the carefully planned and perfectly executed campaign of the Citizens' Union, made up of representatives of all parties and factions, which had used every legitimate method to educate the voters. As for the opposition, they contended themselves with the simple statement: "They rose up and smote us."[5]

The Virginia legislature granted the desired charter, and, in September, 1918, the commission-manager form of government was put into operation. The Council was fortunate in its selection of the first city manager. Charles E. Ashburner, the son of an English army officer, who had been educated in England, France, and Germany, came to the United States to begin his career as an engineer. In 1908, he became the first city manager in the United States when Staunton introduced the new plan of city government as an experiment; after working several years in Richmond, he left in 1914 to become city manager in Springfield, Ohio, where he remained until called to Norfolk. "Quick of thought, indefatigable, he is a man of strong opinions. . . . No one ever doubts his utter honesty. . . . At times pugnacious, again very mellow, always driving for essentials, Charles E. Ashburner, the founder of a new profession, is undoubtedly a personality."[6]

Mr. Ashburner found himself in charge of a city of more than 130,-000 people, whose municipal facilities were designed for a population of fifty or sixty thousand, so that it was necessary to re-equip almost every department to meet the increased demands upon it. His attention was at once directed to the poor condition of the streets. In some

[2] *Ibid.*, Nov. 11, 1917.
[3] *Ibid.*, Nov. 15, 1917.
[4] *Ibid.*, Nov. 2, 1917.
[5] *Ibid.*, Nov. 21, 1917.
[6] *Collier's Weekly*, May 27, 1922; Leonard White, *The City Manager* (Chicago, 1927), pp. 91, 92.

sections of the city automobiles and trucks still had to bump over cobblestones which had done service before the Civil War; elsewhere they were apt to get stuck in the mud. Of the one hundred and seventy-two miles of streets within the city limits, only eighty-two miles were paved. Under the manager's supervision the new director of public works began an intensive program of improvement, in which cobblestones and mud gave way to concrete, business streets were widened, new approaches to the city opened. So vigorously was the work pushed that in the years from 1918 to 1928 the mileage of paved streets was doubled.[7]

Even more pressing was the question of water. For many years it had been evident that the old works, built in 1872-1873, were inadequate, and the Council had frequently considered how best to secure a larger supply. Commercial organizations and public-spirited citizens had urged action; committee after committee had made investigations. In 1917 the city went so far as to purchase Burnt Mills Lake and Lake Phillips, in Nansemond County, together capable of supplying thirty million gallons a day,[8] but there the matter rested. The old government, while waiting for the commission-manager charter to go into operation, would not proceed; the new manager, after taking office, had to get acquainted with the machinery of government before committing himself to a project involving the expenditure of millions.

At this juncture, just as in 1869, a severe drought brought matters to a crisis. In the summer and fall of 1919 one rainless month followed another until the level of the lakes east of the city fell lower and lower, drinking water was at a premium, and personal cleanliness became well-nigh impossible. In January, 1920, the water department was making arrangements to secure drinking water from Portsmouth, for distribution in tank-cars, sprinklers and wagons, when heavy rains brought the famine to an end. This lesson had its effect, and, with the approval by the voters for a six-million-dollar bond issue, work began.

It was a task of great difficulty. A huge dam and basin, with an impressive spillway, was built at Lake Prince.[9] This structure is thirty feet high, 2,150 long, and contains 2,977 cubic yards of reinforced concrete. The reservoir, formed by the dam, has a watershed of 30.2 square miles, and a storage capacity of nearly four billion gallons. More diffi-

[7] *Virginian-Pilot*, Jan. 15, 1928, Sec. 4, p. 1; City Council, *City of Norfolk*, pp. 45-46.
[8] *Virginian-Pilot* Sept. 26, 1917.
[9] Formerly Burnt Mills Lake.

cult even than the building of the dam was the piping of the water many miles across rivers and swamps to Norfolk. In crossing the Nansemond, trestle work carries the pipes over the soft mud flats to the channel, where they are submerged, so as not to interfere with river traffic. When the workers came to the broad Elizabeth, they sank the mains so deep that dredges would have to reach down fifty-eight feet at mean low water to scrape their tops. With the erection of two pumping stations, the new system was complete, and water began to course through the great pipes to the city. The water problem seemed to be permanently solved.[10]

The return of peace found Norfolk solicitous lest a period of deflation follow the intoxicating years of war prosperity. So early as November 4, 1918, Mr. Barton Myers sounded the warning, pointing out, among other things, that Norfolk had not one dock or wharf properly equipped for foreign commerce.[11] True, the great piers at the Army Base had no superior, but they would profit the city little should they remain in the hands of the government, or even fall under the control of one of the great railways. So, immediately after the Armistice, a committee, headed by Mayor Albert L. Roper, requested the War Department to sell or lease the terminal to Norfolk. Mr. Roper made frequent trips to Washington to interview the Secretary of War, the Quartermaster General, Senator Claude A. Swanson, and others, pointing out that the city was entitled to the first consideration because it was Norfolk which had turned the property over to the government when needed for war purposes. Eventually he gained his end, the government consenting to lease to the city one of the great piers, together with some of the adjacent transit sheds. This venture proved an immediate success. Not only did it attract commerce, but it added to the municipal revenue, yielding a net profit of $62,296 in 1921, and $59,077 in 1922.[12] A port commission, appointed to establish cooperation between municipal and private interests, to develop a spirit of community interest among the railways, and to stimulate waterborne commerce, contributed greatly to the fruits of the undertaking.

It soon became evident, however, that if Norfolk was to compete permanently with New York and other great Northern ports, she must have some principal article of export other than coal, tobacco, and cotton. Ships carrying light freight such as tobacco and cotton have to

[10] City Council, *City of Norfolk,* pp. 23-31.
[11] *Virginian-Pilot,* Nov. 5, 1918.
[12] City Council, *City of Norfolk,* pp. 17, 18.

take on in addition grain, ore, steel, or some similarly heavy commodity, to act as a stabilizer. At the piers of Philadelphia, Boston, and New York, not until this "ballast freight" is stored away are other lighter goods added. It is true that coal is a heavy commodity, and that Norfolk shipped it out by the millions of tons, but it is not usually desirable to mix coal with other freight. To the municipal government grain seemed to offer the best solution, and, since for grain loading elevators are necessary, the city had no option save to erect one at its own expense. So, having enlisted the co-operation of several great Chicago grain concerns and having received an assurance from the railroads that there would be no discrimination in rates, they laid the matter before the voters. On February 7, 1922, the people endorsed a bond issue of five million dollars for the elevator and terminal.

A site between the Army Base and the Naval Base was chosen, and the work of construction pushed to completion. The elevator was one of the best and most modern in the United States. It has a capacity of seven hundred and fifty thousand bushels, can deliver grain at the rate of one hundred and twenty-five thousand bushels an hour, and is practically fireproof. "Two wings, or galleries, extend from the main unit, permitting two ships to be loaded at once. The grain is carried on broad belts to the spouts, automatically controlled and electrically operated, so that by the pressing of a button or the flashing of a light, the amount of grain running through each spout can be regulated."[13] The same clear vision of the needs of the future was manifested in the other units of the terminal. A pier was constructed, 1,250 feet long and 494 feet wide, equipped with tractors, trailers, electric and gravity conveyors, lifting devices, cranes, winches, and portable scales. On each side of the pier were built concrete warehouses 100 feet wide and 1,175 feet long, while plans were made for a future giant storage warehouse.[14]

The Army Base terminal and the new city pier were leased in 1925 by the Norfolk Tidewater Terminals, Inc., a link in one of the largest terminal companies in the world. This concern operated them with notable success. In 1926 the number of steamers handled at the piers was 507; in 1927 no less than 632. The cargo tonnage in 1927 was 543,579, of which nearly half was for exportation.[15] The part played by the municipal terminals in stimulating commerce more than compensated the city for a small deficit which their operation entailed.

[13] *Ibid.*, p. 21.
[14] *Ibid.*
[15] *Virginian-Pilot*, Jan. 3, 1928.

Nor did the new government stop here. When the housewives of Norfolk demanded a modern market, the city manager saw that they got it. A building of steel and stone, a masterpiece of its kind, was erected on the block bounded by Monticello Avenue, Brewer, Market, and Tazewell streets, at a cost of half a million dollars. "The walls are like battlements pierced with windows, and the wings, being a story lower than the main building, permit the entire interior to be flooded with light. Sanitation and cleanliness manifestly are watchwords. The stalls border long, wide walks, that extend the entire length of the market, like avenues, with other walks like cross streets." "Here the farmers bring their carts loaded with truck and dairy products," and here are displayed all kinds of pies, jellies, cakes, butter, cheese, and pickles. It was a far cry from the little wooden market house erected at the head of Commercial Place nearly two centuries earlier, to this imposing modern structure.[16]

On January 1, 1923, Norfolk acquired about twenty-seven square miles of territory and thirty thousand additional population, by extending the city bounds across the Lafayette River to include the Army Base, the municipal terminal, the Naval Base, Ocean View, and the suburbs east of the old city and across the Eastern Branch opposite Ohio Creek. In adding this area, the city pledged itself to spend upon it in improvements a sum equal to 12 per cent of the assessed property values; so that sewerage, street paving and lighting, police protection, and schools followed rapidly.

The new city manager did not rest content even with this long list of achievements. With the active support of the Council and the various directors, he broadened and advanced public education, added new libraries, instituted a juvenile and a domestic relations court, extended the parks and playgrounds, introduced a system of food inspection, increased the efficiency of the fire department, built a new armory, and established boulevards to connect with the highways leading into the city.[17] In short, he transformed Norfolk into a modern, "up-to-date" community. But the period of postwar deflation, the reduction of the Army and Navy activities, and the slowing up of shipments for recontruction in Europe combined to produce a reaction in public sentiment against further large expenditures. On September 1, 1923, Mr. Ashburner left to become the manager of Stockton, California, and Colonel W. B. Causey took his place. Causey devoted himself chiefly to an attempt to secure favorable freight service to the municipal

16 City Council, *City of Norfolk*, pp. 65-67.
17 *Ibid*.

docks and grain elevator, and failing in this, after two years of service, resigned. He was succeeded by Major I. Walke Truxtun.

The new manager was described by Professor Leonard D. White, in *The City Manager,* as belonging to an old Southern family, for generations prominent in Norfolk affairs. "He possesses a striking personality, the outstanding feature of which is a high-strung tenacity and nervous power, coupled with a high ideal of public service. He is the personification of nervous force. He speaks rapidly and forcefully, one fist ready at any instant to pound the desk. . . . He is an untiring worker; is sometimes at his desk as early as five o'clock in the morning. He declares that he will support the ideals of council-manager government even though it costs him all of his friends."[18]

When Major Truxtun took office there existed a floating operating deficit of over two hundred and fifty thousand dollars a year. By preparing a sound budget, lengthening office hours, combining the duties of some offices and doing away with others, in two years he converted this deficit into a surplus. Norfolk devoted about 61 per cent of her income to city operation, and 39 per cent to interest and sinking fund on the bonded debt. Of the operating expenses, education constituted a third, public safety nearly another third, and streets, water, lights, sewerage, public welfare, etc., the remainder.[19]

Major Truxtun found conditions in the police force unsatisfactory and at once set himself to the task of reform. Bringing many policemen to trial, he secured the conviction and discharge of those who were found guilty of collusion with bootleggers. This had the desired effect. "The police force is universally admitted to be on a higher plane of efficiency and integrity than ever before. Truxtun has started a school to instruct the patrolmen in handling evidence and giving testimony. . . . He addresses the police once a year, and has told them frankly he would prefer 200 men in whom there was public confidence to 600 men who lacked public confidence."[20]

The efficiency of the police was evidenced, not only in the apprehension of criminals, but in crime prevention. Despite the constant presence of sailors on shore leave and despite the large Negro population, the number of offenses was remarkably small, the homicide rate being far below that of most Southern cities. In 1927, when there were 69.3 homicides for each hundred thousand of population in Memphis,

[18] White, *The City Manager,* p. 100.
[19] J. R. Vandenberry, *Council-Manager Facts.*
[20] White, *The City Manager,* pp. 100, 101.

63 in Birmingham, and 23 in Houston, in Norfolk there were only 7.3. Although the rate jumped to 11.9 in 1928, it was still small compared to 54.9 for Birmingham, 17.6 for Cincinnati, 15.8 for Chicago, and 16.5 for Detroit. Criminals seemed to prefer to pass Norfolk by.[21]

The Fire Department was equally efficient. With forty-five units of modern motor-driven apparatus, with an experienced chief, and a well-trained personnel, the department accomplished wonders in subduing Norfolk's age-old enemy, fire. Prior to 1922 the average fire loss per capita was between seven and eight dollars; in 1926 it was $1.79, and in 1927 slightly less than two dollars. In 1921 there were 450 demerits placed against the city by the fire insurance underwriters; in 1927 the number was only fifty-one. The fireboat *Vulcan* saved waterfront property owners $125,000 in insurance a year, and diminished greatly the risk of a widespread conflagration.[22] The older citizens of Norfolk, when they harked back to the days of the *General B. F. Butler,* or even to those of Chief Kevill and his three steam engines, might well marvel at the contrast.

Public education kept step with other improvements. An extensive building program was carried out, many trained teachers added to the staff, new courses of study introduced, open-air instruction instituted, a division of research and experimentation organized, attention paid to character education, advances made in music, art, physical training, and in the industrial arts. Especially noteworthy was the establishment of the junior high school system, and the resulting revision of courses to permit six years in the elementary schools, three in the junior high schools, and three in the senior high schools. The school system was recognized as one of the most efficient in the country.[23]

Equally important work was done in health and sanitation. A contagious disease hospital was established, war was declared on mosquitoes and flies, schoolchildren were given medical examinations at stated intervals, dental clinics were established. A bacteriological laboratory was erected where milk and meat were daily tested. "No restaurant may serve milk dipped from a can. Every glass comes from a sealed bottle. . . . All fresh meats sold are inspected and stamped. Food manufacturing plants and factories are regularly inspected. . . . Bakeries, ice-cream plants, restaurants" were supervised. As a result

[21] *The Spectator,* April 1, 1928; March, 1929.
[22] *Virginian-Pilot,* Jan. 15, 1928, Sec. IV, p. 1.
[23] The total enrollment in 1927 was 21,800. In 1917-1918 the entire budget for education was $392,936; in 1928 it was $1,470,000 (*Virginian-Pilot,* Jan. 15, 1928, Sec. I, p. 24).

Norfolk had the lowest mortality rate from typhoid of all South Atlantic cities, the number of deaths in 1928 for each hundred thousand of population being 1.6, as compared with 2.1 for Jacksonville, 2.7 for Washington, 3.1 for Richmond, 3.8 for Baltimore, 4.7 for Wilmington, N. C., and 7.4 for Atlanta. The record for diphtheria was equally good, the mortality in 1928 for each hundred thousand people being 3.3, as compared with 3.5 for Jacksonville, 6.2 for Wilmington, 7.6 for Baltimore, and 8.1 for Washington. Thus the city, so long considered an unhealthful spot, might now point with pride to its splendid health work and to its low mortality rate.

The people of Norfolk seemed well satisfied with the progress made in the first twelve years of the commission-manager form of government. The occasional complaints of the high cost of government were met by a reference to statistics, which showed that the burden per capita was one of the lowest in the country for cities of from one hundred to three hundred thousand people. It was generally realized, also, that the people received benefits corresponding to every dollar of taxes. "Norfolk has tried the experiment for ten years," said the *Virginian-Pilot,* on January 15, 1928, "and there is little possibility that Norfolk will desire a change. Political considerations which have hampered municipal and other governments since time immemorial, have been eliminated to a high degree. Service to the public is no longer made secondary to service to some political organization."

At the conclusion of the First World War many predicted that Norfolk would lose the gains made in foreign trade since 1914. "The small exports and insignificant imports of Hampton Roads prior to the war represented our normal trade," it was said, "and we may expect to see the streams shrink once more to the old volume." But the volume, instead of shrinking, continued to expand. In 1918 the exports of Hampton Roads were $134,826,224, in 1919 about $103,000,000, in 1920 they rose to $226,000,000, and in 1921 to $325,000,000. The great ocean liners were kept busy taking on coal at the piers of the Chesapeake and Ohio, the Norfolk and Western, and the Virginian, for shipment to all parts of the world. In 1921 no less than 4,027,996 long tons of cargo were sent out from the Elizabeth alone—to Italy, Great Britain, Brazil, Argentina, Panama, the Canary Islands, France, Chile, even to far-off New Zealand and Australia. That year Great Britain took from Norfolk 507,862 tons of coal and coke, 61,655 tons of tobacco, 20,626 tons of cotton, and 11,983 tons of logs and lumber.[24]

[24] War Department, *Port Series*, No. 15, pp. 268, 269.

Although with the satisfying of Europe's reconstruction needs and the economic depression of 1922, the volume of exports from Hampton Roads fell sharply, it was still ten times as large as in 1914. Obviously it was going to hold its newly acquired rank as one of the most important ports of the country. Exports continued in large volume, amounting in 1924 to $198,000,000, in 1925 to $169,000,000, in 1926 to $200,-000,000, and in 1928 to $182,000,000.

Of great importance was the rapid increase of the exports of grain, so much needed for balanced cargoes. At the same time the shipments of tobacco also mounted until Hampton Roads ranked as the greatest tobacco port of the world. In 1918 the exports of leaf from Norfolk and Newport News was but 10,500,000 pounds; in 1920 they were 105,000,000 pounds; in 1925 no less than 236,000,000 pounds. At the same time cotton held its own, the total number of bales exported being 174,320 in 1922-23; 311,085 in 1925-26, and 384,064 in 1927. Germany was the largest buyer of Norfolk cotton, taking in 1927 nearly 189,000 bales, as compared with 103,000 for Great Britain, 16,500 for Italy, and 12,500 for Japan. Other exports included lumber, flour, starch, glucose, brass, livestock, and cotton cloth, with coal retaining its leading position.[25]

Of vital importance to Norfolk was the steady increase in imports. For a century the port had been hampered by the striking lack of balance between exports and imports, and the loss entailed by the entry of vessels in ballast. Now the State Port Authority was trying to stabilize the commerce by attracting foreign goods, especially from Latin America. It was encouraging to note that in 1928 imports at Hampton Roads were $32,817,774, as compared with $16,500,000 in 1925, and $8,500,000 in 1920. A decade earlier imports had constituted less than 4 per cent of the foreign trade of the port; in 1928 they constituted 15 per cent. Norfolk was not the only great port in the United States that faced the problem of an ill-balanced trade, for at Galveston exports exceeded imports twenty-three times over, while at Boston imports were six times larger than exports, and at Philadelphia nearly three times larger. With the rapid industrial development of the South, and the consequent increased demand for foreign raw materials, it seemed probable that commerce at Hampton Roads would more nearly strike a balance.

[25] *Virginian-Pilot,* Jan. 3, 1928; *Hampton Roads Year Book,* pp. 24, 27, 35.

CHAPTER SIXTEEN

Depression and Recovery

With the opening of Norfolk's two hundred and forty-seventh year, in 1929, its people looked forward to the future with confidence. The stores on Granby Street were crowded with purchasers; long trains of freight cars rolled in from the Virginia and West Virginia mountains to dump their coal on the ships waiting at the piers; at the Navy Yard could be heard the noise of riveting as old vessels were modernized and new submarines and cruisers laid down; out at the Naval Base the construction of new buildings gave work to hundreds; the hotels at Virginia Beach and Ocean View looked forward to another year of thriving business; new industries continued to come to the city.

So there was surprise and dismay when word came in October that the stock market had suffered drastic losses. People could hardly credit their eyes as the financial columns of the newspapers showed that in a few weeks of frantic selling the stocks listed on the New York Stock Exchange had fallen from eighty-seven billion to fifty-five billion dollars.

The Great Depression had begun, a depression unparalleled in American history. Factories were forced to curtail production, or, in many cases, to close their doors; wages were cut; many thousands of laborers were thrown out of work; prices dropped sharply; foreign trade declined; banks went under; construction almost ceased; financial ruin came to thousands; government action and charity alone saved many from hunger.

Many different causes have been assigned for the depression. It was the too rapid expansion of industry, the mechanizing of the farm, the loss of the foreign market which resulted from the high tariff, the expansion of credit and speculation in the stock markets which brought disaster. Perhaps it can be summed up by saying that the nation had not adjusted itself to the industrial and agricultural revolution which had been in progress for some years. The manufacturer had failed to pass on to the consumer the benefits of mass production in lower prices; the farmer was helpless in the face of huge surpluses.

In the three and a half years which followed the crash of October, 1929, when times grew worse and worse, Norfolk fared far better than most American cities. In January, 1931, the *Virginian-Pilot* could report that bread-lines, "the harbingers of business depression," had not made their appearance in the city. "Leaders in community life—in business, in the professions, in commerce, and in the trades—looking upon the record that 1930 has wrought, almost without exception are inclined to the view that Norfolk has much to be thankful for."[1]

When month after month, year after year, production reached even lower levels, when earnings continued to decline, when more thousands were thrown out of work, Norfolk continued to be optimistic. "Norfolk looks on the New Year today with a feeling that the skies are brighter," said the *Virginian-Pilot* in January, 1933. "Norfolk's financial institutions have all remained intact under times which rocked the world."[2] Though local business, like business elsewhere, had suffered from the depression, there had been few failures. Employment held up remarkably well. The city was spared the distressing sight of soup kitchens and sidewalk sale of apples.

Norfolk's marriage to the Navy in large part accounts for the comparative lightness of the impact of the depression on her life. Naval operations brought her an annual income of some $20,000,000. Bluejackets swarmed in the stores and restaurants and theaters; the Navy Yard employed an average of four thousand men, the Naval Base two thousand. And while other industries were forced to curtail their activities, those of the Navy were increased. Many a skilled worker pocketed his wages with thankfulness, after a week's work on the great battleship *Idaho* or the *Mississippi,* which were being modernized at a cost of $12,000,000 each.[3] At the Naval Base the erection of new barracks, a concrete pier, and a half-million dollar general air station provided jobs for hundreds.

---

[1] *Virginian-Pilot,* Jan. 1, 1931.
[2] *Ibid.*
[3] *Ibid.*

But it was the sight of merchant vessels coming and going, or unloading at the piers on the Elizabeth River, which most of all heart-
ened the people of Norfolk. Here was a freighter heading for London,
here another just in from Bremen, here vessels from Cuba, loaded
with sugar, here freighters from Germany, from France, from Italy,
from Turkey, from New York, from New England. "It should be . . .
cause for thankfulness to know that at a time when world commerce is
reduced, our own port shows healthy growth in certain lines," said the
Virginian-Pilot, in January, 1931.

There was some falling off in the exports of coal. Cuba, Italy, and
France had passed tariff laws discriminating against American coal
and favoring English coal. Yet coal dumpings at Hampton Roads in
1932 came to 14,440,000 tons.

The decline in coal exports was offset by the sudden rise in sugar
imports. In 1931 the presence of sugar-laden ships in Hampton
Roads was a common sight. At one time there were 200,000 tons of
Cuban sugar in the warehouses at the Army Base and elsewhere.[4]
Hampton Roads continued to be the premier port for the exportation
of tobacco, chiefly Virginia and North Carolina bright flue-cured tobacco, together with millions of dollars worth of cigarettes. It exported,
also, cotton, cotton cloth, lumber, farm machinery, and grain. Imports
of manganese ore from Africa, fertilizers, coffee, and wood pulp
showed gains.

"Norfolk is not stopping . . . to count her blessings nor ponder
such misfortunes as have befallen her," said the *Virginian-Pilot* in the
Annual Review of January, 1931. "She is engaged in making the most
of her opportunities. Her ship lines she prizes. They use the sea as a
long green path to the ports of the world that are anxious for her
goods. . . . Commerce through this port is a surer thing than it has
ever been before."

It was remarkable that during the dark days of 1931 the city could
boast that it had made "mighty strides" in the field of transportation.
The Baltimore Mail Steamship Line, with five new ships fitted for both
passenger and freight service, was keeping up weekly sailings direct to
Le Havre and Hamburg. As these vessels headed out to sea, with
"full staterooms," people asked each other if the day would not come
when Norfolk would rival New York as the gateway of the United
States.

But as the months passed and the predicted recovery failed to make

[4] *Ibid.,* Jan. 2, 1932.

its appearance, Norfolk began to suffer. It was hopeful thinking for the press to say, "Old Devil Depression is on the run"; the depression became steadily worse. Building fell off, there were some business failures, the number of the unemployed grew, the city fathers found it necessary to practice strict economy.

Norfolk is the market for the farm products, not only of southeastern Virginia, but of the Eastern Shore, and of northeastern North Carolina. A very rich trucking country it is. On the shelves of the grocery stores one finds the soybeans, the spinach, the cabbage, the tomatoes, the onions of Princess Anne, Norfolk, and Nansemond counties; the vegetables and fruits of Northampton and Accomack, and the grain of Gates, Camden, Currituck and other North Carolina counties. But farmers now fell upon hard times. In 1932 bad weather played havoc with their yields. And when they appeared at the Norfolk markets with what cold, or drought, or insect pests had left them, they found prices disastrously low. Princess Anne planters made a little money on sweet potatoes, but on the whole the farmers lost money. Conditions in 1933 were worse. All of this hurt the Norfolk merchants, for it meant fewer purchases of seed, farm machinery, fertilizers, and other goods.

Vacant stores on Granby Street gave mute testimony to the impact of the depression on the city. Purchasers became fewer and fewer, and those who came to buy sought cheapness rather than quality. City finances grew steadily worse, with tax payments falling off and the floating debt mounting. Unemployment increased at an alarming rate.

The city government was forced to make drastic cuts in expenses and curtail expenditures for public works. "A city's activities are limited by the ability of the citizens to pay," wrote City Manager Truxton in January, 1932. "In preparing the budget for 1932 every effort has been made to relieve the stress." A maximum was set for the pay of city employees, the school budget was cut by $175,000, increases of salaries were few and far between.

As the number of the unemployed increased, the problem of relief became acute. Chairman C. Moran Barry, of the Travelers Aid Society of Norfolk, reported that in 1930 it had assisted 20,133 persons. The problems that came before the society were varied and often tragic— runaway children with frantic parents searching for them, foreigners unable to speak English and without employment, old people ill and without funds. All possible aid was given in each case.

But before the end of 1931 it became evident that the resources of the Travelers Aid Society were not sufficient to meet the rapidly increasing demands of the unemployed. So an Emergency Relief Committee was formed, with Robert M. Hughes, Jr., as its chairman. When it was suggested that funds might be raised by means of Sunday theater performances, the Tidewater Ministerial Union protested. The city manager, harassed by the numberless problems of the depression, is said to have retorted that if the union did not like this method of giving hungry men two days' work a week with which to buy food and fuel for their families, they might assume responsibility for an alternative plan of relief.[5]

But it soon became obvious that such makeshift methods of meeting the crisis would be inadequate. So the people of the city in 1932 put forth an extraordinary effort. The Community Fund, as well as independent agencies, found that the demands upon their funds had increased so greatly that it became necessary to make sharp cuts in allocations. When the Community Fund Campaign for 1933 was started, it was hoped that $250,000 would be raised. Great was the disappointment when the campaign, though well-organized and vigorously prosecuted, fell short of its quota by one-third.

But this merely stimulated the people to greater efforts. A commissary at 1008 Granby Street, operated by the Norfolk Relief Association, acted as the clearing house for emergency relief. To it was handed over the emergency funds of the Community Campaign, as well as vast quantities of clothing and other supplies, along with money donated in response to appeals over the radio and in the newspapers.

A Christmas Clearing House cared for the immediate needs of several thousand families. The City Welfare Center opened its doors to the homeless with food and beds. The United Charities, the Salvation Army, Union Missions, though their facilities were overtaxed, gave relief to many families. With the coming of cold weather in 1932 it could be said that "no one in Norfolk was without food and a place to sleep."

It was an inspiring exhibition of community spirit, this wholehearted response to the needs of those in distress. "Thousands of people have contributed their time, means or energy, and have given money, supplies, work," it was said. "Scarcely is there a citizen whose financial situation will permit it, who is not today engaged in some work of charity." Many a leading citizen labored day and night in the cause with no thought of personal return. "Norfolk has developed into a city of giving" was their boast.

[5] *Ibid.*, Sept. 20, 1931.

In the meantime President Hoover had not been idle. Other presidents had taken it for granted that in hard times it was the function of business to fight its way back to recovery. Hoover accepted it as a governmental responsibility. He feared that without the active aid of the government, the capitalistic system might collapse. It was Hoover who first urged Congress to appropriate huge sums for public buildings, public roads, and for improvement of harbors and rivers. Though he favored the administration of relief through the states, municipalities, and voluntary agencies, he set up a national Emergency Relief Organization. By the spring of 1932 this body was distributing to local groups surplus wheat and cotton, and making large loans to the states. In January, 1932, the Reconstruction Finance Corporation was created with a capital of half a billion dollars to make loans to banks, railroads, and life insurance companies. Hoover's Federal Farm Board tried desperately to bring relief to the millions of hard-pressed farmers.

But the people were not satisfied. What they wanted was an end of the depression, and despite Hoover's efforts the depression grew steadily worse. Moreover, since hard times had come during a Republican administration, they held the Republicans responsible for it. So there was no surprise that in the presidential election of 1932, Franklin D. Roosevelt, the Democratic candidate, was elected by an overwhelming majority.

The new President was confronted with the immediate possibility of a collapse in the nation's banking system. Drained of their deposits by frightened customers, with millions of dollars of assets frozen, most of them had been closed by state executive order for a long bank holiday. The day after his inauguration Mr. Roosevelt closed those which remained open, and a few days later pushed through Congress an Emergency Banking Act, which provided for the reopening of all banks found to be sound. By March 13 banks began to open their doors, former depositors were reassured, millions of dollars began to flow back, and business was resumed.

The Norfolk banks weathered the financial storm in a sound condition. They had recognized the seriousness of the crisis, and had taken the necessary steps to meet it. "It has been a source of the greatest satisfaction to the present management," it was stated by the National Bank of Commerce in 1937, "that it approached, experienced, and emerged from the banking holiday without for a single moment needing or desiring the rediscount privileges of the Federal Reserve system, or the subsequent capitalization through the Reconstruction Finance Corporation. These facilities were freely offered, but your management was constantly mindful of its desire to preserve the position and priority of its stockholders."[6] The Seaboard Citizens National Bank reported that its "first dividend was paid January 6, 1868, and dividends have been paid regularly each year since organization."[7]

The banking crisis having passed, the administration set itself the triple task of relief, recovery, and reforms. The most urgent of these was relief. So one of its first acts was to create a new Federal Emergency Relief Administration to make loans and grants to those states whose financial resources were unequal to their relief needs. Yet, despite the millions poured into the FERA by Congress, many months passed before the army of the needy began to dwindle. Labor-saving machinery continued to throw men out of jobs; savings of unemployed men dwindled and disappeared, and private charities broke down as their burdens became too heavy. So an increasing burden rested on the shoulders of the municipalities.

In Norfolk the Community Fund continued its activities. As the months went by and the need for relief mounted, it was decided to conduct another campaign to raise funds to carry it through the first six months of 1934. But, though this campaign was waged with vigor, it fell short of the goal, which had been set at $125,000. It was the general expectation that better times would reduce the number of the needy, and few anticipated that as the year closed, there would be no less than 14,673 persons, or 11.3 per cent of the city's population, on the relief rolls.[8]

New Federal relief policies in 1935 threw an increased burden on the city. When the national government discontinued the Federal Transient Bureau, the care of numberless penniless wanderers was placed on local agencies, the states, and the municipalities. "Those who apply for relief, those who two years ago, or even six months ago, would have been helped with Federal funds without question, are now being refused," stated the Annual Report for 1935. So in Norfolk it became necessary for the Travelers Aid Society, two Union Missions, and the Salvation Army to double their activities. When this proved insufficient, the responsibility for relief fell more and more on the city.

Ten years after the panic of 1929, the problem of relief still remained. "Each year a greater burden has been placed upon the city until now approximately $250,000 is expended for relief purposes," it

[6] *Ibid.*, Jan. 1, 1937.
[7] *Ibid.*
[8] *Ibid.*, Nov. 28, 1934.

was stated in 1939. In addition to general relief, there was special aid to the blind, to dependent children, and to the aged. As before, various organizations—the King's Daughters, Florence Crittenton Home, Union Mission, and others gave welcome assistance. Scores of women were kept busy on a Sewing Room Project, making sheets, mattress covers, garments, towels, curtains, etc., while others gave their time to the Handicraft Project which turned out comforters, bath mats, rugs, brooms, sweaters, and toys.[9]

President Roosevelt's thinking was influenced by those who blamed the depression upon the laissez-faire policy of former administrations. In the complex civilization of today what is needed is a planned economy. The government must take the wheel of the ship of state, and steer it clear of the rocks of overproduction, unemployment, business failures, declining prices. So one of his first acts had been to set up the National Recovery Administration, in a nationwide effort to increase the purchasing power of the people by raising wages and cutting down unemployment.

Brigadier General Hugh S. Johnson, as chief administrator of the NRA, urged manufacturers, merchants, the railroads, and utility corporations to devise "codes of fair competition," raising wages and shortening hours of work. It was a patriotic duty for all to sign, he said, and to those who did he gave a handsome emblem, the Blue Eagle. The store which could not display this emblem was to be shunned by all good people; the products of the manufacturer who had no Blue Eagle were to be boycotted.

Norfolk was selected for the NRA headquarters for Virginia, North Carolina, Maryland, and the District of Columbia, with J. J. Skorup, Jr., the administrator. Immediately Norfolk employers began to fall in line. The shipping companies adopted a code, the upholsterers and decorators worked out a code, the shoe dealers adopted a code, the Retail Dealers Association sent a telegram to President Roosevelt promising their full co-operation. Mr. Skorup was highly gratified. By July 30 about seventy-five Norfolk employers had sent in their agreements.[10] The Blue Eagles began appearing on store windows two days later. Over three hundred employers had signed by that date. On August 3 the number had risen to 586, on August 8 to 1,144. A few days later Mr. Skorup announced that in all Virginia 9,810 signatures had been received to codes affecting 59,066 employees.

Norfolk's good showing was largely due to a committee headed by

[9] *Civic Affairs*, 1939, p. 30.
[10] *Virginian-Pilot*, July 30, 1933.

A. B. Schwarzkopf, president of the Association of Commerce. The committee was directed by General Johnson to organize a campaign of education in speeding "the return of prosperity through the expansion of consumer purchasing power." "It is an inspiring thing to be a part of a great national movement to restore economic security to our people," he telegraphed Mr. Schwarzkopf, "and I appeal to you to marshal all the forces of your community in one united movement to get rid of unemployment."[11] Mr. Schwarzkopf entered upon the task with enthusiasm. He appointed a committee of one hundred leading citizens, who in turn organized a recovery "army." It was to consist of three hundred men and women pledged to battle for prosperity. Winder R. Harris, managing editor of the *Virginian-Pilot,* was elected general; Mrs. E. B. Hodges, president of the Woman's Club, lieutenant-general; Charles L. Kaufman, R. J. Throckmorton, and Leon T. Seawell, colonels. These officers immediately organized their departments and appointed their adjutants. Henry Lewis was made head of the newspaper bureau, Otto Wells head of the bureau of billboards and placards, Saxon W. Holt, Jr., head of the radio bureau. J. Eugene Diggs, Negro lawyer, was made major to organize the Negro work.[12]

"The Blue Eagle began to scream an insistent message of recovery yesterday as the Norfolk NRA campaign forces took to the field," said the *Virginian-Pilot* of August 15. Mason Manghum, of Richmond, head of the Blue Eagle forces in Virginia, at a luncheon gathering at the Fairfax Hotel explained to officers of the "army" the best methods of campaigning, followed by questions and answers. In the evening Mr. Skorup spoke before the members of the American Legion, in the City Council Chamber, and his assistant, Horace K. Dickson, addressed Post 36. Thus started a week's intensive campaign, which was continued with daily radio talks, newspaper articles, and addresses before civic and business organizations.[13]

But even before the "army" campaign got under way it was whispered around the city that certain holders of the Blue Eagle were not playing fair. One employer who signed a code told his employees that their raise in pay was "for the record only," and that anyone who "squealed" would be fired. Others raised wages and then required the employee to hand back the difference in fanciful outlays on his account, such as board for waitresses. To handle complaints of viola-

[11] *Ibid.,* July 22, 1933.
[12] *Ibid.,* Aug. 8, 1933.
[13] *Ibid.,* Aug. 14, 15, 1933.

tions of the codes, a bureau of eight or ten young lawyers was set up, headed by J. J. Beacher.[14] President Roosevelt was confident that public opinion would condemn backsliders and force them into line.

In some cases the codes, so far from reducing unemployment, actually increased it. For unskilled workers, especially for Negroes, the Blue Eagle, instead of being a bird of happiness, turned out to be a bird of prey. Some of the Norfolk restaurants which had long employed Negroes as porters, elevator men, dishwashers, cleaners, etc., at well below the minimum set by the codes, began to dismiss them and hire white workers in their places. "It would be a grim and tragic commentary on the national recovery effort if a business and industrial regimentation directed to lifting the people out of depression, should operate to plunge the most depressed of them in a worse depression still," pointed out the *Virginian-Pilot*.[15]

Despite discouragements of this kind, at the end of the year 1933 the administration claimed that the great NRA experiment had been successful. It had brought about many business reforms, among them the ban on child labor and the sweatshop, and the acceptance of new high standards in advertising. It had restored millions of workers to gainful employment, had reduced working hours, had improved working conditions.

Yet the ultimate results were disappointing. The NRA, while increasing the purchasing power of millions of workers, forced higher prices and so reduced the purchasing power of other millions. It was like trying to lift oneself by one's bootstraps. Some of the leading manufacturers refused to subscribe to a code. A series of disputes followed between employers and the labor unions, marked by strikes which kept thousands of men out of work for weeks. Late in September, 1934, General Johnson resigned, and in the following May a decision by the Supreme Court cut the ground from under the NRA and forced its rapid dismantlement.

The Civil Works Administration, set up in November, 1933, was a far sounder venture than the NRA, and far sounder than the dole. What most men wanted was work, not charity. It restored the self-respect of millions of men who were employed at various tasks, even though many of these tasks were trifling in character, "boondoggling," as they were called in derision. The CWA was dissolved in the spring of 1934.

[14] *Ibid.*, Aug. 5, 7, 18, 1933.
[15] *Ibid.*, Aug. 10, 1933.

But the Civil Works program as administered in Norfolk was far from trifling. Five hundred men were employed in an attempt to eliminate mosquitoes by scientific drainage methods. Others undertook to repair the damage done by recent hurricanes and to build jetties and bulkheads as a precaution against tropical storms in the future. Playgrounds were started at the Larchmont school with football and baseball fields, tennis, hockey, and soccer courts, and a running track. A swimming pool was begun at Lafayette Park, a project was approved for beautifying cemeteries with walks and driveways and general landscaping; another was for repairs on the Museum of Arts and Sciences; still another involved the repairing and painting of school buildings; construction of a wooden bridge on the Ocean View Boulevard; a canning project at the City Home.[16]

Paralleling the CWA was the Public Works Administration, established in the summer of 1933 and headed by Secretary of the Interior, Harold Ickes. Avoiding boondoggling, it devoted its funds to aiding in the building of bridges, dams, sewage systems, hospitals, schools, roads, colleges, libraries, courthouses, parks, and playgrounds. The expenditures were enormous, by the end of 1939 totaling almost six billion dollars.

In Norfolk, when the CWA came to an end, many projects begun under it were continued under the WPA. But new projects were added, some of them of great importance. At first the City Council held back. The policy of spending and even more spending was in direct conflict with the policy of strict economy which had been adopted by the City Council of Norfolk. The Council wanted no Blue Eagle set up on the door of the City Hall. Mayor W. R. L. Taylor criticized his predecessors for extravagance. "In the past the idea of living within our income each year was not considered," he said. "It was the depression that brought us face to face with the necessity of making our cash income and cash outgo meet." He pointed out that this was responsible for a deficit of half a million dollars in one year alone. By strict economy the city had cut this deficit to $50,000 in 1933, and he hoped to show "that our income and outgo are equal."

The CWA and the PWA were not greeted with enthusiasm by the mayor and some of his colleagues of the Council. "I know, and my colleagues know, that there will be no extravagance at City Hall in the future," said Mr. Taylor in January, 1934. "Anybody who thinks

[16] *Ibid.*, Jan. 1, 30; July 19, 1934.

that because we are getting back to normalcy we are going to appropriate money for this and that thing, is going to be mistaken."[17]

This policy led to a bitter conflict in the Council and among the citizens at large. When it was proposed in the Council in November, 1934, to lower taxes, to increase the wages of city employees by 10 per cent, and to add $191,000 to the appropriations for schools, it was voted down by three to two.[18]

But it was becoming obvious that the most immediate need was a new bridge over the Eastern Branch to replace the wooden structure at Campostella Road. As early as 1931 the city was considering means for financing a two-lane bridge by a system of tolls. There followed long delays until in July, 1933, it was announced that $400,000 from the Federal funds allotted for roads in Virginia had been assigned to this project. Elated at this turn of events the City Council voted to add $125,000, so that work could be begun at once. "It turns out that the long delay in solving the pressing Campostella Bridge problem is the thing that will make possible a wider and better bridge than the city could have managed with its own funds," said the editor of the *Virginian-Pilot*. As it was, the steel and concrete structure has four lanes and a walk, and a modern draw span over the river channel.[19]

Not less important than the Campostella Bridge was the construction of a new bridge to replace the old one over the Lafayette River at Hampton Boulevard. The interests of the Federal government, as well as those of the city, were concerned. The bridge was an essential link in the line of communications between the Naval Base and the Marine Hospital and the Norfolk Navy Yard. City Manager Thompson made repeated visits to Washington to appeal to Secretary Ickes for a grant from the PWA funds. After some delay $119,000 was allocated for the project, the remaining $400,000 being financed locally.

When a Citizens' Public Works Committee thought advantage should be taken of the opportunity to secure Federal funds for another bridge over the Lafayette River, for dredging the Southern Branch, and the construction of a sea wall at Ocean View, Mr. Taylor rebuffed them. "I feel that none of these things are absolutely essential, however desirable they may be," he said. "Even though we

[17] *Ibid.*, Jan. 6, 1934.
[18] *Ibid.*, Nov. 28, 1934.
[19] *Ibid.*, July 7 and 8, 1933; Jan. 24, Nov. 10, 18, 1934.

should get thirty per cent of the costs of these projects from the government, the remainder would be a heavy charge on the taxpayers."[20] And the editor of the *Virginian-Pilot* agreed that there ought not to be pressure brought on city officials to raid the treasury for public improvements beyond absolute necessities.[21] But soon there was pressure, pressure too great to be resisted; and it was not long before the City Council was eagerly seeking Federal aid for a number of projects.

Norfolk always has been a city of bridges. Built on a peninsula intersected with bays, rivers, and creeks, traffic has been facilitated in some cases by fillings, in others by ferries, but often by bridges. With the coming of the age of automobiles, it became obvious that the old wooden structures, many of them in a dilapidated condition, were out of date. Their replacement by steel and concrete structures began in 1929 with the construction of the bridge over a branch of the Lafayette River at Colley Avenue. This was followed by the new Granby Street four-lane bridge over the Lafayette River.[22] Construction of the bridge began early in 1935. The structure is 1,800 feet long, and is wide enough for four traffic lanes. There is no draw span since the center is elevated enough to permit the passage of boats using the river. The pushing through of the project, though backed by Senator Byrd and Congressman Colgate Darden and approved by President Roosevelt, was a personal triumph for City Manager Thompson. "I very well know how the city manager has spent time and effort in season and out of season in efforts to get this grant through," said Mayor Taylor.[23]

The Norfolk Division of the College of William and Mary made good use of the PWA to secure a stadium with a seating capacity of 25,000 and a classroom building. At Ocean View, Willoughby, and Brambleton, large sewer projects were started in 1935, largely financed by grants from the PWA. In 1936 we find Mr. Thompson knocking at Secretary Ickes' door to request aid for five important projects: $25,000 toward a junior high school, $45,000 for the Ocean View School, $100,000 for the completion of the Museum of Arts and Sciences, $36,000 for the Berkley School, and $25,000 for the Twenty-sixth Street Bridge.[24] All in all, the CWA and the PWA were of great importance in lifting Norfolk out of the depression. They brought

[20] *Ibid.*, July 26, 1934.
[21] *Ibid.*, Jan. 7, 1934.
[22] *Ibid.*, Nov. 18, 1934.
[23] *Ibid.*, Nov. 10, 1934.
[24] *Ibid.*, Aug. 1, 1936.

much-needed improvements to the city, gave employment to hundreds of men, and helped to restore confidence at a time of discouragement and even despair.

Welcome also was the erection of the long-needed Federal Building. Formerly all the government agencies were housed in the Custom House at Main and Granby streets, with the post office in the basement and the court in the upper stories. When more space became imperative, a new building was erected at Plume and Atlantic streets. But only fifteen years had passed when in 1915 a committee of prominent citizens visited Washington to point out to the Treasury Department that the business of the post office and the courts had outgrown this building and to plead for a new one. This effort failed, but many years later Congressman Menalous Langford succeeded in obtaining an appropriation of $2,000,000 for the new building.

After much discussion a site was selected on the lot formerly occupied in part by the old St. Luke's Church, bounded by Granby Street, Brambleton Avenue, Monticello Avenue, and Bute Street, and construction began. To many this seemed too far "uptown," blocks away from the old post office, the City Hall, and the principal office buildings. The structure, which rises four stories above the street, occupies an entire block and is one of the finest in the South.[25] Its construction was of vital importance to Norfolk in easing the problem of unemployment, and the scores of masons, carpenters, plumbers, and other workmen, as they took home their weekly pay, were grateful to Uncle Sam for keeping them off the relief rolls.

Meanwhile the government had consolidated the various relief agencies under a new agency called the Works Progress Administration, with Harry Hopkins at its head. Although the PWA was continued temporarily, the WPA took over many of its activities, especially those which aided projects for improving streets, building bridges, extending sewer systems, erecting schools and hospitals, etc. All in all, the WPA gave work to eight million persons and spent eleven and a third billion dollars.

Norfolk was alert to this opportunity and many were the projects which the city manager and Council put through in the next few years with WPA and PWA assistance. One of the most important was the development of the Municipal Airport, at Little Creek, on what was formerly a part of Truxton Manor Golf Course, with a handsome administration building, a hangar, and three runways.

[25] *Ibid.*, July 8, 1934.

A grant from the WPA in 1938 made it possible for the city to proceed with the second unit of the Museum of Arts and Sciences, with its fifteen additional galleries, a library, assembly hall, and hall of statuary. The Granby Street High School, which was begun in September, 1938, and opened for classes a year later, cost $500,000, of which the PWA paid $225,000. This lovely building has a large auditorium, gymnasium; art, music, and commercial science rooms; library; and domestic science room.[26] PWA funds aided also in erecting the Ocean View School and in making additions to the Robert Gatewood School. Improvements to the Booker T. Washington High School cost $141,000, of which the WPA paid $60,600.

It was in 1938 that the city in an effort to provide work for Negro women on relief conceived the idea of developing an azalea garden in the wooded area adjacent to the airport. With the aid of the WPA seventy-five acres of woodland were soon cleared and linked by five miles of trails, and 4,200 azaleas, together with hundreds of camellias, rhododendrons, redbuds and other plants added. Today this is one of the most beautiful spots in the United States, rivaling in charm the famous Middleton Place and the Magnolia Gardens of South Carolina.[27]

In 1936 the city decided to make new street construction provide work for persons on the relief rolls, and thus succeeded in getting fifty-eight cents of every dollar from the WPA. In 1939 alone 8.2 miles of new streets and 14.6 miles of curbing and gutters were laid down at a cost of $193,119 to the city and $263,977 to the WPA. Other projects by the PWA and the WPA were the building of the Norfolk Community Hospital for Negroes, the completion of jetties at Ocean View and Willoughby, the extension of the sewage system, the adding of nearly 15,000 feet of water pipes, and the beautifying of the city parks. In 1940 the WPA diverted its funds from many projects of general utility in order to assign all relief labor to defense projects. By that time Norfolk merchants reported that gains in business were from 25 to 50 per cent over 1933. The payment of back taxes was largely responsible for converting the $200,000 deficit of 1933 into a $300,000 surplus. Commercial shipping was the best since 1929. A visit of the United States fleet, with its 40,000 officers and men, brought needed business. Thus year after year the city registered gains, until the great depression became little more than a bad memory.

[26] *Civic Affairs*, 1939, pp. 37-40.
[27] *Ibid.*, 1940, pp. 74, 75.

But the depression and the New Deal had lasting effects which were to be vitally important in shaping the city's development during the next two decades. Prior to the New Deal it was largely taken for granted that the control of American cities was the responsibility of the cities themselves. Why should a municipality turn to the Federal government for aid in paving streets, or building bridges, or laying down sewage pipes? But with the experience of the CWA, the PWA, and the WPA, opinion changed. Begun chiefly to relieve unemployment, these agencies played an ever-increasing part in the development of the cities themselves.

With the return of prosperity there was wide opposition to a return to the old state of affairs. The cities were reluctant to turn their backs on needed improvements for which Federal aid was needed; the Federal government was reluctant to give up a source of local political influence. So Norfolk, when she needed a new schoolhouse, or a hospital, or street paving, or a new bridge, or slum clearance, turned for aid to Uncle Sam. The Norfolk of today, with its fine public buildings, its hospitals, its broad boulevards, its steel and concrete bridges, its lovely parks, its underpasses, its Museum of Arts and Sciences, its modern airport, its sewage system, would not be the same had not Uncle Sam taken her by the hand.

CHAPTER SEVENTEEN

The Second World War

The people of Norfolk wanted their city to grow. But they wanted growth to be gradual, to be the natural result of the advantages offered by their situation and their magnificent harbor. They did not want to repeat the experience of the First World War, with its explosive growth, so they watched with apprehension as the war clouds grew blacker and blacker in the years from 1937 to 1941.

It was in Reconstruction days in South Carolina that a planter was brought before a Freedman's Bureau court, with an all-Negro jury, to be tried for killing a cow which had been turned loose in his garden. The jury returned the verdict, "Not guilty this time, but don't do it again." The people of the United States did not want to be drawn a second time into an overseas war, and so passed a Neutrality Act in 1935 designed to steer the nation clear of the rocks upon which isolationism foundered in 1914. "War is a contagion, whether it is declared or undeclared," said President Roosevelt in October, 1937. "We are determined to keep out of war."

But it became more and more apparent that isolation was impossible in a world aflame. Norfolk celebrated New Year's Day, 1939, with mixed feelings. There was rejoicing at the return of prosperity, with booming industry, full employment, easy money, but alarm at the perilous situation in both Europe and Asia. In Spain General Franco had renewed his smash at the center of the government's lines. In the Far East Japanese war planes were dropping their bombs in a death shower over China. The German press was denouncing Roosevelt and threatening the United States with war; Hitler boasted that he had Aryanized the German people and proclaimed his absorption of Austria and the Sudetenland, which he called, "The richest harvest in our history." London viewed Germany's plan for doubling her submarine strength as the opening of a new race for naval supremacy.[1] The world was shocked and incredulous when word was received that Hitler was seeking to exterminate the Jews in Germany. "I myself could scarcely believe that such things could occur in a twentieth-century civilization," said President Roosevelt.

Though he did not want war, the President thought it wise to prepare for it should it be forced upon the nation. In January, 1938, he asked Congress to appropriate a billion dollars for naval defense, and reluctantly Congress complied. Thereupon Admiral Leahy announced that construction would start on two battleships, four cruisers, eight destroyers, and six or eight submarines.

The effect on Norfolk was electric. At the request of the Navy Department $12,000,000 was set aside for construction at the Naval Base and the Navy Yard. Soon hundreds of men were at work at the Naval Base, replacing the old frame structures built hurriedly during World War I with brick and stone buildings, enlarging the bachelor officers' quarters, repairing the submarine base, dredging at the piers, putting up barracks. At the Naval Air Station over half a million dollars was spent for repair shops, and $395,000 on improvements to the runways and landing field. Down on the Southern Branch at the Navy Yard work started on a 1,000 foot pier, and on rebuilding the ways for the construction of one of the new great battleships. All this meant work for 15,000 men, 5,000 at the Navy Yard alone, with a payroll of $18,000,000 a year.[2] Mars was handing out the gold with a grim smile and a lavish hand.

The hard times of the early thirties were forgotten in the glow of a new prosperity. The stores on Granby Street buzzed with activity. Two new schools had been opened, and the Community Hospital for Negroes was being built. The people boasted of the completion of the beautiful azalea gardens, the new Municipal Airport, new jetties at Ocean View, the growth of suburban areas, the paving of new streets, the Twenty-sixth Street Bridge over the Lafayette River, the expanded water system, the completion of an addition to the Museum of Arts and Sciences.[3]

But elation was tempered by the realization that this was a war boom. "There is no question of tremendous expansion due to Federal activities," warned City Manager Charles B. Borland. Should war

[1] *Virginian-Pilot*, Jan. 1, 1939.
[2] *Ibid.*
[3] *Civic Affairs*, 1939.

come, it would bring temporary inflation, he feared, followed by a new slump. So the people of the city viewed events in Europe with increasing alarm—the continued saber-rattling, the German-Soviet non-aggression pact, Hitler's demand for the return of the Polish Corridor and Danzig. On September 2, 1939, when they picked up the morning paper, they found the first page half covered with blazing headlines. "Britain and France Ready to Enter War"; "Major Hostilities between Germans and Poles"; "Twenty Cities Bombed"; "Poland's Allies to Act Today if Ultimatum Rejected"; "Germany Given Final Warning to Halt Aggressive Action and Recall Troops"; "British and French Standing Firmly Together, Order General Mobilization and Summon Parliaments to Act Immediately."

A roundup of newspaper opinion by the *Virginian-Pilot* showed an overwhelming majority of editorial opinion in favor of American neutrality. "The United States must keep out of this war," was reiterated from coast to coast. But the editor of the *Virginian-Pilot* wisely pointed out that the drive for neutrality had been just as strong in 1914. "The real test will come later," he said. "Then American lives and American homes will be affected. American business will be affected. American thinking will be affected. American emotion will be affected."[4]

But for the moment things seemed to be going as usual. Children were preparing to go back to school after the summer's vacation, visitors began to leave the beaches, the college football teams started practice. But the somber undertone was apparent in the President's proclamation of American neutrality, the cancellation of passports for Europe, and the U-boat sinkings. As the months passed and Germany and Italy won one success after another and it became more and more obvious that American interests were involved, President Roosevelt began to waver on neutrality. "We must strain every nerve, not only to build up our own strength," he said, "but to send aid to Great Britain." In May, 1940, he requested funds from Congress for "at least 50,000 planes a year."

Norfolk now became more and more a center for naval and military activity. The Navy Yard, with 11,000 employees in June, 1940, was adding new workers at the rate of a thousand a month. The Naval Base was planning to double its 8,000 employees. In July, 1940, 1,034 acres of land were taken over by the government for the expansion of the Naval Base and the Naval Air Station. Soon steam shovels ap-

[4] *Virginian-Pilot,* Sept. 3, 1939.

peared on the scene, and two suction dredges began pumping mud and
sand to fill in the low places. Machines began to uproot trees and
stumps. Carpenters and masons set to work constructing barracks,
piers, warehouses, etc. At the Navy Yard work was hastened on the
gigantic battleship *Alabama*.[5]

The Army moved into the Virginia Military Reservation at the
south end of Virginia Beach, which was renamed Camp Pendleton,
and into Fort Story at Cape Henry. Though these bases are several
miles from the city, the soldiers piled into buses at every opportunity
and came in to the movies and to dances. At times the streets were
full of them.

It was on July 29, 1940, that President Roosevelt emphasized the
importance of Hampton Roads as a defense center by choosing it for
an inspection tour. As he came ashore from his yacht *Potomac* at the
Navy Yard, he was greeted by Rear Admiral Joseph K. Taussig, Congressman Colgate W. Darden and others, and conducted through this
hive of activity. Then he was driven to the Naval Base through
cheering crowds, over the Campostella Bridge, through the heart of
the city, up Hampton Boulevard, over the Lafayette River. At the
base he expressed satisfaction at the progress that was being made. "A
year from now we are going to be a lot safer," he said.[6]

The President during his brief stay could not have realized the
many perplexing problems which the sudden increase of defense activities brought to Norfolk. The population was growing by leaps and
bounds, with hundreds of families moving in to take advantage of
boom conditions. By June, 1941, there were 15,559 officers and enlisted
men at the Naval Base and 14,426 more on the ships based there;
while at the Navy Yard civilian workers numbered 20,893 and Navy
personnel 3,716. Altogether sailors and naval employees in the Norfolk
area numbered 71,669 and their wives and children 37,916. It was estimated in November, 1941, that the population of the city had nearly
doubled since the beginning of the defense movement.[7]

The people of Norfolk found it hard to reconcile themselves to this
sudden change. "You know I've been standing here for an hour," a
lifelong citizen said to a passing friend. "I think I've seen 10,000
people and I don't believe I know more than two of them. A few

[5] *Ibid.*, Dec. 28, 1941.
[6] *Ibid.*, July 30, 1940.
[7] *Ibid.*, Dec. 28, 1941.

years ago, watching people walk along here, I would have known half of them, perhaps 90 per cent of them. Now I hardly know any of them."[8]

If the situation was difficult for the people of Norfolk, it was more so for the newcomers. There were not enough houses, not enough hospital beds. The water supply was inadequate; there were too few schools. In going to and from work one might have to stand while bus after bus went by too crowded to squeeze in even one more passenger. There were long lines before the movies, it was hard to find a table at a restaurant, facilities for recreation fell short of needs. "We have a bigger recreation problem here than probably any other place in America," stated former City Manager Thomas P. Thompson. "We have both the Army and Navy with us and there are times when we have 10,000 to 15,000 soldiers and sailors on our streets."[9]

It was the housing situation which caused the most trouble. Admiral Taussig reported that thousands of Navy men were forced to live in disgraceful conditions, as many as three or four often being crowded into a single room, and at times several families sharing a single bath. The term "hot bed" was commonly used to mean a room rented to one person in the daytime and to another at night. Landlords split their houses into several units, and then made more units out of them. Rentals were high.[10]

Private builders were working hard to meet this need, putting up charming small houses here and there, and starting several developments for apartments. But there was some hesitation. Was there any certainty that the shortage would last after the close of the war? People did not want to invest their savings in houses which in a few years might be vacant. "I cannot imagine a greater catastrophe than to have the out-of-town builders construct the thousands of houses they say they are going to build," said the secretary of the Real Estate Board. "They will take their profit and run, leaving our citizens to struggle with a greatly overbuilt community."

But Admiral Taussig was troubled with no such fear. What he wanted was housing for his men, and he wanted it immediately. So he bombarded Washington until it consented to a housing project of 1,042 units for enlisted men, to be located just east of Hampton Boulevard. Benmoreell, the development was called. It was with openly ex-

[8] *Ibid.*
[9] *Ibid.*, July 19, 1941.
[10] *Ibid.*, June 21, 1941.

pressed joy that naval families left their cramped quarters to move in when the first units were thrown open in March, 1942. "We like Norfolk better now!" all agreed.[11]

The city too did its part. In June, 1940, the Council created a Housing Authority, which was to administer a 500-unit housing development, sponsored by the Federal government for married enlisted men in the Navy. In addition to the dwellings, there was a combination community center and administration building with an auditorium, storage room, repair rooms, offices, etc.[12] This project, called Merrimack Park, was located on Mason's Creek, adjoining the extension of the Naval Air Station.

The sudden influx of thousands of families put a heavy strain upon the water supply. New houses would be useless if their occupants remained thirsty and unwashed. A main source of supply was Lake Prince, in Nansemond County, but the old wood pipeline was inadequate to meet the vastly increased needs. So miles of new 30-inch and 36-inch pipe were laid down, at a cost of a third of a million dollars. But after the supply of water had been increased, it was still necessary to facilitate its distribution to outlying districts, and 22,700 feet of 16-inch cast iron pipe were added to supply the northern area, and several miles more to supply the Army forces at Fort Story and Camp Pendleton. To see that the water moved along the pipes, it was necessary to establish new pumping stations and to increase the capacity. Fortunately for the city it was Uncle Sam who had to reach in his pocket to meet most of the cost of these improvements.[13]

The joy of the worker at the Naval Base who succeeded in finding a place to live was often short-lived when he found how difficult it was to get there. When he complained that there should be more streetcars and buses, he was told that more had been ordered. At the gate to the base there were often long lines of stalled cars waiting to get in in the morning and out in the afternoon. And when once out, there might be further delays at grade crossings. Downtown, the narrow streets were often tangled with automobiles, trucks, streetcars, and buses. "This disgusted reader is an expert in the art of exhaling an unnecessary breath from his lungs," wrote one rider, "folding his body into a compact bundle and plunging into the swaying, stumbling mass of humanity hanging from straps, bars, or just balancing them-

[11] *Ibid.*, March 26, 1941, pp. 9, 18.
[12] *Civic Affairs*, 1940, pp. 26-29.
[13] *Civic Affairs*, 1940, pp. 40, 41; *Virginian-Pilot*, Aug. 6, 1940.

selves as best they can."[14] It was not unusual to see a streetcar with
five or six sailors on the roof or hanging on outside the rear platform. One sailor swore that he never knew the cars had seats. A story
went the rounds about the motorman who always succeeded in crowding "just one more on," until it turned out that for every one hauled
in at the front one was being pushed off at the rear.[15]

The Bureau of Traffic Survey, established in 1939, struggled with
this problem. At its advice automatic traffic lights were installed where
most needed; nearly 1,500 new traffic signs were set up; new parking
meters were installed; controls were fixed at Main Street and Commercial Place, and elsewhere. But the main problem was dumped in
the lap of the Federal government, with recommendation for underpasses and new roads.[16] The government, recognizing the folly of having trucks and automobiles foundering in the mud or caught in traffic
jams in northern Norfolk, set aside $530,000 for road improvement.
Workmen began widening, straightening, and paving Sewells Point
Road; widening and resurfacing Hampton Boulevard north of Lafayette River Bridge; and widening and paving Admiral Taussig
Boulevard from the main gate to the east gate of the Naval Base.[17]

With so many sailors and soldiers on the Norfolk streets it was vitally
important that they have facilities to play. Most of them were mere
boys, and if there were not enough playing fields, not enough parks,
not enough social centers, no auditorium, it was inevitable that many
would gravitate to the disreputable houses on East Main Street. It is
true that clean sport beckoned on the beaches stretching from Ocean
View to Virginia Beach, and during the summer months thousands of
servicemen could be seen stretched out on the sand, or diving through
the surf. But with the coming of cold weather they had to look elsewhere.

In solving the recreation problem a fundamental difference of
policy developed between the city and the Navy and Army. Since the
need of the services was urgent and immediate, they pressed for speed;
since the need of the city was permanent, it demanded solidity. The
city recreation committee worked out plans for a combination recreation center, auditorium, and arena, and secured for it an allocation of
$278,000 from the Federal War Agency. But great was City Manager
Borland's disappointment on discovering that the money was to be

[14] *Virginian-Pilot,* July 31, 1941.
[15] *Ibid.,* Jan. 1, 1955.
[16] *Civic Affairs,* 1940, p. 20.
[17] *Virginian-Pilot,* Dec. 28, 1941.

used for a temporary building. "If Secretary Knox is correct in his estimate of Norfolk's future as a permanently enlarged naval center, temporary structures for local defense recreation facilities would hardly seem to qualify as a sound solution of the problem," pointed out the *Virginian-Pilot*.[18]

In the end it was agreed that the city should add $245,000 to the FWA grant, and the auditorium be made permanent. So work was started on a building to include a theater of two thousand seats, and an arena to hold five thousand persons. But it was only in May, 1943, that the building was completed, and Richard D. Cooke, head of the USO Management Committee, began scheduling entertainments. Servicemen were admitted free to the dances and were allotted many tickets to other events, but civilians had to pay.[19]

When a married Navy man moved to Norfolk, after he had secured a place to live, he looked around for a school for his children. He had the choice of many fine schools—the Maury High School, Ruffner Junior High School, Granby Street High School, Blair Junior High School, and others. But, if he lived at or near the Navy Base, some of these schools which were in other parts of the city were too far away for his children to reach. So there was overcrowding in the schools near by, especially in Granby Street High School with 1,698 pupils, Ocean View School with 1,005 children, and Madison, Bay View, and Willard schools.[20]

In some cases the numbers were so great that it became necessary to operate in two shifts. While the new pupils were crowding into schools, the number of qualified teachers decreased because of the temptation of the higher salaries offered by war industries. When the war ended, more than a third of the city's teachers held only emergency certificates.[21] The overflow of population into the suburbs made the school problem especially acute in Norfolk County, where the number of pupils increased from 10,407 in 1940 to 23,893 in 1945. It was only with the construction of additional classrooms at Granby High School and the Titustown schools with grants from Uncle Sam that there was partial relief.

What the servicemen who poured into Norfolk looked for above

18 Oct. 1, 1941.
19 Marvin W. Schlegel, *Conscripted City: Norfolk in World War II* (Norfolk, 1951), p. 312.
20 *Civic Affairs*, 1940, pp. 122, 123.
21 C. F. Marsh, ed., *The Hampton Roads Communities in World War II* (Chapel Hill, 1951), p. 134.

all else was a bit of hospitality. The married men wanted their families to meet old Norfolk families; the single men wanted to meet Norfolk girls. "The fascinating problem is how to bring to individual
soldier and sailor boys and defense workers and their families the decent, pleasant and interesting life of the home town," said Admiral
Taussig.[22] But in the matter of hospitality, as in other things, the city
was swamped. The people might open their homes to a limited number of newcomers, but it would be only a drop in the bucket. And if
here and there friendships were formed, they might be interrupted by
orders for the serviceman to move.

Yet the city did what it could. As early as December, 1940, Saturday
night free dances for sailors and soldiers were organized. The dance
committee, however, found it difficult to recruit enough girls, since
Norfolk girls were wary of sailors, although they responded more
freely when a dance was given for soldiers from the beach camps.
There were Saturday night dances for Negro sailors at the Booker T.
Washington High School. These dances were organized by C. Wiley
Grandy, chairman of the committee on recreation for Negro servicemen.[23]

But it was on Christmas, 1941, that Norfolk really opened its heart.
One hundred sailors were entertained for dinner in the recreation
hall of the Methodist church. All over the city homes were opened to
servicemen, with good Virginia cooking highlighted by "old ham" and
wild goose.[24] The USO on West Freemason Street, operated by the
YWCA, gave a party with a large Christmas tree, with hundreds of
stockings filled with stamps, razor blades, cigarettes, fruits, and candy.[25]
The Navy or Army boy who headed back to his post that night
realized that Norfolk was not the coldhearted place it was reputed
to be.

The people of the city were proud of what had been accomplished
in so short a time to meet the situation suddenly thrust upon them,
despite labor shortages, difficulty in getting essential materials, and
Federal red tape. So they were surprised and angered when a series of
articles appeared in prominent magazines depicting Norfolk as a
place of "confusion, chicanery, ineptitude," with an "air of decrepi-
tude," of "apathy and decay." *Collier's* dwelt on the night life in some
of the trailer camps. The *Architectural Forum* gave the impression

---

[22] *Virginian-Pilot,* March 28, 1941.
[23] *Ibid.,* Jan. 9, 1941.
[24] *Ibid.,* Dec. 25, 1941.
[25] *Ibid.,* Dec. 14, 1941.

that Norfolk was "nothing but a dump." *PM,* the *American Mercury,* and other magazines followed in like vein.[26]

To call their city ugly was especially offensive to the people of Norfolk. These writers must have been blind not to have noticed the architectural gems of Norfolk, that is if they had ever visited the city they were describing. Had they seen the Moses Myers Home, or the old City Hall, or the old Norfolk Academy, or the charming little Adam Thoroughgood House? In speaking of the article in the *Architectural Forum,* the *Virginian-Pilot* accused the writer of "gross exaggerations." "And by dint of completely ignoring certain of the city's physical aspects that are admirable, the portrait painter represents Norfolk as a Rip Van Winkle kind of town—save when war touches its magnificent harbor and electrifies the city's hardened arteries."[27]

Disturbed by the deluge of unfavorable criticism, the Navy Department began an investigation to see whether the city was indeed a modern Jericho. So a committee was sent to Norfolk to question local officials, naval and military officers, and others. Their report stated that the unfavorable conditions had been greatly magnified, and that, despite the extreme difficulties which had faced the city manager and the Council, they had performed their jobs remarkably well.[28]

The people of Norfolk were settling down to a quiet Sunday afternoon on December 7, 1941, when news came that a force of Japanese planes had swept over the American naval base at Pearl Harbor in Hawaii and showered down bombs on the Pacific fleet. As word of this treacherous attack spread throughout the city, there was wild excitement. Automobiles were piled up in long lines before the *Virginian-Pilot* building while newsboys dashed in and out shouting: "Extras! We want extras!"[29] Just how devastating the attack had been was not known for several days, but gradually the news came out that five battleships and three cruisers had been sunk or crippled, with 3,500 casualties. A cry for revenge arose from the American people; Congress promptly declared war on Japan.

In his report on the raid Secretary Knox admitted that the Navy had not been on the alert. "Why were they not?" the editor of the *Virginian-Pilot* wished to know. "It is important that the responsibility for this negligence be fixed."[30] It was only two years later that he had

26 *Ibid.,* June 20, 1942.
27 *Ibid.,* June 21, 1942.
28 *Ibid.,* Jan. 2, 1944.
29 *Ibid.,* Dec. 8, 1941.
30 *Ibid.,* Dec. 16, 1941.

the answer. A White Book, issued by the State Department, then re-vealed that Ambassador Grew had called up from Tokyo less than two weeks before the destruction of the fleet to warn that the Japanese had plans for a "surprise attack at Pearl Harbor." Just why this warn-ing was ignored may never be known.

War with Germany and Italy followed immediately, and Norfolk had to prepare for defense. It was quite unlikely that a fleet could cross the Atlantic to enter the Chesapeake Bay and land a force on Virginia soil, as the British had done in the War of 1812; but, there were new perils unknown in former days. Might not the German U-boats sneak into Hampton Roads to shatter American shipping? Might not a horde of German bombers sweep over the city to lay its buildings in ruins and bring death to thousands of its people?

The city immediately took on a more warlike appearance. Army convoys were seen passing in and out. Antiaircraft batteries and search-lights along the roadsides and at defense centers pointed to the sky. Two hundred men from the Army moved into the Twelfth Street Armory to aid in air raid defense. At the Municipal Airport a squadron of interceptor planes made ready to repel the enemy. "In the present great emergency we have the responsibility of protecting the city in case of air raids and other dangers," one councilman warned the people. Mayor J. D. Wood promised that the citizens would be told how best to combat incendiary bombs. Police and fire officers were given special training at one of the near-by Army posts. Two new fire engines were ordered. Two hundred men and women responded to the appeal for air raid wardens by pledging their serv-ices, and seventy-five women registered for duty at the air defense center.[31] Women volunteers from the American Legion Auxiliary manned a battery of telephones to warn police, firemen, doctors and defense units of the approach of the enemy.[32]

In the meantime, Richard M. Marshall, a civic-minded insurance executive, was made chief air raid warden of the Hampton Roads area, and set up his office in the Pender Building. In October he held a drill, with sirens screeching, and a fire blazing on the roof of a warehouse, to simulate an incendiary bomb.[33] When he tried it again the United States had entered the war, and the blackout took on a grim reality. Everywhere the air raid wardens, with their white helmets and

[31] *Ibid.*, Dec. 10, 1941.
[32] *Ibid.*, Dec. 11, 1941.
[33] *Ibid.*, Oct. 11, 1941.

blue-and-red insignia, could be seen knocking on doors to put out lights and stopping cars and ordering the drivers to seek cover. One merchant who had left his neon sign blazing was dismayed the next morning to find that an angry crowd had smashed it during the night. Other merchants, though they put out their lights, telephoned to know why the Christmas period had been selected. "The Germans and the Japanese won't let us know when they are coming," Mr. Marshall replied. Not satisfied with this trial, Mr. Marshall staged another later in the month. "Our aim is to black this city out as black as ink," he announced. This time the civil defense workers, the Army, and the Navy co-ordinated their efforts; when the sirens sounded, street lights went out, merchants pulled down the store shades, buses came to a stop, and to imaginary bombers the city was invisible.[34]

As the war progressed, the people of Norfolk realized that the time had come to "tighten the belt." As early as January, 1942, there was a sugar shortage, and grocery stores began to ration their customers. Restaurants frowned on persons who insisted on piling four or five heaping teaspoonful of sugar in one cup of coffee. The public resentment against the sugar-hog was illustrated by an incident in a downtown drugstore. When a heavy man expressed resentment because a waitress refused to give him three teaspoonful in his coffee, a smaller man next to him said: "You don't get any sugar, and you don't get any coffee, either, but you do get this." And he landed a blow on the man's face.[35]

Despite the sudden expansion of the population, Norfolk did not suffer for food. The farmers of the Eastern Shore, Nansemond, and Isle of Wight laid out abundant crops and flooded the city markets with meat, poultry, dairy products, potatoes, and other vegetables. And the people of the city and servicemen alike had no reason to complain if they could not get all the coffee they liked.

More serious was the rationing of gasoline and tires, and the ration board office in the old municipal building was often besieged by angry citizens. "How can we get to work without gasoline?" was the complaint. "Without my share, you are forcing me to use the already crowded buses and streetcars, if indeed I can squeeze into them." If the ration board turned them down, they appealed to the local gas dealers not to punch their cards. As a result before the end of June, 1942, more than half the service stations in the city were dry.

34 *Ibid.*, Dec. 30, 1941.
35 *Ibid.*, Feb. 4, 1942.

The outlawing of pleasure driving, which became effective in January, 1943, added to the discontent. The managers of clubs and other places of entertainment wondered whether this restriction would put them out of business. Would a person by driving to a park, or the shore, or a concert, or a movie, or a high school football game be in danger of losing his gasoline ration?[36] But when the ruling was put to the test, the hardship was not as great as many had feared. People discovered that it did them no harm to walk, to use near-by places of amusement, or to use the streetcars or the buses.

The war was brought home to the people on a Sunday in October, 1942, when a seemingly unending stream of military vehicles moved up Hampton Boulevard. They were a part of Task Force A under the command of General George S. Patton, Jr., which sailed from Hampton Roads for North Africa a few days later. "Never before in the history of warfare had an amphibious force set out from one side of the ocean to land and attack an objective 3,000 miles away."[37]

By the end of 1942 Norfolk would have been well on the way toward solving the problems caused by the swelling of the population, had the population not continued to increase. But each day brought new hundreds in search of work in the Navy Yard or the Naval Base, or in stores, or in factories. The large number of naval ships in the harbor greatly added to the "floating population," for not only did the sailors swarm in the streets when on liberty, but wives, sweethearts, mothers, and other relatives came to visit them. This transient population, though it cannot be numbered with any degree of accuracy, placed almost as great a burden on the city facilities as those who came to remain.

And the permanent newcomers increased the population of the city in the years from 1940 to 1944 by about 44,000, of the adjoining Norfolk County by a like number, of Princess Anne County by 5,000, and of Portsmouth by 13,000. Since many of those who came to near-by localities worked, took most of their recreation, and did most of their shopping in Norfolk, they were actually a part of the city's population and added almost as much to its problems as though they resided within its limits.[38]

So to provide water, gas, electricity, hospitals, schools, transportation, recreation, police protection, sewerage, and fire protection for

[36] *Ibid.*, Jan. 7, 1943.
[37] W. R. Wheeler, ed., *The Road to Victory* (2 vols.; Newport News, 1946), I, pp. 65-72.
[38] Marsh, *The Hampton Roads Communities in World War II*, pp. 79-82.

this horde was a constantly increasing headache. Despite the fact that new construction had continued at a record-breaking rate for three years, and that in 1942 alone $8,100,000, exclusive of Federal grants, had been spent on new houses, with the coming of 1943 newcomers still found it difficult to find places to live.[39]

Hundreds of families tried to meet the housing situation by bringing trailers and camping in Princess Anne and Norfolk counties. But when the operators of the camps refused to pay the county taxes, the authorities cut off the electric lights and running water. "These families are not paying taxes to the county, yet are receiving the benefits offered to taxpayers, including police and fire protection and schooling for their children," the City Council pointed out.[40] So concerned was Rear Admiral Gygax, Commandant of the Navy Yard, at the possibility that this impasse might force hundreds of highly skilled workers to leave the area that he sent a fleet of motor trucks to move many of the trailers to sites at a Federal Housing camp. He was determined, he said, to find places for all evicted trailer workmen.[41]

The housing problem remained until the end of the war despite the completion of several vast building projects. By January, 1944, no less than 9,574 permanent and 4,592 temporary dwellings, and 540 dormitories had been added north of the Elizabeth River; and 4,931 permanent homes, 6,472 temporary dwellings, and 2,222 dormitories on the Portsmouth side. Since most of these units were reserved for war workers, none was without a place to lay his head. But servicemen, who continued to pour in by the thousands, found it almost impossible to secure living quarters for their families. One Navy officer, with his wife and small child, spent three nights in an automobile, while four other children were housed with friends.[42] To ease this situation the hotels agreed to reserve some rooms until six in the evening for servicemen and others engaged in war work, and to keep them five days if necessary while they looked for permanent homes.

If for newcomers the finding of places to live was of first importance, an adequate supply of pure water was vital to the entire population. So there was rejoicing when the expansion program for the water system, started in 1941, was pushed to completion. The second pipeline to Lake Prince made 30,000,000 gallons available daily from

[39] *Virginian-Pilot*, June 2, 1943.
[40] *Ibid.*, Jan. 2, 5, and 7, 1943.
[41] *Ibid.*, Jan. 20, 1943.
[42] *Ibid.*, July 28, 1944.

that reservoir; a dam at Lake Burnt Mills was finished; a new water line was laid down to Virginia Beach. The city took over the Nottoway River and Blackwater River lines, which had been built by the Federal government. New filtering units were placed in the Thirty-seventh Street pumping station, doubling its capacity.[43]

Despite a shortage of labor, caused by the shifting of workers to war jobs, great progress was made in solving the traffic problem. A military highway sweeping around the city from the toll-free bridge at Portlock to the intersection of Granby Street and Admiral Taussig Boulevard was completed. Certain streets were widened, sidewalks were installed in others.

When the Office of Defense Transportation in Washington heard that streetcars and buses in Norfolk were jammed, they made a survey of traffic in the city and ordered the rerouting of several of the bus lines. Whatever improvement this made in traffic, it did not mollify those whom the change forced to use their legs on the way to and from their work.[44]

Like other facilities, the hospitals were crowded. So there was much satisfaction when the new 300-bed de Paul Hospital on Granby Street near Talbot Park was ready for occupancy. This structure, built by the Federal government at a cost of $1,750,000, was taken over by St. Vincent's Hospital, which abandoned the old building on Church Street. By the end of 1944 workmen were adding the last touch to a new wing of the Leigh Memorial Hospital, while additions to the Norfolk General Hospital were completed.[45]

With a grant of $42,900 from the Federal government for a program of recreation backed by $37,000 from the city, servicemen found Norfolk a more attractive place to live. Lafayette Park was a favorite spot for officers and men, with dancing in the summer and skating in winter. The new auditorium and arena, which was leased to the United Service Organizations, provided endless pleasure to soldiers and sailors. The first dance, held on July 31, 1943, was followed by boxing matches, wrestling, basketball, lectures, and concerts.

Late in 1943 the old Talbot House on West Freemason Street was remodeled by the Woman's Council of the Navy League and opened as a club for commissioned officers of the United Nations navies. Formerly many an ensign, or lieutenant, or commander, or captain felt that time was hanging heavy on his hands when he came down-town. But now there was a typical old Norfolk home where he could dine and dance, play games, read, write, or just loaf. Here, also, he could join in parties, teas, and dances. "We felt they needed a place to gather and mingle with Norfolk girls," said Mrs. P. N. L. Bellinger, chairman of the council's club committee.[46]

That Norfolk was a hive of industry from the outbreak of war in Europe to the surrender of Japan was due chiefly to one thing—ship-building. And though there were several small private yards, by far the largest part of the work was done by the Norfolk Navy Yard. The chief task of this great establishment had always been to repair war-ships and during this critical period hundreds limped up the South-ern Branch for an overhauling. In addition, forty-two warships were built, among them the mighty *Alabama*.

The work done at the Navy Yard during the war period cost Uncle Sam nearly a billion dollars, one half of which was paid out in wages. Here the demand was for output, output irrespective of cost. On output might depend the result of the war. Workers poured in from near-by farms, from other industries, from states as far off as Cali-fornia. Norfolk itself suffered from the loss of policemen, firemen, garbage collectors, who resigned to take advantage of the higher wages at the Yard. Visitors were astonished to find hundreds of women doing men's work there, some even operating cranes and welding ships. Whereas in January, 1940, there were but 6,520 work-ers at the Yard, in March, 1943, the number had mounted to 43,000.[47]

So spectacular was government shipbuilding that it overshadowed the substantial gains made by private industry. Yet the output of the major firms almost tripled in the years from 1939 to 1944, and the average plant nearly doubled the number of its employees. Food and like products, fertilizers, and furniture continued to be the chief private industries, with shipbuilding forging ahead for the closing months of the war.

Commerce, too, was deeply affected by the war. As news came in of the sinking of colliers from the Hampton Roads ports on their way to New England and New York, coal shipments were often shifted to all-rail routes, free from the submarine menace. But the piers were

---

[46] *Ibid.*
[47] Marsh, *The Hampton Roads Communities in World War II*, pp. 62-65.

even busier than in peace times. A bystander would have seen an endless stream of men, mules and machines going aboard the transports. Here the great cranes lifted hundreds of 1,000-pound demolition bombs and swung them into waiting holds as though they had been tenpins; now a howitzer tank was hoisted aboard; now a mass of 155-millimeter shells; now several carloads of double-decked jeeps; now a line of mules. A few weeks later these men and this equipment would be in the midst of the conflict on the battlefields of North Africa and Europe.

As the U-boat menace slackened in 1944 and 1945, shipments of coal picked up, both to Europe and the North. In addition, as Italy was conquered and the Germans were driven out of France, vast quantities of foodstuffs, livestock, and other goods went out from Hampton Roads for the rehabilitation of those and other war-torn countries. So great was this need that thirty ships that had been lying idle in the James River and elsewhere were brought back into service.[48]

When the news reached Norfolk that Hitler had committed suicide, it was realized that the end was at hand. But it was six days later that the flash came over that Germany had surrendered unconditionally. The next morning, after President Truman confirmed the report in a radio address, the news was received with prayerful dignity and thankfulness. Shopkeepers closed their stores and went home. Laborers in the shipyards paused in their work to exchange congratulations.

That night for the first time in many months lights blazed in store windows and neon signs shone from atop big downtown buildings. Lights glowed in the churches, too, for there people gathered to give thanks to God for victory. But the thoughts of all dwelt on the cost— the loss of sons, of husbands, of fathers. There were thoughts, also, of the task still to be done. Rear Admiral David LeBreton expressed the spirit of the day when he said, "This is the time for thanksgiving and not celebration, which must wait until all our enemies stand under a white flag."[49]

That day was not long delayed. In August, 1945, the world's first atomic bomb laid Hiroshima in ruins and gave warning to the Japanese to surrender or face destruction. At seven in the evening of August 14 word was received that the war was over. This time the

[48] *Virginian-Pilot*, Jan. 9, 1947.
[49] *Ibid.*, May 9, 1945.

celebration was noisy and wild. The streets were soon full of excited people. Sailors and girls joined hands and weaved in and out, snake-dancing between the cars. Others hopped on runningboards, fenders and bumpers. Sailors, realizing that they were the heroes of the day, swung gaily through the crowds, arms encompassing female companions, pausing now and then to steal a kiss. A clanging motorman tried futilely to pilot his trolley, a washtub tied to its rear, through the crowd on Granby Street.[50]

Norfolk emerged from World War II a different place from the city which entered it a few years before. The war had proved a most valuable school of municipal affairs for the city manager, the council, and the citizenry. They took new interest in the city, new pride in the efficiency with which it was run, insisted upon a more adequate water supply, a better system of street lighting, more beautiful parks, finer schools, a more efficient police force, larger hospitals, slum clearances, a better public library, and a local orchestra. Not that these things grew out of the war experience, for some of them had been suggested and some were actually on the way before Pearl Harbor. But it was the war which proved the great stimulus which brought what may be called the laissez-faire period to an end.

Nor can we ignore the tens of thousands of newcomers in accounting for the change. If we include the built-up suburbs just outside the limits of the city we realize that Norfolk had doubled in population. Had the newcomers spent only the war years in Norfolk, their influence would have been small, but tens of thousands became permanent citizens. As such they brought new ideas, new energy, and played a part in arousing interest in the government and local improvements.

The war brought much confusion to Norfolk, it brought crowded living quarters, hasty marriages and other social maladjustments, but it played an important role in the development of the greater, more efficient, more prosperous Norfolk of today.

[50] *Ibid.*, Aug. 15, 1945.

CHAPTER EIGHTEEN

Thinking Big

The surprising result of Norfolk's fifth major war was a remarkable transformation of the spirit of its people. The city had watched the wartime boom begin with wary eyes, remembering painfully the optimistic overexpansion brought on by the First World War and the expensive economic burden it had imposed during the depressed 1930's. To prevent a repetition of the same disaster, local real-estate interests had obtained from the Federal government a promise to make most of the new housing units that had to be constructed of a temporary nature so that they could be removed as soon as the war emergency had passed.

This time, however, the emergency did not pass, and, although the war ended, the boom continued. In 1945, of course, Norfolk could by no means be certain of the fabulous future lying before it, and there was a brief debate between those who favored holding back and those who wanted to push forward. This was settled by the hard-fought municipal election of 1946, when a progressive slate, headed by Pretlow Darden, won control of City Hall. With Darden as mayor, the city launched a program of planned expansion, which brought so much complaint from conservative critics that Darden and his mates refused to run for a second term in 1950. Nevertheless, their program by that time had so demonstrated its success that the new administration under Mayor W. Fred Duckworth continued to display the same progressive attitude.

One of the most hotly argued issues stirred up by the Darden regime was the question of the annexation of land for planned development by the city. The City Planning Commission, given a full-time staff, headed by Donald R. Locke, in 1946 set to work to determine the need for more territory. Its land-use survey, issued in

August, 1948, set forth the need for action. Only 17 per cent of the land inside the city limits was still undeveloped, the report disclosed, as compared with twice that in thirty-nine other cities of comparable size. Putting the figures another way, Norfolk was already overcrowded, with only 5.17 acres for each hundred persons, while forty-eight cities in the same population group had 6.71 acres per hundred. The City Council promptly called in Dr. and Mrs. Thomas H. Reed, well-known annexation experts, to make recommendations on what should be done to provide more living room.

The proposal made by the Reeds was breath-taking in its scope. They suggested that Norfolk should more than double its area by annexing the Tanner's Creek district of Norfolk County and some 25 square miles east of that in Princess Anne County, in addition to 11.9 square miles of the Washington district of Norfolk County, on the south side of the Eastern Branch, as a site for future industrial development. Although much of this territory was still open countryside, the Reeds recommended that it be annexed before it became urbanized so that its development could take place under orderly city planning. Another important reason was that Virginia annexation laws made it much cheaper for the city to acquire rural areas than sections already thickly populated. While admitting that the city would have to spend millions more than it would receive in taxes for some years in order to annex the proposed areas, the Reeds pointed out that the longer Norfolk waited, the more expensive annexation would become.[1]

To no one's surprise, the proposal made by the Reeds touched off a vigorous debate. The officials of the counties involved naturally opposed the program, since under Virginia law the counties would lose all tax revenues from the area lost to the city. South Norfolk, fearful of being swallowed up by its bigger neighbor, prepared to annex the Washington district for itself. Residents of the Tanner's Creek district organized a Council of Civic Leagues to fight against annexation and the higher taxes it would bring them. Inside Norfolk itself the conservative-minded looked critically at a project which would admittedly cost the city millions of dollars. Why should Norfolk spend so much money on annexation, they asked, when the funds were badly needed for improvements inside the existing city limits?

Undeterred by the opposition, the City Council in 1949 adopted an ordinance providing for the annexation of parts of both Norfolk

[1] *The Norfolk Story,* 1948, p. 9.

and Princess Anne counties, only to run into a legal obstacle. The State Supreme Court ruled that Norfolk could proceed against only one county at a time, forcing the city to start over again with a suit aimed at the Tanner's Creek district of Norfolk County. This area would not provide the sought-for room for expansion, since it was already thoroughly urbanized, but under Virginia law it had to be taken before the city could reach out into Princess Anne County. The legal battle was finally settled on May 25, 1954, when the courts awarded the Tanner's Creek district to the city on condition that it pay Norfolk County some eight million dollars in compensation and spend nearly two million more on improvements in the annexed area within the next five years.[2]

Since the residents of Tanner's Creek district had been fighting annexation for six years, the city decided to win over these reluctant annexees by embarking on a good-will program which received national recognition. Calling in the newly organized Public Relations Institute to help, the city formulated a plan to convince its new residents of the value of annexation. Speeches by city officials at public meetings helped to break down the hostility. Soon the Council of Civic Leagues itself had surrendered and agreed to help the city in its campaign of education. A semimonthly newspaper, entitled *Residents of Tomorrow,* was distributed by the city to explain what annexation would mean in both higher taxes and better services, with the result that by the time Tanner's Creek district legally became a part of the city on January 1, 1955, opposition had almost disappeared.[3]

Encouraged by this success, the City Council decided to take the next step in the expansion program by annexing thirty-three square miles of Princess Anne County, going beyond the bounds suggested by the Reeds in 1948 to take in almost all the Kempsville district.[4] Once again opposition appeared, in spite of a unanimous vote by the City Council, and the matter was settled by a referendum on February 7, 1956, with the voters approving by a majority of nearly two to one.[5] The annexation court, however, proved less friendly to the project and ruled that Norfolk could have only the 13.5 square miles of the territory which were already developed. Although the city argued that this would leave it with a smaller percentage of un-

[2] *The Norfolk Story,* 1954, p. 3; *Norfolk* (Official Publication of the Norfolk Chamber of Commerce), Jan., 1959, p. 8.
[3] *American City,* LXX (November, 1955), 126-127.
[4] *The Norfolk Story,* 1955, [p. 8].
[5] New York *Times,* Feb. 8, 1956.

developed land than it already had, an appeal to the State Supreme Court failed to win any further concessions. When the final decree was rendered, Norfolk prepared to pay three million dollars in compensation to Princess Anne County and set about a new campaign of education in the annexed area. This time the task was easier, since there was less opposition; in fact, many of the new Norfolkians welcomed the promised improvements, even though they also meant higher taxes.[6] On January 1, 1959, the annexation went into effect, and Norfolk reached an estimated population of 300,000, making it the eighth largest city in the South and the thirty-eighth in the nation.[7]

As the 1960's dawned, prospects appeared bright for a new era in which Norfolk could abandon its protracted and expensive annexation suits and have instead the friendly co-operation of its sister communities in building a Greater Norfolk. The idea of a metropolitan government, embracing the four cities and the two counties on the south side of Hampton Roads, had been proposed as early as 1953 by Banker John S. Alfriend, and the continued growth in the area during the 1950's had made the plan seem more and more desirable. Political considerations, however, precluded any discussion of the scheme until political conditions were drastically revised during the 1960 session of the General Assembly.

In that session the senators from Norfolk and Princess Anne counties joined in pushing an anti-annexation bill aimed at Norfolk, and the city replied by failing to approve the extension of city water service to several new developments in Princess Anne County. The defeat of the anti-annexation act in the legislature was of great significance, since it was part of an over-all pattern which indicated that the "city boys" had overthrown the traditional dominance of the "country boys" in the General Assembly; the future of the two counties seemed to lie in working with the neighboring cities rather than against them. Shortly after the session ended, Sidney S. Kellam, acknowledged political leader of Princess Anne County, appeared before the Norfolk City Council to propose a study of a metropolitan government for the southern shores of Hampton Roads. The Council willingly accepted his terms of a five-year moratorium on annexations and the extension of water service to the new real-estate developments. The new metropolitan government was still many years in

[6] *Virginian-Pilot*, Jan. 3, 4, 1959.
[7] *Ibid.*, Jan. 1, 1959.

the future, but prospects appeared excellent that by 1980 there would be a Greater Norfolk with a population of more than a million on the south side of Hampton Roads.[8]

One factor promoting greater co-operation in the Hampton Roads communities was the closer physical ties that bound them together. From the time the town was first laid out, Norfolkians had been required to cross water to go anywhere. In the seventeenth century, when waterways were the most convenient transportation routes, that had been an advantage, but by the twentieth century the surrounding water had become a barrier, cutting off Norfolk from the rest of the state. Not until the late 1930's did it become possible to reach the city from the west without paying toll. Even then the toll-free highway was so roundabout that most motorists preferred the inconvenience and expense of the Portsmouth-Norfolk ferries.

Although no bridge between Norfolk and Portsmouth was practicable because of the maritime importance of the Elizabeth River channel, a tunnel under the river was talked about for years, and in 1942 the General Assembly created an Elizabeth River Tunnel Commission to carry out the project. As soon as the war was over, the commission set to work with funds borrowed from the Norfolk City Council. An engineering report was completed early in 1947, and two years later the contracts were let. On May 23, 1952, the tunnel under the Elizabeth River was opened for use, and the ferries, which had been operating for more than two centuries, at last went out of service. A new Berkley bridge, linking the tunnel with downtown Norfolk, was completed at the same time, and the old bridge was torn down.[9]

The ease of communication through the new tunnel increased traffic so rapidly that the revenue predicted for 1970 was almost reached in 1959. At times, in fact, cars jammed the underground highway almost bumper to bumper, and demand arose for another tunnel. Engineers picked out a route for the second tunnel from Pinner's Point in Portsmouth to the foot of Hampton Boulevard and declared that it was economically practicable. A successful bond issue in February, 1960, assured the construction of the new tunnel, with its official opening date scheduled for the first day of 1963.[10]

Meanwhile another tunnel dream had been turned into reality

[8] *Ibid.*, April 13, 14, 1960.
[9] Marvin W. Lee, "The Norfolk-Portsmouth Bridge Tunnel," *Virginia Municipal Review,* XXIX (June, 1952), 105-108.
[10] *Virginian-Pilot,* Feb. 13, 26, 1960.

with the completion of an underwater passage across Hampton Roads. In 1954 the Virginia Department of Highways undertook the construction of a combination bridge-tunnel to span the three miles of water between Willoughby Spit and Old Point Comfort. This $60,-000,000 project involved the construction of the longest trench-type tunnel in the world, 6,860 feet in length, with both ends in the middle of Hampton Roads; this was made possible by the creation of two artificial islands to bring the ends of the tunnel up to the level of the connecting bridges.[11] When the new system was opened on November 1, 1957, it became possible to cross Hampton Roads in five minutes instead of the half hour or more required for the old ferries, and the city provided easier access to downtown Norfolk by extending the new throughway, Tidewater Drive, all the way from the new Berkley bridge to Ocean View. Although the toll which was to be collected until the tunnel was paid for still constituted a significant barrier, the opposite sides of Hampton Roads were being drawn closer together. The new tunnel had been open only a year when the need for a second tube by 1975 was announced.[12] As the 1960's seemed destined to unite the southside cities and counties, perhaps the 1970's would be the decade which would mould both sides of Hampton Roads into a single harmonious community.

The success of the new tunnels led to serious plans for another tunnel so large in scope that it had seemed as fanciful as a trip to the moon a few years earlier. The Chesapeake Bay Ferry Commission, created in 1954 to restore ferry service between the Eastern Shore and Old Point Comfort, hired a firm of experts to report on the possibility of a bridge-tunnel crossing the mouth of the Chesapeake. Finding that sufficient revenue could be expected to cover the cost of the project, the engineers recommended a series of bridges with tunnels under the two ship channels at an estimated cost of $144,-000,000, a proposal approved by the Army Engineers in 1958. Plans were at once made for selling bonds to finance the construction, and the bond issue was successfully floated in the summer of 1960. By the following October the contractors were already at work.

Fundamentally, the fate of the Chesapeake Bay Tunnel, and, indeed, of all the other projects in the area, rested on the assumption that Norfolk would remain prosperous. That prosperity still depended, as it had for decades, on the Navy, and the Navy's operations

---

[11] *Norfolk*, July, 1957, pp. 9-19.
[12] *Virginian-Pilot*, Nov. 10, 1958.

in turn depended on the vagaries of international relations and the progress of military technology, which had already made the battleship as obsolete as the armored knight. Although the defense requirements of the cold war had kept the level of naval activities high at Norfolk, the Navy by 1960 was beginning to disperse its vessels to other bases to make them less vulnerable to H-bomb annihilation.

While Norfolk had no desire to lose the Navy—relations with the sailors, in fact, both collectively and individually, were better than they had ever been—the city was devoting a great deal of energy to broadening its economic base in order to provide greater stability. The most obvious source of new income for the city was through increasing civilian use of the splendid natural port of Hampton Roads, and for this purpose the Norfolk Port Authority was established by the city in 1948. Although Hampton Roads consistently led all North Atlantic ports in export tonnage, most of this tonnage was in coal and other bulk-loaded products, which brought relatively little revenue to the port; the port was low in either exports or imports of the more profitable general cargo. The new city authority devoted itself especially to building up general cargo by seeking ways in which shippers could profit by using Norfolk's port. Its primary job was to sell shippers on the advantages of Norfolk and, incidentally, to sell Norfolk on the advantages of shipping—in the words of its slogan, to "bring the world to Norfolk, and bring Norfolk to the world." It advertised Norfolk at home and abroad, published a monthly magazine, *World Trade,* and solicited trade from individual shippers.

The Norfolk Port Authority proved so valuable that it soon found itself acquiring new functions by a logical extension of the theory on which it was based. Since air travel was closely connected with commerce, it took over the operation of the Municipal Airport in 1950, along with the task of improving air service to the city. When the removal of Broad Creek Village made available 468 acres of land for industrial expansion, the city turned over to the Port Authority the responsibility for developing the site with new plants to increase the port's commerce. The first big project located there was a new $5,000,000 warehouse for Colonial Stores, opened early in 1960. The authority also brought in a new company, the General Mower Corporation, by constructing the necessary factory building on the site and leasing it to the Buffalo firm.[13]

[13] *Ibid.,* Dec. 13, 1959.

Norfolk's planned prosperity also received some help from the state, which in 1952 created the Virginia State Ports Authority. At first the state agency, like the city authority, concentrated on promoting the interests of the Hampton Roads ports, but an engineering survey convinced it that the facilities for handling general cargo would have to be improved in order to increase the ports' business. The engineers reported that there were fourteen general cargo terminals in the three Hampton Roads cities, but that most of the civilian business was handled by four of them, and only one of these met modern standards. All of these piers belonged to the railroads, which operated them at a loss and could not afford to build new facilities, which would serve highway trucks at the railroads' expense. It was therefore proposed that the state authority should purchase and improve these piers and then lease them back to the railroads to operate them.[14] Although the plan was introduced too late for full consideration by the 1958 General Assembly, the necessary legislation was enacted during the 1960 session.

Another example of co-operation for progress was the establishment in 1954 of the Tidewater Virginia Development Council under the leadership of Norfolk Mayor W. Fred Duckworth. It was a corporation supported by contributions from private enterprise and from all the local governments from Isle of Wight County to the Eastern Shore. By 1956 a full-time director, Clarence S. Osthagen, had been obtained, and a year later a full staff was at work promoting the interests of the area.[15]

Not all the changes in the Norfolk scene in the decade of the fifties could be considered progress. Romanticists at the beginning of the decade shed nostalgic tears for the passing of the Chesapeake and Ohio boat, which had ferried passengers from Newport News to the foot of Brooke Avenue for years but finally gave place to a prosaic bus. Railroad bugs felt even sadder at the decade's end when the Norfolk and Western began retiring its steam locomotives, which were among the last in the country. Another railroad passed out of existence at the end of 1959 when the Virginian merged with the Norfolk and Western in an economy measure. A year earlier another economy measure had caused the departure of the headquarters of the Seaboard Air Line from Norfolk to Richmond.

On the biggest change of the decade there was general agreement.

14 Richmond *Times-Dispatch*, Feb. 17, 1958.
15 *Norfolk*, Oct., 1956, pp. 6-8.

That was the incredible face-lifting carried out by the Norfolk Redevelopment and Housing Authority, involving the demolition of buildings on 465 acres of downtown land, an area more than nine times the size of the original town laid out by John Ferebee. The idea of ridding Norfolk of its slums had been proposed as far back as 1937, when a Citizens' Committee on Crime had pointed out the high social cost of slums and recommended a program to eliminate them, and in July, 1940, the Norfolk Housing Authority had been created for that purpose.[16] The wartime emergency, however, had forced the authority to concentrate on defense housing, and it was not until the war was over that it was able to return to its original goal. By that time new legislation had broadened its purpose beyond merely providing new homes for the poor to building a better city for all and had given it a new name, the Norfolk Redevelopment and Housing Authority.

The City Council showed its support of the new program in December, 1948, by appropriating $25,000 to the authority for planning a program of slum clearance. At the same time study was begun on a new minimum housing code to make slums illegal, as well as on a new zoning code to prevent future deterioration of property values. Thus, when the Federal Housing Act of 1949 went into effect, Norfolk was the first city in the country to complete its application for a loan and grant under the national redevelopment program. For this Lawrence M. Cox, executive director of the authority, was congratulated by N. S. Keith, head of the Federal agency. In March, 1950, Norfolk signed a contract for Federal assistance to provide three thousand new homes, and six months later came the necessary grant for acquiring property and demolishing dilapidated buildings.[17]

The area selected for the first project was bounded on the south by Brambleton Avenue, on the north by Broad Creek Road, on the east by Lincoln Street, and on the west by Monticello Avenue. It was a section of tumble-down, rat-infested houses, many without heat or sanitary provisions. It yielded little to the city in taxes, but it cost the city a great deal of money to maintain. The ramshackle wooden houses were a constant threat of fire; the hordes of rats made the area a breeding place of disease; the prevalence of crime demanded special policing. "There is no use fighting illness and distress with

16 Schlegel, *Conscripted City*, pp. 14-16.
17 *American City*, LXIV (May, 1949), 175; *The Norfolk Story*, 1948, pp. 6, 7, 16, 17; 1949-1950, [pp. 10-11].

health education, hospitals, public health nurses, clinics, and the like, if we permit the fever nests of bad housing to generate new foci of infection and spread these diseases more rapidly than we can deal with them," pointed out John M. Huff, Director of Public Health. "In a great many of our dwelling houses right here in Norfolk, we have a perfect set-up for a typhoid epidemic, a dysentery epidemic and perhaps others."[18]

The first step was to provide new homes for the more than two thousand families huddled on the eighty-acre tract. For this purpose substantial two-story brick buildings were erected elsewhere, at Chesterfield Heights, Campostella, and Ballentine Boulevard, as well as at Roberts Park, one of the authority's wartime projects. The tenants in the area scheduled for redevelopment were relocated so rapidly that demolition could begin on December 11, 1951.[19] Two years later the first families had started to move in, and early in 1954 the 752-unit development, named Young Park in honor of one of Norfolk's outstanding Negro citizens, was completed. Even before Young Park was finished, the authority had embarked on the second phase of its program by clearing a new forty-seven-acre site in the Holt Street area, north of City Hall Avenue. By the end of 1955, 626 more low-rent apartments had been erected there, and Tidewater Park, as the new development was called, was completely occupied. The third phase of the program, the construction of another 314 units north of Olney Road, ended what had by now become merely Project Number One.[20]

The net cost of this first phase was $5,699,702, of which only $1,899,901 came out of city taxes, the rest being contributions from the Federal government. For that sum a total of 190 acres of downtown Norfolk had been cleared of slums; about two-thirds of this was used for the new low-rent housing projects, along with the necessary public buildings, schools, playgrounds, fire and police stations. The authority had built 3,428 low-rent homes, in addition to 300 turned over to it by the Federal government, and was contributing over $200,000 every year from the income on these buildings to the city in lieu of taxes. The remaining third of the cleared land was used in part for widening streets and creating new boulevards, but most of it was set aside for resale to private enterprise for business purposes under

[18] *The Norfolk Story*, 1948, p. 17.
[19] *The Norfolk Story*, 1951, p. 11.
[20] *The Norfolk Story*, 1955, [p. 6].

controlled redevelopment.[21] As a site for new factories the authority turned over to the city the Norfolk Industrial Park, the 468-acre tract made available by the removal of Broad Creek Village, one of the demountable wartime housing projects, which lasted so long that its temporary buildings threatened to degenerate into new slums; not until 1955 were the first homes removed from the site.[22]

The disappearance of Broad Creek Village was a sign of the diminished need for low-rent housing, and the authority could now shift its emphasis to redevelopment as it launched Project Number Two. The 135 acres selected for the project lay in a run-down area in Atlantic City, where 64 per cent of the dwellings were substandard, according to a survey made by the authority. The 642 families living in the district were located elsewhere before the wrecking cranes arrived. Future housing in the area was to be of a more luxurious type—tall apartment buildings, located on spacious garden plots, overlooking the water; they would be constructed by private enterprise under controlled redevelopment. Project Number Two would also provide land for a new water-front expressway, but its central feature was the creation of a new Medical Arts Center around the Norfolk General Hospital.[23]

The first step was the expansion of the hospital itself under the direction of the hospital board. The original idea of adding a small building to take care of the institution's most pressing needs, as proposed in April, 1956, expanded so rapidly that by the time construction was finished late in 1958 the addition had become a $5,500,-000, nine-story structure with every modern improvement, and the hospital's capacity had grown from 217 to 475 beds.[24] Meanwhile, work had already been started on a Municipal Public Health Center near-by, intended to bring together the city Health Department, the various public clinics, and the public health agencies associated with the United Fund. Other buildings included in the Medical Arts Center were the King's Daughters' Hospital for children and a privately sponsored Medical Office Tower. Altogether, the center represented a new investment of $10,000,000, only a small part of which was furnished by Norfolk taxpayers, the rest coming from Federal grants, private contributions, and private enterprise.[25]

21 *Norfolk*, March, 1959, p. 18.
22 *The Norfolk Story*, 1955, [p. 6].
23 *Norfolk*, March, 1959, p. 18.
24 *Virginian-Pilot*, Sept. 14, 1958.
25 *Norfolk*, Sept. 1959, p. 8.

Work in the Atlantic City area had scarcely begun before the authority embarked on Project Number Three, the most ambitious program it had yet conceived. It called for a complete remodeling of 140 acres in the heart of downtown Norfolk, tearing down the honky-tonks and flophouses of East Main Street as well as all the shabby buildings north of it, all the way to Brambleton Avenue. The narrow old streets of earlier centuries were to give way to broad boulevards, and new tall office buildings would leave plenty of space for light and for parking.

This wide-sweeping plan had had its beginnings ironically in the need for a new city jail. When that need led to the idea of a new Civic Center, City Manager Thomas F. Maxwell in April, 1956, suggested to the City Council the desirability of an "over-all comprehensive master plan of the central business district." As a result, the council retained Charles K. Agle of Baltimore, who submitted a plan which was approved in 1956. The Redevelopment and Housing Authority then worked out the details of the program and submitted it for public approval in the spring of 1958. The estimated cost of the entire project was some $24,000,000, two-thirds of which would be covered by Federal grants.

There was inevitably some criticism of the plan, especially from the property-owners affected. The businessmen of East Main Street feared that their enterprises would be destroyed, until they were promised help in relocation. Concern was expressed for the six hundred families to be evacuated, since no housing was to be provided in the cleared area, but the authority promised to find new homes for them. Loss of tax revenue was feared, as only twenty acres were to be allocated to taxpaying buildings, and more than three-fourths of the entire area was to remain unbuilt upon.

On the whole, however, there was widespread approval of the project. The board of directors of the Norfolk Chamber of Commerce endorsed it and called on citizens and the City Council to "proceed to its fulfillment at an early date." The board pointed out that it would keep Norfolk "abreast of the nation's leading cities, which are at present making similar redevelopment plans." Mayor W. Fred Duckworth foresaw the city developing rapidly into the hub of a metropolitan area of a million people, partly through the foresight and energy of the Redevelopment and Housing Authority. Albert M. Cole, Administrator of the National Housing and Home Finance Agency, said that Norfolk had been "blessed with three advantages.

These are: imaginative citizens, imaginative officials, and an imaginative press." Richard L. Steiner, Commissioner of the Urban Renewal Administration, thought the Norfolk authority far in the lead of most other communities engaged in urban renewal. "Thanks to the example being set here," he said, "the entire national effort is being quickened."

A typical reaction of the ordinary citizen was expressed by one housewife, who wrote: "I think I can speak for hundreds of other Norfolk women. In recent years I have become so disgusted with the terrible parking and traffic situation in our downtown area that I simply don't go there to shop any more. On many occasions I simply do not buy at all rather than go downtown. If the people of Norfolk don't wake up and realize that the Norfolk Redevelopment and Housing Authority's Project Number 3 would clear up this mess, downtown Norfolk is going to dry up and die on the vine, because more and more people are coming to my way of thinking every day."

As a result of this general support, downtown redevelopment got under way at once. Demolition to clear the site for the new Civic Center began in July, 1958, with the destruction of the old National Hotel on East Main Street. As hundreds of citizens and a few visitors from other cities seated on temporary stands looked on, two giant cranes with a lift capacity of thirty-five tons each ripped into the side walls. Within seconds the walls came tumbling down, and this three-story building was reduced to rubble. It was symbolic of the passing of the old downtown Norfolk and the advent of the new.

As downtown redevelopment progressed gradually towards its goal of completion by 1963, the design of the new Norfolk became steadily more apparent. One by one the tattoo parlors and neon-lighted taprooms of East Main Street disappeared; even the venerable Gaiety, which had provided entertainment in the flesh for a whole generation of sailors, yielded to the redevelopers. East Main Street itself was to be closed to vehicles for the first time since John Ferebee laid it out in 1681, so that it could become a shady pedestrian mall leading to the new Civic Center, just west of the Berkley bridge. The first unit of the $15,000,000 center, the Public Safety Building, got under way in 1959. Farther north in the redevelopment area, across the street from the old courthouse, was to be located the new public library building.

Faith in the bright future envisioned for the city of Norfolk by the redevelopers was shown by private investors who put their capital into the project. Most prominent evidence of this faith was the new

$5,500,000 hotel, rising in 1960 on the "Golden Triangle," between Monticello Avenue and Bank Street, an area cleared during Project Number One and set aside by the authority for a new hotel. A $3,000,000 motel and apartment building was made possible in Ocean View when the City Council sold a municipally owned tract there.[26] On the edge of the redevelopment area private capital put up the $4,000,000 Rennert Building, occupying the site of the old city market on Monticello Avenue; in addition to stores and offices it included a ramp garage providing downtown parking for 650 cars. The structure was prepared to carry a central office tower, rising as high as seventeen stories, if further expansion proved desirable. Private enterprise was also engaged in rehabilitating run-down housing outside the cleared areas to bring it up to the standards set by the minimum housing code of 1951.

As 1959 ended, the news of the Norfolk enlightenment was attracting national attention. A well-known newsmagazine reported, under the title "Vision in Virginia": "The port city of Norfolk, Va., has been called many things in its frowsy past, most of them by sailors, and most of them unprintable. In the coming decade, even the sailors are certain to pipe a happier tune.

"By 1970, if not long before, the new Norfolk will throw an old salt off his bearings. Instead of the dingy slums and flophouses a sailor might remember, he will find a gleaming modern city of new homes and apartment houses, handsome public buildings, attractive shops, and broad new streets and thoroughfares."[27]

Another tribute Norfolk could appreciate came when its veteran rival, Richmond, sent a delegation to learn about urban renewal. The visitors, unprepared for such startling change, could scarcely believe their eyes. One editor summed up their feelings: "One may read of Norfolk's urban renewal projects and get a rough idea of the amazing size of the city's face-lifting undertaking. But the gigantic scope of this almost fantastic program is not fully realized until one visits that city and rides past block and block of rubble where once stood, for the most part, slum dwellings and shabby commercial buildings. . . .

"Richmonders who got a first-hand look at this massive renewal undertaking Wednesday were flabbergasted by the magnitude of Norfolk's physical transformation. . . .

[26] *Virginian-Pilot*, Oct. 21, 30, 1959.
[27] *Newsweek*, Dec. 14, 1959, p. 46.

"As amazing as all this is, some of the Richmonders were almost equally startled at the nigh-incredible word that this immense program has the unanimous backing of City Council and of virtually all the business community. . . .

"They "think big" in Virginia's biggest city."[28]

Early in 1960 Norfolk received the most significant recognition of its achievements. On February 4 Mayor Duckworth raised a blue-and-white flag, bearing the legend "All-America City," over City Hall. Norfolk was one of eleven cities in the United States to receive the award, granted jointly by *Look* Magazine and the National Municipal League. At a huge award luncheon held in the City Arena, *Look's* publisher, Vernon C. Myers, told the audience: "Out of a city whose problems had multiplied almost to the point of disaster, a city plagued by organized vice and disease, branded for its slums by housing authorities, choked by a population boom—out of this dismal picture of a community, Norfolk citizens are creating a city with a bright new character." In reply, Mayor Duckworth said that the award "will only be the starting point for making Norfolk a better place to live."[29]

[28] Richmond *Times-Dispatch*, Oct. 16, 1959.
[29] *Virginian-Pilot*, Feb. 5, March 4, 1960.

CHAPTER NINETEEN

Not By Bread Alone

The culture of a city may be expressed in various ways. One city may boast of its beautiful parks, another of its lovely buildings, another of its libraries, still another of a fine orchestra, or a museum of natural history, or its distinguished painters or writers or sculptors. Early Norfolk could boast of its public buildings—St. Paul's Church, the dignified old Courthouse, the Norfolk Academy, the Custom House. It could also boast of its famous poet, Father Ryan, and its famous sculptor, Alexander Galt. But it was only recently that public-spirited citizens and the city government awoke to the fact that it was their joint responsibility to give Norfolk a widened cultural life, to open new cultural opportunities to the citizens.

A major move in this direction was made in 1905, when the Leache-Wood Alumnae Association set itself the task of working toward an art museum for Norfolk. Twelve years later, when this group became the Norfolk Society of Arts, the same purpose was reiterated and emphasized, and they were greatly encouraged when the City Council granted them a site in the area known as Lee Park, facing the Hague.

Meanwhile the society's art collection, which was being kept in the Norfolk Public Library, was offered a temporary home of its own by a public-spirited citizen, Mrs. William Sloane. Mrs. Sloane lent the society a site on Mowbray Arch and financed the building herself. During World War I the society entertained servicemen there with dances, teas, and open house every night, members of the society acting as hostesses. After the war exhibits were held and the lecture course was resumed; there were poetry readings reminiscent of those given by Edgar Allan Poe a century earlier.

In 1920 the society appointed a music committee, which arranged many fine concerts, some by local artists, some by musicians from other cities. The Sunday concerts of the Wertz String Quartet of Baltimore in 1922 and for several seasons afterwards were especially enjoyed. It was in 1920 also that Mrs. Richard Tucker organized a dramatic club, which became a dramatic committee of the Norfolk Society of Arts. Seven years later, after presenting a number of successful plays, the committee developed into an independent body, the Little Theater.

The Poets' Corner, with Mrs. J. Jett McCormick as the first chairman, was organized in December, 1922. The weekly readings from the poetry and dramatic prose of the times attracted a large and interested group. Three years later permission was given to a number of girls who had formed what they called "The Art Corner" to hold their meetings in the Arts Building and to have exhibitions there. This group later expanded to include artists from the entire area under the name "Tidewater Artists."

The Society of Arts in the meantime renewed its efforts to find a permanent home to replace the temporary quarters on Mowbray Arch. In 1923 Mrs. Sloane took up the matter with the City Council, reminding it of the ordinance of 1917 authorizing a museum in Lee Park; the council confirmed the grant and fixed on a very desirable site facing the Hague. In July, 1924, the city agreed to appropriate $12,500 a year for the maintenance and operation of the museum, if the Society of Arts provided a building to cost not less than $125,000. The title to the building was to be vested in the city, but its custody in the society. Eighteen months later a board of trustees for the proposed museum was appointed, in part by the city and in part by the society.

The first step toward raising the necessary funds was taken in 1923, when the society decided to establish a building fund and voted to set aside a certain amount annually for that purpose. This was a slow process, however, and, in 1926, following the appointment of the board of trustees, Mrs. William Sloane became head of a committee to raise money to bring the museum into existence. The outlook was discouraging. There was no money, no buildings, no fine art or historical collection. But Mrs. Sloane was not discouraged. "If you want something hard enough, I think you get it," she said. "I think the people here are going to want it hard enough to get it." Some months later, when it was known that twenty-three persons or couples had subscribed $104,000, this prediction seemed fully sustained.[1]

Another seven years were to pass, however, before the building came into existence. The most serious difficulty was caused by the panic of 1929, which made it difficult for some of the subscribers to fulfil their pledges. At times construction came to a halt for lack of cash, and Mrs. Sloane had to go out and solicit additional funds before the work could continue.[2]

The building which was completed in 1933 was only part of the over-all project. The plans called for three units, which could be built separately, in Florentine Renaissance style, of tooled stone, concrete, and steel. The first unit, or south wing, contained the administrative quarters, three galleries, and the main stairway. The fact that the new Museum of Arts and Sciences was soon drawing an annual attendance of forty thousand inspired the men and women who had worked so long for it to turn their efforts to completion of the building. Their proposal that the city apply to the Federal Public Works Administration for a grant for that purpose, to be matched by the city, met strong opposition, however. One councilman said that he was not convinced that the museum reached the masses of Norfolk citizens. To this the editor of the *Virginian-Pilot* retorted that the way to spread the benefits of the museum was to provide it with the space and equipment needed to make it a fine arts addition to the city's system of public education.[3] After three years of uncertainty and the election of a new Council, the friends of the museum won. The Federal grant was accepted and matched by a loan, and work was begun on the second unit. Opened in October, 1939, this wing contained fifteen galleries, the library, the assembly hall, and the hall of statuary.

The museum has many notable collections—of rare books, plaster casts, oil paintings, carved ivories, statuary, old coins, and Chinese porcelain dating back to 206 B.C. Especially instructive are the hall of primitive peoples and the hall of natural history. A striking addition, placed at the entrance, is "The Torchbearers," a sculpture in aluminum, showing a falling runner passing the torch on to a man on horse-

---

[1] *Norfolk Museum Bulletin*, Vol. V, No. 3. The large donors were Fergus Reid, William Sloane, Mrs. Sloane, the three brothers, C. Wiley Grandy, W. B. S. Grandy, and Dr. C. R. Grandy, and Miss Caroline Selden.

[2] *Norfolk Museum Bulletin*, Vol. VII, No. 4.

[3] *Virginian-Pilot*, Aug. 1, 1938.

back, as a poetic concept of the progress of man. The museum has been used for numerous exhibitions, Sunday afternoon concerts, lectures on art and literature, and poetry readings.[4] J. D. Hatch, director of the museum until 1960, believed that it should encourage new art as well as preserve and explain the art of past ages. The museum programs were so arranged that art students might regard the masterpieces of other ages as inspiration for their own efforts. It is for this reason, also, that artists are trained by the museum in a series of art and music courses.[5] The Museum of Arts and Sciences took a major step to preserve Norfolk's architectural heritage when it acquired the famous old Myers House and had it restored. The home was refurnished and opened to the public. Of special interest is the kitchen, with its brick floors, its ladder-back chairs, and its old cooking utensils. Another major service to Norfolk was the commissioning of Kenneth Harris, a well-known local water-colorist, to paint a series of Norfolk scenes as a record of the city of 1950.[6]

Another important cultural institution which appeared in the years following the First World War was the first symphony orchestra between Baltimore and Atlanta. In August, 1920, a few devoted music lovers managed to assemble fifty willing and able musicians, and, after a winter of rehearsals, they put on their first concert on April 12, 1921, under the direction of Walter Edward Howe, a local church organist.

One of the leading spirits in founding the Civic Symphony Orchestra, as the group was then known, was Mrs. Marian Carpenter Miles, who had been trained for a concert career by some of the best teachers in America and Germany. So great was her love of music that she expected her guests to bring along to her home whatever instruments they played, no matter how badly, and, whatever the ensemble turned out to be, she would produce a musical score to fit it. Until age forced her retirement, Mrs. Miles served as concertmaster for the symphony and wrote all of the program notes.

Not less important in founding the orchestra was Dr. R. C. Whitehead. His profession was medicine, his passion music. He played a small violoncello, which he referred to as his "late American cigarbox" and lent generously to anyone who wanted to learn how to play it. When viola players were needed, Dr. Whitehead laid aside his

[4] *Civic Affairs*, 1940, pp. 126-128.
[5] *The Norfolk Story*, 1951.
[6] *Virginian-Pilot*, Jan. 20, 1931; *The Norfolk Story*, 1951, pp. 14-15.

cello and took up the viola instead; later he shifted from strings to woodwinds when there was no one else to play the bassoon. As one of the younger members of the orchestra recalled him, "He was business manager, librarian, and janitor for that young orchestra— and he loved every minute of it."[7]

In those early days the symphony led a precarious financial existence. At first Whitehead and the dignified J. A. P. Mottu stood outside the door with collection plates, soliciting a silver offering; later a fifty-cent admission fee became standard. The inevitable deficits were made up by a host of generous music lovers. Conductors departed with alarming frequency, although Frank L. Delpino, a former Navy bandmaster, lasted through most of the 1930's.

It was in the years following the Second World War that the Norfolk Symphony Orchestra, playing in the war-born Municipal Auditorium, reached musical maturity. After the tragic death at thirty-eight of its new conductor, Henry Cowles Whitehead, son of "Doctor Bob," the orchestra found his successor in Edgar Schenkman. A graduate of the Juilliard School of Music, Schenkman had had years of experience in conducting both opera and orchestra before coming to Norfolk in 1948. He also took over the direction of the Norfolk Civic Chorus, which merged its organization with the symphony in 1949 and thus made possible a series of memorable joint concerts. Under Schenkman's leadership the orchestra was converted from a group of amateurs, giving only three concerts a year, to a semi-professional organization of seventy-five, giving annually seven subscription concerts, three children's concerts, and a special performance for Navy personnel. In addition to the children's concerts, it played an important part in the musical education of the young people of Norfolk by sponsoring a youth orchestra through its Women's Auxiliary.[8]

The performance of the orchestra soon won it wide recognition. In 1949 it was invited to Charlottesville to participate in the Virginia Music Festival, and the following year Schenkman was made musical director of the festival. A few years later, when Richmond at last decided to have an orchestra of its own, it borrowed Schenkman to serve as its first conductor. In addition to its concerts at the University of Virginia, the orchestra also played at Mary Washington and at

[7] S. H. Ferebee, "Finger in the Pie, A History of Norfolk's Symphony," *Norfolk*, Oct., 1954, p. 6.
[8] *Ibid.*

Longwood College. Its most important out-of-town performance was at the opening of the Jamestown Festival in 1957. In Phi Beta Kappa Hall at Williamsburg the orchestra and chorus gave the world premiere of Randall Thompson's musical setting of Michael Drayton's "Ode to the Virginian Voyage." Paul Hume, nationally known music critic, said of the performance: "Conductor Schenkman has a large amount of real genius in his handling of both orchestra and chorus."[9]

At the final concert of Schenkman's tenth season as conductor the orchestra showed its appreciation by presenting him with an engrossed award. Of even greater significance was the audience's reaction to the performance of Bach's "Passion according to St. John" on this occasion. A Richmond music critic reported that "the musicians' devoted performance and the audience's standing tribute bore out the deep love and respect their musical leader commands. The memorable discipline and the moving expressiveness of the performance seem to summarize Schenkman's contribution of ten years."[10]

The musical life of Norfolk was invigorated by two new organizations during the postwar years. One was the creation of I. E. Feldman, a former Navy bandmaster, who opened a music studio in Norfolk after the First World War. In 1946 he formed the Feldman Chamber Music Society, which gave an annual series of concerts and had won more than four hundred subscribers by 1959.[11] The other institution was the William and Mary Opera Workshop, established in 1949 by the Norfolk Division of the College.[12]

The theater continued to flourish in Norfolk. In addition to the professional productions in the Municipal Auditorium, the Little Theater put on several plays every year and launched in 1959 an experimental workshop to turn out drama off the beaten track. Another drama group, the Little Creek Players, was made up of members of the armed forces and their families. The city also helped to sponsor an outdoor drama, Paul Green's *The Confederacy*, which was performed at Virginia Beach during 1958 and 1959.

In the art form most popular in Virginia, Norfolk was pre-eminent, largely owing to the enterprise of Frederic Heutte, superintendent of parks and forestry, who turned Norfolk into a city of flowers. Under his guidance Lafayette Park, overlooking Lafayette River, was given new beauty. Making use of WPA labor, he attacked the salt marshes

[9] Washington *Post and Times-Herald*, April 2, 1957.
[10] Richmond *Times-Dispatch*, April 20, 1958.
[11] *Virginian-Pilot*, May 17, 1954.
[12] *Ibid.*, Jan. 4, 1959.

which partially surrounded the park and eliminated this dismal eyesore, at the same time adding twelve fertile acres to the park. On these he planted in a single year over five thousand trees and shrubs, developed a holly garden, and increased the botanical collection by a hundred new varieties. The formal garden, with its thousand hyacinths and five thousand tulips from Holland, its many lovely roses, azaleas, and camellias, attracted thousands of visitors. In 1958 Superintendent Heutte even made Granby Street blossom. With contributions from downtown merchants he was able to set up five hundred flower boxes along the street in the business area.

Heutte's greatest glory, however, was the conception and perfection of an azalea garden which rivaled the famous gardens of the South Carolina low country. A favorable setting was found near the Municipal Airport, amid tall pines, wax myrtle, sweet bay, dogwood, holly, and cypress. The next step was to get the Works Progress Administration to help finance the project and then to put scores of Negro women to work. Within a few months sixty acres had been cleared, rustic fences built, three miles of trail laid out, bridges thrown over little streams, six thousand azaleas and other plants put out. Although the mass of azaleas fixes the character of the garden, Japanese iris, crape myrtle, holly, camellias, and other plants make this a spot of year-round beauty.

In 1947 many additional acres were cleared and planted with azaleas, thousands of rhododendrons, camellias, and daffodils, and several additional miles of trails were cut through the woods. The loblolly pines act as big brothers to the azaleas, for their needles feed the soil which nourishes the flowers. The thousands of picknickers who open their baskets at the rustic tables enjoy the light which is filtered through the trees. They give their hearty approval of the citation of Superintendent Heutte in 1950 by the League of Virginia Municipalities for work in beautifying Norfolk which perhaps will never be erased. Richmond paid its sister city the flattery of imitation in 1952 when it obtained five thousand cuttings from Norfolk to start an azalea garden of its own.

The International Azalea Court in which some girl is crowned queen has become an annual event attracting thousands. In April, 1958, when Miss Patricia Jane LeMay, daughter of Air Force General Curtis LeMay, was escorted across the gold bridge over the pool to the throne, she was greeted with applause from a record crowd of four thousand. The pink gowns of the maids of honor, the mass of azalea blossoms of the queen's dress, and the white uniforms of the midshipmen of the Naval Academy, who formed the escort, made a colorful scene. General LeMay, after placing the crown on his daughter's head, kissed her on both cheeks. There were addresses of welcome by Henry Clay Hofheimer II, president of the Norfolk Chamber of Commerce, and Mayor W. Fred Duckworth.

The side of Norfolk's cultural development which was most neglected was represented by its public library. The building, erected in 1903 with a Carnegie grant, had for years been entirely too small to serve the needs of the expanded city, even though part of the library's collection was dispersed in seven branches. A survey made in 1940 revealed that the branch libraries themselves were overcrowded and understaffed, but nothing was done to improve the situation for more than ten years after the Second World War had ended. In 1956 the Friends of the Norfolk Public Library formed to mobilize public support for a new library, and two years later the impetus for action came in the offer of $100,000 from the Munro Black Fund of the Norfolk Foundation for a new building, provided it were started within three years. When a delegation from the Junior Chamber of Commerce on May 20, 1958, asked the City Council to survey Norfolk's library needs, the council agreed and requested the Public Library Board to suggest the necessary experts.[13]

In August the two recommended experts, Russell Munn, of the Akron Public Library, and Keith Doms, of the Carnegie Library of Pittsburgh, arrived in Norfolk on their first visit to the city. They were enthusiastic about everything they saw in Norfolk—except the library they had come to study. The report they submitted in November declared: "With respect to library service, Norfolk is one of the most under-privileged cities in the United States. . . . based on per capita figures of books owned, books loaned, and dollars spent, Norfolk has about one-third of a library system compared with other cities in its population group. We assume that she wants to correct this situation. The rest of this report is pointed in that direction."[14]

Their report presented a formidable challenge to the city. They proposed capital improvements costing more than $2,500,000 and an annual operating budget of nearly half a million dollars, a figure, they pointed out, which would be only $1.66 per capita, less than the $1.89 per capita average of cities in the same population class. The

13 *Ibid.*, Aug. 18, 1958.
14 *Ibid.*, Nov. 21, 1958.

city was to move three branch libraries to more satisfactory sites and to add three new branches to serve the sections developed in recent years. Most important was the new main library, which the experts urged should be located in the downtown area, where it would be readily accessible to shoppers.[15]

Although the City Council, already deeply involved in the expensive downtown redevelopment program, could not see where the necessary millions were coming from, it authorized the library board to start to work on plans. Then the generous half-million dollar gift of Miss Bessie Kirn made it possible to begin construction in 1960. The site chosen for the modernistic building, the southwest corner of City Hall Avenue and Bank Street, would give Norfolk one of the finest main library locations in the country, City Librarian Arthur M. Kirkby said. Meanwhile, a new branch library was being constructed in Ocean View in the city-owned triangle at the head of Granby Street; in memory of the city librarian from 1917 to 1947, who died in 1959, it was named the Mary Denson Pretlow Branch Library.[16]

Even if Norfolk had lagged behind in developing its library facilities, it could boast that it had created in the field of higher education two four-year degree-granting colleges, the Norfolk Division of the College of William and Mary and the Norfolk Division of Virginia State College, both of them with larger enrollments than their parent institutions. The Negro school had its beginnings in 1935, when a few Norfolk citizens arranged to have Virginia Union University in Richmond offer the first courses at the college level for Negroes. Two rooms at the Hunton Branch YMCA were the only campus the infant institution had, and enrollment was small at first. It received its first public support in 1942, when it became the Norfolk Polytechnic Institute and qualified for aid from the city. Two years later it was taken over by the state and placed under the administration of Virginia State College. With state support it grew rapidly and by 1960 had an enrollment of eighteen hundred in modern buildings on a new campus on Corprew Avenue.[17]

The white school developed from extension courses offered in Norfolk by the College of William and Mary as early as 1919. Ten years later enrollment in these classes had risen to 340, and civic groups asked that a full-time collegiate center be established in the

15 *Ibid.*, Nov. 20, 1958.
16 *Ibid.*, March 9, 1960.
17 *Ibid.*, Dec. 20, 1959.

city.[18] The Norfolk City Council and the school board took a major step in deeding to the college the old Larchmont School building. During the summer of 1930 the building was remodeled to fit it for college purposes, and scientific laboratories were constructed. A capable faculty was engaged, and additional land was purchased for future expansion. In September Norfolk Division opened with 160 students.[19]

The new college grew rapidly. During its second year total enrollment mounted to 455, including 81 registered in the engineering classes sponsored by Virginia Polytechnic Institute. In response to increased demand new programs were added, among them business administration and secretarial science. Although financial aid was hard to come by in the depression years, grants from the Public Works Administration, along with bonds sold by the college, made possible the erection of a new classroom-gymnasium building and a stadium with a seating capacity of 25,000, both completed in 1936.[20] Foreman Field, as the stadium was called, was to be the scene of many exciting football contests, even though Norfolk Division itself abandoned the sport.

Enrollment continued to expand, and the flood of returning veterans, seeking education under the GI Bill of Rights, filled the school to the overflowing point; in fact, from 1946 to 1948, the College of William and Mary was forced to operate a temporary institution, the St. Helena Extension, in the Berkley section of the Navy Yard. The opening of the new Academic Building in 1948, however, provided room for the overflow, and generous state support took care of further expansion. A Science Building was added in 1955, a new and modern library in 1959, and a Fine Arts Building was completed in 1960.

As the number of students mounted steadily to the five thousand mark, the college prepared to stand on its own feet. The first step was permission granted by the parent institution to offer a full four-year program for the first time; the first bachelor's degrees were granted on June 6, 1956, to a graduating class of fifteen students, a number which multiplied each year. Legislation enacted in 1960 set the stage for the Norfolk Division to be accredited independently of

[18] Robert C. McClelland, "Historical Notes on the College and the Community (Revised Issue)," *College of William and Mary in Norfolk General Publications Series*, July, 1955, p. 1.
[19] *Virginian-Pilot*, Jan. 1, 1931.
[20] McClelland, "Historical Notes . . . ," p. 2.

Williamsburg and authorized a new administrative organization to give it equal rank with the mother institution in the William and Mary system. Mayor Duckworth was added to the enlarged board of visitors, and the Norfolk Division began looking for a new name more appropriate to its new status.

The public school system of Norfolk in 1960 was also looking forward to a new era of growth and development after recovering from the severest crisis in its history. The crisis was not of Norfolk's own making, for it originated in decisions made in Washington and Richmond, and Norfolk was faced with the impossibility of obeying conflicting orders. When the historic Supreme Court decision that legally enforced segregation in the public schools was a violation of the Fourteenth Amendment was made final in 1955, the Norfolk School Board announced its intention to abide by the laws of the land. Steps towards desegregation, however, were prohibited by Virginia's "massive resistance" laws of 1956.

Since state law required the closing of any school in which the races were mixed, the school board did its best to postpone the day of reckoning. In endeavoring to comply with a Federal court order issued during the 1956-1957 school year the board adopted an assignment plan. Under that plan 151 Negro children applied for transfer to white schools in the fall of 1958. When the school board in August, 1958, denied all these applications, certain of the Negro students took their case to court, and as a result of the proceedings before U. S. District Judge Walter E. Hoffman it was necessary for the board to report to the court that it would assign seventeen of these Negro children to six white junior and senior high schools. The board re-quested of Judge Hoffman a year's delay in putting such assignments into effect, but the request was denied. Although the decision of the District Court was appealed to the Fourth Circuit Court of Appeals, the Circuit Court upheld the lower court's decision on September 27. At six o'clock that night the school board reluctantly assigned the seventeen Negro children to the white schools beginning Monday, September 29, the date to which the opening of school had been postponed. A few minutes later Governor J. Lindsay Almond, Jr., issued a proclamation taking over the affected schools, and on Monday morning ten thousand Norfolk high school students found the school doors closed to them.[21]

The closing of the high schools found the city sharply divided on

[21] *Virginian-Pilot,* Aug. 20, Sept. 28, 1959.

the proper course to follow. On one side stood those who, opposed as they might be to integration, wanted the schools reopened as soon as possible, even on an integrated basis; on the other were those who preferred segregated private schools to public schools with any degree of integration. The staunchest supporters of public education were the school board and the school teachers, while the Defenders of State Sovereignty and Individual Liberties gave strong backing to the "massive resistance" policy. The Defenders took the lead in organizing the Tidewater Educational Foundation to set up private schools for the displaced pupils but failed to win the co-operation of the idled teachers, who regarded the Foundation as an attempt to undermine support for public education.

The passive resistance of the teachers proved equal to the pressures of massive resistance. Partly as a result of private advice from many of the teachers, only one-fourth of the locked-out students enrolled with the TEF, and even these could not be taught. The TEF had hoped to get the free services of the public school teachers, who were still receiving their salaries from the state. When Colonel James G. Martin, IV, TEF president, appeared before the Norfolk Education Association on October 3 and asked for volunteers, however, he was met with stony silence; only one of the 450 teachers in the closed schools agreed to work for the TEF.

Much as the educators were opposed to any plan for replacing the public schools, they could not stand idly by and let their students go untaught. Many had already joined tutoring groups started before the closing order was issued, and these groups now sprang up all over the city, meeting in Sunday school rooms or parlors; about four thousand of the locked-out pupils received some instruction in this manner. The First Methodist Church organized a school to take care of three hundred in its building. The TEF recruited a dozen teachers from outside the public school system and enrolled 270 students in its classes. South Norfolk came to the rescue by setting up a night school in its high school, providing education for another nine hundred. Other students squeezed into public schools in near-by communities or moved in with relatives in other towns or other states; some sixteen hundred transfers to other schools were recorded. About one-fourth of the exiled students received no education at all; they got married, joined the Army, went to work, or simply stood on street corners. The one survival of the public high schools was the football team. The ghost schools played a full schedule, complete with bands and cheer leaders; the only noticeable difference was the absence of the band uniforms, locked up inside the closed schools.

The plight of the idled students brought Norfolk almost as much national attention as in that harrowing summer of 1942 when the war boom exploded. Norfolk was not the only city affected by the crisis—high schools were also closed in Charlottesville, Warren County, and Little Rock—but its ten thousand students far outnumbered those kept out of the other empty high schools; moreover, many of them were children of Navy families, who took their complaints to Washington. A team of *Life* photographers descended on Norfolk to tell the story of "The Lost Class of 1959." They found a wide range of reaction among the students they interviewed from a group of Norview High boys displaying signs reading, "Nigger Hunting by Permission Only," to the emphatic comment of Brenda Lee Smith, Maury student council member: "I don't care if I'm the only white girl in a whole school of Negroes. I don't care if they're pink or yellow or whatever. I just want to go to school."[22] Out-of-town reporters arrived in numbers to cover the story, and Edward R. Murrow came to film an hour-long television feature for CBS, broadcast on January 21, 1959.

Meanwhile, the fight to reopen the high schools was going on on many different fronts. The Norfolk School Board asked the governor to reopen the schools, even with integration, and the governor replied that he could not do so under state law. The City Council asked the governor to reopen the schools on a segregated basis, and he replied that he could not do that under Federal law. A Norfolk Committee for Public Schools soon numbered several thousand members, but they were admittedly amateurs in politics and seemed to represent no real political strength. When the City Council was asked to request the governor to return the schools to the city for local operation without state support, Mayor Duckworth replied that it would cost the city $2,500,000 a year extra to do this. To get an accurate picture of public opinion, the Council called for a referendum on November 18, 1958. By a predicted 3-2 margin, the voters rejected the idea of returning the schools to local operation, although critics declared that the ballot was "loaded" with a statement that tuition would be charged if the schools were reopened.

With this apparent mandate, the Council set to work on its own

22 *Life*, Nov. 3, 1958, pp. 21-27.

"little massive resistance program." Shortly after the referendum it
adopted a policy of tentatively appropriating school funds and,
beginning January 1, 1959, of making available to the school board
during any one month only so much of such funds as was necessary
for that month's operations, thus retaining control over the city funds
with which the schools were operated and enabling the Council to
close other schools if it became necessary. When Councilman L. L.
Layton at a Council meeting on December 9 made a plea to the
seventeen Negro children to withdraw their application to attend
the white schools, his concluding remarks caused speculation that the
Council intended to close the Negro high schools unless the Negro
applications were withdrawn within the week.[23] Councilman Layton,
however, made clear that this was not intended as an ultimatum,
and the Council decided not to put its plan into effect until the end
of the first semester. It ordained that, beginning February 1, 1959, it
did not propose to make any part of the school funds tentatively
appropriated available to the school board for the operation of any
grade above the sixth.

Before that time could come, however, a series of legal decisions
had made the Council's action unnecessary. Immediately after the
school closing a group of Norfolk parents had asked the Federal
District Court for an injunction ordering the schools reopened. About
the same time Governor Almond had arranged for a suit in the
Virginia Supreme Court of Appeals to test the constitutionality of the
massive resistance laws, and the Federal court waited for the state
court to act before issuing its own ruling. Decision day was January
19, 1959. On that date the State Supreme Court ruled that the massive resistance acts violated the state constitution, and, as soon as the
news reached Norfolk, a special three-judge Federal court ruled that
the state laws violated the U. S. Constitution.[24]

The fight was not quite over. A suit asking for an injunction
against the City Council and the school board to prevent the Council
from putting into effect its proposal to deny funds for the operation
of any high schools had already been filed by a group of Norfolk
parents, and a decision in that case was not handed down until
Tuesday, January 27. That morning a sign of shifting opinion appeared with the publication of "A Public Petition to the Norfolk
City Council," urging the Council to open the schools as soon as

23 *Virginian-Pilot*, Nov. 26, Dec. 10, 1958.
24 New York *Times*, Jan. 20, 1959.

possible. The petition was signed by one hundred prominent businessmen and civic leaders, the first time so many well-known persons had
taken a public stand on the question. Nevertheless, the Council
decided to exhaust its legal defenses so that it could not be accused
of surrendering without a fight. Its attorneys defended it before
District Judge Hoffman, and, when Judge Hoffman granted an injunction against the Council, it appealed the case to the Fourth
Circuit Court of Appeals, which affirmed Judge Hoffman, and then
it applied to the Supreme Court of the United States for a writ of
certiorari, which was denied.[25]

The Council, however, did not ask for a stay of execution, which
might have permitted closing all the high schools at week's end.
Instead the Council announced its willingness to co-operate in opening
all the schools for the beginning of the second semester the following
week. It made clear its position in a statement: "The Council, pur-
suant to the expressed will of the majority of the people whom it
represents, has endeavored to stand against what it considers to be an
abridgment of constitutional rights guaranteed to it and the citizens
of Norfolk. The action of the United States District Court, unless
reversed on appeal, prevents the Council from doing what it deems
to be in the best interests of the City, but, pending the outcome of
the appeal which will be taken, the Council must abide by the order
of the District Court.

"We appeal to every segment of our community to conduct itself
in the same peaceful and law-abiding manner that has been one of the
commendable aspects of this trying time.

"It is our duty and desire to advise every one that no violence or
other unlawful action will be tolerated or condoned. The City's law
enforcement agencies have been alerted to preserve and protect the
property, peace and safety of the City and all of its inhabitants.

"We earnestly and sincerely request the full cooperation of all our
people to this end."[26]

On Monday, February 2, 1959, a crowd of reporters assembled to
watch the first Negro children in Virginia enter a white school. To
their surprise no policemen were visible, for City Manager Thomas F.
Maxwell had such faith in the law-abiding nature of the people of
Norfolk that he kept every uniform out of sight. The white students

[25] *Virginian-Pilot*, Jan. 27, 28, 1959; Letter of Leonard H. Davis to T. F. Maxwell,
Oct. 25, 1960.
[26] *Virginian-Pilot*, Jan. 29, 1959.

Norfolk: Historic Southern Port

themselves were determined that nothing should happen which might close their schools again, and there were no incidents. Most of the locked-out students returned, and the schools operated on a nearly normal basis. When commencement time rolled around in June, more than half the "Lost Class of 1959" was still lost; of the 1,037 seniors who had registered in September at the three city high schools, only 455 were on hand to receive their diplomas at the end of the year. How did it feel to be a member of the Lost Class of 1959? a Maury senior was asked. "That's silly," he replied. "We aren't lost; we know where we're going."[27]

Although the schools were open again, ill feeling created by the crisis still rankled. It was reported that the Council felt the school board had defied the will of the people by its failure to co-operate with the private school movement and that the board should be made more responsive to public opinion. In April, 1959, the Council asked the General Assembly, then in special session, to revise the state law by increasing the size of the school board from six to seven members and shortening their term from three years to two.[28] Under this provision the Council in July named three new members to the board, two of them replacing persons whose terms had expired. Instead of the expected fireworks, however, the new members joined the old in unanimously re-electing as chairman Paul Schweitzer, who had furnished the leadership in defending the public schools.[29]

Meanwhile, the ghost of massive resistance was being quietly laid to rest in the Democratic primary for new elections to the General Assembly. The city's representatives in the assembly had supported Governor Almond's program for acceptance of token integration in the special session and had thus become the target for sharp criticism by the local Defenders. In the race for Norfolk's six seats in the House of Delegates, the Democratic organization endorsed the four incumbents who chose to stand for re-election with their record in favor of public schools, along with two new candidates who attempted to maintain a neutral position. The Defenders put up three men on a massive resistance platform, while two independents ran as enthusiastic supporters of public education. When the primary was held on July 14, 1959, the six nominations went to the six supporters of public schools by a substantial margin. With this demonstration

[27] *Ibid.*, June 7, 1959.
[28] *Ibid.*, April 10, 1959.
[29] *Ibid.*, July 12, 1959.

that public schools were no longer an issue, the Council moved to heal the breach with the school board. Early in 1960 the vacancy on the Council created by the resignation of George R. Abbott was filled by the appointment of none other than school board chairman Paul Schweitzer, erstwhile target of Council criticism. As he was elected by unanimous vote of the City Council, Vice Mayor N. B. Etheridge said, "I hope this clarifies that this council wants the best education money can buy."[30]

At this juncture, when Norfolk stood solidly committed to public education, it was fitting that national recognition in the form of a Pulitzer prize should come to the man who had done as much as anyone to bring about that stand. This was the second time the Pulitzer prize for distinguished editorial writing had come to Norfolk; the first award was made in 1929 to Louis I. Jaffé, editor of the *Virginian-Pilot,* for his 1928 editorials leading to the enactment of a state anti-lynching law. The award in 1960, again for editorials on an issue with racial overtones, went to the man who had succeeded Jaffé ten years earlier, Lenoir Chambers. At a time when it was regarded almost as treason to utter public criticism of the state's massive resistance laws, Chambers' voice had sounded openly and boldly in favor of reopening the public schools, and his editorials through 1959, the crucial year of transition, had helped to guide his city to its firm decision in favor of public education.

The attitude of Editor Chambers, which had become the attitude of the city of Norfolk, was well summed up in the concluding words of his final editorial for 1959, "The Year Virginia Opened the Schools":

"More intelligent handling of problems of great difficulty will continue and increase only if common-sense and courage continue to direct the course of both political leadership and public opinion. The struggles for reasonable solutions are not over. The state may see setbacks of various proportions. It is certain to encounter perplexities not easy to resolve. It may discover demagogues entranced with the thought of exploiting honest doubts and uncertainties as well as old prejudices. It needs sensible cooperation from its Negro citizenship. It needs every ounce of good will it can find from any source.

"But the old years of impracticality, unconstitutionalism, and futility are on the way out. If Virginia can produce more willingness to face the facts and fresh qualities of initiative and leadership in

[30] *Ibid.,* Feb. 18, 1960.

dealing with them, the year the state opened the schools can lead to a New Year of hope."[31]

Standing at the beginning of the 1960's, Norfolk with leadership like this was looking forward, not merely to a New Year, but to a whole new decade, full of hope and confidence in the future.

[31] *Ibid.*, Dec. 31, 1959.

Index

Abbott, George R., 393
Abigail, 90
Abingdon, 175
Abyvon, Mayor, 20
Academy, Norfolk, 92, 132, 137-141, 143, 193, 255-256, 294, 353, 377; Plate VII
Academy of Music, 258, 263-264, 296
Academy Square, 140
Accomac, 226
Accomack County, 331
Acropolis, 119
Adam, 117
Adam and Eve, 81, 123
Adams, John, 90, 91
Adams, John Quincy, 150, 151
Adeona, 87
Admiral Taussig Boulevard, 350, 358
Admiralty, British, 76
Africa, colonizing Negroes in, 127
Agatha, 46
Agle, Charles K., 373
Aid Fire Company, 253
Air raid defense, 354-355
Airplane, first, 291
Aitchinson, Mr., 68
Akron Public Library, 384
Alabama, 176, 229, 260
Alabama, 347, 359
Albemarle, 284
Albemarle cavalry, 111
Albemarle County, N. C., 34
Albemarle County, Va., 83
Albemarle and Chesapeake canal, 185-186, 229, 271, 275
Albemarle and Pantego Railroad, 278
Albemarle Sound, 30-33, 41, 88, 91, 113, 114, 158, 160-163, 167, 185, 210, 211, 216
Albert, 314
Alexander, 87
Alexandria, 44, 79, 82, 158, 176, 184, 222
Alexandria convention, 232, 233
Alexis, Grand Duke, 263, 269
Alfriend, John S., 365
Algeciras, 108
All-America City award, 276
Alleghenies, 178
Allen, William H., and Co., 250
Allen Line, 284

Almond, J. Lindsay, Jr., 387, 390, 392
Alsace, 311
Amelia Island, 108
American Chain Company, 310
American Cousin, The, 262
American Legion, 336
American Legion Auxiliary, 354
American Mercury, 352
Ames and Stevens building, 258
Amherst County, 83
Amsterdam, 109
Anacostian Boat Club, 266
Anderson, Isaac, 93
Andlauer, General, 312
Andrews, Annie M., 193
Andros, Governor Edmund, 36
Anna-Maria, 103
Annapolis Convention, 79
Ann-Elizabeth, 98
Annexation, 261, 323, 362-366
Anniston, Ala., 302
Antelope, 188
Anthony, John, 39
Antifederalists, 78, 79
Antigua, 35, 37, 38, 44-46, 77, 84, 85, 87, 95, 107, 146, 151, 152
Apartment houses, 291-292
Appomattox, surrender at, 232
Appomattox River, 83, 167, 168, 176, 181, 277
Arbuthnot, Admiral, 72
Archer, Edward, 92
Architectural Forum, 352, 353
Argentina, 304, 326
Argonne-Meuse offensive, 312-317
Argus, The Southern, 124, 133, 140, 142, 176, 178, 179, 182, 199, 202, 203
Armistead, Thomas, 87
Armistead, W. A., 92
Armistice, 316
Armstrong, Dr. George D., 193-194, 196-197, 226
Army Base, 306, 321-323, 330
Army Engineers, 367
Army of the Potomac, 213
Arnold, Benedict, 72
Arras, 314
Art Corner, 378
Articles of Confederation, 77, 80

Arts, Norfolk Society of, 264
Arts Building, 377-378
Arundel, 22
Asbury, Francis, 136
Ashburner, Charles E., 319-323
Ashland Hall, 184, 199-204
Assembly, Virginia General, 4, 8, 11, 13, 24, 33, 48, 53, 77, 78, 136, 138, 296, 369, 392
Association of Commerce, 336
Athens, 140
Atlanta, 326, 380
Atlantic, Mississippi, and Ohio Railroad, 272-273, 276; station, 261; *see also* Norfolk and Western Railroad
Atlantic and Danville Railroad, 279, 280
Atlantic and North Carolina Railroad, 274
Atlantic Artillery, 229
Atlantic City, 260, 261, 288, 289, 372, 373
Atlantic Coast Line, 278, 279
Atlantic Hotel, 132, 207, 219, 243, 248, 258, 266, 267, 292, 297
Atlantic Ocean, 30, 32, 37, 38, 40, 354
Atlantic Street, 293, 341
Auditorium, Municipal, 350-351, 358, 381, 382
Augusta, Ga., 120
Austin, Stephen and Moses, 83
Australia, 326
Austria, 344
Automobiles, first, 290-291
Avon Theater, 118-119, 132
Azalea garden, 342, 345, 383

Bacca, 39
Bach, Johann Sebastian, 382
Bachelor's Mill, 56
Back Creek, 4, 15, 92, 131-132, 195, 292, 293; filled in, 251-252
Back Street, 5
Bainbridge, Commodore, 125
Baker, J. C., 266
Baker, Newton D., Secretary of War, 321
Baldwin, Colonel J. P., 271
Balfour, Dr., 188
Balfour and Barraud, 46
Ballance, Samuel, 34
Ballentine Boulevard, 371
Baltimore, 91, 114, 153, 158, 161-163, 165, 166, 168, 169, 172, 176-178, 180, 182, 192, 193, 195, 215, 223, 234, 266, 273, 274, 276, 281, 284, 285, 291, 299, 300, 326, 378, 380; Democratic convention in, 201
Baltimore and Ohio Railroad, 166, 176, 177
Baltimore Mail Steamship Line, 330
Baltimore Steam Packet Company, 179-180

Bandy, 121
Banking crisis, 333-334
Bank of Commerce, 258, 293, 294
Bank Street, 118, 129, 132, 137, 251, 287, 288, 375, 385
Banner of the South, The, 120
Baptist Church, 137, 144, 241
Barbados, 35-37, 39, 84, 147, 277
Barcelona, 277
Barrington, Governor, 34, 35
Barron, Commodore James, 100-101, 124-125
Barry, C. Moran, 331
Barry Brothers, 284
Barry's Row, 192
Baseball, 265-266
Bay View School, 351
Bayne, Thomas, 235-237, 239-244
Beacher, J. J., 337
Beacon, The American, 130, 131, 141, 150, 155, 181
Beardsley's, 248
Beaufort, N. C., 114, 161, 274
Beaufort, 213, 214
Beaumont, 316
Belfast, 277
Belgium, German invasion of, 300
Bell, John, 201-202
Bell Church, 137
Belle Isle, 314
Bellinger, Mrs. P. N. L., 359
Bellona, 102
Belt Line, Norfolk and Portsmouth, 280-281, 306
Ben Franklin, 191
Benmoreell, 348
Benson, C. C., police chief, 254
Beraule, Mr., 138
Berea Church, Great Bridge, 238
Berkeley, Admiral, 103
Berkley, 103, 278, 279
Berkley bridge, 366, 367, 374; approach, Plate XVII
Berkley School, 340
Bermuda, 110, 145, 148, 152
Bermuda Street, 5, 16, 118, 130, 131, 195, 261
Bermudez, Don Pedro, 22
Bernard, Gabriel, 89
Bertie County, N. C., 159
Bethincourt, 314
Betsy, 46
Betty, 39
Biggs, Asa, 267
Biggs, K., 181
Bird, H. D., 179
Birmingham, Ala., 325
Black, Munro, Fund of the Norfolk Foundation, 384
Black-Eyed Susan, 262

Blackouts, 354-355
Blackstone, 284
Blackwater River, 161, 358
Bladensburg, Md., 125
Blair, John, 80
Blair Junior High School, 351
Blake, Peter, 6
Blakely, 172
Blanchard, M., 88
Blanchard, Thomas, 120
Blanchet, François, 89
Bland, William, 138
Blow, General George, 204, 205
Blow, Lula, 267
Blue and Gray Division, 310-313
Blue Eagle, 335-337
Blue Ridge, 311
Board of Public Works, 173
Board of Trade, British, 41
Board of Trade, Norfolk, 297
Boat Club, Norfolk, 267
Bois de Brabant, 313
Bois de Consenvoyne, 313
Bois de Four, 315
Bois de Gerache, 315
Bois de la Grande Montagne, 313
Bois des Ogons, 315, 317
Bois de Septsarges, 315
Boissevain pier, 313
Bonetta, 73
Bonsal, Caleb, bookseller, 134
Bonsal, Caleb, miller, 196
Booker T. Washington High School, 342, 352
Booth, Edwin, 262
Booth, Junius Brutus, 118
Borgia, Lucretia, 262
Borland, Charles B., 345, 350
Borough Tavern, 79, 81, 89, 91
Boston, 18, 25, 50, 91, 95, 107, 115, 158, 163, 165, 166, 178, 179, 198, 214, 223, 299, 300, 322, 327; steamship lines to, 284-285
Boston, 99
Boston Massacre, 236
Boston Port Bill, 50
Botetourt Street, 261
Boush, Samuel, Jr., 6, 8
Boush, Samuel, Sr., 6, 11, 22, 33
Boush Street, 131
Boush's Bluff, 209
Boutakoff, Rear Admiral, 263, 269
Bowden, Henry M., 235-236
Bowden, R., & Co., 87
Boy Scouts, 302
Boykin, W. A., 267
Brabanter Stellung, 312, 313
Bradford lakes, 249
Bramble, George, 261
Brambleton, 260-261, 288, 310, 340

Brambleton Avenue, 261, 341, 370, 373
Branding of livestock, 29-30
Brandywine, 83
Braxton, Carter, 78
Brazil, 260, 326
Breckinridge, John C., 201-202
Bremen, 330
Brewer Street, 323
Brieulles, 312, 315
Briggs' Point, 93, 121, 133, 134
Bristol, England, 3, 35, 46, 51, 182
Bristol, Tenn., 272, 279
British-American Tobacco Co., 310
Broad Creek, 33, 249
Broad Creek Road, 370
Broad Creek Village, 368, 372
Brooke, John M., 213
Brooke Avenue, 293, 369
Brothers, 87
Broughton, R. G., Jr., 254
Broughton, Thomas G., 141
Brown, Francis, 18
Brown, George, 254
Brown, John, of Harpers Ferry, 200, 226
Brown, John, of Norfolk, 51, 63
Bruges, 311
Buchan, schoolmaster, 25
Buchanan, Va., 178
Buchanan, Flag-Officer, 215
Buchanan, James, 200, 204
Buenos Aires, 108
Buffalo, N. Y., 368
Bull, Ole, 117
Bulloch House, 298
Bureau of Traffic Survey, 350
Burnside, General Ambrose E., 210-212, 216, 217
Burnt Mills Lake, 320, 358
Burroughs, W. H., 242
Burton, H. W., 264
Bute Street, 126, 137, 233, 234, 254, 287, 341
Bute Street Baptist Church, 241
Butler, General Benjamin F., 142, 222-231, 255
Butt, Thomas, 6
Byers, Leonora, 93
Byrd, Harry F., 340
Byrd, William, 6, 11, 16, 23, 25, 29, 36, 42, 46

Cabell, Joseph C., 174
Cabell County, 175
Cabin Point, 44, 45
Cádiz, 22, 45, 105, 108, 188
Caesar, 42
Calais, 109, 314
Calhoun, John C., 122, 123
California, 359
Calvert, Christopher, 16, 69

Calvert, John, 95
Calvert, Mayor Maximilian, 49
Calvert's Lane, 118, 126
Calvert's wharf, 87
Calypso, 185
Camden County, N. C., 331
Camp Lee, 303, 313
Camp McClellan, 302, 310, 311
Camp Pendleton, 347, 349
Campamagy, Jean Baptiste, 89
Campbell, A. D., 237
Campbell, Calvin, 14
Campbell, Donald, 25
Campbell, Mrs. Susanna, 25
Campostella, 371
Campostella bridge, 261, 339, 347
Canada, 18, 40, 105, 107, 147, 150
Canal at Richmond, 83-84
Canary Islands, 326
Canby, General E. R. S., 242
Canning, George, 150
Canonicus, 266
Cape Charles, 27
Cape Charles City, 280
Cape Cod, 17, 105
Cape Fear, 40
Cape François, 39
Cape Hatteras, 114, 211
Cape Henry, 27, 30, 31, 55, 71, 99, 100, 103, 347
Cape Henry lighthouse, 296
Cape Lookout, 30, 114
Cape Roman shoals, 114
Capes of the Chesapeake, 37, 60, 67, 70, 72, 76, 77, 83, 89, 90, 96, 99, 100, 110, 215
Capitol, U. S., 140
Capitol, Virginia State, 236
Carnegie, Andrew, 294
Carnegie Library of Pittsburgh, 384
Carolinas, 17, 71; *see also* North *and* South Carolina
Carpenter, 87
Carr, Captain, 111
Carroll, J. C., 266
Carrollton mansion, 298
Carteret, N. C., 286
Cassatt, A. J., 280
Castile, Council of, 174
Castillano, José, 126
Castlereagh, Lord, 147
Catharine Street, 16, 92, 101, 124, 131, 132, 139, 241, 254
Catherine, 38-39
Catherine-Eliza, 97
Catholic Church, 136-137
Catlett, J. Charles, 92
Causey, W. B., 323-324
Cavalier Hotel, 296
Cayuga, 218

Cedar Grove cemetery, 144
Centipede, 113
Central Presbyterian Church, 259
Chabaner, Pierre, 89
Chamber of Commerce, Norfolk, 250, 373, 384
Chamberlin Hotel, 294
Chambers, Lenoir, 393
Chambre, Walter, 51
Champ, 39
Champlitte, France, 311
Chancellorsville, 228-230
Chandler, Lucius H., 239-241, 245-246
Chapel Street, 137
Charles II, 4
Charles Carter, 99
Charles City County, 69
Charles City road, 229
Charleston, S. C., 71, 95, 113, 114, 153, 193, 205, 206, 275; Democratic convention in, 200-201
Charleston, W. Va., 175
Charlotte, N. C., 274, 275
Charlotte County, 161
Charlotte Street, 6, 12, 132, 137, 139, 241
Charlottesville, 175, 183, 381, 389
Charon, 72
Chase, Bishop Philander, 140
Chase, Salmon P., 217
Chattanooga, 272
Cherry, Mr., 126
Chesapeake and Ohio canal, 166
Chesapeake and Ohio Railroad, 277-278, 283, 326; boat discontinued, 369
Chesapeake and Potomac Telephone Company, 310
Chesapeake Bay, 27, 32, 35, 38, 41, 43, 47, 52, 69, 72, 76, 91, 110, 113, 160, 213, 295, 296
Chesapeake Bay bridge-tunnel, 367
Chesapeake Bay Ferry Commission, 367
Chesapeake Bay steamers, 172
Chesapeake Boat Club, 266
Chesapeake-Leopard affair, 100-103, 115, 125
Chesterfield, 229
Chesterfield Heights, 371
Chicago, 322, 325
Chickahominy River, 229
Chile, 305, 326
China, 260, 304, 344
Chisholm, William, 74
Chorus, Norfolk Civic, 381
Chowan and Southern Railway, 278
Chowan precinct, 33-35, 44
Chowan River, 30, 31, 161, 211, 260
Christ Church, 92, 101, 117, 124, 129, 136, 143
Christian, 46
Christmas Clearing House, 332

Chronicle, Norfolk and Portsmouth, 141
Church, Norfolk Parish, 6, 7, 12, 22-24;
  see also St. Paul's Church
Church Street, 5, 6, 9, 11, 13, 22, 33, 54,
  61, 74, 88, 89, 92, 111, 126, 130, 131,
  138-140, 243, 252, 258-260, 287, 288,
  292, 295, 319, 358; Plate XV
Churches, development of, 135-137
Cincinnati, 325
Circuses, 116-117, 268
Citizens' Bank, 258; building, 293
Citizens Public Works Committee, 339
Citizens' Union, 319
City Gas Light Company, 133, 144, 223,
  253
City Hall, 118, 132, 144, 201, 217, 238-
  241, 244, 251, 252, 294, 341, 353, 377;
  Plate XII
City Hall Avenue, 4, 5, 252, 292, 293, 317,
  319, 371, 385; filled in, 132
City Home, 338
City Hotel, 193
City-manager system introduced, 318-
  319
City Point, 83, 179, 240
City Railroad Company, Norfolk, 288
City Welfare Center, 332
Civic center, 373-374; Plate XX
Civil Defense, *see* Air Raid Defense
Civil Rights Bill, 234
Civil War, 165, 207-231
Civil Works Administration, 337-338,
  340, 343
Clarke, Bartholomew, 6
Clarke, Clarence H., 273
Clarksburg, 177
Clarksville, 181
Clay, Henry, 116
Clinton, DeWitt, 166
Clyde, William P., 278
Clyde line, 285
Coal trade, 273-274, 281-283, 304-305,
  330, 359-360
Cobb, General, 230
Cobb, Elijah, 17, 105
Cocke, General John Hartwell, 122
Coffee, Captain, 225
Cold Harbor, 228, 230
Cole, Albert M., 373
College for Young Ladies, Norfolk, 293;
  Plate X
College Place, 293, 294
Colley, John P., 165
Colley Avenue, 267, 289
Collier, Sir George, 70
Collier's, 352
Collinson, Richard, 24
Colmini, 126
Colonial Avenue, 302
Colonial Place, 291

Colonial Stores, 368
Colonial Theatre, 301
Colonization Society, Norfolk, 127
Colorado, 165, 277
Coloradoes rocks, 40
Columbia, 208
Columbia Broadcasting System, 389
Columbia Building, 292
Columbian Bards, 120
Columbus, Ohio, 274
Columbus, 207, 208
Commerce Street, 93
Commercial Place, 5, 7, 291, 292, 323,
  350; Plate XI; *see also* Market Square
Committee of Public Safety, 50-53, 65-66
Committee for Public Schools, 389
Commons, House of, 48, 76
Community Fund, 332, 334
Community Hospital for Negroes, Nor-
  folk, 342, 345
Concord Street, 131
Confederacy, The, 382
Congress, U. S., 77, 81, 95, 97, 99, 104,
  124, 145, 147-150, 301
Congress, 213-215
Conner, Lewis, 6
Conservatory of Music, 264
Constable, Dr., 193
Constantine, Grand Duke, 263, 269
Constellation, 110-113, 115
Constitution, ratification of, 79-81
Constitutional Convention, 79
Constitutional Union party, 201-202
Continental Association, 51, 52
Contrast, The, 118
Convention, French National, 89, 90
Convention, Virginia Revolutionary, 52,
  57, 60, 63, 64, 66
Convoys during colonial wars, 38
Cook, Dr., 224
Cooke, Giles B., 153
Cooke, Richard D., 351
Cooper, John, 91
Corbin, Francis, 80
Cornet, 46
Cornwallis, Lord, 71-73
Corprew, Colonel Thomas J., 229
Corprew Avenue, 385
Cotton Exchange, 258, 276
Cotton trade, 272-276, 287, 327
Council, Colonial, 41
Council of Civic Leagues, 363-364
Couper, William, 107, 128, 190
Court Street, 131
Courthouse, city, *see* City Hall
Courthouse, county, 5, 7, 11, 12, 15
Courthouse, town, 7 n.; *see also* Town
  Hall
Cove Street, 132
Coverley, Mrs. Ann, 18, 31

Covington, 184
Cox, Lawrence M., 370
Cradock, 309
Crampton Gap, battle of, 230
Craney Island, 64, 72, 143, 144, 205, 209, 218; battle of, 111-113; Plate V
Crater, explosion of the, 230
Crawford Street, Portsmouth, 72
Crawford's Point, 33
Creighton baseball club, 265-266
Cretcher, Thomas, 18
Cricket, 121
Cronkhite, General, 316
Cropper, Thomas T., 145
Cross, Betty, 93
Crozet, Claudius, 185
Cuba, 96, 97, 330
Culloden, 21
Culpeper, Thomas, Lord, 4
Culpeper County, 139
Culpeper lock, 160
Cumberland, 207, 208, 213, 214
Cumberland Street, 4, 126, 131, 136, 137
Cumberland Street Baptist Church, 144
Cumberland Street Methodist Church, 144
Cumberland Valley, 182
Cunningham, William, 141
Curaçao, 41
Currituck, 114, 161
Currituck Bridge, 229
Currituck County, N. C., 331
Currituck precinct, 34
Currituck Sound, 31, 163, 185, 268
Custine, Citizen, 89
Custom House: first, 91; of 1824, 122-123, 128; present, 132, 219, 221, 248, 258, 293, 341, 377

Daily Pilot, 256
Dan, 162
Dan River, 161, 181
Dana, Phineas, 124
Dana, Phinehan, 87
Dancing, 122-123
Dane, 39
Dannevoux, 315
Dante's *Inferno*, 315
Danville, 162, 175, 275, 279
Danzig, 346
Darden, Colgate W., Jr., 340, 347
Darden, Mayor Pretlow, 362
Davis, Rev. Mr., 101
Davis, Henry, 212
Davis, Jefferson, 204, 217, 221, 226, 236, 275
Davis, Thomas, 23, 50
Davis, William, 141
Davis, William Wallace, 120
Davis brothers, 125-126

Dawes, S. S., 120
Dawson, James, 16
Day Book, Norfolk, 142, 205-212; suppressed, 219
Dearborn, Henry, 103
Decatur, Commodore Stephen, 101, 125
Declaration of Independence, 301
DeCordy, Mayor Francis, 237, 240, 244
Deep Creek, 134, 159, 161, 250
Deepwater, W. Va., 283
Defenders of State Sovereignty and Individual Liberties, 388, 392
De Grasse, Admiral, 73
Delany, Mayor W. D., 196
Delaware, 198
Delaware, 140, 207, 208; launched, 164
Delaware River, 168
Delegates, Virginia House of, 99, 182, 184, 392
Delisle, Monsieur, 89
Delpino, Frank L., 381
Demerara, 277
Democrats, 200-202
Denan Castle, 39
Denmark, 304
De Paul Hospital, 358
Depression of the 1930's, 328-343
Detroit, 325
Devlin, Mary, 119
Dibbs, Captain John, 6
Dickson, Horace K., 336
Dickson, William C., 266
Dickson place, 293
Diggs, J. Eugene, 336
Dilworth, Peter, 244-245
Dinwiddie, 39
Dinwiddie, Governor Robert, 8-9, 81
Dinwiddie County, 167
Diphtheria mortality rate, 326
Directory, French, 90
Dismal Swamp, 28, 33, 34, 56, 183, 271
Dismal Swamp canal, 158-164, 167, 185, 250; opened, 114
District Court, U. S., 387, 390-391
District of Columbia, 162, 335
Dock Street, 234
Doctor's Creek, 185
Dodson Building, 258, 260, 276
Dolphin, 208
Doms, Keith, 384
Donaldson, balloonist, 268
Donaldson, Thorburn & Co., 87
Donelson, A. J., 200
Dorman, O. M., 237
Dornin, F. B., 266
Douglas, Commodore John E., 101-102
Douglas, Stephen A., 116, 201-202
Douglass, Laura T., 267
Doyle's Lake, 249
Drake, 87

Drayton, Michael, 382
Dred Scott decision, 200, 201
Drudge, Mrs., 24
Drummond, R. Q., 237
Dry dock, 164, 208, 218
Ducamp, Gaspard, 89
Ducking stool, 11, 49
Duckworth, Mayor W. Fred, 362, 369, 373, 376, 384, 387, 389
Dumouriez, Citizen, 89
Dunmore, 62, 65-67
Dunmore, Lady, 20, 21
Dunmore, Lord, 20, 46, 52-68, 71, 141; Plate I
Du Pont de Nemours, E. I., and Co., 310
Durand, Louis, 89
Durant, Lewis E., & Co., 87
Dutchess of Douglas, 39

Eagles' Hall, 319
East Main Street, 350, 373-374; *see also* Main Street
East Street, 5
East Tennessee and Georgia Railroad, 272, 273
Eastern Branch, 4, 5, 33, 54, 103, 144, 183, 185, 267, 281, 282, 323, 339, 363; *see also* Elizabeth River
Eastern Shore, 286, 367, 369
Eastern Shore and Peninsula railroads, 280
Eddy, actor, 262
Edenton, 30, 33, 87, 161
Edmonds, Mr., 139
Education, 6, 24-25, 255-256, 325, 351, 385-394
Eighteenth French Division, 312
Eightieth Division, 313-316
Eilbeck, Jonathan, 63, 74, 92
Eilbeck, Ross & Co., 51
Electric Light Company of Virginia, 252
Eliza, 96, 109
Elizabeth, 46, 51, 90
Elizabeth City, 161
Elizabeth City and Norfolk Railroad, 278
Elizabeth City County, 80
Elizabeth River, 4, 27-29, 31, 33, 42-46, 49, 50, 52, 63-66, 70, 71, 74, 76, 77, 83, 85, 108, 109, 111, 143, 144, 146, 147, 153, 157, 158, 192, 208-210, 213, 216, 218, 266, 269, 271, 272, 274, 276-284, 291, 308, 321, 326, 330, 357; *see also* Eastern, Southern, and Western branches
Elizabeth River parish, 22-24
Elizabeth River tunnels, 366
Elliott, K. B., 285
Elmwood cemetery, 144, 260
Emancipation Proclamation, 220, 233

Emancipator, 197
Embargo, 104-108
Emergency Banking Act, 333
Emergency Relief Committee, 332
Emergency Relief Organization, U. S., 333
Emerson, Captain, 113
Endor, Woman of, 117
England, 14, 45, 51, 76, 188, 319; *see also* Great Britain
Ennes & Hope, 12
Enterprise, 185
Ephesus, 284
Epidemics, 13, 188-197
Episcopal Church, Protestant, 135-136
Ericsson, John, 215
Erie Canal, 153, 160, 166, 174
Etheridge, N. B., 393
Ethiopian Corps, 56, 59
Europe, 3, 68, 83, 85, 87, 105, 113-115, 156, 157, 360
Evans, Captain, 96
Evans, Admiral Robley D., 297
Evansville, Ind., 309
Everett, Edward, 201
Exchange Bank, 196
Exchange Coffee House, 91, 101, 122
Eyre, Littleton, 80

Fair American, 87
Fairfax Hotel, 336
Fairs, 8, 19-20
Falconer, James, 23
Falmouth, 44, 45
Fame, 109
Fanny, 39, 51
Farmers' Bank of Virginia, 139, 165
Farmer's Lane, 131
Fauquier, Governor Francis, 45
Faust, 262, 263
Favorite, 147
Fayette Street, 258
Federal Building, 341
Federal Emergency Relief Administration, 334
Federal Farm Board, 333
Federal Fuel Administration, 306
Federal Housing Act, 370
Federal Transient Bureau, 334
Federal Works Agency, 350-351
Federalist, 79
Federalists, 77, 78, 81, 90
Feldman, I. E., 382
Feldman Chamber Music Society, 382
Fenchurch Street, 5, 92, 118, 130, 131, 136, 139
Ferebee, John, 4, 5, 370, 374
Feret, Alexander, 196
Ferries, 33-34
Ferry Point, 65, 103

Fifty-fourth Regiment, Norfolk militia, 90
Fillmore, Estelle, 267
Fillmore, Millard, 199, 200
Fincastle, 63
Finiken, William, 19
Finland, 311
Fire protection, 12-13, 253, 325
Fireboat *Vulcan,* 325
Fires, 128-129
First American Army, 314
First Baptist Church, 137
First Methodist Church, 388
First National Bank, 235
First Regiment, Virginia Field Artillery, 310
Fisher, Kate, 262
Fiske, Martin, 87
Fiveash, Joseph G., 254
Fleming, Adam, 44
Florence Crittenton Home, 335
Florence, Italy, 120
Florida, 260, 295
Fluvanna County, 83
Folger, Fire Chief, 253
Food Administrator, 307
Fordyce, Captain, 58
Foreman Field, 340, 386
Forrest, W. S., 119, 143, 198, 293
Fort Clark, 211
Fort Fisher, 284
Fort Hatteras, 211, 226
Fort Lee, *see* Camp Lee
Fort Monroe, 122, 213, 216, 233, 253, 294
Fort Nelson, 103, 111, 129, 142, 209
Fort Norfolk, 101, 103, 110, 111, 142, 143, 209, 261
Fort Norfolk Road, 267
Fort Oglethorpe, 302
Fort Story, 296, 347, 349
Fort Sumter, 206
Foster, John, 86
Foster and Moore's store, 221
Fourteenth Amendment, 387
Fourth Circuit Court of Appeals, 387, 391
Fourth Division, 314
Fourth of July celebrations, 80, 123-124
Fourth Virginia Regiment, 302, 310
Fox and Denier, 262
Fox Hunting Club, 268
Fra Diavolo, 263
France, 70, 88, 108, 109, 319, 326, 330, 360; relations with, 88-91
Franco, Francisco, 344
Franklin, General William B., 230
Frazier's Farm, second battle of, 230
Fredericksburg, 44, 149, 176, 213; battle of, 229
Freedmen's Bureau, 241, 344

Freeman, Joseph M., 245
Freemason Street, 92, 101, 124, 130, 131, 133, 136, 248, 251, 252, 254, 264, 287, 293, 294, 352, 358
Freeport Heresy, 200
French Lodge of Wisdom, 89
French Revolution, 84
French Spy, The, 262
French's Hotel, 140; *see also* National Hotel
Friends of the Norfolk Public Library, 384
Friendship, 39
Frying-pan shoals, 114

Gaiety Theater, 374
Gallatin, Albert, 98, 151
Galt, Alexander, postmaster, 196
Galt, Alexander, sculptor, 120-121, 377
Galveston, 275, 327
Garcia, John, 23
Garcia, Manuel, 126
Garnet, Colonel William, 140
Garysville, 170
Gas Light Company, *see* City Gas Light Company
Gaston, 171, 178
Gaston and Weldon Railroad, 181
Gates County, N. C., 331
Gatewood, Rev. R., 256
Gay, John, 18
Gazette and Public Ledger, 96, 100, 102, 103, 104, 106, 110, 125, 141, 157
Gazetteer of Virginia, 165, 167
General B. F. Butler, 253, 325
General Cabell, 170
General Mower Corporation, 368
General Washington, 165
George, 43, 87
George III, 48, 50, 53
George Appold, 284
Georgetown, 266
Georgia, 17, 85, 176, 209, 298
German Club, 269
German-Soviet non-aggression pact, 346
Germantown, 208, 212
Germany, 319, 327, 330, 344, 345, 354, 360, 380
Gettysburg, 229
Ghent, 289
Ghent, Peace of, 145
Girard College, 224
Givens, Mr., 241
Glasford, John, & Co., 42, 44
Glasgow, 35, 44-46, 50, 51, 64, 76, 88
Glennen, Michael, 256
Glenwood, 309
Godfrey, John, 6
Godfrey, Matthew, 6
Godwin, Mr., 116

Goggin, William L., 201
Golden Triangle, 375
Goldsborough, Louis M., 210
Gooch, Governor William, 8, 36, 39, 41, 42
Goode, John, 238
Goodrich, John, 63, 66
Gordan, John D., 196
Gordon, Alexander, 90
Gordon, Dr. Alexander, 14
Gosport, 45, 63, 64, 70, 72, 85, 113, 142, 164, 191-192, 308
Gosport Creek, 72
Graham, Tildsley, 87
Grain elevator built, 322
Grain trade, 44, 82, 321-322, 327
Granby Family Theatre, Plate XVI
Granby Street, 130, 131, 132, 243, 248, 251, 252, 254, 258, 268, 288, 291-294, 316, 317, 319, 328, 331, 332, 341, 345, 358, 361, 383, 385
Granby Street bridge, 92, 119, 132, 251-252, 292
Granby Street High School, 342, 351
Grandy, Captain C. R., 229
Grandy, C. Wiley, 352
Grant, Frederick D., 297
Grant, U. S., 231, 241
Granville County, 181
Gratitude, 316
Graves, William A., Jr. 266
Great Bridge, 54, 55, 65, 66, 103, 185, 229, 238; battle at, 56-59; chapel at, 23
Great Britain, 3, 33, 34, 35, 42, 44, 45, 46, 68, 76, 81, 276, 326, 327, 346; relations with, 98-109, 145-153
Greeley, Horace, 205
Green, Paul, 382
Greenville, N. C., 275
Greensville County, 167
Gregory, 277
Grenada, 37, 46, 90
Grenville, George, 48, 49
Gresham, S. S., Jr., 267
Gresham, W. H., 267
Grew, Joseph, 354
Griffen, George, 254
Grigsby, Hugh Blair, 92, 119-120, 124, 270
Guadeloupe, 39, 40, 84, 85, 87, 190
Guernsey, 41
Guerrière, 164
Guinea, 32, 45
Gwynn's Island, Dunmore's camp at, 66-67
Gygax, Admiral Felix X., 357

Haddington Building, 292; Plate XII
Hagen Stellung, 312
Hague, the, 289, 377, 378

Halifax, 89, 148, 150, 152
Halifax County, N. C., 159, 161, 172, 175, 180
Halstead, F. M., 267
Halstead, Richard, 120
Hamburg, 330
Hamilton, Bermuda, 145
Hamilton, Alexander, 81
Hamilton, Colonel John, 92
Hamlet, 119
Hammond, 63
Hampton, 63, 192, 195, 201
Hampton Boulevard, 339, 347, 348, 350, 356, 366
Hampton Roads, 31, 37, 44, 46, 63, 87, 88, 99, 100-102, 105, 111-113, 151, 210, 214-216, 277, 283, 294-295, 298, 300, 301, 303-307, 326, 327, 330, 347, 354, 356, 359-360, 365-369
Hampton Roads bridge-tunnel, 366-367
Hampton Rough and Ready Club, 199
Handel, Joseph, 117
Hanover Court House, battle of, 230
Hansford, Mrs., 122
Happy Return, 95
Hardy, Fred, 266
Hardy, J. M., 267
Hardy, W. C., 266
Hardy house, 293
Hare Building, 258
Harmony, 218
Harpers Ferry, 176, 230
Harriot, 99
Harris, John, 69
Harris, Kenneth, 380
Harris, Winder R., 336
Harrison, Benjamin, 78
Harrison, William Henry, 199
Harrison, W. T., 237
Harvard College, 224
Hatch, J. D., 380
Hatteras, 284
Hatton, John G. H., 196
Haumont, 313
Havana, 22, 40, 90, 108, 282
Hawaii, 353
Hayne, Colonel Robert Y., 116, 155-156
Health Department, City, 372
Health protection, 325-326
Hebrew, John A., 266
Hebrew Union, 233
Hemenway School, 255
Henrico, 3
Henrico Rifles, 111
Henry, Patrick, 80
Henry Street, 295
Herald and Norfolk and Portsmouth Advertiser, 87, 95, 103, 118, 121, 125, 129, 131, 132, 141, 146, 147, 149-152, 161, 168, 173, 188, 198, 200, 203, 205

Hershaw and Company, 179
Hesdigrieuf, 314
Heslett, William, 6
Heutte, Frederic, 382-383
Hibernian, 276
Hicksford Junction (Emporia), 171
High school, public, opened, 255-256
High Street, Portsmouth, 72, 169, 170
Highways, Virginia Department of, 367
Hill Street, 117
Hinton, Colonel J. W., 238, 266
Hiroshima, 360
History of the Dividing Line, The, 25
Hitler, Adolph, 344, 345, 346, 360
Hoboken, 169, 311
Hodge, 46
Hodges, Mrs. E. B., 336
Hodges, Mary, 6
Hodges, Thomas, 6
Hoffman, Judge Walter E., 387, 391
Hofheimer, Henry Clay, II, 384
Holt, John, 53-54, 141
Holt, Mayor John E., 122
Holt, Saxon W., Jr., 336
Holt Street, 137, 139, 254, 371
Holt Street bridge, 261
Holt's Lane, 131
Homicide rate, 324-325
Hook and Ladder Company, 253
Hoover, Herbert C., 333
Hope, James Barron, 256
Hope Hose Company, 253
Hopkins, Mr., 66
Hopkins, Harry, 341
Hornet, 17
Horse racing, *see* Racing
Horton, Minnie, 267
Hosmer, Jean, 262
Hospital expansion, 358, 372
Hospital Point, 209
Housing and Home Finance Agency, 373
Housing Authority, Norfolk, 349, 370
Housing projects, 371
Housing shortage, in First World War, 309; in Second World War, 348, 349, 355-357
Houston, 325
Howard, General O. O., 241
Howard Association, 195, 196, 223
Howe, Colonel Robert, 52, 57, 59-61, 63-64
Howe, Walter Edward, 380
Hubard, James R., 204
Hudson River, 166
Huff, John M., 371
Huger, General Benjamin, 210, 216
Huger Battery, 229
Hughes, Robert M., Jr., 332
Humble Sons of God, 233
Hume, Paul, 382

Humphrey, Captain, 100
Hunchback, 119
Hunter, John, 63
Hunter, Dr. William, 14
Hunter's shipyard, 131
Huntersville, 260, 288
Hunting, 268
Huntington, Collis P., 277
Hunton Branch, Y. M. C. A., 385
Hustings, James, 19
Hutchings, John, 69
Hutchings, Zachariah, 39
Hygeia hotel, 294-295

Iago, 262
Ickes, Harold, 338-340
Idaho, 329
Illinois, 140
Imecourt, 315
Immigrants, opposition to, 199-200
Impressment of American sailors, 98-100, 103
Independence Hall, 298
Independent Grays, 229
Independent Society, 233
Independent Volunteers, 123
Indian Creek, 42
Indian Pole Bridge, 268
Industrial Park, Norfolk, 372
Industry, 42
Inman, John H., 278, 279
Inoculation, 13
International Azalea Court, 383-384
Irish Widow, The, 117
Isaac Bell, 284
Isle of Pines, 96, 109
Isle of Wight County, 80, 285, 355, 369
Italy, 260, 326, 327, 330, 354, 360

Jack, slave, 10
Jack Cade, 262
Jackson, Andrew, 115, 151
Jackson, T. J., 230
Jackson Street, 252
Jacksonville, 326
Jacobin Clubs, 90
Jacobins, 65
Jaffé, Louis I., 393
Jail, county, 5, 11, 15; town, 11, 75; city, 132, 373, 374
Jamaica, 38, 40, 41, 44-46, 51, 77, 84, 85, 87, 95-97, 107, 108, 146, 151, 152, 277
James, Charles E., 254
James River, 25, 27, 38, 42, 43, 46, 57, 60, 76, 83, 114, 158, 162, 167, 174, 176, 178, 179, 182, 213, 214, 216-218, 229, 277, 278, 360
James River and Kanawha canal, 272, 281

James River and Kanawha Company, 174-175, 177, 182
Jamestown, 4, 48, 213, 215
Jamestown, 165
Jamestown Exposition of 1907, 296-298, 308
Jamestown Festival, 382
Jamestown Flats, 218
Jamieson, Niel, 37, 44, 45, 63, 66, 74
Janauschek, Fannie, 262-263
Japan, 327, 353
Jarrett, Henry C., 119
Jay, John, 81-82
Jay Treaty, 81-82
J. E. Coffee, 195
Jefferson, Joseph, 119, 263
Jefferson, Thomas, 25, 102, 103, 104, 109, 120
Jenkins, Henry, 19
Jenner, Edward, 188
Jenny, 39
Jeremiah, Negro, 127
Jericho, 353
John Adams, 164
John Barrett, 170
Johnson, Mrs., 25
Johnson, Andrew, 232, 233, 235
Johnson, George, 93
Johnson, George W., 277
Johnson, Herschel V., 201
Johnson, Hugh S., 335-337
Johnson, James, 80
Johnston, Joseph E., 216, 219
Jones, George, 118
Jones, Hugh, 3
Jones, John, 12
Jordan, J. Parker, 240, 244
Josslin, Richard, 18, 19
Journal, Norfolk, 88, 180, 238, 242-245, 249, 251, 256, 275, 281
Journal, Norfolk and Portsmouth, 79, 141
Joyce, John, 46
Juilliard School of Music, 381
Juliet, 263
Junior Chamber of Commerce, 384
Junior Volunteers, 101, 123, 229
Juniper baseball club, 265
Juniper water, 249-250

Kanawha River, 174, 176
Kansas, 200, 309
Kaufman, Charles L., 336
Keeling, R. James, 120
Keene, Laura, 262
Keith, N. S., 370
Kellam, Sidney S., 365
Kellogg Opera Troupe, 263
Kelsall, Roger, 23
Kemps, 33, 54, 55, 58, 65, 66, 103

Kempsville, 59, 114, 185
Kempsville district, 364
Kentucky, 274, 309
Kevill, Thomas, fire chief, 253, 325
Kimball, Vice-president of N. & W., 282
King, George, 254
King, Miles, 80, 92
Kingbird, 39
Kingfisher, 62
King's Daughters, 335; hospital, 372
King's Lane, 117
Kingston, 40
Kingston, Jamaica, 41, 87, 88
Kirkby, Arthur M., 385
Kirn, Bessie, 385
Knight, Thomas, 93
Knott, Captain William, 5, 6, 16
Know-Nothing party, 199-200
Knowles, dramatist, 119
Knox, Frank, 351, 353
Koerner, Anton F., 264
Kriemhild Stellung, 312

La Badine, 95
Labor shortages, 307, 309, 359
Lady Walterstoff, 83
Lafayette, General, 116, 122-123
Lafayette Park, 338, 358, 382
Lafayette River, 291, 323, 345, 347, 382
Lafayette River bridge: at Colley Avenue, 340; at Granby Street, 339-340; at Hampton Boulevard, 339, 350
Lagaudette, Peter, 126
Lake Drummond, 116, 134, 159, 249, 250
Lake Phillips, 320
Lake Prince, 320, 349, 357
Lamb, W. W., Supt. of schools, 255
Lamb, William, exporter, 284
Lamb, Mayor William W., 210, 217, 282
Lambert, Hillary, 87
Lamberts Point, 111, 126, 193, 209, 283, 289, 291; coal pier established at, 282
Lancastershire Witch, 40
Landmark, Norfolk, 256, 277
Lane, Joseph, 201
Langford, Menalous, 341
Lankford, Jesse, 169
Laperouse, Jean Pierre, 89
Larchmont, 291
Larchmont School, 338, 386
La Rochefoucauld, 11, 16, 28, 65, 76, 83, 85, 89, 128, 138, 159
Lawrence's oyster house, 292
Lawson, Colonel, 54, 55
Lawson, Lieutenant Colonel Anthony, 5
Layton, L. L., 390
Leache, Irene, 264
Leache-Wood Alumnae Association, 377
Leache-Wood School, 264
League of Virginia Municipalities, 383

Leahy, Admiral William D., 345
LeBreton, Admiral David, 360
Ledger-Dispatch, 256
Lee, Arthur, 138
Lee, General Charles, 65-66
Lee, Fitzhugh, 296
Lee, H. Richard, 92
Lee, Mayor Richard E., 101-102
Lee, Richard H., 138
Lee, Robert E., 210, 216, 219, 230; visits Norfolk, 268-269
Lee Parade, 291, 297, 298
Lee Park, 377, 378
Lee's wharf, 118
Leftwich, General Joel, 110
Le Havre, 330
Leigh, Mrs. James Y., 269
Leigh Memorial Hospital, 358
Leleivie, Gabriel, 88
Lemasurier, Mary, 88
LeMay, General Curtis, 383, 384
LeMay, Patricia Jane, 383
Leonard, Abram F., 120
Leonidas, 109
Leopard, attacks *Chesapeake*, 100-101
Le Page, E. B., 266
Lepage, Louis, 89
Leslie, Captain, 54, 58, 59
Leslie, General, 71
Lesner's Garden, 259
Lester, Thomas, 87
Letcher, Governor John, 210
Letters of a South Carolinian, 119
Lewis, General Andrew, 67
Lewis, Armistead, 93
Lewis, Henry, 336
Liberty Loans, 303
Library, Norfolk Public, 264, 294, 377, 384-385; Plate XX
Library Association, Norfolk, 294
Library of Congress, 141
Life, 389
Light Artillery Blues, 123, 229, 302, 310, 316
Lincoln, Abraham, 202, 205, 213, 221, 222; visits Norfolk, 217
Lincoln-Douglas debates, 200
Lincoln Street, 370
Linde Air Products Corporation, 310
Lindsay, William, 91
Lindsay's Retreat, 121
Linkhorn Bay, 296
Linsey's Gardens, 240
Lisbon, 45
Literature, 119-120
Little Creek, 249, 341
Little Creek Players, 382
Little Rock, 389
Little Theater, 378, 382
Little Water Street, 93, 190, 253, 254

Liverpool, 46, 51, 75, 87, 88, 115, 156, 157, 276, 277, 284
Liverpool, 61, 62, 65
Livestock, 29-30
Locke, Donald R., 362
Loftland, John, 18
London, 3, 12, 21, 42, 45, 46, 75, 81, 86, 87, 97, 115, 147, 156, 168, 260, 330, 344
London Assurance, 119
Longwood College, 382
Look Magazine, 376
Lorillard Steamship wharf; 252
Louisiana, 152, 153
Lovitt, E. H. C., 261
Lovitt Avenue, 255
Lovitt's New Bridge, 261
Loyal Hunter, 46
Loyall, Captain B. P., 269
Loyall, Mayor Paul, 17, 53
Loyall's Lane, 126
Lowell, Mass., 223, 224
Lowenburg, M. D., 297
Lowenburg stores, 258
Lower Norfolk County, 4, 5
Ludlow, Mayor John R., 237
Lyme, 32
Lynch, Francis, 87
Lynch, J. C., 266
Lynchburg, 162, 174, 175, 178, 182, 183, 272
Lynnhaven Bay, 113

McAlpine, William J., 249-250
McCarrick, James, 277
McCartney, Captain John, 53
McCauley, Commodore Charles S., 207
McClellan, General George B., 213, 216, 229, 230
McClurg, Dr. D. W., 14
McCormick, Mrs. J. Jett, 378
McCullough, A. A., 251
McCullough, F. W., 290-291
McCullough Lumber Company, 292
McCullough's wharf, 282
MacDonald, Robert, 101
Mace, 9, 81, 140
Macgill, N., 87
McIntosh, George, 87, 266
McIntosh home, 293
Mackenzie, John, 93
McLean, A., 141
McLean, J., 141
McLean, Louis, 151
Maclure, Alexander, 93
McMenamin, James, 266
McMoran, James, 23
McPherson, Duncan, 90
Madden and Whitehurst, 87
Madeira, 14, 45, 87
Madeleine Farm, 315, 317

Madison, 165
Madison, James, 25, 76, 77, 78, 79, 109, 145
Madison School, 351
Magnin, Hilarus, 141
Magnolia Gardens, 342
Magruder, General John B., 214, 217
Maguire, Mr., 138
Mahone, William, 183, 229, 230, 272-273
Main Street, 4-7, 9, 11, 13, 15, 16, 31, 32, 35, 53, 61, 74, 87, 88, 91, 93, 115, 117, 118, 122, 125, 127, 183, 190-193, 220, 233, 235, 248, 252, 254, 263, 268, 276, 287, 288, 291, 294, 316, 319, 341, 350; in 1887, 257-258; Plate XIV; *see also* East Main Street
Maitland, Robert, 93
Malaga, 98
Malbone, Peter, 18
Malbrouck Hill, 313
Mallory, Stephen R., 212
Malvern Hill, 230
Manassas, 213
Manassas, second battle of, 229, 230
Manchester, 229
Manghum, Mason, 336
Manhattan, 166
Mann, General, 234
Manufacturing, 198-199
Margarettsville, 170, 172
Maria, 87, 95
Marine Bank, 258
Marine Hospital, 142, 144, 339
Mariner Street, 133
Market house, 7, 12, 75, 91, 129; new house built, 323, torn down, 375
Market Square, 11, 14, 87, 89, 101, 115, 122, 127, 129, 131, 133, 190, 234, 253, 269, 288; in 1887, 258-260; *see also* Commercial Place
Market Street, 131, 323
Markets, 134-135
Marmont Farm, 312
Marne, battle of the, 300
Mars, 109
Mars Hill, 119
Marsden, John, 23
Marshall, Major, 57
Marshall, Richard M., 354-355
Martha Johnson, 87
Martin, Colonel James G., IV, 388
Martin, Joseph, dancing master, 122
Martin, Joseph, gazetteer, 130, 131, 165, 167
Martin, William, 254
Martinique, 40, 84, 85
Mary and Jane, 51
Mary Washington College, 381
Maryland, 27, 43, 44, 45, 47, 77, 78, 113, 157, 176, 198, 228, 298, 330, 335

Maryland baseball club, 266
Mason, George, 79
Mason, Stephen T., 82
Mason County, 175
Mason's Creek, 348
Mason's store, 47
Massachusetts, 78, 298
Massachusetts charter, overriding of, 50-51
Mathews, Thomas, 79, 80, 90
Mathews County, 66, 192
Matone's Garden, 117
Maury, Walker, 136
Maury High School, 319, 351, 389, 392
Maxwell, Captain, 80
Maxwell, Mrs., 24
Maxwell, James, 16, 56, 69
Maxwell, Thomas F., 373, 391
Maxwell, William, 149
Maxwell, William, poet, 120
Maxwell Street, 131
Mayflower, 297
Mechanics Hall, 117, 132, 144, 205
Mecklenburg County, Va., 161, 181
Medical Arts Center, 372
Medical Office Tower, 372
Meherrin River, 161
Memphis, Tenn., 251, 274, 324
Memphis and Charleston Railroad, 272
Mercer, Joseph, 18
Mercer, Thomas, 18
Merchant Street, 92
Merchants and Miners line, 285
Mercury, 53
Merrimac, 207, 208, 212, 213; *see also Virginia*
Merrimack Park, 349
Metcalf Lane, 131
Methodist Church, 133, 136, 137, 144, 155
Methuselah, 160
Meuse River, 312, 315, 316
Middle Street, Portsmouth, 72
Middlesex County, 80
Middleton Place, 342
Miles, Mrs. Marian Carpenter, 380
Military highway, 358
Miller, Dr. William, 13
Minnesota, 309
Minnesota, 214-216
Minute Men, 203
Mississippi, 329
Mississippi Inlet, 261
Mississippi River, 182
Mitchell, Joseph, 23
Mitchell, Maggie, 119, 263
Mitchell's Lane, 129
Mobile, 193
Molasses Act, 48
Molly, 40, 46, 51

Monitor, 215-216
Monroe, James, 124, 149
Montague, Captain, 21
Montague, Andrew J., 297
Montaign Farm, 314
Montgomery, Ala., 204
Monticello, 209
Monticello Avenue, 323, 341, 370, 375
Monticello Hotel, 293; Plate XIII
Moore, shortstop, 265
Moore, P. T., 266
Moore, Tom, 128
Moore's Bridges, 249, 250; Plate VIII
Morgan, Captain Jeremiah, 17
Morris, Gouverneur, 81
Morton, Major General Charles G., 311
Moscow, burning of, 218
Moseley, 46
Moseley, Edward, 6
Moseley, Edward H., 49
Mosley, Colonel, 20, 21
Mottu, J. A. P., 381
Mowbray Arch, 377, 378
Municipal Airport, 341, 345, 354, 368, 383
Municipal government, establishment of first, 7-8
Municipal Public Health Center, 372
Munn, Russell, 384
Murdoch, James E., 119
Murdock, Ferguson, 37
Murrow, Edward R., 389
Murray, K. C., superintendent of schools, 255
Museum of Arts and Sciences, 338, 340, 342, 343, 345, 377-380
Museum of Nature, 121
Music Festival, Virginia, 381
Muter, George, 69
Myers, Mayor Barton, 278, 279, 283, 321
Myers, Moses, 92, 93, 124, 163
Myers, Vernon C., 376
Myers house, 256, 353, 380

Nag's Head, 185, 211
Nancy, 39
Nansemond County, 3, 61, 80, 106, 167, 285, 320, 331, 349, 355
Nansemond River, 33, 112, 216, 249, 321
Nantes, 70
Nantillois, 315
Napoleon, 95, 104, 109
Napoleon, Louis, 116
Nash, Thomas, 6
Nash, Thomas, Jr., 18
Nashville, 279
National Bank of Commerce, 333
National Guard, 302-303
National Hotel, 132, 196, 201, 248, 374; *see also* French's Hotel

National Municipal League, 376
National Recovery Administration, 335-337
Nautilus, 127
Naval Academy, 384
Naval Air Station, 345, 346, 349
Naval Base, 307-308, 309, 322, 323, 328, 329, 339, 345-347, 350, 351, 356
Naval Board of Virginia, 69
Naval Hospital, Portsmouth, 111, 132, 143, 144, 309
Naval Overseas Transportation Service, 305-306
Navigation Acts, 41
Navy Department, U. S., 104, 307, 345, 353
Navy Yard, 192, 211-213, 308, 309, 328, 329, 339, 345-347, 356, 357, 359; founded, 164-165; seized by Confederacy, 207-209; evacuated by Confederacy, 217-218
Navy Yard of Virginia, 69
Nebraska Street, 11, 248
Ned, Negro, 127
Negroes: regulation of, 10; uprising by, 126-127; as soldiers, 219-220, 225; in Reconstruction, 233-246; *see also* Slavery
Neilson, Lillian Adelaide, 263
Neuse River, 185
Neutrality Act, 344
Nevada, 301
Nevis, 35, 37, 38, 84, 95, 151, 152
New Bedford, 115
New England, 87, 146, 283, 304, 330, 359; trade, 35, 37, 41
New Orleans, 158, 193, 275; battle of, 115; Butler's rule in, 222, 223
New Régime, The, 142
New River Railway, 273, 281
New York, 67, 68, 71, 78, 83, 91, 95, 97, 107, 115, 146, 156-158, 162, 163, 165, 166, 168, 176, 178, 191-193, 207, 208, 214-216, 260, 285, 289, 299, 303, 304, 322, 330, 359; steamship lines to, 284-285; trade rivalry with, 153-157
New York *Evening Post,* 282, 286-287
New York, Philadelphia, and Norfolk Railroad, 280
New York *Tribune,* 212
New Zealand, 326
Newburn, 165
Newcombe, John F., 278
Newell, John, Jr., 124
Newport, R. I., 72
Newport News, 110, 213, 214, 277, 283, 297, 300, 301, 304, 307, 313, 316, 327, 369
Newspapers, 141-142, 256
Newsweek, 375

Newton, George, 6, 122
Newton, Nathaniel, 6, 19
Newton, Thomas, Jr., 65, 69, 71, 124, 138, 148, 149, 150, 153
Newton, 54
Newton home, 293, 294
Newton home, old, 292
Newton's Creek, 4, 5, 33, 92, 260, 261
Niagara, 284
Nivison, John, 91
Nixon's circus, 268
Noe's Bridge, 261
Non-Intercourse Act, 108-109
Norfolk and Carolina Railroad, 278, 279
Norfolk and Great Western Railroad, 279, 281
Norfolk and Petersburg Railroad, 182-185, 209, 216, 261, 268, 271, 272
Norfolk and Southern Railroad, 278, 296
Norfolk and Western Railroad, 4, 185, 258, 273, 281-283, 289, 326, 369; grade crossing at Colonial Avenue, 302; *see also* Atlantic, Mississippi, and Ohio Railroad
Norfolk County, 5, 22, 27, 61, 66, 68, 71, 80, 167, 285, 331, 351, 356, 357, 363-365
Norfolk Division, College of William and Mary, 340, 382, 385-387
Norfolk Division, Virginia State College, 385
Norfolk Education Association, 388
Norfolk General Hospital, 358, 372
Norfolk–Hampton Roads Company, 297
Norfolk Knitting and Cotton Manufacturing Company, 261
Norfolk National Bank, 258
Norfolk Rough and Ready Club, 199
Norfolk Shipbuilding and Dry Dock Company, 310
Norma, 262
North Africa, invasion of, 356, 360
North Anna River, battle of, 230
North Carolina, 18, 26, 29, 40, 47, 61, 88, 113, 114, 156, 176, 198, 209, 210, 225, 229, 278, 280, 283, 285, 286, 330, 331, 335; annexation to, 178-179, 183, 184; trade with, 30-35, 76, 91, 158, 164; troops from, 57, 59
North Carolina, 165
North Carolina Railway, 274, 275
North Carolina Supreme Court, 173
North Landing, 114
North River, 114, 185
North West River, 34
Northampton County, N. C., 167
Northampton County, Va., 80, 331
Northumberland County, 286
Northwestern Virginia Railway, 177
Norview High School, 389
Norway, 304

Nottoway, 170
Nottoway River, 161, 358

Oak Grove, 192, 229, 230
Obolinski, Prince, 269
Ocean View, 217, 249, 289, 323, 328, 340, 350, 367, 375, 385; development of, 295
Ocean View Boulevard, 338
Ocean View Elementary School, 340, 342, 351
Ocean View Hotel, 295
Ocean View jetty, 339, 342, 345
Ocean View Railroad Company, 295
Ocracoke inlet, 30, 32, 33, 41
Odd Fellows' Hall, 259, 261
"Ode to the Virginian Voyage," 382
Odum, J. B., 181
Office of Defense Transportation, 358
Ohio Creek, 323
Ohio River, 174-177, 198
Old Coffee House, 122
Old Dominion line, 285
Old Point Comfort, 3, 201, 209, 214-216, 224, 262, 294, 295, 367
Oliver, T. S., 290
Olney Road, 289, 371
O'Neale, Captain, 157
One-hundred-eleventh Field Artillery, 310, 316
One-hundred-fifteenth Infantry Regiment, 312
One-hundred-sixteenth Infantry Regiment, 310-313, 316
Opera, 262
Opera House, 119, 201, 209, 261, 263, 267
Orataro, 36
Orinoco tobacco, 3, 27
Ormont Farm, 313
Ornes, 312
O'Rourke, James, 266
Osborne's warehouse, 45
Osthagen, Clarence S., 369
Otter, 53, 62, 65, 67

Page, Thomas Nelson, 297
Page and Allen's shipyard, 165, 191
Pakenham, General, 115
Pamlico Sound, 30, 32, 33, 41, 114, 160, 185, 210, 211, 286
Panama, 326
Panchon, pitcher, 265
Paradise Creek, 309
Paris, 168, 260
Park Avenue, 255, 261
Park Place, 291
Parker Street, 92
Parkersburg, 175, 177
Parks, Hattie, 269
Parliament, 41, 64, 149
Pasquotank precinct, 34

Pasquotank River, 29, 34, 159, 167
Pasteur, James, 23, 24
Patapsco River, 168
Patrick Henry, 169, 213-215
Patti, Adelina, 117
Patton, General George S., Jr., 356
Paulding, Rear Admiral, 208
Pawnee, 208
Peace and Plenty, 63
Peanut growing, 285
Pearl Harbor, 353, 354, 361
Pearl of Savoy, The, 263
Pearle, 32
Pedrick, John, 10
Peggy, 39, 46, 50
Peirpoint, Francis H., 221-225, 227, 232-235, 271
Pender Building, 354
Peninsula, invasion of the, 216, 229
Pennock, William, 93, 124, 163
Pennsylvania, 27, 83, 176, 198, 228, 298
Pennsylvania, 207, 208
Pennsylvania Railroad, 280, 286
Pepper's, 271
Pericles, 118
Perquimans precinct, 35
Perquimans River, 31, 33
Perry, 165
Pershing, General John J., 312, 313
Petersburg, 44, 76, 78, 79, 82, 83, 91, 101, 111, 114, 122, 149, 158, 162, 164, 168-169, 175, 176, 183, 192, 207, 229, 240, 265, 277, 303, 313; siege of, 229
Petersburg, 161
Petersburg and Roanoke Railroad, 167, 171-173, 179, 182
Petersburg *Intelligencer*, 168, 181
Phaeton, 18
Phi Beta Kappa Hall, 382
Phidias, 118
Philadelphia, 25, 40, 79, 81, 83, 86, 88, 91, 130, 140, 146, 163, 165, 166, 168, 193, 281, 284, 285, 299, 310, 322, 327
Philharmonic Association, 117
Philipia bay, 97
Phillips, General, 72
Philips, Daniel, 10
Phillips, Josiah, 71
Phoebus, Mr., 294
Phoenix, 87
Phripp, Matthew, 54
Piedmont railway, 275
Pierce, Franklin, 199
Pierce, Thomas W., 245
Pilot Boy, 218
Pine Beach, 308
Pineapple, 40
Pinner's Point, 209, 278-280, 289, 366
Pioneer, 164
Pitt, William, 50, 76

Pittsylvania County, 175
Piracy, 32-33
Planning Commission, 362-363
Planter, 109
Platt, James H., 239-243
Pleasant Valley, Md., 230
Pleasure-driving ban, 356
Plume, William, 124
Plume & Company's Rope and Oakum Works, 144
Plume Street, 131, 251, 293, 341
Plymouth, 208, 212, 218
Pocahontas, 3, 298
Pocahontas coal region, 273, 281, 282
Poe, Edgar Allan, 117, 377
Poems, Patriotic, Religious and Miscellaneous, 120
Poetry, 120
Poets' Corner, 378
Point Peter, 190
Point Pleasant, battle of, 67
Poland, Hitler's attack on, 346
Police protection, 9-10, 253-255, 324, 325
Polish Corridor, 346
Pollard, Joseph A., police chief, 255
Polly, 39
Polytechnic Institute, Norfolk, 385
PM, 352
Pope, General John, 230
Port Authority, Norfolk, 368
Port Authority, Virginia State, 327, 369
Port Republic, 87
Port-au-Prince, 96
Porten, William, county clerk, 5
Porter, John L., 213
Porter and Dyson, 165
Portland, Me., 282
Portlock, 358
Portsmouth, 22, 33, 53, 61, 65, 66, 68, 70-73, 75, 84-86, 91, 97, 113, 126, 142, 144, 154, 165, 168-171, 180-182, 192, 201, 202, 207, 209, 224, 226, 227, 229, 230, 260, 266, 268, 275, 280, 289, 300, 304, 305, 309, 320, 356, 357, 366
Portsmouth and Weldon Railroad, *see* Seaboard and Roanoke Railroad
Portsmouth Baptist Church, 137
Portsmouth Grays, 170
Portsmouth parish, 23
Portsmouth Rough and Ready Club, 199
Portugal, 107
Poscaty region, 34
Post, Norfolk, 158, 248, 254, 256, 264
Potomac, 347
Potomac Boat Club, 266
Potomac River, 3, 27, 38, 43, 67, 76, 158, 177, 230, 266, 286
Powell, Grace, 18
Powell's Point, 31

Powhatan, 157, 165
Powtomac creek, 157
Presbyterian Church, 132, 137, 139, 144
Pretlow, Mary Denson, Branch Library, 385
Price, Mr., 190, 191
Price, Thomas, 16
Prince of Wales, 87
Princess Anne Country Club, 296
Princess Anne County, 5, 14, 20, 27, 30, 54, 55, 61, 66, 68, 71, 80, 121, 135, 199, 217, 225, 229, 249, 261, 285, 331, 356, 357, 363-365
Princess Anne Hotel, 296
Princess Anne Road, 61, 89, 111, 289
Prison, *see* Jail
Privateering, 38-40, 90, 95-97
Proby, Paul, 16
Providence, R. I., 130, 285
Public Ledger, 256; for earlier newspaper, *see Gazette and Public Ledger*
Public Library, *see* Library, Norfolk Public
Public Relations Institute, 364
Public Safety Building, 374; Plate XX
Public schools, 255, 325, 351, 387-394
Public Works Administration, 338-343, 379, 386
Pulitzer prize, 393
Purcell House, 258

Quarles, C. H., 267
Quartermaster General, 321
Quashabee, cook, 20
Quebec, 40, 107
Queen Street causeway, 261
Quigley, Chief Yeoman, 302

Race riots, 233-235
Racing, 121, 267-268
Railroads, 166-187, 271-283, 369
Raleigh, N. C., 178, 213, 274
Raleigh and Augusta Railroad, 275
Raleigh and Gaston Railroad, 180-181, 274, 275
Raleigh Square, 298
Ramsey, Dr. George, 14
Randolph, Edward, 28
Randolph, George W., 217
Randolph, Sir John, 8
Randolph, John, of Roanoke, 120
Ranger, 39, 90
Rannie, Mr., 117
Rappahannock River, 43, 44, 76
Rationing, 355-356
Ravanche de Cerf, 109
Ravin de Molleville, 313
Real Estate Board, 348
Reams, E. H., 282
Reconstruction, 232-246

Reconstruction Finance Corporation, 333
Recreation, for servicemen, 351-352
Red Italia, 314
Redevelopment and Housing Authority, Norfolk, 369-376; Plates XVIII and XIX
Redwood, John, 6
Reed, Dr. and Mrs. Thomas H., 363, 364
Reed, Walter, 189, 197
Reed Street, 92
Reid, Governor, 181
Reid, Charles, 184
Reid, William, 181, 196
Reid and Soulter, 181
Relief Association, Norfolk, 332
Relief for the unemployed, 332-335
Rennert Building, 375; Plate XIX
Republican Blues, 101
Republicans, 201-202
Resolution, 95
Retail Dealers Association, 335
Reval, 276, 277
Revenge, 97
Revolution, American, 40, 48-73, 103
Reynolds Brothers, 284; warehouse, 276
Rhode Island, 36, 79
Rhonnald, Alexander, 23
Richard III, 118
Richmond, 44, 76, 82, 88, 91, 108, 110, 111, 114, 123, 149, 157, 158, 161, 162, 165, 167, 174, 175-177, 182, 184, 186, 192, 193, 195, 210, 213, 216-218, 232, 273, 275, 277, 278, 296, 319, 326, 336, 369, 381-383, 385, 387; evacuation of, 121; secession convention in, 205-206; trade rivalry with, 167-175, 272; trolley cars in, 288
Richmond, 164
Richmond, Earl of, 64
Richmond and Danville Railroad, 182, 272, 274, 278, 279
Richmond and Petersburg Railroad, 179, 180
Richmond *Dispatch,* 210, 256
Richmond *Enquirer,* 277
Richmond, Fredericksburg, and Potomac Railroad, 172, 179, 180
Richmond Grays, 207
Richmond Light Infantry Blues, 101, 164
Richmond *Times,* 176
Richmond *Times-Dispatch,* 375-376
Ricks and Milhado, 284
Riddick, Willis, 80
Ridgeway, 181
Riffand's Garden, 116
Rip Van Winkle, 263, 353
Rives, Captain Francis E., 172-173
Roanoke, 162, 165, 214

Roanoke dock, 253
Roanoke inlet, 30
Roanoke Island, 211, 212, 229
Roanoke River, 34, 114, 160-162, 167, 169, 170-172, 181, 182, 271
Roanoke Sound, 30
Roanoke Square, 234
Roanoke Valley Railroad, 181
Robert Gatewood School, 342
Roberts, William D., 196
Roberts Park, 371
Robertson, Moses, 23
Robertson and Sully, 116
Robinson, Patrick, 72
Robinson, Captain William, 5
Rochambeau, General, 73
Rochelle and Smith, 172
Rocketts, 84, 178, 277
Roebuck, 67
Rogers, Colonel George T., 229
Rogers, H. H., 282-283
Rogers, Samuel, 19
Rolfe, John, 3
Roosevelt, Franklin D., 333, 335, 340, 344, 346, 347
Roosevelt, Theodore, 297
Roper, Mayor Albert L., 321
Rosainville's Bower, 121
Roscoe, William, 120
Ross, Alexander, 18
Rothery's Lane, 87
Rouke, Johnny, 134
Rowing, 266-267
Royall, Mrs. Anne, 127, 129, 134, 142
Royster Building, 293, 294, 314
Rudd, William, 23
Ruffner Junior High School, 351
Rush, Richard, 147
Russia, 304
Russians, visit of, 263, 269
Ryan, Abram Joseph, Father, 120, 377
Ryan and Gayle, 165

Sable Island, 284
St. Augustine, 55, 68
St. Bartholomew's, 108
St. Christopher, 37, 39
St. George, Bermuda, 145
St. Helena Extension, College of William and Mary, 386
St. Jago de Cuba (Santiago), 108
St. James Hotel, 258
St. John's, 148, 150, 152
St. Lawrence, 164, 214
St. Luke's Church, 341
St. Martin's, 39
St. Mary's, 27, 137
St. Mihiel salient, 314
St. Nazaire, 311, 314
St. Patrick's Church, 144

St. Paul's Church, 92, 135-136, 143, 259, 377; Plate VI; *see also* Church, Norfolk Parish
St. Thomas, 41, 191
St. Vincent de Paul Hospital, 259, 358
St. Vincent's, 46
Salisbury, N. C., 274
Sally, 40
Salusbury, L. C., 267
Salvation Army, 332, 334
Sammer, France, 314
Samogneux, 312, 313
Sampson, Captain, 51
San Domingo, 37, 40, 41, 85, 96, 137; refugees from, 88-89
San Francisco, 300
Sanborn, Lieutenant, killed, 221
Sandwich, Earl of, 64
Sangster's, 248
Sanspareil, 90
Santegan, Louis, 88
Sapin, 107
Sarah, 96
Saratoga, 284
Sardo and Company, 262
Savannah, 109, 193, 275, 285
Sawtelle, Colonel, 227
Sawyer's ferry, 34
Sayer's Point, 33, 35
Schenkman, Edgar, 381-382
Schiller, J. C. F. von, 263
Schofield, General John M., 235, 237, 241
School of Scandal, 117
Schools, Public, *see* Public Schools
Schwarzkopf, A. B., 336
Schweitzer, Paul, 392-393
Scotland, 25, 45, 46, 190
Scotland Neck, 114, 160
Scott, John P., 140
Sculpture, 120-121
Seaboard Air Line, 369
Seaboard and Roanoke Railroad, 167-173, 179-184, 209, 211, 216, 271, 274, 275, 278; station, 268
Seaboard Boat Club, 266
Seaboard Citizens National Bank, 334
Sea-Horse, 164
Seawell, Leon T., 336
Secession movement, 202-205
Second Infantry Division, 315
Secret of Guilde Court, 263
Segar, A. S., 242, 243
Seine River, 168
Selden, Dr. Samuel, 294
Selden, Dr. William, 294
Selma, N. C., 279, 280
Senate, U. S., 82
Senate, Virginia, 184
Seven Pines, 229

Seventy-ninth Division, 313
Seventy-seventh Infantry Division, 315
Sewells Point, 209, 213, 214, 218, 283, 289, 297, 304, 306, 308
Sewells Point Road, 350
Sewerage, 250-251
Shakespeare, William, 119
Shallote island, 40
Sharp, Charles, 277
Sharpsburg, 229, 230
Shaw, John, 53
She Stoops to Conquer, 262
Sheffield, George W., 141
Shenandoah Valley, 175-177, 230
Shepherd, Solomon, 80
Shipbuilding, 41-43, 77, 85, 86, 146, 164-165, 308, 359
Shockoes, 83
Shortages, in First World War, 306-307; in Second World War, 355-359
Sicily, 87
Sikes, Levi, 61
Simpson, Francis, 6
Sims, Admiral W. S., 301
Sixteenth Irish Division, 314
Sixth Virginia Regiment, 229-231
Sizemore, Samuel, 6
Sketches of Norfolk, 198
Skorup, J. J., Jr., 335, 336
Slaughter, Dr. Augustine, 139
Slave trade, 38
Slavery, in Norfolk, 127, 197-198
Sloane, Mrs. William, 377-379
Slum clearance, 370-373
Smallpox, 13; inoculation against, 188-189
Smith, Mr., 241
Smith, Mr., of the Borough Tavern, 81
Smith, Brenda Lee, 389
Smith, Charles, 13, 23
Smith, Captain John, 298
Smith, Meriwether, 78
Smith, Peter, first resident, 5
Smith, Peter, and Company's store, 288
Smith, Samuel, 6
Smith, W. A., 274
Smith, Captain William, 49
Smith Harbor, 298
Smith's Creek, 111, 260-261, 287-289
Socials, 265
Society of Arts, Norfolk, 377-378
Society of Constitutional and Governmental Support, 90
Sons of Houn, 233
Sons of Liberty, 49
Sophia, 87
South Carolina, 40, 85, 155, 203, 210, 229, 260, 342, 383
South Mountain, 230
South Norfolk, 289, 363, 388

Southampton, 165
Southampton County, 167
Southern Branch, 33-35, 53, 54, 56, 57, 103, 114, 159, 163, 164, 183, 212, 250, 339, 345, 350; *see also* Elizabeth River
Southern Department, Continental Army, 65
Southern Literary Messenger, 119
Southern Railway, 279, 280
Southern Rights Association, 203
Southgate, John, 93
Southgate's wharf, 190
Southside Railroad, 182-184, 272, 273
Spain, 14, 25, 344
Spangenberg, Bishop, 35
Spaniards, riot over, 22
Sparrows, Smith, 42
Spaulding, James, 11
Speddin, Robert, 63, 66
Sports, 121, 265-268
Spotswood, Governor Alexander, 23, 32-33, 41
Spotsylvania, 228-230
Springfield, 254
Springfield, Ohio, 319
Sprowle, Andrew, 40, 53, 63, 66
Stamp Act, 49-50, 52
Standard Oil Company, 310
Standish, 266
Stanhope, Major F. W., 235
Stanton, Edwin M., 213, 217, 222, 225
Stapleton, Mr., 193
State Department, U. S., 354
Staunton, 175, 291, 319
Staunton River, 161, 181
Steamboats, effect on trade, 157-158
Steiner, Richard L., 374
Stephens, Colonel, 59
Sterling, Maggie, 267
Stewart, Robert, 71
Stevens, Ebenezer, 9
Stevens, S. A., furniture house, 292; *see also* Ames and Stevens
Stevens, Thaddeus, 232, 235
Stock market crash of 1929, 328-329
Stockley Gardens, 261
Stockton, Cal., 323
Strange, John D., 141
Strasburg, 276
Street lights, 133, 252-253
Streetcars, 288-290; Plate IX
Streets, maintenance of, 9, 130, 252, 319-320, 342
Stringer, John, 80
Stuyvesant, Peter, 298
Styx, 262
Suburban and City Railway, 288
Suburban development, 6, 287-291
Sudetenland, 344

Suffolk, 33, 44, 57, 61, 70, 106, 169, 170, 171, 183, 192, 239, 240, 265, 278, 300, 313
Sugar Act, resistance to, 48-49
Sugar trade, 35-38, 153-154, 330
Sukey and Juno, 87
Sully, Mr., 118
Sumner, 97
Supreme Court, U. S., 337, 387
Supreme Court of Appeals, Virginia, 364, 390
Surry County, 44
Susan, 109
Susanna, 39
Sussex County, 167
Swallow, 46
Swanson, Claude A., 297, 321
Sweden, 108, 304
Sweetscented tobacco, 3, 27
Swetlana, 269
Swift and Co., 290
Swindell, James H., 117
Sykes, Mr., 241
Symphony, Norfolk, 380-382
Syracuse, N. Y., 193

Tabb, Mayor Thomas, 232, 234, 248, 271
Tabb, Thomas C., superintendent of schools, 255
Tabor, Dr. Thomas, 6
Talbot, Isaac, 165
Talbot, Captain Thomas, 15
Talbot House, 358
Talbot Park, 358
Talbot Street, 15, 117, 129
Taliaferro, General William B., 207, 209
Talou Hill, 312
Taming of the Shrew, The, 262
Tanner's Creek, 64, 65, 111, 209, 217, 289, 291; *see also* Lafayette River
Tanner's Creek district, 363-364
Tar River, 185
Tarboro, 278
Tar-burning, 28
Tariff, 152-153
Tasso, Torquato, 93
Tatnall, Flag-Officer Josiah, 216, 218
Tatum, Captain Nathaniel, 12, 42
Taussig, Admiral Joseph K., 347-348, 352
Taverns, 18-19, 91
Taylor, James, 80, 87
Taylor, Dr. James, 92
Taylor, Jennie, 267
Taylor, General Robert B., 91, 111, 122, 124, 270; Plate IV
Taylor, Colonel W. H., 242
Taylor, Mayor W. R. L., 338-340
Taylor, Zachary, 199
Taylor Building, 292; Plate XII

Tazewell, L. W., 266
Tazewell, Littleton W., 91, 102, 124, 138, 270
Tazewell house, 143, 293
Tazewell Street, 293, 323
Tea Act, 50; Norfolk's opposition to, 51
Teach, William (Blackbeard), 32-33
Teneriffe, 87
Tennessee, 260, 280
Terminal development, 322, 369
Texas, 309
Thames, 168
Theater, 117-119, 261-264, 382
Theseus, temple of, 140
Third British Army, 314
Thirtieth Illinois Regiment, 248
Thirtieth Regiment, 234
Thirty-fourth English Division, 314
Thirty-ninth Illinois Regiment, 265
Thirty-seventh Street pumping station, 358
Thirty-third Division, 312, 314
Thomas, Charles, 39
Thomas and Sarah, 46
Thompson, Fergus, 6
Thompson, John, 39
Thompson, Philip R., 139
Thompson, Randall, 382
Thompson, Thomas P., city manager, 339, 340, 348
Thorne, Jennie, 267
Thoroughgood, Adam, House, 353
Thorowgood's Farm, 121
Three Blind Mice, 262
Three-hundred-eighteenth Infantry Regiment, 313-316
Throckmorton, R. J., 336
Thruston, Malachi, 6
Thuillier, Mr., 122
Tidewater Artists, 378
Tidewater Drive, 367
Tidewater Educational Foundation, 388
Tidewater Ministerial Union, 332
Tidewater Park, 371
Tidewater Terminals, Norfolk, Inc., 322
Tidewater Virginia Development Council, 369
Timber cutting, 29
Timberlake, James B., & Co., 87
Titustown schools, 351
Tobacco trade, 3, 27-28, 43-44, 82-83, 327, 330
Tobago, 95
Tokyo, 354
Toomer, Captain James H., 230
Toomoth, James, 11
Toomoth, Mary, 11
Topham, Augustus, 99
Tories in Norfolk, 52-63, 69-73
Tournaments, 267

Town Bridge, 8, 9, 12, 131
Town Hall, 79, 90, 99, 100, 122, 149, 152
Town Point, 52, 62, 80, 81, 87, 128, 183, 190, 191, 194, 248
Towns, acts to create, 4
Townshend, Charles, 50, 52
Trade, 27-47, 75-87, 104-109, 113-115, 145-171, 186-187, 271-287, 300-301, 303-306, 326-327, 330, 368-369
Traffic problems, in Second World War, 349-350
Travelers Aid Society, 331-332, 334
Travis, Lieutenant, 58
Trinidad, 277
Tripoli, 125
Triumphant, 90
Trolley cars introduced, 288-289
Truck farming, 285-287, 307, 331
Truman, Harry S, 360
Truxton, 309
Truxton, I. Walke, 324, 331
Truxton Manor Golf Course, 341
Tschudi, Richard B., 141
Tucker, Captain, 12
Tucker, John, 42, 47
Tucker, Mrs. Richard, 378
Tucker, Robert, 15, 23
Tucker's Mill, 72; Dunmore's camp at, 65-66
Tully, Cornelius, 6
Tunis and Park, lumber company, 294
Tunis and Serpell Lumber Co., 278
Tunstall, Alexander, 153
Tunstall, Robert W., 256
Turf Association, Norfolk, 267
Turkey, 25, 330
Turkey Ridge, battle of, 230
Turks Island, 45, 46
Turner, Henry L., 267
Tuttle's soda fountain, 248
Twelfth Street Armory, 354
Twelfth Virginia Infantry Regiment, 229
Twentieth New York Infantry, 233, 234
Twenty-ninth Division, 310-313, 316
Twenty-seventh Massachusetts Infantry, 226
Twenty-sixth French Division, 312
Twenty-sixth Street Bridge, 340, 345
Two Friends, 39
Two Penny Point, 268
Tyler, Mr., 246
Tyler, John, 79
Tyler, President John, 155, 181
Typhoid mortality rate, 326

Uncle Tom's Cabin, 198
Underwood, John C., 232
Undine Boat Club, 266
Union, Norfolk, 220

Union, steamboat, 165
Union League, 236
Union Missions, 332, 334, 335
Union Street, 128, 129, 234, 252, 253
United Artillery, 229
United Charities, 332
United Fire Company, 253, 268
United Fund, 372
United Service Organizations, 352, 358; management committee, 351
United States Bank, 165
University of Virginia, 120, 256, 381
Upton Street, 190
Urban Renewal Administration, 374

Vacherauville, 312
Valmy, battle at, 89
Vauxhall Gardens, 121
Venice, 93
Venus, 109
Verdun, battle of, 303
Verpel, 315
Vestry, Elizabeth River parish, 22-24
Vewby's ferry, 34
Victory Loan, 303
Viele, General Egbert L., 217, 220-222
Vigilant, 109
Virginia (Merrimac), 212-219
Virginia, propeller steamship, 284
Virginia, steamboat, 164
Virginia and North Carolina Transportation Company, 161
Virginia and Tennessee Railroad, 182, 184, 272, 273
Virginia Bank, 165, 191
Virginia Beach, 295-296, 328, 347, 350, 358, 382
Virginia Central Railroad, 178, 184
Virginia Chronicle and Norfolk and Portsmouth General Advertiser, 141
Virginia Club, 302
Virginia Coal and Navigation Company, 310
Virginia Company, 3
Virginia Federal Convention of 1788, 119
Virginia Gazette, 25, 39, 46, 141
Virginia Military Institute, 298
Virginia Military Reservation, 347
Virginia Polytechnic Institute, 298, 386
Virginian, 316
Virginian-Pilot, 256, 292, 301, 304, 306, 309, 310, 319, 326, 329, 330, 336, 337, 339, 340, 346, 351, 353, 393
Virginia Railway, 282-283, 326, 369
Virginia State College, 385
Virginia Union University, 385
Vizenneau, Peter, 88
Volker Stellung, 312
Voss, Israel, 6

Wainwaring, Captain, 22
Waiting for the Verdict, 262
Wakefield, 313
Walcott, 120
Walke, Anthony, 14, 80
Walke, Thomas, 6, 80
Walker, Gilbert C., 235, 238, 241-243, 272
Walker, Thomas, 18
Walker Street, 133
Waller, D. W., 119
Waller, William, 266
Walter, Thomas U., 140
Walters, Bray B., 196
Walters, Harry, 278
Walthall, 179
Walthall, Byron, 120
War Board, 305
War Department, U. S., 103, 321
War of 1812, 109-115, 141, 159-160, 165, 354
Ward, Dr., 188
Warren, Admiral, 113
Warren County, N. C., 161
Warren County, Va., 389
Warren's wharf, 190
Washington, 157, 165
Washington, George, 25, 69, 72-73, 79, 81, 82, 174
Washington, D. C., 106, 113, 140, 157, 172, 175, 192, 213-215, 223, 230, 266, 274, 292, 300, 326, 339, 341, 348, 363, 387, 388
Washington Point, 142, 144
Washington Street, 91
Washington's birthday balls, 122
Water Street, 4, 92, 93, 115, 118, 122, 125, 126, 127, 129, 131, 183, 252, 276, 282, 292
Water supply, 11-12, 133-134, 247-250, 320-321, 349
Waverly, 313
Webb, James, 80
Webb, Mollie, 267
Webber, William, 266
Webster, Daniel, 155
Weisdorf's band, 243
Weld, Isaac, 33, 88
Weldon, 161, 167, 170-172, 178, 180, 181, 192, 217, 271
Weldon and Wilmington Railroad, 171-172, 180, 279
Wells, H. H., 238, 242, 243
Wells, Otto, 336
Wertz String Quartet, 378
Wescott, Wright, 16, 69
West, Mrs., 92
West Ghent, 292

West Indies, 14, 35-47, 48, 49, 64, 68, 70, 76-82, 84-91, 95, 105-107, 110, 145-153, 157, 188, 304
West Point, Va., 277, 279, 280
West Virginia, 222, 273, 274, 280, 281, 283, 304, 328
Western Branch, 285
Western Branch Belt Railroad, 278
Westham, 83
Westwood, Worlick, 80
Wheat trade, *see* Grain trade
Wheeling, 175, 177
Whigs, 199-201
White, Captain and Mrs., 225
White, Fuller, 9
White, Leonard D., 324
White Hardware Company, 291
Whitehaven, 51
Whitehead, Alexander, 136, 138
Whitehead, Henry Cowles, 381
Whitehead, James, 136, 138-139
Whitehead, John B., 244-245
Whitehead, Dr. N. C., 124
Whitehead, Dr. R. C., 380-381
Whitehurst, killed, 234-235
Whittle, Conway and Fortescue, 96
Wide-Water Street, 115
Wigwam Gardens, 93, 121
Wilcox's Farm, 230
Wild, General E. A., 225, 227, 229
Wilderness, battle of the, 229, 230
Willard School, 351
William and Mary, 87
William and Mary, College of, 24, 385-387
William and Mary Opera Workshop, 382
William Kennedy, 284
William Lawrence, 284
William Selden, 218
Williams, Captain, 98
Williams, John, 237
Williamsburg, 25, 54, 57, 382, 387
Williamson, William P., 213
Willock's Lane, 129
Willoughby jetty, 342
Willoughby Spit, 289, 340, 367
Wills, Josiah, 181, 196
Wilmington, Del., 185, 288
Wilmington, N. C., 113, 114, 172, 274, 326
Wilmington and Shelby Railroad, 275
Wilson, Woodrow, 300, 301, 308
Wimble, Nancy, 21
Winchester, 175
Winchester and Potomac Railroad, 176
Wing, Dr. W. W., 235, 236
Wingfield, Rev. S. H., 227
Winthrope, Mrs. Munroe, 228
Wirt, William, 124, 135

Wise, Captain George, 112
Wise, Henry A., 192, 200, 201, 211, 229
Wise, Nicholas, 4, 5
Withers, R. E., 238-239, 242
Wolfe Street, 93, 205
Woman's Club, 336
Woman's Council of the Navy League, 358-359
Wonycott, Nicholas, 69
Wood, Anna Cogswell, 264
Wood, Mayor J. D., 354
Woodford, Colonel William, 57-61, 63-64
Woodis, Mayor Hunter, 193, 196, 270
Woodis Rifles, 229
Woodside's Lane, 93, 190, 191
Woodworth, Rev. C. L., 226
Wool, General John E., 217, 220, 222
Works Progress Administration, 338, 341-343, 382, 383
World War, First, 300-317, 362, 377
World War, Second, 344-361
Wright, Dr. David M., 221
Wright, Penelope, 221

Wright, William, 87
Wyatt, Governor Francis, 3
Wythe, George, 80

X. Y. Z. affair, 90, 95

Yale College, 119
Yellow fever, 13, 188-197
Y. M. C. A., 258, 264, 294
Yoncq, 315, 316
York County, 80
York River, 25, 27, 43, 46, 83, 213, 216, 278, 279
York Street, 261
Yorktown, 233, 308; surrender at, 72-73
Yorktown, 165
Yorktown centennial, 256
Young Park, 371
Youthful Days of Richelieu, 262
Y. W. C. A., 352

Zion's Sons, 233

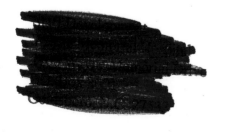

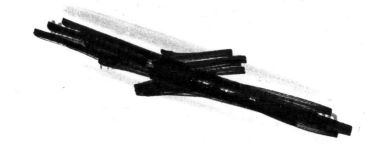

Bradley's Neurology in Clinical Practice

Staff Development
Wayne Memorial Hospital
2700 Wayne Memorial Drive
P.O. Box 8001
Goldsboro, N.C. 27533

We dedicate this book to our families in acknowledgement of their understanding and support.

Bradley's Neurology in Clinical Practice

VOLUME I

SEVENTH EDITION

ROBERT B. DAROFF, MD
Professor, and Chair Emeritus
Department of Neurology
Case Western Reserve School of Medicine
University Hospitals Case Medical Center
Cleveland, OH, USA

JOSEPH JANKOVIC, MD
Professor of Neurology
Distinguished Chair in Movement Disorders
Director of Parkinson's Disease Center and Movement
   Disorders Clinic
Department of Neurology
Baylor College of Medicine
Houston, TX, USA

JOHN C. MAZZIOTTA, MD, PhD
Vice Chancellor of UCLA Health Sciences
Dean, David Geffen School of Medicine
CEO UCLA Health
University of California, Los Angeles
Los Angeles, CA, USA

SCOTT L. POMEROY, MD, PhD
Bronson Crothers Professor of Neurology
Director, Intellectual and Developmental Disabilities
   Research Center
Harvard Medical School
Chair, Department of Neurology
Neurologist-in-Chief
Boston Children's Hospital
Boston, MA, USA

For additional online content visit expertconsult.com

ELSEVIER   London, New York, Oxford, Philadelphia, St Louis, Sydney, Toronto

---

Notices

Knowledge and best practice in this field are constantly changing. As new research and experience broaden our understanding, changes in research methods, professional practices, or medical treatment may become necessary.

Practitioners and researchers must always rely on their own experience and knowledge in evaluating and using any information, methods, compounds, or experiments described herein. In using such information or methods they should be mindful of their own safety and the safety of others, including parties for whom they have a professional responsibility.

With respect to any drug or pharmaceutical products identified, readers are advised to check the most current information provided (i) on procedures featured or (ii) by the manufacturer of each product to be administered, to verify the recommended dose or formula, the method and duration of administration, and contraindications. It is the responsibility of practitioners, relying on their own experience and knowledge of their patients, to make diagnoses, to determine dosages and the best treatment for each individual patient, and to take all appropriate safety precautions.

To the fullest extent of the law, neither the Publisher nor the authors, contributors, or editors, assume any liability for any injury and/or damage to persons or property as a matter of products liability, negligence or otherwise, or from any use or operation of any methods, products, instructions, or ideas contained in the material herein.

ISBN: 978-0-323-28783-8
eISBN: 978-0-323-33916-2

Content Strategist: Charlotta Kryhl
Content Development Specialist: Joanne Scott
Content Coordinators: Humayra Rahman Khan, Samuel Crowe
Project Manager: Andrew Riley
Design: Miles Hitchen
Illustration Manager: Karen Giacomucci
Illustrator: Joe Chovan
Marketing Manager: Michele Milano

Printed in China

Last digit is the print number: 9 8 7 6 5 4 3 2

Working together to grow libraries in developing countries

www.elsevier.com • www.bookaid.org

Contents

Dedication, ii

Foreword, ix

Preface, x

List of Contributors, xi

Video Table of Contents, xviii

Volume 1: Principles of Diagnosis

PART I
Common Neurological Problems

1 **Diagnosis of Neurological Disease, 1**
Robert B. Daroff, Joseph Jankovic, John C. Mazziotta,
Scott L. Pomeroy

2 **Episodic Impairment of Consciousness, 8**
Joseph Bruni

3 **Falls and Drop Attacks, 17**
Bernd F. Remler, Robert B. Daroff

4 **Delirium, 23**
Mario F. Mendez, Claudia R. Padilla

5 **Stupor and Coma, 34**
Joseph R. Berger

6 **Brain Death, Vegetative State, and Minimally
Conscious States, 51**
Jennifer E. Fugate, Eelco F.M. Wijdicks

7 **Intellectual and Memory Impairments, 57**
Howard S. Kirshner, Brandon Ally

8 **Global Developmental Delay and
Regression, 66**
Tyler Reimschisel

9 **Behavior and Personality Disturbances, 73**
HyungSub Shim, Amanda Miller, Carissa Gehl,
Jane S. Paulsen

10 **Depression and Psychosis in Neurological
Practice, 92**
David L. Perez, Evan D. Murray, Bruce H. Price

11 **Limb Apraxias and Related Disorders, 115**
Mario F. Mendez, Mariel B. Deutsch

12 **Agnosias, 122**
Howard S. Kirshner

13 **Aphasia and Aphasic Syndromes, 128**
Howard S. Kirshner

14 **Dysarthria and Apraxia of Speech, 145**
Howard S. Kirshner

15 **Neurogenic Dysphagia, 148**
Ronald F. Pfeiffer

16 **Visual Loss, 158**
Matthew J. Thurtell, Robert L. Tomsak

17 **Abnormalities of the Optic Nerve and
Retina, 163**
Sashank Prasad, Laura J. Balcer

18 **Pupillary and Eyelid Abnormalities, 179**
Matthew J. Thurtell, Janet C. Rucker

19 **Disturbances of Smell and Taste, 190**
Richard L. Doty, Steven M. Bromley

20 **Cranial and Facial Pain, 197**
J. D. Bartleson, David F. Black, Jerry W. Swanson

21 **Brainstem Syndromes, 205**
Matthew J. Thurtell, Michael Wall

22 **Ataxic and Cerebellar Disorders, 217**
S.H. Subramony, Guangbin Xia

23 **Diagnosis and Assessment of Parkinson
Disease and Other Movement
Disorders, 223**
Joseph Jankovic, Anthony E. Lang

24 **Gait Disorders, 250**
Philip D. Thompson, John G. Nutt

25 **Hemiplegia and Monoplegia, 262**
Karl E. Misulis, E. Lee Murray

26 **Paraplegia and Spinal Cord
Syndromes, 273**
Bruce H. Dobkin

27 **Proximal, Distal, and Generalized
Weakness, 279**
David C. Preston, Barbara E. Shapiro

28 **Muscle Pain and Cramps, 296**
Leo H. Wang, Glenn Lopate, Alan Pestronk

29 **Hypotonic (Floppy) Infant, 305**
W. Bryan Burnette

30 **Sensory Abnormalities of the Limbs, Trunk,
and Face, 314**
Karl E. Misulis, E. Lee Murray

31 **Arm and Neck Pain, 324**
Michael Ronthal

32 **Lower Back and Lower Limb Pain, 332**
Karl E. Misulis, E. Lee Murray

PART II
Neurological Investigations and Related Clinical Neurosciences

SECTION A   General Principles,   343

33   Laboratory Investigations in Diagnosis and Management of Neurological Disease,   343
Robert B. Daroff, Joseph Jankovic, John C. Mazziotta, Scott L. Pomeroy

SECTION B   Clinical Neurophysiology,   348

34   Electroencephalography and Evoked Potentials,   348
Cecil D. Hahn, Ronald G. Emerson

35   Clinical Electromyography,   366
Bashar Katirji

36   Neuromodulation and Transcranial Magnetic Stimulation,   391
Young H. Sohn, David H. Benninger, Mark Hallett

37   Deep Brain Stimulation,   401
Valerie Rundle-González, Zhongxing Peng-Chen, Abhay Kumar, Michael S. Okun

38   Intraoperative Monitoring,   407
Marc R. Nuwer

SECTION C   Neuroimaging,   411

39   Structural Imaging using Magnetic Resonance Imaging and Computed Tomography,   411
Bela Ajtai, Joseph C. Masdeu, Eric Lindzen

40   Vascular Imaging: Computed Tomographic Angiography, Magnetic Resonance Angiography, and Ultrasound,   459
Peter Adamczyk, David S. Liebeskind

41   Functional Neuroimaging: Functional Magnetic Resonance Imaging, Positron Emission Tomography, and Single-Photon Emission Computed Tomography,   486
Philipp T. Meyer, Michel Rijntjes, Sabine Hellwig, Stefan Klöppel, Cornelius Weiller

42   Chemical Imaging: Ligands and Pathology-Seeking Agents,   504
Vijay Chandran, A. Jon Stoessl

SECTION D   Clinical Neurosciences,   511

43   Neuropsychology,   511
Benjamin D. Hill, Justin J.F. O'Rourke, Leigh Beglinger, Jane S. Paulsen

44   Neuro-ophthalmology: Ocular Motor System,   528
Patrick J.M. Lavin

45   Neuro-ophthalmology: Afferent Visual System,   573
Matthew J. Thurtell, Robert L. Tomsak

46   Neuro-otology: Diagnosis and Management of Neuro-otological Disorders,   583
Kevin A. Kerber, Robert W. Baloh

47   Neurourology,   605
Jalesh N. Panicker, Ranan DasGupta, Amit Batla

48   Sexual Dysfunctions in Neurological Disorders,   622
Frédérique Courtois, Dany Cordeau

49   Neuroepidemiology,   635
Mitchell T. Wallin, John F. Kurtzke

50   Clinical Neurogenetics,   648
Brent L. Fogel, Daniel H. Geschwind

51   Neuroimmunology,   676
Tanuja Chitnis, Samia J. Khoury

52   Neuroendocrinology,   696
Paul E. Cooper, Stan H.M. van Uum

Volume 2: Neurological Disorders and Their Management

PART III
Neurological Diseases and Their Treatment

SECTION A   Principles of Management,   713

53   Management of Neurological Disease,   713
Robert B. Daroff, Joseph Jankovic, John C. Mazziotta, Scott L. Pomeroy

54   Principles of Pain Management,   720
Pradeep Dinakar

55   Principles of Neurointensive Care,   742
Alejandro A. Rabinstein, Jennifer E. Fugate

56   Principles of Neurointerventional Therapy,   758
Marc A. Lazzaro, Osama O. Zaidat

57   Neurological Rehabilitation,   784
Bruce H. Dobkin

SECTION B   Neurological Complications of Systemic Disease,   814

58   Neurological Complications of Systemic Disease: Adults,   814
S. Andrew Josephson, Michael J. Aminoff

59   Neurological Complications of Systemic Disease: Children,   835
Aline I. Hamati

SECTION C   Trauma of the Nervous System,   850

60   Basic Neuroscience of Neurotrauma,   850
W. Dalton Dietrich, Helen M. Bramlett

61   Sports and Performance Concussion,   860
Andrea A. Almeida, Jeffrey S. Kutcher

62 Craniocerebral Trauma, 867
Martina Stippler

63 Spinal Cord Trauma, 881
Laura A. Snyder, Lee Tan, Carter Gerard, Richard G. Fessler

64 Trauma of the Nervous System: Peripheral Nerve Trauma, 903
Bryan Tsao, Nicholas Boulis, Brian Murray

SECTION D Vascular Diseases of the Nervous System, 920

65 Ischemic Cerebrovascular Disease, 920
José Biller, Sean Ruland, Michael J. Schneck

66 Intracerebral Hemorrhage, 968
Carlos S. Kase, Ashkan Shoamanesh

67 Intracranial Aneurysms and Subarachnoid Hemorrhage, 983
Viktor Szeder, Satoshi Tateshima, Gary R. Duckwiler

68 Stroke in Children, 996
Meredith R. Golomb, José Biller

69 Spinal Cord Vascular Disease, 1007
Michael J. Lyerly, Asim K. Bag, David S. Geldmacher

70 Central Nervous System Vasculitis, 1015
James W. Schmidley

SECTION E Cancer and the Nervous System, 1018

71 Epidemiology of Brain Tumors, 1018
Dominique S. Michaud

72 Pathology and Molecular Genetics, 1026
Jason T. Huse

73 Clinical Features of Brain Tumors and Complications of Their Treatment, 1045
Mikael L. Rinne, Lakshmi Nayak

74 Primary Nervous System Tumors in Adults, 1049
Joachim M. Baehring, Fred H. Hochberg

75 Primary Nervous System Tumors in Infants and Children, 1065
Matthias A. Karajannis, Sharon L. Gardner, Jeffrey C. Allen

76 Nervous System Metastases, 1084
Robert Cavaliere, David Schiff, Patrick Wen, Kristin Huntoon

SECTION F Infections of the Nervous System, 1102

77 Neurological Manifestations of Human Immunodeficiency Virus Infection in Adults, 1102
Ashok Verma, Joseph R. Berger

78 Viral Encephalitis and Meningitis, 1121
J. David Beckham, Marylou V. Solbrig, Kenneth L. Tyler

79 Bacterial, Fungal and Parasitic Diseases of the Nervous System, 1147
Nicolaas C. Anderson, Anita A. Koshy, Karen L. Roos

SECTION G Neurological Disorders, 1159

80 Multiple Sclerosis and Other Inflammatory Demyelinating Diseases of the Central Nervous System, 1159
Michelle T. Fabian, Stephen C. Krieger, Fred D. Lublin

81 Paraneoplastic Disorders of the Nervous System, 1187
Myrna R. Rosenfeld, Josep Dalmau

82 Autoimmune Encephalitis with Antibodies to Cell Surface Antigens, 1196
Myrna R. Rosenfeld, Josep Dalmau

83 Anoxic-Ischemic Encephalopathy, 1201
Jennifer E. Fugate, Eelco F.M. Wijdicks

84 Toxic and Metabolic Encephalopathies, 1209
Karin Weissenborn, Alan H. Lockwood

85 Deficiency Diseases of the Nervous System, 1226
Yuen T. So

86 Effects of Toxins and Physical Agents on the Nervous System, 1237
Michael J. Aminoff, Yuen T. So

87 Effects of Drug Abuse on the Nervous System, 1254
John C.M. Brust

88 Brain Edema and Disorders of Cerebrospinal Fluid Circulation, 1261
Gary A. Rosenberg

89 Developmental Disorders of the Nervous System, 1279
Harvey B. Sarnat, Laura Flores-Sarnat

90 Autism and Other Developmental Disabilities, 1301
Ruth Nass, Reet Sidhu, Gail Ross

91 Inborn Errors of Metabolism and the Nervous System, 1324
K. M. Gibson, Phillip L. Pearl

92 Neurodegenerative Disease Processes, 1342
Roger A. Barker

93 Mitochondrial Disorders, 1349
Chris Turner, Anthony H.V. Schapira

94 Prion Diseases, 1365
Michael D. Geschwind

95 Alzheimer Disease and Other Dementias, 1380
Ron Peterson, Jonathan Graff-Radford

96 Parkinson Disease and Other Movement Disorders, 1422
Joseph Jankovic

97 Disorders of the Cerebellum, Including the Degenerative Ataxias, 1461
S.H. Subramony, Guangbin Xia

98 Disorders of Upper and Lower Motor
Neurons,   1484
Conor Fearon, Brian Murray, Hiroshi Mitsumoto

99 Channelopathies: Episodic and Electrical
Disorders of the Nervous System,   1519
Geoffrey A. Kerchner, Louis J. Ptáček

100 Neurocutaneous Syndromes,   1538
Monica P. Islam, E. Steve Roach

101 Epilepsies,   1563
Bassel W. Abou-Khalil, Martin J. Gallagher, Robert L. Macdonald

102 Sleep and Its Disorders,   1615
Sudhansu Chokroverty, Alon Y. Avidan

103 Headache and Other Craniofacial Pain,   1686
*Ivan Garza, Todd J. Schwedt, Carrie E. Robertson,
Jonathan H. Smith*

104 Cranial Neuropathies,   1720
Janet C. Rucker, Matthew J. Thurtell

105 Disorders of Bones, Joints, Ligaments, and
Meninges,   1736
Michael Devereaux, David Hart

106 Disorders of Nerve Roots and Plexuses,   1766
David A. Chad, Michael P. Bowley

107 Disorders of Peripheral Nerves,   1791
Bashar Katirji

108 Disorders of the Autonomic Nervous
System,   1867
Thomas Chelimsky, Gisela Chelimsky

109 Disorders of Neuromuscular
Transmission,   1896
Donald B. Sanders, Jeffrey T. Guptill

110 Disorders of Skeletal Muscle,   1915
Anthony A. Amato

111 Neurological Problems of the
Newborn,   1956
Elke Roland, Alan Hill

112 Neurological Problems of Pregnancy,   1973
D. Malcolm Shaner

113 Functional and Dissociative (Psychogenic)
Neurological Symptoms,   1992
Jon Stone, Alan Carson

Index,   I1

Foreword

In the foreword to the sixth edition of *Neurology in Clinical Practice*, I described the early history of the development of this textbook. I emphasized that we, the founding editors, considered it very important that experienced neurologists should teach the next generation the skills and art of diagnosis of neurological diseases. Much of neurological diagnosis rests on pattern recognition that comes from seeing many cases. However, that does not mean that it cannot be taught to neurologists who are still gaining experience in their profession. We all remember the clinical pearls that our mentors passed on to us. "If you see a patient with a sensory neuropathy and cerebellar syndrome, think paraneoplastic."

"A patient with funny eye movements and episodes of impaired consciousness is likely to have a mitochondriopathy." And the aphorism that I never ceased to emphasize to my residents: "You diagnose psychogenic disorder at your own peril and that of your patient!" This is still relevant today despite all the new investigative techniques; psychogenic disorders should be diagnosed on positive criteria and the possibility of a psychogenic overlay to an underlying organic condition considered. Part I of the seventh edition provides the experience of senior neurologists who have specialized in each subdiscipline. It has been expanded with two new chapters and provides a wealth of clinical wisdom.

As the current editors say in the preface to the seventh edition, in the quarter of a century since we conceptualized this textbook we have witnessed an astounding expansion in the clinical and basic neurosciences. The advances that have come in the last few years and that are of importance to the practicing neurologist will be found in the chapters in Parts II and III of this seventh edition. Five new chapters have been added to highlight new areas of understanding. The editors have maintained the freshness of the text by the addition of 60 new authors. They have expanded the electronic experience with an exciting online version with an impressive list of videos.

My old friend, Gerry Fenichel, who started *Neurology in Clinical Practice* with me, Bob Daroff and David Marsden, has now retired from the editorial board. He is ably succeeded as the lead editor for pediatric neurology by Scott Pomeroy, who is Neurologist-in-Chief at the Boston Children's Hospital.

It is now time to take stock of the changes that have occurred in the field of neurology in the last few years and to consider what we can hope for in the coming decade. The diagnosis and treatment of many of the neurological diseases, like stroke, epilepsy, MS and neurotrauma, have already improved greatly, and we can expect to see yet further advances in the coming years. We may not be able to cure or prevent these conditions, but we can do a great deal to eleviate their effect. Advances in neurogenetics have already expanded our understanding of the mechanisms of inherited neurological diseases, particularly those of infancy and childhood. In the next decade, we shall see that knowledge expand to provide effective new treatments based upon manipulation of the underlying DNA and RNA mechanisms. We may hope that in the next decade we will see similar advances in the understanding and ability to prevent and treat the developmental disorders of childhood, including autism.

What is most urgently needed in the next decade is a breakthrough in the neurodegenerative diseases of late adult life, like Alzheimer disease, Parkinson disease, amyotrophic lateral sclerosis, progressive supranuclear palsy, and frontotemporal degeneration. Here, let me insert a personal, and possibly heretical, comment. I believe that all these diseases are syndromes. Each is not a single diseases with a single cause, but rather a disease phenotype, where the same clinical and pathological features are caused by numerous noxious factors. Though in some patients these diseases are clearly inherited, in most cases they are sporadic. All are likely to be due to interplay between as yet unknown environmental factors and genetic changes that predispose individuals to suffer undue sensitivity to those environmental factors. Moreover, I believe it is quite likely that "when we know everything" we shall discover that several of these diseases share common causes.

Breakthroughs in discovering the causes of the age-related neurodegenerations are desperately needed, not only because they are fast becoming the greatest scourge of the elderly after cancer, but also because, despite major advances in the inherited forms of these diseases, we still have little understanding of the causes of the much commoner sporadic forms. We need to know the underlying environmental and genetic factors in order to be able to prevent or at least ameliorate these progressive neurological degenerations.

Walter G. Bradley DM, FRCP
Founding Editor, *Neurology in Clinical Practice*
Department of Neurology
Miller School of Medicine
University of Miami
Miami, Florida

Preface

Neurology in Clinical Practice is a practical textbook of neurology that covers all the clinical neurosciences and provides not only a description of neurological diseases and their pathophysiology but also a practical approach to their diagnosis and management. In the preface to the 1991 first edition of this book, we forecast that major technological and research advances would soon reveal the underlying cause and potential treatment of an ever-increasing number of neurological diseases.

The near quarter century since that prediction has been filled with the excitement of new discoveries resulting from the blossoming of neurosciences. Genetics and molecular biology have revolutionized our understanding of neurological disorders; targeted therapies that treat the basis of disease have improved outcomes and changed the course of many neurological diseases such as multiple sclerosis and other neuroimmune disorders and tumors associated with tuberous sclerosis. Advances in neuroimaging now enable the precise identification of functional regions and fine neuroanatomy of the human brain in health and disease. The important and challenging problem of neuroprotection is being addressed in both neurodegenerative disorders and acute injuries to the nervous system, such as stroke, hypoxic brain injury, and trauma. In line with this effort, basic science progress in areas of neuroplasticity and neural repair is yielding important results that should translate into clinical utility in the near future. When the first edition of this textbook was published, there was essentially no effective means of treating acute ischemic stroke. Today we have numerous opportunities to help such patients, and a campaign has begun to educate the general public about the urgency of seeking treatment when stroke symptoms occur. These and other advances have changed neurology to a field in which interventions are increasingly improving the outcomes of disorders previously considered to be untreatable.

The advent of teleneurology is also beginning to provide treatment for patients who lack access to neurological specialists or whose problems are too complicated for routine management in the community. Teleneurology consults are beginning to be provided nationwide across all subspecialties of our discipline, with a particular emphasis on patients who need intraoperative monitoring, critical care neurology, and stroke interventions.

To the benefit of patients, clinical neuroscience has partnered with engineering. Neuromodulation has become an important part of clinical therapy for patients with movement disorders and has applications in pain management and seizure control. Along these same lines, brain-controlled devices will soon help provide assistance to individuals whose mobility or communication skills are compromised. Recent advances in optogenetics have led to development of techniques that allow exploration and manipulation of neural circuitry, which may have therapeutic applications in a variety of neurologic disorders.

Finally, a search for biomarkers that reliably identify a preclinical state and track progression of disease is a promising goal in many neurodegenerative disorders. Age-related neurodegenerative diseases, such as Alzheimer disease and Parkinson disease, are increasingly prevalent and represent a growing health and socioeconomic burden. The costs in terms of suffering and hardship for patients and their families are too immense to quantify. As such, there is an urgent need for basic and clinical neuroscience to make progress in finding ways to delay the onset and slow progression of neurodegenerative disorders and, ultimately, prevent them.

There are startling new advances changing the neurosciences. The engineering of nanotechnologies into strategies to treat patients with neurological disorders is just beginning. Advances in genetics, including whole genome and whole exome sequencing, will undoubtedly result not only in discoveries of new genes but also new disease mechanisms. Novel imaging techniques provide insights into connectivity deficits in sensory and motor networks that have been associated with several neurological disorders. Innovative neurosurgical techniques and robotics are increasingly being utilized in enhancing function and optimizing quality of life of patients with neurological disorders.

We still have a long way to go to reach the ultimate goal of being able to understand and treat all neurological diseases. Neurology remains an intellectually exciting discipline, both because of the complexity of the nervous system and because of the insight that the pathophysiology of neurological disease provides into the workings of the brain and mind. Accordingly, we offer the seventh edition of *Neurology in Clinical Practice* as the updated comprehensive and most authoritative presentation of both the art and the science of neurology.

For this edition, the text has been rewritten and updated, and over 60 new authors have been added to the cadre of contributors. New chapters have been added covering brain death, deep brain stimulation, sexual function in degenerative disorders, concussion, drug abuse, and mechanisms of neurodegenerative disorders. The seventh edition includes an interactive online version housed on *www.expertconsult.com*, which can be also downloaded for offline use on phones or tablets. The electronic version of the text contains video and audio material, as well as additional illustrations and references. A work of this breadth would not have been possible without the contributions of many colleagues throughout the world. We are deeply grateful to them for their selfless devotion to neurological education. We are also grateful to our Elsevier counterparts, Lotta Kryhl, Senior Content Strategist; Joanne Scott, Deputy Content Development Manager; and Humayra Rahman Khan, Senior Content Coordinator, who were key in drawing this project together. Additionally, we thank Andrew Riley, Project Manager, without whose energy and efficiency the high quality of production and rapidity of publication of this work would not have been achieved. We also gratefully acknowledge the contributions of our readers, whose feedback regarding the print and online components of *Neurology in Clinical Practice* has been invaluable in refining and enhancing our educational goals. Finally, we wish to express our deep appreciation to our families for their support throughout this project and over the many decades of our shared lives.

Robert B. Daroff, MD

Joseph Jankovic, MD

John C. Mazziotta, MD, PhD

Scott L. Pomeroy, MD, PhD

List of Contributors

Bassel W. Abou-Khalil, MD
Professor of Neurology
Director of Epilepsy Division,
   Neurology
Vanderbilt University Medical Center
Nashville, TN, USA

Peter Adamczyk, MD
Vascular Neurology Fellow
Department of Neurology University of
   California–Los Angeles Medical
   Center
Los Angeles, CA, USA

Bela Ajtai, MD, PhD
Attending Neurologist
DENT Neurologic Institute
Amherst, NY, USA

Jeffrey C. Allen, MD
Director, Pediatric Neuro-oncology and
   Neurofibromatosis Programs
Department of Pediatrics, Division of
   Pediatric Hematology-Oncology
NYU Langone Medical Center
New York, NY, USA

Brandon Ally, PhD
Assistant Professor
Department of Neurology
Vanderbilt University
Nashville, TN, USA

Andrea A. Almeida, MD
BA Sports Neurology Fellow
Clinical Lecturer, Neurology
University of Michigan
Ann Arbor, MI, USA

Anthony A. Amato, MD
Vice-Chairman Neurology
Brigham and Women's Hospital;
Professor of Neurology
Harvard Medical School
Boston, MA, USA

Michael J. Aminoff, MD, DSc, FRCP
Distinguished Professor
Department of Neurology
School of Medicine
University of California
San Francisco, CA, USA

Nicolaas C. Anderson, DO, MS
Chief Resident
Department of Neurology
University of Arizona College of
   Medicine
Tucson, AZ, USA

Alon Y. Avidan, MD, MPH
Director, UCLA Sleep Disorders Center
Director, UCLA Neurology Clinic
University of California at Los Angeles
David Geffen School of Medicine at
   UCLA
Los Angeles, CA, USA

Joachim M. Baehring, MD, DSc
Associate Professor, Departments of
   Neurology, Neurosurgery and
   Medicine;
Chief
Section of Neuro-Oncology
Yale Cancer Center
Yale School of Medicine
New Haven, CT, USA

Asim K. Bag, MD
Assistant Professor, Department of
   Radiology
University of Alabama at Birmingham
Birmingham, AL, USA

Laura J. Balcer, MD, MSCE
Professor of Neurology and Population
   Health;
Vice Chair, Department of Neurology
NYU Langone Medical Center
New York, NY, USA

Robert W. Baloh, MD
Professor, Department of Neurology
Division of Head and Neck Surgery
University of California School of
   Medicine
Los Angeles, CA, USA

**Roger A. Barker, BA, MBBS, MRCP
PhD**
Professor of Clinical Neuroscience
Honorary Consultant Neurologist
Department of Clinical Neurosciences
University of Cambridge
Addenbrooke's Hospital
Cambridge, UK

J. D. Bartleson, MD, FAAN
Associate Professor of Neurology
Mayo Clinic
Rochester, MN, USA

Amit Batla, MD
Clinical Teaching Fellow
Institute of Neurology
London, UK

John David Beckham, MD
Assistant Professor
Division of Infectious Diseases
Departments of Medicine, Neurology &
   Microbiology;
Director, Infectious Disease Fellowship
   Training Program
University of Colorado Anschutz
   Medical Campus
Aurora, CO, USA

Leigh Beglinger, PhD
Neuropsychologist
Elks Rehab System
Boise, ID, USA

David H. Benninger, PD Dr.
Senior Consultant and Lecturer in
   Neurology
Department of Clinical Neurosciences
University Hospital of Lausanne
   (CHUV)
Lausanne, Switzerland

**Joseph R. Berger, MD, FACP, FAAN,
FANA**
Professor of Neurology; Chief of the
   Multiple Sclerosis Division
Department of Neurology
Perelman School of Medicine
University of Pennsylvania
Philadelphia, PA, USA

José Biller, MD, FACP, FAAN, FAHA
Professor and Chairman
Department of Neurology
Loyola University Chicago Stritch
   School of Medicine
Maywood, IL, USA

David F. Black, MD
Assistant Professor of Neurology and
   Radiology
Mayo Clinic
Rochester, MN, USA

Nicholas Boulis, MD
Associate Professor
Department of Neurosurgery, Emory
   University
Atlanta, GA, USA

Michael P. Bowley, MD, PhD
Instructor, Neurology
Massachusetts General Hospital
Boston, MA, USA

Helen M. Bramlett, PhD
Associate Professor, Neurological
  Surgery
University of Miami Miller School of
  Medicine;
Research Health Scientist, Research
  Service
Bruce W. Carter Department of Veterans
  Affairs Medical Center
Miami, FL, USA

Steven M. Bromley
Director
Bromley Neurology
Audubon, NJ, USA

Joseph Bruni, MD, FRCPC
Consultant Neurologist
St. Michael's Hospital;
Associate Professor of Medicine
University of Toronto
Toronto, ON, Canada

John C. M. Brust, AB, MD
Professor of Neurology
Columbia University College of
  Physicians & Surgeons
New York, NY, USA

W. Bryan Burnette, MD, MS
Associate Professor
Pediatrics and Neurology
Vanderbilt University School of
  Medicine,
Nashville, TN, USA

**Alan Carson, MB, ChB, MD,
FRCPsych, FRCP, MPhil**
Consultant Neuropsychiatrist;
Senior Lecturer in Psychological
  Medicine
Department of Clinical Neurosciences
University of Edinburgh
Edinburgh, UK

Robert Cavaliere, MD
Assistant Professor
The Ohio State University
Columbus, OH, USA

David A. Chad, MD
Staff Neurologist
Massachusetts General Hospital;
Associate Professor Neurology
Harvard Medical School
Boston, MA, USA

Vijay Chandran, MBBS, DM
Clinical Fellow
Pacific Parkinson's Research Centre
University of British Columbia
Vancouver, BC, Canada

Gisela Chelimsky, MD
Professor of Paediatrics
The Medical College of Wisconsin
Milwaukee, WI, USA

Thomas Chelimsky, MD
Professor of Neurology
The Medical College of Wisconsin
Milwaukee, WI, USA

Tanuja Chitnis, MD
Neurologist, Partners MS Center
Brigham and Women's Hospital;
Associate Professor of Neurology
Harvard Medical School
Boston, MA, USA

Sudhansu Chokroverty, MD, FRCP
Professor and Co-Chair;
Program Director of Clinical
  Neurophysiology and Sleep Medicine
NJ Neuroscience Institute at JFK;
Clinical Professor, Robert Wood
  Johnson Medical School
New Brunswick, NJ, USA

Paul E. Cooper, MD, FRCPC, FAAN
Professor of Neurology
London Health Sciences Centre,
  University Hospital
London, ON, Canada

Dany Cordeau, RN, PhD(c)
Registered Nurse
Department of Sexology
Université du Québec à Montréal
Montreal, QC, Canada

Frédérique Courtois, PhD
Chair, Full Professor
Department of Sexology
Université du Québec à Montréal
Montreal, QC, Canada

Josep Dalmau, MD, PhD
ICREA Research Professor
Hospital Clinic, IDIBAPS/University of
  Barcelona, Barcelona, Spain
Adjunct Professor, Neurology
University of Pennsylvania,
  Philadelphia, PA, USA

Robert B. Daroff, MD
Professor and Chair Emeritus
Department of Neurology
Case Western Reserve School of
  Medicine
University Hospitals Case Medical
  Center
Cleveland, OH, USA

**Ranan DasGupta, MBBChir, MA, MD,
FRCS(Urol)**
Consultant Urological Surgeon
Department of Urology
Imperial College Healthcare NHS Trust
London, UK

Mariel B. Deutsch, MD
Behavioral Neurology and
  Neuropsychiatry Fellow V.A. Greater
  Los Angeles Healthcare System
David Geffen School of Medicine at
  UCLA
Los Angeles, CA, USA

Michael Devereaux, MD
Professor of Neurology, University
  Hospitals Case Medical Center
Case Western Reserve University
Cleveland, OH, USA

W. Dalton Dietrich, PhD
Scientific Director, The Miami Project to
  Cure Paralysis
Kinetic Concepts Distinguished Chair
  in Neurosurgery
Senior Associate Dean for Discovery
  Science
Professor of Neurological Surgery,
  Neurology and Cell Biology and
  Anatomy
University of Miami
Leonard M. Miller School of Medicine
Lois Pope LIFE Center
Miami, FL, USA

Pradeep Dinakar, MD, MS
Instructor, Anesthesiology & Neurology
Harvard Medical School
Boston Children's Hospital
Brigham and Women's Hospital
Boston, MA, USA

Bruce H. Dobkin, MD
Professor of Neurology
University of California Los Angeles
Los Angeles, CA, USA

Richard L. Doty, BS, MA, PhD
Director, Smell and Taste Center
Hospital of the University of
  Pennsylvania;
Professor, Otorhinolaryngology: Head
  and Neck Surgery
University of Pennsylvania, Perelman
  School of Medicine
Philadelphia, PA, USA

Gary R. Duckwiler, MD
Professor and Director Interventional
  Neuroradiology;
Director, INR Fellowship Program
Co-Director UCLA HHT Center of
  Excellence
David Geffen School of Medicine at
  UCLA
Los Angeles, CA, USA

Ronald G. Emerson, MD
Attending Neurologist
Hospital for Special Surgery
New York, NY, USA

Michelle T. Fabian, MD
Assistant Professor
Icahn School of Medicine at Mount
  Sinai
New York, NY, USA

Conor Fearon, BE, MB, BCh, BAO
Specialist Registrar, Neurology
Dublin Neurological Institute
Mater Misericordiae University Hospital
Dublin, Ireland

Richard G. Fessler, MD, PhD
Professor, Neurosurgery
Rush University Medical Center,
Chicago, IL, USA

Laura Flores-Sarnat, MD
Adjunct Research Professor of Clinical
  Neurosciences and Paediatrics
University of Calgary and Alberta
  Children's Hospital Research Institute
Calgary, AB, Canada

Brent L. Fogel, MD, PhD
Assistant Professor of Neurology
David Geffen School of Medicine
University of California, Los Angeles
Los Angeles, CA, USA

Jennifer E. Fugate, DO
Assistant Professor of Neurology
Divisions of Critical Care and
  Cerebrovascular Neurology
Mayo Clinic
Rochester, MN, USA

Martin J. Gallagher, MD, PhD
Associate Professor
Vanderbilt University School of
  Medicine
Nashville, TN, USA

Sharon L. Gardner, MD
Associate Professor, Pediatrics
New York University Langone Medical
  Center
New York, NY, USA

Ivan Garza, MD
Assistant Professor of Neurology
Department of Neurology
Mayo Clinic
Rochester, MN, USA

Carissa Gehl, PhD
Staff Neuropsychologist
Iowa City Veterans Affairs Medical
  Center
Iowa City, IA, USA

David S. Geldmacher, MD
Professor
Department of Neurology
University of Alabama at Birmingham
Birmingham, AL, USA

Carter Gerard, MD
Neurosurgery Resident
Rush University Medical Center
Chicago, IL, USA

Daniel H. Geschwind, MD, PhD
Professor, Neurology
University of California, San Francisco
San Francisco, CA, USA

Michael David Geschwind, MD, PhD
Associate Professor, Neurology
University of California
San Francisco, CA, USA

K. M. Gibson, PhD, FACMG
Allen I. White Distinguished Professor
  and Chair, Department of
  Experimental and Systems
  Pharmacology College of Pharmacy
Washington State University
Spokane, WA, USA

Meredith R. Golomb, MD, MSc
Associate Professor
Division of Child Neurology,
  Department of Neurology
Indiana University School of Medicine
Indianapolis, IN, USA

Jonathan Graff-Radford, MD
Assistant Professor of Neurology
Mayo Clinic College of Medicine
Rochester, MN, USA

Jeffrey T. Guptill, MD, MA, MHS
Assistant Professor of Neurology
Associate Medical Director
Duke Clinical Research Unit
Duke Clinical Research Institute
Durham, NC, USA

Cecil D. Hahn, MD, MPH
Assistant Professor
Paediatrics (Neurology)
University of Toronto;
Director
Critical Care EEG Monitoring Program
The Hospital for Sick Children
Toronto, ON, Canada

Mark Hallett, MD
Chief, Human Motor Control Section
National Institute of Neurological
  Disorders and Stroke, NIH
Bethesda, MD, USA

Aline I. Hamati, MD
Clinical Assistant Professor of Pediatric
  Neurology
Indiana University School of Medicine
Riley Hospital for Children
Indianapolis, IN, USA

David Hart, MD
Director, Neurosurgery Spine
The Neurological Institute
University Hospitals Case Medical
  Center
Associate Professor of Neurological
  Surgery
Department of Neurological Surgery
Case Western Reserve University
Cleveland, OH, USA

Sabine Hellwig, MD
Neurologist
Assistant in Psychiatry
Department of Psychiatry and
  Psychotherapy
University Hospital Freiburg
Freiburg, Germany

Alan Hill, MD, PhD
Professor, Pediatrics
University of British Columbia,
Child Neurologist
British Columbia's Children's Hospital
Vancouver, BC, Canada

Benjamin D. Hill, PhD
Assistant Professor
Psychology Department/CCP
University of South Alabama
Mobile, AL, USA

Fred H. Hochberg, MD
Visiting Scientist, Neurosurgery
University of California at San Diego
San Diego, CA, USA

Kristin Huntoon, PhD, DO
Clinical Housestaff and Instructor
Department of Neurological Surgery
The Ohio State University Wexner
  Medical Center
Columbus, OH, USA

Jason T. Huse, MD, PhD
Assistant Member
Department of Pathology
Human Oncology and Pathogenesis
  Program
Memorial Sloan-Kettering Cancer
  Center
New York, NY, USA

Monica P. Islam, MD
Assistant Professor, Clinical Pediatrics
The Ohio State University College of
  Medicine;
Pediatric Neurologist
Nationwide Children's Hospital
Columbus, OH, USA

Joseph Jankovic, MD
Professor of Neurology
Distinguished Chair in Movement
  Disorders
Director of Parkinson's Disease Center
  and Movement
Disorders Clinic
Department of Neurology
Baylor College of Medicine
Houston, TX, USA

S. Andrew Josephson, MD
Acting Chair, UCSF Department of
  Neurology
Director, Neurohospitalist Program
Medical Director, Inpatient Neurology
University of California, San Francisco
San Francisco, CA, USA

Matthias A. Karajannis, MD, MS
Associate Professor of Pediatrics and
  Otolaryngology
Division of Pediatric Hematology/
  Oncology
NYU Langone Medical Center
The Stephen D. Hassenfeld Children's
  Center for Cancer and Blood
  Disorders
New York, NY, USA

Carlos S. Kase, MD
Professor of Neurology
Boston University School of Medicine;
Neurologist-in-Chief
Boston Medical Center
Boston, MA, USA

Bashar Katirji, MD
Director, Neuromuscular Center and
  EMG Laboratory
University Hospitals Case Medical
  Center;
Professor, Neurology
Case Western Reserve University School
  of Medicine
Cleveland, OH, USA

Kevin A. Kerber, MD
Associate Professor
University of Michigan Health System
Ann Arbor, MI, USA

Geoffrey A. Kerchner, MD, PhD
Consulting Associate Professor
Neurology and Neurological Sciences
Stanford University School of Medicine
Stanford, CA, USA

Samia J. Khoury, MD
Co-director, Partners MS Center
Brigham and Women's Hospital;
Jack, Sadie, and David Breakstone
  Professor of Neurology
Harvard Medical School
Boston, MA, USA

Howard S. Kirshner, BA, MD
Professor and Vice Chairman
Department of Neurology
Vanderbilt University Medical Center
Nashville, TN, USA

Stefan Klöppel, MD
Head of Memory Clinic
Department of Psychiatry and
  Psychotherapy
University Medical Center Freiburg
Freiburg, Germany

Anita A. Koshy, MD
Assistant Professor
Department of Neurology, Department
  of Immunobiology
University of Arizona, College of
  Medicine
Tucson, AZ, USA

Stephen C. Krieger, MD
Assistant Professor of Neurology
Corinne Goldsmith Dickinson Center
  for MS
Icahn School of Medicine at Mount
  Sinai
New York, NY, USA

Abhay Kumar, MD
Assistant Professor
Neurology
Saint Louis University
Saint Louis, MO, USA

John F. Kurtzke, MD, FACP, FAAN
Professor Emeritus, Neurology
Georgetown University;
Consultant, Neurology
Veterans Affairs Medical Center
Washington, DC, USA

Jeffrey S. Kutcher, MD
Associate Professor of Neurology
Director
Michigan NeuroSport
University of Michigan Health System
Ann Arbor, MI, USA

Anthony E. Lang, MD, FRCPC
Professor
Department of Medicine, Neurology
University of Toronto
Director of Movement Disorders Center
  and the Edmond J. Safra Program in
  Parkinson's Disease
Toronto Western Hospital
Toronto, ON, Canada

**Patrick J. M. Lavin, MB, BCh, BAO,
MRCPI**
Professor, Neurology and
  Ophthalmology
Department of Neurology
Vanderbilt University Medical School
Nashville, TN, USA

Marc A. Lazzaro, MD
Assistant Professor of Neurology and
  Neurosurgery
Director, Neurointerventional
  Fellowship Training Program
Medical Director, Telestroke Program
Medical College of Wisconsin and
  Froedtert Hospital
Milwaukee, WI, USA

David S. Liebeskind, MD, FAAN, FAHA
Professor of Neurology
Neurology Director, Stroke Imaging;
Co-Director, UCLA Cerebral Blood Flow
  Laboratory;
Director, UCLA Vascular Neurology
  Residency Program;
Associate Neurology Director, UCLA
  Stroke Center
UCLA Department of Neurology
Los Angeles, CA, USA

Eric Lindzen, MD, PhD
Jacobs Neurological Institute School of
  Medicine and Biomedical Sciences
State University of New York at Buffalo
Buffalo, NY, USA

Alan H. Lockwood, MD, FAAN, FANA
Emeritus Professor
Neurology and Nuclear Medicine
University at Buffalo
Buffalo, NY, USA

Glenn Lopate, MD
Professor of Neurology
Department of Neurology
Washington University School of
  Medicine
Saint Louis, MO, USA

Fred D. Lublin, MD
Saunders Family Professor of
  Neurology;
Director, The Corinne Goldsmith
  Dickinson Center for MS
Icahn School of Medicine at Mount
  Sinai
New York, NY, USA

Michael J. Lyerly, MD
Assistant Professor
Director, Birmingham VA Medical
  Center Stroke Center
Department of Neurology
University of Alabama at Birmingham
Birmingham, AL, USA

Robert L. Macdonald, MD, PhD
Gerald M. Fenichel Professor and Chair
  of Neurology
Vanderbilt University Medical Center
Nashville, TN, USA

Joseph C. Masdeu, MD, PhD
Graham Family Distinguished Chair in
  Neurological Sciences;
Director, Nantz National Alzheimer
  Center and Neuroimaging
Houston Methodist Neurological
  Institute
Houston Methodist Hospital
Houston, TX, USA

John C. Mazziotta, MD, PhD
Vice Chancellor of UCLA Health
  Sciences
Dean, David Geffen School of Medicine
CEO UCLA Health
University of California, Los Angeles
Los Angeles, CA, USA

Mario F. Mendez, MD, PhD
Director, Behavioral Neurology
  Program, and Professor Neurology
  and Psychiatry
David Geffen School of Medicine at
  UCLA;
Director, Neurobehavior
V.A. Greater Los Angeles Healthcare
  System
Los Angeles, CA, USA

Philipp T. Meyer, MD, PhD
Chair, Department of Nuclear Medicine
University Hospital Freiburg
Freiburg, Germany

Dominique S. Michaud, ScD
Professor, Department of Public Health
  and Community Medicine
Tufts University School of Medicine
Boston, MA, USA

Amanda Miller, L.M.S.W.
Social Worker
University of Iowa Huntington's
  Disease Society of America Center of
  Excellence
University of Iowa Carver College of
  Medicine
Iowa City, IA, USA

Karl E. Misulis, MD, PhD
Clinical Professor, Neurology
Vanderbilt University School of
    Medicine;
Chief Medical Information Officer
West Tennessee Healthcare
Nashville, TN, USA

Hiroshi Mitsumoto, MD, DSc
Director
Eleanor and Lou Gehrig MDA/ALS
    Research Center
The Neurological Institute
New York, NY, USA

Brian Murray, MB, BCh, BAO, MSc
Consultant Neurologist
Department of Neurology
Mater Misericordiae University Hospital
Dublin, Ireland

E. Lee Murray, MD
Clinical Assistant Professor of
    Neurology
University of Tennessee Health Science
    Center
Memphis, TN;
Attending Neurologist
West Tennessee Neuroscience
Jackson, TN, USA

Evan D. Murray, MD
Assistant in Neurology/ Instructor in
    Neurology
Department of Neurology
McLean Hospital/ Massachusetts
    General Hospital/ Harvard Medical
    School
Belmont, MA;
Director, Traumatic Brain Injury Service
Manchester VA Medical Center
Manchester, NH, USA

Ruth Nass, MD
Professor of Child Neurology, Child
    and Adolescent Psychiatry, and
    Pediatrics
New York University Langone Medical
    Center
New York, NY, USA

Lakshmi Nayak, MD
Assistant Professor of Neurology,
    Harvard Medical School,
Center for Neuro-Oncology, Dana-
    Farber/Brigham and Women's Cancer
    Center,
Boston, MA, USA

John G. Nutt, MD
Professor of Neurology
Oregon Health & Science University
Portland, OR, USA

Marc R. Nuwer, MD, PhD
Department Head, Clinical
    Neurophysiology
Ronald Reagan UCLA Medical Center;
Professor, Neurology
David Geffen School of Medicine at
    UCLA
Los Angeles, CA, USA

Michael S. Okun, MD
Adelaide Lackner Professor of
    Neurology and Neurosurgery
UF Center for Movement Disorders and
    Neurorestoration
Gainesville, FL, USA

Justin J. F. O'Rourke, PhD
Clinical Neuropsychologist
South Texas Veterans Healthcare System
San Antonio, TX, USA

Claudia R. Padilla, MD
Behavioral Neurology and
    Neuropsychiatry Fellow
David Geffen School of Medicine
University of California at Los Angeles
Neurobehavior Unit, VA Greater Los
    Angeles Healthcare System
Los Angeles, CA, USA

**Jalesh N. Panicker, MD, DM,
MRCP(UK)**
Consultant and Honorary Senior
    Lecturer
Department of Uroneurology
The National Hospital for Neurology
    and Neurosurgery
UCL Institute of Neurology
London, UK

Jane S. Paulsen, PhD
Roy J. Carver Chair for Neuroscience
    and Professor
Psychiatry, Neurology, Neurosicences
    and Psychology Research
The University of Iowa
Iowa City, IA, USA

Phillip L. Pearl, MD
Director of Epilepsy and Clinical
    Neurophysiology
Boston Children's Hospital
William G. Lennox Chair and Professor
    of Neurology
Harvard Medical School
Boston, MA, USA

Zhongxing Peng-Chen, MD
Neurologist, Movement Disorders
    Specialist
Hospital Padre Hurtado;
Movement Disorders Specialist
Fundación de Trastornos del
    Movimiento ATIX
Santiago, Chile

David L. Perez, MD
Assistant in Neurology and Psychiatry/
    Clinical Fellow in Neurology
Department of Neurology, Cognitive
    Behavioral Neurology and
    Frontotemporal Disorders Units
Department of Psychiatry, Division of
    Neuropsychiatry
Massachusetts General Hospital/
    Harvard Medical School
Boston, MA, USA

Alan Pestronk, MD
Professor
Department of Neurology, Immunology
    and Pathology
Director
Neuromuscular Clinical Laboratory
Washington University School of
    Medicine
Saint Louis, MO, USA

Ronald C. Peterson, PhD, MD
Professor of Neurology
Cora Kanow Professor of Alzheimer's
    Disease Research
Mayo Clinic College of Medicine
Rochester, MN, USA

Ronald F. Pfeiffer, MD
Professor and Vice Chair
Department of Neurology
University of Tennessee Health Science
    Center
Memphis, TN, USA

Scott L. Pomeroy, MD, PhD
Bronson Crothers Professor of
    Neurology
Director, Intellectual and
    Developmental Disabilities
Research Center
Harvard Medical School
Chair, Department of Neurology
Neurologist-in-Chief
Boston Children's Hospital
Boston, MA, USA

Sashank Prasad, MD
Assistant Professor of Neurology
Harvard Medical School
Department of Neurology
Division of Neuro-Ophthalmology
Brigham and Women's Hospital
Boston, MA, USA

David C. Preston, MD
Professor of Neurology
Case Western Reserve University School
    of Medicine;
Vice Chairman, Neurology
University Hospitals Case Medical
    Center
Cleveland, OH, USA

Bruce H. Price, MD
Chief of Neurology
McLean Hospital
Belmont;
Associate Neurologist/ Associate
    Professor of Neurology
Massachusetts General Hospital/
    Harvard Medical School
Boston, MA, USA

Louis J. L. Ptáček, MD
Investigator
Howard Hughes Medical Institute
John C. Coleman Distinguished
    Professor of Neurology
University of California
San Francisco, CA, USA

Alejandro A. Rabinstein, MD
Professor of Neurology
Divisions of Critical Care and
   Cerebrovascular Neurology
Mayo Clinic
Rochester, MN, USA

Tyler Reimschisel, MD
Assistant Professor of Pediatrics and
   Neurology
Vanderbilt University Medical Center
Nashville, TN, USA

Bernd F. Remler, MD
Professor of Neurology and
   Ophthalmology
Medical College of Wisconsin;
Zablocki VA Medical Center
Milwaukee, WI, USA

Michel Rijntjes, MD
Senior Physician
Department of Neurology
University Medical Center
Freiburg, Germany

Mikael L. Rinne, MD, PhD
Instructor in Neurology, Harvard
   Medical School,
Center for Neuro-Oncology, Dana-
   Farber/Brigham and Women's Cancer
   Center,
Boston, MA, USA

E. Steve Roach, MD
Professor, Pediatrics and Neurology
Ohio State University College of
   Medicine,
Nationwide Children's Hospital
   Columbus
Columbus, OH, USA

Carrie E. Robertson, MD
Assistant Professor of Neurology
Mayo Clinic
Rochester, MN, USA

Elke Roland, MD
Associate Professor
University of British Columbia;
Child Neurologist
British Columbia's Children's Hospital,
Vancouver, BC, Canada

**Michael Ronthal, MbBCh, FRCP,
FRCPE, FCP(SA)**
Professor of Neurology
Harvard Medical School
Beth Israel Deaconess Medical Center
Boston, MA, USA

Karen L. Roos, MD
John and Nancy Nelson Professor of
   Neurology;
Professor of Neurological Surgery
Indiana University School of Medicine
Indianapolis, IN, USA

Gary A. Rosenberg, MD
Professor and Chair
University of New Mexico Health
   Sciences Center
Albuquerque, NM, USA

Myrna R. Rosenfeld, MD, PhD
Senior Researcher
Hospital Clinic-IDIBAPS
Barcelona, Spain;
Adjunct Professor Neurology
University of Pennsylvania
Philadelphia, PA, USA

Gail Ross, PhD
Associate Professor of Psychology
Weill Cornell Medical College
Department of Pediatrics
New York, NY, USA

Janet C. Rucker, MD
Bernard A. and Charlotte Marden
   Professorship of Neurology Division
   and Fellowship Director,
   Neuro-Ophthalmology;
Associate Professor, Department of
   Neurology
NYU Langone Medical Center
New York, NY, USA

Sean Ruland, DO
Associate Professor
Loyola-Stritch School of Medicine
Maywood, IL, USA

Valerie Rundle-González, MD
Adjunct Clinical Postdoc Associate
Department of Neurology
UF Center for Movement Disorders and
   Neurorestoration
Gainesville, FL, USA

Donald B. Sanders, MD
Professor
Duke University Medical Center
Durham, NC, USA

Harvey B. Sarnat, MS, MD, FRCPC
Professor of Paediatrics, Pathology
   (Neuropathology) and Clinical
   Neurosciences
University of Calgary Faculty of
   Medicine
Alberta Children's Hospital Research
   Institute
Calgary, AB, Canada

**Anthony H. V. Schapira, MD, DSc,
FRCP, FMedSci**
Professor and Chair
Department of Clinical Neurosciences
UCL Institute of Neurology
London, UK

David Schiff, MD
Harrison Distinguished Teaching
   Professor
Neurology, Neurological Surgery, and
   Medicine
University of Virginia
Charlottesville, VA, USA

James W. Schmidley, MD
Professor
Virginia Tech Carilion School of
   Medicne
Roanoke, VA, USA

Michael J. Schneck, MD
Professor, Neurology and Neurosurgery
Loyola University Chicago Stritch
   School of Medicine
Maywood, IL, USA

Todd J. Schwedt, MD
Associate Professor
Department of Neurology
Mayo Clinic
Phoenix, AZ, USA

D. Malcolm Shaner, MD
Chief, Kaiser Permanente West Los
   Angeles Medical Center;
Clinical Professor
David Geffen School of Medicine
Los Angeles, CA, USA

Barbara E. Shapiro, MD, PhD
Associate Professor of Neurology
University Hospitals Case Medical
   Center
Cleveland, OH, USA

HyungSub Shim, MD
Clinical Assistant Professor
Department of Neurology
University of Iowa Carver College of
   Medicine
Iowa City, IA, USA

Ashkan Shoamanesh, MD, FRCPC
Marta and Owen Boris Chair in Stroke
   Research and Care
Assistant Professor of Neurology,
   McMaster University
Hamilton, ON, Canada

Reet Sidhu, MD
Assistant Professor of Neurology
Department of Neurology, Division of
   Child Neurology
Columbia University College of
   Physicians & Surgeons,
Columbia University Medical Center
New York, NY, USA

Jonathan H. Smith, MD
Assistant Professor, Department of
   Neurology
Director, Adult Neurology Residency
University of Kentucky College of
   Medicine
Lexington, KY, USA

Laura A. Snyder, MD
Neurosurgery Resident
Barrow Neurological Institute
Phoenix, AZ, USA

Yuen T. So, MD, PhD
Professor
Department of Neurology and
   Neurological Sciences
Stanford University
Stanford, CA, USA

Young H. Sohn, MD, PhD
Professor
Yonsei University Health System
Seoul, South Korea

Marylou V. Solbrig, MD
Professor Medicine (Neurology) and
    Medical Microbiology
University of Manitoba
Health Sciences Centre
Winnipeg, MB, Canada

Martina Stippler, MD, MS
Assistant Professor
Beth Israel Deaconess Medical Center
Boston, MA, USA

A. Jon Stoessl, CM, MD, FRCPC, FCAHS
Professor and Head
University of British Columbia
Vancouver, BC, Canada

Jon Stone, MBChB, PhD, FRCP
Consultant Neurologist and Honorary
    Senior Lecturer
Department of Clinical Neurosciences
University of Edinburgh
Edinburgh, UK

S.H. Subramony, MD
Professor
McKnight Brain Institute at University
    of Florida
Gainesville, FL, USA

Jerry W. Swanson, MD
Professor of Neurology
Mayo Clinic College of Medicine
Rochester, MN, USA

Viktor Szeder, MD, PhD, MSc
Assistant Clinical Professor
Division of Interventional
    Neuroradiology
David Geffen School of Medicine at
    UCLA
Los Angeles, CA, USA

Lee Tan, MD
Neurosurgery Resident
Rush University Medical Center
Chicago, IL, USA

Satoshi Tateshima, MD, DMSc
Associate Professor
Division of Interventional
    Neuroradiology
David Geffen School of Medicine at
    UCLA
Los Angeles, CA, USA

Philip D. Thompson, MB, BS, PhD, FRACP
Professor of Neurology
Discipline of Medicine and Department
    of Neurology
University of Adelaide and Royal
    Adelaide Hospital
Adelaide, SA, Australia

Matthew J. Thurtell, MBBS, FRACP
Assistant Professor
Department of Ophthalmology &
    Visual Sciences;
Department of Neurology
University of Iowa
Iowa City, IA, USA

Robert L. Tomsak, MD, PhD
Professor of Ophthalmology and
    Neurology
Wayne State University School of
    Medicine;
Specialist in Neuro-ophthalmology
Kresge Eye Institute
Detroit, MI, USA

Bryan Tsao, MD
Chair, Department of Neurology
Associate Professor of Neurology
Loma Linda University School of
    Medicine
Loma Linda, CA, USA

Chris Turner, BSc (Hons) MBChB (Oxon), FRCP, PhD
Consultant Neurologist and Honorary
    Senior Lecturer
MRC Centre for Neuromuscular Disease
National Hospital for Neurology and
    Neurosurgery
London, UK

Kenneth L. Tyler, MD
Reuler-Lewin Family Professor and
    Chair
University of Colorado School of
    Medicine;
Professor of Medicine and Microbiology
Denver VA Medical Center
Aurora, CO, USA

Stan H. M. van Uum, MD, PhD, FRCPC
Associate Professor
Schulich School of Medicine and
    Dentistry
Western University
London, ON, Canada

Ashok Verma, MD, DM, MBA
Professor, Neurology
University of Miami Miller School of
    Medicine;
Medical Director
Kessenich Family MDA ALS Center,
    University of Miami,
Miami, FL, USA

Michael Wall, MD
Professor, Neurology and
    Ophthalmology;
Staff Physician
University of Iowa
Iowa City, IA, USA

Mitchell T. Wallin, MD, MPH
Clinical Associate Director, VA MS
    Center of Excellence, East
Associate Professor of Neurology,
    Georgetown University School of
    Medicine
Washington, DC, USA

Leo H. Wang, MD, PhD
Assistant Professor
Department of Neurology
University of Washington
Seattle, WA, USA

Cornelius Weiller, MD
Professor, Neurology
University Clinic
Freiburg, Germany

Karin Weissenborn, MD
Professor, Department of Neurology
Hannover Medical School
Hannover, Germany

Patrick Y. Wen, MD
Director, Center for Neuro-Oncology
Dana-Farber Cancer Institute;
Director, Division of Neuro-Oncology,
    Department of Neurology
Brigham and Women's Hospital
Boston, MA, USA

Eelco F. M. Wijdicks, MD, PhD, FACP, FNCS, FANA
Professor of Neurology, Mayo College
    of Medicine;
Chair, Division of Critical Care
    Neurology;
Consultant, Neurosciences Intensive
    Care Unit
Mayo Clinic Campus, Saint Marys
    Hospital
Rochester, MN, USA

Guangbin Xia, MD, PhD
Assistant Professor, Neurology and
    Neuroscience
University of Florida
Gainesville, FL, USA

Osama O. Zaidat, MD, MS
Professor of Neurology, Neurosurgery
    and Radiology
Director Comprehensive Stroke
    Program
Chief Neuro-Interventional Division
Medical College of Wisconsin /
    Froedtert Hospital
Milwaukee, WI, USA

Video Table of Contents

Seizure 1
Chapter 34, Video 1

Seizure 2
Chapter 34, Video 2

Seizure 3
Chapter 34, Video 3

End-Plate Noise
Chapter 35, Video 1

End-Plate Spikes
Chapter 35, Video 2

Fibrillation Potential
Chapter 35, Video 3

Fasciculation Potential
Chapter 35, Video 4

Myotonic Discharges
Chapter 35, Video 5

Myokymic Discharge
Chapter 35, Video 6

Complex Repetitive Discharge
Chapter 35, Video 7

Clinical Electromyography: Neuromyotonic Discharge
Chapter 35, Video 8

Clinical Electromyography: Cramp Discharge
Chapter 35, Video 9

Normal Potential at Slight Concentration
Chapter 35, Video 10

Polyphasic Motor Unit Action Potential with Satellite Potentials
Chapter 35, Video 11

Brief Duration, Short Amplitude and Polyphasic Motor Unit Action Potentials
Chapter 35, Video 12

Chronic Reinnervation – Long Duration and Increased Amplitude
Chapter 35, Video 13

Unstable Motor Unit Action Potentials
Chapter 35, Video 14

Moderately Decreased Recruitment
Chapter 35, Video 15

Poor Activation
Chapter 35, Video 16

(Clips 35.1–16 From Preston D. C., Shapiro B. E. Electromyography and Neuromuscular Disorders: Clinical–Electrophysiologic Correlations, 3rd edn. © 2013, Elsevier Inc.)

"Off" Stimulation Evaluation in Parkinson Disease
Chapter 37, Video 1

"On" Stimulation Evaluation in Parkinson Disease
Chapter 37, Video 2

Pre-surgical Evaluation in Essential Tremor
Chapter 37, Video 3

Post-surgical Evaluation in Essential Tremor
Chapter 37, Video 4

Internuclear Ophthalmoplegia
Chapter 44, Video 1

Acute Peripheral Vestibular Nystagmus
Chapter 46, Video 1

Forced Ductions
Chapter 44, Video 2

Ocular Flutter
Chapter 46, Video 2

Gaze-Evoked Nystagmus
Chapter 44, Video 3

Gaze-Evoked Nystagmus and Impaired Smooth Pursuit
Chapter 46, Video 3

Upbeat Nystagmus
Chapter 44, Video 4

Gaze-Evoked Downbeating Nystagmus
Chapter 46, Video 4

Downbeat Nystagmus
Chapter 44, Video 5

Hypermetric Saccades
Chapter 46, Video 5

Ocular Flutter
Chapter 44, Video 6

Head-Thrust Tests
Chapter 46, Video 6

Opsoclonus
Chapter 44, Video 7

Benign Paroxysmal Positional Vertigo
Chapter 46, Video 7

Square Wave Jerks
Chapter 44, Video 8

Epley Maneuver
Chapter 46, Video 8

Parkinson Disease: Marked Flexion of the Trunk (Camptorcormia Because of PD-Related Skeletal Deformity)
Chapter 96, Video 1

Progressive Supranuclear Palsy; Marked Vertical Ophthalmoparesis, Perseveration of Gaze to Left even though the Body Faces Forward
Chapter 96, Video 8

Patient with Parkinson Disease and Anterocollis and Camptocormia
Chapter 96, Video 2

Progressive Supranuclear Palsy; Typical Facial Expression with Deep Facial Folds, Square Wave Jerks on Primary Gaze, Slow Saccades, Inappropriate Laughter (Pseudobulbar Palsy), Right Arm Levitation
Chapter 96, Video 9

Patient with Parkinsonism and Striatal Hand Deformities
Chapter 96, Video 3

Progressive Supranuclear Palsy; Deep Facial Folds, Vertical Ophthalmoplegia, Marked Postural Instability, Slumps into a Chair
Chapter 96, Video 10

Parkinson Disease; Patient with Young-Onset Parkinson Disease and Gait Difficulty Due to Freezing (Motor Blocks)
Chapter 96, Video 4

Progressive Supranuclear Palsy; Deep Facial Folds, Apraxia of Eyelid Opening, in Addition to Vertical Ophthalmopareses, Patient Demonstrates Evidence of Internuclear Ophthalmoplegia, the Presence of Right Arm Tremor (Atypical for Progressive Supranuclear Palsy) Suggests the Co-Existence of Parkinson Disease
Chapter 96, Video 11

Parkinson Disease; Patient Describes Levodopa-Induced Visual Hallucinations (e.g., Seeing and Picking Worms)
Chapter 96, Video 5

Multiple System Atrophy; Patient Describes Symptoms of Dysautonomia, Demonstrates Flexion of the Neck and Apraxia of Eyelid Opening, Typical of MSA
Chapter 96, Video 12

Parkinson Disease; Levodopa-Induced Dyskinesia
Chapter 96, Video 6

Corticobasal Degeneration; Patient Describes Apraxia of Left Leg, Demonstrates Ideomotor Apraxia in Left More than Right Hand and Marked Left Leg and Foot Apraxia
Chapter 96, Video 13

Progressive Supranuclear Palsy; Typical Worried, Frowning Facial Expression (Procerus Sign), Apraxia of Eyelid Opening, Although Vertical (Downward) Gaze is Preserved, Vertical Optokinetic Nystagmus is Absent, When Walking Patient Pivots on Turning (in Contrast to Patients with Parkinson Disease Who Turn En Bloc)
Chapter 96, Video 7

Corticobasal Degeneration; Patient Describes Alien Hand Phenomenon in the Right Arm, Demonstrates Marked Apraxia in the Right More than Left Hand, Spontaneous and Evoked Myoclonus in the Right Hand, Markedly Impaired Graphesthesia
Chapter 96, Video 14

Corticobasal Degeneration; Evoked Hand and Arm Myoclonus
Chapter 96, Video 15

Corticobasal Degeneration; Patient Describes Right Alien Hand Phenomenon, Right Hand Myoclonus, Marked Ideomotor Apraxia in the Right More than Left Hand
Chapter 96, Video 16

Vascular Parkinsonism; Broad-Based Gait, Freezing on Turning (Lower Body Parkinsonism) Associated with Binswanger's Disease
Chapter 96, Video 17

Vascular Parkinsonism; Gait Initiation Failure (Pure Freezing)
Chapter 96, Video 18

Essential Tremor; Marked Improvement in Right Hand Tremor with Contralateral Deep Brain Stimulation of the VIM Thalamus
Chapter 96, Video 19

Cerebellar Outflow Tremor Because of Multiple Sclerosis; Markedly Improved with Deep Brain Stimulation of the VIM Thalamus
Chapter 96, Video 20

Orthostatic Tremor; Patient Describes Problems with Standing, Demonstrates High Frequency (16 Hz) Tremor in Legs Present Only upon Standing, Leg Tremor Disappears When Leaning Against Table
Chapter 96, Video 21

Wilson Disease; Slow Tremor (Myorrhythmia) in the Left Hand
Chapter 96, Video 22

Herditary Spastic Paraparesis
Chapter 98, Video 1

Fasciculations
Chapter 98, Video 2

Kennedy Disease (X-Linked Recessive Bulbospinal Neuronopathy)
Chapter 98, Video 3

Amyotrophic Lateral Sclerosis
Chapter 98, Video 4

C9orf72 Mutation
Chapter 98, Video 5

(Clip 98.5 Adapted from Movement Disorders, 2012; http://www.ncbi.nlm.nih.gov/pmc/articles/PMC3516857/)

NREM Parasomnia (Confusional Arousal)
Chapter 102, Video 1

NREM Parasomnia (Confusional Arousal)
Chapter 102, Video 2

(Clips 102.1 and 102.2 From Pincherle, A. et al. Epilepsy and NREM-parasomnia: A complex and reciprocal relationship. Sleep Medicine. 13(4), 2012. Pages 442–444. © Elsevier. doi:10.1016/S1389-9457(12)00144-X.)

Large Left Hypertropia Secondary to Right Oculomotor Nerve Palsy
Chapter 104, Video 1

Left Appendicular Ataxia
Chapter 104, Video 2

Prominent Left Ptosis
Chapter 104, Video 3

**Cranial Neuropathies/Impaired
Adduction, Elevation, And
Depression with Intact Abduction
of the Left Nerve**
Chapter 104, Video 4

**Bilateral Abduction Deficits
Secondary to Demyelinating
Bilateral Abducens Palsies**
Chapter 104, Video 5

Esotropia
Chapter 104, Video 6

**Facial Nerve Function in a Patient
with a History of Right Facial
Palsy Two Years Ago and Current
Left Facial Palsy**
Chapter 104, Video 7

Other Babinski Sign
Chapter 104, Video 8

*(Clips 104.1–2 from Leigh R. J., Zee, D. S. The Neurology of
Eye Movements, 5th Edition, 2015. © Oxford University Press;
Clip 104.8 Courtesy of Joseph Jankovic, MD)*

Tensilon Test
Chapter 109, Video 1

"Curtain" Sign
Chapter 109, Video 2

**Patient Describing Dissociation at
Onset of Functional Left
Hemiparesis and Functional Left
Facial Spasm**
Chapter 113, Video 1

**Longstanding Functional Left
Arm and Leg Weakness and
Sensory Disturbance**
Chapter 113, Video 2

**Right Sided Functional Leg
Weakness with a Positive
Hoover Sign**
Chapter 113, Video 3

**Functional Facial Spasm Showing
Contraction of Platysma on the
Right with Jaw Deviation to the
Right**
Chapter 113, Video 4

**Bilateral Functional Ankle/Foot
Dystonia Showing Fixed Nature
of Deformity During Gait**
Chapter 113, Video 5

**Sedation Used Therapeutically for Treatment of
Functional Paralysis and Functional**
Chapter 113, Video 6

*(Clip 113.6 From Stone J, Hoeritzauer I, Brown K, Carson A.
Therapeutic Sedation for Functional (Psychogenic) Neurological
Symptoms. J Psychosom Res 2014;76:165–8.)*

TABLE 1.1 Outline of the Screening Neurological Examination

Examination component	Description/observation/maneuver
MENTAL STATUS	Assessed while recording the history
CRANIAL NERVES:	
CN I	Should be tested in all persons who experience spontaneous loss of smell, in patients suspected to have Parkinson disease, and in patients who have suffered head injury
CN II	*Each eye:* Gross visual acuity Visual fields by confrontation Fundoscopy
CN III, IV, VI	Horizontal and vertical eye movements Pupillary response to light Presence of nystagmus or other ocular oscillations
CN V	Pinprick and touch sensation on face, corneal reflex
CN VII	Close eyes, show teeth
CN VIII	Perception of whispered voice in each ear or rubbing of fingers; if hearing is impaired, look in external auditory canals, and use tuning fork for lateralization and bone-versus-air sound conduction
CN IX, X	Palate lifts in midline, gag reflex present
CN XI	Shrug shoulders
CN XII	Protrude tongue
LIMBS	*Separate testing of each limb:* Presence of involuntary movements Muscle mass (atrophy, hypertrophy) and look for fasciculations Muscle tone in response to passive flexion and extension Power of main muscle groups Coordination Finger-to-nose and heel-to-shin testing Performance of rapid alternating movements Tendon reflexes Plantar responses Pinprick and light touch on hands and feet Double simultaneous stimuli on hands and feet Joint position sense in hallux and index finger Vibration sense at ankle and index finger
GAIT AND BALANCE	Spontaneous gait should be observed; stance, base, cadence, arm swing, tandem gait should be noted Postural stability should be assessed by the pull test
ROMBERG TEST	Stand with eyes open and then closed

of a limb may result from a corticospinal tract lesion, sensory defect, or cerebellar lesion. If the limb incoordination is due to a cerebellar lesion, findings will include ataxia on finger-to-nose and heel-to-shin testing, abnormal rapid alternating movements of the hands (dysdiadochokinesia), and often nystagmus and ocular dysmetria. If some of these signs of cerebellar dysfunction are missing, examination of joint position sense, limb strength, and reflexes may demonstrate that this incoordination is due to something other than a cerebellar lesion. At the end of the neurological examination, the abnormal physical signs should be classified as definitely abnormal (*hard signs*) or equivocally abnormal (*soft signs*). The hard

signs, when combined with symptoms from the history, allow the neurologist to develop a hypothesis about the anatomical site of the lesion or at least about the neurological pathways involved. The soft signs can then be reviewed to determine whether they conflict with or support the initial conclusion. An important point is that the primary purpose of the neurological examination is to reveal functional disturbances that localize abnormalities. The standard neurological examination is less effective when used to monitor the course of a disease or its temporal response to treatment. Measuring changes in neurological function over time requires special quantitative functional tests and rating scales.

General Physical Examination

The nervous system is damaged in so many general medical diseases that a general physical examination is an integral part of the examination of patients with neurological disorders. Atrial fibrillation, valvular heart disease, or an atrial septal defect may cause embolic strokes in the central nervous system. Hypertension increases the risk for all types of stroke. Signs of malignancy raise the possibility of metastatic lesions of the nervous system or paraneoplastic neurological syndromes such as a subacute cerebellar degeneration or sensory peripheral neuropathy. In addition, some diseases such as vasculitis and sarcoidosis affect both the brain and other organs.

ASSESSMENT OF THE CAUSE OF THE PATIENT'S SYMPTOMS
Anatomical Localization

Hypotheses about lesion localization, neurological systems involved, and pathology of the disorder can be formed once the history is complete (see Fig. 1.1). The neurologist then uses the examination findings to confirm the localization of the lesion before trying to determine its cause. The initial question is whether the disease is in the brain, spinal cord, peripheral nerves, neuromuscular junctions, or muscles. Then it must be established whether the disorder is focal, multifocal, or systemic. A *system disorder* is a disease that causes degeneration of one part of the nervous system while sparing other parts of the nervous system. For instance, degeneration of the corticospinal tracts and spinal motor neurons with sparing of the sensory pathways of the central and peripheral nervous systems is the hallmark of the system degeneration termed *motor neuron disease*, or *amyotrophic lateral sclerosis*. Multiple system atrophy is another example of a system degeneration characterized by slowness of movement (parkinsonism), ataxia, and dysautonomia.

The first step in localization is to translate the patient's symptoms and signs into abnormalities of a nucleus, tract, or part of the nervous system. Loss of pain and temperature sensation on one half of the body, excluding the face, indicates a lesion of the contralateral spinothalamic tract in the high cervical spinal cord. A left sixth nerve palsy, with weakness of left face and right limbs, points to a left pontine lesion. A left homonymous hemianopia indicates a lesion in the right optic tract, optic radiations, or occipital cortex. The neurological examination plays a crucial role in localizing the lesion. A patient complaining of tingling and numbness in the feet initially may be thought to have a peripheral neuropathy. If examination shows hyper-reflexia in the arms and legs and no vibration sensation below the clavicles, the lesion is likely to be in the spinal cord, and the many causes of peripheral neuropathy can be dropped from consideration. A patient with a history of weakness of the left arm and leg who is found on examination to have a left homonymous hemianopia has a right cerebral lesion, not a cervical cord problem.

The neurologist must decide whether the symptoms and signs could all arise from one focal lesion or whether several anatomical sites must be involved. The *principle of parsimony*, or *Occam's razor*, requires that the clinician strive to hypothesize only one lesion. The differential diagnosis for a single focal lesion is significantly different from that for multiple lesions. Thus, a patient complaining of left-sided vision loss and left-sided weakness is likely to have a lesion in the right cerebral hemisphere, possibly caused by stroke or tumor. On the other hand, if the visual difficulty is due to a central scotoma in the left eye, and if the upper motor neuron weakness affects the left limbs but spares the lower cranial nerves, two lesions must be present: one in the left optic nerve and one in the left corticospinal tract below the medulla—as seen, for example, in multiple sclerosis. If a patient with slowly progressive slurring of speech and difficulty walking is found to have ataxia of the arms and legs, bilateral extensor plantar responses, and optic atrophy, the lesion must be either multifocal (affecting brainstem and optic nerves, and therefore probably multiple sclerosis) or a system disorder, such as a spinocerebellar degeneration. The complex vascular anatomy of the brain can sometimes cause multifocal neurological deficits to result from one vascular abnormality. For instance, a patient with occlusion of one vertebral artery may suffer a stroke that produces a midbrain lesion, a hemianopia, and an amnestic syndrome.

Synthesis of symptoms and signs for anatomical localization of a lesion requires a good knowledge of neuroanatomy, including the location of all major pathways in the nervous system and their inter-relationships at different levels. In making this synthesis, the neurologist trainee will find it helpful to refer to diagrams that show transverse sections of the spinal cord, medulla, pons, and midbrain; the brachial and lumbosacral plexuses; and the dermatomes and myotomes. Knowledge of the functional anatomy of the cerebral cortex and the blood supply of the brain and spinal cord also is essential.

Symptoms and signs may arise not only from disturbances caused at the focus of an abnormality—*focal localizing signs*—but also at a distance. One example is the damage that results from the shift of intracranial contents produced by an expanding supratentorial tumor. This may cause a palsy of the third or sixth cranial nerve, even though the tumor is located far from the cranial nerves. Clinical features caused by damage far from the primary site of abnormality sometimes are called *false localizing signs*. This term derives from the era before neuroimaging studies when clinical examination was the major means of lesion localization. In fact, these are not false signs but rather signs that the intracranial shifts are marked, alerting the clinician to the large size of the space-occupying lesion within the skull.

Differential Diagnosis

Once the likely site of the lesion is identified, the next step is to generate a list of diseases or conditions that may be responsible for the patient's symptoms and signs—the differential diagnosis (see Fig. 1.1). The experienced neurologist automatically first considers the most likely causes, followed by less common causes. The beginner is happy to generate a list of the main causes of the signs and symptoms in whatever order they come to mind. Experience indicates the most likely causes based on specific patient characteristics, the portions of the nervous system affected, and the relative frequency of each disease. An important point is that *rare presentations of common diseases are more common than common presentations of rare diseases*. Equally important, the neurologist must be vigilant in including in differential diagnosis less likely disorders that if overlooked can cause significant morbidity and/or mortality. A proper differential diagnosis list should include the most likely causes of the patient's signs and symptoms as well as the most ominous.

Sometimes only a single disease can be incriminated, but usually several candidate diseases can be identified. The list of possibilities should take into account both the temporal features of the patient's symptoms and the pathological processes known to affect the relevant area of the nervous system. For example, in a patient with signs indicating a lesion of the internal capsule, the cause is likely to be stroke if the hemiplegia was of sudden onset. With progression over weeks or months, a more likely cause is an expanding tumor. As another example, in a patient with signs of multifocal lesions whose symptoms have relapsed and remitted over several years, the diagnosis is likely to be multiple sclerosis or multiple strokes (depending on the patient's age, sex, and risk factors). If symptoms appeared only recently and have gradually progressed, multiple metastases should be considered.

Again, the principle of parsimony or Occam's razor should be applied in constructing the differential diagnostic list. An example is that of a patient with a 3-week history of a progressive spinal cord lesion who suddenly experiences aphasia. Perhaps the patient had a tumor compressing the spinal cord and has incidentally incurred a small stroke. The principle of parsimony, however, would suggest a single disease, probably cancer with multiple metastases. Another example is that of a patient with progressive atrophy of the small muscles of the hands for 6 months before the appearance of a pseudobulbar palsy. This patient could have bilateral ulnar nerve lesions and recent bilateral strokes, but amyotrophic lateral sclerosis is more likely. Nature does not always obey the rules of parsimony, however.

The differential diagnosis generally starts with pathological processes such as a stroke, a tumor, or an abscess. Each pathological process may result from any of several different diseases. Thus, a clinical diagnosis of an intracranial neoplasm generates a list of the different types of tumors likely to be responsible for the clinical manifestations in the affected patient. Similarly, in a patient with a stroke, the clinical history may help discriminate among hemorrhage, embolism, thrombosis, vascular spasm, and vasculitis. The skilled diagnostician is justly proud of placing the correct diagnosis at the top of the list, but it is more important to ensure that all possible diseases are considered. If a disease is not even considered, it is unlikely to be diagnosed. Treatable disorders should always be kept in mind, even if they have a very low probability. This is especially true if they may mimic more common incurable neurological disorders such as Alzheimer disease or amyotrophic lateral sclerosis.

Laboratory Investigations

Sometimes the neurological diagnosis can be made without any laboratory investigations. This is true for a clear-cut case of Parkinson disease, myasthenia gravis, or multiple sclerosis. Nevertheless, even in these situations, appropriate laboratory documentation is important for other physicians who will see the patient in the future. In other instances, the cause of the disease will be elucidated only by the use of laboratory tests. These tests may in individual cases include hematological and biochemical blood studies; neurophysiological testing (Chapters 34–38); neuroimaging (Chapters 39–42); organ biopsy; and bacteriological and virological studies. The use of laboratory tests in the diagnosis of neurological diseases is considered more fully in Chapter 33.

MANAGEMENT OF NEUROLOGICAL DISORDERS

Not all diseases are curable. Even if a disease is incurable, however, the physician will be able to reduce the patient's discomfort and assist the patient and family in managing the disease. Understanding a neurological disease is a science. Diagnosing a neurological disease is a combination of science and experience. Managing a neurological disease is an art, an introduction to which is provided in Chapter 53.

EXPERIENCED NEUROLOGIST'S APPROACH TO THE DIAGNOSIS OF COMMON NEUROLOGICAL PROBLEMS

The skills of a neurologist are learned. Seeing many cases of a disease teaches us which symptoms and signs *should* be present and—just as important—which *should not* be present in a given neurological disease. Although there is no substitute for experience and pattern recognition, the trainee can learn the clues used by the seasoned practitioner to reach a correct diagnosis. Part 1 of this book covers the main symptoms and signs of neurological disease. These chapters describe how an experienced neurologist approaches common presenting problems such as a movement disorder, a speech disturbance, or diplopia to arrive at the diagnosis. Part 2 of this book comprises the major fields of investigation and management of neurological disease. Part 3 provides a compendium of the neurological diseases themselves.

2 Episodic Impairment of Consciousness

Joseph Bruni

CHAPTER OUTLINE

SYNCOPE
History and Physical Examination
Causes of Syncope
Investigations of Patients with Syncope
SEIZURES
History and Physical Examination
Absence Seizures
Tonic-Clonic Seizures
Complex Partial Seizures
Investigations of Seizures
Psychogenic or Pseudoseizures (Nonepileptic Seizures)
MISCELLANEOUS CAUSES OF ALTERED CONSCIOUSNESS

Temporary loss of consciousness may be caused by impaired cerebral perfusion (syncope, fainting), cerebral ischemia, migraine, epileptic seizures, metabolic disturbances, sudden increases in intracranial pressure (ICP), or sleep disorders. Anxiety attacks, psychogenic seizures, panic disorder, and malingering may be difficult to distinguish from these conditions. Detailed laboratory examinations and prolonged periods of observation may not always clarify the diagnosis.

Syncope may result from cardiac causes and several noncardiac causes. Often, no cause is determined. Specific causes include decreased cardiac output secondary to cardiac arrhythmias, outflow obstruction, hypovolemia, orthostatic hypotension, or decreased venous return. Cerebrovascular disturbances from transient ischemic attacks of the posterior or anterior cerebral circulations, or cerebral vasospasm from migraine, subarachnoid hemorrhage, or hypertensive encephalopathy, may result in temporary loss of consciousness. Situational syncope may occur in association with cough, micturition, defecation, swallowing, Valsalva maneuver, or diving. Metabolic disturbances due to hypoxia, drugs, anemia, and hypoglycemia may result in frank syncope or, more frequently, the sensation of an impending faint (presyncope).

Absence seizures, generalized tonic-clonic seizures, and complex partial seizures are associated with alterations of consciousness and are usually easily distinguished from syncope. Epileptic seizures may be difficult to distinguish from nonepileptic (psychogenic seizures), panic attacks, and malingering. In children, breath-holding spells, a form of syncope (discussed later under "Miscellaneous Causes of Altered Consciousness"), can cause a transitory alteration of consciousness that may mimic epileptic seizures. Although rapid increases in ICP (which may result from intermittent hydrocephalus, severe head trauma, brain tumors, intracerebral hemorrhage, or Reye syndrome) may produce sudden loss of consciousness, affected patients frequently have other neurological manifestations that lead to this diagnosis.

In patients with episodic impairment of consciousness, diagnosis relies heavily on the clinical history described by the patient and observers. Laboratory investigations, however, may provide useful information. In a small number of patients, a cause for the loss of consciousness may not be established, and these patients may require longer periods of observation. Table 2.1 compares the clinical features of syncope and seizures.

SYNCOPE

The pathophysiological basis of syncope is the gradual failure of cerebral perfusion, with a reduction in cerebral oxygen availability. *Syncope* refers to a symptom complex characterized by lightheadedness, generalized muscle weakness, giddiness, visual blurring, tinnitus, and gastrointestinal (GI) symptoms. The patient may appear pale and feel cold and "sweaty." The onset of loss of consciousness generally is gradual but may be rapid if related to certain conditions such as a cardiac arrhythmia or in the elderly. The gradual onset may allow patients to protect themselves from falling and injury. Factors precipitating a simple faint are emotional stress, unpleasant visual stimuli, prolonged standing, or pain. Although the duration of unconsciousness is brief, it may range from seconds to minutes. During the faint, the patient may be motionless or display myoclonic jerks, but never tonic-clonic movements. Urinary incontinence is uncommon. The pulse is weak and often slow. Breathing may be shallow and the blood pressure barely obtainable. As the fainting episode corrects itself by the patient becoming horizontal, normal color returns, breathing becomes more regular, and the pulse and blood pressure return to normal. After the faint, the patient experiences some residual weakness, but unlike the postictal state, confusion, headaches, and drowsiness are uncommon. Nausea may be noted when the patient regains consciousness. The causes of syncope are classified by their pathophysiological mechanism (Box 2.1), but cerebral hypoperfusion is always the common final pathway. Rarely, vasovagal syncope may have a genetic component suggestive of autosomal dominant inheritance (Klein et al., 2013). Wieling et al. (2009) reviewed the clinical features of the successive phases of syncope.

History and Physical Examination

The history and physical examination are the most important components of the initial evaluation of syncope. Significant age and sex differences exist in the frequency of the various types of syncope. Syncope occurring in children and young adults is most frequently due to hyperventilation or vasovagal (vasodepressor) attacks and less frequently due to congenital heart disease (Lewis and Dhala, 1999). Fainting associated with benign tachycardias without underlying organic heart disease also may occur in children. Syncope due to basilar migraine is more common in young females. Although vasovagal syncope can occur in older patients (Tan et al., 2008), when repeated syncope begins in later life, organic disease of the cerebral circulation or cardiovascular system usually is responsible.

A careful history is the most important step in establishing the cause of syncope. The patient's description usually establishes the diagnosis. The neurologist should always obtain as full a description as possible of the first faint. The clinical

TABLE 2.1 Comparison of Clinical Features of Syncope and Seizures

Features	Syncope	Seizure
Relation to posture	Common	No
Time of day	Diurnal	Diurnal or nocturnal
Precipitating factors	Emotion, injury, pain, crowds, heat, exercise, fear, dehydration, coughing, micturition	Sleep loss, drug/alcohol withdrawal
Skin color	Pallor	Cyanosis or normal
Diaphoresis	Common	Rare
Aura or premonitory symptoms	Long	Brief
Convulsion	Rare	Common
Other abnormal movements	Minor twitching	Rhythmic jerks
Injury	Rare	Common (with convulsive seizures)
Urinary incontinence	Rare	Common
Tongue biting	No	Can occur with convulsive seizures
Postictal confusion	Rare	Common
Postictal headache	No	Common
Focal neurological signs	No	Occasional
Cardiovascular signs	Common (cardiac syncope)	No
Abnormal findings on EEG	Rare (generalized slowing may occur during the event)	Common

EEG, Electroencephalogram.

BOX 2.1 Classification and Etiology of Syncope

Cardiac:
   Arrhythmias:
      Bradyarrhythmias
      Tachyarrhythmias
      Reflex arrhythmias
   Decreased cardiac output:
      Outflow obstruction
      Inflow obstruction
      Cardiomyopathy
Hypovolemic
Hypotensive:
   Vasovagal attack
   Drugs
   Dysautonomia
Cerebrovascular:
   Carotid disease
   Vertebrobasilar disease
   Vasospasm
   Takayasu disease
Metabolic:
   Hypoglycemia
   Anemia
   Anoxia
Hyperventilation
Multifactorial:
   Vasovagal (vasodepressor) attack
   Cardiac syncope
   Situational: Cough, micturition, defecation, swallowing, diving
      Valsalva maneuver

features should be established, with emphasis on precipitating factors, posture, type of onset of the faint (including whether it was abrupt or gradual), position of head and neck, the presence and duration of preceding and associated symptoms, duration of loss of consciousness, rate of recovery, and sequelae. If possible, question an observer about clonic movements, color changes, diaphoresis, pulse, respiration, urinary incontinence, and the nature of recovery.

Clues in the history that suggest cardiac syncope include a history of palpitations or a fluttering sensation in the chest before loss of consciousness. These symptoms are common in arrhythmias. In vasodepressor syncope and orthostatic hypotension, preceding symptoms of lightheadedness are common. Episodes of cardiac syncope generally are briefer than vasodepressor syncope, and the onset usually is rapid. Episodes due to cardiac arrhythmias occur independently of position, whereas in vasodepressor syncope and syncope due to orthostatic hypotension the patient usually is standing.

Attacks of syncope precipitated by exertion suggest a cardiac etiology. Exercise may induce arrhythmic syncope or syncope due to decreased cardiac output secondary to blood flow obstruction, such as may occur with aortic or subaortic stenosis. Exercise syncope also may be due to cerebrovascular disease, aortic arch disease, congenital heart disease, pulseless

disease (Takayasu disease), pulmonary hypertension, anemia, hypoxia, and hypoglycemia. A family history of sudden cardiac death, especially in females, suggests the long QT-interval syndrome. Postexercise syncope may be secondary to situational syncope or autonomic dysfunction. A careful and complete medical and medication history is mandatory to determine whether prescribed drugs have induced either orthostatic hypotension or cardiac arrhythmias. To avoid missing a significant cardiac disorder, consider a comprehensive cardiac evaluation in patients with exercise-related syncope. Particularly in the elderly, cardiac syncope must be distinguished from more benign causes because of increased risk of sudden cardiac death (Anderson and O'Callaghan, 2012).

The neurologist should inquire about the frequency of attacks of loss of consciousness and the presence of cerebrovascular or cardiovascular symptoms between episodes. Question the patient whether all episodes are similar, because some patients experience more than one type of attack. In the elderly, syncope may cause unexplained falls lacking prodromal symptoms. With an accurate description of the attacks and familiarity with clinical features of various types of syncope, the physician should correctly diagnose most patients (Brignole et al., 2006; Shen et al., 2004). Seizure types that must be distinguished from syncope include orbitofrontal complex partial seizures, which can be associated with autonomic changes, and complex partial seizures that are associated with sudden falls and altered awareness, followed by confusion and gradual recovery (temporal lobe syncope). Features that distinguish syncope from seizures and other alterations of consciousness are discussed later in the chapter.

After a complete history, the physical examination is of next importance. Examination during the episode is very informative but frequently impossible unless syncope is reproducible by a Valsalva maneuver or by recreating the circumstances of the attack, such as by position change. In the patient with suspected cardiac syncope, pay particular attention to the vital signs and determination of supine and erect blood pressure. Normally, with standing, the systolic blood pressure *rises* and the pulse rate may *increase*. An orthostatic drop in blood pressure greater than 15 mm Hg may suggest autonomic dysfunction. Assess blood pressure in both arms when suspecting cerebrovascular disease, subclavian steal, or Takayasu arteritis.

During syncope due to a cardiac arrhythmia, a heart rate faster than 140 beats per minute usually indicates an ectopic cardiac rhythm, whereas a bradycardia with heart rate of less than 40 beats per minute suggests complete atrioventricular (AV) block. Carotid sinus massage sometimes terminates a supraventricular tachycardia, but this maneuver is not advisable because of the risk of cerebral embolism from atheroma in the carotid artery wall. In contrast, a ventricular tachycardia shows no response to carotid sinus massage. Stokes-Adams attacks may be of longer duration and may be associated with audible atrial contraction and a first heart sound of variable intensity. Heart disease as a cause of syncope is more common in the elderly patient. The patient should undergo cardiac auscultation for the presence of cardiac murmurs and abnormalities of the heart sounds. Possible murmurs include aortic stenosis, subaortic stenosis, or mitral valve origin. An intermittent posture-related murmur may be associated with an atrial myxoma. A systolic click in a young person suggests mitral valve prolapse. A pericardial rub suggests pericarditis.

All patients should undergo observation of the carotid pulse and auscultation of the neck. The degree of aortic stenosis may be reflected at times in a delayed carotid upstroke. Carotid, ophthalmic, and supraclavicular bruits suggest underlying cerebrovascular disease. Carotid sinus massage may be useful in older patients suspected of having carotid sinus syncope, but it is important to keep in mind that up to 25% of asymptomatic persons may have some degree of carotid sinus hypersensitivity. Carotid massage should be avoided in patients with suspected cerebrovascular disease, and when performed, it should be done under properly controlled conditions with electrocardiographic (ECG) and blood pressure monitoring. The response to carotid massage is vasodepressor, cardioinhibitory, or mixed.

Causes of Syncope
Cardiac Arrhythmias

Both bradyarrhythmias and tachyarrhythmias may result in syncope, and abnormalities of cardiac rhythm due to dysfunction from the sinoatrial (SA) node to the Purkinje network may be involved. Always consider arrhythmias in all cases in which an obvious mechanism is not established. Syncope due to cardiac arrhythmias generally occurs more quickly than syncope from other causes. Cardiac syncope may occur in any position, is occasionally exercise induced, and may occur in both congenital and acquired forms of heart disease.

Although palpitations sometimes occur during arrhythmias, others are unaware of any cardiac symptoms. Syncopal episodes secondary to cardiac arrhythmias may be more prolonged than benign syncope. The most common arrhythmias causing syncope are AV block, SA block, and paroxysmal supraventricular and ventricular tachyarrhythmias. *AV block* describes disturbances of conduction occurring in the AV conducting system, which include the AV node to the bundle of His and the Purkinje network. *SA block* describes a failure of consistent pacemaker function of the SA node. *Paroxysmal tachycardia* refers to a rapid heart rate secondary to an ectopic

focus outside the SA node; this may be either supra- or intraventricular. In patients with implanted pacemakers, syncope can occur because of pacemaker malfunction.

Atrioventricular Block

Atrioventricular block is probably the most common cause of arrhythmic cardiac syncope. The term *Stokes-Adams attack* describes disturbances of consciousness occurring in association with a complete AV block. Complete AV block occurs primarily in elderly patients. The onset of a Stokes-Adams attack generally is sudden, although a number of visual, sensory, and perceptual premonitory symptoms may be experienced. During the syncopal attack, the pulse disappears and no heart sounds are audible. The patient is pale and, if standing, falls down, often with resultant injury. If the attack is sufficiently prolonged, respiration may become labored, and urinary incontinence and clonic muscle jerks may occur. Prolonged confusion and neurological signs of cerebral ischemia may be present. Regaining of consciousness generally is rapid.

The clinical features of complete AV block include a slow-collapsing pulse and elevation of the jugular venous pressure, sometimes with cannon waves. The first heart sound is of variable intensity, and heart sounds related to atrial contractions may be audible. An ECG confirming the diagnosis demonstrates independence of atrial P waves and ventricular QRS complexes. During Stokes-Adams attacks, the ECG generally shows ventricular standstill, but ventricular fibrillation or tachycardia also may occur.

Sinoatrial Block

Sinoatrial block may result in dizziness, lightheadedness, and syncope. It is most frequent in the elderly. Palpitations are common, and the patient appears pale. Patients with SA node dysfunction frequently have other conduction disturbances, and certain drugs (e.g., verapamil, digoxin, beta-blockers) may further impair SA node function. On examination, the patient's pulse may be regular between attacks. During an attack, the pulse may be slow or irregular, and any of a number of rhythm disturbances may be present.

Paroxysmal Tachycardia

Supraventricular tachycardias include atrial fibrillation with a rapid ventricular response, atrial flutter, and the Wolff–Parkinson–White syndrome. These arrhythmias may suddenly reduce cardiac output enough to cause syncope. Ventricular tachycardia or ventricular fibrillation may result in syncope if the heart rate is sufficiently fast and if the arrhythmia lasts longer than a few seconds. Patients generally are elderly and usually have evidence of underlying cardiac disease. Ventricular fibrillation may be part of the long QT syndrome, which has a cardiac-only phenotype or may be associated with congenital sensorineural deafness in children. In most patients with this syndrome, episodes begin in the first decade of life, but onset may be much later. Exercise may precipitate an episode of cardiac syncope. Long QT syndrome may be congenital or acquired and manifests in adults as epilepsy. Acquired causes include cardiac ischemia, mitral valve prolapse, myocarditis, and electrolyte disturbances as well as many drugs. In the short QT syndrome, signs and symptoms are highly variable, ranging from complete absence of clinical manifestations to recurrent syncope to sudden death. The age at onset often is young, and affected persons frequently are otherwise healthy. A family history of sudden death indicates a familial short QT syndrome inherited as an autosomal dominant mutation. The ECG demonstrates a short QT interval and a tall and peaked T wave, and electrophysiological studies may induce ventricular fibrillation. Brugada syndrome may produce syncope as a result of ventricular tachycardia or ventricular fibrillation (Brugada et al., 2000). The ECG demonstrates an incomplete right bundle-branch block in leads V_1 and V_2, with ST-segment elevation in the right precordial leads.

Reflex Cardiac Arrhythmias

A hypersensitive carotid sinus may be a cause of syncope in the elderly, most frequently men. Syncope may result from a reflex sinus bradycardia, sinus arrest, or AV block; peripheral vasodilatation with a fall in arterial pressure; or a combination of both. Although 10% of the population older than 60 years of age may have a hypersensitive carotid sinus, not all such patients experience syncope. Accordingly, consider this diagnosis only when the clinical history is compatible. Carotid sinus syncope may be initiated by wearing a tight collar or by carotid sinus massage on clinical examination. When syncope occurs, the patient usually is upright, and the duration of the loss of consciousness generally is a few minutes. On regaining consciousness, the patient is mentally clear. Unfortunately, no accepted diagnostic criteria exist for carotid sinus syncope, and the condition is overdiagnosed.

Syncope in certain patients can be induced by unilateral carotid massage or compression or by partial occlusion (usually atherosclerotic) of the contralateral carotid artery or a vertebral artery or by the release of atheromatous emboli. Because of these risks, carotid artery massage is contraindicated.

The rare syndrome of glossopharyngeal neuralgia is characterized by intense paroxysmal pain in the throat and neck accompanied by bradycardia or asystole, severe hypotension, and, if prolonged, seizures. Episodes of pain may be initiated by swallowing but also by chewing, speaking, laughing, coughing, shouting, sneezing, yawning, or talking. The episodes of pain always precede the loss of consciousness (see Chapter 20). Rarely, cardiac syncope may be due to bradyarrhythmias consequent to vagus nerve irritation caused by esophageal diverticula, tumors, and aneurysms in the region of the carotid sinus or by mediastinal masses or gallbladder disease.

Decreased Cardiac Output

Syncope may occur as a result of a sudden and marked decrease in cardiac output. Causes are both congenital and acquired. Tetralogy of Fallot, the most common congenital malformation causing syncope, does so by producing hypoxia due to right-to-left shunting. Other congenital conditions associated with cyanotic heart disease also may cause syncope. Ischemic heart disease and myocardial infarction (MI), aortic stenosis, idiopathic hypertrophic subaortic stenosis, pulmonary hypertension, and other causes of obstruction of pulmonary outflow, atrial myxoma, and cardiac tamponade may sufficiently impair cardiac output to cause syncope. Exercise-induced or effort syncope may occur in aortic or subaortic stenosis and other states in which there is reduced cardiac output and associated peripheral vasodilatation induced by the exercise. Exercise-induced cardiac syncope and exercise-induced cardiac arrhythmias may be related.

In patients with valvular heart disease, the cause of syncope may be arrhythmias. Syncope also may be due to reduced cardiac output secondary to myocardial failure, to mechanical prosthetic valve malfunction, or to thrombus formation. Mitral valve prolapse generally is a benign condition, but rarely, cardiac arrhythmias can occur. The most significant arrhythmias are ventricular. In atrial myxoma or with massive pulmonary embolism, a sudden drop in left ventricular output may occur. In atrial myxoma, syncope frequently is positional and occurs when the tumor falls into the AV valve opening

during a change in position of the patient, thereby causing obstruction of the left ventricular inflow.

Decreased cardiac output also may be secondary to conditions causing an inflow obstruction or reduced venous return. Such conditions include superior and inferior vena cava obstruction, tension pneumothorax, constrictive cardiomyopathies, constrictive pericarditis, and cardiac tamponade. Syncope associated with aortic dissection may be due to cardiac tamponade but also may be secondary to hypotension, obstruction of cerebral circulation, or a cardiac arrhythmia.

Hypovolemia

Acute blood loss, usually due to GI tract bleeding, may cause weakness, faintness, and syncope if sufficient blood is lost. Blood volume depletion by dehydration may cause faintness and weakness, but true syncope is uncommon except when combining dehydration and exercise.

Hypotension

Several conditions cause syncope by producing a fall in arterial pressure. Cardiac causes were discussed earlier. The common faint (synonymous with *vasovagal* or *vasodepressor syncope*) is the most frequent cause of a transitory fall in blood pressure resulting in syncope. It often is recurrent, tends to occur in relation to emotional stimuli, and may affect 20% to 25% of young people. Less commonly, it occurs in older patients with cardiovascular disease.

The common faint may or may not be associated with bradycardia. The patient experiences impairment of consciousness, with loss of postural tone. Signs of autonomic hyperactivity are common, including pallor, diaphoresis, nausea, and dilated pupils. After recovery, patients may have persistent pallor, sweating, and nausea; if they get up too quickly, they may black out again. Presyncopal symptoms of lethargy and fatigue, nausea, weakness, a sensation of an impending faint, yawning, and blurred vision may occur. It is more likely to occur in certain circumstances such as in a hot crowded room, especially if the affected person is tired or hungry and upright or sitting. Venipuncture, the sight of blood, or a sudden painful or traumatic experience may precipitate syncope. When the patient regains consciousness, there usually is no confusion or headache, although weakness is frequent. As in other causes of syncope, if the period of cerebral hypoperfusion is prolonged, urinary incontinence and a few clonic movements may occur (convulsive syncope).

Orthostatic syncope occurs when autonomic factors that compensate for the upright posture are inadequate. This can result from a variety of clinical disorders. Blood volume depletion or venous pooling may cause syncope when the affected person assumes an upright posture. Orthostatic hypotension resulting in syncope also may occur with drugs that impair sympathetic nervous system function. Diuretics, antihypertensive medications, nitrates, arterial vasodilators, sildenafil, calcium channel blockers, monoamine oxidase inhibitors, phenothiazines, opiates, L-dopa, alcohol, and tricyclic antidepressants all may cause orthostatic hypotension. Patients with postural tachycardia syndrome (POTS) frequently experience orthostatic symptoms without orthostatic hypotension, but syncope can occur occasionally. Data suggest that there is sympathetic activation in this syndrome (Garland et al., 2007). Autonomic nervous system dysfunction resulting in syncope due to orthostatic hypotension may be a result of primary autonomic failure due to Shy–Drager syndrome (multiple system atrophy) or Riley–Day syndrome. Neuropathies that affect the autonomic nervous system include those of diabetes mellitus, amyloidosis, Guillain–Barré syndrome, acquired immunodeficiency syndrome (AIDS), chronic alcoholism, hepatic porphyria, beriberi, and autoimmune subacute autonomic neuropathy and small fiber neuropathies. Rarely, subacute combined degeneration, syringomyelia, and other spinal cord lesions may damage the descending sympathetic pathways, producing orthostatic hypotension. Accordingly, conditions that affect both the central and peripheral baroreceptor mechanisms may cause orthostatic hypotension (Benafroch, 2008).

Cerebrovascular Ischemia

Syncope occasionally may result from reduction of cerebral blood flow in either the carotid or vertebrobasilar system in patients with extensive occlusive disease. Most frequently, the underlying condition is atherosclerosis of the cerebral vessels, but reduction of cerebral blood flow due to cerebral embolism, mechanical factors in the neck (e.g., severe osteoarthritis), and arteritis (e.g., Takayasu disease or cranial arteritis) may be responsible. In the subclavian steal syndrome, a very rare impairment of consciousness is associated with upper extremity exercise and resultant diversion of cerebral blood flow to the peripheral circulation. In elderly patients with cervical skeletal deformities, certain head movements such as hyperextension or lateral rotation can result in syncope secondary to vertebrobasilar arterial ischemia. In these patients, associated vestibular symptoms are common. Occasionally, cerebral vasospasm secondary to basilar artery migraine or subarachnoid hemorrhage may be responsible. Insufficiency of the cerebral circulation frequently causes other neurological symptoms, depending on the circulation involved.

Reduction in blood flow in the carotid circulation may lead to loss of consciousness, lightheadedness, giddiness, and a sensation of an impending faint. Reduction in blood flow in the vertebrobasilar system also may lead to loss of consciousness, but dizziness, lightheadedness, drop attacks without loss of consciousness, and bilateral motor and sensory symptoms are more common. Dizziness and lightheadedness alone, however, are not symptoms of vertebrobasilar insufficiency. Syncope due to compression of the vertebral artery during certain head and neck movements may be associated with episodes of vertigo, disequilibrium, or drop attacks. Patients may describe blackouts on looking upward suddenly or on turning the head quickly to one side. Generally, symptoms persist for several seconds after the movement stops.

In Takayasu disease, major occlusion of blood flow in the carotid and vertebrobasilar systems may occur; in addition to fainting, other neurological manifestations are frequent. Pulsations in the neck and arm vessels usually are absent, and blood pressure in the arms is unobtainable. The syncopal episodes characteristically occur with mild or moderate exercise and with certain head movements. Cerebral vasospasm may result in syncope, particularly if the posterior circulation is involved. In basilar artery migraine, usually seen in young women and children, a variety of brainstem symptoms also may be experienced, and it is associated with a pulsating headache. The loss of consciousness usually is gradual, but a confusional state may last for hours (see Chapter 65).

Metabolic Disorders

A number of metabolic disturbances including hypoglycemia, anoxia, and hyperventilation-induced alkalosis may predispose affected persons to syncope, but usually only lightheadedness and dizziness are experienced. The abruptness of onset of loss of consciousness depends on the acuteness and reversibility of the metabolic disturbances. Syncope due to hypoglycemia usually develops gradually. The patient has a sensation of hunger; there may be a relationship to fasting, a history of

diabetes mellitus, and a prompt response to ingestion of food. Symptoms are unrelated to posture but may increase with exercise. During the syncopal attack, no significant change in blood pressure or pulse occurs. Hypoadrenalism may give rise to syncope by causing orthostatic hypotension. Disturbances of calcium, magnesium, and potassium metabolism are other rare causes of syncope. Anoxia may produce syncope because of the lack of oxygen or through the production of a vasodepressor type of syncope. A feeling of lightheadedness is common, but true syncope is less common. Patients with underlying cardiac or pulmonary disease are susceptible. In patients with chronic anemia or certain hemoglobinopathies that impair oxygen transport, similar symptoms may occur. Syncopal symptoms may be more prominent with exercise or physical activity.

Hyperventilation-induced syncope usually has a psychogenic origin. During hyperventilation, the patient may experience paresthesia of the face, hands, and feet, a buzzing sensation in the head, lightheadedness, giddiness, blurring of vision, mouth dryness, and occasionally tetany. Patients often complain of tightness in the chest and a sense of panic. Symptoms can occur in the supine or erect position and are gradual in onset. Rebreathing into a paper bag relieves the symptoms. During hyperventilation, a tachycardia may be present, but blood pressure generally remains normal.

Miscellaneous Causes of Syncope

More than one mechanism may be responsible in certain types of syncope. Both vasodepressor and cardioinhibitory factors may be operational in common syncope. In cardiac syncope, a reduction of cardiac output may be due to a single cause such as obstruction to inflow or outflow or a cardiac arrhythmia, but multiple factors are frequent.

Situational syncope, such as is associated with cough (tussive syncope) and micturition, are special cases of reflex syncope. In cough syncope, loss of consciousness occurs after a paroxysm of severe coughing. This is most likely to occur in obese men, usually smokers or patients with chronic bronchitis. The syncopal episodes occur suddenly, generally after repeated coughing but occasionally after a single cough. Before losing consciousness, the patient may feel lightheaded. The face often becomes flushed secondary to congestion, and then pale. Diaphoresis may be present, and loss of muscle tone may occur. Syncope generally is brief, lasting only seconds, and recovery is rapid. Several factors probably are operational in causing cough syncope. The most significant is blockage of venous return by raised intrathoracic pressure. In weight-lifting syncope, a similar mechanism is operational.

Micturition syncope most commonly occurs in men during or after micturition, usually after arising from bed in the middle of the night to urinate in the erect position. There may be a history of drinking alcohol before going to bed. The syncope may result from sudden reflex peripheral vasodilatation caused by the release of intravesicular pressure and bradycardia. The relative peripheral vasodilatation from recent alcohol use and a supine sleeping position is contributory because blood pressure is lowest in the middle of the night. The syncopal propensity may increase with fever. Rarely, micturition syncope with headache may result from a pheochromocytoma in the bladder wall. Defecation syncope is uncommon, but it probably shares the underlying pathophysiological mechanisms responsible for micturition syncope. Convulsive syncope is an episode of syncope of any cause that is sufficiently prolonged to result in a few clonic jerks; the other features typically are syncopal and should not be confused with epileptic seizures. Other causes of situational syncope include diving and the postprandial state. Syncope during sexual activity may be due to neurocardiogenic syncope, coronary artery disease, or the use of erectile dysfunction medications. Rare intracranial causes of syncope include intermittent obstruction to CSF flow such as with a third ventricular mass. Rarely, syncope can occur with Arnold Chiari malformations, but these patients usually have other symptoms of brainstem dysfunction.

Investigations of Patients with Syncope

In the investigation of the patient with episodic impairment of consciousness, the diagnostic tests performed depend on the initial differential diagnosis. Individualize investigations, but some measurements such as hematocrit, blood glucose, and ECG are always appropriate. A resting ECG may reveal an abnormality of cardiac rhythm or the presence of underlying ischemic or congenital heart disease. In the patient suspected of cardiac syncope, a chest radiograph may show evidence of cardiac hypertrophy, valvular heart disease, or pulmonary hypertension. Other noninvasive investigations include radionuclide cardiac scanning, echocardiography, and prolonged Holter monitoring for the detection of cardiac arrhythmias. Echocardiography is useful in the diagnosis of valvular heart disease, cardiomyopathy, atrial myxoma, prosthetic valve dysfunction, pericardial effusion, aortic dissection, and congenital heart disease. Holter monitoring detects twice as many ECG abnormalities as those discovered on a routine ECG and may disclose an arrhythmia at the time of a syncopal episode. Holter monitoring typically for a 24-hour period is usual, although longer periods of recording may be required. Implantable loop recordings can provide long-term rhythm monitoring in patients suspected of having a cardiac arrhythmia (Krahn et al., 2004).

Exercise testing and electrophysiological studies are useful in selected patients. Exercise testing may be useful in detecting coronary artery disease, and exercise-related syncopal recordings may help localize the site of conduction disturbances. Consider tilt-table testing in patients with unexplained syncope in high-risk settings or with recurrent faints in the absence of heart disease (Kapoor, 1999). False positives occur, and 10% of healthy persons may faint. Tilt testing frequently employs pharmacological agents such as nitroglycerin or isoproterenol. The specificity of tilt-table testing is approximately 90%, but the sensitivity differs in different patient populations. In patients suspected to have syncope due to cerebrovascular causes, noninvasive diagnostic studies including Doppler flow studies of the cerebral vessels and magnetic resonance imaging (MRI) or magnetic resonance angiography may provide useful information. The American Academy of Neurology recommends that carotid imaging not be performed unless there are other focal neurologic symptoms (Langer-Gould et al., 2013). Cerebral angiography is sometimes useful. Electroencephalography (EEG) is useful in differentiating syncope from epileptic seizure disorders. An EEG should be obtained only when a seizure disorder is suspected and generally has a low diagnostic yield (Poliquin-Lasnier and Moore, 2009). A systematic evaluation can establish a definitive diagnosis in 98% of patients (Brignole et al., 2006). Neurally mediated (vasovagal or vasodepressor) syncope was found in 66% of patients, orthostatic hypotension in 10%, primary arrhythmias in 11%, and structural cardiopulmonary disease in 5%. Initial history, physical examination, and a standard ECG established a diagnosis in 50% of patients. A risk score such as the San Francisco Syncope Rule (SFSR) can help identify patients who need urgent referral. The presence of cardiac failure, anemia, abnormal ECG, or systolic hypotension helps identify these patients (Parry and Tan, 2010). A systematic review of the SFSR rule accuracy

(Saccilotto et al., 2011) found that the rule cannot be applied safely to all patients and should only be applied to patients for whom no cause of syncope is identified. The rule should only be used in conjunction with clinical evaluation, particularly in elderly patients. The ROSE study is another risk stratification evaluation of patients who present to the emergency department (Reed et al., 2010). Independent predictors of one month serious outcome were brain natriuretic peptide concentration, positive fecal occult blood, hemoglobin $\leq$ 90 g/L, oxygen saturation $\leq$ 94%, and Q-wave on the ECG. Serious outcome or all-cause death occur in 7.1% but this study also requires further validation.

SEIZURES

Epileptic seizures cause sudden, unexplained loss of consciousness in a child or an adult (see Chapter 101). Seizures and syncope are distinguishable clinically; pallor is not associated with seizures.

History and Physical Examination

The most definitive way to diagnose epilepsy and the type of seizure is clinical observation of the seizure, although this often is not possible, except when seizures are frequent. The history of an episode, as obtained from the patient and an observer, is of paramount importance. The neurologist should obtain a family history and should inquire about birth complications, central nervous system (CNS) infection, head trauma, and previous febrile seizures, because they all may have relevance.

The neurologist should obtain a complete description of the episode and inquire about any warning before the event, possible precipitating factors, and other neurological symptoms that may suggest an underlying structural cause. Important considerations are the age at onset, frequency, and diurnal variation of the events. Seizures generally are brief and have stereotypical patterns, as described previously. With complex partial seizures and tonic-clonic seizures, a period of postictal confusion is highly characteristic. Unlike some types of syncope, seizures are unrelated to posture and generally last longer. In a tonic-clonic seizure, cyanosis frequently is present, pallor is uncommon, and breathing may be stertorous. In children with autonomic seizures (Panayiotopoulos syndrome) syncope-like epileptic seizures can occur (Koutroumanidis et al., 2012).

Tonic-clonic and complex partial seizures may begin at any age from infancy to late adulthood, although young infants may not demonstrate the typical features because of incomplete development of the nervous system.

The neurological examination may reveal an underlying structural disturbance responsible for the seizure disorder. Birth-related trauma may result in asymmetries of physical development, cranial bruits may indicate an arteriovenous malformation, and space-occupying lesions may result in papilledema or in focal motor, sensory, or reflex signs. In the pediatric age group, mental retardation occurs in association with birth injury or metabolic defects. The skin should be examined for abnormal pigment changes and other dysmorphic features characteristic of some of the neurodegenerative disorders.

If examination is immediately after a suspected tonic-clonic seizure, the neurologist should search for abnormal signs such as focal motor weakness and reflex asymmetry and for pathological reflexes such as a Babinski sign. Such findings may help confirm that the attack was a seizure and suggest a possible lateralization or location of the seizure focus.

Absence Seizures

The onset of absence seizures is usually between the ages of 5 and 15 years, and a family history of seizures is present in 20% to 40% of patients. The absence seizure is a well-defined clinical and EEG event. The essential feature is an abrupt, brief episode of decreased awareness without any warning, aura, or postictal symptoms. At the onset of the absence seizure, there is an interruption of activity. A simple absence seizure is characterized clinically only by an alteration of consciousness. Characteristic of a complex absence seizure is an alteration of consciousness and other signs such as minor motor automatisms. During a simple absence seizure, the patient remains immobile, breathing is normal, skin color remains unchanged, postural tone is not lost, and no motor manifestations occur. After the seizure, the patient immediately resumes the previous activities and may be unaware of the attack. An absence seizure generally lasts 10 to 15 seconds, but it may be shorter or as long as 40 seconds.

Complex absence seizures have additional manifestations such as diminution of postural tone that may cause the patient to fall, an increase in postural tone, minor clonic movements of the facial musculature or extremities, minor face or extremity automatisms, or autonomic phenomena such as pallor, flushing, tachycardia, piloerection, mydriasis, or urinary incontinence.

If absence seizures are suspected, office diagnosis is frequently possible by having the patient hyperventilate for 3 to 4 minutes, which often induces an absence seizure.

Tonic-Clonic Seizures

The tonic-clonic seizure is the most dramatic manifestation of epilepsy and characterized by motor activity and loss of consciousness. Tonic-clonic seizures may be the only manifestation of epilepsy or may be associated with other seizure types. In a primary generalized tonic-clonic seizure, the affected person generally experiences no warning or aura, although a few myoclonic jerks may occur in some patients. The seizure begins with a tonic phase, during which there is sustained muscle contraction lasting 10 to 20 seconds. Following this phase is a clonic phase that lasts approximately 30 seconds and is characterized by recurrent muscle contractions. During a tonic-clonic seizure, a number of autonomic changes may be present, including an increase in blood pressure and heart rate, apnea, mydriasis, urinary or fecal incontinence, piloerection, cyanosis, and diaphoresis. Injury may result from a fall or tongue biting. In the postictal period, consciousness returns slowly, and the patient may remain lethargic and confused for a variable period. Pathological reflexes may be elicitable.

Some generalized motor seizures with transitory alteration of consciousness may have only tonic or only clonic components. Tonic seizures consist of an increase in muscle tone, and the alteration of consciousness generally is brief. Clonic seizures have a brief impairment of consciousness and bilateral clonic movements. Recovery may be rapid, but if the seizure is more prolonged, a postictal period of confusion may be noted.

Complex Partial Seizures

In a complex partial seizure, the first seizure manifestation may be an alteration of consciousness, but the patient frequently experiences an aura or warning symptom. The seizure may have a simple partial onset that may include motor, sensory, visceral, or psychic symptoms. The patient initially may experience hallucinations or illusions, affective symptoms such as fear or depression, cognitive symptoms such as a sense of depersonalization or unreality, or aphasia.

The complex partial seizure generally lasts 1 to 3 minutes but may be shorter or longer. It may become generalized and evolve into a tonic-clonic convulsion. During a complex partial seizure, automatisms, generally more complex than those in absence seizures, may occur. The automatisms may involve continuation of the patient's activity before the onset of the seizure, or they may be new motor acts. Such new automatisms are variable but frequently consist of chewing or swallowing movements, lip smacking, grimacing, or automatisms of the extremities, including fumbling with objects, walking, or trying to stand up. Rarely, patients with complex partial seizures have drop attacks; in such cases, the term *temporal lobe syncope* often is used. The duration of the postictal period after a complex partial seizure is variable, with a gradual return to normal consciousness and normal response to external stimuli. Table 2.2 provides a comparison of absence seizures and complex partial seizures.

Investigations of Seizures

In the initial investigations of the patient with tonic-clonic or complex partial seizures, perform a complete blood cell count, urinalysis, biochemical screening, and determinations of blood glucose level and serum calcium concentration. Laboratory investigations generally are not helpful in establishing a diagnosis of absence seizures. In infants and children, consider biochemical screening for amino acid disorders.

MRI is the imaging modality of choice for the investigation of patients with suspected seizures. It is superior to computed tomography and increases the yield of focal structural disturbances. Cerebrospinal fluid examination is not necessary in every patient with a seizure disorder and should be reserved for those in whom a recent seizure may relate to an acute CNS infection.

TABLE 2.2 Comparison of Absence and Complex Partial Seizures

Feature	Absence seizure	Complex partial seizure
Neurological status	Normal	May have positive history or examination
Age at onset	Childhood or adolescence	Any age
Aura or warning	No	Common
Onset	Abrupt	Gradual
Duration	Seconds	Up to minutes
Automatisms	Simple	More complex
Provocation by hyperventilation	Common	Uncommon
Termination	Abrupt	Gradual
Frequency	Possibly multiple seizures per day	Occasional
Postictal phase	No	Confusion, fatigue
Electroencephalogram	Generalized spike and wave	Focal epileptic discharges or nonspecific abnormalities
Neuroimaging	Usually normal findings	May demonstrate focal lesions

An EEG provides laboratory support for a clinical impression and helps classify the type of seizure. Epilepsy is a clinical diagnosis; therefore, an EEG study cannot confirm the diagnosis with certainty unless the patient has a clinical event during the recording. Normal findings on the EEG do not exclude epilepsy, and minor nonspecific abnormalities do not confirm epilepsy. Some patients with clinically documented seizures show no abnormality even after serial EEG recordings, sleep recordings, and special activation techniques. The EEG is most frequently helpful in the diagnosis of absence seizures. EEG supplemented with simultaneous video monitoring documents ictal events, allowing for a strict correlation between EEG changes and clinical manifestations. Simultaneous EEG and video monitoring also is useful in distinguishing epileptic seizures from nonepileptic phenomena.

In most patients, an accurate diagnosis requires only the clinical history and the foregoing investigations. Others present a diagnostic dilemma. A 24-hour ambulatory EEG recording differentiates an epileptic seizure from nonepileptic phenomena and also helps classify the specific type of seizure.

Psychogenic (Nonepileptic) Seizures

Nonepileptic seizures are paroxysmal episodes of altered behavior that superficially resemble epileptic seizures but lack the expected EEG epileptic changes (Ettinger et al., 1999). However, as many as 40% of patients with pseudo- or nonepileptic seizures also experience true epileptic seizures.

A diagnosis often is difficult to establish based on the initial history alone. Establishing the correct diagnosis often requires observation of the patient's clinical episodes, but complex partial seizures of frontal lobe origin may be difficult to distinguish from nonepileptic seizures. Nonepileptic seizures occur in children and adults and are more common in females. Most frequently, they superficially resemble tonic-clonic seizures. They generally are abrupt in onset, occur in the presence of other people, and do not occur during sleep. Motor activity is uncoordinated, but urinary incontinence and physical injury are uncommon. Nonepileptic seizures tend to be more prolonged than true tonic-clonic seizures. Pelvic thrusting is common. Ictal eye closing is common in nonepileptic seizures, whereas the eyes tend to be open in true epileptic seizures (Chung et al., 2006). During and immediately after the seizure, the patient may not respond to verbal or painful stimuli. Cyanosis does not occur, and focal neurological signs and pathological reflexes are absent. The clinical characteristics of nonepileptic seizures in children may be different than in adults (Patel et al., 2007). In younger children there is less of a gender difference and motor activity may be more subtle. Risk factors in children include depressive illnesses, concomitant epilepsy, and cognitive dysfunction.

Episodes without prominent motor activity resembling syncope are more appropriately referred to as psychogenic pseudosyncope (Tannemaat et al., 2013). The apparent loss of consciousness in these patients may be longer than in syncope. The diagnosis can be distinguished from syncope if tilt-table testing fails to document a decrease in heart rate or blood pressure.

In the patient with known epilepsy, consider the diagnosis of nonepileptic seizures when previously controlled seizures become medically refractory. The patient should undergo psychological assessments because most affected persons are found to have specific psychiatric disturbances. In this patient group, a high frequency of hysteria, depression, anxiety, somatoform disorders, dissociative disorders, and personality disturbances is recognized. A history of physical or sexual abuse is also more prevalent in nonepileptic seizure patients. At times, a secondary gain is identifiable. In some patients

with psychogenic seizures, the clinical episodes frequently precipitate by suggestion and by certain clinical tests such as hyperventilation, photic stimulation, intravenous saline infusion, tactile (vibration) stimulation, or pinching the nose to induce apnea. Hyperventilation and photic stimulation also may induce true epileptic seizures, but their clinical features usually are distinctive. Some physicians avoid the use of placebo procedures, because this could have an adverse effect on the doctor–patient relationship (Parra et al., 1998).

Findings on the interictal EEG in patients with pseudoseizures are normal and remain normal during the clinical episode, demonstrating no evidence of a cerebral dysrhythmia. It is important to note, however, that a number of organic conditions may present with similar behavioral and motor symptoms and a nonepileptiform EEG (Caplan et al., 2011). The term pseudopseudoseizures is frequently used to describe these paroxysmal events. These may include conditions such as frontal lobe seizures, limb shaking transient ischemic attacks, and paroxysmal dyskinesias. With the introduction of long-term ambulatory EEG monitoring, correlating the episodic behavior of a patient with the EEG tracing is possible, and psychogenic seizures are distinguishable from true epileptic seizures. Table 2.3 compares the features of psychogenic seizures with those of epileptic seizures.

As an auxiliary investigation of suspected psychogenic seizures, plasma prolactin concentrations may provide additional supportive data. Plasma prolactin concentrations frequently are elevated after tonic-clonic seizures, peaking in 15 to 20 minutes, and less frequently after complex partial seizures. Serum prolactin levels almost invariably are normal after psychogenic seizures, although such a finding does not exclude the diagnosis of true epileptic seizures (Chen et al., 2005). Elevated prolactin levels, however, also may be present after syncope and with the use of drugs such as antidepressants, estrogens, bromocriptine, ergots, phenothiazines, and antiepileptic drugs.

Although several procedures are employed to help distinguish epileptic from nonepileptic seizures, none of these procedures have both high sensitivity and high specificity. No procedure attains the reliability of EEG-video monitoring, which remains the standard diagnostic method for distinguishing between the two (Cuthill and Espie, 2005).

MISCELLANEOUS CAUSES OF ALTERED CONSCIOUSNESS

In children, alteration of consciousness may accompany breath-holding spells and metabolic disturbances. Breath-holding spells and seizures are easily distinguished. Most spells start at 6 to 28 months of age, but they may occur as early as the first month of life; they usually disappear by 5 or 6 years of age. Breath-holding spells may occur several times per day and appear as either cyanosis or pallor.

The trigger for cyanotic breath-holding spells is usually a sudden injury or fright, anger, or frustration. The child initially is provoked, cries vigorously for a few breaths, and stops breathing in expiration, whereupon cyanosis rapidly develops. Consciousness is lost because of hypoxia. Although stiffening, a few clonic movements, and urinary incontinence occasionally are observed, these episodes can be clearly distinguished from epileptic seizures by the history of provocation and by noting that the apnea and cyanosis occur before any alteration of consciousness. In these children, findings on the neurological examination and the EEG are normal.

The provocation for pallid breath-holding is often a mild painful injury or a startle. The infant cries initially and then becomes pale and loses consciousness. As in the cyanotic type, stiffening, clonic movements, and urinary incontinence may

TABLE 2.3 Comparison of Psychogenic and Epileptic Seizures

Attack feature	Psychogenic seizure	Epileptic seizure
Stereotypy of attack	May be variable	Usually stereotypical
Onset or progression	Gradual	More rapid
Duration	May be prolonged	Brief
Diurnal variation	Daytime	Nocturnal or daytime
Injury	Rare	Can occur with tonic-clonic seizures
Tongue biting	Rare (tip of tongue)	Can occur with tonic-clonic seizures (sides of tongue)
Ictal eye closure	Common	Rare (eyes generally open)
Urinary incontinence	Rare	Frequent
Vocalization	May occur	Uncommon
Motor activity	Prolonged, uncoordinated; pelvic thrusting	Automatisms or side-to-side head movements, flailing, coordinated tonic-clonic activity
Prolonged loss of muscle tone	Common	Rare
Postictal confusion	Rare	Common
Postictal headache	Rare	Common
Postictal crying	Common	Rare
Relation to medication changes	Unrelated	Usually related
Relation to menses in women	Uncommon	Occasionally increased
Triggers	Emotional disturbances	No
Frequency of attacks	More frequent, up to daily	Less frequent
Interictal EEG findings	Normal	Frequently abnormal
Reproduction of attack by suggestion	Sometimes	No
Ictal EEG findings	Normal	Abnormal
Presence of secondary gain	Common	Uncommon
Presence of others	Frequently	Variable
Psychiatric disturbances	Common	Uncommon

EEG, electroencephalogram.

rarely occur. In the pallid infant syndrome, loss of consciousness is secondary to excessive vagal tone, resulting in bradycardia and subsequent cerebral ischemia, as in a vasovagal attack.

Breath-holding spells do not require treatment, but when intervention is required, levetiracetam (Keppra) is effective for prophylaxis at ordinary anticonvulsant doses.

Several pediatric metabolic disorders may have clinical manifestations of alterations of consciousness, lethargy, or seizures (see Chapter 91).

REFERENCES

The complete reference list is available online at https://expertconsult .inkling.com/.

3 Falls and Drop Attacks

Bernd F. Remler, Robert B. Daroff

CHAPTER OUTLINE

DROP ATTACKS WITH LOSS OF CONSCIOUSNESS
Syncope
Seizures
DROP ATTACKS WITHOUT LOSS OF CONSCIOUSNESS
Transient Ischemic Attacks
Third Ventricular and Posterior Fossa Abnormalities
Otolith Crisis
FALLS
Neuromuscular Disorders and Myelopathy
Other Cerebral or Cerebellar Disorders
Cryptogenic Falls in the Middle-Aged
Aging, Neurodegeneration, and the Neural Substrate of
Gait and Balance
SUMMARY

Everyone occasionally loses balance and sometimes falls, but unprovoked and repeated falls signal a potentially serious neurological problem. Considering the large number of potential etiologies, it is helpful to determine whether a patient has suffered a drop attack or an accidental fall. The term drop attack describes a sudden fall occurring without warning that may or may not be associated with loss of consciousness. Falls, on the other hand, reflect an inability to remain upright during a postural challenge. This most commonly affects individuals with chronic neurological impairment. Drop attacks, when associated with loss of consciousness, are likely due to a syncopal (cardiogenic) or epileptic event. Patients with preserved consciousness during a drop attack may have Meniere disease and fall as a result of otolith dysfunction. They may be narcoleptics experiencing a cataplectic attack, or harbor midline tumors in the posterior fossa or in the third ventricle. Transient ischemic attacks (TIAs) involving the posterior circulation or the anterior cerebral artery distribution can manifest in the same monosymptomatic manner. Chronic neurologic deficits such as lower-extremity weakness, spasticity, rigidity, sensory loss, or ataxia predispose to repetitive falls. Middle-aged women may fall with no discernible cause. Finally, the elderly, with their inevitable infirmities, fall frequently and with potentially disastrous consequences. These associations permit a classification of falls and drop attacks, presented in Box 3.1.

The medical history is essential in evaluating patients with falls and drop attacks. The situational and environmental circumstances of the event must be ascertained. To help establish a diagnosis from the wide range of possible causes, a detailed interview of the patient or of a witness to the fall is required. Aside from the patient's gender and age, which affect fall risk, answers to the following basic questions should be elicited:

What were the circumstances of the fall and has the patient fallen before?
Did the patient lose consciousness? If so, for how long?

Did lightheadedness, vertiginous sensations, or palpitations precede the event?
Is there a history of a seizure disorder, startle sensitivity, or falls precipitated by strong emotions?
Has the patient had excessive daytime sleepiness?
Does the patient have headaches or migraine attacks associated with weakness?
Does the patient have vascular risk factors, and were there previous symptoms suggestive of TIAs?
Are there symptoms of sensory loss, limb weakness, or stiffness?
Is there a history of visual impairment, hearing loss, vertigo, or tinnitus?

The neurological examination is as important and can establish whether falls may be related to a disorder of the central or peripheral nervous system. Specific abnormalities include motor or sensory deficits in the lower limbs; the rigidity, tremor, and ocular motor abnormalities associated with Parkinson disease (PD) or progressive supranuclear palsy (PSP); ataxia, spasticity, cognitive impairment, and other signs suggestive of a neurodegenerative disorder or multiple sclerosis. Patients with normal findings on the neurological examination and no history of associated neurological or cardiac symptoms present a special challenge. In such patients, magnetic resonance imaging (MRI) and vascular imaging can be considered to rule out a clinically silent midline cerebral neoplasm, hindbrain malformation, or vascular occlusive disease. The workup is otherwise tailored to the clinical circumstance and may include cardiac and autonomic studies, nocturnal polysomnography, and in rare circumstances, genetic and metabolic testing if related conditions are suspected. Patients who frequently experience near-falls without injuries may have a psychogenic disorder of station and gait.

DROP ATTACKS WITH LOSS OF CONSCIOUSNESS

Syncope

The manifestations and causes of syncope are described in Chapter 2. Severe ventricular arrhythmias and hypotension lead to cephalic ischemia and falling. With sudden-onset third-degree heart block (Stokes-Adams attack), the patient loses consciousness and falls without warning. Less severe causes of decreased cardiac output, such as bradyarrhythmias or tachyarrhythmias, are associated with prodromal faintness before loss of consciousness. Elderly patients with cardioinhibitory sinus syndrome ("sick sinus syndrome"), however, may describe dizziness and falling rather than faintness, because of amnesia for the presyncopal symptoms. Thus, the history alone may not reveal the cardiovascular etiology of the fall. By contrast, cerebral hypoperfusion due to peripheral loss of vascular tone usually is associated with a presyncopal syndrome of progressive lightheadedness, faintness, dimming of vision, and "rubbery"-feeling legs. But even in the context of positive tilt-table testing up to 37% of patients report a clinically misleading symptom of true, "cardiogenic" vertigo (Newman-Toker et al., 2008). Vertigo and downbeat nystagmus may also occur with asystole (Choi et al., 2010). Orthostatic hypotension conveys a markedly increased risk of falling

---

BOX 3.1 Causes and Types of Falls and Drops

DROP ATTACKS

With loss of consciousness:
  Syncope
  Seizures

Without loss of consciousness:
  Transient ischemic attacks:
    Vertebrobasilar insufficiency
    Anterior cerebral artery ischemia
  Third ventricular and posterior fossa tumors
  Chiari malformation
  Otolithic crisis

FALLS

Neuromuscular disorders (neuropathy, radiculopathy, and
  myopathy)
Cerebral or cerebellar disorders
Cryptogenic falls in the middle-aged
Aging, neurodegeneration and the neural substrate of gait and
  balance:
  Basal ganglia disorders:
    Parkinson disease
    Progressive Supranuclear Palsy and other parkinsonian
      syndromes
  The aged state

---

in the elderly (see also the section "Aged State"). Sudden drops in young persons, particularly when engaged in athletic activities, suggest a cardiac etiology. Exertional syncope requires a detailed cardiac evaluation to rule out valvular disease, right ventricular dysplasia, and other cardiomyopathies.

Seizures

Epileptic drop attacks are caused by several mechanisms, including asymmetrical tonic contractions of limb and axial muscles, loss of tone of postural muscles, and seizure-related cardiac arrhythmias. Arrhythmia-related epileptic drop attacks mimic cardiogenic syncope and, like temporal lobe drop attacks, typically are associated with a period of altered consciousness after the drop. Video-EEG monitoring of epileptic patients with a history of falls permits characterization of the various motor phenomena that cause loss of posture. For the clinician, however, the precise nature of these events is less important than establishing a diagnosis of seizures. This is straightforward in patients with long-standing epilepsy, but falls in patients with poststroke hemiparesis may be falsely attributed to motor weakness rather than to new-onset seizures. Destabilizing extensor spasms of spasticity can also be difficult to distinguish from focal seizures. In children and adolescents with a history of drop attacks, a tilt-table test should be considered to avoid overdiagnosing epilepsy (Sabri et al., 2006). True epileptic drop attacks in young patients with severe childhood epilepsies may respond favorably to callosotomy (Sunaga et al., 2009). The injury potential of epileptic drops associated with Lennox–Gastaut syndrome can be reduced with adjunctive use of clobazam and rufinimide (VanStraten and Ng, 2012), and with vagal nerve stimulation in some. Falling as a consequence of the tonic axial component of startle-induced seizures may be controllable with lamotrigine. Paradoxically, some antiseizure drugs can precipitate drop attacks, such as carbamazepine in rolandic epilepsy.

DROP ATTACKS WITHOUT LOSS OF CONSCIOUSNESS

Transient Ischemic Attacks

Drop attacks secondary to TIAs are sudden falls occurring without warning or obvious explanation such as tripping. Loss of consciousness either does not occur or is only momentary; the sensorium and lower limb strength are intact immediately or shortly after the patient hits the ground. Between episodes the neurological examination should not reveal lower limb motor or sensory dysfunction. The vascular distributions for drop attacks from TIAs are the posterior circulation and the anterior cerebral arteries.

Vertebrobasilar Insufficiency

Drop attacks caused by posterior circulation insufficiency result from transient ischemia to the corticospinal tracts or the paramedian reticular formation. They are rarely an isolated manifestation of vertebrobasilar insufficiency, as most patients have a history of TIAs that include the more common signs and symptoms of vertigo, diplopia, ataxia, weakness, and hemisensory loss. Occasionally, however, a drop attack is the ominous precursor of severe neurological deficits due to progressive thrombosis of the basilar artery, and may precede permanent ischemic damage only by hours.

Anterior Cerebral Artery Ischemia

Anterior cerebral artery ischemia causes drop attacks by impairing perfusion of the parasagittal premotor and motor cortex controlling the lower extremities. Origination of both anterior cerebral arteries from the same root occurs in approximately 20% of the population and predisposes to ischemic drop attacks from a single embolus. Paraparesis and even tetraparesis can result from simultaneous infarctions in bilateral ACA territories (Kang and Kim, 2008). Rare cases of drop attacks arising in the context of carotid dissection (Casana et al., 2011) and frontal AV fistulas (Oh et al., 2011) have been described.

Third Ventricular and Posterior Fossa Abnormalities

Drop attacks can be a manifestation of colloid cysts of the third ventricle, Chiari malformation ("Chiari drop attack"), or mass lesions within the posterior fossa. With colloid cysts, unprovoked falling is the second most common symptom, after position-induced headaches. This history may be the only clinical clue to the diagnosis because the neurological examination can be entirely normal. Abrupt neck flexion may precipitate drop attacks in otherwise asymptomatic patients who are harboring posterior fossa tumors. Drop attacks occur in 2% to 3% of patients with Chiari malformation. These may be associated with loss of consciousness and often resolve after decompression surgery (Straus et al., 2009). Drops induced by rapid head turning were considered pathognomonic of cysticercosis of the fourth ventricle in the early twentieth century (Brun sign). The contemporary maneuver of cervical spine manipulation is rarely associated with a drop attack (Sweeney and Doody, 2010). Intracranial mass lesions such as parasagittal meningiomas, foramen magnum tumors, or subdural hematomas can also be associated with sudden drops. However, baseline abnormalities of gait and motor functions coexist, and falling may occur consequent to these impairments rather than to acute loss of muscle tone.

4 Delirium

Mario F. Mendez, Claudia R. Padilla

CHAPTER OUTLINE

CLINICAL CHARACTERISTICS
  Acute Onset with Fluctuating Course
  Cognitive and Related Abnormalities
  Behavioral and Emotional Abnormalities
PATHOPHYSIOLOGY
DIAGNOSIS
  Predisposing and Precipitating Factors
  Mental Status Examination
  Diagnostic Scales and Criteria
  Physical Examination
  Laboratory Tests
DIFFERENTIAL DIAGNOSIS
  Common Causes of Delirium
  Special Problems in Differential Diagnosis
PREVENTION AND MANAGEMENT
PROGNOSIS

Delirium is an acute mental status change characterized by abnormal and fluctuating attention. There is a disturbance in level of awareness and reduced ability to direct, focus, sustain, and shift attention (APA, 2013). These difficulties additionally impair other areas of cognition. The syndrome of delirium can be a physiological consequence of a medical condition or stem from a primary neurological cause.

Delirium is by far the most common behavioral disorder in a medical-surgical setting. In general hospitals, the prevalence ranges from 15% to 24% on admission. The incidence ranges between 6% and 56% of hospitalized patients, 11% to 51% postoperatively in elderly patients, and 80% or more of intensive care unit (ICU) patients (Alce et al., 2013; Inouye et al., 2014). The consequences of delirium are serious: they include prolonged hospitalizations, increased mortality, high rates of discharges to other institutions, severe impact on caregivers and spouses, and between $143 billion and $152 billion annually in direct healthcare costs in the United States (Kerr et al, 2013; Leslie and Inouye, 2011).

Physicians have known about this disorder since antiquity. Hippocrates referred to it as *phrenitis*, the origin of our word *frenzy*. In the first century AD, Celsus introduced the term *delirium*, from the Latin for "out of furrow," meaning derailment of the mind, and Galen observed that delirium was often due to physical diseases that affected the mind "sympathetically." In the nineteenth century, Gowers recognized that these patients could be either lethargic or hyperactive. Bonhoeffer, in his classification of organic behavioral disorders, established that delirium is associated with clouding of consciousness. Finally, Engel and Romano (1959) described alpha slowing with delta and theta intrusions on electroencephalograms (EEGs) and correlated these changes with clinical severity. They noted that treating the medical cause resulted in reversal of both the clinical and EEG changes of delirium.

Despite this long history, physicians, nurses, and other clinicians often fail to diagnose delirium (Wong et al., 2010), and up to two-thirds of delirium cases go undetected or misdiagnosed (O'Hanlon et al., 2014). Healthcare providers often miss this syndrome more from lack of recognition than misdiagnosis. The elderly in particular may have a "quieter," more subtle presentation of delirium that may evade detection. Adding to the confusion about delirium are the many terms used to describe this disorder: acute confusional state, altered mental status, acute organic syndrome, acute brain failure, acute brain syndrome, acute cerebral insufficiency, exogenous psychosis, metabolic encephalopathy, organic psychosis, ICU psychosis, toxic encephalopathy, toxic psychosis, and others.

Clinicians must take care to distinguish delirium from dementia, the other common disorder of cognitive functioning. Delirium is acute in onset (usually hours to a few days) whereas dementia is chronic (usually insidious in onset and progressive). The definition of delirium must emphasize an acute behavioral decompensation with fluctuating attention, regardless of etiology or the presence of baseline cognitive deficits or dementia. Complicating this distinction is the fact that underlying dementia is a major risk factor for delirium.

Clinicians must also take care to define the terms used with delirium. *Attention* is the ability to focus on specific stimuli to the exclusion of others. *Awareness* is the ability to perceive or be conscious of events or experiences. *Arousal*, a basic prerequisite for attention, indicates responsiveness or excitability into action. *Coma*, *stupor*, *wakefulness*, and *alertness* are states of arousal. *Consciousness*, a product of arousal, means clarity of awareness of the environment. *Confusion* is the inability for clear and coherent thought and speech.

CLINICAL CHARACTERISTICS

The essential elements of delirium are summarized in Boxes 4.1 and 4.2. Among the revised American Psychiatric Association's criteria (APA, 2013) for this disorder is a disturbance that develops over a short period of time; tends to fluctuate; and impairs awareness, attention, and other areas of cognition. In general, awareness, attention, and cognition fluctuate over the course of a day. Furthermore, delirious patients have disorganized thinking and an altered level of consciousness, perceptual disturbances, disturbance of the sleep/wake cycle, increased or decreased psychomotor activity, disorientation, and memory impairment. Other cognitive, behavioral, and emotional disturbances may also occur as part of the spectrum of delirium. Delirium can be summarized into the 10 clinical characteristics that follow.

Acute Onset with Fluctuating Course

Delirium develops rapidly over hours or days, but rarely over more than a week, and fluctuations in the course occur throughout the day. There are lucid intervals interspersed with the daily fluctuations. Gross swings in attention and awareness, arousal, or both occur unpredictably and irregularly and become worse at night. Because of potential lucid intervals, medical personnel may be misled by patients who exhibit improved attention and awareness unless these patients are evaluated over time.

BOX 4.1 Clinical Characteristics of Delirium

Acute onset of mental status change with fluctuating course
Attentional deficits
Confusion or disorganized thinking
Altered level of consciousness
Perceptual disturbances
Disturbed sleep/wake cycle
Altered psychomotor activity
Disorientation and memory impairment
Other cognitive deficits
Behavioral and emotional abnormalities

Cognitive and Related Abnormalities
Attentional Deficits

A disturbance of attention and consequent altered awareness is the cardinal symptom of delirium. Patients are distractible, and stimuli may gain attention indiscriminately, trivial ones often getting more attention than important ones. All components of attention are disturbed, including selectivity, sustainability, processing capacity, ease of mobilization, monitoring of the environment, and the ability to shift attention when necessary. Although many of the same illnesses result in a spectrum of disturbances from mild inattention to coma, delirium is not the same as disturbance of arousal.

BOX 4.2 DSM-5 Diagnostic Criteria: Delirium*

A. A disturbance in attention (i.e. reduced ability to direct, focus, sustain, and shift attention) and awareness (reduced orientation to the environment).
B. The disturbance develops over a short period of time (usually hours to a few days), represents a change from baseline attention and awareness, and tends to fluctuate in severity during the course of a day.
C. An additional disturbance in cognition (e.g., memory deficit, disorientation, language, visuospatial ability, or perception).
D. The disturbances in Citeria A and C are not better explained by another pre-existing, established, or evolving neurocognitive disorder and do not occur in the context of a severely reduced level of arousal, such as coma.
E. There is evidence from the history, physical examination, or laboratory findings that the disturbance is a direct physiological consequence of another medical condition, substance intoxication or withdrawal (i.e., due to a drug of abuse or to a medication), or exposure to a toxin, or is due to multiple etiologies.

Specify whether:

Substance intoxication delirium: This diagnosis should be made isntaed of substance intoxication when the symptoms in

Criteria A and C predominate in the clinical picture and when they are sufficiently severe to warrant clinical attention.
- **Coding note:** The ICD-9-CM and ICD-10CM codes for the [specific substance] intoxication delirium are indicated in the table below. Note that the ICD-10-CM code depends on whether or not there is a comorbid substance use disorder present for the same class of substance. If a mild substance use disorder is comorbid with the substance intoxication delirium, the 4th position character is "1," and the clinician should record "mild [substance] use disorder," before the substance intoxication delirium (e.g., "mild cocaine use disorder is comorbid with the substance intoxication delirium"). If a moderate or severe substance use disorder is comorbid with the substance intoxication delirium, the 4th position character is "2,"and the clinician should record "moderate [substance] use disorder" or "severe [substance] use disorder," depending on the severity of the comorbid substance use disorder. If there is no comorbid substance use disorder (e.g., after a one0time heavy use of the substance), then the 4th position character is "9,"and the clinician should record only the substance intoxication delirium.

		ICD-10-CM		
	ICD-9-CM	With use disorder, mild	With use disorder, moderate or severe	Without use disorder
Alcohol	291.0	F10.121	F10.221	F10.921
Cannabis	292.81	F12.121	F12.221	F12.921
Phencyclidine	292.81	F16.121	F16.221	F16.921
Other hallucinogen	292.81	F16.121	F16.221	F16.921
Inhalent	292.81	F18.221	F18.221	F18.921
Opiod	292.81	F11.121	F11.221	F11.921
Sedative, hypnotic, or anxiolytic	292.81	F13.121	F13.221	F13.921
Amphetamine (or other stimulant)	292.81	F15.121	F15.221	F15.921
Cocaine	292.81	F14.121	F14.221	F14.921
Other (or unknown) substance	292.81	F19.221	F19.221	F19.921

Substance withdrawal delirium: This diagnosis should be made instead of substance withdrawal when the symptoms in Criteria A and C predominate in the clinical picture and when they are sufficiently severe to warrant clinical attention.
- **Code** [specific substance] withdrawal delirium: **291.0 (F10.231)** alcohol; **292.0 (F11.23)** opioid; 292.0 (F13.231) sedative, hypnotic, or anxiolytic; **292.0 (F19.231)** other (or unknown) substance/medication.

Medication-induced delirium: This diagnosis applies when the symptoms in Criteria A and C arise as a side effect of a medication taken as prescribed.

- **Coding note:** The ICD-9-CM code for [specific medication]-induced delirium is **292.81**. The ICD-10-CM code depends on the type of medication. If the medication is an opioid taken as prescribed, the code is **F11.921**. If the medication is a sedative, hypnotic, or anxiolytic taken as prescribed, the code is **F13.921**. If the medication is an amphetamine-type or other stimulant taken as prescribed, the code is **F15.921**. For medications that do not fit into any of the classes (e.g., dexamethasone) and in cases in which a substance is judged to be an etiological factor but the specific class of substance is unknown, the code is **F19.921**.

BOX 4.2 DSM-5 Diagnostic Criteria: Delirium (Continued)

293.0 (F05) Delirium due to another medical condition: There is evidence from the history, physical examination, or laboratory findings that the disturbance is attributable to the physiological consequences of another medical condition.
- **Coding note:** Use multiple spate codes reflecting specific delirium etiologies (e.g., 572.2 [K72.90] hepatic encephalopathy, 293.0 [F05] delirium due to hepatic encephalopathy). The other medical condition should also be coded and listed separately immediately before the delirium due to another medical condition (e.g., 572.2 [K72.90] hepatic encephalopathy; 293.0 [F05] delirium due to hepatic encephalopathy).

293.0 (F05) Delirium due to multiple etiologies:
There is evidence from the history physical examination, or laboratory findings that the delirium has more than one etiology (e.g., more than one etiological medical condition; another medical condition plus substance intoxication or medication side effect).
- **Coding note:** Use multiple separate codes reflecting specific delirium etiologies (e.g., 572.2 [K72.90] hepatic

encephalopathy, 293.0 [F05] delirium due to hepatic failure; 291/0 [F10.231] alcohol withdrawal delirium). Note that the etiological medical condition both appears as a separate code that precedes the delirium code and is substituted into the delirium due to another medical condition rubric.

Specify if:
Acute: Lasting a few hours or days.
Persistent: lasting weeks or months.

Specify if:
Hyperactive: The individual has a hyperactive level of psychomotor activity that may be accompanied by mood lability, agitation, and/or refusal to cooperate with medical care.
Hypoactive: The individual has a hypoactive level of psychomotor activity that may be accompanied by sluggishness and lethargy that approaches stupor.
Mixed level of activity: The individual has a normal level of psychomotor activity even though attention and awareness are disturbed. Also includes individuals whose activity level rapidly fluctuates.

*Previously referred to in DSM-IV as "dementia, delirium, amnestic, and other cognitive disorders."
Note: The following supportive features are commonly present in delirium but are not key diagnostic features: sleep/wake cycle disturbance, psychomotor disturbance, perceptual disturbances (e.g., hallucinations, illusions), emotional disturbances, delusions, labile affect, dysarthria, and EEG abnormalities (generalized slowing of background activity).

Confusion or Disorganized Thinking

Delirious patients are unable to maintain the stream of thought with accustomed clarity, coherence, and speed. There are multiple intrusions of competing thoughts and sensations, and patients are unable to order symbols, carry out sequenced activity, and organize goal-directed behavior.

The patient's speech reflects this jumbled thinking. Speech shifts from subject to subject and is rambling, tangential, and circumlocutory, with hesitations, repetitions, and perseverations. Decreased relevance of the speech content and decreased reading comprehension are characteristic of delirium. Confused speech is further characterized by an abnormal rate, frequent dysarthria, and nonaphasic misnaming, particularly of words related to stress or illness, such as those referable to hospitalization.

Altered Level of Consciousness

Consciousness, or clarity of awareness, may be disturbed. Most patients have lethargy and decreased arousal. Others, such as those with delirium tremens, are hyperalert and easily aroused. In hyperalert patients, the extreme arousal does not preclude attentional deficits because patients are indiscriminate in their alertness, are easily distracted by irrelevant stimuli, and cannot sustain attention. The two extremes of consciousness may overlap or alternate in the same patient or may occur from the same causative factor.

Perceptual Disturbances

The most common perceptual disturbance is decreased perceptions per unit of time; patients miss things that are going on around them. Illusions and other misperceptions result from abnormal sensory discrimination. Perceptions may be multiple, changing, or abnormal in size or location. Hallucinations also occur, particularly in younger patients and in

those in the hyperactive subtype. They are most common in the visual sphere and are often vivid, three-dimensional, and in full color. Patients may see lilliputian animals or people that appear to move about. Hallucinations are generally unpleasant, and some patients attempt to fight them or run away with fear. Some hallucinatory experiences may be release phenomena, with intrusions of dreams or visual imagery into wakefulness. Psychotic auditory hallucinations with voices commenting on the patient's behavior are unusual.

Disturbed Sleep/Wake Cycle

Disruption of the day/night cycle causes excessive daytime drowsiness and reversal of the normal diurnal rhythm. "Sundowning"—with restlessness and confusion during the night—is common, and delirium may be manifest only at night. Nocturnal peregrinations can result in a serious problem when the delirious patient, partially clothed in a hospital gown, has to be retrieved from the hospital lobby or from the street in the middle of the night. This is one of the least specific symptoms and also occurs in dementia, depression, and other behavioral conditions. In delirium, however, disruption of circadian sleep cycles may result in rapid eye movement or dream-state overflow into waking.

Altered Psychomotor Activity

There are three subtypes of delirium, based on changes in psychomotor activity. The hypoactive subtype is characterized by psychomotor retardation. These are the patients with lethargy and decreased arousal. The hyperactive subtype is usually hyperalert and agitated, and has prominent overactivity of the autonomic nervous system. Moreover, the hyperactive type is more likely to have delusions and perceptual disorders such as hallucinations. About half of patients with delirium manifest elements of both subtypes, called mixed subtype, alternating between hyperactive and hypoactive. Only about 15% are strictly hyperactive. In addition to the patients being younger, the hyperactive subtype has more drug-related causes, a shorter hospital stay, and a better prognosis.

Disorientation and Memory Impairment

Disturbances in orientation and memory are related. Patients are disoriented first to time of day, followed by other aspects of time, and then to place. They may perceive abnormal juxtapositions of events or places. Disorientation to person—in the sense of loss of personal identity—is rare. Disorientation is one of the most common findings in delirium but is not specific for delirium; it occurs in dementia and amnesia as well. Among patients with delirium, recent memory is disrupted in large part by the decreased registration caused by attentional problems.

In delirium, reduplicative paramnesia, a specific memory-related disorder, results from decreased integration of recent observations with past memories. Persons or places are "replaced" in this condition. In general, delirious patients tend to mistake the unfamiliar for the familiar. For example, they tend to relocate the hospital closer to their homes. In a form of reduplicative paramnesia known as *Capgras syndrome*, however, a familiar person is mistakenly thought to be an unfamiliar impostor.

Other Cognitive Deficits

Disturbances occur in visuospatial abilities and in writing. Higher visual-processing deficits include difficulties in visual object recognition, environmental orientation, and organization of drawings and other constructions.

Writing disturbance may be the most sensitive language abnormality in delirium. The most salient characteristics are abnormalities in the mechanics of writing: The formation of letters and words is indistinct, and words and sentences sprawl in different directions (Fig. 4.1). There is a reluctance to write, and there are motor impairments (e.g., tremors, micrographia) and spatial disorders (e.g., misalignment, leaving insufficient space for the writing sample). Sometimes the writing shows perseverations of loops in aspects of the writing. Spelling and syntax are also disturbed, with spelling errors particularly involving consonants, small grammatical words (prepositions and conjunctions), and the last letters of words. Writing is easily disrupted in these disorders, possibly because it depends on multiple components and is the least used language function.

Behavioral and Emotional Abnormalities

Behavioral changes include poorly systematized delusions, often with persecutory and other paranoid ideation and personality alterations. Delusions, like hallucinations, are probably release phenomena and are generally fleeting, changing, and readily affected by sensory input. These delusions are most often persecutory. Some patients exhibit facetious humor and playful behavior, lack of concern about their illness, poor insight, impaired judgment, and confabulation.

There can be marked emotional lability. Sometimes patients are agitated and fearful or depressed or quite apathetic. Dysphoric (unpleasant) emotional states are the more common, and emotions are not sustained. Up to half of elderly delirious patients display symptoms of depression with low mood, loss of interests, fatigue, decreased appetite and sleep, and other feelings related to depression. There may be mood-congruent delusions and hallucinations. The mood changes of delirium are probably due to direct effects of the confusional state on the limbic system and its regulation of emotions.

Finally, more elementary behavioral changes may be the principal symptoms of delirium. This is especially the case in

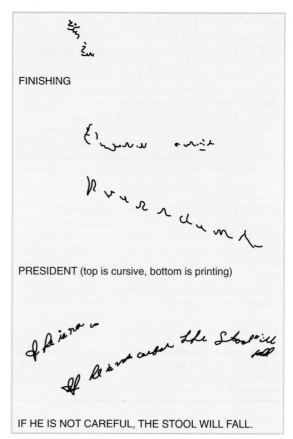

Fig. 4.1 Writing disturbances in delirium. Patients were asked to write indicated words to dictation. *(Reprinted with permission from Chédru, J., Geschwind, N., 1972. Writing disturbances in acute confusional states. Neuropsychologia 10, 343–353.)*

the elderly, in whom decreased activities of daily living, urinary incontinence, and frequent falls are among the major manifestations of this disorder.

PATHOPHYSIOLOGY

The pathophysiology of delirium is not entirely understood, but it depends on widely distributed neurological dysfunction. Delirium is the final common pathway of many pathophysiological disturbances that reduce or alter cerebral oxidative metabolism. These metabolic changes result in diffuse impairment in multiple neuronal pathways and systems.

Several brain areas involved in attention are particularly disturbed in delirium. Dysfunction of the anterior cingulate cortex is involved in disturbances of the management of attention (Reischies et al., 2005). Other areas include the bilateral or right prefrontal cortex in attentional maintenance and executive control, the temporoparietal junction region in disengaging and shifting attention, the thalamus in engaging attention, and the upper brainstem structures in moving the focus of attention. The thalamic nuclei are uniquely positioned to screen incoming sensory information, and small lesions in the thalamus may cause delirium. In addition, there is evidence that the right hemisphere is dominant for attention. Cortical blood flow studies suggest that right hemisphere cortical areas and their limbic connections are the "attentional gate" for sensory input through feedback to the reticular nucleus of the thalamus.

Another explanation for delirium is alterations in neurotransmitters, particularly a cholinergic-dopaminergic imbalance.

There is extensive evidence for a cholinergic deficit in delirium (Alce et al., 2013). Anticholinergic agents can induce the clinical and EEG changes of delirium, which are reversible with the administration of cholinergic medications such as physostigmine. The beneficial effects of donepezil, rivastigmine, and galantamine—acetylcholinesterase-inhibitor medications used for Alzheimer disease—may be partly due to an activating or attention-enhancing role. Moreover, cholinergic neurons project from the pons and the basal forebrain to the cortex and make cortical neurons more responsive to other inputs. A decrease in acetylcholine results in decreased perfusion in the frontal cortex. Hypoglycemia, hypoxia, and other metabolic changes may differentially affect acetylcholine-mediated functions. Other neurotransmitters may be involved in delirium, including dopamine, serotonin, norepinephrine, γ-aminobutyric acid, glutamine, opiates, and histamine. Dopamine has an inhibitory effect on the release of acetylcholine, hence the delirium-producing effects of L-dopa and other anti-parkinsonism medications (Martins and Fernandes, 2012; Trzepacz and van der Mast, 2002). Opiates may induce the effects by increasing dopamine and glutamate activity. Polymorphisms in genes coding for a dopamine transporter and two dopamine receptors have been associated with the development of delirium (van Munster et al., 2010).

Inflammatory cytokines such as interleukins, interferon, and tumor necrosis factor alpha (TNF-α) may contribute to delirium by altering blood–brain barrier permeability and further affecting neurotransmission (Cole, 2004; Fong et al., 2009; Inouye, 2006; Martins and Fernandes, 2012). The combination of inflammatory mediators and dysregulation of the limbic–hypothalamic–pituitary axis may lead to exacerbation or prolongation of delirium (Maclullich et al., 2008; Martins and Fernandes, 2012). Finally, secretion of melatonin, a hormone integral to circadian rhythm and the sleep/wake cycle, may be abnormal in delirious patients compared to those without delirium (Fitzgerald et al., 2013).

DIAGNOSIS

Diagnosis is a two-step process. The first step is the recognition of delirium, which requires a thorough history, a bedside mental status examination focusing on attention, and a review of established diagnostic scales or criteria for delirium. The second step is to identify the cause from a large number of potential diagnoses. Because the clinical manifestations offer few clues to the cause, crucial to the differential diagnosis are the general history, physical examination, and laboratory assessments.

The general history assesses several elements. An abrupt decline in mentation, particularly in the hospital, should be presumed to be delirium. Although patients may state that they cannot think straight or concentrate, family members or other good historians should be available to describe the patient's behavior and medical history. The observer may have noted early symptoms of delirium such as inability to perform at a usual level, decreased awareness of complex details, insomnia, and frightening or vivid dreams. It is crucial to obtain accurate information about systemic illnesses, drug use, recent trauma, occupational and environmental exposures, malnutrition, allergies, and any preceding symptoms leading to delirium. Furthermore, the clinician should thoroughly review the patient's medication list.

Predisposing and Precipitating Factors

The greater the number of predisposing factors, the fewer or milder are the precipitating factors needed to result in delirium (Anderson, 2005) (Box 4.3). Four factors independently

---

BOX 4.3 Predisposing and Precipitating Factors for Delirium

- Elderly, especially 80 years or older
- Dementia, cognitive impairment, or other brain disorder
- Fluid and electrolyte disturbances and dehydration
- Other metabolic disturbance, especially elevated BUN level or hepatic insufficiency
- Number and severity of medical illnesses including cancer
- Infections, especially urinary tract, pulmonary, and AIDS
- Malnutrition, low serum albumin level
- Cardiorespiratory failure or hypoxemia
- Prior stroke or other nondementia brain disorder
- Polypharmacy and use of analgesics, psychoactive drugs, or anticholinergics
- Drug abuse, alcohol or sedative dependency
- Sensory impairment, especially visual
- Sensory overstimulation and "ICU psychosis"
- Sensory deprivation
- Sleep disturbance
- Functional impairment
- Fever, hypothermia
- Physical trauma or severe burns
- Fractures
- Male gender
- Depression
- Specific surgeries:
  - Cardiac, especially open heart surgery
  - Orthopedic, especially femoral neck and hip fractures, bilateral knee replacements
  - Ophthalmological, especially cataract surgery
  - Noncardiac thoracic surgery and aortic aneurysmal repairs
  - Transurethral resection of the prostate

AIDS, Acquired immunodeficiency syndrome; *BUN*, blood urea nitrogen; *ICU*, intensive care unit.

---

predispose to delirium: vision impairments (<20/70 binocular), severity of illness, cognitive impairment, and dehydration (high ratio of blood urea to creatinine) (Inouye, 2006). Among these, cognitive impairment or dementia is worth emphasizing. Elderly patients with dementia are five times more likely to develop delirium than those without dementia and it is associated with increased cognitive decline, admission to institutions, and mortality (Elie et al., 1998; Inouye et al., 2014). Patients with dementia may develop delirium after minor medication changes or other relatively insignificant precipitating factors (Inouye et al., 2014). Moreover, premorbid impairment in executive functions may be independently associated with greater risk of developing delirium (Rudolph et al., 2006). Other important predisposing factors for delirium are advanced age, especially older than 80 years, and the presence of chronic medical illnesses (Johnson, 2001). Many of these elderly patients predisposed to delirium have cerebral atrophy or white matter and basal ganglia ischemic changes on neuroimaging. Additional predisposing factors are the degree of physical impairment, hip and other bone fractures, serum sodium changes, infections and fevers, and the use of multiple drugs, particularly those with narcotic, anticholinergic, or psychoactive properties. The predisposing factors for delirium are additive, each new factor increasing the risk considerably. Moreover, frail elderly patients often have multiple predisposing factors, the most common being functional dependency, multiple medical comorbidities, depression, and polypharmacy (Laurila et al., 2008).

In most cases, the cause of delirium is multifactorial, resulting from the interaction between patient-specific predisposing factors and multiple precipitating factors (Inouye et al., 2014; Inouye and Charpentier, 1996; Laurila et al., 2008). Five specific factors that can independently precipitate delirium are use of physical restraints, malnutrition or weight loss (albumin levels less than 30 g/L), use of indwelling bladder catheters, adding more than three medications within a 24-hour period, and an iatrogenic medical complication (Inouye and Charpentier, 1996). Other precipitating factors for incident delirium, which is the term used to describe a delirium that newly occurs during the course of a stay in a clinical setting, include electrolyte disturbances (hyponatremia, hypercalcemia, etc.), major organ system disease, occult respiratory failure, occult infection, pain, specific medications such as sedative-hypnotics or histamine-2 blockers, sleep disturbances, and alterations in the environment. Novel situations and unfamiliar surroundings contribute to sensory overstimulation in the elderly, and sensory overload may be a factor in producing "ICU psychosis." Ultimately, delirium occurs in patients from a synergistic interaction of predisposing factors with precipitating factors.

In addition to the risk factors already discussed, heritability of delirium is an area of investigation. The presence of genes such as apolipoprotein E (APOE), dopamine receptor genes DRD2 and DRD3, and the dopamine transporter gene, SLC6A3, are possible pathophysiological vulnerabilities for delirium (van Munster et al., 2009, 2010). Despite conflicting data, there is evidence for an association between APOE ε4 carriers and a longer duration of delirium (van Munster et al., 2009). Polymorphisms in SLC6A3 and DRD2 have occurred in association with delirium from alcohol and in elderly delirious patients with hip fractures (van Munster et al., 2009, 2010).

Mental Status Examination

Initial general behavioral observations are an important part of the neurological mental status examination. The most important are observations of attentiveness and arousability. Attention may wander so much that it must constantly be brought back to the subject at hand. General behavior may range from falling asleep during the interview to agitation and combativeness. Slow and loosely connected thinking and speech may be present, with irrelevancies, perseverations, repetitions, and intrusions. Patients may propagate their errors in thinking and perception by elaboration or confabulation. Finally, the examiner should evaluate the patient's general appearance and grooming, motor activity and spontaneity, mood and affect, propriety and witticisms, and the presence of any special preoccupations or inaccurate perceptions.

Bedside tests of attention can be divided into serial recitation tasks, continuous performance tasks, and alternate response tasks. The digit span test is a serial recitation task in which a series of digits is presented, one digit per second, and the patient is asked to repeat the entire sequence immediately after presentation. Perceptual clumping is avoided by the use of random digits and a regular rhythm of presentation. Correct recitation of seven (plus or minus two) digits is considered normal. The serial reversal test is a form of recitation task in which the patient recites backward a digit span, the spelling of a word such as *world*, or the results of counting by ones, threes, or sevens from a predetermined number. Continuous performance tasks include the *A* vigilance test, in which the patient must indicate whenever the letter *A* is heard among random letters presented one per second. This can also be done visually by asking the patient to cross out every instance of a particular letter in a magazine or newspaper paragraph. Alternate response tasks are exemplified by the repetition of a

three-step motor sequence (palm-side-fist), which is also a test of frontal functions. These attentional tests are not overly sensitive or specific, and they can be affected by the patient's educational background, degree of effort, or presence of other cognitive deficits. In sum, the best assessment of attention may be general behavioral observations and an appraisal of how "interviewable" the patient is.

Attentional or arousal deficits may preclude the opportunity to pursue the mental status examination much further, but the examiner should attempt to assess orientation and other areas of cognition. Patients who are off 3 days on the date, 2 days on the day of the week, or 4 hours on the time of day may be significantly disoriented to time. The examiner should inquire whether the patient knows where he or she is, what kind of place it is, and in what circumstances he or she is there. Disturbed recent memory is demonstrated by asking the patient to retain the examiner's name or three words for 5 minutes. A language examination should distinguish between the language of confusion and that of a primary aphasia (see Special Problems in Differential Diagnosis, later in this chapter). Attempts at simple constructions such as copying a cube may be unsuccessful. Hallucinations can sometimes be brought out by holding a white piece of paper or an imaginary string between the fingers and asking the patient to describe what he or she sees.

Diagnostic Scales and Criteria

The usual mental status scales and tests may not help in differentiating delirium from dementia and other cognitive disturbances. Specific criteria and scales are available for the diagnosis of delirium. Foremost among these are the *Diagnostic and Statistical Manual of Mental Disorders*, fifth edition (DSM-V; APA, 2013), criteria for delirium (see Box 4.2). The confusion assessment method (CAM) is a widely used instrument for screening for and diagnosing delirium (Ely et al., 2001) (Box 4.4). The Delirium Rating Scale-Revised-98 (DRS-R-98), a revision of the earlier delirium rating scale (DRS), is a 16-item scale with 13 severity items and three diagnostic items that reliably distinguish delirium from dementia, depression, and schizophrenia (Trzepacz et al., 2001). Both the CAM and the DRS-R-98 are best used in combination with a cognitive test (Adamis et al., 2010). The Memorial Delirium Assessment Scale (MDAS) is a 10-item scale designed to quantify the

---

BOX 4.4 Diagnosis of Delirium by the Confusion Assessment Method

The diagnosis of delirium by the confusion assessment method (CAM) requires the presence of features 1, 2 and either 3 or 4 (Inouye et al., 1990).

Feature 1: Acute onset and fluctuating course
Was there an acute change from the patient's baseline? Did the (abnormal) behavior fluctuate in severity?
Feature 2: Inattention
Did the patient have difficulty keeping track of what was being said?
Feature 3: Disorganized thinking
Was the patient's thinking disorganized or incoherent (rambling conversation, unclear or illogical flow of ideas)?
Feature 4: Altered level of consciousness
Overall, would you rate this patient's level of consciousness as alert (normal), vigilant (hyperalert), lethargic (drowsy, easily aroused), stupor (difficulty to arouse), or coma (unarousable)?

severity of delirium in medically ill patients (Breitbart et al., 1997). While it may also be useful as a diagnostic tool, it is best used after the initial delirium diagnosis is made (Adamis et al., 2010). The delirium symptom interview is also a valuable instrument but may not distinguish delirium from dementia. The Neelon and Champagne (NEECHAM) Confusion Scale (Neelon et al., 1996) is an easily administered screening tool widely used in the nursing community. It combines behavioral and physiological signs of delirium, but it has been suggested that the NEECHAM measures acute confusion rather than delirium (Adamis et al., 2010). The confusion assessment method for ICU (CAM-ICU) and the intensive care delirium screening checklist (ICDSC) are two validated critical care assessment tools used to easily and relatively quickly screen for delirium in the ICU (Alce et al., 2013).

The diagnosis of delirium is facilitated by the use of the CAM, DRS-R-98, MDAS, the delirium symptom interview, the delirium index (McCusker et al., 2004), or the NEECHAM, along with the history from collateral sources such as family and nursing notes, a mental status examination focusing on attention, and specific tests such as a writing sample.

Physical Examination

The physical examination should elicit any signs of systemic illness, focal neurological abnormalities, meningismus, increased intracranial pressure (ICP), extracranial cerebrovascular disease, or head trauma. In delirium, less specific findings include an action or postural tremor of high frequency (8–10 Hz), asterixis or brief lapses in tonic posture (especially at the wrist), multifocal myoclonus or shock-like jerks from diverse sites, choreiform movements, dysarthria, and gait instability. Patients may manifest agitation or psychomotor retardation, apathy, waxy flexibility, catatonia, or carphologia ("lint-picking" behavior). The presence of hyperactivity of the autonomic nervous system may be life threatening because of possible dehydration, electrolyte disturbances, or tachyarrhythmias.

Laboratory Tests

Despite false-positive and false-negative rates on single tracings (Inouye, 2006), EEG changes virtually always accompany delirium when several EEGs are obtained over time (see Chapter 34). Disorganization of the usual cerebral rhythms and generalized slowing are the most common changes, as illustrated in Engel and Romano's classic paper (1959). The mean EEG frequency or degree of slowing correlates with the degree of delirium. Both hypoactive and hyperactive subtypes of delirium have similar EEG slowing; however, predominant low-voltage fast activity is also present on withdrawal from sedative drugs or alcohol. Additional EEG patterns from intracranial causes of delirium include focal slowing, asymmetric delta activity, and paroxysmal discharges (spikes, sharp waves, and spike–wave complexes). Periodic complexes such as triphasic waves and periodic lateralizing epileptiform discharges may help in the differential diagnosis (see Chapter 34). EEGs are of value in deciding whether confusional behavior may be due to an intracranial cause, in making the diagnosis of delirium in patients with unclear behavior, in evaluating demented patients who might have a superimposed delirium, in differentiating delirium from schizophrenia and other primary psychiatric states, and in following the course of delirium over time.

Other essential laboratory tests include a complete blood cell count; measurements of glucose, electrolytes, blood urea nitrogen, creatinine, transaminase, and ammonia levels; thyroid function tests; arterial blood gas studies; chest radiographs; electrocardiogram; urinalysis; and urine drug screening. Less routine tests, such as antibody tests against Hu or NMDA receptors, should be considered when routine labs are unrevealing and there is a suspicion for malignancy. Although they are nonspecific, evoked potential studies often show prolonged latencies.

Since most cases of delirium are due to medical conditions, lumbar puncture and neuroimaging are needed in only a minority of delirious patients (Inouye, 2006). The need for a lumbar puncture, however, deserves special comment. This valuable test, which is often neglected in the evaluation of delirious patients, should be performed as part of the workup when the cause is uncertain. The lumbar puncture should be preceded by a computed tomographic (CT) or magnetic resonance imaging (MRI) scan of the brain, especially if there are focal neurological findings or suspicions of increased ICP, a space-occupying lesion, or head trauma. The yield of functional imaging is variable, showing global increased metabolism in patients with delirium tremens and global decreased metabolism or focal frontal hypoactivity in many other delirious patients.

DIFFERENTIAL DIAGNOSIS
Common Causes of Delirium

The following discussion is a selective commentary that illustrates some basic principles and helps organize the approach to working through the large differential diagnosis. Almost any sufficiently severe medical or surgical illness can cause delirium, and the best advice is to follow all available diagnostic leads (Table 4.1). (For further discussion of individual entities, the reader should refer to corresponding chapters in this book.) The confusion-inducing effects of these disturbances are additive, and there may be more than one causal factor, the individual contribution of which cannot be elucidated. Nearly half of elderly patients with delirium have more than one cause of their disorder, and clinicians should not stop looking for causes when a single one is found. Of the causes for delirium, the most common among the elderly are metabolic disturbances, infection, stroke, and drugs, particularly anticholinergic and narcotic medications. The most common causes among the young are drug abuse and alcohol withdrawal.

Metabolic Disturbances

Metabolic disturbances are the most common causes of delirium (see Chapters 58 and 83–86). Fortunately, the examination and routine laboratory tests screen for most acquired metabolic disturbances that might be encountered. Because of the potential for life-threatening or permanent damage, some of these conditions—particularly hypoxia and hypoglycemia—must be considered immediately. Also consider dehydration, fluid and electrolyte disorders, and disturbances of calcium and magnesium. The rapidity of change in an electrolyte level may be as important a factor as its absolute value for the development of delirium. For example, some people tolerate chronic sodium levels of 115 mEq/L or less, but a rapid fall to this level can precipitate delirium, seizures, or even central pontine myelinolysis, particularly if the correction of hyponatremia is too rapid. Hypoxia from low cardiac output, respiratory insufficiency, or other causes is another common source of delirium. A cardiac encephalopathy may ensue from heart failure, increased venous pressure transmitted to the dural venous sinuses and veins, and increased ICP (Caplan, 2006). Also consider other major organ failures such as liver and kidney failure, including the possibility of unusual causes such as undetected portocaval shunting or acute pancreatitis

TABLE 4.1 Major Causes of Delirium

METABOLIC	Electrolytes: hypo/hypernatremia, hypo/hypercalcemia, hypo/hypermagnesemia, hypo/hyperphosphatemia Endocrine: hypo/hyperthyroidism, hypo/hypercortisolism, hypo/hyperglycemia Cardiac encephalopathy, hepatic encephalopathy, uremic encephalopathy Hypoxia and hypercarbia Vitamin deficiencies: thiamine, vitamin B$_{12}$, nicotinic acid, folic acid Toxic and industrial exposures: carbon monoxide, organic solvent, lead, manganese, mercury, carbon disulfide, heavy metals Porphyria
TOXIC	Intoxication and overdose Withdrawal: alcohol, benzodiazepines, barbiturates, amphetamines, cocaine, coffee, phencyclidine, hallucinogens, inhalants, meperidine, and other narcotics Drugs: anticholinergic, benzodiazepines, opiates, antihistamines, antiepileptics, muscle relaxants, dopamine agonists, monoamine oxidase inhibitors, levodopa, corticosteroids, fluoroquinolone and cephalosporin antibiotics, beta-blockers, digitalis, lithium, clozapine, tricyclics antidepressants, calcineurin inhibitors
INFECTIOUS	Urinary tract infection, pneumonia, sepsis, meningitis, encephalitis
NEUROLOGIC	Vascular: ischemic stroke, intracerebral or subarachnoid hemorrhage, vasculitis Neoplastic: brain tumors, carcinomatous meningitis, paraneoplastic limbic encephalitis Seizure-related: postictal state, nonconvulsive status epilepticus Trauma: concussion, subdural hematoma
PERIOPERATIVE	Surgery: thoracic (cardiac and noncardiac), vascular, and hip replacement, anesthetic and drug effects, hypoxia and anemia, hyperventilation, fluid and electrolyte disturbances, hypotension, embolism, infection or sepsis, untreated pain, fragmented sleep, sensory deprivation or overload
MISCELLANEOUS	Hyperviscosity syndromes

with the release of lipases. Delirium due to endocrine dysfunction often has prominent affective symptoms such as hyperthyroidism and Cushing syndrome. Delirium occasionally results from toxins including industrial agents, pollutants, and heavy metals such as arsenic, bismuth, gold, lead, mercury, thallium, and zinc. Other considerations are inborn errors of metabolism such as acute intermittent porphyria. Finally, it is particularly important to consider thiamine deficiency. In alcoholics and others at risk, thiamine must be given immediately to avoid precipitating Wernicke encephalopathy with the administration of glucose.

Drugs

Drug intoxication and drug withdrawal are among the most common causes of delirium. Approximately 50% of patients over the age of 65 take five or more chronic medications daily, and medications contribute to delirium in up to 39% of these patients (Inouye and Charpentier, 1996). Drug effects are additive, and drugs that are especially likely to cause delirium are those with anticholinergic properties, including many over-the-counter cold preparations, antihistamines, antidepressants, and neuroleptics. Patients with anticholinergic intoxication present "hot as a hare, blind as a bat, dry as a bone, red as a beet, and mad as a hatter," reflecting fever, dilated pupils, dry mouth, flushing, and delirium. Other important groups of drugs associated with delirium, especially in the elderly, are sedative hypnotics such as long-acting benzodiazepines, narcotic analgesics and meperidine, and histamine-2 receptor blockers. Anti-parkinsonism drugs result in confusion with prominent hallucinations and delusions in patients with Parkinson disease who are particularly susceptible. Corticosteroid psychosis may develop in patients taking the equivalent of 40 mg/day or more of prednisone. The behavioral effects of corticosteroids often begin with euphoria and hypomania and proceed to a hyperactive delirium. Any drug administered intrathecally, such as metrizamide, is prone to induce confusional behavior. Drug withdrawal syndromes can be caused by many agents including barbiturates and other minor tranquilizers, sedative hypnotics, amphetamines, cocaine or "crack," and alcohol. Delirium tremens begins 72 to 96 hours after alcohol withdrawal, with profound agitation, tremulousness, diaphoresis, tachycardia, fever, and frightening visual hallucinations.

Excited delirium syndrome, also known as agitated delirium is a drug-related alteration in mental status with combativeness or aggressiveness (Vilke et al., 2012). Similar to delirium tremens, these patients can develop severe psychomotor agitation, anxiety, hallucinations, elevated body temperature, tachycardia, diaphoresis, tolerance to significant pain, violent and bizarre behavior, and "superhuman strength." Excited delirium patients are commonly found to have acute drug intoxication or history of drug abuse. Most patients with excited delirium syndrome will survive, although there still is a high fatality rate around 10% (Vilke et al., 2012). Awareness among medical personnel regarding this syndrome is crucial for intervention and proactive treatment to prevent deaths.

Infections

Infections and fevers often produce delirium. The main offenders are urinary tract infections, pneumonia, and septicemia. In a sporadic encephalitis or meningoencephalitis, important causal considerations are herpes simplex virus, Lyme disease, and acquired immunodeficiency syndrome (AIDS) (see Chapter 77). Patients with AIDS may be delirious because of the human immunodeficiency virus (HIV) itself or because of an opportunistic infection. Immunocompromised patients are at greater risk of infection, and any suspicion of infection should prompt culture of urine, sputum, blood, and cerebrospinal fluid.

Strokes

Delirium can be the nonspecific consequence of any acute stroke, but most postinfarct confusion usually resolves in 24 to 48 hours (see Chapters 65 and 66). Sustained delirium can result from specific strokes, including right middle cerebral artery infarcts affecting prefrontal and posterior parietal areas, and posterior cerebral artery infarcts resulting in either bilateral or left-sided occipitotemporal lesions (fusiform gyrus). The latter lesions can lead to agitation, visual field changes, and even Anton syndrome (see Chapter 16). Delirium may also follow occlusion of the anterior cerebral artery or rupture of an anterior communicating artery aneurysm with involvement of the anterior cingulate gyrus and septal region. Thalamic or posterior parietal cortex strokes may present with severe delirium, even with small lesions.

Other cerebrovascular conditions that can produce delirium include high-grade bilateral carotid stenosis, hypertensive

parenterally, preferably intravenously, in doses of 0.4 to 2.0 mg if opiate overdose is the suspected cause of coma. An abrupt and complete reversal of narcotic effect may precipitate an acute abstinence syndrome in persons who are physically dependent on opiates.

An initial examination should include a check of general appearance, blood pressure, pulse, temperature, respiratory rate and breath sounds, best response to stimulation, pupil size and responsiveness, and posturing or adventitious movements. The neck should be stabilized in all instances of trauma until cervical spine fracture or subluxation can be ruled out. The airway should be protected in all comatose patients, and an intravenous line placed. In coma, however, the classic sign of an acute condition in the abdomen—namely, abdominal rigidity—may be subtle in degree or absent. In addition, the diagnosis of blunt abdominal trauma is difficult in patients with a change in mental status. Therefore, in unconscious patients with a history of trauma, CT scan of the abdomen or peritoneal lavage by an experienced surgeon may be warranted. Hypotension, marked hypertension, bradycardia, arrhythmias causing depression of blood pressure, marked hyperthermia, and signs of cerebral herniation mandate immediate therapeutic intervention. Hyperthermia or meningismus prompts consideration of urgent lumbar puncture. Examination of the fundus of the eye for papilledema and a computed tomography (CT) scan of the brain should be performed before lumbar puncture in any comatose patient. Infection over the site of the lumbar puncture, papilledema, and decerebrate posturing are contraindications to lumbar puncture and, even in their absence, medicolegal considerations may render a CT scan of the head preferable before proceeding to lumbar puncture. To avoid a delay in therapy when acute bacterial meningitis is strongly suspected, antibiotics and adjunctive corticosteroids should be administered within one hour of hospital admission (Brouwer et al., 2010) even if CSF collection cannot be obtained in a timely fashion. Corticosteroid administration should be avoided in the presence of septic shock. Blood cultures and throat swabs should be obtained on these patients prior to antibiotic administration. The risk of herniation from a lumbar puncture in patients with evidence of increased intracerebral pressure is difficult to ascertain from the literature; estimates range from 1% to 12%, depending on the series (Posner et al., 2007). It is important to recognize that both central and tonsillar herniation may increase neck tone. Despite an elevated intracranial pressure (ICP), sufficient cerebrospinal fluid (CSF) should always be obtained to perform the necessary studies. The performance of bacterial culture and cell count, essential in cases of suspected bacterial meningitis, requires but a few milliliters of fluid. Intravenous access and intravenous mannitol should be ready in the event that unexpected herniation begins after the lumbar puncture. When the CSF pressure is greater than 500 mm H_2O, some authorities recommend leaving the needle in place to monitor the pressure and administering intravenous mannitol to lower the pressure. If focal signs develop during or after the lumbar puncture, immediate intubation and hyperventilation also may be necessary to reduce intracerebral pressure urgently until more definitive therapy is available.

Ecchymosis, petechiae, or evidence of ready bleeding on general examination may indicate coagulation abnormality or thrombocytopenia. This increases the risk of epidural hematoma after a lumbar puncture, which may cause devastating spinal cord compression. Measurements of prothrombin time, partial thromboplastin time, and platelet count should precede lumbar puncture in these cases, and the coagulation abnormality or thrombocytopenia should be corrected before proceeding to lumbar puncture.

Common Presentations

Coma usually manifests in one of three ways. Most commonly, it occurs as an expected or predictable progression of an underlying illness. Examples are focal brainstem infarction with extension; chronic obstructive pulmonary disease in a patient who is given too high a concentration of oxygen, thereby decreasing respiratory drive and resulting in carbon dioxide narcosis; and known barbiturate overdose when the ingested drug cannot be fully removed and begins to cause unresponsiveness. Second, coma occurs as an unpredictable event in a patient whose prior medical conditions are known to the physician. The coma may be a complication of an underlying medical illness, such as in a patient with arrhythmia who suffers anoxia after a cardiac arrest. Alternatively, an unrelated event may occur, such as sepsis from an intravenous line in a cardiac patient or a stroke in a hypothyroid patient. Finally, coma can occur in a patient whose medical history is totally unknown to the physician. Sometimes this type of presentation is associated with a known probable cause, such as head trauma incurred in a motor vehicle accident, but often the comatose patient presents to the physician without an obvious associated cause. Thorough objective systematic assessment must be applied in every comatose patient. Special care must be taken not to be lulled or misled by an apparently predictable progression of an underlying illness or other obvious cause of coma.

History

Once the patient is relatively stable, clues to the cause of the coma should be sought by briefly interviewing relatives, friends, bystanders, or medical personnel who may have observed the patient before or during the decrease in consciousness. Telephone calls to family members may be helpful. The patient's wallet or purse should be examined for lists of medications, a physician's card, or other information. Attempts should be made to ascertain the patient's social background and prior medical history and the circumstances in which the patient was found. The presence of drug paraphernalia or empty medicine bottles suggests a drug overdose. Newer recreational drugs, such as γ-hydroxybutyrate and bath salts, must be considered in the differential diagnosis. An oral hypoglycemic agent or insulin in the medicine cabinet or refrigerator implies possible hypoglycemia. Antiarrhythmic agents such as procainamide or quinidine suggest existing coronary artery disease with possible myocardial infarction or warn that an unwitnessed arrhythmia may have caused cerebral hypoperfusion, with resulting anoxic encephalopathy. Warfarin, typically prescribed for patients with deep venous thrombosis or pulmonary embolism, those at risk for cerebral embolism, and those with a history of brainstem or cerebral ischemia, may be responsible for massive intracerebral bleeding. In patients found to be unresponsive at the scene of an accident, the unresponsive state may be due to trauma incurred in the accident, or sudden loss of consciousness may have precipitated the accident.

The neurologist often is called when patients do not awaken after surgery or when coma supervenes following a surgical procedure. Postoperative causes of coma include many of those mentioned in Box 5.1. In addition, the physician also must have a high index of suspicion for certain neurological conditions that occur in this setting, including fat embolism, Addisonian crisis, and hypothyroid coma (precipitated by acute illness or surgical stress); Wernicke encephalopathy from carbohydrate loading without adequate thiamine stores; and iatrogenic overdose of a narcotic analgesic. Attempts should be made to ascertain whether the patient complained of symptoms before onset of coma. Common signs and symptoms include headache preceding subarachnoid hemorrhage, chest pain with aortic dissection or myocardial infarction, shortness of breath from hypoxia, stiff neck in meningoencephalitis, and vertigo in brainstem stroke. Nausea and vomiting are common in poisonings. Coma also may be secondary to increased ICP. Observers may have noted head trauma, drug abuse, seizures, or hemiparesis. Descriptions of falling to one side, dysarthria or aphasia, ptosis, pupillary dilatation, or disconjugate gaze may help localize structural lesions. The time course of the disease, as noted by family or friends, may help differentiate the often relatively slow, progressive course of toxic-metabolic or infectious causes from abrupt, catastrophic changes that are seen most commonly with vascular events. Finally, family members or friends may be invaluable in identifying psychiatric causes of unresponsiveness. The family may describe a long history of psychiatric disease, previous similar episodes from which the patient recovered, current social stresses on the patient, or the patient's unusual, idiosyncratic response to stress. Special care must be taken with psychiatric patients because of the often biased approach to these patients, which may lead to incomplete evaluation. Psychiatric patients are subject to all of the causes of coma listed in Box 5.1.

General Examination

A systematic, detailed general examination is especially helpful in the approach to the comatose patient, who is unable to describe prior or current medical problems. This examination begins in the initial rapid examination with evaluation of blood pressure, pulse, respiratory rate, and temperature.

Blood Pressure Evaluation

Hypotension. Cerebral hypoperfusion secondary to hypotension may result in coma if the mean arterial pressure falls below the value for which the brain is able to autoregulate (normally 60 mm Hg). This value is substantially higher in chronically hypertensive persons, in whom the cerebral blood flow–mean arterial pressure curve is shifted to the right. Among the causes of hypotension are hypovolemia, massive external or internal hemorrhage, myocardial infarction, cardiac tamponade, dissecting aortic aneurysm, intoxication with alcohol or other drugs (especially barbiturates), toxins, Wernicke encephalopathy, Addison disease, and sepsis. Although most patients with hypotension are cold because of peripheral vasoconstriction, patients with Addison disease or sepsis may have warm shock due to peripheral vasodilation. Medullary damage also may result in hypotension because of damage to the pressor center.

Hypertension. Hypertension is the cause of alterations in arousal in hypertensive crisis and is seen secondarily as a response to cerebral infarction, in subarachnoid hemorrhage, with certain brainstem infarctions, and with increased intracerebral pressure. The Kocher-Cushing (or Claude Bernard) reflex is the development of hypertension associated with bradycardia and respiratory irregularity due to increased ICP. This response occurs more commonly in the setting of a posterior fossa lesion and in children. It results from compression or ischemia of the pressor area lying beneath the floor of the fourth ventricle. Hypertension is a common condition and thus may be present but unrelated to the cause of coma.

Heart Rate

In addition to the Kocher-Cushing reflex, bradycardia can result from myocardial conduction blocks, with certain

poisonings, and from effects of drugs such as the beta-blockers. Tachycardia is a result of hypovolemia, hyperthyroidism, fever, anemia, and certain toxins and drugs, including cocaine, atropine, and other anticholinergic medications.

Respiration

The most common causes of decreased respiratory rate are metabolic or toxic, such as carbon dioxide narcosis or drug overdose with central nervous system (CNS) depressants. Increased respiratory rate can result from hypoxia, hypercapnia, acidosis, hyperthermia, hepatic disease, toxins or drugs (especially those that produce a metabolic acidosis, such as methanol, ethylene glycol, paraldehyde, and salicylates), sepsis, and pulmonary embolism (including fat embolism) and sometimes is seen in psychogenic unresponsiveness. Brainstem lesions causing hypopnea or hyperpnea are discussed later in the chapter. Changes in respiratory rate or rhythm in a comatose patient may be deceiving, because a metabolic disorder may coexist with a CNS lesion.

Temperature

Core temperature is best measured with a rectal probe in a comatose patient, because oral or axillary temperatures are unreliable. Pyrexia most often is a sign of infection. Accordingly, any evidence of fever in a comatose patient warrants strong consideration of lumbar puncture. Absence of an elevated temperature does not rule out infection. Immunosuppressed patients, elderly patients, and patients with metabolic or endocrine abnormalities such as uremia or hypothyroidism may not experience an increase in temperature in response to overwhelming infection. Pure neurogenic hyperthermia is rare and usually is due to subarachnoid hemorrhage or diencephalic (hypothalamus) lesions. A clue to brainstem origin is shivering without sweating. Shivering in the absence of sweating, particularly when unilateral in nature, also may be observed with a deep intracerebral hemorrhage. Other causes of increased temperature associated with coma are heatstroke, thyrotoxic crisis, and drug toxicity. (Atropine and other anticholinergics elevate core temperature but decrease diaphoresis, resulting in a warm, dry patient with dilated pupils and diminished bowel sounds.)

Except in heatstroke and malignant hyperthermia, fever does not result in stupor or coma by itself. Conversely, hypothermia, regardless of cause, is anticipated to lead to altered consciousness. Hypothermia causes diminished cerebral metabolism and, if the temperature is sufficiently low, may result in an isoelectric electroencephalogram. Hypothermia usually is metabolic or environmental in cause; however, it also is seen with hypotension accompanied by vasoconstriction and may occur with sepsis. Other causes of hypothermia associated with coma are hypothyroid coma, hypopituitarism, Wernicke encephalopathy, cold exposure, drugs (barbiturates), and other poisonings. Central lesions causing hypothermia are found in the posterior hypothalamus. The absence of shivering or vasoconstriction, or the presence of sweating, is a clue to the central origin of these lesions.

General Appearance

The general appearance of the patient may provide further clues to the diagnosis. Torn or disheveled clothing may indicate prior assault. Vomiting may be a sign of increased ICP, drug overdose, or metabolic or other toxic cause. Urinary or fecal incontinence suggests an epileptic seizure or may result from a generalized autonomic discharge resulting from the same cause as for the coma. Examination of body habitus may reveal cushingoid patients at risk for an acute Addisonian crisis with abrupt withdrawal of their medications or additional stress from intercurrent illness. Cachexia suggests cancer, chronic inflammatory disorders, Addison disease, hypothyroid coma, or hyperthyroid crisis. The cachectic patient also is subject to Wernicke encephalopathy in association with carbohydrate loading. Gynecomastia, spider nevi, testicular atrophy, and decreased axillary and pubic hair are common in the alcoholic with cirrhosis.

Head and Neck Examination

The head and neck must be carefully examined for signs of trauma. Palpation for depressed skull fractures and edema should be attempted, although this means of evaluation is not very sensitive. Laceration or edema of the scalp is indicative of head trauma. The term *raccoon eyes* refers to orbital ecchymosis due to anterior basal skull fracture. *Battle's sign* is a hematoma overlying the mastoid, originating from basilar skull fracture extending into the mastoid portion of the temporal bone. The ecchymotic lesions typically are not apparent until 2 to 3 days after the traumatic event.

Meningismus or neck stiffness may be a sign of infectious or carcinomatous meningitis, subarachnoid hemorrhage, or central or tonsillar herniation. Neck stiffness may be absent, however, in coma from any cause but is likely to be present in less severe alterations in arousal. Scars on the neck may be from endarterectomy, implying vascular disease, or from thyroidectomy or parathyroidectomy, suggesting concomitant hypothyroidism, hypoparathyroidism, or both. Goiter may be found with hypothyroidism or hyperthyroidism.

Eye Examination

Examination of the eyes includes observation of the cornea, conjunctiva, sclera, iris, lens, and eyelids. Edema of the conjunctiva and eyelids may occur in congestive heart failure and nephrotic syndrome. Congestion and inflammation of the conjunctiva may occur in the comatose patient from exposure. Enophthalmos indicates dehydration. Scleral icterus is seen with liver disease, and yellowish discoloration of the skin without scleral involvement may be due to drugs such as rifampin. Band keratopathy is caused by hypercalcemia, whereas hypocalcemia is associated with cataracts. Kayser-Fleischer rings are seen in progressive lenticular degeneration (Wilson disease). Arcus senilis is seen in normal aging but also in hyperlipidemia. Fat embolism may cause petechiae in conjunctiva and eye grounds.

Funduscopic examination may demonstrate evidence of hypertension or diabetes. Grayish deposits surrounding the optic disc have been reported in lead poisoning. The retina is congested and edematous in methyl alcohol poisoning, and the disc margin may be blurred. Subhyaloid hemorrhage appears occasionally as a consequence of a rapid increase in ICP due to subarachnoid hemorrhage (Terson's syndrome). Papilledema results from increased ICP and may be indicative of an intracranial mass lesion or hypertensive encephalopathy.

Otoscopic Examination

Otoscopic examination should rule out hemotympanum or CSF otorrhea from a basilar skull fracture involving the petrous ridge, as well as infection of the middle ear. Infections of the middle ear, mastoid, and paranasal sinuses constitute the most common source of underlying infection in brain abscess. CSF rhinorrhea, which appears as clear fluid from the nose, may depend on head position. The presence of glucose in the watery discharge is virtually diagnostic, although false-positive results are possible.

Oral Examination

Alcohol intoxication, diabetic ketoacidosis (acetone odor), uremia, and hepatic encephalopathy (musty odor of cholemia or *fetor hepaticus*) may be suspected from the odor of the breath. Arsenic poisoning produces the odor of garlic. Poor oral hygiene or oral abscesses may be a source of sepsis or severe pulmonary infection with associated hypoxemia. Pustules on the nose or upper lip may seed the cavernous sinus with bacteria by way of the angular vein. Lacerations on the tongue, whether old or new, suggest seizure disorder. Thin, blue-black pigmentation along the gingival margin may be seen in certain heavy metal poisonings (bismuth, mercury, and lead).

Integument Examination

Systematic examination of the integument includes inspection of the skin, nails, and mucous membranes. A great deal of information can be gained by a brief examination of the skin (Table 5.2). Hot, dry skin is a feature of heatstroke. Sweaty skin is seen with hypotension or hypoglycemia. Drugs may cause macular-papular, vesicular, or petechial-purpuric rashes or bullous skin lesions. Bullous skin lesions most often are a result of barbiturates but also may be caused by imipramine, meprobamate, glutethimide, phenothiazine, and carbon monoxide. Kaposi sarcoma, anogenital herpetic lesions, or oral candidiasis should suggest the acquired immunodeficiency syndrome (AIDS), with its plethora of CNS abnormalities.

Examination of Lymph Nodes

Generalized lymphadenopathy is nonspecific, because it may be seen with neoplasm, infection (including AIDS), collagen vascular disease, sarcoid, hyperthyroidism, Addison disease, and drug reaction (especially that due to phenytoin). Local lymph node enlargement or inflammation, however, may provide clues to a primary tumor site or source of infection.

Cardiac Examination

Cardiac auscultation will confirm the presence of arrhythmias such as atrial fibrillation, with its inherent increased risk of emboli. Changing mitral murmurs are heard with atrial myxomas and papillary muscle ischemia, which is seen with current or impending myocardial infarction. Constant murmurs indicate valvular heart disease and may be heard with the valvular vegetation of bacterial endocarditis.

Abdominal Examination

Possibly helpful findings on abdominal examination include abnormal bowel sounds, organomegaly, masses, and ascites. Bowel sounds are absent in an acute abdominal condition, as well as with anticholinergic poisoning. Hyperactive bowel sounds may be a consequence of increased gastrointestinal motility from exposure to an acetylcholinesterase inhibitor (a common pesticide ingredient). The liver may be enlarged as a result of right heart failure or tumor infiltration. Nodules or a rock-hard liver may be due to hepatoma or metastatic disease. The liver may be small and hard in cirrhosis. Splenomegaly is caused by portal hypertension, hematological malignancies, infection, and collagen vascular diseases. Intra-abdominal masses may indicate carcinoma. Ascites occurs with liver disease, right heart failure, neoplasms with metastasis to the liver, or ovarian cancer.

Miscellaneous Examinations

Examination of the breasts in the female and of the testicles in the male and rectal examination may reveal common

TABLE 5.2 Skin Lesions and Rashes in Coma

Lesion or rash	Possible cause
Antecubital needle marks	Opiate drug abuse
Pale skin	Anemia or hemorrhage
Sallow, puffy appearance	Hypopituitarism
Hypermelanosis (increased pigment)	Porphyria, Addison disease, chronic nutritional deficiency, disseminated malignant melanoma, chemotherapy
Generalized cyanosis	Hypoxemia or carbon dioxide poisoning
Grayish-blue cyanosis	Methemoglobin (aniline or nitrobenzene) intoxication
Localized cyanosis	Arterial emboli or vasculitis
Cherry-red skin	Carbon monoxide poisoning
Icterus	Hepatic dysfunction or hemolytic anemia
Petechiae	Disseminated intravascular coagulation, thrombotic thrombocytopenic purpura, drugs
Ecchymosis	Trauma, corticosteroid use, abnormal coagulation from liver disease or anticoagulants
Telangiectasia	Chronic alcoholism, occasionally vascular malformations of the brain
Vesicular rash	Herpes simplex, varicella, Behçet disease, drugs
Petechial-purpuric rash	Meningococcemia, other bacterial sepsis (rarely), gonococcemia, staphylococcemia, *Pseudomonas*, subacute bacterial endocarditis, allergic vasculitis, purpura fulminans, Rocky Mountain spotted fever, typhus, fat emboli
Macular-papular rash	Typhus, *Candida, Cryptococcus,* Toxoplasmosis, Subacute bacterial endocarditis, Staphylococcal toxic shock, typhoid, leptospirosis, *Pseudomonas* sepsis, immunological disorders: Systemic lupus erythematosus Dermatomyositis Serum sickness
OTHER SKIN LESIONS	
Ecthyma gangrenosum	Necrotic eschar often seen in the anogenital or axillary area in *Pseudomonas* sepsis
Splinter hemorrhages	Linear hemorrhages under the nail, seen in subacute bacterial endocarditis, anemia, leukemia, and sepsis
Osler's nodes	Purplish or erythematous painful, tender nodules on palms and soles, seen in subacute bacterial endocarditis
Gangrene of digits' extremities	Emboli to larger peripheral or arteries

Data on diseases associated with rashes from Corey, L., and Kirby, P., 1987, Rash and fever, in: Braunwald, E., Isselbacher, K. J., and Petersdorf, R. G. (Eds.), Harrison's Principles of Internal Medicine, 11th edn., McGraw-Hill, New York, pp. 240–244.

primary tumors. A positive result on tests for blood in stool obtained at rectal examination is consistent with gastrointestinal bleeding and, possibly, bowel carcinoma. Large amounts of blood in the gastrointestinal tract may be sufficient to precipitate hepatic encephalopathy in the patient with cirrhosis.

Neurological Examination

Neurological signs may vary depending on the cause of the impaired consciousness and its severity, and they may be partial or incomplete. For example, the patient may have a partial third nerve palsy with pupillary dilation, rather than a complete absence of all third nerve function, or muscle tone may be decreased but not absent. This concept is especially important in the examination of the stuporous or comatose patient because the level of arousal may also influence the expression of neurological signs. In the stuporous or comatose patient, even slight deviations from normal should not be dismissed as unimportant. Such findings should be carefully considered to discover their pattern or meaning.

The neurological examination of a comatose patient serves three purposes: (1) to aid in determining the cause of coma, (2) to provide a baseline, and (3) to help determine the prognosis. For prognosis and localization of a structural lesion, the following components of the examination have been found

to be most helpful: state of consciousness, respiratory pattern, pupillary size and response to light, spontaneous and reflex eye movements, and skeletal muscle motor response.

State of Consciousness

The importance of a detailed description of the state of consciousness is worth reemphasizing. It is imperative that the exact stimulus and the patient's specific response be recorded. Several modes of stimulation should be used, including auditory, visual, and noxious. Stimuli of progressively increasing intensity should be applied, with the maximal state of arousal noted and the stimuli, the site of stimulation, and the patient's exact response described. The examiner should start with verbal stimuli, softly and then more loudly calling the patient's name or giving simple instructions to open the eyes. If there is no significant response, more threatening stimuli, such as taking the patient's hand and advancing it toward the patient's face, are applied. However, a blink response to visual threat need not indicate consciousness. Finally, painful stimuli may be needed to arouse the patient. All patients in apparent coma should be asked to open or close the eyes and to look up and down; these voluntary movements are preserved in the locked-in syndrome but cannot be elicited in coma—an important distinction.

Supraorbital pressure evokes a response even in patients who may have lost afferent pain pathways as a result of

TABLE 5.3 The Glasgow Coma Scale

Best motor response	M
Obeys	6
Localizes	5
Withdraws	4
Abnormal flexion	3
Extensor response	2
Nil	1
Verbal response	**V**
Oriented	5
Confused conversation	4
Inappropriate words	3
Incomprehensible sounds	2
Nil	1
Eye opening	**E**
Spontaneous	4
To speech	3
To pain	2
Nil	1

peripheral neuropathy or spinal cord or some brainstem lesions. Nail bed pressure or pinching the chest or extremities may help localize a lesion when it evokes asymmetrical withdrawal responses. Care must be taken to avoid soft tissue damage. Purposeful movements indicate a milder alteration in consciousness. Vocalization to pain in the early hours of a coma, even if only a grunt, indicates relatively light alteration in consciousness. Later, primitive vocalization may be a feature of the vegetative state.

The Glasgow Coma Scale (Table 5.3) is used widely to assess the initial severity of traumatic brain injury. This battery assesses three separate aspects of a patient's behavior: the stimulus required to induce eye opening, the best motor response, and the best verbal response. Degrees of increasing dysfunction are scored. Its reproducibility and simplicity make the Glasgow Coma Scale an ideal method of assessment for non-neurologists involved in the care of comatose patients, such as neurological intensive care nurses. Its failure to assess other essential neurological parameters, however, limits its utility. Additionally, in patients who are intubated or who have suffered facial trauma, assessment of certain components of the Glasgow Coma Scale, such as eye opening and speech, may be difficult or impossible. An alternative scale referred to as the FOUR Score has been proposed (Wijdicks et al., 2005) and is based on eye response, motor response, brainstem reflexes (pupillary reaction, corneal reflex, and cough reflex), and respirations.

Respiration

Normal breathing is quiet and unlabored. The presence of any respiratory noise implies airway obstruction, which must be dealt with immediately to prevent hypoxia. Normal respiration depends on (1) a brainstem mechanism, located between the midpons and cervical medullary junction, that regulates metabolic needs; and (2) forebrain influences that subserve behavioral needs such as speech production. The organization and function of brainstem mechanisms responsible for respiratory rhythm generation, as well as forebrain influences, are

complex and beyond the scope of this chapter. Neuropathological correlates of respiration are presented in Fig. 5.1.

Respiratory patterns that are helpful in localizing levels of involvement include Cheyne–Stokes respiration, central neurogenic hyperventilation, apneustic breathing, cluster breathing, and ataxic respiration. *Cheyne–Stokes respiration* is a respiratory pattern that slowly oscillates between hyperventilation and hypoventilation. In 1818, Cheyne described his patient as follows: "For several days his breathing was irregular; it would entirely cease for a quarter of a minute, then it would become perceptible, though very low, then by degrees it became heaving and quick and then it would gradually cease again. This revolution in the state of his breathing occupied about a minute during which there were about 30 acts of respiration." Cheyne–Stokes respiration is associated with bilateral hemispheric or diencephalic insults, but it may occur as a result of bilateral damage anywhere along the descending pathway between the forebrain and upper pons. It also is seen with cardiac disorders that prolong circulation time. Alertness, pupillary size, and heart rhythm may vary during Cheyne–Stokes respiration (Posner et al., 2007). Patients are more alert during the waxing portion of breathing. A continuous pattern of Cheyne–Stokes respiration is a relatively good prognostic sign, usually implying that permanent brainstem damage has not occurred. However, the emergence of Cheyne–Stokes respiration in a patient with a unilateral mass lesion may be an early sign of herniation. A change in pattern from Cheyne–Stokes respiration to certain other respiratory patterns, described next, is ominous.

Two breathing patterns similar to Cheyne–Stokes respiration should not be confused with it. *Short-cycle periodic breathing* is a respiratory pattern with a cycle (faster rhythm) shorter than Cheyne–Stokes respiration, with one or two waxing breaths, followed by two to four rapid breaths, then one or two waning breaths. It is seen with increased ICP, lower pontine lesions, or expanding lesions in the posterior fossa (Posner et al., 2007). A similar type of respiration, in which there are short bursts of seven to ten rapid breaths, then apnea without a waning and waxing prodrome, has been erroneously referred to as Biot breathing. Biot, in fact, described an ataxic respiratory pattern, which is described later.

Central neurogenic hyperventilation refers to rapid breathing, from 40 to 70 breaths per minute, usually due to central tegmental pontine lesions just ventral to the aqueduct or fourth ventricle (Posner et al., 2007). This type of breathing is rare and must be differentiated from reactive hyperventilation due to metabolic abnormalities of hypoxemia secondary to pulmonary involvement. Large CNS lesions may cause neurogenic pulmonary edema, with associated hypoxemia and increased respiratory rate. Increased intracerebral pressure causes spontaneous hyperpnea. Hyperpnea cannot be ascribed to a CNS lesion when arterial oxygen partial pressure is less than 70 to 80 mm Hg or carbon dioxide partial pressure is greater than 40 mm Hg.

Kussmaul breathing is a deep, regular respiration observed with metabolic acidosis. *Apneustic breathing* is a prolonged inspiratory gasp with a pause at full inspiration. It is caused by lesions of the dorsolateral lower half of the pons (Posner et al., 2007). *Cluster breathing*, which results from high medullary damage, involves periodic respirations that are irregular in frequency and amplitude, with variable pauses between clusters of breaths.

Ataxic breathing is irregular in rate and rhythm and usually is due to medullary lesions. The combination of ataxic respiration and bilateral sixth nerve palsy may be a warning sign of brainstem compression from an expanding lesion in the posterior fossa. This is an important sign because brainstem compression due to tonsillar herniation (or other causes) may

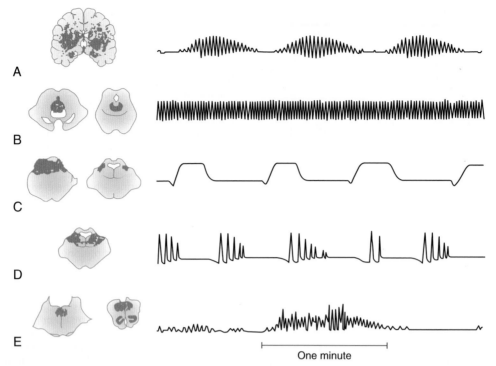

Fig. 5.1 Abnormal respiratory patterns associated with pathologic lesions (*shaded areas*) at various levels of the brain. The tracings were obtained by chest-abdomen pneumograph; inspiration reads up. **A,** Cheyne-Stokes respiration—diffuse forebrain damage. **B,** Central neurogenic hyperventilation—lesions of low midbrain ventral to aqueduct of Sylvius and of upper pons ventral to the fourth ventricle. **C,** Apneusis—dorsolateral tegmental lesion of middle and caudal pons. **D,** Cluster breathing—lower pontine tegmental lesion. **E,** Ataxic breathing—lesion of the reticular formation of the dorsomedial part of the medulla. *(Reprinted from Plum, F., Posner, J.B., 1995, The Diagnosis of Stupor and Coma, 3rd edn., Oxford University Press, New York. Copyright 1966, 1972, 1980, 1996, Oxford University Press, Inc. Used by permission of Oxford University Press, Inc.)*

result in abrupt loss of respiration or blood pressure. Ataxic and gasping respirations are signs of lower brainstem damage and often are preterminal respiratory patterns.

Pupil Size and Reactivity

Normal pupil size in the comatose patient depends on the level of illumination and the state of autonomic innervation. The sympathetic efferent innervation consists of a three-neuron arc. The first-order neuron arises in the hypothalamus and travels ipsilaterally through the posterolateral tegmentum to the ciliospinal center of Budge at the T1 level of the spinal cord. The second-order neuron leaves this center and synapses in the superior cervical sympathetic ganglion. The third-order neuron travels along the internal carotid artery and then through the ciliary ganglion to the pupillodilator muscles. The parasympathetic efferent innervation of the pupil arises in the Edinger-Westphal nucleus and travels in the oculomotor nerve to the ciliary ganglion, from which it innervates the pupillosphincter muscle (Fig. 5.2).

Afferent input to the pupillary reflex depends on the integrity of the optic nerve, optic chiasm, optic tract, and projections into the midbrain tectum and efferent fibers through the Edinger-Westphal nucleus and oculomotor nerve. Abnormalities in pupil size and reactivity help delineate structural damage between the thalamus and pons (Fig. 5.3), act as a warning sign heralding brainstem herniation, and help differentiate structural causes of coma from metabolic causes.

Thalamic lesions cause small, reactive pupils, which often are referred to as *diencephalic pupils*. Similar pupillary findings are noted in many toxic-metabolic conditions resulting in coma. Hypothalamic lesions or lesions elsewhere along the sympathetic pathway result in *Horner syndrome*. Midbrain lesions produce three types of pupillary abnormality, depending on where the lesion occurs: (1) Dorsal tectal lesions interrupt the pupillary light reflex, resulting in *midposition pupils*, which are fixed to light but react to near vision; the latter is impossible to test in the comatose patient. Spontaneous fluctuations in size occur, and the ciliospinal reflex is preserved. (2) Nuclear midbrain lesions usually affect both sympathetic and parasympathetic pathways, resulting in *fixed, irregular midposition pupils*, which may be unequal. (3) Lesions of the third nerve fascicle in the brainstem, or after the nerve has exited the brainstem, cause *wide pupillary dilation*, unresponsive to light. Pontine lesions interrupt sympathetic pathways and cause small, so-called *pinpoint pupils*, which remain reactive, although magnification may be needed to observe this feature. Lesions above the thalamus and below the pons should leave pupillary function intact, except for Horner syndrome in medullary or cervical spinal cord lesions. The pathophysiology of pupillary response is discussed further in Chapters 18 and 45.

Asymmetry in pupillary size or reactivity, even of minor degree, is important. Asymmetry of pupil size may be due to dilation (mydriasis) of one pupil, such as with third nerve palsy, or contraction (miosis) of the other, as in Horner syndrome. This may be differentiated by the pupillary reactivity to light and associated neurological signs. A dilated pupil due to a partial third nerve palsy is less reactive and usually is associated with extraocular muscle involvement. The pupil in Horner syndrome is reactive; if the syndrome results from a lesion in the CNS, it may be associated with anhidrosis of the entire ipsilateral body. Cervical sympathetic chain lesions produce anhidrosis of only face, neck, and arm. A partial or complete third nerve palsy causing a dilated pupil may result

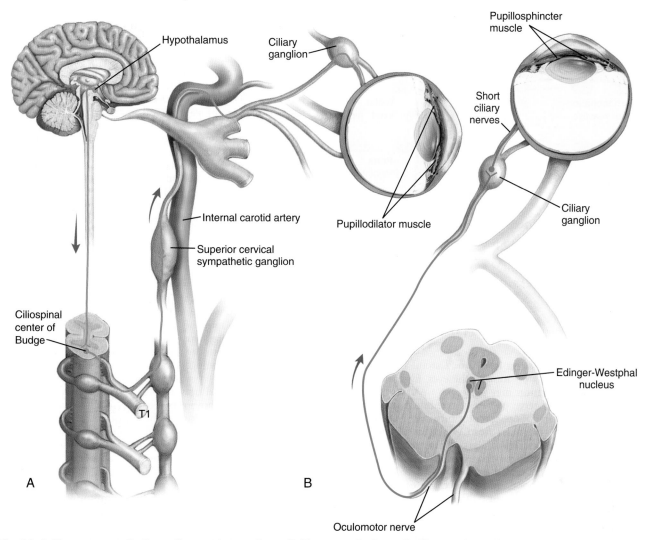

Fig. 5.2 A, The parasympathetic pupilloconstrictor pathway. **B,** The sympathetic pupillodilator pathway. *(Reprinted from Plum, F., Posner, J.B., 1995, The Diagnosis of Stupor and Coma, 3rd edn., Oxford University Press, New York. Copyright 1966, 1972, 1980, 1996, Oxford University Press, Inc. Used by permission of Oxford University Press, Inc.)*

from an intramedullary lesion, most commonly in the midbrain, such as an intramedullary glioma or infarction; uncal herniation compressing the third nerve; or a posterior communicating artery aneurysm. A sluggishly reactive pupil may be one of the first signs of uncal herniation, followed soon thereafter by dilation of that pupil and, later, complete third nerve paralysis.

Several caveats are important in examining the pupil or assessing pupillary reflexes. A common mistake is the use of insufficient illumination. The otoscope may be useful in this regard, because it provides both adequate illumination and magnification. Rarely, pre-existing ocular or neurological injury may fix the pupils or result in pupillary asymmetry. Seizures may cause transient anisocoria. Local and systemic medications may affect pupillary function. Topical ophthalmological preparations containing an acetylcholinesterase inhibitor, used in the treatment of glaucoma, produce miosis. The effect of a mydriatic agent placed by the patient or a prior observer may wear off unevenly, resulting in pupillary asymmetry. Some common misleading causes of a unilateral dilated pupil include prior mydriatic administration, old

ocular trauma or ophthalmic surgery, and, more rarely, carotid artery insufficiency.

Ocular Motility

Normal ocular motility (see Chapters 16 and 44) depends on the integrity of a large portion of the cerebrum, cerebellum, and brainstem. Preservation of normal ocular motility implies that a large portion of the brainstem from the vestibular nuclei at the pontomedullary junction to the oculomotor nucleus in the midbrain is intact. Voluntary ocular motility cannot be judged in the comatose patient, so the examiner must rely on reflex eye movements that allow for assessment of the ocular motor system. The eye movements normally are conjugate and eyes are in the midposition in the alert person. Sleep or obtundation alone may unmask a latent vertical or horizontal strabismus, resulting in dysconjugacy; therefore, patients must be examined when maximally aroused. The eyes return to the midposition in brain-dead patients. Evaluation of ocular motility consists of (1) observation of the resting position of the eyes, including eye deviation; (2) notation of

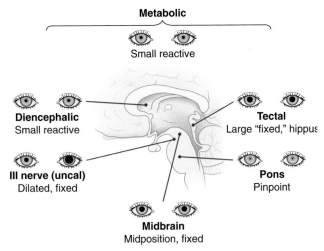

Fig. 5.3 Pupils in comatose patients. *(Reprinted from Plum, F., Posner, J.B., 1995, The Diagnosis of Stupor and Coma, 3rd edn., Oxford University Press, New York. Copyright 1966, 1972, 1980, 1996, Oxford University Press, Inc. Used by permission of Oxford University Press, Inc.)*

spontaneous eye movements; and (3) testing of reflex ocular movements.

Abnormalities in Resting Position. Careful attention must be paid to the resting position of the eyes. Even a small discrepancy in eye position may represent a partial extraocular nerve palsy. Partial nerve palsies or combined nerve palsies predictably result in a more complex picture on examination. Unilateral third nerve palsy from either an intramedullary midbrain lesion or extramedullary compression causes the affected eye to be displaced downward and laterally. A sixth nerve palsy produces inward deviation. Isolated sixth nerve palsy, however, is a poor localizer because of the extensive course of the nerve and because this palsy may be caused by nonspecific increases in ICP, presumably from stretching of the extramedullary portion of the nerve. A fourth nerve palsy is difficult to assess in the comatose patient because of the subtle nature of the deficit in ocular motility. Extraocular nerve palsies often become more apparent with the "doll's eye maneuver" or cold caloric testing in the comatose patient.

Eye Deviation. Spontaneous eye deviation may be conjugate or dysconjugate. Conjugate lateral eye deviation usually is due to an ipsilateral lesion in the frontal eye fields but may be due to a lesion anywhere in the pathway from the ipsilateral eye fields to the contralateral parapontine reticular formation (see Chapter 44). Dysconjugate lateral eye movement may result from a sixth nerve palsy in the abducting eye, a third nerve palsy in the adducting eye, or an internuclear ophthalmoplegia. An internuclear ophthalmoplegia may be differentiated from a third nerve palsy by the preservation of vertical eye movements. Downward deviation of the eyes below the horizontal meridian usually is due to brainstem lesions (most often from tectal compression); however, it also may be seen in metabolic disorders such as hepatic coma. Thalamic and subthalamic lesions produce downward and inward deviation of the eyes. Patients with these lesions appear to be looking at the tip of the nose. Sleep, seizure, syncope, apnea of Cheyne–Stokes respiration, hemorrhage into the vermis, and brainstem ischemia or encephalitis cause upward eye deviation, making this a poor localizing sign. Skew deviation is a maintained deviation of one eye above the other (hypertropia) that is not due to a peripheral neuromuscular lesion or a local extracranial problem in the orbit. It usually indicates a posterior fossa lesion (brainstem or cerebellar). Dysconjugate vertical eye position sometimes may occur in the absence of a brainstem lesion in the obtunded patient.

Spontaneous Eye Movements. Spontaneous eye movements (see Chapter 44) are of many types. Purposeful-appearing eye movements in a patient who otherwise seems unresponsive should lead to consideration of the locked-in syndrome, catatonia, pseudocoma, or PVS. *Roving eye movements* are slow, conjugate, lateral to-and-fro movements. For roving eye movements to be present, the ocular motor nuclei and their connections must be intact. Generally, when roving eye movements are present, the brainstem is relatively intact and coma is due to a metabolic or toxic cause or bilateral lesions above the brainstem. Detection of roving eye movements may be complicated by ocular palsies or internuclear ophthalmoplegia. These superimposed lesions produce relatively predictable patterns but often obscure the essential roving nature of the movement for the inexperienced observer.

Nystagmus occurring in comatose patients suggests an irritative or epileptogenic supratentorial focus. An epileptogenic focus in one frontal eye field causes contralateral conjugate eye deviation. Nystagmus due to an irritative focus may rarely occur alone, without other motor manifestations of seizures. In addition, inconspicuous movements of the eye, eyelid, face, jaw, or tongue may be associated with electroencephalographic status epilepticus. An electroencephalogram (EEG) is required to ascertain the presence of this condition.

Spontaneous conjugate vertical eye movements are separated into different types according to the relative velocities of their downward and upward phases. In *ocular bobbing*, rapid downward jerks of both eyes are observed, followed by a slow return to the midposition. In the typical form, there is associated paralysis of both reflex and spontaneous horizontal eye movements. *Monocular* or *paretic bobbing* occurs when a coexisting ocular motor palsy alters the appearance of typical bobbing. The term *atypical bobbing* refers to all other variations of bobbing that cannot be explained by an ocular palsy superimposed on typical bobbing. Most commonly, this term is used to describe ocular bobbing when lateral eye movements are preserved. *Typical ocular bobbing* is specific but not pathognomonic for acute pontine lesions. Atypical ocular bobbing occurs with anoxia and is nonlocalizing. *Ocular dipping*, also known as *inverse ocular bobbing*, refers to spontaneous eye movements in which an initial slow downward phase is followed by a relatively rapid return. Reflex horizontal eye movements are preserved. It usually is associated with diffuse cerebral damage. In *reverse ocular bobbing* there is a slow initial downward phase, followed by a rapid return that carries the eyes past the midposition into full upward gaze. Then the eyes slowly return to the midposition. Reverse ocular bobbing is nonlocalizing.

Vertical nystagmus, due to an abnormal pursuit or vestibular system, is slow deviation of the eyes from the primary position, with a rapid (saccadic), immediate return to the primary position. It is differentiated from bobbing by the absence of latency between the corrective saccade and the next slow deviation. *Ocular-palatal myoclonus* (the palatal movement also is called *palatal tremor*) occurs after damage to the lower brainstem involving the Guillain-Mollaret triangle, which extends between the cerebellar dentate nucleus, red nucleus, and inferior olive. It consists of a pendular vertical nystagmus, in synchrony with the palatal movements. Ocular flutter is back-to-back saccades in the horizontal plane and usually is a manifestation of cerebellar disease.

Reflex Ocular Movements. Examination of ocular movement is not complete in the comatose patient without assessment of reflex ocular movements, including the oculocephalic reflex (doll's eye phenomenon) and, if necessary, the caloric (thermal) testing. In practice, the terms *doll's eye phenomenon* and *doll's eye maneuver* are used synonymously to refer to the *oculocephalic reflex*, which is the preferred term for the description of the response. This reflex is tested by observation of the motion of the eyes during sudden rotation of the head, by the examiner, in both directions laterally and then with flexion and extension of the neck, also performed by the examiner. When supranuclear influences on the ocular motor nerves are removed, the eyes move in the orbit opposite to the direction of the head turn, and maintain their position in space. *This maneuver should not be performed on any patient until the stability of the neck has been adequately assessed.* If there is any question of neck stability, a neck brace should be applied and caloric testing substituted. In the normal oculocephalic reflex (normal or positive doll's eye phenomenon), the eyes move conjugately in a direction opposite to the direction of movement of the head. Cranial nerve palsies predictably alter the response to this maneuver (Table 5.4).

Clinical caloric testing (as distinct from quantitative calorics, used to assess vestibular end-organ disorders; see Chapter 46) is commonly done by applying cold water to the tympanic membrane. With the patient supine, the head should be tilted forward 30 degrees to allow maximal stimulation of the lateral semicircular canal, which is most responsible for reflex lateral eye movements. After the ear canal is carefully checked to ensure that it is patent and the tympanic membrane is free of defect, 10 mL of ice-cold water is slowly instilled into one ear canal. For purposes of the neurological examination, irrigation of each ear with 10 mL of ice water generally is sufficient.

Cold water applied to the tympanic membrane causes currents to be set up in the endolymph of the semicircular canal. This results in a change in the baseline firing of the vestibular nerve and slow (tonic) conjugate deviation of the eyes toward the stimulated ear. In an awake person, the eye deviation is corrected with a resulting nystagmoid jerking of the eye toward the midline (fast phase). Warm-water irrigation produces reversal of flow of the endolymph, which causes conjugate eye deviation with a slow phase away from the stimulated ear and a normal corrective saccadic fast phase toward the ear. By tradition, the nystagmus is named by the direction of the fast phase. The mnemonic COWS (cold *o*pposite, *w*arm *s*ame) refers to the fast phases. Simultaneous bilateral cold water application results in slow downward deviation, whereas simultaneous bilateral warm water application causes upward deviation.

Oculocephalic or caloric testing may elicit subtle or unsuspected ocular palsies. Abnormal dysconjugate responses occur with cranial nerve palsies, intranuclear ophthalmoplegia, or restrictive eye disease. Movements may be sluggish or absent. Sometimes reinforcement of cold caloric testing with superimposed passive head turning after injection of cold water into the ear may reveal eye movement when either test alone shows none.

False-negative or misleading responses on caloric testing occur with pre-existing inner ear disease, vestibulopathy such as that due to ototoxic drugs such as streptomycin, vestibular paresis caused by illnesses such as Wernicke encephalopathy, and drug effects. Subtotal labyrinthine lesions decrease the response; there is no response when the labyrinth is destroyed. Lesions of the vestibular nerve cause a decreased or absent response. Drugs that suppress either vestibular or ocular motor function, or both, include sedatives, anticholinergics, anticonvulsants, tricyclic antidepressants, and neuromuscular blocking agents. If the response from one ear is indeterminate, both cold- and warm-water stimuli should be applied to the other ear. If the test remains equivocal, superimposition of the doll's

TABLE 5.4 Oculocephalic Reflex*

Method	Response	Interpretation
Lateral head rotation	Eyes remain conjugate, move in direction opposite to head movement and maintain position in space	Normal
	No movement in either eye on rotating head to left or right	Bilateral pontine gaze palsy, bilateral labyrinthine dysfunction, drug intoxication, anesthesia
	Eyes move appropriately when head is rotated in one direction but do not move when head is rotated in opposite direction	Unilateral pontine gaze palsy
	One eye abducts, the other eye does not adduct	Third nerve palsy
		Internuclear ophthalmoplegia
Vertical head flexion and extension	Eyes remain conjugate, move in direction opposite to head movement and maintain position in space	Normal
	No movement in either eye	Bilateral midbrain lesions
	Only one eye moves	Third nerve palsy
	Bilateral symmetrical limitation of upgaze	Aging

*To be performed only after neck stability has been ascertained.

eye maneuver is recommended. The interpretation of abnormal cold caloric responses is summarized in Table 5.5.

An unusual ocular reflex that has been observed in the setting of PVS is reflex opening of both eyes triggered by flexion of an arm at the elbow. This reflex is distinct from reflex eye opening in the comatose patient induced by raising the head or turning it from side to side.

Motor System

Examination of the motor system of a stuporous or comatose patient begins with a description of the resting posture and adventitious movements. Purposeful and nonpurposeful movements are noted and the two sides of the body compared. Head and eye deviation to one side, with contralateral hemiparesis, suggests a supratentorial lesion, whereas ipsilateral paralysis indicates a probable brainstem lesion. External rotation of the lower limb is a sign of hemiplegia or hip fracture.

Decerebrate posturing is bilateral extensor posture, with extension of the lower extremities and adduction and internal rotation of the shoulders and extension at the elbows and wrist. Bilateral midbrain or pontine lesions usually are responsible for decerebrate posturing. Less commonly, deep metabolic encephalopathies or bilateral supratentorial lesions involving the motor pathways may produce a similar pattern.

Decorticate posturing is bilateral flexion at the elbows and wrists, with shoulder adduction and extension of the lower extremities. It is a much poorer localizing posture, because it may result from lesions in many locations, although usually

TABLE 5.5 Caloric Testing

Method	Response	Interpretation
Cold water instilled in right ear	Slow phase to right, fast (corrective) phase to the left	Normal
	No response (make sure canal is patent, apply warm-water stimulus to opposite ear)	Obstructed ear canal, "dead" labyrinth, eighth nerve or nuclear dysfunction, false-negative result (see text)
	Slow phase to right, no fast phase	Toxic-metabolic disorder, drugs, structural lesion above brainstem
	Downbeating nystagmus	Horizontal gaze palsy
Cold water instilled in left ear	Responses should be opposite those for right ear	Peripheral eighth nerve or labyrinth disorder on right (provided that right canal is patent)
Warm water instilled in left ear after no response from cold water in right ear	Slow phase to right, fast phase to left	

above the brainstem. Decorticate posture is not as ominous a sign as decerebrate posture because the former occurs with many relatively reversible lesions.

Unilateral decerebrate or decorticate postures also are less ominous. Lesions causing unilateral posturing may be anywhere in the motor system from cortex to brainstem. Unilateral extensor posturing is common immediately after a cerebrovascular accident, followed in time by a flexor response.

Posturing may occur spontaneously or in response to external stimuli such as pain, or may even be set off by such minimal events as the patient's own breathing. These postures, though common, may also be variable in their expression because of other associated brainstem or more rostral brain damage. Special attention should be given to posturing because it often signals a brainstem herniation syndrome. Emergency room personnel and inexperienced physicians may mistake these abnormal postures for convulsions (seizures) and institute anticonvulsant therapy, resulting in an unfortunate delay of appropriate therapy for the patient.

Adventitious movements in the comatose patient may be helpful in separating metabolic from structural lesions. Tonic-clonic or other stereotyped movements signal seizure as the probable cause of decreased alertness. *Myoclonic jerking*, consisting of nonrhythmic jerking movements in single or multiple muscle groups, is seen with anoxic encephalopathy or other metabolic comas, such as hepatic encephalopathy. *Rhythmic myoclonus*, which must be differentiated from epileptic movements, usually is a sign of brainstem injury. Tetany occurs with hypocalcemia. *Cerebellar fits* result from intermittent tonsillar herniation and are characterized by deterioration of level of arousal, opisthotonos, respiratory rate slowing and irregularity, and pupillary dilatation.

The motor response to painful stimuli should be tested, but the pattern of response may vary depending on the site stimulated. Purposeful responses may be difficult to discriminate from more primitive reflexes. Flexion, extension, and adduction may be either voluntary or reflex in nature. In general, abduction is most reliably voluntary, with shoulder abduction stated to be the only definite nonreflex reaction. This is tested in the comatose patient with noxious stimuli, such as pinching the medial aspect of the upper arm. Reflex flexor response to pain in the upper extremity consists of adduction of the shoulder, flexion of the elbow, and pronation of the arm. The *triple flexion response* in the lower extremities refers to reflex withdrawal, with flexion at the hip and knee and dorsiflexion at the ankle, in response to painful stimulation on the foot or lower extremity. Such reflexes seldom are helpful in localizing a lesion.

Spinal reflexes are reflexes mediated at the level of the spinal cord and do not depend on the functional integrity of the brain or brainstem. Most patients with absent cortical or brainstem function have some form of spinal reflex. The *plantar reflex* may be extensor in coma from any cause, including drug overdoses and postictal states. It becomes flexor on recovery of consciousness if there is no underlying structural damage. Muscle tone and asymmetry in muscle tone are helpful in localizing a focal structural lesion and may help differentiate metabolic from structural coma. Acute structural damage above the brainstem usually results in decreased or flaccid tone. In older lesions, tone usually is increased. Metabolic insults generally cause a symmetrical decrease in tone. Finally, generalized flaccidity is ultimately seen after brain death.

Coma and Brain Herniation

Knowledge of some of the clinical signs of brain herniation is especially important in the clinical approach to coma. Traditional signs of herniation due to supratentorial masses usually are variations of either an uncal or a central pattern. Classically, the uncal pattern includes early signs of third nerve and midbrain compression. The pupil initially dilates as a result of third nerve compression but later returns to the midposition with midbrain compression that involves the sympathetic as well as the parasympathetic tracts. In the central pattern, the earliest signs are mild impairment of consciousness, with poor concentration, drowsiness, or unexpected agitation; small but reactive pupils; loss of the fast component of cold caloric testing; poor or absent reflex vertical gaze; and bilateral corticospinal tract signs, including increased tone of the body ipsilateral to the hemispheric mass lesion responsible for herniation (Posner et al., 2007).

Signs of herniation tend to progress generally in a rostro-caudal manner. An exception occurs when intraventricular bleeding extends to the fourth ventricle and produces a pressure wave compressing the area around the fourth ventricle. Also, when a lumbar puncture reduces CSF pressure suddenly, in the face of a mass lesion that produced increased ICP, sudden herniation of the cerebellar tonsils through the foramen magnum may result (Posner et al., 2007). Both of these clinical scenarios may be associated with sudden, unexpected failure of medullary functions that support respiration or blood pressure. In patients with herniation syndromes, the clinical picture may be confusing because of changing signs or the expression of scattered, isolated signs of dysfunction in separate parts of the brain. In addition, certain signs may be more prominent than others.

Increased ICP invariably accompanies brainstem herniation and may be associated with increased systolic blood pressure, bradycardia, and sixth nerve palsies. These signs, however, as well as many of the traditional signs of herniation as described, actually occur relatively late. Earlier signs of potential herniation are decreasing level of arousal, slight change in

6 Brain Death, Vegetative State, and Minimally Conscious States

Jennifer E. Fugate, Eelco F. M. Wijdicks

CHAPTER OUTLINE

BRAIN DEATH
PROLONGED DISORDERS OF CONSCIOUSNESS
Vegetative State
Minimally Conscious State
IMAGING IN DISORDERS OF CONSCIOUSNESS
DECISION-MAKING AND BIOETHICS

Consciousness refers to normal wakefulness with awareness of self and the external environment. Explanations and descriptions of consciousness are complex and cross the disciplines of neuroscience, psychology, and philosophy. In medicine, the assessment of consciousness is a clinical assessment done by observing a patient's arousal, interaction to stimuli, and thought content as expressed by language. Consciousness implies there is the possibility of expressing a considered thought and not just a reflexive response. Consciousness can change through a continuum from full wakefulness and awareness, to drowsiness, disorientation, loss of meaningful communication, and coma. Terms such as "stupor," "semi-coma," "somnolence," "altered mental status," "encephalopathy," and "quiet delirium" are unfortunately often vaguely applied. A precise description of examination findings is required and more useful.

Consciousness is traditionally dichotomized into two components in a simplistic—but conceptually useful—approach. The *content* of consciousness includes all cognitive functions, emotions, and intuitions of the brain. The *level* of consciousness refers to global alertness and behavioral responsivity. Several key anatomical structures control the conscious state: the ascending reticular activating system (ARAS) in the midbrain and upper pons, the diencephalon (thalamus and hypothalamus), and the cortex (Fig. 6.1). The neurochemistry driving this complex system consists of several important neurotransmitters: norepinephrine (originating from the locus ceruleus and pontine lateral tegmentum), dopamine (ventral tegmentum), serotonin (raphe nuclei), acetylcholine (basal forebrain), histamine (posterior hypothalamus), and orexin-hypocretin (lateral hypothalamus) (McClenathan et al., 2013). As the target of all incoming signals, the thalamus is central in governing consciousness and relays and gates information diffusely to brain networks.

Most of the knowledge of the physiology and neurochemistry underpinning consciousness has been derived from animal studies with some links to humans, but lately more often in humans during normal wakefulness or sleep states (Wijdicks, 2014). The pathophysiology and changes in neurotransmission that occur in comatose patients with acute brain injury have not been explicitly studied. Still, extrapolation has useful and practical implications for the care of such patients. Major mechanisms of coma involve destructive lesions of the thalamus or diffuse connections to the cortex or ARAS. These structures can be directly damaged or injured by compression or shifts, and the changes often alter consciousness permanently. More selective lesions involving a unilateral hemisphere or thalamus will not substantially impair long-term consciousness. Coma is typically a transient state and one of several distinct clinical states emerges within days to weeks (Fig. 6.2).

BRAIN DEATH

Deeply comatose patients who lose *all* clinical signs of brain and brainstem function due to a major destructive lesion should be clearly distinguished from other comatose states. Before proceeding with a brain death evaluation, it is crucial that the irreversible cause of coma is established and there are no potential factors confounding the neurological examination. In most cases, the patient should have been treated aggressively with measures such as administration of hyperosmolar agents, surgical evacuation of space-occupying lesions producing brainstem displacement, ventriculostomy, or other ICP-lowering therapies. Once an untreatable catastrophic neurologic structural injury has been proven while in this supported state, recovery does not occur and there is no known effective medical or surgical intervention. Irreversibility is determined by absent motor responses, loss of all brainstem reflexes, and the apnea test (described later). Death by these neurologic criteria is a medically and legally accepted way of determining a person's death (Wijdicks, 2011). Brain death is relatively uncommon because the brainstem is very resilient to injury. When it does occur, the most common causes are severe traumatic brain injury (TBI), aneurysmal subarachnoid hemorrhage (aSAH), massive intraparenchymal hemorrhage, or on rare occasion anoxic-ischemic brain injury. Neurologic criteria for determining death first took shape in the 1950s and have been refined and developed throughout the world. The American Academy of Neurology has issued guidelines for brain death determination based on a thorough review of existing evidence (Wijdicks et al., 2010). Brain death is based on a detailed and thorough clinical evaluation (Fig. 6.3) and in most countries (including the United States) confirmatory tests are not required if the clinical examination—including a formal apnea test—can be completed.

It is essential that certain prerequisites be met prior to the clinical examination. The main confounding factors that need to be excluded are hypothermia (core body temperature should be $\geq 36\,°C$); drug intoxication or poisoning; lingering effects of sedatives, analgesics, and neuromuscular blockers; and severe electrolyte or acid–base disturbances (Table 6.1). Once the cause of coma has been established by the history and neuroimaging, and all prerequisites are met, the clinical examination is performed. A period of time, usually hours, should have passed after the onset of brain injury to exclude the possibility of recovery. Because the history early in the course is often fragmentary, and the use of sedative and analgesic medications is often unknown, brain death should not be determined within hours of Emergency Department evaluation or transfer from an outside facility.

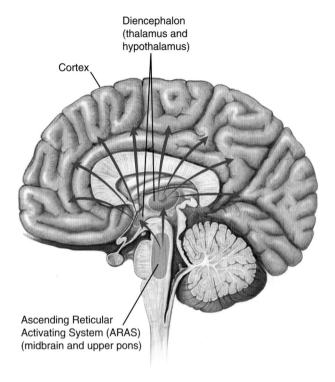

Fig. 6.1 Anatomical structures involved in governing consciousness and the awake state (see text). *(Modified from Wijdicks, E.F., 2011. Brain Death, 2nd edn. Oxford University Press, Oxford.)*

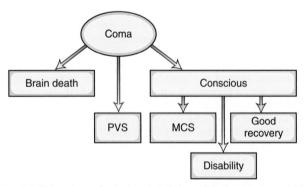

Fig. 6.2 This schematic depicts the distinct clinical states into which acutely comatose patients may transition.

A detailed examination of brainstem reflexes is the crux of the clinical assessment. Most pupils in brain death have a 4- to 6-mm diameter and the pupillary response to bright light should be absent in both eyes. Constricted pupils should not be seen and should raise the concern of medication effect (often opioids). Clinical findings not consistent with a diagnosis of brain death are shown in Box 6.1. Corneal reflexes should be absent bilaterally. Caloric testing of the oculovestibular reflexes is performed with the head elevated to 30 degrees so that the horizontal semicircular canal becomes vertical. A small suction catheter is connected to a 50-mL syringe filled with ice water. In brain death, the reflex is absent, and after irrigation of the tympanum on each side, there are no eye movements. In a comatose, non-brain dead patient with intact oculovestibular reflexes, the eyes slowly deviate toward the side of the cold stimulus. The eyes should be observed for at least one full minute after injection and the time between stimulation of each side should be at least 5 minutes. The gag reflex in response to stimulation of the

TABLE 6.1 Ensuring a Lack of Confounders for Brain Death Determination

Confounder	Prerequisite target	Action
Hypothermia	T ≤ 32°C	Warm to ≥36°C
Sedative drug effect	None present	Wait 5 half-lives* Obtain serum drug levels if available (e.g., barbituates)
Paralytic drug effect	None present	Wait 5 half-lives* Use peripheral nerve stimulator
Hypotension	SBP ≥ 100 mm Hg	Vasopressor/ inotrope infusions
Severe acid–base disturbance	Normal arterial pH $PaCO_2$ 35–45 mm Hg	Adjust ventilator settings Obtain urine drug and toxin screen
Hypoxemia	PaO_2 ≥ 200 mm Hg	Pre-oxygenate with FiO_2 1.0

*Assumes normal hepatic and renal function and no prior hypothermia.
T, temperature; *SBP*, systolic blood pressure.

BOX 6.1 Clinical Findings not Compatible with Brain Death

Nystagmus or other spontaneous eye movements
Conjugate eye deviation
Pinpoint pupils
Grimacing to noxious stimulation
Decerebrate or decorticate motor posturing

posterior oropharynx should be absent and can be tested by inserting a finger deep into the oral cavity and actually feeling the absence of contraction. The lack of a cough response is demonstrated by passing a suction catheter through the endotracheal tube and providing suctioning pressure all the way to the level of the carina.

The application of deep pressure on both condyles at the temporomandibular joint, supraorbital notch, fingernail beds, or sternal rubbing should elicit no grimacing and no motor response in the extremities. Decerebrate and decorticate posturing (see Chapter 5) are motor responses that are not compatible with brain death, but some limb movements may be produced by spinally mediated reflexes.

Following the confirmation of absent motor responses, lack of respiratory drive is documented by an apnea test. This is most commonly performed using the apneic oxygenation-diffusion technique and involves preoxygenation with 100% oxygenation. A systolic blood pressure of 90–100 mm Hg is needed prior to the apnea test and most often vasopressors are already required to meet that goal (Fugate et al., 2011). Doses of vasopressors might need to be increased if persistent hypotension is problematic. A baseline arterial blood gas should show adequate oxygenation (PaO_2 ≥ 200 mm Hg) and normal $PaCO_2$ (35–45 mm Hg). Artificial ventilation is then removed for a period of 8–10 minutes, allowing buildup of arterial tension of carbon dioxide and the pH to be lowered, which under normal circumstances would stimulate respiratory centers. After disconnection from the ventilator, the patient is observed for breathing efforts (chest expansion,

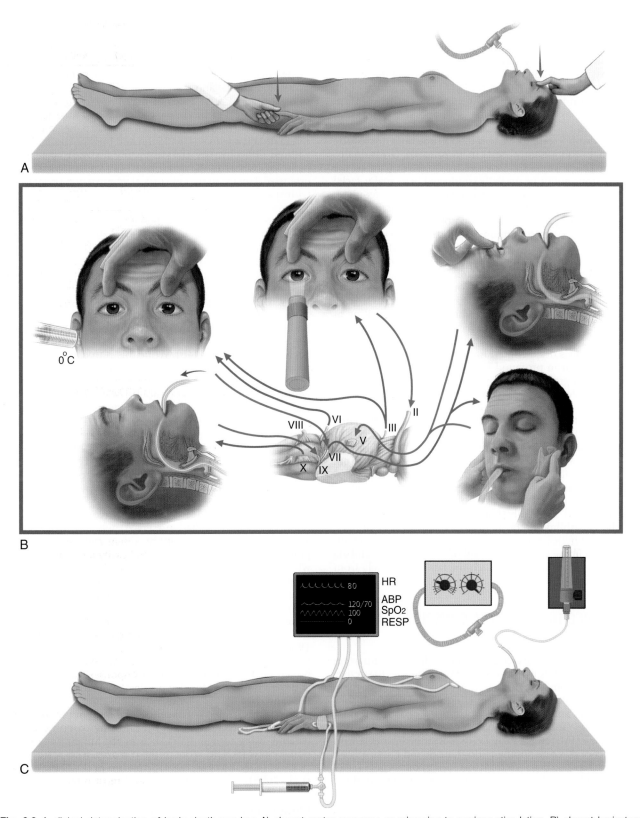

Fig. 6.3 A clinical determination of brain death requires A) absent motor response or grimacing to noxious stimulation, B) absent brainstem reflexes, and C) no respiratory effort despite adequate CO_2 challenge during formal apnea testing (see text). *(Modified from Wijdicks EF. Brain Death, 2nd edn. Oxford University Press 2011.)*

abdominal excursion, or gasping). The lack of respiratory drive is demonstrated when there have been no breathing efforts despite a rise in $PaCO_2$ to 60 mm Hg or an increase ≥ 20 mm Hg from a normal baseline $PaCO_2$. The apnea test using oxygen diffusion with oxygen insufflation at the level of the carina is very safe (Datar et al., 2014) but the acidosis may reduce myocardial contractility, causing transient hypotension and there may be a need for a temporary increase in vasopressors.

Brain death is a clinical determination and does not require additional "confirmatory" tests in most cases. Occasionally, there are times when these are needed if certain parts of the examination cannot be properly conducted (e.g., major facial trauma that precludes a reliable assessment). When required, electrophysiologic tests include electroencephalogram (EEG), auditory evoked potentials, and somatosensory evoked potentials. The EEG (with minimum of eight scalp electrodes and an interelectrode distance of at least 10 cm) should show electrocerebral silence, which necessitates no electrical potentials of more than 2 mV during a 30-minute recording. Artifacts created by the ventilator, pulse, or surrounding electrical devices are often seen and may lead to uncertainty in the interpretation. The clinical examination and the excluding of confounders remains the foundation of brain death determination. It should be noted that unresponsive patients could have "flat" EEGs despite intact brainstem reflexes (Heckmann et al., 2003), or in profound hypothermia or drug overdose. Cerebral angiography, cerebral perfusion scintigraphy, or transcranial Doppler have been used to demonstrate the cessation of cerebral blood flow as ancillary tests, but there are technical pitfalls with these methods and they have not been validated (Wijdicks, 2010).

When the determination of brain death is made clinically, and the apnea test is the last component of the examination, the time of brain death is the time that the arterial PCO_2 reached the target value in the absence of respiratory effort. The family is told that their loved one has died. After adequate time has passed, the family should then be approached regarding the possibility of organ transplantation. Federal laws require the physician to contact an organ procurement organization, and in the United States and other countries, members of this organization will approach the family separately from the medical team.

PROLONGED DISORDERS OF CONSCIOUSNESS
Vegetative State

The advent of intensive care units and mechanical ventilation has allowed patients with devastating brain injuries to survive. While deeply comatose during the acute phase, some of these patients transition to a different clinical state in which they regain awake and sleep cycles, but remain unaware of their surroundings. This clinical syndrome—named persistent vegetative state (PVS) in the early 1970s—described patients with no evidence of a functioning mind (Jennett and Plum, 1972). This state has also been referred to as "unresponsiveness wakefulness syndrome" because of the negative connotation of the word "vegetative" (Laureys et al., 2010). After prolonged coma, patients begin to have periods of spontaneous eye-opening but do not visually fixate or track objects with their eyes. The key feature is that patients show "no evidence of sustained, reproducible, purposeful, or voluntary behavioral responses" to external stimuli (Multi-Society Task Force, 1994a). A patient's eyes may open wide but consistently demonstrated visual pursuit and fixation are absent. A large mirror held in front of the patient—to track their own face—is a useful test—and probably the best stimulus—to assess whether visual

fixation and pursuit occur. A startle response is often present and may manifest as myoclonus, head flexion, or a decorticate response (Wijdicks and Cranford, 2005). Primitive reflexes such as snout, glabella, and palmomental reflexes may be easily elicited. Random movements of the limbs and trunk, occasional grunts, and even occasional tears or smiles are all signs consistent with PVS but may provoke uncertainty for family members or inexperienced clinicians. Autonomic and brainstem functions are preserved so that patients generally can maintain adequate circulation and breathe spontaneously without difficulty. The clinical picture fits with what is seen pathologically, with the majority of brains at autopsy showing extensive damage to the subcortical white matter or thalamus, with sparing of the brainstem (Adams et al., 2000).

At what point can a vegetative state (VS) be considered permanent? When is there a high degree of clinical certainty that the clinical state is irreversible and the chance of regaining consciousness is exceedingly unlikely? The clinical course of PVS depends in large part on the underlying etiology and the duration of unconsciousness. The most common causes are traumatic brain injury (TBI) and hypoxic-ischemic brain injury. Patients in post-traumatic VS are unlikely to regain consciousness after 12 months, while those with anoxic brain injury have even less potential for improvement and very rarely recover consciousness after 3 months (Multi-Society Task Force, 1994b). While this is true for the majority of patients, a minority of patients may recover from PVS beyond these cut-offs (Matsuda et al., 2003). For patients with post-traumatic VS, at 6 months about 50% are still vegetative, 33% are dead, 16% are conscious, and 4% are independent (Multi-Society Task Force, 1994a). The outcomes for postanoxic PVS are even worse, with none regaining consciousness or independence at 6 months, 72% remaining in PVS, and 28% dead (Multi-Society Task Force, 1994a). A more recent but small prospective study of patients with anoxic VS found that 7/43 patients (16%) recovered responsiveness and were living at 2 years, 12 (28%) remained vegetative, and 24 (56%) died (Estraneo et al., 2013). All responsive survivors had preserved pupillary light reflexes and present cortical responses with somatosensory-evoked potentials during the acute phase of injury. Notably, those who do become aware again often find themselves severely disabled. Age also plays a key role, particularly in TBI, with younger patients showing better recovery rates. In one report, the rates of recovering independence at one year were 0% for patients older than 40 years, 9% for patients aged 20–29, and 21% for patients less than 20 years old (Braakman et al., 1988).

The clinical assessment of a patient who is unconscious can be very challenging. The examination may need to be repeated at different times of the day because of fluctuations in awareness and circadian oscillations affecting arousal. Some studies suggest a misdiagnosis in a substantial minority of patients in PVS and a reclassification of 13–28% of supposedly vegetative patients using formal scales such as the *full outline of unresponsiveness* (FOUR) score or the coma recovery scale-revised (CRS-R) (Giacino et al., 2004; Schnakers et al., 2009; Wijdicks et al., 2005).

Minimally Conscious State

In the 1990s, clinicians involved in the care of brain-injured patients began to recognize that some patients previously diagnosed as vegetative showed subtle and partial awareness of their environment. This emerging clinical state was characterized and defined as the minimally conscious state (MCS) by expert consensus of members of a multidisciplinary work group in 2002 (Giacino et al., 2002). The distinguishing

Recent research has linked the right frontal cortex to the sense of self. Keenan and colleagues (2001) studied patients undergoing the Wada test, in which a barbiturate is injected into the carotid artery to determine cortical language dominance. They presented subjects with a self-photograph and a photograph of a famous person, followed by a "morphed" photograph of a famous person and the patient. When the left hemisphere was anesthetized, the subjects said that the morphed photograph represented the subject himself, whereas with right hemisphere anesthesia, the subject selected the famous face. Patients with frontotemporal dementia also indicate a relationship between the right frontal lobe and self-concept. In the series by Miller and colleagues (2001), six of the seven patients who developed a major change in self-concept during their illness had predominant atrophy in the nondominant frontal lobe. A last example of the sense of self is the so-called Theory of Mind, which alludes to the understanding of another person as a conscious human being. Keenan and colleagues (2005) cite evidence that the right hemisphere frontotemporal cortex is dominant for both the sense of self and the recognition of other people.

The frontal lobes, as the executive center of the brain and the determining agent for attention and motor planning, are the origin of several critical networks for cognition and action. Cummings (1993) described five frontal networks for consciousness and behavior. The frontal cortex projects to the basal ganglia, then to thalamic nuclei, and back to the cortex.

Clinical neurology provides important information about how lesions in the brain impair consciousness. The functioning of the awake mind requires the ascending inputs referred to as the *reticular activating system*, with its way stations in the brainstem and thalamus, as well as an intact cerebral cortex. Bilateral lesions of the brainstem or thalamus produce coma. Very diffuse lesions of the hemispheres produce an "awake" patient who shows no responsiveness to the environment, a state sometimes called *coma vigil* or *persistent vegetative state*, as in the well-known Terri Schiavo case (Bernat, 2006; Perry et al., 2005). Patients with very slight responses to environmental stimuli are said to be in a *minimally conscious state* (Wijdicks and Cranford, 2005). Recently, functional brain imaging studies have suggested that at least in a few patients labeled as having persistent vegetative state or minimally conscious state after traumatic brain injury, patients can think of playing tennis or standing in their home and seeing the other rooms, and the brain areas activated are similar to those of normal subjects. These same subjects, a small minority of patients with chronically impaired consciousness secondary to traumatic brain injury, showed evidence of conscious modulation of brain activity to indicate "yes" or "no" responses (Monti et al., 2010). This report has engendered controversy over our ability to determine when a patient truly lacks consciousness. In an accompanying editorial, Ropper noted that activation on brain imaging studies does not equal conscious awareness, and the concept that "I have brain activation, therefore I am … would seriously put Descartes before the horse" (Ropper, 2010).

Still less severe diffuse abnormalities of the association cortex produce encephalopathy, delirium, or dementia. These topics involve very common syndromes of clinical neurology. Stupor and coma are discussed in Chapter 5, and encephalopathy, or delirium, is covered in Chapter 4.

Focal lesions of the cerebral cortex generally produce deficits in specific cognitive systems. A detailed listing of such disorders would include much of the subject matter of behavioral neurology. Examples include Broca aphasia from a left frontal lesion, Wernicke aphasia from a left temporal lesion, Gerstmann syndrome (acalculia, left-right confusion, finger agnosia, and agraphia) from a left parietal lesion, visual agnosia or failure to recognize visual objects (usually from bilateral posterior lesions), apraxia from a left parietal lesion, and constructional impairment from a right parietal lesion. Multiple focal lesions can affect cognitive function in a more global fashion, as in the dementias (Chapter 66). Some authorities separate "cortical" dementias such as Alzheimer disease, in which combinations of cortical deficits are common, from "subcortical" dementias, in which mental slowing is the most prominent feature.

The frontal lobes are heavily involved in integration of the functions provided by other areas of cortex, and lesions there may affect personality and behavior in the absence of easily discernible deficits of specific cognitive, language, or memory function. In severe form, extensive lesions of the orbitofrontal cortex may leave the individual awake but staring, unable to respond to the environment, a state called *akinetic mutism*. With lesser lesions, patients with frontal lobe lesions may lose their ability to form mature judgments, reacting impulsively to incoming stimuli in a manner reminiscent of animal behavior. Such patients may be inappropriately frank or disinhibited. A familiar example is the famous case of Phineas Gage, a worker who sustained a severe injury to the frontal lobes. Gage became irritable, impulsive, and so changed in personality that coworkers said he was "no longer Gage." Bedside neurological testing and even standard neuropsychological tests of patients with frontal lobe damage may reveal normal intelligence except for concrete or idiosyncratic interpretation of proverbs and similarities. Experimentally, subjects with frontal lobe lesions can be shown to have difficulty with sequential processes or shifting of cognitive sets, as tested by the Wisconsin Card Sorting Test or the Category Test of the Halstead-Reitan battery. Luria introduced a simple bedside test of sequential shapes (Fig. 7.1). In contrast to the subtlety of these deficits to the examiner, the patient's family may state that there is a dramatic change in the patient's personality.

Another clinical window into the phenomena of consciousness comes from surgery to separate the hemispheres by cutting the corpus callosum. In split-brain or commissurotomized patients, each hemisphere seems to have a separate consciousness. The left hemisphere, which has the capacity for speech and language, can express this consciousness in words. For example, a split-brain patient can report words or pictures that appear in the right visual field. The right hemisphere cannot produce verbal accounts of items seen in the left visual field, but the subject can choose the correct item by pointing with the left hand; at the same time, the subject claims to have no conscious knowledge of the item. In terms of the speaking left hemisphere, the right hemisphere has "unconscious" visual knowledge, or *blindsight*. At times, the left hand of the patient may seem to operate under a different agenda from the right hand. A split-brain patient may select a dress from a rack with the right hand while the left hand puts it back or selects a more daring fashion. This rivalry of the left hand with the right is called the *alien hand syndrome*, a striking example of the

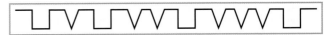

Fig. 7.1 Luria's test of alternating sequences. *(Adapted from Luria, A.R., 1969. Frontal lobe syndromes, In: Vynken, P., Bruyn, G.W. (Eds.), Handbook of Clinical Neurology, vol. 2, Elsevier, New York. Reprinted with permission from Kirshner, H.S., 2002. Behavioral Neurology: Practical Science of Mind and Brain, second ed. Butterworth Heinemann, Boston.)*

separate consciousnesses of the two divided hemispheres (Gazzaniga, 1998). Callosal syndromes, including the alien hand syndrome, have also been described in patients with strokes involving the corpus callosum (Chan and Ross, 1997).

MEMORY
Forms and Stages of Declarative Memory

Generally defined, *memory* refers to the ability of the brain to store and retrieve information, the necessary prerequisite for all learning. Some memories are so vivid they seem like a reliving of a prior experience, as in Marcel Proust's sudden recollections of his youth on biting into a madeleine pastry. Other memories are more vague or bring up a series of facts rather than a perceptual experience. Memory has been divided into several types and stages, leading to a confusing set of terms and concepts. Clinical neurologists have historically divided memory into three temporal stages. These stages can be helpful when conceptualizing diagnosis and difficulties in independent living and have a general correspondence to the stages and concepts of memory proposed by cognitive neuroscientists. The first stage, referred to as *immediate memory* by clinicians, corresponds to Baddeley's concept of *working memory* (Baddeley, 2010). *Immediate or working memory* refers to the system that actively holds pieces of transitory information in conscious awareness, where it can be subsequently manipulated or used to perform a task. There has been recent debate over the true capacity of working memory, but the general consensus is that the normal adult human being can retain 5 to 9 meaningful items in working memory (Miller, 1956). This information can generally reside in conscious awareness indefinitely with attention and rehearsal. However, without rehearsal, this information is lost in approximately 18 to 20 seconds (Brown, 1958; Peterson and Peterson, 1959). As an example, most people can hear or see a telephone number, walk across the room, and dial the number without difficulty. Once the number is dialed and conversation is started, the number fades from working memory. Relying primarily on prefrontal brain regions, working memory declines with normal aging. Further, disorders of attention, focal lesions of the superior frontal neocortex affecting Brodmann areas 8 and 9, and patients with aphasia secondary to left frontal lesions can show profound impairment in working memory (Goldman-Rakic, 1996).

The second stage of memory, referred to by clinicians as *short-term* or *recent memory*, involves the ability to encode and retrieve specific items, such as words or events, after a delay of minutes or hours. Some of the aforementioned confusion over terminology comes from the fact that cognitive psychologists posit that working memory underlies short-term memory and consider it distinct from episodic learning and memory. In clinical parlance, short-term memory is synonymous with recent episodic memory. Short-term or recent episodic memory requires the function of the hippocampus and parahippocampal areas of the medial temporal lobe for both encoding and storage. The amygdala, a structure adjacent to the medial temporal cortex, is not essential for episodic memory but seems crucial for the encoding of emotional or social contexts of specific events (Markowitsch and Staniloiu, 2011). In contrast, the retrieval of recent episodic memories tends to rely on a delicate interaction between prefrontal regions and medial temporal regions. Budson and Price (2005) provide a simple analogy for remembering the anatomical organization of recent episodic memory. In this analogy, the frontal lobes are considered the "filing clerk" of the memory system, deciding what memories to retrieve and from where to retrieve them. The medial temporal lobes are the "recent memory filing

cabinet," where recent memories are stored. Patients with medial temporal lobe damage (e.g., Alzheimer disease) have a damaged file cabinet, in which memories are unable to be stored. In contrast, patients with frontal lobe damage (e.g., stroke, tumor) have difficulty in properly organizing the files in the cabinet or difficulty locating them during retrieval. Finally, in patients with subcortical white matter pathology (e.g., ischemic disease, multiple sclerosis), the file clerk has difficulty gaining access to the file cabinet, which makes retrieval difficult. However, once given an option between multiple files—through a recognition or multiple choice test—the file clerk can correctly identify the needed file. The commonly used bedside test of recalling three unrelated items at 5 minutes assesses recent episodic memory, as do questions about this morning's breakfast. It is relatively easy to test for impairment in recent episodic memory by including general questions about recent events in one's life or the news in rapport building and interview.

The third stage, referred to as *remote* or *long-term* episodic memory, refers to the ability to retrieve specific items, such as words or events, after a delay of weeks, months, or years. An example of this would be asking the patient about the last movie they have seen or what they did on their last birthday. Retrieval of remote episodic memories tends to require less hippocampal and medial temporal lobe involvement (Dudai, 2004). Consolidation of long-term memories can occur at the synaptic and systems levels. Synaptically, consolidation occurs through long-term potentiation and protein synthesis in the hippocampus during the first few hours of learning (Roediger et al., 2007). In contrast, on a systems level, consolidation occurs over long periods of time where hippocampal-dependent memory representations are stored in the neocortex. Recent work has shown a relatively linear decline in hippocampal activation as time passes (Frankland and Bontempi, 2005). In other words, the older the memory, the less the hippocampus and medial temporal regions are needed for retrieval. This was previously demonstrated through patient H.M. and patients with Alzheimer disease who cannot retrieve recent information or events, but can easily recall events from many years ago. Similarly to short-term episodic memory, the frontal lobes are required to retrieve memories, but rather than the hippocampus, the file clerk must access memories in cortical regions.

Remaining within the realm of long-term declarative memory, there appears to be overlap in the type of information retrieved for remote memories. In addition to episodic memory, which according to Tulving (1985) requires some type of "mental time travel" to revisit the original experience, *semantic memories* can be retrieved. Semantic memory is referred to as factual knowledge that includes memory of meanings, understandings, and other concept-based knowledge as well as general knowledge about the world. Recall of famous figures or events, such as presidents or wars, and knowledge of semantic information, such as the definitions of words and the differences between words, are examples of semantic memory. Semantic memory differs from personal long-term memory in that the subject can continuously replenish such knowledge by reading and conversation.

Semantic memory is thought to reside in multiple cortical regions such as the visual association cortex for visual memories and the temporal cortex for auditory memories. This concept of multiple localizations of semantic memory is supported by functional brain imaging research (Cappa, 2008). Specific semantic knowledge of word meanings is thought to reside in the left lateral temporal cortex. Remote memory, as we shall see later, resists the effects of medial temporal damage; once memory is well stored in the neocortex, it can be retrieved without use of the hippocampal system.

TABLE 7.1 Memory Stages

Traditional term	Cognitive neuroscience term	Awareness level	Anatomy
Immediate memory	Working memory	Explicit	Prefrontal cortex
Short-term memory	Episodic memory	Explicit	Medial temporal lobe
Long-term memory	Semantic memory	Explicit	Lateral temporal and other cortices
Motor memory	Procedural memory	Implicit	Basal ganglia, cerebellum

Other nondeclarative categories of memory, such as motor and procedural memories, will be discussed later in this chapter. Table 7.1 is a classification of memory stages.

Formation and Retrieval of Episodic Memories

Recently, use of functional brain imaging in healthy human subjects and computational modeling has contributed to knowledge of the anatomy of episodic memory function. A network of structures has been identified in the encoding or formation of episodic memory. While the hippocampus and all of its subregions are critical to the encoding of information, it is highly connected (both structurally and functionally) to the amygdala, entorhinal cortex, perirhinal cortex, temporal pole, insula, ventromedial prefrontal cortex, anterior and posterior cingulate, precuneus, and inferior parietal cortex (Kier et al., 2004; Poppenk and Moscovitch, 2011), which have all been implicated in the role of episodic memory. When sensory information is processed by specific sensory cortices (e.g., the occipital lobe for visual information), prefrontal regions attend and select important information to be encoded into memory. To-be-remembered information passes through the entorhinal cortex and into the hippocampus through the dentate gyrus (Rolls, 2007). The dentate gyrus acts as a "pattern separator" creating unique memory representations as it passes information to hippocampal subregion CA3 (Yassa and Stark, 2011). Subregion CA3 acts as its own autoassociation network whereby recurrent projections onto itself work to temporarily store a memory representation for later recall (Hunsaker and Kesner, 2013).

According to early positron emission tomography (PET) work, several brain regions show consistent activation in healthy subjects during memory retrieval. These brain regions include (1) the prefrontal cortex, especially on the right; (2) the hippocamus and adjacent medial temporal regions; (3) the anterior cingulate cortex; (4) the posterior midline regions of the cingulate, precuneate, and cuneate gyri; (5) the inferior parietal cortex, especially on the right; and (6) the cerebellum, particularly on the left (Cabeza et al., 1997). A model for the functions of these areas in memory is as follows: the prefrontal cortex appears to relate to attention, retrieval activation, and memory search; the hippocampi, particularly subregions CA3 and CA1, to conscious recollection of recently learned information; the cingulate cortex to the activation of memory and selection of a specific response; the posterior midline regions to visual imagery; the parietal cortex to spatial and memory awareness; and the cerebellum to voluntary self-initiated retrieval (Cabeza et al., 1997; Dickerson and Eichenbaum, 2010; Wagner et al., 1998). In subjects asked to recognize previously presented pairs of associated words, the right prefrontal cortex, anterior cingulate cortex, and inferior parietal region were the most activated. When the subject had to recall the words, the basal ganglia and left cerebellum also became active. In similar studies using functional MRI, Wagner and colleagues (1998) found that the left prefrontal region was predominantly involved when words were semantically encoded in memory; the right frontal activations seen in the previous study reflected nonverbal memory stimuli. Even in the hippocampus, words elicited activation of the left hippocampus, objects evoked activation in both hippocampi, and faces mainly activated the right hippocampus (Fliessbach et al., 2010; Rosazza et al., 2009). In studies of the recognition of visual designs, Petersson and colleagues (1997) found that the medial temporal cortex activates more during new learning tasks than during previously trained and practiced memory tasks. Other areas activated during the new learning task included the prefrontal and anterior cingulate areas, more on the right side, and the parieto-occipital lobes bilaterally. Trained tasks activated the hippocampi much less but did activate the right infero-occipitotemporal region. This finding correlates with human studies indicating that overlearned memories gradually become less dependent on the hippocampus. Rugg and colleagues (1997) also found greater activation of the left medial temporal cortex in tasks in which the subject remembered words by "deep encoding" of their meaning compared to simpler "shallow" encoding of the specific word. Other studies have shown that the deeper the encoding of a word's meaning, the better the subject remembers it (Schacter, 1996). Finally, the amygdala appears necessary for affective aspects of memory items, such as recall of fear associated with a specific stimulus (Knight et al., 2009).

Basic research on animals has begun to unravel the fundamental biochemical processes involved in memory. Bailey and colleagues (1996) have studied memory formation in the giant snail, *Aplysia*. Development of long-term facilitation, a primitive form of memory, requires activation of a gene called CREB (cyclic adenosine monophosphate response element-binding protein) in sensory neurons. In this system and also in similar studies on the fruit fly, *Drosophila*, gene activation and protein synthesis are necessary for memory formation. Injection of protein-synthesis inhibitors into the hippocampus can prevent consolidation of memories (McGaugh, 2000). Although similar studies have not been performed in humans, it is likely that similar gene activation and protein synthesis, perhaps beginning in the hippocampi but proceeding through its neocortical connections, is necessary for the transition from immediate working memory to longer-term storage of memory (Bear, 1997). This field of research may hold promise for the development of drugs to enhance memory storage.

Amnestic Syndrome

The amnestic syndrome (Box 7.1) refers to profound loss of recent or short-term episodic memory. These patients, most of whom have bilateral hippocampal damage, have normal immediate and working memory span and largely normal ability to recall remote and semantic memories such as their childhood upbringing and education. Other cognitive or higher cortical functions may be completely intact (e.g., attention, executive functioning, language), which distinguishes these patients from those with dementias such as Alzheimer disease. Procedural or motor memory (see Other Types of Memory) tends to remain preserved in patients with amnestic syndrome, who may be taught to perform a new motor skill

BOX 7.1 Amnestic Syndrome Features

Impaired recent memory (anterograde, retrograde)
Global amnesia
Spared procedural memory
Preserved immediate memory
Preserved remote memory
Intact general cognitive function
Disorientation to time or place
Confabulation

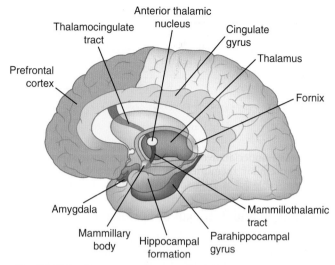

Fig. 7.2 Episodic memory. The medial temporal lobes, including the hippocampus and parahippocampus, form the core of the episodic memory system. Other brain regions are also necessary for episodic memory to function correctly. (*Adapted from Budson, A.E., Price, B.H., 2005. Memory dysfunction, N Engl J Med 352, 692–699.*)

such as mirror writing. When asked to perform the newly learned skill again, the patient will typically not recall knowing how to do it, but the motor skill remains and the patient can easily demonstrate the skill. Other more variable features of the amnestic syndrome include potential disorientation to time and place. Further, the amnestic syndrome can include *confabulation*, or making up information the memory system does not supply. Amnestic patients live in an eternal present in which they can interact, speak intelligently, and reason appropriately, but they do not remember anything about the interaction a few minutes after it ends. An amnestic patient may complete an IQ test within the normal or even above normal range, but not recall taking the examination minutes later. These patients are condemned to repeat the same experiences without learning from them.

The registration of short-term episodic memory involves a consolidation period during which a blow to the head, as in a football injury, can prevent memories from being stored or recalled. The recognition or recall of newly learned information appears to require the hippocampus. The site of storage of memories, as noted earlier, likely involves large areas of the neocortex specialized for specific cognitive functions such as auditory or visual analysis. Once processed in the neocortex and stored for a long period of time, items can be recalled even in the presence of hippocampal damage, as in the case of remote or semantic memories. After an injury producing hippocampal damage, a retrograde period of memory loss may extend back from minutes to years, and the subject cannot form new anterograde memories. As the ability to form new memories returns, the period of retrograde amnesia shortens or "shrinks" ("shrinking retrograde amnesia"). After a minor head injury, the permanent amnestic period may involve a few minutes of retrograde amnesia and a few hours or days of anterograde amnesia. In experimental studies in which amnestic subjects are shown famous people from past decades, a temporal gradient has been found in which subjects have excellent memory for remote personages but recall progressively less from periods dating up to the recent past.

The neuroanatomy of the amnestic syndrome is one of the best-studied areas of cognitive neuropsychology. In animal models, bilateral lesions of the hippocampus, parahippocampal gyrus, and entorhinal cortex produce profound amnesia (Squire and Zola, 1996). Human patients undergoing temporal lobectomy for epilepsy have shown very similar syndromes. In the early period of this surgery, a few patients were deliberately subjected to bilateral medial temporal ablations, with disastrous results for memory, as seen in the famous patient, H.M. (Corkin, 2002; Squire, 2009). In other cases, unilateral temporal lobectomy caused severe amnesia. In one such case, an autopsy many years later showed pre-existing damage to the contralateral hippocampus. Patients currently receive extensive evaluation (e.g., the Wada intracarotid barbiturate infusion test) to ensure that ablation of one hippocampus will not result in an amnestic syndrome, although partial memory

deficits still occur. Other common causes of the amnestic syndrome involving bilateral medial temporal lesions include bilateral strokes in the posterior cerebral artery territory, involving the hippocampus, and herpes simplex encephalitis, which has a predilection for the orbitofrontal and medial temporal cortices. Gold and Squire (2006) described three new cases of the amnestic syndrome with detailed neurobehavioral testing in life and neuropathology at autopsy. One had bilateral hippocampal damage, one had Wernicke–Korsakoff syndrome with damage in the mammillary bodies and dorsomedial thalamus, and one had bilateral thalamic infarctions. We will return to these other anatomic substrates of memory later.

Although the neuroanatomy of memory storage and retrieval has been known for many years, numerous recent refinements have been made. Figure 7.2 shows a simplified diagram of the memory system in the human brain. The hippocampus on each side projects via the fornix to the septal areas, then to the mammillary bodies, which in turn project to the anterior nucleus of the thalamus and on to the cingulate gyrus of the frontal lobe, which projects back to the hippocampus. This circuit (Papez circuit) is critical for short-term memory registration and retrieval. Disease processes that affect extrahippocampal parts of this circuit also cause amnesia. One well-studied example is the Wernicke–Korsakoff syndrome induced by thiamine deficiency, usually in the setting of alcoholism, with damage to the mammillary bodies and dorsomedial thalamic nuclei (Gold and Squire, 2006). A second clinical example is that of patients with ruptured aneurysms of the anterior communicating artery, which are associated with damage to the deep medial frontal areas such as the septal nuclei. These two amnestic syndromes are commonly associated with confabulation. The anterior communicating artery aneurysm syndrome also involves frontal executive dysfunction (Diamond et al., 1997). Traumatic brain injuries commonly produce memory loss, probably because the most common sites of damage are in the frontal and temporal lobes, but other deficits besides memory frequently occur. Of course, memory loss can be seen in several other neurological conditions, including brain tumors of the thalamus or temporal lobes, white matter diseases such as multiple sclerosis, and dementing diseases such as Alzheimer disease, which has a predilection for the entorhinal cortex, perirhinal cortex, hippocampus, basal frontal nuclei, and neocortex (Braak and Braak, 1991). In these other disorders, memory loss is usually not as isolated a deficit as in the amnestic syndrome.

Syndromes of Partial Memory Loss

In contrast to the global amnesia seen in amnestic syndrome, patients who have memory loss for selected classes of items have been described. For example, patients who undergo left temporal lobectomy for intractable epilepsy usually have detectable impairment of short-term verbal memory, whereas those undergoing right temporal resection have impairment only of nonverbal memory. Isolated sensory-specific memory loss syndromes have also been described, such as pure visual or tactile memory loss. Ross (1980) described two patients with bilateral occipital lesions that disconnected the visual cortex from the memory structures. These patients could draw a diagram of their homes but could not learn new spatial layouts. Ross postulated that diagnosis of a selective visual recent memory deficit requires documentation of normal visual perception, absence of aphasia sufficient to impair testing, intact immediate visual memory, intact remote visual memory, and normal recent memory in other modalities. A similar syndrome of isolated tactile memory loss has also been described.

Transient Amnesia

Transient amnesia is a temporary version of amnestic syndrome. The most striking example of transient amnesia is the syndrome of transient global amnesia, lasting from several to 24 hours. In this syndrome, an otherwise cognitively intact individual suddenly loses memory for recent events, asks repetitive questions about his or her environment, and sometimes confabulates. During the episode, the patient has both anterograde and retrograde amnesia, as in the permanent amnestic syndrome. As recovery occurs, however, the retrograde portion "shrinks" to a short period, leaving a permanent gap in memory of the brief retrograde amnesia before the episode and the period of no learning during the episode. The syndrome is of unknown cause but can be closely imitated by disorders of known etiology such as partial complex seizures, migraine, and possibly transient ischemia of the hippocampus on one or both sides. Strupp and colleagues (1998) reported that 7 of 10 patients imaged during episodes of transient global amnesia showed abnormal diffusion MRI signal in the left hippocampus; 3 of these had bilateral hippocampal abnormalities. Permanent infarctions were not found. Yang and colleagues (2008) reported similar hippocampal lesions in the lateral or CA1 region in 17 of 20 cases of TGA. Other investigators have found frontal lobe abnormalities by diffusion-weighted MRI or PET. Gonzalez-Martinez and colleagues (2010) recently reported a case in which a small left thalamic infarction found by diffusion-weighted MRI was associated with hypometabolism in the left thalamic region, seen on FDG-PET. These studies do not prove an ischemic etiology for transient global amnesia; rather, they indicate transient dysfunction in the hippocampus or its connections. The last several patients with transient global amnesia observed at our hospital have had normal diffusion-weighted MRI studies, except for two patients who had incomplete recovery; these patients both had left medial temporal infarctions. Confusional migraine, partial epilepsy (Bilo et al., 2009), drug intoxication, alcoholic "blackouts," and minor head injuries can also produce transient amnesia.

TABLE 7.2 Types of Memory and Their Localization

Types of recent memory	Localization
DECLARATIVE (EXPLICIT)	
Facts, events	Medial temporal lobe
NONDECLARATIVE (IMPLICIT)	
Procedural skills	Basal ganglia, frontal lobes
Classical conditioning	Cerebellum (+ amygdala)
Probabilistic classification learning	Basal ganglia
Priming	Neocortex

OTHER TYPES OF MEMORY (NONDECLARATIVE OR IMPLICIT MEMORY)

A confusing array of memory classifications and terminology has arisen, as shown in Table 7.2. Several aspects of memory do not involve the conscious recall involved in the three temporal memory stages. A simple example is motor memory, such as the ability to ride a bicycle, which is remarkably resistant to hippocampal damage. Such motor memories probably reside in the basal ganglia and cerebellum. In Squire and Zola's (1996) classification, motor memories of this type are called *procedural* or *implicit nondeclarative memories*; note that all three of the temporal stages of memory—working (immediate) memory, episodic (short-term) memory, and semantic (long-term) memory—are *declarative, explicit*.

Another term for the class of memories for which subjects have no conscious awareness is *implicit* or *nondeclarative memory* (in contrast to the explicit declarative memory of episodic events). Implicit memories have in common storage and retrieval mechanisms that do not involve the hippocampal system; perhaps for this reason, the subject has no conscious knowledge of them. These procedural memories involve "knowing how" rather than "knowing that." Amnestic patients can learn new motor memories such as mirror drawing, which they can perform once started, although they have no recollection of knowing the task. Motor learning likely involves the supplementary motor cortex, basal ganglia, and cerebellum. Strokes in the territory of the recurrent artery of Heubner (affecting the caudate nucleus) can affect procedural memory (Mizuta and Motomura, 2006). Another type of memory localized to the cerebellum is *classical conditioning*, in which an unconditioned stimulus becomes associated with a reward or punishment given when the conditioned stimulus is presented (Clark et al., 2002; Thompson and Kim, 1996). The conditioning itself clearly involves the cerebellum, but the emotional aspect of the reward or punishment stimulus may reside in the amygdala. Classical conditioning can continue to function after bilateral hippocampal damage. Squire and Zola (1996) outlined other types of nondeclarative memory that take place independent of the hippocampal system. Probabilistic classification learning (e.g., predicting the weather from a combination of cues that are regularly associated with sunny or rainy weather) is unaffected by hippocampal damage but impaired in diseases of the basal ganglia such as Huntington and Parkinson diseases (Gluck et al., 2002; Thompson and Kim, 1996). Learning artificial grammar can also take place in the presence of amnestic syndrome, with functional imaging showing activation in the left parietal and occipital lobes (Skosnik et al., 2002). In all these memory experiments, the subject has no awareness of how he or she is able to answer the questions. The last form of nondeclarative memory is called *priming*, the presentation of a stimulus associated with the word or idea to be remembered, which then aids in retrieval of the item (e.g., recalling the word *doctor* when *nurse* appears on a priming list). Priming appears to involve the neocortex (Levy et al., 2004; Thompson and Kim, 1996). Schacter and Buckner (1998) have shown that deliberate use of priming can help amnestic patients compensate for their memory loss in everyday life.

BEDSIDE TESTS OF MEMORY AND COGNITIVE FUNCTION

The most important point to be made about bedside evaluations of cognition and memory is that they are an integral part of the neurological examination and a tool by which the neurologist localizes lesions affecting the higher cortical functions, just as the motor or cerebellar examinations localize neurological deficits. The most common error made by neurologists is to omit a systematic evaluation of mental function in patients who seem "alert and oriented." Deficits of memory, deficits in fund of knowledge, or focal deficits such as apraxia, agnosia, acalculia, or constructional impairment can be missed. Some patients have a "cocktail party" conversational pattern that belies such deficits; others become expert at deferring questions to a spouse or family member. Every neurologist has the task of deciding which patients need formal cognitive testing and whether to make up an individual test routine or to rely on one of the standard tests. Again, it is more important to make the assessment than to follow a specific format.

Several versions of bedside mental status testing have been published. Perhaps the most widely used is Folstein's Mini-Mental State Examination (MMSE). The MMSE consists of 30 points: 5 for orientation to time (year, season, month, date, and day), 5 for orientation to place (state, county, town, hospital, and floor), 5 for attention (either serial 7's with 1 point for each of the first five subtractions or "spell *world* backward"), 3 for registration of three items, 3 for recall of three items after 5 minutes, 2 for naming a pencil and a watch, 1 for repeating "no ifs, ands, or buts," 3 for following a three-stage command, 1 for following a printed command ("close your eyes"), 1 for writing a sentence, 1 for copying a diagram of two intersecting pentagons.

The advantages of the MMSE are short time of administration and quantitation, useful in documentation for insurance benefits, such as rehabilitative therapies or drug therapy, and for disability assessment. Several disadvantages of the MMSE have been identified. First, the normal range of scores depends on education. The low-normal cutoff is estimated by Crum and colleagues (1993) to be 19 for uneducated people, 23 for graduates of elementary or junior high school, 27 for high school graduates, and 29 for college graduates. Age is also a factor. In addition, the test is weighted toward orientation and language, and results can be normal in patients with right hemisphere or frontal lobe damage. Finally, even an abnormal score does not distinguish a focal lesion from a more diffuse disorder such as an encephalopathy or dementia.

One answer to the dilemma of mental status testing is to use the MMSE as a screening test and then supplement it with more focused tests. Box 7.2 lists the key elements of a mental status examination, whether the examiner chooses to adopt the MMSE or one of the other bedside cognitive instruments, or to create an individual test battery. Several texts provide further detail on such a battery. Although the mental status examination is the most neglected area of the neurological examination, it generally requires only a few minutes, and its cost-effectiveness compares well with brain imaging studies such as MRI or PET.

BOX 7.2 Bedside Mental Status Examination

Orientation (time, place, person, situation)
Memory (immediate, short term, long term)
Fund of information
Speech and language
Praxis
Calculations
Visual–constructional abilities
Abstract reasoning, sequential processes

An experienced examiner can learn much about the subject's mental status by careful observation during the history. Considerable insight can be gained into the subject's recent memory, orientation, language function, affect or mood, insight, and judgment. Affect and mood are best assessed in this fashion; if there is doubt, the examiner should consider how the patient makes the examiner feel: a depressed patient often makes the examiner feel depressed, whereas a manic patient makes the examiner feel happy and amused.

The formal mental status examination should always include explicit testing of orientation including the date, place, and situation. Memory testing should include an immediate attention test, of which the most popular are forward digit span, serial-7 subtractions from 100, or the MMSE test "spell *world* backward." Short-term memory should include recall of three unrelated words at 5 minutes. The subject should always be asked to say them back after presentation to make sure the three items have registered. At times, nonverbal short-term memory, such as recalling the locations of three hidden coins or reproducing drawings, can be useful to test. Remote memory can be tested by having the subject name children or siblings. Fund of information can be tested with recent presidents or other political figures. For patients who do not pay attention to politics, use of athletic stars or television celebrities may be more appropriate. Language testing should include spontaneous speech, naming, repetition, auditory comprehension, reading, and writing (the bedside language test is described in more detail in Chapter 13). In our practice, we like to show subjects more difficult naming items such as the drawings from the NIH Stroke Scale or body parts such as the thumb or the palm of the hand. Praxis testing should include the use of both imaginary and real (e.g., saw, hammer, pencil) objects. Both hands should be tested separately. Calculation tasks include the serial-7 subtraction test and simple change-making problems. Visual-spatial-constructional tasks can include line bisection, copying a cube or other design, and drawing a clock or a house (Fig. 7.3). The MMSE contains only one constructional task, the copying of intersecting pentagons. Many neurologists supplement this with the clock-drawing test. Insight and judgment are probably best tested by assessing the patient's understanding of his own illness. Artificial tests include interpretation of proverbs (e.g., "Those who live in glass houses should not throw stones") or stating why an apple and an orange are similar. An artificial test sometimes used to test frontal lobe processing is the copying and continuation of Luria's test of alternating sequences (sequential squares and triangles; see Fig. 7.1). With these tests, preliminary localization can be made in the deep memory structures of the medial temporal lobes, the frontal lobes (insight and judgment, proverbs, similarities, Luria's sequence test), the left hemisphere language cortex in the frontal and temporal lobes, the left parietal region (calculations), and the right parietal lobe (visual-constructional tasks).

In conclusion, this chapter considers the areas of neurology that most physicians find the most abstruse—namely, the

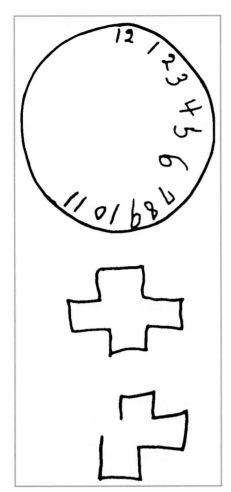

Fig. 7.3 Spontaneous clock drawing and copying of a cross by a patient with a right parietal infarction. The patient had only mild hemiparesis but dense left hemianopia and neglect of the left side of the body. The neglect of the left side of space is evident in both drawings. *(Reprinted with permission from Kirshner, H.S., 2002. Behavioral Neurology: Practical Science of Mind and Brain, second ed. Butterworth Heinemann, Boston.)*

higher cortical functions, intellect, and memory. As stated at the outset, this area of neurology can be treated as a series of specific functions to be analyzed at the bedside and localized, just like other functions of the nervous system. In fact, the rapidly increasing knowledge of cognitive neuroscience and our vastly improved ability to image the brain both at rest and during functional activities promise a new era of practical diagnosis of higher cognitive disorders.

REFERENCES

The complete reference list is available online at https://expertconsult .inkling.com/.

8 Global Developmental Delay and Regression

Tyler Reimschisel

CHAPTER OUTLINE

TYPICAL AND ATYPICAL DEVELOPMENT
Child Development Concepts
GLOBAL DEVELOPMENTAL DELAY
Developmental History
Neurological and Other Medical History
Physical Examination
Diagnostic Testing
MANAGEMENT
PROGNOSIS
RECURRENCE RISK
REGRESSION

Developmental delay occurs in approximately 1% to 3% of children. Since developmental delay is common, monitoring a child's development is an essential component of well-child care. Ongoing assessment of the child's development at each well-child visit creates a pattern of development that is more useful than measuring the discrete milestone achievements at a single visit; therefore, developmental screening should be completed at each well-child visit (Council on Children with Disabilities, 2006). Identification of a child with developmental delays should be accomplished as early as possible, because the earlier a child is identified, the sooner the child can receive a thorough evaluation and begin therapeutic interventions that can improve the child's outcome. Developmental delay is common and one of the most frequent presenting complaints to a pediatric neurology clinic; therefore, neurologists should have a systematic approach to the child with developmental delay.

This chapter begins with a brief discussion of child development concepts related to typical and atypical development. Next, the clinical evaluation and management of developmental delay is reviewed. The chapter closes with a discussion of neurological regression.

TYPICAL AND ATYPICAL DEVELOPMENT
Child Development Concepts

Child development is a continuous process of acquiring new and advanced skills. This development depends on maturation of the nervous system. Although typical child development follows a relatively consistent sequence, it is not linear. Instead, there are spurts and lags. For example, motor development in the first year of life proceeds relatively rapidly. Babies typically mature from being completely immobile to walking in just over 12 months, but then motor development progresses less dramatically during the second year of life. Conversely, language development in the first year of life occurs slowly, but there is an explosion of language acquisition between a child's first and second birthdays.

On average, most children achieve each developmental milestone within a defined and narrow age range (Table 8.1).

Usually physicians learn the average age for acquiring specific skills. However, since each developmental skill can be acquired within an age range, it is much more useful clinically to know when a child's development falls outside this range. These so-called red flags are important because they can be used to identify when a child has developmental delay for specific skills. For example, although the average age of walking is approximately 13 months, a child may walk as late as 17 months and still be within the typical developmental range. In this example, the red flag for independent walking is 18 months, and a child who is not walking by 18 months of age is delayed.

GLOBAL DEVELOPMENTAL DELAY
Developmental History

Child development is classically divided into five interdependent domains or streams: gross motor, fine motor and problem-solving, receptive language, expressive language, and socialization/adaptive. The approach to a child with possible developmental delays is based on a working knowledge of these domains and the typical age ranges for acquiring specific milestones within each domain. Therefore, the clinician should begin the evaluation of a child with developmental concerns by obtaining a developmental history, and emphasis should be placed on the pattern of milestone acquisition as well as the child's current developmental skills. Clinicians working in a busy clinical setting may need to base this history primarily on the caregiver's report of the child's developmental abilities. Clinicians may also use standardized tools to aid in this portion of the history, including the Ireton Child Development Inventory (CDI), the Ages and Stages Questionnaire (ASQ), and the Parents' Evaluation of Developmental Status (PEDS). However, if the clinician's history confirms a developmental disability, standardized testing by a developmental specialist or clinical psychologist should be strongly considered; this formal evaluation will provide a much better assessment of the child's developmental abilities.

When there is concern about developmental delay in a child, a developmental quotient should be calculated. The *developmental quotient* is the ratio of the child's developmental age over the chronological age. The developmental quotient should be calculated for each developmental stream. Typical development is a developmental quotient greater than 70%, and atypical development is a developmental quotient less than 70%. Toddlers and young children with atypical development are at risk for lifelong developmental problems. The term *global development delay* is used if a child younger than 5 to 6 years of age has a developmental quotient less than 70% in two or more domains. Children with global developmental delay should receive a thorough medical evaluation to try to determine the cause of the delay and begin management for their developmental disabilities.

Neurological and Other Medical History

For children with global developmental delay, the clinician should obtain a thorough medical history, including a detailed neurological history. Pertinent aspects of the history include

Additional diagnostic tests are not typically warranted in children with nonspecific global developmental delay. However, depending on the presentation, the clinician may consider more invasive tests such as CSF analysis, electromyography (EMG) and nerve conduction studies, muscle and/or nerve biopsies, and cell culture for enzyme analysis or other biochemical testing. However, these studies are rarely indicated until the mentioned routine studies have been completed.

MANAGEMENT

Medical management of global developmental delay begins with a disclosure to the family of the clinician's concern for the diagnosis. As with any situation in which the physician discloses difficult news, this must be done gently but clearly. The clinician should be prepared to respond to a full range of emotions including doubt, denial, sorrow, and anger. Furthermore, the family will usually need time to process the information that their child has or is at risk for having lifelong developmental problems. Therefore, a follow-up appointment should be scheduled to review the diagnosis and address additional questions or concerns the family may have.

In addition, any comorbid conditions should be treated, or the clinician should refer the patient to the appropriate subspecialist who can provide treatment for the comorbid condition. The clinician can also help facilitate social, community, or educational supports for the family. These may include family support groups, national parent organizations, and other resources in the community for families of children with developmental disabilities.

One of the most important aspects of the management of a child with global developmental delay is ensuring that the child receives early and appropriate therapeutic and educational interventions. Children younger than 3 years of age with developmental delays can be enrolled in early intervention programs. Each state's program includes a multidisciplinary team of therapists who complete a comprehensive assessment and provide appropriate interventions. Their assessment is summarized in a report called the *Individualized Family Service Plan*; this plan serves as the basis for provision of therapeutic services.

Children who are older than 3 years of age receive services through the special education program within the local school district. These services are usually provided by a multidisciplinary team of therapists as well as a psychologist. They also complete an assessment and summarize their findings in a report called the *Individualized Education Plan* (IEP). The IEP serves as the basis for the services that will be provided to the child within the school system. Federal law mandates that children receive the special services they need in the least restrictive environment possible. Therefore, many children with developmental disabilities are now educated in the regular ("mainstream") classroom with an aide instead of being placed in a separate classroom. However, some children with more significant intellectual or behavioral problems may require placement in a special education classroom for part or all of the day.

PROGNOSIS

Once a child is diagnosed with global developmental delay, the family will inquire about the child's ultimate developmental outcome, including cognitive and motor abilities, future level of independence, and life expectancy. In young children with mild developmental delay, it is not prudent to predict a developmental outcome with certainty. Instead, the potential range of outcomes should be discussed. Depending on the severity of the delays and associated medical problems, this range may include typical development once the child is school-aged. In an otherwise healthy individual with developmental delay, the life expectancy is normal. Children with significantly impaired mobility or other neurological impairments may have a shortened life expectancy.

Though some toddlers and young children with developmental delay may "catch up" and ultimately have typical development, global developmental delay is associated with an increased risk for having a *developmental disability*—a lifelong and chronic condition due to mental and/or physical impairments that impacts major life activities such as language function, learning, mobility, self-help, and independent living. Several types of developmental disabilities exist, including cerebral palsy, learning disabilities like dyslexia, intellectual disability, autism spectrum disorders, attention deficit-hyperactivity disorder, hearing impairment, and vision impairment.

These developmental disabilities are predominantly impairments in a specific subset of the developmental domains. For example, cerebral palsy is primarily an impairment of gross and fine motor skills; intellectual disability is primarily an impairment of language, problem-solving, and social-adaptive abilities; and autism spectrum disorders are primarily disorders of social-adaptive behaviors with or without language and communication impairments.

Developmental disabilities are common. Approximately 16% to 18% of children have a developmental disability that includes behavior problems, and 1% to 3% of the population has an intellectual disability. Approximately 1% of children have an autism spectrum disorder.

Toddlers or preschool children who are diagnosed with global developmental delay are at highest risk for being diagnosed with intellectual disability at an older age, especially as the developmental quotient worsens. *Intellectual disability* is defined as significantly subaverage general intellectual functioning (IQ less than 70) with limitations in adaptive functioning in at least two of the following skill areas: communication, self-help, social skills, academic skills, work, leisure, and health and/or safety. The incidence of intellectual disability is 1% to 3% in the general population. Males are more likely to be affected than females; occurrence rates are 1:4000 males and only 1:6000 females.

In general, the diagnosis of intellectual disability is not made in a toddler or preschool child unless they have been diagnosed with a specific genetic condition associated with intellectual disability. In the absence of a specific genetic diagnosis, the diagnosis of intellectual disability in most children is made once they are able to complete formal psychology testing at approximately 5 years of age.

In our practice, when the developmental delays of a child younger than four are very severe, we will occasionally tell the family that the child will likely have intellectual disability. In these situations, we may share this concern even if the child does not have a formal diagnosis of a genetic syndrome or before the child is old enough to complete formal psychology testing. Children with severe developmental delays may in fact be too impaired to perform formal psychology testing.

RECURRENCE RISK

Many couples are interested in knowing what their risk is for having another child with similar developmental concerns. A recurrence risk can only be provided with certainty if a specific etiology has been confirmed. Despite extensive genetic testing and other evaluations, the majority of children with developmental delays will not be diagnosed with a specific named genetic condition or other etiology for the delays.

Consequently, the clinician can only provide an empirical recurrence risk based on population data and family history information. Though each case is unique, the most prudent approach is to remind the family that 1% to 3% of the population has intellectual disability, and their risk for having another child with global developmental delay and subsequent intellectual disability is greater than the population risk. It is helpful to double frame the risk by also stating that it is more likely that they would have an *unaffected* child than an *affected* child.

REGRESSION

A regressive or neurodegenerative disease should be suspected when a child has ongoing and relentless loss of developmental skills. In addition, a regressive disease may begin to manifest itself as the development of a new neurological problem, such as a new-onset seizure disorder or movement disorder, development of a different type of seizure in a child with epilepsy, vision impairment, behavior problems, and dementia or cognitive decline.

In a child with neurological regression, a thorough neurological history and examination is warranted. The history should focus on any modifiable factors that could contribute to neurological decline, including worsening of another medical problem, recent modification to an existing medication regimen or initiation of a new medication, recovery from a prolonged acute illness or surgery, or a psychosocial stressor. All children with neurological decline should receive an extensive physical examination, with attention to those aspects of the examination that could provide clues to an underlying neurodegenerative disease (see Table 8.5). A pediatric ophthalmologist should also examine the patient for ocular stigmata of a neurodegenerative disease (see Table 8.4). A brain MRI should be performed to assess for changes that can be seen in many regressive diseases—atrophy, ventriculomegaly, white matter changes, and infarcts. Additional studies should be considered based on the patient's clinical presentation: comprehensive metabolic panel, lipid panel, creatine kinase,

EEG, EMG and nerve conduction studies, echocardiogram, and hearing test.

The need for genetic testing is based on the patient's presentation and results of the recommended studies. Categories of genetic diseases that should be considered include aminoacidopathies, organic acidurias, fatty acid oxidation defects, glycogen storage diseases, mitochondrial cytopathies, lysosomal storage diseases, neuronal ceroid lipofuscinoses, peroxisomal disorders, neurotransmitter synthesis disorders, spinal muscular atrophy syndromes, creatine synthesis disorders, congenital disorders of glycosylation, metal metabolism disorders (Menkes, Wilson, pantothenate kinase-associated neurodegeneration), and purine and pyrimidines disorders. Testing for most conditions can be done on blood, urine, and/or CSF samples. Alternatively, if the presentation is nonspecific and not pathognomonic for one of the above conditions, it may be most prudent and productive to perform whole exome sequencing as a first-line test. It is now very rare that more invasive procedures are warranted, including biopsies of the skin, muscle, liver, nerve, bone marrow, or conjunctiva.

Many reasons exist for aggressively pursuing a diagnosis of an underlying neurodegenerative disease. Most regressive disorders are irreversible, and the treatment is symptomatic. However, early diagnosis can reverse the neurological impairment or prevent future morbidity is some conditions such as Wilson disease, homocystinuria, and glutaric aciduria type I. Occasionally, pharmaceutical trials may be available to patients. Furthermore, a correct diagnosis can help the clinician provide better information about prognosis and life expectancy. Recurrence risk information and prenatal diagnosis may also be offered to families. For those conditions that are progressive and life limiting, the clinician should collaborate with a pediatric palliative care team to discuss end-of-life goals of care with the family.

REFERENCES

The complete reference list is available online at https://expertconsult
.inkling.com/.

9 Behavior and Personality Disturbances

HyungSub Shim, Amanda Miller, Carissa Gehl, Jane S. Paulsen

CHAPTER OUTLINE

FRONTOSUBCORTICAL CIRCUITRY

ASSESSING BEHAVIOR AND PERSONALITY DISTURBANCES IN PATIENTS WITH CEREBRAL DYSFUNCTION

Classification of Neurobehavioral Symptoms and Disorders

Assessment of Depression

Assessment of Other Behavioral and Personality Disturbances

BEHAVIOR AND PERSONALITY DISTURBANCES ASSOCIATED WITH CEREBRAL DYSFUNCTION

Alzheimer Disease

Frontotemporal Dementia

Vascular Dementia

Parkinson Disease

Dementia with Lewy Bodies

Huntington Disease

Tourette Syndrome

Multiple Sclerosis

Amyotrophic Lateral Sclerosis

Epilepsy

Stroke

Traumatic Brain Injury

Behavioral and personality disturbances commonly occur in individuals with neurological disease or injury (Table 9.1). Identification and treatment of behavioral disturbances are critical because they are frequently associated with reduced functional capacity, decreased quality of life, and greater economic cost, caregiver burden, and morbidity. Dysfunction of various brain circuits, most notably the frontosubcortical and amygdaloid circuits, as well as psychological factors may contribute to increased rates of disturbances.

Historically, clear divisions between the fields of psychiatry and neurology have existed. Psychiatry focused on disruptions of behavior and personality resulting from "nonorganic" or psychological causes, whereas neurology focused on disease and injury with "organic" causes. The division between psychiatry and neurology has become blurred over the past few decades, however, because research shows neuroanatomic and biochemical correlates of behavior and personality disturbances. As a response, increased collaboration and partnership between these two fields has emerged. An example of this collaboration is the creation of the American Neuropsychiatric Association (ANPA), established in 1988. In fact, the United Council for Neurologic Subspecialties offers accreditation for behavioral neurology and neuropsychiatry as a single fellowship.

The aim of this chapter is threefold. First, theoretical information linking brain circuitry to behavioral and personality disturbances is described. Second, assessment methods for behavior and personality in persons with cerebral dysfunction are detailed. Finally, information regarding the prevalence, phenomenology, and treatment of behavior and personality disturbances in dementia, movement disorders, epilepsy, stroke, and traumatic brain injury (TBI) is presented.

FRONTOSUBCORTICAL CIRCUITRY

The frontosubcortical circuits provide a unifying framework for understanding the behavioral changes that accompany cortical and subcortical brain dysfunction. In the past 3 decades, a number of significant advances have been made in our understanding of the neuroanatomy, neurophysiology, and chemoarchitecture of the frontosubcortical circuits. An increasingly broad spectrum of neuropsychiatric phenomenology is now being interpreted in the context of dysfunction in this region. A brief overview of the frontosubcortical circuits and their signature behavioral syndromes is offered as a strategy to better understand the behavior and personality changes that accompany neurological conditions. Alexander and colleagues described five discrete parallel circuits linking regions of the frontal cortex to the striatum, the globus pallidus and substantia nigra, and the thalamus (Alexander, DeLong and Strick, 1996). These circuits consist of "direct" and "indirect" pathways. In general, the direct pathway facilitates the flow of information, and the indirect pathway inhibits it. The overall model for the frontosubcortical circuits can be observed in Fig. 9.1.

Five frontosubcortical circuits were initially described as motor, oculomotor, dorsolateral prefrontal, lateral orbitofrontal, and anterior cingulate gyrus. Table 9.2 gives descriptions of specific neuroanatomic pathways for these circuits. Efforts to link functional domains to this brain circuitry have been developed and revised over the past few decades. Disruption of dorsolateral prefrontal, lateral orbitofrontal, and anterior cingulate gyrus circuits is associated with behavioral and personality disruptions. Specific behavioral syndromes have been attributed to dysfunction in these circuits (Box 9.1) (Mega and Cummings, 2001). Disruptions at any point in the circuit (e.g., the frontal cortex, corpus striatum, globus pallidus) may result in alterations of behavior.

Disruption of the dorsolateral circuit (Fig. 9.2) is associated with executive dysfunction, including poor planning and organization skills, memory retrieval deficits, and poor set shifting. Table 9.3 lists neurological disorders associated with disruption of this circuit. The orbitofrontal circuit (see Fig. 9.2) is associated with increased irritability, impulsivity, mood lability, tactlessness, and socially inappropriate behavior, whereas disruptions of the latter part of the orbitofrontal circuit may also result in a mood disorder, obsessive-compulsive disorder (OCD), or both. Finally, the anterior cingulate gyrus circuit is associated with decreased motivation, apathy, decreased speech, and akinesia. Although these models may be heuristic in developing function-structure hypotheses, it is unlikely that any current model is sufficient to explain the complex interface between behavior and brain circuitry.

Additionally, the role of the amygdala in behavior and personality disturbances is an area of increased interest and research. The amygdala exhibits a number of interconnections with the previously described frontosubcortical circuitry via the frontal cortex, thalamus, and ventromedial striatum (for a

TABLE 9.1 Prevalence of Behavioral and Psychiatric Disturbances in Neurological Disorders

	Depression	Apathy	Anxiety	Psychosis	Aggression	PBA
AD	0%–86%	Up to 92%	—	10%–73%	33%–67%	—
ALS	40%–50%	—	—	—	—	10%–49%
FTD	—	95%	—	20% del., 7% hall.	—	—
VaD	32%	—	19%–70%	33% del., 13%–25% hall.	—	—
PD	40%–50%	16.5%–40.0%	—	16% del., 30% hall.	—	4%–6%
HD	Up to 63%	59%	—	3%–12%	19%–59%	—
TS	73%	—	—	—	—	—
MS	37%–54%	—	9.2%–25.0%	—	—	10%
Epilepsy	8%–63%	—	19%–50%	0.6%–7.0%	4.8%–50.0%	—
Stroke	30%–40%	—	Up to 27%	—	Up to 32%	11%–34%
TBI	6%–77%	10%–60%	11%–70%	2%–20%	11%–98%	5%–11%

AD, Alzheimer disease; *ALS*, amyotrophic lateral sclerosis; *del.*, delusions; *FTD*, frontotemporal dementia; *hall.*, hallucinations; *HD*, Huntington disease; *MS*, multiple sclerosis; *PD*, Parkinson disease; *PBA*, pseudobulbar affect; *TS*, Tourette syndrome; *TBI*, traumatic brain injury; *VaD*, vascular dementia.

TABLE 9.2 Frontal-Subcortical Circuitry

Circuit	Frontal lobe	Striatum	GPi and SNr	Thalamus
Dorsolateral	Dorsolateral PFC	Dorsolateral CN	Lateral Mediodorsal GPi Rostrolateral SNr	VA nucleus
Orbitofrontal	Orbitofrontal PFC	Ventromedial CN	Mediodorsal GPi Rostromedial SNr	VA nucleus
Anterior cingulate	Supracallosal anterior cingulate	Ventral striatum	Rostromedial GPi Ventral pallidum Rostrodorsal SNr	Mediodorsal nucleus

CN, Caudate nucleus; *GPi*, internal segment of the globus pallidus; *PFC*, prefrontal cortex; *SNr*, substantia nigra pars reticulata; *VA*, ventral anterior; *ventral striatum*, ventromedial caudate nucleus, ventral putamen, nucleus accumbens, and olfactory tubercle.

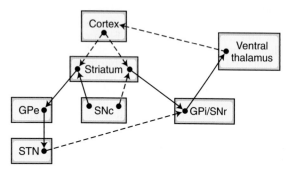

Fig. 9.1 Frontosubcortical circuit general model. The solid line represents inhibitory neurons and dotted lines represent excitatory neurons. *GPe*, External segment of the globus pallidus; *GPi*, internal segment of the globus pallidus; *SNc*, substantia nigra pars compacta; *SNr*, substantia nigra pars reticulata; *STN*, subthalamic nucleus.

BOX 9.1   Behavioral Syndromes Associated with Dysfunction of the Motor Circuits

SYMPTOMS ASSOCIATED WITH DISRUPTION OF THE DORSOLATERAL CIRCUIT

Poor organizational strategies
Poor memory search strategies
Stimulus-bound behavior
Environmental dependency
Impaired set-shifting and maintenance

SYMPTOMS ASSOCIATED WITH DISRUPTION OF THE ORBITOFRONTAL CIRCUIT

Emotional incontinence
Tactlessness
Irritability
Undue familiarity
Antisocial behavior
Environmental dependency
Mood disorders (depression, lability, mania)
Obsessive-compulsive disorder

SYMPTOMS ASSOCIATED WITH DISRUPTION OF THE ANTERIOR CINGULATE CIRCUIT

Impaired motivation
Akinetic mutism
Apathy
Poverty of speech
Psychic emptiness
Poor response inhibition

review, see Price and Drevets, 2010). Classic studies linking the amygdala and behavior include Kluver and Bucy's (1997) early work of bitemporal lesions in primates. Following selective lesions to the amygdala, monkeys exhibited less caution and fear when exposed to unfamiliar stimuli. Human case studies of individuals with amygdala lesions have also been described and have revealed similar findings. One individual with bilateral amygdala damage exhibited difficulty in recognition of fear and exhibited increased social interactions with features of disinhibition (Adolphs, 2010). Researchers have long implicated the amygdala in anxiety and fear. For example,

TABLE 9.3 Disorders Associated with Disruptions of Frontal-Subcortical Circuitry

Syndrome	Disruption of dorsolateral frontal-subcortical circuit	Disruption of orbitofrontal frontal-subcortical circuit	Disruption of anterior cingulate frontal-subcortical circuit
Alzheimer disease			X
Corticobasal degeneration	X		
Frontotemporal dementia	X	X	X
HIV dementia	X		
Huntington disease	X	X	X
Multiple sclerosis		X	X
Multiple symptom atrophy	X		
Obsessive-compulsive disorder		X	
Parkinson disease	X		X
Progressive supranuclear palsy	X		
Schizophrenia	X		X
Tourette syndrome		X	
Vascular dementia	X		

Modified with permission from Chow, T.W., Cummings, J.L., 1999. Frontal-subcortical circuits, in: Miller, B.L., Cummings, J.L. (Eds.), The Human Frontal Lobes: Functions and Disorders. Guilford, New York. Reproduced with permission of Guilford Publications, Inc.

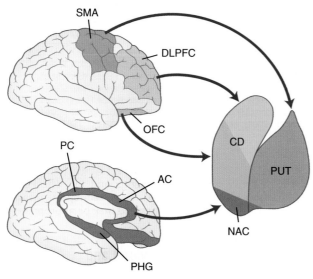

Fig. 9.2 Frontostriatal projections. *AC*, Anterior cingulate gyrus; *CD*, caudate nucleus; *DLPFC*, dorsal lateral prefrontal cortex; *NAC*, nucleus accumbens; *OFC*, orbital frontal cortex; *PC*, posterior cingulate gyrus; *PHG*, parahippocampal gyrus; *PUT*, putamen; *SMA*, supplementary motor area. *(Reprinted with permission from Brody, A.L., Saxena, S., 1996. Brain imaging in obsessive-compulsive disorder: evidence for the involvement of frontal-subcortical circuitry in the mediation of symptomatology. CNS. Spectr. 1, 27–41. Copyright 1996 by MBL Communications. Reproduced with permission.)*

changes in amygdala volume and functioning have been observed in post-traumatic stress disorder (PTSD) (Shin et al., 2006). More recently, research has suggested the amygdala in a wider range of emotional and behavioral responses and syndromes. Although findings have been somewhat mixed, the amygdala has been implicated in mood disorders including depression and bipolar disorder (Hamidi et al., 2004).

The current chapter focuses on behavioral and psychiatric changes in neurological disease and injury. Please see Chapter 43 for detailed information on assessment and description of

common cognitive changes observed in neurological disease and injury.

ASSESSING BEHAVIOR AND PERSONALITY DISTURBANCES IN PATIENTS WITH CEREBRAL DYSFUNCTION

There is evidence that appropriate treatment of behavior and personality disturbances in patients with acquired brain disease can prevent hospitalizations (Chang and Troyer, 2011; Davydow et al., 2013, 2014). Clinical research and practice with behavioral and personality disturbances in patients with neurological disease and injury is laden with challenges and complexity. Some limitations of the available research are as follows:

1. Treatment of other symptoms (such as a movement disorder) may mask psychiatric and behavioral symptoms;
2. Most available neuropsychiatric assessment tools use conventional psychiatric terminology based on idiopathic psychiatric illness, which sometimes fails to distinctly reflect the symptoms associated with acquired disease and/or trauma;
3. There is overlap between symptoms of cerebral dysfunction and symptoms of behavior and personality disturbances; for example, psychomotor retardation or reduced energy, libido, or appetite might reflect an underlying syndrome (Parkinson disease (PD)), an acquired injury (i.e., TBI), or a major depressive episode;
4. Cognitive impairments may confound the detection of behavioral changes. For example, language and memory deficits occurring in individuals with cerebral dysfunction can limit self-reports and can restrict the ability to assess changes in mood or insight; and
5. The validity of the behavioral dysfunction assessed can vary depending upon the source. Ample research shows that clinical ratings acquired from the patient, a collateral or spouse, and a healthcare worker can vary widely (see, for example, Hoth et al., 2007). Patients with cerebral dysfunction may have impaired insight; thus, they may underreport behavioral difficulties. Similarly, caregivers may also provide biased information, as their current mood or

degree of caregiver burden may influence their reporting of behavioral symptoms.

Nevertheless, clinically meaningful and objective measures of behavior symptoms are very important. In the clinic, an unstructured but targeted interview with the patient and the caregivers separately can be useful. Inventories and scales based on semi-structured interviews give valuable insight when used with appropriate training.

Classification of Neurobehavioral Symptoms and Disorders

Neurocognitive disorders (NCD), which include delirium, mild cognitive impairment, and dementia, are characterized by the presence of acquired cognitive decline from a previously attained level of functioning. Methods to classify these disorders have been diverse, with distinct expert consensus groups having determined criteria for disorders with different etiologies. The specific approaches resulted in varying terminology to describe the cognitive syndromes, many definitions for the same syndrome, and often more than one set of criteria for a specific etiology. The recently published fifth revision of the *Diagnostic and Statistical Manual of Mental Disorders* (DSM-V) by the American Psychiatric Association provides a common framework for the diagnosis of these diverse disorders. DSM-V first defines the cognitive syndromes of delirium and mild and major neurocognitive disorder (or dementia) and then describes criteria to delineate specific etiologic subtypes of mild and major neurocognitive disorders. The DSM-V approach builds on the expectation that investigators and clinicians will embrace a common language to share knowledge regarding neurocognitive disorders. As the use of these criteria becomes more widespread and is shared by the International Classification of Diseases in its 11th revision (ICD-11), a common international classification for these disorders could emerge for the first time, promoting effective communication among clinicians and researchers.

Assessment of Depression

Symptoms of neurological illness or injury may manifest as depression. In fact, depression is frequently a very early symptom or precedes onset of illness in many neurodegenerative disorders (Green et al., 2003; Ishihara and Brayne, 2006). There are several scales available for the assessment of mood disorders that might be useful in patients with acquired cerebral dysfunction. When clinicians think time is limited, self-report scales can be helpful in determining which symptoms are present and how bothersome or severe each symptom is. Table 9.4 offers additional information regarding some appropriate scales. Individuals scoring highly on these self-report measures may benefit from referral for additional evaluation and possible intervention by mental health professionals.

Domains assessed by the different measures vary such that certain scales may not detect some symptoms of depression. Two of the most commonly used measures are the Beck Depression Inventory (BDI) and the Hamilton Depression Rating Scale (HDRS). Research suggests that the BDI may be a useful screening tool in PD and Tourette syndrome, and the HDRS may be an appropriate screening tool in PD. However, these measures assess several symptoms such as psychomotor retardation and reduced energy that are common in neurological illness and injury. Thus, care must be taken to be certain that these measures do not suggest the person is depressed based on symptoms of neurological syndrome or injury. The Geriatric Depression Scale (GDS) was developed for use in elderly populations and may be a useful screening

TABLE 9.4 Common Measures of Depression Symptom Severity

Scale	Method	Items	Domains assessed
BDI-II	Self-administered	21	Cognitive symptoms Performance impairments Somatic symptoms
CES-D	Self-administered	20	Somatic symptoms Depressed affect Positive affect Interpersonal problems
GDS	Self-administered	30	Sad mood Lack of energy Positive mood Agitation/anxiety Social withdrawal
HADS	Self-administered	14	General depression Anxiety
HDRS	Interview	21	Anxiety General depression Insomnia Somatic symptoms
PHQ-9	Self-administered	9	Cognitive symptoms Somatic symptoms Level of functional impairment
ZDS	Self-administered	20	Positive affect Negative symptoms Somatic symptoms

BDI-II, Beck Depression Inventory, second edn. (Beck et al., 1996); *CES-D*, Center for Epidemiologic Studies Depression Scale (Radloff, 1997); *GDS*, Geriatric Depression Scale (Brink et al., 1982); *HADS*, Hospital Anxiety and Depression Scale (Zigmond and Smith, 1983); *HDRS*, Hamilton Depression Rating Scale (Hamilton, 1960); *PHQ-9*, Patient Health Questionnaire (Kroenke et al., 2001); *ZDS*, Zung Depression Scale (Zung, 1965).

tool for patients with early dementia and PD. The Patient Health Questionnaire (PHQ-9) is a self-report measure designed for primary care settings and may be appropriate in neurological settings.

Assessment of Other Behavioral and Personality Disturbances

In addition to depression, other behavioral and personality disturbances occur in patients with cerebral dysfunction, and several measures have been created to assess them (Table 9.5). These measures were specifically designed to assess behavioral symptoms in AD: Alzheimer Disease Assessment Scale (ADAS); Behavioral Pathology in Alzheimer Disease Rating Scale (BEHAVE-AD); CERAD Behavior Rating Scale for Dementia (C-BRSD); general dementia: Neuropsychiatric Inventory (NPI); frontal lobe dementia: Frontal Behavior Inventory (FBI); TBI: Neurobehavioral Rating Scale-Revised (NRS-R); and damage to frontal regions: Frontal Systems Behavior Scale (FrSBe). Some measures such as the NPI and the FrSBe have been implemented in diverse conditions including AD, PD, Huntington Disease (HD), and multiple sclerosis (MS). In addition, the NPI, which is available in an interview and a questionnaire format, has been frequently used as an outcome measure in clinical trials. Most recently efforts to better assess apathy have emerged (Agüera-Ortiz et al., 2013; Radakovic and Abrahams, 2014). Many of these measures might be useful ways to screen for a wide variety of potential behavioral disruptions among patients with neurological illness or injury.

TABLE 9.5 Common Measures for Assessing Behavior and Personality in Patients with Cerebral Dysfunction

Scale	Administration			Behaviors assessed				
	Source	Time (Minutes)		Depression	Apathy	Anxiety	Psychosis	Aggression
ADAS	Patient and caregiver Trained examiner	45		Yes	No	No	Yes	No
BEHAVE-AD	Caregiver interview	20		Yes	No	Yes	Yes	Yes
C-BRSD	Caregiver interview	20–30		Yes	Yes	No	Yes	Yes
FBI	Caregiver interview	10–15		No	Yes	No	No	Yes
FrSBe	Patient questionnaire Caregiver questionnaire	10		No	Yes	No	No	No
NPI	Caregiver interview	10		Yes	Yes	Yes	Yes	Yes
NPI-Q	Caregiver	5		Yes	Yes	Yes	Yes	Yes
NRS-R	Patient/caregiver interview	15–20		Yes	No	Yes	No	Yes

ADAS, Alzheimer Disease Assessment Scale; *BEHAVE-AD*, Behavioral Pathology in Alzheimer Disease Rating Scale; *C-BRSD*, CERAD (Consortium to Establish a Registry for Alzheimer Disease) Behavior Rating Scale for Dementia; *FBI*, Frontal Behavior Inventory; *FrSBe*, Frontal Systems Behavior Scale; *NPI*, Neuropsychiatric Inventory; *NPI-Q*, Neuropsychiatric Inventory-Questionnaire; *NRS-R*, Neurobehavioral Rating Scale-Revised.

BEHAVIOR AND PERSONALITY DISTURBANCES ASSOCIATED WITH CEREBRAL DYSFUNCTION
Alzheimer Disease

Based on data from the Centers for Disease Control and Prevention (CDC), it is estimated that AD affects 4 million individuals in the United States (Tejada-Vera, 2013). Current projections estimate that by 2050 the number of people living with AD in the US will rise to 13.8 million (Hebert et al., 2013). Patients with AD experience a wide range of behavioral disturbances, including affective symptoms, agitation, aggression, and psychosis. Behavioral disturbances in AD are associated with increased caregiver burden, patient and caregiver abuse, greater use of psychotropic medications, more rapid cognitive decline, and earlier institutionalization. The relationship between behavioral changes in AD and neuropathological markers is equivocal. Some researchers report a correlation between behavioral changes in AD and increased white matter hyperintensities (WMH) (Berlow et al., 2009), while others have not observed this relationship (Staekenborg et al., 2008). Many studies do not document a correlation between the presence or absence of behavioral symptoms and whole brain or hippocampal volume (Berlow et al., 2009; Staekenborg et al., 2008). In contrast to frontotemporal dementia (FTD), social comportment is relatively spared in AD.

Use of atypical antipsychotic medications has historically been the preferred method of treatment for behavioral disturbances in AD including irritability, aggression, and psychosis. However, use of atypical antipsychotic medications in elderly adults may be associated with a nearly twofold increase in risk for mortality (Kuehn, 2005). Additionally, a multisite study of atypical antipsychotics (olanzapine, quetiapine, and risperidone) showed no significant difference in Clinical Global Impression Scale scores for any antipsychotic medication over a placebo group (Schneider et al., 2006). Moreover, more participants found the side effects of the atypical antipsychotic medications to be intolerable compared to the placebo group (Schneider et al., 2006). In a retrospective observational study, behavioral symptoms were reduced in over 20% of patients following treatment with antipsychotics, while a full half of participants exhibited worsening of symptoms (Kleijer et al., 2009). However, other retrospective observational studies have reported improvements in 33% to 43% of individuals with AD and behavioral disturbances treated with

atypical antipsychotics (Rocca et al., 2007). Additionally, a retrospective cohort study showed that men display higher risk than women of developing a serious adverse event when started on an oral atypical antipsychotic (Rochon et al., 2013). The U.S. Food and Drug Administration (FDA) have issued a black-box warning on the use of antipsychotics in elderly persons with dementia. Antipsychotics may be beneficial in a small subgroup of individuals, but care must be taken in prescribing such medications, owing to the potential side effects in the context of questionable effectiveness. A review of the clinical trial literature for cholinesterase inhibitors and memantine suggests that individuals treated with these pharmaceuticals typically do experience a reduction in behavioral symptoms, including improved mood and abatement of apathy (Cummings et al., 2008).

Although the neurodegenerative process itself can be the cause of behavioral disturbances in AD, other causes such as medication side effects or medical comorbidities must be explored. In many situations, behavioral disturbances may reflect an individual with impaired cognitive and language abilities attempting to communicate information to their care providers (Sutor et al., 2006). Given the nature of these behavioral disturbances and the limited availability of pharmacological interventions, behavioral interventions and environmental modifications may be among the most helpful strategies in managing undesired behaviors. Detailed discussion of such behavioral interventions is beyond the scope of this chapter, but for more detailed information, readers may wish to review Sutor and colleagues (2006).

Clinicians may wish to refer patients to geriatric psychiatry and/or neuropsychology providers for identification and implementation of behavioral and environmental interventions. Common environmental interventions include use of familiar and personal belongings readily viewable in the environment to reduce confusion and agitation. Similarly, minimizing background distracters and establishing a standard predictable routine may also be helpful in reducing confusion and agitation. It is not uncommon for undesired behaviors (e.g., aggression) to receive significant attention while preferred behaviors (e.g., working on quiet activity) receive no reinforcement. To successfully reduce undesired activities, individuals need to increase desired activities through reinforcing preferred behavior, offering desired activities, and reducing reinforcement of undesired behavior. Finally, redirection is frequently attempted in individuals with cognitive

TABLE 9.6 Multistep Approach for Redirecting Patients with Dementia

Step	Description and example
Validate	Validation of the individual's emotional state to establish rapport *Example:* "You look worried."
Join	Join the patient's behavior. *Example:* "You're looking for your children? Well, I'm trying to find something too. Let's look together."
Distract	Distraction is easier after establishing a common goal. This works best when individuals have significant cognitive impairment. *Example:* "Let's look over there where they are having coffee."
Redirect	At this stage, redirection may be possible. *Example:* "That coffee smells good; do you want a cup?"

Adapted from Sutor, B., Nykamp, L.J., Smith, G.E., 2006. Get creative to manage dementia-related behaviors. Curr Psychiatry 5, 81–96.

TABLE 9.7 Clinical Aspects Differentiating Dementia from Depression

Major depression	Dementia
Acute, nonprogressive	Insidious and progressive
Affective before cognitive	Cognitive before affective
Attention impaired	Memory impaired
Orientation intact	Orientation impaired
Complains of memory	Minimizes/normalizes memory
Gives up on testing	Obvious effort on testing
Language intact	Aphasic errors
Better at night	Sundowning
Self-referred	Referred by others

impairment who are engaging in undesired activities. Redirection is likely to be most successful if done in a multistep process involving validation of emotion, joining of behavior, distraction, and only then followed by redirection (Sutor et al., 2006; see Table 9.6).

Depression

The true prevalence of depression in AD is controversial, with estimates up to 86%. One reason for the mixed findings lies in the different methods employed to assess depression in AD, such as family interviews and patient self-report. Some symptoms of depression are confounded with components of AD (e.g., concentration, energy, interest). The probability of depression in AD appears to be greater if there is a history of depression either in the patient or in the family. Table 9.7 suggests differences between the signs of depression and confounding signs of dementia. Interestingly, there does not appear to be a clear relationship between depressive symptoms and severity of AD (Verkaik et al., 2007). Depression is associated with greater social and functional impairments in patients with AD (Starkstein et al., 2005), although others have not observed a correlation between depression and functional impairment (Landes et al., 2005).

Selective serotonin reuptake inhibitors (SSRIs) remain the preferred mode of treatment for depression in AD and although sertraline and citalopram have been shown to be effective (Lyketsos et al., 2000), findings are mixed. Although

discontinuation of current antidepressant treatment shows worsening (Bergh et al., 2012), one review (Banerjee et al., 2011) suggests that secondary to the absence of benefit compared with placebo and the increased risk of adverse events (Rosenberg et al., 2010), the use of antidepressants for first-line treatment of depression in Alzheimer disease should be reconsidered. One recent paper formulated recommendations for future work:

1. It remains both ethical and essential for trials of new medication for depression in dementia to have a placebo arm.
2. Further research is required to evaluate the impact that treatments for depression in dementia have on carers in terms of quality of life and the time they spend caregiving.
3. Alternative biological and psychological therapies for depression in dementia should be considered, including new classes of antidepressants (such as venlafaxine) or antidementia medication (e.g., cholinesterase inhibitors).
4. Research is needed to investigate the natural history of depression in dementia in the community when patients are not referred to secondary care services.
5. Further work is needed to investigate the costs of depression in dementia including caregiver burden and moderators to the treatment effects (Banerjee et al., 2013). A recent publication suggests that antidementia medication and nonpharmacological interventions can be potential choices (Chi et al., 2014).

Apathy

Apathy, defined as diminished motivation not attributable to decreased level of consciousness, cognitive impairment, or emotional distress, is among the most common behavioral changes noted in AD. Assessment of apathy in AD may be difficult because it may be unclear whether decreased activity is due to apathy or inability to perform activities. Consistent with expectations based on frontal-subcortical circuitry, apathy in AD has been shown to be associated with bilateral reductions in gray matter volume in the anterior cingulate cortex, orbitofrontal cortex, dorsolateral prefrontal cortex, and putamen (Bruen et al., 2008). Apathy in AD is associated with greater functional and cognitive impairment (Landes et al., 2005) as well as lower quality of life (Hurt et al., 2008).

Aggression

Aggressive verbalizations and acts are common in AD. Reported prevalence rates range from 25% to 67%; studies have indicated that verbal aggression is more common in men and in individuals with delusions or agitation (Eustace et al., 2001) and is associated with increased placement in skilled nursing facilities. Sertraline has been associated with a 38% response rate for the treatment of aggression and irritability in AD (Lanctot et al., 2002).

Psychosis

Prevalence rates of psychotic symptoms in AD range from 10% to 73%, with rates in clinical populations exceeding community-based samples. Interestingly, hallucinations and delusions are significantly less common among individuals with early-onset AD (Toyota et al., 2007). Once present, delusions recur or persist for several years in most patients with AD (Fig. 9.3). The presence of hallucinations is associated with increased placement in skilled nursing centers.

Previously it was believed that individuals with AD experienced delusions secondary to significant cognitive difficulties. However, more recent research has identified additional correlates and biological markers of psychosis. Evidence from

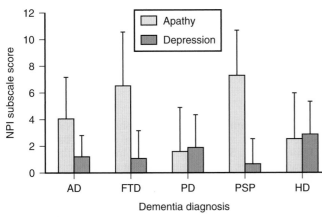

Fig. 9.3 Incidence of psychosis in patients with Alzheimer disease. *AD*, Alzheimer disease; *FTD*, frontotemporal dementia; *HD*, Huntington disease; *NPI*, neuropsychiatric inventory; *PD*, Parkinson disease; *PSP*, progressive supranuclear palsy. *(Reprinted with permission from Paulsen, J.S., Salmon, D.P., Thal, L.J., et al., 2000. Incidence of and risk factors for hallucinations and delusions in patients with probable AD. Neurology 54, 1965–1971.)*

TABLE 9.8 Psychotic Symptoms in Alzheimer Disease versus Schizophrenia in Elderly Patients

	Psychosis in Alzheimer disease	Schizophrenia in the elderly
Incidence	30%–50%	<1%
Bizarre or complex delusions	Rare	Common
Misidentification of caregivers	Common	Rare
Common form of hallucinations	Visual	Auditory
Schneiderian first-rank symptoms	Rare	Common
Active suicidal ideation	Rare	Common
History of psychosis	Rare	Very common
Eventual remission of psychosis	Common	Uncommon
Need for many years of maintenance on antipsychotics	Uncommon	Very common
Average optimal daily dose of an antipsychotic	15%–25% of that in young adult with schizophrenia	40%–60% of that in a young adult with schizophrenia

Reprinted with permission from Jeste, D.V., Finkel, S.I., 2000. Psychosis of Alzheimer's disease and related dementias. Am J Geriatr Psychiatry 8, 29–34.

neuropsychological investigations suggests more executive and frontal dysfunction in AD with psychotic symptoms than AD without these symptoms. For example, delusions have been associated with reduced gray matter volume in the inferior right frontal gyrus and the inferior parietal lobule (Bruen et al., 2008). The presence of delusions in AD is associated with poorer performance on the Frontal Assessment Battery (FAB) but was not related to global measures of cognitive impairment (i.e., MMSE) (Nagata et al., 2009). Persons with AD and hallucinations (but not delusions) are at significantly increased risk for mortality (Wilson et al., 2005).

The delusions reported in AD are typically paranoid-type, nonbizarre, and simple. Complex or bizarre delusions seen in patients with schizophrenia are conspicuously absent in patients with AD. Misidentification phenomena, however, are common in AD. Whereas hallucinations in AD are more often visual than auditory, the reverse is true for schizophrenia (Table 9.8).

Frontotemporal Dementia

Frontotemporal dementia is a heterogeneous group of syndromes including primary progressive aphasia (PPA) and behavioral variant frontotemporal dementia (bvFTD). Consensus criteria for diagnosis of FTD have been described, with presence of behavioral change an important feature, especially in bvFTD. Behavioral changes may also be present in PPA, particularly later in the course. Caregiver distress is greater among individuals with FTD and behavioral changes, particularly apathy and disinhibition, versus those with primarily aphasic difficulties (Massimo et al., 2009).

Behavioral Disruption

Atrophy within the frontal lobes leads to disruption of the frontosubcortical circuits and the characteristic behavioral syndromes in FTD. Two classic behavioral syndromes have been described among individuals with FTD: an apathetic and a disinhibited subtype. Apathy is a very common symptom in individuals with FTD. Individuals may show little concern for personal hygiene and may appear unkempt. Moreover, symptoms of orbitofrontal syndrome, such as disinhibition, poor impulse control, tactlessness, and poor judgment

are common. Loss of empathy, mental inflexibility, and stereotyped behaviors are also common. Symptoms similar to those observed in Klüver–Bucy syndrome, such as hyperorality and hypersexuality, may occur in late stages. Frequently the family members and caregivers are the ones who report these behavioral disturbances, as many patients with FTD experience reduced insight into their current difficulties. Behavioral change to varying degrees has been described in all FTD syndromes, including PPA (Grossman, 2012; Kertesz et al., 2010), although they frequently are less severe and/or occur later in the progression of the illness.

No curative treatments exist for FTD. However, there has been some success with pharmacological intervention for behavioral dyscontrol. Although few large-scale studies have been completed, evidence suggests that behavioral disturbances such as disinhibition, overeating, and compulsions may show some response to treatment with SSRIs (Huey et al., 2006).

Anosognosia

As noted in the consensus criteria, individuals with FTD frequently exhibit anosognosia. This loss of insight may manifest as an inability to perceive symptoms or a lack of concern for their current difficulties. Among individuals with frontotemporal lobar degeneration (FTLD), individuals with bvFTD exhibit greater anosognosia than individuals with the aphasic subtypes of FTLD (Zamboni et al., 2010). Patients with FTD frequently describe significantly fewer problems with cognition and behavior than what their caregivers describe. Moreover, this observed discrepancy between patient and caregiver report is greater among individuals with FTD than in individuals with AD, particularly for language, behavior, and functioning difficulties (Salmon et al., 2008). Severity of anosognosia is not typically associated with severity of dementia (Zamboni et al., 2010). The relationship between impaired awareness and specific neuropathology is somewhat unclear. Some studies have shown an association between impaired awareness and right frontal disruptions (Mendez and Shapira, 2005) while others have shown a link between anosognosia and involvement of the right temporoparietal cortex (Zamboni et al., 2010).

Relationship to Anatomy

From a pathological perspective, individuals with FTD vary with regard to the degree to which the frontal versus temporal lobes and right versus left hemispheres are affected. Significant research has looked at the relationship between patterns of behavioral syndromes and underlying neuropathology (see Josephs, 2007 for a review). Individuals with bvFTD typically exhibit greater frontal versus temporal atrophy, which is typically symmetrical. Evidence shows that individuals with bvFTD and primarily apathetic behavioral changes show greater frontal involvement, particularly from/in the right dorsolateral prefrontal cortex (Massimo et al., 2009; Zamboni et al., 2008). Individuals with primarily disinhibited behavioral change show greater involvement of the right mediotemporal limbic and temporal lobe (Zamboni et al., 2008), although others have described increased atrophy within the left dorsolateral prefrontal cortex (Massimo et al., 2009). Individuals with semantic dementia (SD), a variant of PPA, most typically exhibit atrophy and dysfunction within the left anterior temporal lobe, while individuals with SD and behavioral changes are more likely to also exhibit changes in the ventromedial and superior frontal lobes. Individuals with progressive non-fluent aphasia (PNFA), another PPA variant, are more likely to show changes in left frontal and perisylvian areas.

Vascular Dementia

Dementia secondary to vascular changes is among the most common causes of dementia in older adults. NINDS-AIREN diagnostic criteria for vascular dementia include the presence of dementia and cerebrovascular disease, including evidence of such disease on imaging, with a documented relationship between these two criteria (see Sachdev et al., 2014, for a recent review). Pathologically, vascular dementia (VaD) frequently involves small-vessel disease involving white matter hyperintensities and/or lacunar strokes, most commonly affecting subcortical regions; therefore, frontosubcortical circuits are frequently disrupted, and behavioral disturbances are common. Apathy, depression, and behavioral changes are common in VaD. The presence of significant cerebrovascular changes is observed among individuals with AD, suggesting that both pathologies may be present among a large subgroup of individuals with dementia.

Depression

The mean reported prevalence of depression in VaD is 32%, although rates vary widely between studies (Ballard and O'Brien, 2002). Sample source likely influences the reported prevalence rates, with community samples endorsing lower rates of depression than clinic samples. Individuals with VaD and depression are less likely to have had a stroke and are more likely to have a prior history of depression and impairments in memory or attention than patients with VaD without depression. The relationship between age and depression in VaD is unclear, with increased rates of depression being reported in both younger and older samples.

Additional Behavioral and Psychiatric Disorders

Apathy in VaD is associated with increased impairment in both basic and instrumental activities of daily living (Zawacki et al., 2002). This relationship is particularly apparent in patients with VaD who have also experienced a stroke. Rates of psychotic symptoms are similar in AD and VaD. Delusions (33%) and visual hallucinations (13% to 25%) are reported in VaD and are associated with impaired cognitive functioning (Ballard and O'Brien, 2002). Care must be taken in the assessment of delusions in VaD and in dementia in general. It is important to differentiate delusions from confabulation or thought processes based on impaired cognitive functioning.

Parkinson Disease

Behavioral changes are common in PD, and while research has adequately characterized these difficulties, little controlled research has assessed the effectiveness of various interventions. The majority of neuropsychiatric symptoms in PD are more common in patients with mild cognitive decline or dementia, possibly related to shared underlying pathologies (Aarsland et al., 2014). Accurate diagnosis of neuropsychiatric syndromes in PD is important but can be difficult, due to overlapping of motor signs of parkinsonism: cognitive impairment, mood disorders and apathy. Table 9.9 offers more

TABLE 9.9 Neuropsychiatric Features and Treatment in Parkinson Disease

Syndrome	Subtype	Key feature	Treatment
Depression	Major depression	Low mood or loss of interest/pleasure	No large controlled trials published to date. Nonpharmacological (counseling), dopamine agonists (pramipexole, ropinirole), antidepressants (tricyclics, trazodone, SSRIs, SSNRI, SNRI, mirtazapine)
	Minor depression	Low mood and/or loss of interest/pleasure	No available evidence
	Dysthymia	Low mood ≥ 2 years	No available evidence
Anxiety	Panic attacks	Episodic panic attacks	Poor evidence for benzodiazepines, clomipramine, nonpharmacological
	GAD	Excessive, often irrational anxiety or worry	Same as above
Psychosis	Hallucinations	Seeing imaginary people or animals	Clozapine: two randomized trials showing improvement
	Delusions	False, fixed idiosyncratic beliefs, maintained despite contrary evidence	Same as above
Apathy		Lack of initiative, motivation	Limited evidence: dopamine agonists, stimulants, modafinil

Modified with permission from Aarsland, D., Marsh, L., Schrag, A., 2009. Neuropsychiatric symptoms in Parkinson's disease. Mov Disord 24, 2175–2186.

detailed information regarding characteristics of behavioral change observed in PD as well as recent reviews of neurotherapeutic methods (Connolly and Fox, 2014; Tan, 2012).

Depression

Depression is the most common psychiatric disturbance in persons with PD. Depending on the threshold for diagnosis and sample assessed, reported rates vary. Depression may predate the onset of motor symptoms in PD (Ishihara and Brayne, 2006). Risk factors for depression in PD include greater cognitive impairment, earlier disease onset, and family history of depression. Depression is *not* associated with increased motor symptom severity (Holroyd et al., 2005). The correlation between depression and disability is equivocal. Although the precise etiology is unknown, it is believed that depression in PD results from disruptions in dopamine (D2), noradrenaline, and serotonin pathways (Veazey et al., 2005).

Very few well-controlled studies have assessed antidepressant therapy in PD. Available research suggests that SSRIs are well tolerated and likely effective in the treatment of depression in PD (see McDonald et al., 2003, for a review). SSRIs are frequently implemented as a first-line therapy for depression in patients with PD, although SSRIs may worsen motor symptoms. In such cases, tricyclic antidepressants may be an effective alternative. Successful treatment of depressive symptoms with an SSRI may also result in reductions in anxiety and decreased disability.

Psychosis

Hallucinations, typically visual, occur in up to 40% of patients with PD, with 16% reporting delusions (Fenelon et al., 2000). Psychotic symptoms are very uncommon early in the course of PD. Other diagnoses such as dementia with Lewy bodies (DLB) should be considered in patients exhibiting hallucinations early in the course of the disease. Table 9.10 summarizes important distinctions between psychosis in PD and DLB. Psychotic symptoms are more common in PD patients with greater cognitive impairment, longer duration of illness, greater daytime somnolence, and older age and in those who are institutionalized. Psychotic symptoms are strong predictors of nursing home placement and mortality in PD (Fenelon et al., 2000).

Historical accounts of PD rarely described psychotic symptoms, and it has been postulated that psychosis occurred secondary to dopamine agonist use. While dopamine agonists may contribute to the development of psychosis, additional factors are also important. For example, individuals with psychosis are more likely to exhibit cholinergic deficits and have Lewy bodies in the temporal lobe observed at autopsy (Aarsland et al., 2009).

Intervention for remediation of psychotic symptoms in PD can involve several processes. Discontinuation of anticholinergics, selegiline, and amantadine before reducing L-dopa is recommended. Following these discontinuations, reduction and simplification of dopamine agonists may be beneficial. Atypical antipsychotics are added only when a reduction of other medications has not resulted in improvement, as even atypical antipsychotics have been associated with worsening of PD motor symptoms (Goetz et al., 2000).

Apathy

Individuals with PD often experience increased rates of apathy. Estimates of apathy in PD have ranged from 16.5% to 40.0%. Individuals with apathy exhibit greater cognitive impairment (Dujardin et al., 2007). Controlled clinical trials for apathy in PD are very limited. Environmental and other behavioral interventions including establishment of a routine, structured schedule, and cuing from others can be helpful in some settings. Dopamine agonists, psychostimulants, modafinil, dopamine agonists, and testosterone have been reported to be helpful in decreasing apathy (see Aarsland et al., 2009, for more detailed information).

Impulse Control Disorders

Among the most difficult-to-treat patients with PD are those with impulse control disorders (ICDs) or dopamine dysregulation syndrome (DSS). ICDs include compulsive gambling as well as compulsive sexual, spending, and eating behaviors and DDS includes compulsive PD medication use, particularly short-acting agents. Patients are often unaware of the severity and impact of these behaviors and can be reluctant to try recommended treatments (Okun and Weintraub, 2013). Although evidence in support of pharmacological treatments and behavioral therapy for management of these symptoms is accruing, some have suggested deep brain stimulation and intestinal levodopa. Research is needed to compare and document the efficacy of suggested treatments for ICDs in PD (Weintraub et al., 2010).

Neuropsychiatric Effects of Deep Brain Stimulation

Deep brain stimulation (DBS) is a well-recognized treatment for motor complications of levodopa therapy in patients with

TABLE 9.10 Differentiating Psychosis in Parkinson Disease and Dementia with Lewy Bodies

Psychosis in Parkinson disease	Psychosis in dementia with Lewy bodies
• Psychosis occurs in many but not all patients.	• Psychosis is a core feature for diagnosis.
• Visual hallucinations are more common than delusions.	• Visual hallucinations and delusions occur at similar frequencies.
• Psychosis is generally medication induced.	• Psychosis occurs in the absence of antiparkinsonian medications.
• Hallucinations are usually fleeting and nocturnal.	• Hallucinations are generally persistent/recurrent.
• Fluctuating level of consciousness represents onset of delirium.	• Fluctuating level of consciousness can be a core feature.
• Dementia may or may not accompany psychosis.	• Presence of dementia is required for a diagnosis of DLB.
• Motor impairment virtually always precedes psychosis.	• Motor impairment may occur after psychosis.
• Neuroleptics worsen motor function, but "neuroleptic sensitivity" associated with DLB is not a feature of PD.	• Neuroleptic sensitivity characterized by dramatic motor and cognitive worsening and associated with increased morbidity and mortality has been reported.
• Disordered dopaminergic (and possibly serotonergic) transmissions are the most frequently hypothesized underlying mechanisms.	• Disordered cholinergic transmission may be the most important underlying mechanism.

DLB, Dementia with Lewy bodies; *PD*, Parkinson disease.
From Ismail, M.S., Richard, I.H., 2004. A reality test: how well do we understand psychosis in Parkinson's disease? J Neuropsychiatry Clin Neurosci 16, 8–18. Copyright 2004 by American Psychiatric Press Inc. Reproduced with permission.

TABLE 9.12 Percentage of Patients with Huntington Disease Endorsing Psychiatric Symptoms by TFC Stage

Symptom	Stage 1 (n = 432)	Stage 2 (n = 660)	Stage 3 (n = 520)	Stage 4 (n = 221)	Stage 5 (n = 84)
Depression	57.5%	62.9%	59.3%	52.1%	42.2%
Suicide	6.0%	9.7%	10.3%	9.9%	5.5%
Aggression	39.5%	47.7%	51.8%	54.1%	54.4%
Obsessions	13.3%	16.9%	25.5%	28.9%	13.3%
Delusions	2.4%	3.5%	6.1%	9.9%	2.2%
Hallucinations	2.3%	4.2%	6.3%	11.2%	3.3%

Data provided by the Huntington Study Group.

PD. Although patient selection, surgical procedure, mechanisms of DBS, postoperative management, and motor outcomes have been extensively reviewed, details regarding nonmotor aspects of DBS are still emerging. A recent review evaluated five randomized clinical trials comparing DBS with the best available medical treatment (Castrioto et al., 2014). Although non-motor symptoms were not systematically assessed, eTable 9.11 summarizes changes in depression, suicidal ideation, fatigue, apathy, anxiety, lability, impulse control, and psychosis. Although firm conclusions are not possible due to nonstandard methodology, the following summary might suffice: (1) anxiety was improved, (2) outcomes for impulse-control were mixed, (3) weight gain secondary to increased eating behaviors was consistent, (4) depressive episodes were more frequent although less severe, (5) apathy worsened, and (6) no conclusion could be reached from suicidal ideation assessment. Given the lack of standard methodology used across studies, interpretations are difficult to make and further research is warranted to better characterize behavioral and personality changes following DBS. Authors provided prevention and management recommendations for clinicians to use to provide the best clinical care for PD patients undergoing DBS (see eBox 9.3).

Dementia with Lewy Bodies

Dementia with Lewy bodies is increasingly being recognized as a common cause of dementia in older adults. DLB is associated with fluctuating cognitive difficulties, parkinsonism, and hallucinations. Clinical presentation overlap occurs between the presentation of DLB with AD and PD. Research has observed greater overall behavioral symptoms among individuals with DLB than in individuals with AD, particularly with regard to hallucinations and apathy (Ricci et al., 2009). Recent imaging research suggests that depressive symptoms in mild AD and DLB are associated with cortical thinning in prefrontal and temporal areas, suggesting a need to re-evaluate antidepressants in these patients (Lebedev et al., 2014; Lebedeva et al., 2014).

Psychosis

Psychotic symptoms, particularly hallucinations, are a hallmark feature of DLB. Insight is typically poor. Unlike patients with AD or PD, patients with DLB exhibit hallucinations early in the course of the illness. Delusions are also common in DLB. The neuropathological correlates of hallucinations in DLB are somewhat unclear. It has been suggested that hallucinations are likely due to decreased acetylcholine as well as to changes in the basal forebrain and the ventral temporal lobe (Ferman and Boeve, 2007).

Hallucinations are correlated with poorer functioning with regard to instrumental activities of daily living (Ricci et al.,

TABLE 9.13 Ratings by Nursing Home Staff of Problematic Behaviors in Patients with Huntington Disease

Behavior problem	Percentage	Rank
Agitation	76	2.0
Irritability	72	2.9
Disinhibition	59	3.3
Depression	51	4.2
Anxiety	50	4.4
Appetite	54	5.1
Delusions	43	5.5
Sleep disorders	50	5.5
Apathy	32	6.8
Euphoria	40	6.9

From Paulsen and Hamilton, unpublished data.

2009). Typical neuroleptics are avoided in DLB, because patients exhibit high sensitivity to these drugs and may experience severe parkinsonian symptoms and other side effects. In contrast, atypical neuroleptics such as clozapine and quetiapine, as well as cholinesterase inhibitors, are associated with improved cognition and decreased psychotic symptoms (McKeith, 2002).

Huntington Disease

Up to 79% of individuals with HD report psychiatric and behavioral symptoms as the presenting manifestation of the disease. Symptom presentation varies across stage of illness in HD (Table 9.12). Behavioral symptoms are commonly observed among institutionalized patients with HD (Table 9.13). The behavioral difficulties can lead to placement difficulties in these patients.

Depression

Depression is one of the most common concerns for individuals and families with HD, occurring in up to 69% of patients (van Duijn et al., 2008). Depression in HD is associated with worse cognitive performance (Smith et al., 2012), contributes to significant morbidity (Beglinger et al., 2010) as well as early mortality due to suicide (Fiedorowicz et al., 2011). Depression may precede the onset of neurological symptoms in HD by 2 to 20 years, although large-scale empirical research has been minimal. Depression is common immediately before diagnosis, when neurological soft signs and other subtle abnormalities become evident (Epping et al., 2013). Following a definite diagnosis of HD, however, depression is most prevalent in the middle stages of the disease (i.e., Shoulson-Fahn stages 2 and 3) and may diminish in the later stages (Paulsen et al., 2005b). Positron emission tomography (PET) studies indicate that patients with HD with depression have hypermetabolism in the inferior frontal cortex and thalamus relative to nondepressed patients with HD or normal age-matched controls. Recent efforts to understand the cellular and molecular mechanisms underlying behavioral disorders in patients with HD have suggested that dysfunctional HTT affects cellular pathways that are involved in mood disorders or in the response to antidepressants, including BDNF/TrkB and serotonergic signaling. Thus, the pathogenic polyQ expansion in HTT could lead to mood disorders not only by the gain of a new toxic function but also by the perturbation of its normal function (Pla et al., 2014).

Suicide

Suicide is more common in HD than in other neurological disorders with high rates of depression such as stroke and PD. Most studies have found a four- to sixfold increase of suicide in HD, with reports as high as 8 to 20 times greater than the general population. Two "critical periods" during which suicidal ideation in HD increases dramatically have been identified. First, frequency of suicidal ideation doubles from 10.4% in at-risk persons with a normal neurological examination to 20.5% in at-risk persons with soft neurological signs. Second, in persons with a diagnosis of HD, 16% had suicidal ideation in stage 1, whereas nearly 21% had suicidal ideation in stage 2. Although the underlying mechanisms for suicidal risk in HD are poorly understood, it may be beneficial for healthcare providers to be aware of periods during which patients may be at an increased risk of suicide (Paulsen et al., 2005a). A history of suicide attempts and the presence of depression were strongly predictive of suicidal behavior in a large sample of prodromal HD (*n* = 735; Fiedorowicz et al., 2011).

Psychosis

Psychosis occurs with increased frequency in HD, with estimates ranging from 3% to 12%. Psychosis is more common among early adulthood-onset cases than among those whose disease begins in middle or late adulthood. Psychosis in HD is more resistant to treatment than psychosis in schizophrenia. Huntington Study Group data suggest that psychosis may increase as the disease progresses (see Table 9.12), although psychosis can become difficult to measure in the later stages of disease.

Obsessive-Compulsive Traits

Although true OCD is rare in HD, obsessive and compulsive behaviors are prevalent (13% to 30%). Obsessive thinking often increases with proximity to disease onset and then remains stable throughout the illness. Obsessive thinking associated with HD is reminiscent of perseveration, such that individuals get "stuck" on a previous occurrence or need and are unable to shift.

Aggression

Aggressive behaviors ranging from irritability to intermittent explosive disorders occur in 19% to 59% of patients with HD. Although aggressive outbursts are often the principal reason for admission to a psychiatric facility, research on the prevalence and incidence of irritability and aggressive outbursts in HD is sparse. The primary limitation in summarizing these symptoms in HD is the varied terminology used to describe this continuum of behaviors. Clinicians and HD family members report that difficulty with placement attributable to

the patient's aggression was among the principal obstacles to providing placement, although recent research demonstrates that problematic behaviors are evident in a minority of HD patients in nursing homes (Zarowitz et al., 2014).

Apathy

Early signs of HD may include withdrawal from activities and friends, decline in personal appearance, lack of behavioral initiation, decreased spontaneous speech, and constriction of emotional expression. Frequently, these symptoms are considered reflective of depression. Though difficult to distinguish, apathy is defined as diminished motivation not attributable to cognitive impairment, emotional distress, or decreased level of consciousness. Depression involves considerable emotional distress evidenced by tearfulness, sadness, anxiety, agitation, insomnia, anorexia, feelings of worthlessness and hopelessness, and recurrent thoughts of death. Both apathy (59%) and depression (70%) are common in HD. However, 53% of individuals experienced only one of these symptoms rather than the two combined. Furthermore, depression and apathy were not correlated. Recent reports suggest that apathy is one of the most common symptoms reported in HD (van Duijn et al., 2014) and severity of apathy may progress with disease duration.

Tourette Syndrome

Tourette syndrome (TS) is associated with disinhibition of frontosubcortical circuitry; as a result, it is not surprising that increased rates of psychiatric and behavioral symptoms are observed. These behavioral difficulties are more strongly associated with psychosocial functioning than the presence of tics (Zinner and Coffey, 2009). Rates of psychiatric disorders vary widely; significantly higher rates of psychiatric disorders are reported when samples are drawn from psychiatric clinics than from movement disorder clinics. Given the correlation between psychiatric symptoms and changes in psychosocial functioning, treatments in TS that consider psychiatric and behavioral symptoms are encouraged (Shprecher et al., 2014).

Approximately 20% to 40% of individuals with TS meet criteria for OCD, while up to 90% of individuals in a clinic referred sample may exhibit subthreshold levels of obsessive-compulsive symptoms (Zinner and Coffey, 2009). The frequency and severity of tics often decrease as individuals enter adulthood, but the comorbid obsessive-compulsive symptoms are more likely to continue into adulthood and are associated with difficulties in psychosocial functioning (Cheung et al., 2007). Mood and anxiety symptoms are common in TS. The relationship between severity of depression and presence/prevalence of tics is unclear. The comorbid presence of obsessive-compulsive symptoms is associated with increased risk for depressive symptoms (Zinner and Coffey, 2009).

Multiple Sclerosis

The assessment of behavioral symptoms in MS is complicated because one of the hallmark symptoms of MS is variability of symptoms across time. Additionally, there is significant heterogeneity within patients with MS. Finally, a disconnection between the experience of emotion and the expression of emotion has historically been observed in individuals with MS.

Depression

Depression is the most common behavioral symptom in MS, occurring at rates of 37% to 54%. Patients with MS may report symptoms of depression even with outward signs of euphoria. While depression is frequently associated with reduced quality of life, the correlation between depressive symptoms and disability in MS is equivocal. Depression in MS is *not* consistently associated with increased rates of stressful events, disease duration, sex, age, or socioeconomic status. Among the subtypes of MS, depression may be most common in those with relapsing-remitting MS (Beiske et al., 2008). Fatigue is a strong predictor of depression among individuals with MS (Beiske et al., 2008). Depression in MS is largely chronic and may require intervention at various times throughout the course of disease (Koch et al., 2014).

Increased rates of suicidal ideation, suicide attempts, and completed suicides have been observed in individuals with MS. Suicide rates in MS are between two and seven times higher than in the general population (Bronnum-Hansen et al., 2005). Risk factors for suicidal ideation in MS include social isolation, current depression, and lifetime diagnosis of alcohol abuse disorder. Although suicide attempts occur throughout the progression of the disease, some have suggested that increased risk may be particularly high in the year following diagnosis (Bronnum-Hansen et al., 2005).

Biological factors likely contribute to depressive symptoms in MS. It has been hypothesized that the inflammatory process associated with MS may directly lead to depressive symptoms. Similarly, demyelination lesions in MS may directly contribute to the etiology of depression. Imaging studies in MS, however, have failed to show clear neuropathological correlates of depression. Disruptions have been observed in right parietal, right temporal, and right frontal areas (Zorzon et al., 2001) as well as the limbic cortex, implying disruption of frontosubcortical circuitry. It is likely that depression in MS results from a combination of psychosocial and biological factors.

Although controversial, depression may be a side effect for some individuals treated with interferon beta-1b (IFN-β-1b) (Feinstein, 2000). Patients with severe depression should be closely monitored while receiving IFN-β-1b. The relationship between depression and IFN-β-1a and interferon-alpha (IFN-α) is equivocal, as conflicting results have been reported. In contrast, glatiramer acetate has not been associated with increased depressive symptoms (Feinstein, 2000). Because of the potential relationship between depression and treatment for MS, as well as the high rates of depression in MS, it is critical that physicians take care to thoroughly assess a patient's current and past history of depression. This may be particularly important prior to beginning IFN interventions, as patients with histories of depression may be more likely to experience symptoms of depression following IFN treatment.

Few randomly assigned clinical trials have been conducted for the treatment of depression in MS. Several open-label trials of SSRIs have been conducted, which suggest that SSRIs may be effective in the treatment of depression in MS (Siegert and Abernethy, 2005). In addition, psychotherapy, particularly that focusing on coping skills, is efficacious in the reduction of depressive symptoms.

Anxiety

Although common, anxiety is often overlooked because anxiety symptoms may be viewed as a result of poor coping skills. Some strategies to minimize anxiety in individuals with MS are described in Box 9.2. Comorbid anxiety and depression are associated with greater somatic complaints, social difficulties, and suicidal ideation than either anxiety or depression alone. Predictors of anxiety in individuals with MS include fatigue, pain, and younger age of onset (Beiske et al., 2008).

BOX 9.2 Strategies to Minimize Anxiety in Patients with Multiple Sclerosis

- Respect adaptive denial as a useful coping mechanism.
- Provide referrals to the National Multiple Sclerosis Society (1-800-Fight-MS) early in disease.
- Help patients to live "one day at a time," and restrict predictions regarding the future.
- Help patients manage stress with relaxation techniques.
- Involve occupational therapists for energy conservation techniques.
- Focus on the patient's abilities, not disabilities.
- Consider patient's educational and financial background when giving explanations and referrals.
- Realize that patients have access to the Internet, self-help groups, and medical journals, and may ask "difficult" questions.
- Expect grief reactions to losses.
- Deal with losses one at a time.
- Attend to the mental health needs of patients' families and caregivers.
- Respect the patient's symptoms as real.
- Avoid overmedicating.
- Focus supportive psychotherapy on concrete, reality-based cognitive and educational issues related to multiple sclerosis.
- Provide targeted pharmacotherapy.
- Refer appropriate patients for cognitive remediation training.
- Ask about sexual problems, as well as bowel and bladder dysfunction.
- Keep an open dialogue with the patient about suicidal thoughts.

Modified with permission from Riether, A.M., 1999. Anxiety in patients with multiple sclerosis. Semin Neuropsychiatry 4, 103–113.

Euphoria

Increased rates of cheerfulness, optimism, and denial of disability may occur in MS. Early studies suggested that over 70% of individuals with MS experienced periods of euphoria. However, more recent studies suggest that prevalence rates of euphoria are between 10% and 25%. Euphoria frequently co-occurs with disinhibition, impulsivity, and emotional lability. Individuals with euphoria are more likely to have cerebral involvement, enlarged ventricles, poorer cognitive and neurological function, and increased social disability.

Pseudobulbar Affect

Pseudobulbar affect (PBA) occurs when there is disparity between an individual's emotional *experience* and his or her emotional *expression*; affected individuals are unable to control laughter or crying. Approximately 10% of individuals with MS exhibit periods of PBA (Parvizi et al., 2009). PBA is more common in MS patients who have entered the chronic-progressive disease course, have high levels of disability, and have cognitive dysfunction. The neuropathological substrate for PBA is believed to involve several aspects of the frontosubcortical circuits as well as the cerebellum (Parvizi et al., 2009). Table 9.14 gives more detailed information. Dextromethorphan/quinidine may be effective in treating such symptoms (Panitch et al., 2006; Pioro et al., 2010), and is FDA-approved. Additionally, tricyclic and SSRI antidepressant medications may be helpful in reducing PBA symptoms (Parvizi et al., 2009).

TABLE 9.14 Neuroanatomical Structures and Pseudobulbar Affect

Structure	Neuroanatomical significance
Prefrontal cortex and anterior cingulate	A major component of the limbic lobe, with motor efferents to the brainstem structures involved in emotional expression.
Internal capsule	A white matter structure consisting of pathways descending from the brain to the brainstem and spinal cord. Some of these pathways are related to the brainstem nuclei, some to the cerebellum (via basis pontis), and some reach the spinal cord.
Thalamus	A node in the pathways to the cortex originated from the brainstem, cerebellum, and basal ganglia.
Subthalamic nucleus	A crucial node in the indirect pathways that carry signals from the striatum to the frontal lobe via the thalamus.
Basis pontis	Relay center for pathways entering the cerebellum.
Cerebellar white and gray matter	Receives inputs from many parts of the nervous system and sends its signals to the spinal cord, brainstem, and cerebral cortex (mostly frontal lobe and some to somatomotor parietal cortical areas) through the thalamus.

Modified with permission from Parvizi, J., Coburn, K.L., Shillcutt, S.D., et al., 2009. Neuroanatomy of pathological laughing and crying: a report of the American Neuropsychiatric Association Committee on Research. J Neuropsychiatry. Clin Neurosci 21, 75–87. Copyright 2009, American Psychiatric Association.

Amyotrophic Lateral Sclerosis

Historically, amyotrophic lateral sclerosis (ALS) has been largely viewed as a pure motor neuron disease. Increased awareness of cognitive and behavioral changes in individuals with ALS has burgeoned over the past few years. Mutations in the gene C9orf72, which causes TDP-43 positive inclusions, have been implicated in a large number of cases of both conditions. In fact, the two can coexist in the same family or in the same individual with a single mutation (Bennion Callister and Pickering-Brown, 2014; Seelaar et al., 2007). Patients with ALS and the C9orf72 repeat expansion seem to present a recognizable phenotype characterized by earlier disease onset, the presence of cognitive and behavioral impairment, specific neuroimaging changes, a family history of autosomal dominant neurodegeneration, and reduced survival (Byrne et al., 2012). It is now well understood that behavioral and cognitive disturbances occur in a substantial proportion of patients, a subgroup of whom present with frontotemporal dementia. Deficits are characterized by executive and working memory impairments extending to changes in language and social cognition. Behavior and social cognition deficits closely resemble those reported in the behavioral variant of frontotemporal dementia, and consensus criteria for diagnosis of cognitive and behavioral syndromes related to ALS are reprinted in Table 9.15.

Depression

Depressive symptoms occur in 40% to 50% of individuals with ALS (Kubler et al., 2005), although most individuals exhibit subsyndromal depression. Depression in ALS has historically been thought to be associated with increased physical impairment, although these results are increasingly overturned

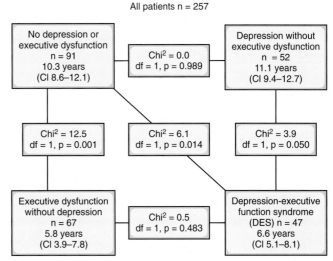

Fig. 9.4 Poststroke survival by presence or absence of depression and executive dysfunction (endpoint, all causes of death). NOTE: determined by Kaplan Meier Logistic-Rank Analysis. *(Reprinted with permission from Melkas, S., Vataja R., Oksala N.K., et al., 2010. Depression-executive dysfunction syndrome relates to poor poststroke survival. Am J Geriatr Psychiatry 18, 1007–1016.)*

(Kubler et al., 2005; Lule et al., 2008). Individuals with low psychological well-being were at increased risk of mortality (Fig. 9.4). Mortality risk was more strongly associated with psychological distress than age and was similar to the association of risk associated with severity of illness. Depression is correlated with duration of illness; however, depression is not associated with ventilator use or tube feeding (Kubler et al., 2005). Quality of life is highly impacted by presence of depressive symptoms, more so than the presence of physical limitations, indicating that physicians should be aware of available treatments for depressive symptoms (Lule et al., 2008).

Pseudobulbar Affect

Up to 50% of individuals with ALS, most often those with pseudobulbar syndrome, report PBA (Parvizi et al., 2009). Individuals with PBA may be more likely to exhibit behavioral changes similar to those observed among individuals with FTD (Gibbons et al., 2008). Little research has assessed treatment of pseudobulbar affect. Potential pharmacological interventions include use of tricyclic and SSRI antidepressant medications (Parvizi et al., 2009). Dextromethorphan/ quinidine may also be an effective treatment for PBA (Parvizi et al., 2009), and is now FDA-approved. Reduction in PBA symptoms was associated with improved quality of life and quality of relationships.

Personality Change

With recognition of the correlation between ALS and FTD, increased interest has been placed on assessing for potential behavioral changes in ALS. Minimal research has fully explored this question. Gibbons and colleagues (2008) assessed behavioral changes among a small group of individuals with ALS by using a structured interview of close family members of those with ALS. In this small study, 14/16 individuals with ALS exhibited behavioral changes. Of those with behavioral changes, 69% exhibited reduced concern for others, 63% exhibited increased irritability, and 38% exhibited increased

TABLE 9.15 Consensus Criteria (Strong et al., 2009) for Diagnosis of Cognitive and Behavioural Syndromes Related to Amyotrophic Lateral Sclerosis and Their Potential Limitations

	Features listed by Strong and colleagues (Strong et al., 2009)	Comments
Relevant background characteristics for assessment of cognitive impairment	Premorbid intellectual ability; bulbar dysfunction; motor weakness; neurological comorbidities; systemic disorders (e.g., diabetes, hypothyroidism); drug effects (e.g., substance use, narcotic analgesics, psychotropics); psychiatric disorders (eg, severe anxiety or depression, psychosis); respiratory dysfunction (measured by forced vital capacity, maximum inspiratory force, nocturnal oximetry or carbon dioxide readings); disrupted sleep; delirium; pain; fatigue; low motivation to undertake tests	A comprehensive list of potential confounds that might underlie or affect the presentation of cognitive impairment and behavioural change and that should be considered on a case-by-case basis
Background characteristics to be taken into account in diagnosis of behavioural impairment	Psychiatric disorders; psychological reaction to diagnosis of amyotrophic lateral sclerosis; premorbid diagnosis of personality disorder; pseudobulbar affect/emotional lability/pathological laughing and crying should be differentiated from depression.	A comprehensive list of potential confounds that might underlie or affect the presentation of cognitive impairment and behavioural change and that should be considered on a case-by-case basis
Amyotrophic lateral sclerosis–cognitive impairment	Patient should have impaired scores (i.e., ≤5th percentile) on standardised neuropsychological tests compared with age-matched and education matched norms, on two or more separate neuropsychological tests that are sensitive to executive dysfunction; domains other than executive functions should be assessed	Full assessments should control adequately for motor dysfunction and speech difficulties or use of assistive communication; examination of executive dysfunction only might underestimate prevalence of cognitive impairment; (Taylor et al., 2012) no data yet as to whether inclusion of measures of social cognition or theory of mind would affect detection; should ensure that impairments cannot be better explained by the potential confounds
Amyotrophic lateral sclerosis–behavioural impairment	Patient should meet two or more non-overlapping supportive diagnostic features from established criteria for behavioural variant frontotemporal dementia (Neary et al., 1998; Rascovsky et al., 2007) (presence of only one feature might lead to overdiagnosis); presence of two behavioural abnormalities necessitates support obtained from two or more sources selected from interview or observation of the patient, report from a carer, or structured interview or questionnaire; reports from family or friends are essential; need to clarify that changes in behaviour should be new, disabling, and not better accounted for by physical limitations that result from the disease	Tests of social cognition or the theory of mind might corroborate informants' reports; questionnaires specific to amyotrophic lateral sclerosis might improve correct identification of behavioural change (most available tests do not take into account the physical and resulting functional restrictions imposed by the disease); should ensure that impairments cannot be better explained by the potential confounds
Amyotrophic lateral sclerosis–frontotemporal dementia	Three categories are commonly recognised111—behavioural variant frontotemporal dementia (progressive behavioural change characterised by insidious onset, changed social behaviour, impaired self-control of interpersonal behaviour, emotional blunting, and loss of insight), progressive non-fluent aphasia (progressively non-fluent speech accompanied by magrammatism, paraphasias, or anomia), and semantic dementia (fluent speech but impaired comprehension of word meaning or object identity, or both)	Criteria for frontotemporal lobar degeneration syndromes (of which behavioural variant frontotemporal dementia, progressive non-fluent aphasia, and semantic dementia are subtypes) were not originally defined for amyotrophic lateral sclerosis; should ensure that impairments cannot be better explained by the potential confounds For behavioural variant frontotemporal dementia, diagnosis is mainly based on behavioural symptoms—thus the illness will not be diagnosed in patients without behavioural change but with primary executive dysfunction; diagnosis does not place main emphasis on evidence of executive dysfunction as measured with cognitive tests (although such evidences does contribute)
Amyotrophic lateral sclerosis–comorbid dementia	Association with a dementia not typical of frontotemporal dementia (e.g., Alzheimer disease, vascular dementia, mixed dementias)	Alzheimer pathological changes might be noted in patients presenting with behavioural variant frontotemporal dementia, (Snowden et al., 2011) so this possible classification should not be discounted in amyotrophic lateral sclerosis

With permission from Goldstein, LH and Abrahams, S 2013, Changes in cognition and behaviour in amyotrophic lateral sclerosis: nature of impairment and implications for assessment. Lancet Neurology, 12, 368–80.

apathy. A questionnaire to assess behavioral change has been developed specifically for ALS to minimize exaggerations of behavior related to motor dysfunction (Raaphorst et al., 2012). Additional screening instruments for the detection and tracking of these syndromes in ALS are provided in Table 9.16.

Epilepsy

Behavioral and personality disturbances occur in up to 50% of individuals with epilepsy. Identification and treatment of these behavioral disturbances remain inadequate, with less than half of individuals with epilepsy and major depressive

TABLE 9.20 Core Features of Behavioral Symptoms in Traumatic Brain Injury

Core features	Depression	Apathy	Anxiety	Dysregulation
Mood (Intensity, scope)	Sad, irritable, frustrated (constant, global)	Flat, unexcited (constant, global)	Worried, distressed (frequent, situational)	Angry, tense (frequent, global)
Activity level	Low activity	Lack of initiative, behavior	Restless, "keyed up"	Impulsive, physically aggressive, argumentative
Attitude	Loss of interest, pleasure	Lack of concern	Overconcern	Argumentative
Awareness	Overestimates problems	Does not notice problems	Overestimates problems	Underestimates problems
Cognitions	Rumination on loss, failures	Unresponsive to events	Rumination on harm, danger	Rumination on tension, arousal
Physiological	Under- or hyperaroused	Underaroused	Hyperaroused	Underaroused or agitated
Coping style	Avoidance, social withdrawal	Compliant, dependent	Avoidance, checking behaviors	Uncontrolled outbursts

Modified from Seel, R.T., Macciocchi, S., Kreutzer, J.S., 2010. Clinical considerations for the diagnosis of major depression after moderate to severe TBI. J Head Trauma Rehabil 25, 99–112.

failed to replicate this finding. Other factors associated with post-TBI depression include poor coping styles, social isolation, and increased stress (Kim et al., 2007). Depression in TBI is associated with increased suicidality, increased cognitive problems, greater disability, and aggression. See Table 9.20 for additional information regarding differentiating features associated with depression in TBI.

Suicidal ideation (65%) and attempts (8.1%) are common following TBI (Silver et al., 2001). In contrast to sex differences reported in the general population, women with TBI are more likely to commit suicide than men with TBI. Furthermore, suicide was more common in individuals with more severe injury and those younger than 21 years or older than 60 years at the time of injury.

No large class I studies of use of antidepressant medications, particularly SSRIs, in TBI have been completed, but small studies provide preliminary support for their use to treat depressive symptoms following TBI. Care must be taken in certain situations, because some antidepressants (i.e., bupropion) are associated with increased risk of seizures. Close monitoring following the beginning of a trial of antidepressant medication is encouraged; in some settings, such medications can increase agitation or anxiety in individuals with TBI. Please see Alderfer and colleagues (2005) for more details regarding recommendations for treatment of depression following TBI.

Anxiety

Less research has assessed the prevalence of anxiety disorders in TBI; however, studies suggest that 11% to 70% of individuals meet criteria for an anxiety disorder. A meta-analysis suggested that the mean prevalence of anxiety disorders following TBI is 29%. Panic disorder occurs in 3.2% to 9.0% of individuals with a TBI (Silver et al., 2001).

Apathy

Symptoms of apathy are reported in 10% to 60% of individuals with a TBI. Among individuals with TBI referred to a behavioral management program, lack of initiation was among the most commonly reported problems, occurring in approximately 60% of the sample (Kelly et al., 2008). Apathy in TBI is often associated with depressive symptoms, although a significant number of individuals (28%) report experiencing apathy but not depression. Lesions affecting the right hemisphere and subcortical regions are more strongly associated with apathy than lesions affecting the left hemisphere.

Personality Change

Personality change following TBI is common secondary to frequent injury to the frontal lobe and disruption of the frontosubcortical circuitry. Common changes include increased irritability, aggression, disinhibition, and inappropriate behavior. Although these difficulties can be among the most disabling for individuals with TBI, research in these areas is limited, and no uniform, agreed-upon diagnostic criteria for these behavioral changes exist.

Aggression within 6 months of TBI has been reported in up to 60% of individuals with TBI (Baguley et al., 2006). Among individuals referred to a TBI behavior management service, verbal aggression and inappropriate social behavior were among the most commonly reported behavioral difficulties and occurred in more than 80% of individuals (Kelly et al., 2008). Aggression following TBI is associated with depression, poorer psychosocial functioning, and greater disability (Rao et al., 2009).

A number of pharmacological interventions have been used to reduce and remediate behavioral changes following brain injury. See Nicholl and LaFrance (2009) for a review. One class of medication used in these settings is AEDs, now routinely used to treat aggression, disinhibition, and mania following TBI. Again, few large-scale studies have assessed the effectiveness of AEDs in the treatment of behavioral change following TBI. Historically, neuroleptic drugs were used in high doses to treat behavioral dyscontrol in individuals with cognitive impairment. More recently, there has been increased interest in the use of atypical neuroleptics to treat both psychosis and behavioral changes following TBI.

In addition to pharmacological interventions, behavioral and environmental interventions have been shown to be effective at remediating behavioral dyscontrol following TBI. The discussion of behavioral and environmental techniques aimed at decreasing behavioral dyscontrol, including aggression and irritability, is beyond the scope of this chapter (see Sohlberg and Mateer, 2001 for more information). Providers may find referrals for such interventions within rehabilitation programs. Briefly, interventions may seek to reduce stimulation in the environment, increase structure and predictability, reinforce good behavior with limited response to undesired behavior, and use structured problem-solving strategies.

REFERENCES

The complete reference list is available online at https://expertconsult .inkling.com/.

10 Depression and Psychosis in Neurological Practice

David L. Perez, Evan D. Murray, Bruce H. Price

CHAPTER OUTLINE

PRINCIPLES OF DIFFERENTIAL DIAGNOSIS

PRINCIPLES OF NEUROPSYCHIATRIC EVALUATION

COGNITIVE-AFFECTIVE-BEHAVIORAL BRAIN BEHAVIOR RELATIONSHIPS
Cortical Networks

BIOLOGY OF PSYCHOSIS

BIOLOGY OF DEPRESSION

CLINICAL SYMPTOMS AND SIGNS SUGGESTING NEUROLOGICAL DISEASE

PSYCHIATRIC MANIFESTATIONS OF NEUROLOGICAL DISEASE
Stroke and Cerebral Vascular Disease
Infectious
Metabolic and Toxic
Neoplastic
Degenerative
Traumatic Brain Injury
Depression-Related Cognitive Impairment
Delirium
Catatonia

TREATMENT MODALITIES
Electroconvulsive Therapy
Vagus Nerve Stimulation
Repetitive Transcranial Magnetic Stimulation
Psychiatric Neurosurgery or Psychosurgery

TREATMENT PRINCIPLES

The most widely recognized nomenclature used for discussion of mental disorders derives from the classification system developed for the *Diagnostic and Statistical Manual of Mental Disorders* (DSM). The American Psychiatric Association introduced the DSM in 1952 to facilitate psychiatric diagnosis through improved standardization of nomenclature. There have been consecutive revisions of this highly useful and relied-upon document since its inception, with the last revision being in 2013. Discussion about the potential secondary causes of depression and psychosis requires a familiarity with the most salient features of the primary psychiatric conditions. A brief outline of selected conditions is included in eBoxes 10.1 and 10.2, along with other content in this chapter marked "online only."

PRINCIPLES OF DIFFERENTIAL DIAGNOSIS

Emotional and cognitive processes are based on brain structure and physiology. Abnormal behavior can be attributable to the complex interplay of neural physiology, social influences, and physical environment (Andreasen, 1997). Psychosis, mania, depression, disinhibition, obsessive compulsive behaviors, and anxiety all can occur as a result of neurological

disease and can be virtually indistinguishable from the idiopathic forms (Rickards, 2005; Robinson and Travella, 1996). Neurological conditions must be considered in the differential diagnosis of any disorder with psychiatric symptoms.

Neuropsychiatric abnormalities can be associated with altered functioning in anatomical regions. Any disease, toxin, drug, or process that affects a particular region can be expected to show changes in behavior mediated by the circuits within that region. The limbic system and the frontosubcortical circuits are most commonly implicated in neuropsychiatric symptoms. This neuroanatomical conceptual framework can provide useful information for localization and thus differential diagnosis. For example, the Klüver–Bucy syndrome, which consists of placidity, apathy, visual and auditory agnosia, hyperorality, and hypersexuality, occurs in processes that cause injury to the bilateral medial temporoamygdalar regions. A few of the most common causes of this syndrome include herpes encephalitis, traumatic brain injury (TBI), frontotemporal dementias (FTDs), and late-onset or severe Alzheimer disease (AD). Disinhibition, a particularly common neuropsychiatric symptom, may be observed in patients with brain trauma, cerebrovascular ischemia, demyelination, abscesses, or tumors, as well as degenerative dementias. Damage to any portion of the cortical and subcortical portions of the orbitofrontal-striatal-pallidal-thalamic circuit can result in disinhibition (Bonelli and Cummings, 2007).

Mood disorders, paranoia, disinhibition, and apathy derive, in part, from dysfunction in the limbic system and basal ganglia, which are phylogenetically more primitive (Mesulam, 2000). In some cases, the behavioral changes represent a psychological response to the underlying disability; in others, neuropsychiatric abnormalities manifest as a result of intrinsic neurocircuit alterations caused by the disease itself. For example, studies have shown that apathy in Parkinson disease (PD) is probably related to the underlying disease process, rather than being a psychological reaction to disability or to depression, and is closely associated with cognitive impairment (Kirsch-Darrow et al., 2006). Positron emission tomographic (PET) and single-photon emission computed tomographic (SPECT) studies suggest similar regions of abnormality in acquired (secondary) forms of depression, mania, obsessive compulsive disorder (OCD), and psychosis, compared with their primary psychiatric presentations (Milad and Rauch, 2012; Rubinsztein et al., 2001). Table 10.1 summarizes neuropsychiatric symptoms and their anatomical correlates. Additionally, the developmental phase during which a neurological illness occurs influences the frequency with which some neuropsychiatric syndromes are manifested. Adults with post-TBI sequelae tend to exhibit a higher rate of depression and anxiety. In contrast, post-TBI sequelae in children often involve attention deficits, hyperactivity, irritability, aggressiveness, and oppositional behavior (Max, 2014). When temporal lobe epilepsy or Huntington disease (HD) begins in adolescence, a higher incidence of psychosis is noted than when their onset occurs later in life. Earlier onset of multiple sclerosis (MS) and stroke are associated with a higher incidence of depression (Rickards, 2005).

Patients with AD, PD, HD, and FTDs can develop multiple coexisting symptoms such as irritability, agitation, impulse-control disorders, apathy, depression, delusions, and psychosis

TABLE 10.1 Neuropsychiatric Symptoms and Corresponding Neuroanatomy

Symptom	Neuroanatomical region
Depression	Prefrontal cortex (particularly left anterior regions, anterior cingulate gyrus, subgenu of the corpus callosum, orbitofrontal cortex), basal ganglia, left caudate
Mania	Inferomedial and ventromedial frontal cortex, right inferomedial frontal cortex, anterior cingulate, caudate nucleus, thalamus, and temporothalamic projections
Apathy	Anterior cingulate gyrus, nucleus accumbens, globus pallidus, thalamus
OCD	Orbital or medial frontal cortex, caudate nucleus, globus pallidus
Disinhibition	Orbitofrontal cortex, hypothalamus, septum
Paraphilia	Mediotemporal cortex, hypothalamus, septum, rostral brainstem
Hallucinations	Unimodal association cortex, orbitofrontal cortex, paralimbic cortex, limbic cortex, striatum, thalamus, midbrain
Delusions	Orbitofrontal cortex, amygdala, striatum, thalamus

OCD, Obsessive-compulsive disorder.

TABLE 10.2 Neurological Disorders and Associated Prominent Behavioral Features

Neurological disorder	Associated behavioral disturbances
Alzheimer disease	Depression, irritability, anxiety, apathy, delusions, paranoia, psychosis
Lewy body dementia	Fluctuating confusion, hallucinations, delusions, depression, RBD
Vascular dementia	Depression, apathy, psychosis
Parkinson disease	Depression, anxiety, drug-associated hallucinations and psychosis, RBD
FTD	Early impaired judgment, disinhibition, apathy, loss of empathy, depression, delusions, psychosis
PSP	Disinhibition, apathy
TBI	Depression, disinhibition, apathy, irritability, psychosis (uncommon)
HD	Depression, irritability, delusions, mania, apathy, obsessive-compulsive tendencies, psychosis
Corticobasal degeneration	Depression, irritability, RBD, alien hand syndrome
Epilepsy	Depression, psychosis
HIV infection	Apathy, depression, mania, psychosis
MS	Depression, irritability, anxiety, euphoria, psychosis, pseudobulbar affect
ALS	Depression, disinhibition, apathy, impaired judgment

ALS, Amyotrophic lateral sclerosis; *FTD*, frontotemporal dementia; *HD*, Huntington disease; *HIV*, human immunodeficiency virus; *MS*, multiple sclerosis; *OCD*, obsessive-compulsive disorder; *PSP*, progressive supranuclear palsy; *RBD*, rapid eye movement behavior disorder; *TBI*, traumatic brain injury.

that may be exacerbated by medications used to treat the underlying disorder (Table 10.2). For example, in patients with PD dopamine agonists such as pramipexole and ropinirole have been found to increase the risk of pathological gambling, compulsive shopping, hypersexuality, and other impulse-control disorders, sometimes referred to as *dopamine dysregulation* (Voon et al., 2006; Weintraub et al., 2006). Management outcome can be influenced by multiple factors. For instance, the complex relationship between behavioral changes and the caregiver's ability to cope play a role in illness management and nursing home placement (de Vugt et al., 2005). Behavioral disturbances in patients with neurological illness have also been related to the severity of caregiver distress.

PRINCIPLES OF NEUROPSYCHIATRIC EVALUATION

A number of important principles must be taken into account when evaluating and treating a patient for behavioral disturbances.

1. A normal neurological examination does not exclude neurological conditions. Lesions in the limbic, paralimbic, and prefrontal regions may manifest with cognitive-affective-behavioral changes in the absence of elemental neurological abnormalities.
2. Normal routine laboratory testing, brain imaging, electroencephalography, and cerebral spinal fluid analysis do not necessarily exclude diseases of neurological origin.
3. New neurological complaints or behavioral changes that are atypical for a coexisting primary psychiatric disorder should not be dismissed as being of psychiatric origin in a person with a pre-existing psychiatric history.
4. The possibility of iatrogenically induced symptoms such as lethargy with benzodiazepines, parkinsonism with neuroleptics, or hallucinations with dopaminergic medications must be taken into account. Medication side effects can significantly complicate the clinical history and physical examination in both the acute and long-term setting.

Medication side effects can also potentially be harbingers of underlying pathology or progression of illness. For example, marked parkinsonism occurring after neuroleptic exposure can be a feature of PD and dementia with Lewy bodies (Aarsland et al., 2005) before the underlying neurodegenerative condition becomes clinically apparent. PD patients may develop hallucinations as a side effect of dopaminergic medications (Starkstein et al., 2012).

5. Treatments of primary psychiatric and neurological behavioral disturbances share common principles. A response to therapy does not constitute evidence for a primary psychiatric condition.

The medical evaluation of affective and psychotic symptoms must be individualized based on the patient's family history, social environment, habits, risk factors, age, gender, clinical history, and examination findings. A careful review of the patient's medical history and a general physical examination as well as a neurological examination (Murray and Price, 2008; Ovsiew, 2008) should be performed to assess for possible neurological and medical causes. The most basic evaluation should include vital signs (blood pressure, pulse, respirations, and temperature) and a laboratory evaluation that minimally includes a complete blood cell count (CBC), electrolyte panel, serum glucose, blood urea nitrogen (BUN), creatinine, calcium, total protein, and albumin, liver function assessment and thyroid function assessment. Additional laboratory testing may be considered according to the clinical history and risk factors. These studies might include a toxicology screen, cobalamin (B_{12}), homocysteine, methylmalonic acid, folate, human immunodeficiency virus (HIV) serology, rapid plasma regain (RPR), antinuclear antibodies (ANA), erythrocyte sedimentation rate (ESR), c-reactive protein (CRP), ceruloplasmin, heavy metal screen, ammonia, serum and cerebrospinal fluid paraneoplastic panel, urine porphobilinogen, number of CAG repeats for Huntington disease, and other specialized rheumatologic, metabolic, and genetic tests. Consideration should also be given to checking the patient's oxygen saturation on room air (especially in the elderly). Neurological abnormalities suggested by the clinical history or identified on examination, especially those attributable to the central nervous system (CNS), should prompt further evaluation for neurological and medical causes of psychiatric illness. A clear consensus has not been reached as to when neuroimaging is indicated as part of the evaluation of new-onset depression in patients without focal neurological complaints and a normal neurological examination. This must be individualized based on clinical judgment. Treatment-resistant depression should prompt reassessment of the diagnosis and evaluation to rule out secondary causes of depressive illness including cerebrovascular (small-vessel) disease. A careful history to rule out a primary sleep disorder such as obstructive sleep apnea should be considered in the evaluation of refractory depressive symptoms (Haba-Rubio, 2005) or cognitive complaints. When new-onset atypical psychosis presents in the absence of identifiable infectious/inflammatory, metabolic, toxic, or other causes, we recommend that magnetic resonance imaging (MRI) of the brain be incorporated into the evaluation. In our experience, 5% to 10% of such patients have MRI abnormalities that identify potential neurological contributions (particularly in those 65 years of age and older). The MRI will help exclude lesions (e.g., demyelination, ischemic disease, neoplasm, congenital structural abnormalities, evidence of metabolic storage diseases) in limbic, paralimbic, and frontal regions, which may not be clearly associated with neurological abnormalities on elemental examination (Walterfang et al., 2005). An electroencephalogram (EEG) should be considered to evaluate for complex partial seizures if there is a history of intermittent, discrete, or abrupt episodes of psychiatric dysfunction (e.g., confusion, spells of lost time, psychotic symptoms), stereotypy of hallucinations, automatisms (e.g., lip smacking, repetitive movements) associated with episodes of psychiatric dysfunction (or confusion), or a suspicion of encephalopathy (or delirium). Sensitivity of the EEG for detecting seizure activity is highest when the patient has experienced the specific symptoms while undergoing the study. Selected cases may require 24-hour or prolonged EEG monitoring to capture a clinical event to clarify whether a seizure disorder is present.

COGNITIVE-AFFECTIVE-BEHAVIORAL BRAIN BEHAVIOR RELATIONSHIPS

We begin with a brief overview of cortical functional anatomy related to perceptual, cognitive, affective, and behavioral processing, after which will follow a synopsis of frontal network functional anatomy describing the distinct frontosubcortical circuits subserving important cognitive-affective-behavioral domains.

The cerebral cortex can be subdivided into five major functional subtypes: primary sensory-motor, unimodal association, heteromodal association, paralimbic, and limbic (Fig. 10.1). The primary sensory areas are the point of entry for sensory information into the cortical circuitry. The primary motor cortex conveys complex motor programs to motor neurons in the brainstem and spinal cord. Processing of sensory information occurs as information moves from primary sensory areas to adjacent unimodal association areas. The unimodal and heteromodal cortices are involved in perceptual processing and motor planning. The complexity of processing increases as information is then transmitted to heteromodal association areas which receive input from more than one sensory modality. Examples of heteromodal association cortex include the prefrontal cortex, posterior parietal cortex, parts of the lateral temporal cortex, and portions of the parahippocampal gyrus. These cortical regions have a six-layered cytoarchitecture. Further cortical processing occurs in areas designated as *paralimbic*. These regions demonstrate a gradual transition of cortical architecture from the six-layered to the more primitive and simplified allocortex of limbic structures. The paralimbic regions, implicated in idiopathic and secondary neuropsychiatric symptoms, consist of orbitofrontal cortex (OFC), cingulate cortex, insula, temporal pole, and parahippocampal cortex. Cognitive, emotional, and visceral inputs merge in these regions. The limbic subdivision is composed of the hippocampus, amygdala, substantia innominata, prepiriform olfactory cortex, and septal area (Fig. 10.2). Limbic structures are to a great extent reciprocally interconnected with the hypothalamus. Limbic regions are intimately involved with processing and regulation of emotion, memory, motivation, autonomic, and endocrine function. The highest level of cognitive processing occurs in regions referred to as *transmodal areas*. These areas are composed of heteromodal, paralimbic, and limbic regions, which are collectively linked, in parallel, to other transmodal regions. Interconnections among transmodal areas (e.g., Wernicke area, posterior parietal cortex, hippocampal-enterorhinal complex) allow integration of distributed perceptual processing systems, resulting in perceptual recognition such as scenes and events becoming experiences and words taking on meaning (Mesulam, 2000).

Cortical Networks

Classically, five distinct cortical networks have been conceptualized as governing various aspects of cognitive functioning:

1. the language network, which includes transmodal regions or "epicenters" in Broca and Wernicke areas located in the pars opercularis/triangular portions of the inferior frontal gyrus and posterior aspect of the superior temporal gyrus, respectively;
2. spatial awareness, based in transmodal regions in the frontal eye fields and posterior parietal cortex;
3. the memory and emotional network, located in the hippocampal-enterorhinal region and amygdala;
4. the executive function–working memory network, based in transmodal regions in the lateral prefrontal cortex and possibly the inferior parietal cortices; and
5. the face-object recognition network, based in the temporopolar and middle temporal cortices (Mesulam, 1998).

Lesions of transmodal cortical areas result in global impairments such as hemineglect, anosognosia, amnesia, and multimodal anomia. Disconnection of transmodal regions from a specific unimodal input will result in selective perceptual impairments such as category-specific anomias, prosopagnosia, pure word deafness, or pure word blindness.

The emergence of functional neuroimaging technologies including task-based (Pan et al., 2011) and resting-state functional connectivity analyses (Zhang and Raichle, 2010) has over the past several decades allowed for the *in vivo* inspection of brain networks. Apart from the five networks already described, several additional networks have emerged as particularly important to the understanding of brain-behavior relationships in behavioral neurology and neuropsychiatry:

positively correlated with plasma cortisol levels (Drevets et al., 2002), suggesting a link between elevated amygdalar activity and hypothalamic–pituitary–adrenal axis dysfunction.

Prefrontal cortex dysfunction also plays an important role in the pathophysiology of depression. The subgenual ACC has been implicated in the modulation of negative mood states (Hamani et al., 2011). Several neuroimaging studies characterized elevated baseline subgenual activation in depression (Dougherty et al., 2003; Gotlib et al., 2005; Konarski et al., 2009; Mayberg et al., 2005), while other investigations have described reduced subgenual activations (Drevets et al., 1997). Mayberg and colleagues have suggested that depression can be potentially defined phenomenologically as "the tendency to enter into, and inability to disengage from, a negative mood state" (Holtzheimer and Mayberg, 2011). Subgenual ACC dysfunction may play a critical role in the inability to effectively modulate mood states. In addition to the ACC, the OFC and DLPFC exhibit abnormalities in depression. Consistent with OFC lesions linked to increased depression risk, depression severity is inversely correlated with medial and posterior-lateral OFC activity in neuroimaging studies (Drevets, 2007; Price and Drevets, 2010). Reduced OFC activations may lead to amygdalar disinhibition in depression. Meanwhile, the DLPFC potentially exhibits a lateralized dysfunctional pattern in depression. While not consistently identified, depressed patients have shown left DLPFC hypoactivity and right DLPFC hyperactivity (Grimm et al., 2008); left DLPFC hypoactivity was linked to negative emotional judgments, while right DLPFC hyperactivity was associated with attentional deficits. Subcortically, decreased ventral striatum/nucleus accumbens activation has been linked to anhedonia (Epstein et al., 2006; Keedwell et al., 2005; Pizzagalli et al., 2009). In neurologic disorders, damage to the prefrontal cortex from stroke or tumor, or to the striatum from degenerative diseases such as PD and HD, is associated with depression (Charney and Manji, 2004). Functional imaging studies of subcortical disorders such as these reveal hypometabolism in paralimbic regions, including the anterotemporal cortex and anterior cingulate, correlated with depression (Bonelli and Cummings, 2007). Depression in PD, HD, and epilepsy has been associated with reduced metabolic activity in the orbitofrontal cortex and caudate nucleus.

Functional imaging studies of untreated depression have been extended to evaluate responses to pharmacological, cognitive-behavioral, and surgical treatments. Clinical improvement after treatment with serotonin-specific reuptake inhibitors such as fluoxetine correlates with increased activity on PET in brainstem and dorsal cortical regions including the prefrontal, parietal, anterior, and posterior cingulate areas, and with decreased activity in limbic and striatal regions including the subgenual cingulate (Hamani et al., 2011), hippocampus, insula, and pallidum. These findings are consistent with the prevailing model for involvement of a limbic-cortical-striatal-pallidal-thalamic circuit in major depression. The same group has shown that imaging can be used to identify patterns of metabolic activity predictive of treatment response. Hypometabolism of the rostral anterior cingulate characterized patients who failed to respond to antidepressants, whereas hypermetabolism characterized responders. Dougherty and co-workers (2003) used PET to search for neuroimaging profiles that might predict clinical response to anterior cingulotomy in patients with treatment-refractory depression. Responders displayed elevated preoperative metabolism in the left prefrontal cortex and the left thalamus. A combination of functional imaging and pharmacogenomic technologies might allow subsets of treatment responders to be classified and predicted more precisely than with either technology alone. Goldapple and co-investigators (2004) used PET to study the clinical response of cognitive-behavioral therapy in patients with unipolar depression and found increases in hippocampus and dorsal cingulate and decreases in dorsal, ventral, and medial frontal cortex (Goldapple et al., 2004). The authors speculate that the same limbic-cortical-striatal-pallidal-thalamic circuit is involved but that differences in the direction of metabolic changes may reflect different underlying mechanisms of action of cognitive-behavioral therapy (CBT) and selective serotonin reuptake inhibitors (SSRIs). Recently, PET resting-state right anterior insula metabolism has also been identified as a potential treatment selective biomarker in depression for cognitive behavioral therapy and SSRI treatment response (McGrath et al., 2013).

CLINICAL SYMPTOMS AND SIGNS SUGGESTING NEUROLOGICAL DISEASE

Many neurological conditions have associated psychiatric symptoms. Psychiatrists and neurologists need to be intimately acquainted with features of the clinical history and examination that indicate the need for further investigation. Box 10.3 outlines some key features that have historically suggested an underlying neurological condition. eBox 10.4 reviews some key areas of the review of systems that can be helpful when assessing for neurological and medical causes of psychiatric symptoms. eTable 10.3 reviews abnormalities in the elemental neurological examination associated with diseases that can exhibit significant neuropsychiatric features.

PSYCHIATRIC MANIFESTATIONS OF NEUROLOGICAL DISEASE

Virtually any process that affects the neurocircuits described earlier can result in behavioral changes and psychiatric symptoms at some point. Psychiatric symptoms may be striking and precede any neurological manifestation by years. eTable 10.4 lists conditions that can be associated with psychosis or depression. Box 10.5 summarizes some key points from the preceding discussion. A general overview and discussion of a number of major categories of neurological and systemic conditions with prominent neuropsychiatric features follows. More detailed information regarding the evaluation, natural history, pathology, and specific treatment recommendations for these conditions is beyond the scope of this chapter.

Stroke and Cerebral Vascular Disease

Stroke is the leading cause of neurological disability in the United States and one of the most common causes of acquired behavioral changes in adults. The neuropsychiatric consequences of stroke depend on the location and size of the stroke, pre-existing brain pathology, baseline intellectual capacity and functioning, age, and premorbid psychiatric history. Neuropsychiatric symptoms may occur in the setting of first strokes and multi-infarct dementia. In general, interruption of bilateral frontotemporal lobe function is associated with an increased risk of depressive and psychotic symptoms. Specific stroke-related syndromes such as aphasia and visuo-spatial dysfunction are beyond the scope of this chapter, so only the abnormalities in mood and emotion after stroke will be discussed. A common misconception is that depressive symptoms can be explained as a response to the associated neurological deficits and impairment in function. Evidence supports a higher incidence of depression in stroke survivors than occurs in persons with other equally debilitating diseases. Minor depression is more closely related to the patient's elemental deficits. Emotional and cognitive disorders may

---

BOX 10.3 Historical Features Suggesting Neurological Disease in Patients with Psychiatric Symptoms

PRESENCE OF ATYPICAL PSYCHIATRIC FEATURES

Late or very early age of onset
Acute or subacute onset
Lack of significant psychosocial stressors
Catatonia
Diminished comportment
Cognitive decline
Intractability despite adequate therapy
Progressive symptoms

HISTORY OF PRESENT ILLNESS INCLUDES

New or worsening headache
Inattention
Somnolence
Incontinence
Focal neurological complaints such as weakness, sensory changes, incoordination, or gait difficulty
Neuroendocrine changes
Anorexia/weight loss

PATIENT HISTORY

Risk factors for cerebrovascular disease, or central nervous system infections
Malignancy
Immunocompromise
Significant head trauma
Seizures
Movement disorder
Hepatobiliary disorders
Abdominal crises of unknown cause
Biological relatives with similar diseases or complaints

UNEXPLAINED DIAGNOSTIC ABNORMALITIES

Screening laboratories
Neuroimaging studies or possibly imaging of other systems
Electroencephalogram
Cerebrospinal fluid

BOX 10.5 Key Points

1. Affective and psychotic disorders may occur as a result of neurological disease and be indistinguishable from the idiopathic forms.
2. Neuropsychiatric and cognitive dysfunction can be correlated with altered functioning in anatomical regions.
3. Cortical processing of sensory information proceeds from its point of entry through association areas with progressively more complex interconnections with other regions having sensory, memory, cognitive, emotional, and autonomic information, resulting ultimately in perceptual recognition and emotional meaning for experiences.
4. Frontosubcortical circuits are heavily involved in cognitive, affective, and behavioral functioning. Disruption of frontal circuits at the cortical or subcortical level by various processes can be associated with similar neuropsychiatric symptoms.
5. Features of the patient's clinical history and examination can be suggestive of a medical or neurological cause of psychiatric symptoms.

Many medical and neurological conditions are associated with neuropsychiatric symptoms. Each condition may carry unique implications for prognosis, treatment, and long-term management.

---

occur independently of or in association with sensorimotor dysfunction in stroke. Poststroke depression (PSD) is the most common neuropsychiatric syndrome, occurring in 30% to 50% of survivors at 1 year, with irritability, agitation, and apathy often present as well. About half of patients with depressive symptoms will meet criteria for a major depressive episode. Although somewhat controversial, onset of depression within the first few weeks after a stroke is most commonly associated with lesions affecting the frontal lobes, especially the prefrontal cortex and head of the caudate (Starkstein et al., 1987). The frequency and severity of depression increase with closer proximity to the frontal poles. Left prefrontal lesions are more commonly associated with acute depression and may be complicated by aphasia, resulting in the patient's inability to express the symptoms. Mania is much less common but occurs usually in relation to lesions of the right hemisphere, particularly with involvement of the OFC-subcortical circuit and medial temporal structures (Perez et al., 2011). Single manic events as well as recurrent manic and depressive episodes have been reported. Nondominant hemispheric strokes may also result in aprosody without associated depression. Currently, the standard treatment of PSD remains supportive psychotherapy and pharmacotherapy.

Apart from the association between large territory strokes and depression, the "vascular depression" hypothesis denotes the potential increased association between cerebrovascular disease and late-life depression (Alexopoulos, 2005; Alexopoulos et al., 1997). Clinically, vascular or late-life-depression is characterized by executive deficits, slowed processing speed, psychomotor retardation, lack of insight, and disability out of proportion to depressive symptoms. Cerebrovascular white matter T2 MRI hyperintensities from diabetes, hyperlipidemia, cardiac disease, and hypertension have been linked to this condition. Some studies have localized white matter lesions to the prefrontal cortex and temporal lobe, including particular fiber tracts (e.g., cingulum bundle, uncinate fasciculus (Sheline et al., 2008)). Vascular depression has been associated with poor antidepressant response and higher relapse rates (Alexopoulos et al., 2000). Frontolimbic disconnection and cerebrovascular hypoperfusion are some of the theorized mechanisms linking cerebrovascular disease to late-life depression.

Psychosis or psychotic features may present as a rare complication of a single stroke, but the prevalence of these features is not well established. Manifestations may include paranoia, delusions, ideas of reference, hallucinations, or psychosis. Paranoia and psychosis have been reported in association with left temporal strokes that result in Wernicke aphasia. Other regions producing similar neuropsychiatric symptoms include the right temporoparietal region and the caudate nuclei. Right hemispheric lesions may also be more associated with visual hallucinations and delusions. Reduplicative paramnesia and misidentifications syndromes such as Capgras syndrome and Fregoli syndrome have also been reported. Reduplicative paramnesia is a syndrome in which patients claim that they are simultaneously in two or more locations. It has been observed to occur in patients with combined lesions of frontal and right temporal lobes but has also been described as due to temporal-limbic-frontal dysfunction (Politis and Loane, 2012). Capgras syndrome is the false belief that someone familiar, usually a family member or close friend, has been replaced by an identical-appearing imposter. It has been proposed that this results from right temporal-limbic-frontal disconnection resulting in a disturbance in recognizing familiar people and places (Feinberg et al., 1999). A role for the left hemisphere in generating a fixed, false narrative in the context of right lateralized perceptual deficits has also been postulated (Devinsky, 2009). In Fregoli syndrome, the patient believes a persecutor is able to take on a variety of faces, like an actor. Psychotic episodes can also be a manifestation of complex partial seizures secondary to stroke. Patients with poststroke psychosis are more prone to have comorbid epilepsy than poststroke patients without associated psychosis. Lesions or infarcts of the ventral midbrain can result in a syndrome characterized by well-formed and complex visual hallucinations referred to as *peduncular hallucinosis*. Obsessive-compulsive features have also been reported with strokes. These symptoms have been postulated to be due to dysfunction in the orbitofrontal-subcortical circuitry.

Consensus criteria for accurately diagnosing vascular cognitive impairments and dementia are lacking (Gorelick et al., 2011; Wiederkehr et al., 2008). The vascular cognitive impairments can be conceptualized as being made up of three groups: vascular dementia, mixed vascular dementia and AD pathology, and vascular cognitive impairment not meeting criteria for dementia. These conditions may have variable contributions from mixed forms of small-vessel disease, large-vessel disease, and cardioembolic disease, which accounts for the clinical phenotypic heterogeneity. AD pathology is commonly found in association with cerebrovascular disease pathology, leading to uncertainty with respect to the relative contributions of each in some cases. A temporal relationship between a stroke and the onset of dementia or a stepwise progression of cognitive decline with evidence of cerebrovascular disease on examination and neuroimaging are considered most helpful. No specific neuroimaging profile exists that is diagnostic for pure cerebrovascular disease-related dementia. Vascular dementia may present with prominent cortical, subcortical, or mixed features. Cortical vascular dementia may manifest as unilateral sensorimotor dysfunction, abrupt onset of cognitive dysfunction and aphasia, and difficulties with planning, goal formation, organization, and abstraction. Subcortical vascular dementia often affects frontosubcortical circuitry, resulting in executive dysfunction, cognitive and psychomotor slowing, difficulties with abstraction, apathy, memory problems (recognition and cued recognition relatively intact), working memory impairment, and decreased ability to perform activities of daily living. Memory difficulties tend to be less severe than in AD. Limited data suggest that cholinesterase inhibitors are beneficial for treatment of vascular dementia, as demonstrated by improvements in cognition, global functioning, and performance of activities of daily living.

Infectious

An expansive list of infections that result in behavioral changes during early, middle, or late phases of illness or as a result of treatments or subsequent opportunistic infections could be generated. This portion will only focus on a few salient examples with contemporary relevance and illustrative complexity.

Human Immunodeficiency Virus

Individuals infected with HIV can be affected by a variety of neuropsychiatric and neurological problems independent of opportunistic infections and neoplasms. These include cognitive impairment, behavioral changes, and sensorimotor disturbances. Neurologists and psychiatrists must anticipate a spectrum of psychiatric phenomena that can include depression, paranoia, delusions, hallucinations, psychosis, mania, irritability, and apathy. *HIV-associated dementia* (HAD) is the term given to the syndrome that presents with bradyphrenia, memory decline, executive dysfunction, impaired concentration, and apathy. These features are compatible with a subcortical dementia with prominent dysfunction in the frontal-basal ganglia circuitry (Woods et al., 2004). *Minor cognitive motor disorder* (MCMD) refers to a milder form of this syndrome that has become more common since the advent of highly active antiretroviral therapy (HAART). HAD may be the acquired immunodeficiency virus syndrome (AIDS)-defining illness in up to 10% of patients. It has been estimated to occur in 20% to 30% of untreated adults. HAART has reduced its frequency by approximately 50%, but the frequency of pathologically proven HIV encephalitis remains high.

Lifetime prevalence of depression in HIV-infected individuals is 22% to 45%, with depressed individuals demonstrating reduced compliance with antiretroviral therapy and increased HIV-related morbidity. Antidepressants have been efficacious in treating HAD (Himelhoch and Medoff, 2005). Psychostimulants may also be a helpful adjunct in treating HAD. Evidence suggests that HIV-infected patients with new-onset psychosis usually respond well to typical neuroleptic medications, but they are more sensitive to the side effects of these medications, particularly extrapyramidal symptoms and tardive dyskinesias. This sensitivity is thought to be due to HIV's effect on the basal ganglia, resulting in a loss of dopaminergic neurons. When prescribing typical neuroleptics, caution is warranted owing to this sensitivity and the additional possible pharmacological interactions with antiretroviral medications. Atypical neuroleptics are favored.

HAART and other medications used in HIV patients can have neuropsychiatric side effects. For example, the nucleoside reverse transcriptase inhibitor zidovudine (AZT) may lead to mania, delirium, or depression. Moreover, many medications used in the treatment of HIV inhibit or induce the cytochrome P450 system, thereby altering psychotropic drug levels. Therefore, drug interactions in HIV patients with psychiatric disorders are common and require close monitoring.

Creutzfeldt–Jakob Disease

Prion diseases are a group of fatal degenerative disorders of the nervous system caused by a conformational change in the prion protein, a normal constituent of cell membranes. They are characterized by long incubation periods followed by relatively rapid neurological decline and death (Johnson, 2005). Creutzfeldt–Jakob disease (CJD) is the most common human prion disease but is rare, with an incidence of between 0.5 and 1.5 cases per million people per year. The sporadic form of the disease accounts for about 85% of cases, typically occurs later in life (mean age, 60 years), and manifests with a rapidly progressive course characterized by cerebellar ataxia, dementia, myoclonus, exaggerated startle reflex, seizures, and psychiatric symptoms progressing to akinetic mutism and complete disability within months after disease onset. Cerebrospinal fluid analysis may be positive for 14-3-3 protein, which has been shown to have a sensitivity of 92% and a specificity of 80% (Muayqil et al., 2012). Diffusion-weighted imaging may show posterior cortical ribbon or striatal hyperintensities, while middle to late stage sporadic CJD may show periodic sharp wave complexes on EEG (Geschwind et al., 2008). Psychiatric symptoms such as personality changes, anxiety, depression, paranoia, obsessive-compulsive features, and psychosis occur in about 80% of patients during the first 100 days of illness (Wall et al., 2005). About 60% present with symptoms compatible with a rapidly progressive dementia. The mean duration of the illness is 6 to 7 months.

The autosomal dominant familial form of CJD accounts for 10% to 15% of cases, and iatrogenically caused cases account for about 1%. New-variant CJD is a new form of acquired spongiform encephalopathy that emerged in 1994 in the United Kingdom. This form has been linked with consumption of infected animal products. Patients with the new variant have a different course characterized by younger age at onset (mean age, 29 years), prominent psychiatric and sensory symptoms, and a longer disease course. Spencer and colleagues reported that 63% demonstrated purely psychiatric symptoms at onset (dysphoria, anxiety, anhedonia), 15% had purely neurological symptoms, and 22% had features of both (Spencer et al., 2002). New-variant CJD may be distinguished from sporadic CJD by hyperintensities in the pulvinar on MRI. Median duration of illness was 13 months, and by the time of death, prominent neurological and psychiatric manifestations were universal.

Neurosyphilis

A resurgence of neurosyphilis has accompanied the AIDS epidemic in the industrialized world. Neurosyphilis may occur in any stage of syphilis. Early neurosyphilis, seen in the first weeks to years of infection, is primarily a meningitic process in which the parenchyma is not typically involved. It can coexist with primary or secondary syphilis and be asymptomatic. Inadequate treatment of early syphilis and coinfection with HIV predispose to early neurosyphilis. Epidemiological studies in HIV-infected patients have documented increased HIV shedding associated with genital ulcers, suggesting that syphilis increases the susceptibility of infected persons to HIV acquisition and transmission (Lynn and Lightman, 2004). Symptomatic early neurosyphilis may present with meningitis, with or without cranial nerve involvement or ocular changes, meningovascular disease, or stroke. Late neurosyphilis affects the meninges, brain, or spinal cord parenchyma and usually occurs years to decades after primary infection. Manifestations of late neurosyphilis include tabes dorsalis, a rapidly progressive dementia with psychotic features, or general paresis (a.k.a. general paralysis of the insane), or both. Pupillary abnormalities are common, the most classic being Argyll Robertson pupils: miotic, irregular pupils showing light-near dissociation (Berger and Dean, 2014). Dementia as a symptom of neurosyphilis is unlikely to improve significantly with treatment, yet the course of the illness can be arrested. Presenting psychiatric symptoms of neurosyphilis can include personality changes, hostility, confusion, hallucinations, expansiveness, delusions, and dysphoria. Symptoms also reported in association with neurosyphilis include explosive temper, emotional lability, anhedonia, social withdrawal, decreased attention to personal affairs, unusual giddiness, histrionicity, hypersexuality, and mania. A significant incidence of depression has been associated with general paresis.

There is no uniform consensus for the best approach to diagnosing neurosyphilis. Diagnosis usually depends on various combinations of reactive serological tests, cerebral spinal fluid (CSF) cell count or protein, CSF Venereal Disease Research Laboratories (VDRL) testing, and clinical manifestations. Some authorities argue that all patients with syphilis should have CSF examination, since asymptomatic neurosyphilis can only be identified by changes in the CSF. The CSF VDRL is the standard serological test for CSF and is highly specific but insensitive. When reactive in the absence of substantial contamination of CSF with blood, it is usually considered diagnostic. Its titer may be used to assess the activity of the disease and response to treatment. Two tests of CSF may be used to confirm a diagnosis of neurosyphilis: *Treponema pallidum* hemagglutination assay (TPHA) and fluorescent

treponemal antibody absorption (FTA-ABS) assay. No single serology screen is perfect for diagnosing neurosyphilis. Other indicators of disease activity include CSF abnormalities such as elevated white blood cell count, elevated protein, and increased gamma globulin (IgG) levels. Treatment of neurosyphilis consists of a regimen of aqueous penicillin G, 18 to 24 million units/day, administered as 3 to 4 million units intravenously (IV) every 4 hours, or continuous infusion for 10 to 14 days. An alternative treatment is procaine penicillin G, 2 to 4 million units intramuscularly (IM) daily, with probenecid, 500 mg orally (PO), both daily for 10 to 14 days. A common recommendation to ensure an adequate response and cure is to repeat CSF studies 6 months after treatment.

Metabolic and Toxic

Essentially any metabolic derangement, if severe enough or combined with other conditions, can adversely affect behavior and cognition (eTable 10.5). Metabolic disorders should remain within the differential diagnosis when evaluating patients with psychiatric symptoms.

Thyroid Disease

Hypothyroidism results from a deficiency in circulating thyroxine (T_4). It can result from impaired function at the level of the hypothalamus (tertiary hypothyroidism), the anterior pituitary (secondary hypothyroidism), or the thyroid gland (primary hypothyroidism, the most common cause of hypothyroidism). Neurological symptoms and signs can include headache, fatigue, apathy, inattention, slowness of speech and thought, sensorineural hearing loss, sleep apnea, and seizures. Some of these symptoms may mimic depression. Hypothyroidism can worsen or complicate the course of depression, resulting in a seemingly refractory depression. More rare findings include polyneuropathy, cranial neuropathy, muscle weakness, psychosis (referred to as *myxedema madness*), dementia, coma, and death. Psychosis typically presents with paranoid delusions and auditory hallucinations.

Hyperthyroidism may be due to a number of causes that produce increased serum T_4. With mild hyperthyroidism, patients are typically anxious, irritable, emotionally labile, tachycardic, and tremulous. Other symptoms can include apathy, depression, panic attacks, feelings of exhaustion, inability to concentrate, and memory problems. When apathy and depression are present, the term *apathetic hyperthyroidism* is often used. Thyroid storm results from an abrupt elevation in T_4, often provoked by a significant stress such as surgery. It can be associated with fever, tachycardia, seizures, and coma; if untreated, it is often fatal. Psychosis and paranoia frequently occur during thyroid storm but are rare with milder hyperthyroidism, as is mania. Many patients usually will experience complete remission of symptoms 1 to 2 months after a euthyroid state is obtained, with a marked reduction in anxiety, sense of exhaustion, irritability, and depression. Some authors, however, report an increased rate of anxiety in patients, as well as persistence of affective and cognitive symptoms for several months to up to 10 years after a euthyroid state is established.

Steroid-responsive encephalopathy associated with autoimmune thyroiditis (STREAT), also known as Hashimoto encephalopathy, is a rare disorder involving thyroid autoimmunity (Castillo et al., 2006). Antibodies associated with this condition include antithyroid peroxidase antibodies (previously known as *antithyroid microsomal antibodies*) and antithyroglobulin antibodies. The clinical syndrome may manifest with a progressive or relapsing and remitting course consisting of tremor, myoclonus, transient aphasia, stroke-like episodes, psychosis, seizures, encephalopathy, hypersomnolence, stupor, or coma. Encephalopathy usually develops over 1 to 7 days. The underlying mechanism of Hashimoto encephalopathy remains under investigation, and importantly, thyroid-stimulating hormone levels can be normal in this disorder. CSF most often shows an elevated protein level with almost no nucleated cells, whereas oligoclonal bands are often present. The EEG is abnormal in almost all cases, showing generalized slowing or frontal intermittent rhythmic delta activity. Triphasic waves, focal slowing, and epileptiform abnormalities may also be seen. MRI of the brain is often normal but may reveal hyperintensities on T2-weighted or fluid-attenuated inversion recovery (FLAIR) imaging in the subcortical white matter or at the gray/white matter junction. SPECT may show regions of hypoperfusion. The neurological and psychiatric symptoms respond well to treatment, which generally involves high-dose steroids. The associated abnormal findings on EEG, and often the MRI abnormalities, resolve with effective treatment.

Wilson Disease

Wilson disease (WD), also known as *hepatolenticular degeneration*, is an autosomal recessive disorder produced by a mutation on chromosome 13. The gene encodes a transport protein, the mutation of which causes abnormal deposition of copper in the liver, brain (especially the basal ganglia), and the cornea of the eyes. WD typically begins in childhood but in some cases has its onset as late as the fifth or sixth decade. About one-third of patients present with psychiatric symptoms, one-third present with neurological features, and one-third present with hepatic disease. Neurological manifestations are largely extrapyramidal, including chorea, tremor (infrequently including wing-beating like characteristics), and dystonia. Other symptoms include dysphagia, dysarthria, ataxia, gait disturbance, and a fixed (sardonic) smile. Seizures may also occur in a minority of patients. Potential neuropsychiatric symptoms are numerous, with at least half of patients manifesting symptoms early in the disease course. Personality and mood changes are the most common neuropsychiatric features, with depression occurring in approximately 30% of patients. Bipolar spectrum symptoms occur in about 20% of patients. Suicidal ideation is recognized in about 5% to 15%. WD patients can present with increased sensitivity to neuroleptics. Other symptoms include irritability, aggression, and psychosis. Cognitively, the profile is consistent with disturbance of frontosubcortical networks. Even long-term-treated WD patients develop psychiatric symptoms in about 70% of cases (Srinivas et al., 2008; Svetel et al., 2009).

Diagnosis is suggested by identification of Kayser–Fleischer (KF) rings in patients with the appropriate clinical picture. The KF ring is a yellow-brown discoloration of the Descemet membrane in the limbic area of the cornea, best visualized with slit-lamp examination. A KF ring is present in 98% of patients with neurological disease and in 80% of all cases of WD. Reduced serum ceruloplasmin levels and elevated 24-hour urine copper excretion are consistent with this disorder. A liver biopsy is sometimes necessary to make the diagnosis. MRI studies may show abnormal T2 signal in the putamen, midbrain, pons, thalamus, cerebellum, and other structures. Atrophy is commonly present. The initial treatment for symptomatic patients is chelation therapy with either penicillamine or trientine. An estimated 20% to 50% of patients with neurological manifestations treated with penicillamine experience an acute worsening of their symptoms. A portion of these patients do not recover to their pretreatment neurological baseline. Alternatives that may have a lower incidence of neurological worsening include trientine or tetrathiomolybdate.

Both may be used in combination with zinc therapy. Treatment of presymptomatic patients or maintenance therapy of successfully treated symptomatic patients can be accomplished with a chelating agent or zinc. Early treatment may result in partial improvement of the MRI changes as well as most of the neurological and psychiatric symptoms.

Vitamin B$_{12}$ and Folic Acid Deficiency

The true prevalence of vitamin B$_{12}$ deficiency in the general population is unknown. The Framingham study demonstrated a prevalence of 12% among elderly persons living in the community. Other studies have suggested that the incidence may be as high as 30% to 40% among the sick and institutionalized elderly. The most common sign of vitamin B$_{12}$ deficiency is macrocytic anemia. However, signs and symptoms attributed to the nervous system are diverse and can occur in the absence of anemia or macrocytosis. Furthermore, a normal serum cobalamin level does not exclude the possibility of a clinical deficiency. Serum homocysteine levels, which are elevated in more than 90% of deficiency states, and serum methylmalonic acid levels can be used to verify deficiency states in the appropriate settings.

Subacute combined degeneration (SCD) refers to the combination of spinal cord and peripheral nerve pathology associated with vitamin B$_{12}$ deficiency. Patients often complain of unsteady gait and distal paresthesias. The examination may demonstrate evidence of posterior column, pyramidal tract, and peripheral nerve involvement. Cognitive, behavioral, and psychiatric manifestations can occur in isolation or together with the elemental signs and symptoms. Personality change, cognitive dysfunction, mania, depression, and psychosis have been reported. Prominent psychotic features include paranoid or religious delusions and auditory and visual hallucinations. Dementia is often comorbid with cobalamin deficiency; however, the causative association is unclear. There are few research data to support the existence of reversible dementia due to B$_{12}$ deficiency. Cobalamin deficiency-associated cognitive impairment is more likely to improve when impairment is mild and of short duration. Folate deficiency can produce a clinical picture similar to cobalamin deficiency, although some investigators report that folate deficiency tends to produce more depression, whereas vitamin B$_{12}$ deficiency tends to produce more psychosis. Elevated serum homocysteine is also seen with a functional folate deficiency state wherein folate utilization is impaired. Repletion of folate if comorbid vitamin B$_{12}$ deficiency is not first corrected can result in an acute exacerbation of the neuropsychiatric symptoms.

Porphyrias

The porphyrias are caused by enzymatic defects in the heme biosynthetic pathway. Porphyrias with neuropsychiatric symptoms include acute intermittent porphyria (AIP), variegated porphyria (VP), hereditary mixed coproporphyria (HMP), and plumboporphyria (extremely rare and autosomal recessive), which may give rise to acute episodes of potentially fatal symptoms such as neurovisceral crisis, abdominal pain, delirium, psychosis, neuropathy, and autonomic instability. AIP, the most common type reported in the United States, follows an autosomal dominant pattern of inheritance and is due to a mutation in the gene for porphobilinogen deaminase. The disease is characterized by attacks that may last days to weeks, with relatively normal function between attacks. Infrequently, the clinical course may exhibit persisting clinical abnormalities with superimposed episodes of exacerbation. The episodic nature, clinical variability, and unusual features may cause symptoms to be misattributed to somatoform, functional (psychogenic) or other psychiatric disorders. Attacks may be spontaneous but are typically precipitated by a variety of factors such as infection, alcohol use, pregnancy, anesthesia, and numerous medications that include antidepressants, anticonvulsants, and oral contraceptives.

Porphyric attacks usually manifest with a triad consisting of abdominal pain, peripheral neuropathy, and neuropsychiatric symptoms. Seizures may also occur. Abdominal pain is the most common symptom, which can result in surgical exploration if the diagnosis is unknown. A variety of cognitive and behavioral changes can occur, including anxiety, restlessness, insomnia, depression, mania, hallucinations, delusions, confusion, catatonia, and psychosis. The diagnosis can be confirmed during an acute attack of AIP, HMP, or VP by measuring urine porphobilinogens. Acute attacks are treated with avoidance of precipitating factors (e.g., medications), IV hemin, IV glucose, and pain control.

Drug Abuse

Common neurological manifestations are broad and include the direct effects of intoxication, side effects, and withdrawal syndromes, as well as indirect effects. Direct effects can range from somnolence with sedatives to psychosis from hallucinogens and stimulants. Side effects may be as severe as stroke or vasculitis from stimulant abuse. Withdrawal may be lethal as in the case of alcohol withdrawal and delirium tremens. Indirect effects can occur as a result of trauma, such as head injury, suffered while under the influence. Substance abuse has a high comorbidity with a variety of psychiatric conditions. Neuropsychiatric manifestations occur with abuse of all classes of drugs and are summarized in eBox 10.6. The behavioral and cognitive manifestations of substance abuse may be transient but in a vulnerable subset of individuals may be chronic. Growing evidence suggests that drug use (e.g., 3,4-methylenedioxymethamphetamine (MDMA, "ecstasy")) may promote the development of chronic neuropsychiatric states such as depression and impaired cognition due to changes in structural and functional neuroanatomy (Parrott, 2013). Although *cannabis* use seems to be neither a sufficient nor a necessary cause of psychosis, it does confer an increased relative risk for developing schizophrenia later in life (Radhakrishnan et al., 2014).

Systemic Lupus Erythematosus

Systemic lupus erythematosus (SLE, lupus) is a multisystem inflammatory disorder that affects all ages, although young females are at a significantly elevated risk. CNS involvement is common, with clinical manifestations seen at some point during their disease course in up to 90% of patients. Primary neurological and psychiatric manifestations of SLE are likely due to a mixture of pathogenic mechanisms that include vascular abnormalities, autoantibodies, and the local production of inflammatory mediators. Secondary neurological and psychiatric manifestations occur as a result of various therapies (e.g., immunosuppression with steroids) or complications of the disease.

Neuropsychiatric symptoms are common, often episodic, and may occur in association with steroid treatment, which creates significant dilemmas in management. Depression and anxiety each occur in approximately 25% of SLE patients. Reports of the prevalence of overall mood disturbances range between 16% and 75%, and reports of anxiety disorders occur in 7% to 70%. Psychosis is more rare and tends to occur in the context of confusional states. Its overall prevalence has been reported to range from 5% to 8%. The incidence of psychotic symptoms in patients receiving prednisone doses between 60 and 100 mg/day is approximately 30%. These symptoms are reported to respond favorably to reduction in

steroid dose and psychotropic management. Focal or generalized seizures may occur in the setting of active generalized SLE or as an isolated event. The prevalence of seizures ranges from 3% to 51%. Cognitive manifestations of SLE including temporary, fluctuating, or relatively stable characteristics eventually occur in up to 75% of patients; these manifestations range from mild attentional difficulties to dementia. In some patients, cognitive performance improves with resolution of any concurrent psychiatric disturbances. Cerebrovascular disease may underlie nonreversible cognitive dysfunction and when progressive may cause atrophy and multi-infarct dementia. Many patients with cognitive impairment have no demonstrable vascular lesions on neuroimaging. Cognitive impairment may manifest as subcortical features with deficits in processing speed, attention, learning and memory, conceptual reasoning, and cognitive flexibility. Reports of the prevalence of subclinical cognitive impairment range from 11% to 54% of patients. A number of brain-specific antibodies have been studied as potential diagnostic markers of psychosis associated with neuropsychiatric SLE (NPSLE), but none appear to be specific (Kimura et al., 2010). SLE patients identified as having a persistently positive immunoglobulin (Ig)G anticardiolipin antibody over a 5-year period have been demonstrated to have a greater reduction in psychomotor speed than antibody-negative SLE patients. Patients with a persistently elevated IgA anticardiolipin antibody level have been demonstrated to have poorer performance on tests of conceptual reasoning and executive function than antibody-negative SLE patients. Elevated IgG and IgA anticardiolipin antibody levels may be causative or a marker of long-term subtle deterioration in cognitive function in SLE patients. However, their role in routine evaluation and management remains controversial. Cerebrovascular disease is a well-known cause of neuropsychiatric dysfunction and is reported to occur in 5% to 18% of SLE patients.

The criteria set most widely used for diagnosing SLE is that developed by the American College of Rheumatology (ACR). An antinuclear antibody (ANA) titer to 1:40 or higher is the most sensitive of the ACR criteria and is present in up to 99% of persons with SLE at some point in their illness. The ANA, however, is not specific. It can be positive in several other rheumatological conditions as well as in relation to some medication exposures. There is also a significant incidence of false-positive tests. Anti–double-stranded DNA and anti-Smith antibodies, particularly in high titers, have high specificity for SLE, although their sensitivity is low. The rapid plasma reagin (RPR) test, a syphilis serology, may be falsely positive.

Treatment of NPSLE includes corticosteroids and immunosuppressive therapy, including pulse IV cyclophosphamide or plasmapheresis when NPSLE is thought to occur secondary to an inflammatory process. Anticoagulation is used in patients with thrombotic disease in the setting of antiphospholipid antibody syndrome.

Multiple Sclerosis

Multiple sclerosis is an inflammatory demyelinating disease that manifests the pathological hallmark findings of multifocal demyelinated plaques in the brain and spinal cord. MS lesions are typically disseminated throughout the CNS, with a predilection for the optic nerves, brainstem, spinal cord, cerebellum, and periventricular white matter. Its cause remains unknown but is thought to be an immune-mediated disorder affecting individuals with a genetic predisposition. The heterogeneity of clinical, pathological, and MRI findings suggest involvement of more than one pathological mechanism. It is the leading cause of nontraumatic disability among young adults. Socioepidemiological studies indicate that MS leads to unemployment within a 10-year disease course in as many as 50% to 80% of patients. Females are more affected than males at a 2 : 1 ratio. It is characterized either by attacks of neurological deficits with variable remittance or by a steady progressive course of neurological decline. Neuropsychiatric manifestations of MS are common, occurring in up to 60% of patients at some point in their disease. The lifetime prevalence of major depression in MS is approximately 50%. The lifetime prevalence of bipolar disorder is twice the prevalence in the general population. Euphoria may be present in more advanced MS, usually in association with cognitive deficits. *Pseudobulbar affect*—defined as outbursts of involuntary, uncontrollable, stereotypical episodes of laughing or crying—occurs in varying degrees of severity in approximately 10% of patients. Other symptoms include anxiety, sleep disorder, emotional lability/irritability, apathy, mania, suicidality, and rarely psychosis. Occasionally, psychiatric symptoms may present as the major manifestation of an episode of demyelination. The presence of psychiatric symptomatology does not preclude the use of steroids to abbreviate clinical attacks of MS. There is at present ongoing debate about whether interferon therapy is associated with a higher incidence of depression in MS patients. Clinically, pharmacological and behavioral treatment mirrors the management of depression and psychosis in patients without MS. Recently published guidelines for the management of psychiatric symptoms of MS suggested that there is insufficient evidence to refute or support the use of antidepressants for depression or anxiety disorders in this population, though a combination of dextromethorphan and quinidine may be considered for the treatment of pseudobulbar affect (Minden et al., 2014).

Cognitive impairment is found in approximately 40% of patients. Deficits have been described in working, semantic, and episodic memory as well as in the person's ability to accurately assess his or her own memory function. Patients may also suffer from impaired attention, cognitive slowing, reduced verbal fluency, and difficulties with abstract reasoning and concept formation. Correlations between cognitive impairment and MRI location of lesions and indices of total lesion area are actively under investigation (Charil et al., 2003; Reuter et al., 2011). There are few data on the treatment of cognitive dysfunction in MS (Amato et al., 2013). The disease-modifying agent interferon beta-1a was noted to be associated with improvements in information-processing and problem-solving abilities over a 2-year longitudinal study. A small trial demonstrated an improvement in complex attention, concentration, and visual memory in a group of patients treated for 1 year with interferon beta-1b compared with controls (Barak and Achiron, 2002). Donepezil, 10 mg daily, has been reported to improve verbal learning and memory in some MS patients.

Neoplastic

A variety of neoplasms cause cognitive and behavioral disorders. Of particular relevance are mass lesions and paraneoplastic syndromes. Mass lesions can be single or multiple and can be primary to the CNS or metastatic. The most common intracranial primary tumors are astrocytomas (e.g., glioblastoma multiforme), meningiomas, pituitary tumors, vestibular schwannomas, and oligodendrogliomas. Common metastatic tumors include primary lung and breast tumors, melanoma, and renal and colon cancers. The number of patients presenting with a primary psychiatric diagnosis secondary to an unidentified brain tumor is likely to be less than 5%. However, 15% to 20% of patients with intracranial tumors may present with neuropsychiatric manifestations before the development of primary neurological problems such as motor or sensory deficits. The behavioral manifestations of mass lesions are diverse and related to a number of factors including direct disruption of local structures or circuits, rate of growth, seizures, and increased intracranial pressure. A relationship between tumor location and specific psychiatric symptoms has not been established. Meningiomas, given their slow growth over years, are classic examples of tumors that can present solely with behavioral manifestations. Common locations include the olfactory groove and sphenoid wings, which can disrupt adjacent limbic structures such as the orbital frontal gyri and medial temporal lobes.

Paraneoplastic syndromes represent remote nonmetastatic manifestations of malignancy. Neurological paraneoplastic syndromes are primarily immune-mediated disorders that may develop as a result of antigens shared between the nervous system and tumor cells. The most common primary malignancies that promote neurological paraneoplastic syndromes are ovarian and small-cell lung cancer (SCLC). These syndromes generally develop subacutely, often before the primary malignancy is identified, and may preferentially involve selected regions of the CNS. Typical sites of involvement include muscle, neuromuscular junction, peripheral nerve, cerebellum, and limbic structures. Limbic encephalitis, associated with SCLC, testicular cancer, and ovarian teratomas among other pathologies, produces a significant amnestic syndrome and neuropsychiatric symptoms including agitation, depression, personality changes, apathy, delusions, hallucinations, psychosis and complex partial and generalized seizures. Anti N-methyl-D-aspartate (NMDA) receptor encephalitis associated with antibodies against the NR1-NR2 heterodimer of the receptor has been increasingly recognized as presenting commonly in young women with ovarian teratomas and psychiatric symptoms including anxiety, agitation, bizarre behavior, paranoid delusions, visual or auditory hallucinations, and/or memory loss. Additional frequently encountered symptoms include seizures, decreased consciousness, dyskinesias, autonomic instability, and hypoventilation (Dalmau and Rosenfeld, 2008; Dalmau et al., 2008). Elevated markers in paraneoplastic syndromes may include: (1) intracellular paraneoplastic antigens such as Hu, associated with SCLC, and Ta and Ma-2 (Hoffmann et al., 2008), associated with testicular cancer; and (2) cell membrane antigens such as the NMDA receptor and voltage-gated potassium channels. Paraneoplastic disorders are often progressive and refractory to therapy, although in some cases significant improvement follows tumor resection and early initiated immunotherapy interventions. Significant neuropsychiatric sequelae can arise from the various chemotherapeutic and radiation therapies used for cancer treatment.

Degenerative

Neuropsychiatric symptoms are common in most degenerative disorders that produce significant dementia. The individual presentations of such symptoms are related to a number of factors specific to the disease: location of lesion burden, rate of progression of disease, and factors specific to the individual (e.g., premorbid personality, education level, psychiatric history, social support system, and coping skills). Neurodegenerative diseases are increasingly recognized as involving abnormalities of protein metabolism. About 70% of dementias in the elderly and more than 90% of neurodegenerative dementias can be linked to abnormalities of three proteins: β-amyloid, α-synuclein, and tau. Disorders of protein metabolism have associated neuroanatomical regions of vulnerable cell populations that are related to the clinical manifestations. AD, for example, has associated disorders of β-amyloid and tau. PD, dementia with Lewy bodies (DLB), and multisystem atrophies are synucleinopathies. α-Synuclein is the main component of Lewy bodies, which are a major histological marker seen in PD and DLB. In these disorders, Lewy bodies may be found in the substantia nigra, locus coeruleus, nucleus basalis, limbic system, and transitional and neocortex. Frontotemporal dementia, progressive supranuclear palsy (PSP), and corticobasal ganglionic degeneration implicate abnormal tau metabolism in their pathogenesis. Tauopathies are associated with selective involvement of the frontal and temporal cortex and frontosubcortical circuitry.

Alzheimer Disease and Mild Cognitive Impairment

Neuropsychiatric symptoms of AD may include agitation, aggression, delusions including paranoia, hallucinations, anxiety, apathy, social withdrawal, reduced speech output, reduction or alteration of long-standing family relationships, and loss of sense of humor. With disease progression, patients often lose awareness (insight) into the nature and severity of their deficits. A review of 100 cases of autopsy-proven AD demonstrated that 74% of patients had behavioral symptoms detected at the time of the initial evaluation. Symptoms included apathy (51%), hallucinations (25%), delusions (20%), depressed mood (6.6%), verbal aggression (36.8%), and physical aggression (17%). The presence of behavioral symptoms at the initial evaluation was associated with greater functional impairment not directly related to their cognitive impairments. Depressive symptoms, dysphoria, or major depression eventually occur in approximately half of patients. Psychosis has been reported to occur in 30% to 50% of patients at some time during the course of the illness, more commonly in the later stages. Mania occurs in less than 5%. Behavioral changes have been shown to be problematic and to precipitate earlier nursing home placement. Social comportment has been viewed as being relatively spared in AD, but subtle personality changes occur in nearly every individual over time. Significant impairment in the ability to recognize facial expressions of emotion and an inability to repeat, comprehend, and discriminate affective elements of language have been reported. It has been hypothesized that 15% of AD patients may have a frontal variant wherein they present with difficulties attributable to frontal lobe circuitry rather than an amnestic syndrome. Impairments in driving ability (Dawson et al., 2009) and decision-making abilities such as medical decision-making (Okonkwo et al., 2008) and financial management (Marson et al., 2009) may be present even in early AD.

Atypical antipsychotic drugs are widely used to treat psychosis, aggression, and agitation in patients with AD. Their benefits are uncertain, and concerns about safety have emerged, including increased risk of mortality, cerebrovascular events, metabolic derangements, extrapyramidal symptoms, falls, cognitive worsening, cardiac arrhythmia, and pneumonia among other symptoms (Steinberg and Lyketsos, 2012). Adverse effects may offset advantages in the efficacy of atypical antipsychotic drugs for the treatment of psychosis, aggression, or agitation in AD patients, particularly if used chronically. Limited evidence suggests that electroconvulsive therapy (ECT) may be effective for management of agitation (Sutor and Rasmussen, 2008).

The concept of mild cognitive impairment (MCI) was developed to characterize a population of individuals exhibiting symptoms that are between normal age-related cognitive decline and dementia. These patients have a very slight degree of functional impairment and minimal decline from their prior level of functioning and therefore do not meet criteria for dementia. MCI (*amnestic single domain*) was initially defined as a condition of memory impairment beyond what was expected for age, in the absence of impairments in other domains of cognitive functioning such as working memory, executive function, language, and visual-spatial ability. This concept has since evolved and now includes a total of four subtypes of impairment that are not of sufficient severity to warrant the diagnosis of dementia. The second type of MCI, called *amnestic multiple domain*, is associated with memory impairment plus impairment in one or more other cognitive domains. The third subtype is called *nonamnestic single domain*, and the fourth is known as *nonamnestic multiple domain* MCI. In many cases, the natural history of these subtypes leads to different endpoint conditions. Combining the clinical syndrome with the presumed cause may allow for reliable prediction of outcome of the MCI syndrome. When associated with only memory impairment, MCI may represent normal aging or depression or progress to AD. Amnestic MCI–multiple domains have a higher association with depression or progression to AD or vascular dementia. Nonamnestic single-domain MCI may have a higher likelihood of progression to frontal temporal dementia. Nonamnestic multiple-domain MCI may have a higher likelihood of progression to Lewy body dementia or vascular dementia (Petersen and Negash, 2008).

In 2008, it was estimated that more than 5 million people in the United States older than age 71 had MCI. The prevalence of MCI among persons younger than age 75 has been estimated to be 19% and for those older than 85 years, 29%. Almost a third of these individuals have amnestic MCI which may progress to AD at a rate of 10% to 15% per year. The conversion rate of amnestic MCI to dementia over a 6-year period may be as high as 80%. Neuropsychiatric symptoms are common in persons with MCI. Depression occurs in 20%, apathy in 15%, and irritability in 15%. Increased levels of agitation and aggression are also present. Almost half of MCI patients demonstrate one of these neuropsychiatric symptoms coincident with the onset of cognitive impairment. Impaired awareness of memory dysfunction may also be present to a degree comparable to that found in persons with early AD. Evidence suggests that persons with MCI have an increased risk of motor vehicle accidents when risk factors such as having a history of driving citations, crashes, reduced driving mileage, situational avoidance, or aggression or impulsivity are present. Difficulties with medical decision-making have also been identified in some individuals with MCI (Okonkwo et al., 2008).

Frontotemporal Dementia

Frontotemporal dementia (FTD), the most common progressive focal cortical syndrome, is characterized by atrophy of the frontal and anterotemporal lobes. Age at presentation is usually between 45 and 65 years (almost invariably before age 65), and reports of its incidence range from being equal in males and females to (more recently) predominating in males by a ratio of 14:3. The prevalence of FTD is equal to that of AD for early-onset (age < 65) dementia. Features of behavioral variant FTD may include apathy, social withdrawal, loss of empathy or sympathy, disinhibition, impulsivity, poor insight, anosognosia, ritualistic or obsessive tendencies, and inappropriate sexual behavior; infrequently, particularly in the early stages of the disease, agitation, delusions, hallucinations, and psychosis may also occur (Rascovsky et al., 2011). Elements of the Klüver–Bucy syndrome may be present. Memory and language are usually spared during the early disease course. Depressive symptoms occur in 30% to 40% of patients. SSRIs are somewhat effective in treating behavioral symptoms including disinhibition but are less effective in treating cognitive symptoms. About 30% of patients with FTD have a positive family history, and first-degree relatives of patients have a 3.5 times higher risk of developing dementia. Genes known to be mutated in this disorder include those encoding microtubule-associated protein tau and progranulin; the gene C9ORF72 is a common genetic cause of both FTD and amotrophic lateral sclerosis.

Idiopathic Parkinson Disease

Neuropsychiatric manifestations of PD are common. Depression is the most common psychiatric symptom, with a reported prevalence of 25% to 50%. Establishing the diagnosis of depression is complicated by the presence of comorbid confounding symptoms including dementia, facial masking, bradykinesia, apathy, and hypophonia. Menza et al. (2009) conducted a placebo-controlled trial in PD patients with depression and found that nortriptyline was efficacious, but paroxetine was not. Psychosis is also particularly prevalent and generally related to dopaminergic agents (Menza et al., 2009). The onset of motor impairment almost always precedes that of psychosis. Hallucinations, usually fleeting and nocturnal, are typically visual and occur in 30% of treated patients. Auditory and olfactory hallucinations, however, are rare. Visual hallucinations are associated with impaired cognition, use of anticholinergic medications, and impaired vision. In contrast to the hallucinations associated with DLB, patients with PD generally have at least partial insight into the nature of their hallucinations. Delusions occur less commonly and are often persecutory in nature. Management is complicated by neuroleptic sensitivity to both typical and atypical agents. Typical neuroleptics should be avoided. Novel atypical neuroleptics with potentially more favorable pharmacological properties, such as quetiapine and clozapine, may have theoretical advantages over other agents for treating PD. Evidence suggests that clozapine is effective, quetiapine may be effective, and olanzepine is not effective. Impulse-control disorders including pathological gambling, binge-eating, and compulsive sexual behavior and buying are associated with dopamine agonist treatment in PD (Weintraub et al., 2010).

Many PD patients will develop dementia 10 years or more after the onset of motor symptoms. Up to 80% of PD patients will eventually develop frank dementia, a majority of whom will show comorbid AD pathology. Initial deficits may include cognitive slowing, memory retrieval deficits, attentional difficulties, visual-spatial deficits, and mild executive impairments. In advanced disease, memory encoding and storage can become impaired. Primary language difficulties are not involved until the disease has significantly progressed. Some evidence suggests that patients with an akinetic-dominant form of PD with hallucinations are at higher risk of developing dementia than patients with a tremor-dominant form who have no hallucinations. Dementia is a major prognostic factor for progressive disability and nursing home placement. In a placebo-controlled trial, rivastigmine (a cholinesterase inhibitor) has been shown to produce moderate but significant improvements in global ratings of dementia, cognition, and behavioral symptoms in patients with mild to moderate PD. Open-label drug data suggest that all three cholinesterase inhibitors may be effective.

Dementia with Lewy Bodies

By some accounts, DLB is the second most common cause of dementia. The revised consensus criteria for the clinical diagnosis of DLB reiterate dementia as an essential feature for the diagnosis of DLB occurring before or concurrently with parkinsonism. Criteria developed for research purposes to distinguish DLB from PD with dementia use an arbitrary period of 1 year within which the occurrence of dementia and extrapyramidal symptoms suggests the diagnosis of possible DLB. If the clinical history of parkinsonism is longer than 1 year

before dementia occurs, a diagnosis of PD with dementia is more accurate. Deficits of attention, executive function, and visuospatial ability may be prominent. These deficits may be worse in DLB than in patients with AD. Prominent or persistent memory impairment may not necessarily occur in the early stages but is usually evident with progression. Memory impairment is a less prominent feature than in AD. According to the revised consensus criteria, two core features are sufficient for the diagnosis of probable DLB and one feature for the diagnosis of possible DLB. Core features include fluctuating cognition, recurrent visual hallucinations, and spontaneous features of parkinsonism. Other suggestive and supportive features associated with DLB include delusions, hallucinations in other modalities, rapid eye movement (REM) sleep behavior disorder, depression, severe neuroleptic sensitivity, autonomic dysfunction, repeated falls/syncope, and episodes of unexplained transient loss of consciousness.

Hallucinations are characteristically seen early in the disease course and are persistent and recurrent. Visual hallucinations tend to occur early in the illness, are typically well formed and complex, and occur in 50% to 80% of patients. Auditory hallucinations occur in approximately 30% of patients and olfactory hallucinations in 5% to 10% of patients. Delusions may be systematized and are present in 50% of patients over the course of the disease. Depression is estimated to be nearly as common as that in AD. Treatment is complicated by hypersensitivity to the adverse effects of antidopaminergic neuroleptic agents (both typical and atypical). Typical agents should be avoided. Atypical neuroleptics with potentially more favorable pharmacological properties (e.g., quetiapine and clozapine) may have theoretical advantages over other agents in treating DLB as with PD. Cholinesterase inhibitors are helpful for managing neuropsychiatric symptoms and may be beneficial for treating fluctuating cognitive impairment and improving global functioning and activities of daily living.

Huntington Disease

Huntington Disease is a degenerative disorder of autosomal dominant inheritance resulting from an expanded trinucleotide (cytosine-adenine-guanine [CAG]) repeat on chromosome 4. Symptoms typically develop during the fourth or fifth decade, initially manifesting with neurological features, psychiatric features, or both. Neurologically, patients often demonstrate generalized chorea, motor impersistence, and oculomotor dysfunction. In the juvenile form, the Westphal variant, early parkinsonian features are prominent, as are seizures, ataxia, and myoclonus. Significant cognitive impairment is inevitable and is often present early in the disease. Features of a subcortical dementia are present with involvement of frontosubcortical circuits. Common features include cognitive slowing, memory retrieval deficits, attentional difficulties, and executive dysfunction. Patients often lack awareness of their chorea and their cognitive and emotional deficits. Psychiatric features such as personality changes, apathy, irritability, and depression are common. Depression may be exacerbated by tetrabenazine used for the treatment of chorea, since this drug is a dopamine-depleting agent. Psychosis may occur in up to 25% of patients with HD. Anxiety and obsessive tendencies also occur (Phillips et al., 2008).

Epilepsy

Behavioral and cognitive dysfunction is frequently observed in patients with epilepsy and represents an important challenge in treating these patients. A complex array of factors influence the neuropsychiatric effect of epilepsy: cause, location of epileptogenic focus, age at onset, duration of epilepsy, nature of the epilepsy syndrome, seizure type, frequency, medications used for treatment, and psychosocial factors. Epilepsies that develop subsequent to brain trauma and stroke may be associated with cognitive and behavioral changes due to brain injury quite apart from those associated with the secondary seizures. The localization of an epileptogenic focus is also an important determinant of cognitive deficits. For example, temporal lobe epilepsy may be associated with memory defects, and frontal lobe epilepsy may be associated with performance deficits in executive functioning. Behavioral disturbances are most common with complex partial seizures and seizures involving foci in the temporolimbic structures. The age of onset can affect cognitive and behavioral functioning; onset of epilepsy before 5 years of age appears to be a risk factor for a lower intelligence quotient (IQ). Attention-deficit hyperactivity disorder, inattentive type, has been observed to be 2.5 times more common in children younger than 16 years with newly diagnosed unprovoked seizures than in controls. Behavioral symptoms may be more prominent in later-onset seizures. Duration of epilepsy and seizure type and frequency are other factors that affect cognition and behavior. Individuals with generalized tonic-clonic seizures may have greater associated cognitive impairment than that observed in persons with partial seizures, and compared with patients experiencing fewer seizures, those who experience repeated generalized tonic-clonic seizures generally have increased cognitive impairment. A single seizure can be associated with postictal attentional deficits lasting 24 hours or longer. Antiepileptic medications add another level of complexity to management by introducing their associated side effects, which may include impairment of working memory, slowed cognitive processing, language disturbances, and behavioral changes. Anticonvulsants have been reported to be associated with a host of effects on sleep such as insomnia, alterations of sleep architecture, and in some cases, worsening of sleep disordered breathing (barbiturates and benzodiazepines). These may all adversely affect cognition. On the other hand, anticonvulsants may reduce seizure activity, interictal activity, and arousals from sleep, thereby contributing to improved cognitive function.

Cognitive adverse side effects are more prominent in patients receiving polytherapy and have been noted to improve with a switch to monotherapy. It is estimated that more than 60% of patients with epilepsy meet diagnostic criteria for at least one psychiatric disorder during their lifetime. Depression is the most common symptom, occurring with an estimated prevalence of 11% to 44%. The prevalence of psychosis is estimated at between 2% and 8%. Other prominent psychiatric symptoms associated with epilepsy include anxiety, aggression, personality disorders, and panic disorders. Mania is considered rare. When evaluating mood disorder symptoms or psychosis in a patient with epilepsy, it is important to take into account the chronological relationship of the seizures with the symptoms. Conceptually, these symptoms can be classified into peri-ictal or preictal, ictal, postictal, and interictal. Paradoxically, depression or psychosis can follow remission of epilepsy, either after epilepsy surgery or the initiation of effective antiepileptic drug therapy, as part of the phenomenon of forced normalization. Peri-ictal or preictal dysphoric or depressive syndromes frequently precede a seizure. They may last hours to days and resolve with the occurrence of the seizure or persist for hours to days afterward. Peri-ictal depressive symptoms are more common in focal seizures than in generalized seizures. Ictal depressive symptoms occur in approximately 10% of temporal lobe epilepsy patients. Ictal depression is most often characterized by a sudden onset of symptoms independent of external stressors. No associated hemispheric lateralization of the epileptic focus has been clearly demonstrated. Anxiety is the most common ictal

psychiatric symptom, with ictal panic being a mimic for idiopathic panic disorder. Treatment of preictal and ictal depressive symptoms does not usually require antidepressant therapy. Treatment should be directed at reducing the frequency of seizures.

The prevalence of postictal depression has not been established. Patients with poorly controlled simple focal seizures have been reported to have postictal depressive symptoms averaging approximately 37 hours. After a seizure, depressive symptoms have been known to last up to 2 weeks with some reports, suggesting increased suicide risk. Investigation of patients with postictal depression has revealed unilateral frontal or temporal foci without hemispheric predominance. Interictal depression is considered the most common type of depression in epileptic patients. Its estimated prevalence ranges from 20% to 70%, depending on the patient group characteristics. Episodic major depression and dysthymia are common, whereas bipolar affective symptoms are rare. Interictal depressive symptoms are often chronic and less prominent than those with a frank major depressive disorder (MDD), resulting in patients not reporting their symptoms and healthcare providers not recognizing them. Treatment may be required for postictal depressive symptoms and usually is required for interictal depressive symptoms. Treatment should consist of an antidepressant medication and optimized seizure control. SSRIs have a lower risk of associated seizures and should be considered as first-line pharmacotherapy. Electroconvulsive therapy is not contraindicated in patients with epilepsy and should be considered for severe or treatment-refractory depression. The incidence of seizures in epilepsy patients after ECT is not increased compared to that in patients without epilepsy.

Psychosis is a rare primary manifestation of a seizure focus. When present, it is best treated by controlling the ictus and thus by antiepileptic medications. Psychosis may commonly manifest as a postictal phenomenon (representing approximately 25% of all psychosis associated with epilepsy). Diagnostic criteria for postictal psychosis (PIP) include (1) an episode of psychosis emerging within 1 week after the return of normal mental function following a seizure; (2) an episode length between 24 hours and 3 months; and (3) no evidence of EEG-supported nonconvulsive status epilepticus, anticonvulsant toxicity, previous history of interictal psychosis, recent head injury, or alcohol or drug intoxication. PIP may manifest affect-laden symptomatology. Commonly, there is a prompt response to low-dose antipsychotics or benzodiazepines. The annual incidence of PIP among patients who undergo inpatient video EEG monitoring was estimated to be approximately 6%. The prevalence of having experienced PIP among treatment-resistant partial epilepsy outpatients has been reported to be 7%. PIP is most commonly associated with temporal lobe epilepsy. Psychotic symptoms may include auditory, visual, or olfactory hallucinations. Abnormalities of thought content or form may include ideas of reference, paranoia, delusions, grandiosity, religious delusions, thought blocking, tangentiality, or loose associations. Manic symptoms may briefly occur in a minority of patients but are usually not of sufficient duration to meet criteria for a manic episode. In patients with temporal lobe epilepsy and PIP, studies have shown a higher incidence of bilateral cerebral injury or dysfunction, bilateral independent temporal region EEG discharges, and bifrontal and bitemporal hyperperfusion patterns on SPECT. These data suggest that bilateral cerebral abnormalities may be an important feature of PIP.

There has been speculation that PIP may sometimes be caused by complex partial (limbic) status (Elliott et al., 2009). When this is thought to be the case, acute therapy with antiepileptic medications would be advised, possibly in

TABLE 11.1 Testing in Limb Apraxias

	Ideomotor, parietal	Ideomotor, disconnection*	Dissociation*	Ideational*	Conceptual*	Limb-kinetic
Pantomime to verbal command	**Abnormal**[†]	**Abnormal**[†]	**Abnormal**[‡]	Normal[§]	**Abnormal**[‖]	Normal
Imitation of gestures	**Abnormal**[†]	**Abnormal**[†]	Normal	Normal[§]	Normal	Normal[¶]
Gesture knowledge	**Abnormal**	Normal	Normal	Normal	Normal	Normal
Sequential actions	Normal[†]	Normal	**Abnormal**	**Abnormal**	**Abnormal**	Normal
Conceptual knowledge of tool use	Normal	Normal	Normal	**Abnormal**/normal[§]	**Abnormal**	Normal
Limb-kinetic movement	Normal	Normal	Normal	Normal	Normal	**Abnormal**
Real object use	Normal/**abnormal**[#]	Normal/**abnormal**[#]	Normal	Normal/**abnormal**[#]	**Abnormal**[‖]	Normal/**abnormal**[#]

*Callosal apraxia, which is limited to the nondominant limb, can present as disconnection-variant ideomotor apraxia, a dissociative apraxia, or (rarely) a conceptual apraxia.
[†]Spatiotemporal production errors on single, individual ideomotor tasks.
[‡]Unrecognizable movements or attempts.
[§]Errors on performing sequential actions only (i.e., individual actions and their conceptual knowledge are normal).
[‖]Content and tool use errors on individual ideomotor tasks.
[¶]Decreased dexterity in fine finger movements.
[#]Errors depend on severity. In general, errors are worse with verbal commands>imitation>real spontaneous object use and worse for transitive than intransitive actions.

and index finger on each hand. Disturbed meaningless gestures indicate either an inability to apprehend spatial relationships involving the hands and arms in parietal-variant ideomotor apraxia or a basic disturbances in idiokinetic movements (Goldenberg, 2013). Third, for gesture knowledge, the examiner performs the same transitive and intransitive gestures and asks the patient to identify the gesture. The patient must identify the gesture and discriminate between those that are well and poorly performed. Fourth, the patient must perform tasks that require several motor acts in sequence, such as making a sandwich or preparing a letter for mailing. Fifth, the examiner shows the patient pictures of tools or objects or the actual tools or objects themselves. The examiner then requests that the patient pantomime the action associated with the tool or object. Finally, the examiner checks for fine finger movements by asking the patient to do repetitive tapping, picking up a coin with a pincer grasp, and twirling the coin. Additional impairment in the patient's ability to use real objects indicates marked severity of the limb apraxia. The pattern of deficits will determine the types of apraxia (Table 11.1). Specialists in occupational therapy, physical therapy, speech pathology, and neuropsychology can further assess and quantify the deficits in limb apraxia using instruments like the Apraxia Battery for Adults-2, the Florida Apraxia Battery, the Cologne Apraxia Screening, the Test of Upper Limb Apraxia, and others (Dovern et al., 2012; Power et al., 2010; Vanbellingen et al., 2010).

Testing for Ideomotor Apraxia, Parietal and Disconnection Variants

Patients with the ideomotor apraxias cannot pantomime to command or imitate the examiner's gestures. These patients improve only partially with intransitive acts, imitation, and real object use. Ideomotor apraxia results in spatiotemporal

errors in the positioning and orientation of the arm, hand, and fingers to the target and in the timing of the movements, but the goal of the action is still recognizable. In addition to poor positioning of the limb in relation to an imagined object, patients with ideomotor apraxia have an incorrect trajectory of their limb through space owing to poor coordination of multiple joint movements. Patients with ideomotor apraxia also have hesitant, stuttered movements rather than smooth, effortless ones. The difference between parietal variant and disconnection types of ideomotor apraxia is that patients with the disconnection variant can comprehend gestures and pantomimes and discriminate between correctly and incorrectly performed pantomimes.

On attempting to pantomime, patients with ideomotor apraxia may substitute a body part for the tool or object (Raymer et al., 1997). For example, when attempting to pantomime combing their hair or brushing their teeth, they substitute their fingers for the comb or toothbrush. Normal subjects may make the same errors, so the examiner should ask patients not to substitute their fingers or other body parts but to pantomime using a "pretend tool." Patients with ideomotor apraxia may not improve with these instructions and continue to make body-part substitution errors. The persistent substitution of a body part for a tool or object activates the right inferior parietal lobe; hence, patients with ideomotor apraxia with left parietal injury appear to be using their normal right parietal lobe in order to pantomime gestures (Ohgami et al., 2004).

Testing for Dissociation Apraxia

The testing for dissociation apraxia is the same as for ideomotor apraxia. An important feature of dissociation apraxia when attempting to pantomime is the absence of recognizable movements. When asked to pantomime to verbal command, these patients may look at their hands but fail to perform any pertinent actions. Unlike patients with ideomotor apraxia, however, they can imitate the examiner's actions. Given the language–motor disconnection, it is important to evaluate the patient for language disorders and to exclude aphasia. Similar defects in other modalities are possible as well. For example, some patients who are asked to pantomime in response to visual or tactile stimuli may be unable to do so but can correctly pantomime to verbal command.

Testing for Ideational Apraxia

The test for ideational apraxia involves pantomiming multistep sequential tasks to verbal command. Examples are asking the patient to demonstrate how to prepare a letter for mailing or a sandwich for eating. The examiner instructs the patient that the imaginary elements needed for the task are laid out in front of them; the patient is then observed to see whether the correct sequence of events is performed. Ideational apraxia manifests as a failure to perform each step in the correct order. If disturbed, the examiner can repeat this testing with a real object, such as providing the patient with a letter and stamp.

Testing for Conceptual Apraxia

Patients with conceptual apraxia make content errors and demonstrate the actions of tools or objects other than the one they were asked to pantomime. For example, the examiner shows the patient either pictures or the actual tools or objects and asks the patient to pantomime or demonstrate their use or function. Patients with conceptual apraxia pantomime the wrong use or function, but they are able to imitate gestures without spatiotemporal errors (see Table 11.1).

Testing for Limb-Kinetic Apraxia

For limb-kinetic apraxia testing, the examiner asks the patient to perform fine finger movements and looks for evidence of incoordination. For example, the examiner asks the patient to pick up a small coin such as a dime from the table with the thumb and the index finger only. Normally, people use the pincer grasp to pick up a dime by putting a forefinger on one edge of the coin and the thumb on the opposite edge. Patients with limb-kinetic apraxia will have trouble doing this without sliding the coin to the edge of the table or using multiple fingers. Another test involves the patient rotating a nickel between the thumb, index, and middle fingers 10 times as rapidly as they can. Patients with limb-kinetic apraxia are slow and clumsy at these tasks (Hanna-Pladdy et al., 2002). In addition, they may also have disproportionate problems with meaningless gestures.

Testing for Callosal Apraxia

The examination for callosal apraxias is the same as for the other limb apraxias except that the abnormalities are limited to the nondominant hand. The testing for callosal apraxia may reveal a disconnection-variant ideomotor apraxia, a dissociative apraxia, or even a conceptual apraxia in the non-dominant limb (Heilman et al., 1997).

PATHOPHYSIOLOGY OF LIMB APRAXIAS

Ideomotor apraxia is associated with lesions in a variety of structures including the inferior parietal lobe, the frontal lobe, and the premotor areas, particularly the SMA. There are reports of ideomotor apraxia due to subcortical lesions in the basal ganglia (caudate-putamen), thalamus (pulvinar), and associ-ated white-matter tracts including the corpus callosum. Limb apraxias can be caused by any central nervous system disorder that affects these regions. The different forms of limb apraxia result from cerebrovascular lesions, especially left middle cerebral artery strokes with right hemiparesis and apraxia evident in the left upper extremity. Right anterior cerebral artery strokes and paramedian lesions could produce ideomotor apraxia, disconnection variant. Ideomotor apraxia and limb-kinetic apraxia can be the initial or presenting manifestation of disorders such as corticobasal syndrome, primary progressive aphasia, or parietal-variant Alzheimer disease (Rohrer et al., 2010). Tumors, traumatic brain injury, infections, and other pathologies can also lead to limb apraxias.

There are important considerations of hemispheric specialization and handedness on praxis. Early investigators proposed that handedness was related to the hemispheric laterality of the movement formulas. Studies using functional imaging have provided converging evidence that in people who are right-handed, it is the left inferior parietal lobe that appears to store the movement representation needed for learned skilled movements (Muhlau et al., 2005). Left-handed people, however, may demonstrate an ideomotor apraxia from a right hemisphere lesion, because their movement formulas can be stored in their right hemisphere. It is not unusual to see right-handed patients with large left hemisphere lesions who are not apraxic, and there are rare reports of right-handed patients with right hemisphere lesions and limb apraxia. These findings suggest that hand preference is not entirely determined by the laterality of the movement formulas, and praxis and handedness can be dissociated.

REHABILITATION FOR LIMB APRAXIAS

Because many instrumental and routine ADLs depend on learned skilled movements, patients with limb apraxia usually have impaired functional abilities. The presence of limb apraxia, more than any other neuropsychological disorder, correlates with the level of caregiver assistance required six months after a stroke, whereas the absence of apraxia is a significant predictor of return to work after a stroke (Saeki et al., 1995). The treatment of limb apraxia is therefore important for improving the quality of life of the patient.

Even though many apraxia treatments have been studied, none has emerged as the standard. There are no effective pharmacotherapies for limb apraxia, and treatments primarily involve rehabilitation strategies. Buxbaum and associates (2008) surveyed the literature on the rehabilitation of limb apraxia and identified 10 studies with 10 treatment strategies: multiple cues, error type reduction, six-stage task hierarchy, conductive education, strategy training, transitive/intransitive gesture training, rehabilitative treatment, error completion, exploration training, and combined error completion and exploration training. Most of these approaches emphasize cueing with multiple modalities, with verbal, visual, and tactile inputs, repetitive learning, and feedback and correction of errors. Patients with post-stroke apraxia have had generalization of cognitive strategy training to other activities of daily living (Geusgens et al., 2006), but others have not (Bickerton et al., 2006). One novel study uses sensors embedded in household tools and objects to detect apraxic errors and guide rehabilitation (Hughes et al., 2013). In sum, patients can learn and produce new gestures, but the newly learned gestures may not generalize well to contexts outside the rehabilitation setting. Nevertheless, some patients with ideomotor apraxia have improved with gesture-production exercises (Smania et al., 2000), with positive effects lasting two months after completion of gesture training (Smania et al., 2006), and patients with apraxia would benefit from referral to a rehabilitation specialist with experience in treating apraxias (Cantagallo et al., 2012; Dovern et al., 2012).

Additional practical interventions for the management of limb apraxias involve making environmental changes. This includes removing unsafe tools or implements, providing a limited number of tools to select from, replacing complex tasks with simpler ones that require few or no tools and fewer steps, as well as similar modifications.

RELATED DISORDERS

Other movement disturbances may be related to or confused with the limb apraxias. The *alien limb phenomenon*, a potential result of callosal lesions, is the experience that a limb feels foreign and has involuntary semipurposeful movements, such as spontaneous limb levitation. This disorder can occur from neurodegenerative conditions, most notably corticobasal syndrome. *Akinesia* is the inability to initiate a movement in the absence of motor deficits, and *hypokinesia* is a delay in initiating a response. Akinesia and hypokinesia can be directional, with decreased initiation of movement in a specific spatial direction or hemifield. Akinesia and hypokinesia result from a failure to activate the corticospinal system due to Parkinson disease and diseases that affect the frontal lobe cortex, basal ganglia, and thalamus.

Several other movement disturbances are associated with frontal lobe dysfunction. *Motor impersistence* is the inability to sustain a movement or posture and occurs with dorsolateral frontal lesions. *Magnetic grasp and grope reflexes* with automatic reaching for environmental stimuli are primitive release signs. In *echopraxia*, some patients automatically imitate observed movements. Along with utilization behavior, echopraxia may be part of the environmental dependency syndrome of some patients with frontal lesions. *Catalepsy* is the maintenance of a body position into which patients are placed (waxy flexibility). Two related terms are *mitgehen* ("going with"), where patients allow a body part to move in response to light pressure, and *mitmachen* ("doing with"), where patients allow a body part to be put into any position in response to slight pressure, then return the body part to the original resting position after the examiner releases it. *Motor perseveration* is the inability to stop a movement or a series of movements after the task is complete. In recurrent motor perseveration, the patient keeps returning to a prior completed motor program, and in afferent or continuous motor perseveration, the patient cannot end a motor program that has just been completed.

SUMMARY

Limb apraxia, or the disturbance of learned skilled movements, is an important but often missed or unrecognized impairment. Clinicians may misattribute limb apraxia to weakness, hemiparesis, clumsiness, or other motor, sensory, spatial, or cognitive disturbance. Apraxia may only be evident on fine, sequential, or specific movements of the upper extremities and requires a systematic praxis examination (Zadikoff and Lang, 2005). Apraxia is an important cognitive disturbance and a salient sign in patients with strokes, Alzheimer disease, corticobasal syndrome, and other conditions. The model of left parietal movement formulas and disconnection syndromes introduced by Liepmann over 100 years ago continues to be compelling today. This model, in the context of a dedicated apraxia examination and analysis for spatiotemporal or content errors, clarifies and classifies the limb apraxias. Although more effective treatments need to be developed, rehabilitation strategies can be helpful interventions for these disturbances. Fortunately, recent advances in technology and rehabilitation continue to enhance our understanding and management of the limb apraxias.

REFERENCES

The complete reference list is available online at https://expertconsult .inkling.com/.

12 Agnosias

Howard S. Kirshner

CHAPTER OUTLINE

VISUAL AGNOSIAS
   Cortical Visual Disturbances
   Cortical Visual Distortions
   Balint Syndrome and Simultanagnosia
   Visual Object Agnosia
   Optic Aphasia
   Prosopagnosia
   Klüver-Bucy Syndrome
AUDITORY AGNOSIAS
   Cortical Deafness
   Pure Word Deafness
   Auditory Nonverbal Agnosia
   Phonagnosia
   Amusia
TACTILE AGNOSIAS
   Tactile Aphasia
SUMMARY

Agnosias are disorders of recognition. The general public is familiar with agnosia from Oliver Sacks' patient, who not only failed to recognize his wife's face but also mistook it for a hat. Sigmund Freud originally introduced the term *agnosia* in 1891 to denote disturbances in the ability to recognize and name objects, usually in one sensory modality, in the presence of intact primary sensation. Another definition, that of Milner and Teuber in 1968, referred to agnosia as a "normal percept stripped of its meaning." The agnosic patient can perceive and describe sensory features of an object yet cannot recognize or identify the object.

Criteria for the diagnosis of agnosia include: (1) failure to recognize an object; (2) normal perception of the object, excluding an elementary sensory disorder; (3) ability to name the object once it is recognized, excluding anomia as the principal deficit; and (4) absence of a generalized dementia. In addition, agnosias usually affect only one sensory modality, and the patient can identify the same object when presented in a different sensory modality. For example, a patient with visual agnosia may fail to identify a bell by sight but readily identifies it by touch or by the sound of its ring.

Agnosias are defined in terms of the specific sensory modality affected—usually visual, auditory, or tactile—or they may be selective for one class of items within a sensory modality, such as color agnosia or prosopagnosia (agnosia for faces). To diagnose agnosia, the examiner must establish that the deficit is not a primary sensory disorder, as documented by tests of visual acuity, visual fields, auditory function, and somatosensory functions, and not part of a more general cognitive disorder such as aphasia or dementia, as established by the bedside mental status examination. Naming deficits in aphasia or dementia are, with rare exceptions, not restricted to a single sensory modality.

Clinically, agnosias seem complex and arcane, yet they are important in understanding the behavior of neurological patients, and they provide fascinating insights into brain mechanisms related to perception and recognition. Part of their complexity derives from the underlying neuropathology; agnosias frequently result from bilateral or diffuse lesions such as hypoxic encephalopathy, multiple strokes, and major head injuries, and agnosic phenomena also play a role in neurodegenerative disorders and dementias, despite the definitions earlier.

Agnosias have aroused controversies since their earliest descriptions. Some authorities have attributed agnosic deficits to primary perceptual loss in the setting of general cognitive dysfunction or dementia. Abundant case studies, however, argue in favor of true agnosic deficits. In each sensory modality, a spectrum of disorders can be traced from primary sensory dysfunction to agnosia. We approach agnosias by sensory modality, with progression from primary sensory deficits to disorders of recognition.

VISUAL AGNOSIAS
Cortical Visual Disturbances

Patients with bilateral occipital lobe damage may have complete "cortical" blindness. Some patients with cortical blindness are unaware that they cannot see, and some even confabulate visual descriptions or blame their poor vision on dim lighting or not having their glasses (Anton syndrome, originally described in 1899). Patients with Anton syndrome may describe objects they "see" in the room around them but walk immediately into a wall. The phenomena of this syndrome suggest that the thinking and speaking areas of the brain are not consciously aware of the lack of input from visual centers. Anton syndrome can still be thought of as a perceptual deficit rather than a visual agnosia, but one in which there is unawareness or neglect of the sensory deficit. Such visual unawareness is also frequently seen with hemianopic visual field defects (e.g., in patients with R hemisphere strokes), and it even has a correlate in normal people; we are not conscious of a visual field defect behind our heads, yet we know to turn when we hear a noise from behind. In contrast to Anton syndrome, some cortically blind patients actually have preserved ability to react to visual stimuli, despite the lack of any conscious visual perception, a phenomenon termed *blindsight* or *inverse Anton syndrome* (Leopold, 2012; Ro and Rafal, 2006). Blindsight may be considered an agnosic deficit, because the patient fails to recognize what he or she sees. Residual vision is usually absent in blindness caused by disorders of the eyes, optic nerves, or optic tracts. Patients with cortical vision loss may react to more elementary visual stimuli such as brightness, size, and movement, whereas they cannot perceive finer attributes such as shape, color, and depth. Subjects sometimes look toward objects they cannot consciously see. One study reported a woman with postanoxic cortical blindness who could catch a ball without awareness of seeing it. Blindsight may be mediated by subcortical connections such as those from the optic tracts to the midbrain.

Lesions causing cortical blindness may also be accompanied by visual hallucinations. Irritative lesions of the visual

specific to word classes. Proper names of persons are often affected severely. The examiner should ask questions to be sure that the patient recognizes the items or people that he or she cannot name.

Auditory comprehension is tested first by asking the patient to follow a series of commands of one, two, and three steps. An example of a one-step command is "stick out your tongue"; a two-step command is "hold up your left thumb and close your eyes." Successful following of commands ensures adequate comprehension, at least at this simple level, but failure to follow commands does not automatically establish a loss of comprehension. The patient must hear the command, understand the language the examiner speaks, and possess the motor ability to execute it, including the absence of apraxia. *Apraxia* (see Chapter 11 for full discussion) is defined operationally as the inability to carry out a motor command despite normal comprehension and normal ability to carry out the motor act in another context, such as to imitation or with use of a real object. Because apraxia is difficult to exclude with confidence, it is advisable to test comprehension by tasks that do not require a motor act, such as yes-no questions, or by commands that require only a pointing response. The responses to nonsense questions (e.g., "Do you vomit every day?") quickly establish whether the patient comprehends. Nonsense questions often produce surprising results, given the tendency of some aphasics to cover up comprehension difficulty with social chatter.

Repetition of words and phrases should be deliberately tested. Dysarthric patients have difficulty with rapid sequences of consonants, such as "Methodist Episcopal," whereas aphasics have special difficulty with grammatically complex sentences. The phrase "no ifs, ands, or buts" is especially challenging for aphasics. Often, aphasics can repeat familiar or "high-probability" phrases much better than unfamiliar ones.

Reading should be tested both aloud and for comprehension. The examiner should carry a few printed commands to facilitate a rapid comparison of auditory to reading comprehension. Of course, the examiner must have some idea of the patient's premorbid reading ability.

Writing, the element of the bedside examination most often omitted, not only provides a further sample of expressive language but also allows an analysis of spelling, which is not possible with spoken language. A writing specimen may be the most sensitive indicator of mild aphasia, and it provides a permanent record for future comparison. Spontaneous writing, such as a sentence describing why the patient has come for examination, is especially sensitive for the detection of language difficulty. When spontaneous writing fails, writing to dictation and copying should be tested as well.

Finally, the neurologist combines the results of the bedside language examination with those of the rest of the mental status examination and of the neurological examination in general. These "associated signs" help to classify the type of aphasia and to localize the responsible brain lesion.

DIFFERENTIAL DIAGNOSIS OF APHASIC SYNDROMES
Broca Aphasia

In 1861, the French physician Paul Broca described two patients, establishing the aphasia syndrome that now bears his name. The speech pattern is nonfluent; on bedside examination, the patient speaks hesitantly, often producing the principal, meaning-containing nouns and verbs but omitting small grammatical words and morphemes. This pattern is called *agrammatism* or telegraphic speech. An example is "wife come hospital." Patients with acute Broca aphasia may be

mute or may produce only single words, often with dysarthria and apraxia of speech. They make many phonemic errors, inconsistent from utterance to utterance, with substitution of phonemes usually differing only slightly from the correct target (e.g., p for b). Naming is deficient, but the patient often manifests a "tip of the tongue" phenomenon, getting out the first letter or phoneme of the correct name. Paraphasic errors in naming are more frequently of literal than verbal type. Auditory comprehension seems intact, but detailed testing usually reveals some deficiency, particularly in the comprehension of complex syntax. For example, sentences with embedded clauses involving prepositional relationships cause difficulty for Broca aphasics in comprehension as well as in expression ("The rug that Bill gave to Betty tripped the visitor"). A recent PET study in normals (Caplan et al., 1998) showed activation of the Broca area in the frontal cortex during tests of syntactic comprehension. Repetition is hesitant in these patients, resembling their spontaneous speech. Reading is often impaired despite relatively preserved auditory comprehension. Benson termed this reading difficulty of Broca aphasics the "third alexia," in distinction to the two classical types of alexia (see Aphasic Alexia, later in this chapter). Patients with Broca aphasia may have difficulty with syntax in reading, just as in auditory comprehension and speech. Writing is virtually always deficient in Broca aphasics. Most patients have a right hemiparesis, necessitating use of the nondominant, left hand for writing, but this left-handed writing is far more abnormal than the awkward renditions of a normal right-handed subject. Many patients can scrawl only a few letters.

Associated neurological deficits of Broca aphasia include right hemiparesis, hemisensory loss, and apraxia of the oral apparatus and the nonparalyzed left limbs. Apraxia in response to motor commands is important to recognize because it may be mistaken for comprehension disturbance. Comprehension should be tested by responses to yes-no questions or commands to point to an object. The common features of Broca aphasia are listed in Table 13.1.

An important clinical feature of Broca aphasia is its frequent association with depression (Robinson 1997). Patients with Broca aphasia are typically aware of and frustrated by their deficits. At times they become withdrawn and refuse help or therapy. Usually, the depression lifts as the deficit recovers, but it may be a limiting factor in rehabilitation.

The lesions responsible for Broca aphasia usually include the traditional Broca area in the posterior part of the inferior frontal gyrus, along with damage to adjacent cortex and subcortical white matter. Most patients with lasting Broca aphasia, including Broca's original cases, have much larger

TABLE 13.1 Bedside Features of Broca Aphasia

Feature	Syndrome
Spontaneous speech	Nonfluent, mute, or telegraphic, usually dysarthric
Naming	Impaired
Comprehension	Intact (mild difficulty with complex grammatical phrases)
Repetition	Impaired
Reading	Often impaired ("third alexia")
Writing	Impaired (dysmorphic, dysgrammatical)
Associated signs	Right hemiparesis Right hemisensory loss ± Apraxia of left limbs

left frontoparietal lesions, including most of the territory of the upper division of the left middle cerebral artery. Such patients typically evolve from global to Broca aphasia over weeks to months. Patients who manifest Broca aphasia immediately after their strokes, by contrast, have smaller lesions of the inferior frontal region, and their deficits generally resolve quickly. In computed tomography (CT) scan analyses at the Boston Veterans Administration Medical Center, lesions restricted to the lower precentral gyrus produced only dysarthria and mild expressive disturbance. Lesions involving the traditional Broca area (Brodmann areas 44 and 45) resulted in difficulty initiating speech, and lesions combining Broca area, the lower precentral gyrus, and subcortical white matter yielded the full syndrome of Broca aphasia. In studies by the same group, damage to two subcortical white matter sites—the rostral subcallosal fasciculus deep to the Broca area and the periventricular white matter adjacent to the body of the left lateral ventricle—were required to cause permanent nonfluency. Figure 13.3 shows a magnetic resonance imaging (MRI) scan from a case of Broca aphasia.

Aphemia

A rare variant of Broca aphasia is *aphemia*, a nonfluent syndrome in which the patient is initially mute and then able to speak with phoneme substitutions and pauses. All other language functions are intact, including writing. This rare and usually transitory syndrome results from small lesions of the Broca area or its subcortical white matter or of the inferior precentral gyrus. Because written expression and auditory comprehension are normal, aphemia is not a true language disorder; aphemia may be equivalent to pure apraxia of speech.

Wernicke Aphasia

Wernicke aphasia may be considered a syndrome opposite to Broca aphasia, in that expressive speech is fluent but comprehension is impaired. The speech pattern is effortless and sometimes even excessively fluent (logorrhea). A speaker of a foreign language would notice nothing amiss, but a listener who shares the patient's language detects speech empty of meaning, containing verbal paraphasias, neologisms, and jargon productions. Neurolinguists refer to this pattern as *paragrammatism*. In milder cases, the intended meaning of an utterance may be discerned, but the sentence goes awry with paraphasic substitutions. Naming in Wernicke aphasia is deficient, often with bizarre, paraphasic substitutions for the correct name. Auditory comprehension is impaired, sometimes even for simple nonsense questions. Deficient semantics is the major cause of the comprehension disturbance in Wernicke aphasia, along with disturbed access to the internal lexicon. Repetition is impaired; whispering a phrase in the patient's ear, as in a hearing test, may help cue the patient to attempt repetition. Reading comprehension is usually affected similarly to auditory comprehension, but occasional patients show greater deficit in one modality versus the other. The discovery of spared reading ability in Wernicke aphasics is important in allowing these patients to communicate. In addition, neurolinguistic theories of reading must include access of visual language images to semantic interpretation, even in the absence of auditory comprehension. Writing is also impaired, but in a manner quite different from that of Broca aphasia. The patient usually has no hemiparesis and can grasp the pen and write easily. Written productions are even more abnormal than oral ones, however, in that spelling errors are also evident. Writing samples are especially useful in the detection of mild Wernicke aphasia.

Associated signs are limited in Wernicke aphasia; most patients have no elementary motor or sensory deficits, although a partial or complete right homonymous hemianopia may be present. The characteristic bedside examination findings in Wernicke aphasia are summarized in Table 13.2.

The psychiatric manifestations of Wernicke aphasia are quite different from those of Broca aphasia. Depression is less common; many Wernicke aphasics seem unaware of or unconcerned about their communicative deficits. With time, some patients become angry or paranoid about the inability of family members and medical staff to understand them. This behavior, like depression, may hinder rehabilitative efforts.

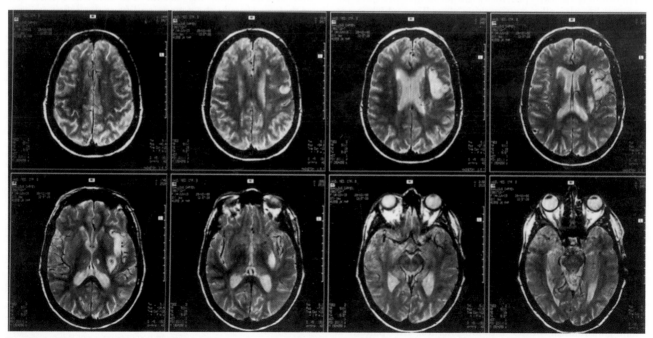

Fig. 13.3 Magnetic resonance imaging scan from a patient with Broca aphasia. In this patient, the cortical Broca area, subcortical white matter, and the insula were all involved in the infarction. The patient made a good recovery.

TABLE 13.2 Bedside Features of Wernicke Aphasia

Feature	Syndrome
Spontaneous speech	Fluent, with paraphasic errors Usually not dysarthric Sometimes logorrheic
Naming	Impaired (often bizarre paraphasic misnaming)
Comprehension	Impaired
Repetition	Impaired
Reading	Impaired for comprehension, reading aloud
Writing	Well-formed, paragraphic
Associated signs	± Right hemianopia Motor, sensory signs usually absent

The lesions of patients with Wernicke aphasia usually involve the posterior portion of the superior temporal gyrus, sometimes extending into the inferior parietal lobule. Figure 13.4 shows a typical example. The exact confines of the Wernicke area have been much debated. Damage to the Wernicke area (Brodmann area 22) has been reported to correlate most closely with persistent loss of comprehension of single words, although others (Kertesz et al., 1993) have found only larger temporoparietal lesions in patients with lasting Wernicke aphasia. In the acute phase, the ability to match a spoken word to a picture is quantitatively related to decreased perfusion of the Wernicke area on perfusion-weighted MRI, indicating less variability during the acute phase than after recovery has taken place (Hillis et al., 2001). Electrical stimulation of the Wernicke area produces consistent interruption of auditory comprehension, supporting the importance of this region for decoding auditory language. A receptive speech area in the left inferior temporal gyrus has also been suggested by electrical stimulation studies and by a few descriptions of patients with seizures involving this area (Kirshner et al., 1995), but aphasia has not been recognized with destructive lesions of this area. Extension of the lesion into the inferior parietal region may predict greater involvement of reading comprehension. In terms of vascular anatomy, the Wernicke area lies within the territory of the inferior division of the left middle cerebral artery.

Pure Word Deafness

Pure word deafness is a rare but striking syndrome of isolated loss of auditory comprehension and repetition, without any abnormality of speech, naming, reading, or writing. Hearing for pure tones and for nonverbal noises, such as animal cries, is intact. Most cases have mild aphasic deficits, especially paraphasic speech. Classically, the anatomical substrate is a bilateral lesion, isolating Wernicke's area from input from the primary auditory cortex, in the bilateral Heschl's gyri. Pure word deafness is thus an example of a "disconnection syndrome," in which the deficit results from loss of white matter connections rather than of gray matter language centers. Some cases of pure word deafness, however, have unilateral, left temporal lesions. These cases closely resemble Wernicke aphasia with greater impairment of auditory comprehension than of reading.

Global Aphasia

Global aphasia may be thought of as a summation of the deficits of Broca aphasia and Wernicke aphasia. Speech is nonfluent or mute, but comprehension is also poor, as are naming, repetition, reading, and writing. Most patients have dense right hemiparesis, hemisensory loss, and often hemianopia, although occasional patients have little hemiparesis. Milder aphasic syndromes in which all modalities of language are affected are often called *mixed aphasias*. The lesions of patients with global aphasia are usually large, involving both the inferior frontal and superior temporal regions, and often much of the parietal lobe in between. This lesion represents most of the territory of the left middle cerebral artery. Patients in whom the superior temporal gyrus is spared tend to recover their auditory comprehension and to evolve toward the syndrome of Broca aphasia. Recovery in global aphasia may be prolonged; global aphasics may recover more during the second 6 months than during the first 6 months after a stroke. Characteristics of global aphasia are presented in Table 13.3.

Conduction Aphasia

Conduction aphasia is an uncommon but theoretically important syndrome that can be remembered by its striking deficit of repetition. Most patients have relatively normal spontaneous speech, although some make literal paraphasic errors and hesitate frequently for self-correction. Naming may be impaired, but auditory comprehension is preserved. Repetition may be disturbed to seemingly ridiculous extremes, such that a patient who can express himself at a sentence level and comprehend conversation may be unable to repeat even single words. One such patient could not repeat the word "boy" but said "I like girls better." Reading and writing are somewhat variable, but reading aloud may share some of the same difficulty as repeating. Associated deficits include hemianopia in some patients; right-sided sensory loss may be present, but right hemiparesis is usually mild or absent. Some patients have limb apraxia, creating a misimpression that comprehension is impaired. Bedside examination findings in conduction aphasia are summarized in Table 13.4.

The lesions of conduction aphasia usually involve either the superior temporal or inferior parietal regions. Benson and associates suggested that patients with limb apraxia have parietal lesions, whereas those without apraxia have temporal lesions (Benson et al., 1973). Conduction aphasia may represent a stage of recovery in patients with Wernicke aphasia in whom the damage to the superior temporal gyrus is not complete.

Conduction aphasia has been advanced as a classical disconnection syndrome. Wernicke originally postulated that a lesion disconnecting the Wernicke and Broca areas would produce this syndrome; Geschwind later pointed to the arcuate fasciculus, a white matter tract traveling from the deep temporal lobe, around the sylvian fissure to the frontal lobe, as the site of disconnection. Anatomical involvement of the arcuate fasciculus is present in most, if not all, cases of conduction aphasia, but some doubt has been raised about the importance of the arcuate fasciculus to conduction aphasia or even to repetition (Bernal and Ardila, 2009). In cases of conduction aphasia, there is usually also cortical involvement of the supramarginal gyrus or temporal lobe. The supramarginal gyrus appears to be involved in auditory immediate memory and in phoneme perception related to word meaning, as well as phoneme generation (Hickok and Poeppel, 2000). Lesions in this area are associated with conduction aphasia and phonemic paraphasic errors. Others have pointed out that lesions of the arcuate fasciculus do not always produce conduction aphasia. Another theory of conduction aphasia has involved a defect in auditory verbal

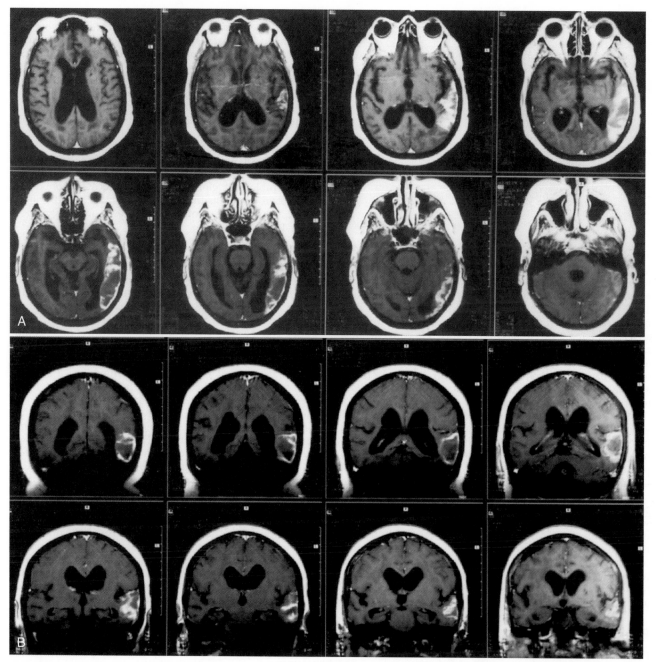

Fig. 13.4 Axial and coronal magnetic resonance imaging slices **(A and B)**, and an axial positron emission tomographic (PET) scan view **(C)** of an elderly woman with Wernicke aphasia. There is a large left superior temporal lobe lesion. The onset of the deficit was not clear, and the PET scan was useful in showing that the lesion had reduced metabolism, favoring a stroke over a tumor.

short-term (or what most neurologists would call immediate) memory.

Anomic Aphasia

Anomic aphasia refers to aphasic syndromes in which naming, or access to the internal lexicon, is the principal deficit. Spontaneous speech is normal except for the pauses and circumlocutions produced by the inability to name. Comprehension, repetition, reading, and writing are intact, except for the same word-finding difficulty in written productions. Anomic aphasia is common but less specific in localization than other aphasic syndromes. Isolated, severe anomia may indicate focal

left hemisphere pathology. Alexander and Benson (1997) refer to the angular gyrus as the site of lesions producing anomic aphasia, but lesions there usually produce other deficits as well, including alexia and the four elements of Gerstmann syndrome: agraphia, right-left disorientation, acalculia, and finger agnosia, or inability to identify fingers. Isolated lesions of the temporal lobe can produce pure anomia, and positron emission tomography (PET) studies of naming in normal subjects have also shown consistent activation of the superior temporal lobe. Inability to produce nouns is characteristic of temporal lobe lesions, whereas inability to produce verbs occurs more with frontal lesions (Damasio, 1992). Even specific classes of nouns may be selectively affected in some

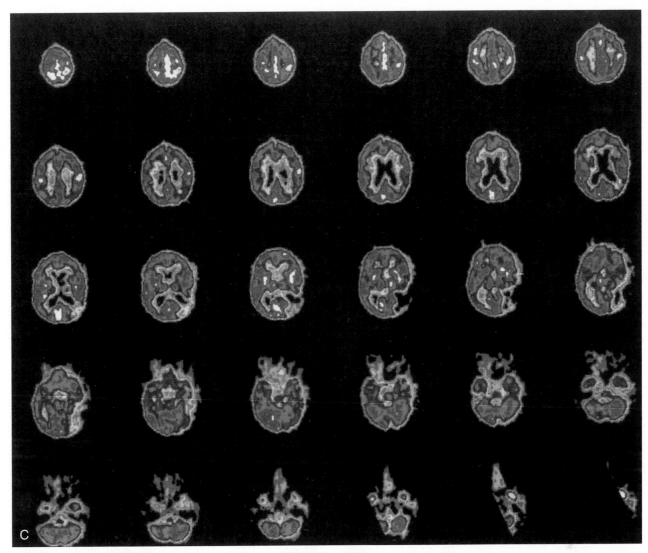

Fig. 13.4, cont'd

TABLE 13.3 Bedside Features of Global Aphasia

Feature	Syndrome
Spontaneous speech	Mute or nonfluent
Naming	Impaired
Comprehension	Impaired
Repetition	Impaired
Reading	Impaired
Writing	Impaired
Associated signs	Right hemiparesis Right hemisensory loss Right hemianopia

TABLE 13.4 Bedside Features of Conduction Aphasia

Feature	Syndrome
Spontaneous speech	Fluent, some hesitancy, literal paraphasic errors
Naming	May be moderately impaired
Comprehension	Intact
Repetition	Severely impaired
Reading	+ Inability to read aloud; some reading comprehension
Writing	Variable deficits
Associated signs	+ Apraxia of left limbs + Right hemiparesis, usually mild + Right hemisensory loss + Right hemianopia

cases of anomic aphasia. Anomia is also seen with mass lesions elsewhere in the brain, and in diffuse degenerative disorders, such as Alzheimer disease. Anomic aphasia is also a common stage in the recovery of many aphasic syndromes. Anomic aphasia thus serves as an indicator of left hemisphere or diffuse brain disease, but it has only limited localizing value. The typical features of anomic aphasia are presented in Table 13.5.

Transcortical Aphasias

The transcortical aphasias are syndromes in which repetition is normal, presumably because the causative lesions do not disrupt the perisylvian language circuit from the Wernicke area through the arcuate fasciculus to the Broca area. Instead, these

TABLE 13.5 Bedside Features of Anomic Aphasia

Feature	Syndrome
Spontaneous speech	Fluent, some word-finding pauses, circumlocution
Naming	Impaired
Comprehension	Intact
Repetition	Intact
Reading	Intact
Writing	Intact, except for anomia
Associated signs	Variable or none

TABLE 13.6 Bedside Features of Transcortical Aphasias

Feature	Isolation syndrome	Transcortical motor	Transcortical sensory
Speech	Nonfluent, echolalic	Nonfluent	Fluent, echolalic
Naming	Impaired	Impaired	Impaired
Comprehension	Impaired	Intact	Impaired
Repetition	Intact	Intact	Intact
Reading	Impaired	+ Intact	Impaired
Writing	Impaired	+ Intact	Impaired

lesions disrupt connections from other cortical centers into the language circuit (hence the name "transcortical"). The transcortical syndromes are easiest to think of as analogues of the syndromes of global, Broca, and Wernicke aphasias, with intact repetition.

Mixed transcortical aphasia, or the syndrome of the isolation of the speech area, is a global aphasia in which the patient repeats, often echolalically, but has no propositional speech or comprehension. This syndrome is rare, occurring predominantly in large, watershed infarctions of the left hemisphere or both hemispheres that spare the perisylvian cortex, or in advanced dementias.

Transcortical motor aphasia is an analogue of Broca aphasia in which speech is hesitant or telegraphic, comprehension is relatively spared, but repetition is fluent. This syndrome occurs with lesions in the frontal lobe, anterior to the Broca area, in the deep frontal white matter, or in the medial frontal region, in the vicinity of the supplementary motor area. All of these lesion sites are within the territory of the anterior cerebral artery, separating this syndrome from the aphasia syndromes of the middle cerebral artery (Broca, Wernicke, global, and conduction).

The third transcortical syndrome, transcortical sensory aphasia, is an analogue of Wernicke aphasia in which fluent, paraphasic speech, paraphasic naming, impaired auditory and reading comprehension, and abnormal writing coexist with normal repetition. This syndrome is relatively uncommon, occurring in strokes of the left temporo-occipital area and in dementias. Bedside examination findings in the transcortical aphasias are summarized in Table 13.6.

Subcortical Aphasias

A current area of interest in aphasia research involves the "subcortical" aphasias. Although all the syndromes discussed so far are defined by behavioral characteristics that can be diagnosed on the bedside examination, the subcortical aphasias are defined by lesion localization in the basal ganglia or deep cerebral white matter. As knowledge about subcortical aphasia has accumulated, two major groups of aphasic symptomatology have been described: aphasia with thalamic lesions and aphasia with lesions of the subcortical white matter and basal ganglia.

Left thalamic hemorrhages frequently produce a Wernicke-like fluent aphasia, with better comprehension than cortical Wernicke aphasia. A fluctuating or "dichotomous" state has been described, alternating between an alert state with nearly normal language and a drowsy state in which the patient mumbles paraphasically and comprehends poorly. Luria has called this a quasi-aphasic abnormality of vigilance, in that the thalamus plays a role in alerting the language cortex. Thalamic aphasia can occur even with a right thalamic lesion in a left-handed patient, indicating that hemispheric language dominance extends to the thalamic level (Kirshner and Kistler, 1982). Whereas some skeptics have attributed thalamic aphasia to pressure on adjacent structures and secondary effects on the cortex, cases of thalamic aphasia have been described with small ischemic lesions, especially those involving the paramedian or anterior nuclei of the thalamus, in the territory of the tuberothalamic artery. Because these lesions produce little or no mass effect, such cases indicate that the thalamus and its connections play a definite role in language function (Carrerra and Bogousslavsky, 2006).

Lesions of the left basal ganglia and deep white matter also cause aphasia. As in thalamic aphasia, the first syndromes described were in basal ganglia hemorrhages, especially those involving the putamen, the most common site of hypertensive intracerebral hemorrhage. Here the aphasic syndromes are more variable but most commonly involve global or Wernicke-like aphasia. As in thalamic lesions, ischemic strokes have provided better localizing information. The most common lesion is an infarct involving the anterior putamen, caudate nucleus, and anterior limb of the internal capsule. Patients with this lesion have an "anterior subcortical aphasia syndrome" involving dysarthria, decreased fluency, mildly impaired repetition, and mild comprehension disturbance (Mega and Alexander, 1994). This syndrome most closely resembles Broca aphasia, but with greater dysarthria and less language dysfunction. Figure 13.5 shows an example of this syndrome. More restricted lesions of the anterior putamen, head of caudate, and periventricular white matter produce hesitancy or slow initiation of speech but little true language disturbance. More posterior lesions involving the putamen and deep temporal white matter, referred to as the *temporal isthmus*, are associated with fluent, paraphasic speech and impaired comprehension resembling Wernicke aphasia (Naeser et al., 1990). Small lesions in the posterior limb of the internal capsule and adjacent putamen cause mainly dysarthria, but mild aphasic deficits may occasionally occur. Finally, larger subcortical lesions involving both the anterior and posterior lesion sites produce global aphasia. A wide variety of aphasia syndromes can thus be seen with subcortical lesion sites. Nadeau and Crosson (1997) presented an anatomical model of basal ganglia involvement in speech and language, based on the known motor functions and fiber connections of these structures. Evidence from PET indicates that basal ganglia lesions affect language, both directly and indirectly, via decreased activation of cortical language areas.

The insula, a cortical structure that shares a deep location with the subcortical structures, may also be important to speech and language function. Dronkers (1996) reported that involvement of this area is closely associated with the presence of apraxia of speech in aphasic patients. Hillis and colleagues (2004), however, in MRI studies of acute stroke patients,

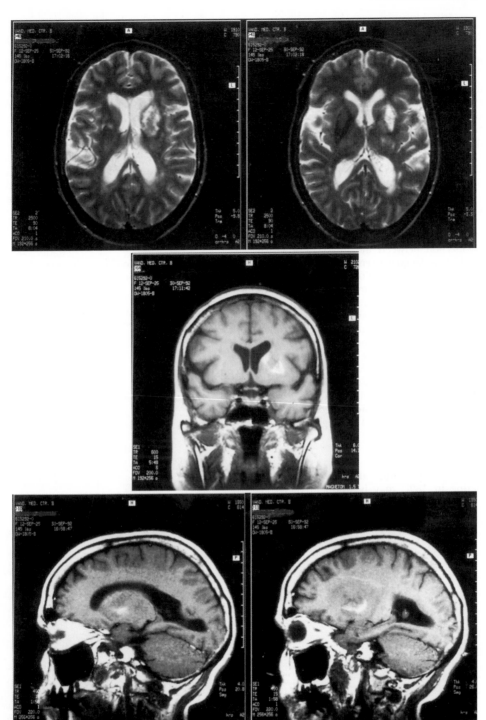

Fig. 13.5 Magnetic resonance imaging (MRI) scan slices in the axial, coronal, and sagittal planes from a patient with subcortical aphasia. The lesion is an infarction involving the anterior caudate, putamen, and anterior limb of the left internal capsule. The patient presented with dysarthria and mild, nonfluent aphasia with anomia, with good comprehension. The advantage of MRI in permitting visualization of the lesion in all three planes is apparent.

found that the left frontal cortex correlates more with speech apraxia than the insula.

In clinical terms, subcortical lesions do produce aphasia, although less commonly than cortical lesions do, and the language characteristics of subcortical aphasias are often atypical. The presentation of a difficult-to-classify aphasic syndrome, in the presence of dysarthria and right hemiparesis, should lead to suspicion of a subcortical lesion.

Pure Alexia without Agraphia

Alexia, or acquired inability to read, is a form of aphasia, according to the definition given at the beginning of this chapter. The classic syndrome of alexia, pure alexia without agraphia, was described by the French neurologist Dejerine in 1892. This syndrome may be thought of as a linguistic blindfolding: patients can write but cannot read their own writing.

On bedside examination, speech, auditory comprehension, and repetition are normal. Naming may be deficient, especially for colors.

Patients initially cannot read at all; as they recover, they learn to read letter by letter, spelling out words laboriously. They cannot read words at a glance, as normal readers do. By contrast, they quickly understand words spelled orally to them, and they can spell normally. Some patients can match words to pictures, indicating that some subconscious awareness of the word is present, perhaps in the right hemisphere. Associated deficits include a right hemianopia or right upper quadrant defect in nearly all patients and, frequently, a deficit of short-term memory. There is usually no hemiparesis or sensory loss.

The causative lesion in pure alexia is nearly always a stroke in the territory of the left posterior cerebral artery, with infarction of the medial occipital lobe, often the splenium of the corpus callosum, and often the medial temporal lobe. Dejerine postulated a disconnection between the intact right visual cortex and left hemisphere language centers, particularly the angular gyrus. (Figure 13.6 is an adaptation of Dejerine's original diagram.) Geschwind later rediscovered this disconnection hypothesis. Although Damasio and Damasio (1983) found splenial involvement in only two of 16 cases, they postulated a disconnection within the deep white matter of the left occipital lobe. As in the disconnection hypothesis for conduction aphasia, the theory fails to explain all the behavioral phenomena, such as the sparing of single letters. A deficit in short-term memory for visual language elements, or an inability to perceive multiple letters at once (simultanagnosia), can also explain many features of the syndrome. Typical findings of pure alexia without agraphia are presented in Table 13.7 (Fig. 13.7).

Alexia with Agraphia

The second classic alexia syndrome, alexia with agraphia, described by Dejerine in 1891, may be thought of as an acquired illiteracy, in which a previously educated patient is rendered unable to read or write. The oral language modalities of speech, naming, auditory comprehension, and repetition are largely intact, but many cases manifest a fluent, paraphasic speech pattern with impaired naming. This syndrome thus overlaps Wernicke aphasia, especially in cases in which reading is more impaired than auditory comprehension. Associated deficits include right hemianopia and elements of Gerstmann syndrome: agraphia, acalculia, right-left disorientation, and finger agnosia. The lesions typically involve the inferior parietal lobule, especially the angular gyrus. Etiologies include strokes in the territory of the angular branch of the left middle cerebral artery or mass lesions in the same region. Characteristic features of the syndrome of alexia with agraphia are summarized in Table 13.8.

Aphasic Alexia

In addition to the two classic alexia syndromes, many patients with aphasia have associated reading disturbance. Examples

TABLE 13.7 Bedside Features of Pure Alexia without Agraphia

Feature	Syndrome
Spontaneous speech	Intact
Naming	+ Impaired, especially colors
Comprehension	Intact
Repetition	Intact
Reading	Impaired (some sparing of single letters)
Writing	Intact
Associated signs	Right hemianopia or superior quadrantanopia Short-term memory loss Motor, sensory signs usually absent

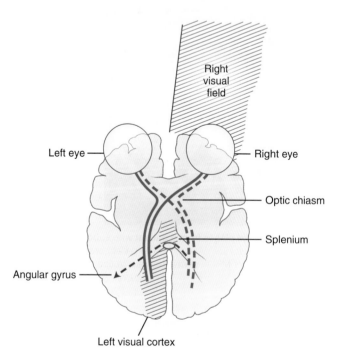

Fig. 13.6 Horizontal brain diagram of pure alexia without agraphia, adapted from that of Dejerine in 1892. Visual information from the left visual field reaches the right occipital cortex but is "disconnected" from the left hemisphere language centers by the lesion in the splenium of the corpus callosum.

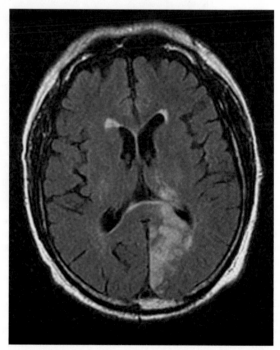

Fig. 13.7 FLAIR MRI image of an 82-year-old male patient with alexia without agraphia. The infarction involves the medial occipital lobe and the splenium of the corpus callosum, within the territory of the left posterior cerebral artery.

TABLE 13.8 Bedside Features of Alexia with Agraphia

Feature	Syndrome
Spontaneous speech	Fluent, often some paraphasia
Naming	+ Impaired
Comprehension	Intact, or less impaired than reading
Repetition	Intact
Reading	Severely impaired
Writing	Severely impaired
Associated signs	Right hemianopia Motor, sensory signs often absent

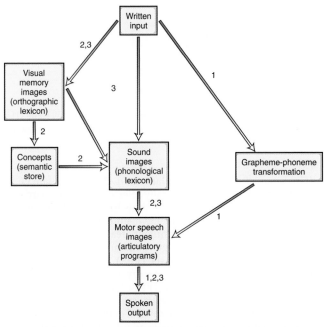

Fig. 13.8 Neurolinguistic model of the reading process. According to evidence from the alexias, there are three separate routes to reading: 1 is the phonological (or grapheme-phoneme conversion) route; 2 is the semantic (or lexical-semantic-phonological) route; and 3 is the nonlexical phonological route. In deep dyslexia, only route 2 can operate; in phonological dyslexia, 3 is the principal pathway; in surface dyslexia, only 1 is functional. *(Adapted with permission from D.I. Margolin. Cognitive neuropsychology. Resolving enigmas about Wernicke's aphasia and other higher cortical disorders. Arch Neurol 1991;48:751–765.)*

already cited are the "third alexia" syndrome of Broca aphasia and the reading deficit of Wernicke aphasia. Neurolinguists and cognitive psychologists have divided alexias according to breakdowns in specific stages of the reading process. The linguistic concepts of surface structure versus the deep meanings of words have been instrumental in these new classifications. Four patterns of alexia (or dyslexia, in British usage) have been recognized: letter-by-letter, deep, phonological, and surface dyslexia. Figure 13.8 diagrams the steps in the reading process and the points of breakdown in the four syndromes. Letter-by-letter dyslexia is equivalent to pure alexia without agraphia. Deep dyslexia is a severe reading disorder in which patients recognize and read aloud only familiar words, especially concrete, imageable nouns and verbs. They make semantic or visual errors in reading and fail completely in reading

nonsense syllables or nonwords. Word reading is not affected by word length or by regularity of spelling; one patient, for example, could read *ambulance* but not *am*. Most cases have severe aphasia, with extensive left frontoparietal damage.

Phonological dyslexia is similar to deep dyslexia, with poor reading of nonwords, but single nouns and verbs are read in a nearly normal fashion, and semantic errors are rare. Patients appear to read words without understanding. The fourth type, surface dyslexia, involves spared ability to read laboriously by grapheme-phoneme conversion but inability to recognize words at a glance. These patients can read nonsense syllables but not words of irregular spelling, such as *colonel* or *yacht*. Their errors tend to be phonological rather than semantic or visual (e.g., pronouncing *rough* and *though* alike).

Agraphia

Like reading, writing may be affected either in isolation (pure agraphia) or in association with aphasia (aphasic agraphia). In addition, writing can be impaired by motor disorders, by apraxia, and by visuospatial deficits. Isolated agraphia has been described with left frontal or parietal lesions.

Agraphias can be analyzed in the same way as the alexias (Fig. 13.9). Thus, phonological agraphia involves the inability to convert phonemes into graphemes or to write pronounceable nonsense syllables, in the presence of ability to write familiar words. Deep dysgraphia is similar to phonological agraphia, but the patient can write nouns and verbs better than articles, prepositions, adjectives, and adverbs. In lexical or surface dysgraphia, patients can write regularly spelled words and pronounceable nonsense words but not irregularly spelled words. These patients have intact phoneme-grapheme conversion but cannot write by a whole-word or "lexical" strategy.

LANGUAGE IN RIGHT HEMISPHERE DISORDERS

Language and communication disorders are important even in patients with right hemisphere disease. First, left-handed patients may have right hemisphere language dominance and may develop aphasic syndromes from right hemisphere lesions. Second, right-handed patients occasionally become aphasic after right hemisphere strokes, a phenomenon called *crossed aphasia* (Bakar et al., 1996). These patients presumably have crossed or mixed dominance. Third, even right-handed persons with typical left hemisphere dominance for language have subtly altered language function after right hemisphere damage. Such patients are not aphasic, in that the fundamental mechanisms of speech production, repetition, and comprehension are undisturbed. Affective aspects of language are impaired, however, such that the speech sounds flat and unemotional; the normal prosody, or emotional intonation, of speech is lost. Syndromes of loss of emotional aspects of speech are termed aprosodias. Motor aprosodia involves loss of expressive emotion with preservation of emotional comprehension; sensory aprosodia involves loss of comprehension of affective language, also called *affective agnosia*. More than just emotion, stress and emphasis within a sentence are also affected by right hemisphere dysfunction. More importantly, such vital aspects of human communication as metaphor, humor, sarcasm, irony, and related constituents of language that transcend the literal meaning of words are especially sensitive to right hemisphere dysfunction. These deficits significantly impair patients in the pragmatics of communication. In other words, right hemisphere-damaged patients understand what is said, but not how it is said. They may have difficulty following a complex story (Rehak et al., 1992). Such higher level language deficits are related to the right

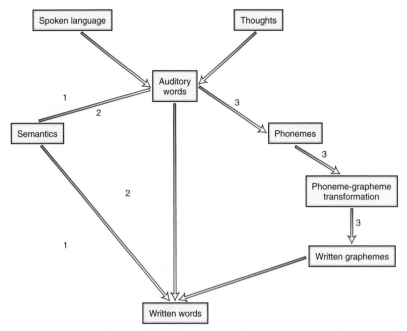

Fig. 13.9 Neurolinguistic model of writing and the agraphias. In deep agraphia, only the semantic (phonological-semantic-lexical) route (1) is operative; in phonological agraphia, route 2, the nonlexical phonological route produces written words directly from spoken words; in surface agraphia, only route 3, the phoneme-grapheme pathway, can be used to generate writing.

hemisphere disorders of inattention and neglect, discussed in Chapters 4 and 45.

LANGUAGE IN DEMENTING DISEASES

Language impairment is commonly seen in patients with dementia. Despite considerable variability from patient to patient, two patterns of language dissolution can be described. The first, the common presentation of Alzheimer disease (AD), involves early loss of memory and general cognitive deterioration. In these patients, mental status examinations are most remarkable for deficits in short-term memory, insight, and judgment, but language impairments can be found in naming and in discourse, with impoverished language content and loss of abstraction and metaphor. The mechanics of language—grammatical construction of sentences, receptive vocabulary, auditory comprehension, repetition, and oral reading—tend to remain preserved until later stages. By aphasia testing, patients with early AD have anomic aphasia. In later stages, language functions become more obviously impaired. In terms of the components of language mentioned earlier in this chapter, the semantic aspects of language tend to deteriorate first, then syntax, and finally phonology. Reading and writing—the last-learned language functions—are among the first to decline. Auditory comprehension later becomes deficient, whereas repetition and articulation remain normal. The language profile may then resemble that of transcortical sensory or Wernicke aphasia. In terminal stages, speech is reduced to the expression of simple biological wants; eventually, even muteness can develop. By this time, most patients are institutionalized or bedridden.

The second pattern of language dissolution in dementia, less common than the first, involves the gradual onset of a progressive aphasia, often without other cognitive deterioration. Auditory comprehension is involved early in the illness, and specific aphasic symptoms are evident, such as paraphasic or nonfluent speech, misnaming, and errors of repetition. These deficits worsen gradually, mimicking the course of a brain tumor or mass lesion rather than a typical dementia

(Grossman et al., 1996; Mesulam, 2001, 2003; Mesulam et al., 2014). The syndrome is generally referred to as "primary progressive aphasia." CT scans may show focal atrophy in the left perisylvian region, whereas EEG studies may show focal slowing. PET has shown prominent areas of decreased metabolism in the left temporal region and adjacent cortical areas.

Primary progressive aphasia (PPA) is now considered a variant of a more general category of dementing illnesses called *frontotemporal dementia* (FTD; Neary et al., 1998). For recent reviews of these disorders, see Mesulam et al. (2014) and Kirshner (2014). Frontotemporal dementia is now divided into four subgroups: behavioral variant FTD (Roskovsky et al., 2011); progressive nonfluent aphasia (Mesulam, 2003, Rohrer et al., 2010); semantic dementia (Hodges and Patterson, 2007; Snowden et al., 1989); and logopenic primary progressive aphasia. Mesulam's original cases of PPA had largely the progressive nonfluent aphasia, a Broca-like pattern of aphasia involving agrammatism and apraxia of speech (Mesulam, 2001, 2003). Progressive nonfluent aphasia usually reflects a "tauopathy," with mutations in familial cases found in the tau gene on Chromosome 17 (Heutink et al., 1997). Semantic dementia (Hodges and Patterson, 2007; Snowden et al., 1989) is a progressive fluent aphasia with impaired naming and loss of understanding of even single words. In reading, they may have a surface alexia pattern. Semantic dementia is usually not a tauopathy, but most cases have ubiquitin staining and evidence of a progranulin mutation, also on Chromosome 17, with production of an abnormal protein called TDP-43 (Baker et al., 2006; Cruts et al., 2006). Rarely, patients with this syndrome have Alzheimer disease at autopsy. The third variant of primary progressive aphasia, logopenic progressive aphasia, involves anomia and some repetition difficulty, with intact single word comprehension. This variant is most commonly associated with Alzheimer disease, with an unusual focal onset (Gorno-Tempini et al., 2008, 2011). These three patterns of primary progressive aphasia are associated with different patterns of atrophy on MRI and hypometabolism on PET: progressive nonfluent aphasia is associated with left frontal and insular atrophy; semantic dementia is associated with bilateral anterior temporal atrophy; logopenic progressive aphasia is associated with posterior temporal and inferior parietal atrophy, often bilateral but sometimes more obvious on the left side (Diehl et al., 2004; Josephs et al., 2010).

Other variants of FTD include corticobasal degeneration, which can also present with language abnormalities (Kertesz et al., 2000), and FTD with motor neuron disease. In one study of 10 patients with primary progressive aphasia followed prospectively until they became nonfluent or mute, Kertesz and Munoz (2003) found that at autopsy all had evidence of frontotemporal dementia: CBD in four, Pick body dementia in three, and tau and synuclein negative ubiquinated inclusions of the motor neuron disease in three. Imaging studies have shown that primary progressive aphasia is often associated with atrophy in the left frontotemporal region and other areas such as the fusiform and precentral gyri and intrapariatal sulcus are activated, possibly as a compensatory neuronal strategy (Sonty et al., 2003). Whitwell and colleagues (2006) have used voxel-based MRI morphometry to delineate different patterns of atrophy in FTD associated with motor neuron disease versus ubiquitin pathology. Cases of isolated aphasia secondary to Creutzfeldt–Jakob disease have been reported, but these usually progress to dementia over a period of months.

INVESTIGATION OF THE APHASIC PATIENT
Clinical Tests

The bedside language examination is useful in forming a preliminary impression of the type of aphasia and the localization of the causative lesion. Follow-up examinations are also helpful; as in all neurological diagnosis, the evolution of a neurological deficit over time is the most important clue to the specific disease process. For example, an embolic stroke and a brain tumor might both produce Wernicke aphasia, but strokes occur suddenly, with improvement thereafter, whereas tumors produce gradually worsening aphasia.

In addition to the bedside examination, a large number of standardized aphasia test batteries have been published. The physician should think of these tests as more detailed extensions of the bedside examination. They have the advantage of quantitation and standardization, permitting comparison over time and, in some cases, even a diagnosis of the specific aphasia syndrome. Research on aphasia depends on these standardized tests.

For neurologists, the most helpful battery is the Boston Diagnostic Aphasia Examination, or its Canadian adaptation, the Western Aphasia Battery. Both tests provide subtest information analogous to the bedside examination, and therefore meaningful to neurologists, as well as aphasia syndrome classification. The Porch Index of Communicative Ability quantitates performance in many specific functions, allowing comparison over time. Other aphasia tests are designed to evaluate specific language areas. For example, the Boston Naming Test evaluates a wide variety of naming stimuli, whereas the Token Test evaluates higher-level comprehension deficits. Further information on neuropsychological tests can be found in Chapter 43.

Further diagnosis of the aphasic patient rests on the confirmation of a brain lesion by neuroimaging (Fig. 13.10). The CT brain scan (discussed in Chapter 40) revolutionized the localization of aphasia by permitting "real-time" delineation of a focal lesion in a living patient; previously, the physician had to outlive the patient to obtain a clinical-pathological correlation at autopsy. MRI scanning provides better resolution of areas difficult to see on CT, such as the temporal cortex adjacent to the petrous bones, and more sensitive detection of tissue pathology, such as early changes of infarction. The

anatomical distinction of cortical from subcortical aphasia is best made by MRI. Acute strokes are visualized early on diffusion-weighted MRI.

The EEG is helpful in aphasia in localizing seizure discharges, interictal spikes, and slowing seen after destructive lesions, such as traumatic contusions and infarctions. The EEG can provide evidence that aphasia is an ictal or postictal phenomenon and can furnish early clues to aphasia secondary to mass lesions or to herpes simplex encephalitis. In research applications, electrophysiological testing via subdural grid and depth electrodes, or stimulation mapping of epileptic foci in preparation for epilepsy surgery, have aided in the identification of cortical areas involved in language.

Cerebral arteriography is useful in the diagnosis of aneurysms, arteriovenous malformations (AVMs), arterial occlusions, vasculitis, and venous outflow obstructions. In preparation for epilepsy surgery, the Wada test, or infusion of amobarbital through an arterial catheter, is useful in the determination of language dominance. Other, related studies by language activation with functional MRI (fMRI) or PET now rival the Wada test for the study of language dominance (Abou-Khalil and Schlaggar, 2002).

Single-photon emission CT (SPECT), PET, and functional MRI (see Chapter 40) are contributing greatly to the study of language. Patterns of brain activation in response to language stimuli have been recorded, mainly in normal persons, and these studies have largely confirmed the localizations based on pathology such as stroke over the past 140 years (Posner et al., 1988). In addition, these techniques can be used to map areas of the brain that activate during language functions after insults such as strokes, and the pattern of recovery can be studied. Some such studies have indicated right hemisphere activation in patients recovering from aphasia (Cappa et al., 1997), whereas others have found that only left hemisphere activation is associated with full recovery (Heiss et al., 1999; Thompson and den Ouden, 2008; Winhuisen et al., 2007). Inhibiting these areas by transcranial magnetic stimulation also seems to support the importance of left hemisphere regions in the recovery of language function (Winhuisen et al., 2007). An fMRI study (Saur et al., 2006) has suggested hypometabolism in the language cortex shortly after an ischemic insult, followed by increased activation of homologous areas in the contralateral hemisphere, and then a shift back to the more normal pattern of left hemisphere activation. Subcortical contributions to aphasia and language under degenerative conditions have been studied with PET. These techniques provide the best correlation between brain structure and function currently available and should help advance our understanding of language disorders and their recovery.

DIFFERENTIAL DIAGNOSIS

Vascular lesions, especially ischemic strokes, are the most common causes of aphasia. Historically, most research studies in aphasia have used stroke patients because stroke is an "experiment" of nature in which one area of the brain is damaged while the rest remains theoretically intact. Strokes are characterized by the abrupt onset of a neurological deficit in a patient with vascular risk factors. The precise temporal profile is important: most embolic strokes are sudden and maximal at onset, whereas thrombotic strokes typically wax and wane or increase in steps. The bedside aphasia examination is helpful in delineating the vascular territory affected. For example, the sudden onset of Wernicke aphasia nearly always indicates an embolus to the inferior division of the left middle cerebral artery. Global aphasia may be caused by an embolus to the middle cerebral artery stem, thrombosis of the internal carotid artery, or even a hemorrhage into the deep basal

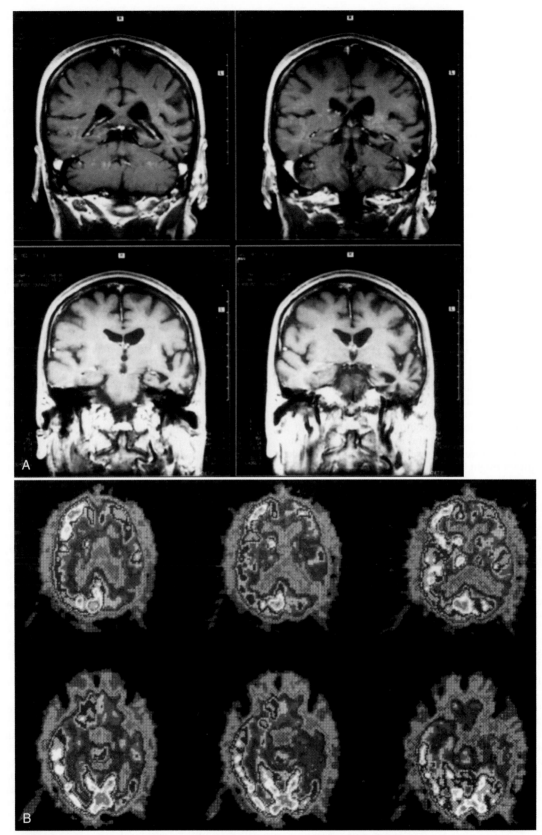

Fig. 13.10 Coronal T1-weighted magnetic resonance imaging scan of a patient with primary progressive aphasia. Note the marked atrophy of the left temporal lobe. **(A)** Axial fluorine-2-deoxyglucose positron emission. **(B)** Tomographic scan showing extensive hypometabolism in the left cerebral hemisphere, especially marked in the left temporal lobe.

ganglia. Whereas most aphasic syndromes involve the territory of the left middle cerebral artery, transcortical motor aphasia is specific to the anterior cerebral territory, and pure alexia without agraphia is specific to the posterior cerebral artery territory. The clinical features of the aphasia are thus of crucial importance to the vascular diagnosis.

Hemorrhagic strokes are also an important cause of aphasia, most commonly the basal ganglionic hemorrhages associated with hypertension. The deficits tend to worsen gradually over minutes to hours, in contrast to the sudden or stepwise onset of ischemic strokes. Headache, vomiting, and obtundation are more common with hemorrhages. Because hemorrhages compress cerebral tissue without necessarily destroying it, the ultimate recovery from aphasia is often better in hemorrhages than in ischemic strokes, although hemorrhages are more often fatal. Other etiologies of intracerebral hemorrhage include anticoagulants, head injury, blood dyscrasias, thrombocytopenia, and bleeding into structural lesions, such as infarctions, tumors, AVMs, and aneurysms. Hemorrhages from AVMs mimic strokes, with abrupt onset of focal neurological deficit. Ruptured aneurysms, on the other hand, present with severe headache and stiff neck or with coma; most patients have no focal deficits, but delayed deficits (e.g., aphasia) may develop secondary to vasospasm. Lobar hemorrhages may occur in elderly patients without hypertension. These hemorrhages occur near the cortical surface, sometimes extending into the subarachnoid space, and they may be recurrent. Pathological studies have shown amyloid deposition in small arterioles, or amyloid angiopathy. A final vascular cause of aphasia is cerebral vasculitis (see Chapter 70).

Traumatic brain injury is a common cause of aphasia. Cerebral contusions, depressed skull fractures, and hematomas of the intracerebral, subdural, and epidural spaces all cause aphasia when they disrupt or compress left hemisphere language structures. Trauma tends to be less localized than ischemic stroke, and thus aphasia is often admixed with the general effects of the head injury, such as depressed consciousness, encephalopathy or delirium, amnesia, and other deficits. Head injuries in young people may be associated with severe deficits but excellent long-term recovery. Language deficits, especially those involving discourse organization, can be found in most cases of significant closed head injury (Chapman et al., 1992). Gunshot wounds produce focal aphasic syndromes, which rival stroke as a source of clinical-anatomical correlation. Subdural hematomas are infamous for mimicking other neurological syndromes. Aphasia is occasionally associated with subdural hematomas overlying the left hemisphere, but it may be mild and may be overlooked because of the patient's more severe complaints of headache, memory loss, and drowsiness.

Tumors of the left hemisphere frequently present with aphasia. The onset of the aphasia is gradual, and other cognitive deficits may be associated because of edema and mass effect. Aphasia secondary to an enlarging tumor may thus be difficult to distinguish from a diffuse encephalopathy or early dementia. Any syndrome of abnormal language function should therefore be investigated for a focal, dominant hemisphere lesion.

Infections of the nervous system may cause aphasia. Brain abscesses can mimic tumors in every respect, and those in the left hemisphere can present with progressive aphasia. Chronic infections, such as tuberculosis or syphilis, can result in focal abnormalities that run the entire gamut of central nervous system symptoms and signs. Herpes simplex encephalitis has a predilection for the temporal lobe and orbital frontal cortex, and aphasia can be an early symptom, along with headache, confusion, fever, and seizures. Aphasia is often a permanent sequela in survivors of herpes encephalitis. Acquired immunodeficiency syndrome (AIDS) has become a common cause of language disorders. Opportunistic infections can cause focal lesions anywhere in the brain, and the neurotropic human immunodeficiency virus agent itself produces a dementia (AIDS dementia complex), in which language deficits play a part.

Aphasia is frequently caused by the degenerative central nervous system diseases. Reference has already been made to the focal, progressive aphasia in patients with frontotemporal dementia, as compared with the more diffuse cognitive deterioration characteristic of Alzheimer disease.

Language dysfunction in Alzheimer disease may be more common in familial cases and may predict poor prognosis. Cognitive deterioration in patients with Parkinson disease may also include language deterioration similar to that of Alzheimer disease, although Parkinson disease tends to involve more fluctuation in orientation and greater tendency to active hallucinations and delusions. Corticobasal degeneration is also associated with primary progressive aphasia and FTD, as noted earlier. A striking abnormality of speech (i.e., initial stuttering followed by true aphasia and dementia) has been described in the dialysis dementia syndrome. This disorder may be associated with spongiform degeneration of the frontotemporal cortex, similar to Creutzfeldt–Jakob disease. Paraphasic substitutions and nonsense speech are also occasionally encountered in acute encephalopathies, such as hyponatremia or lithium toxicity.

Another cause of aphasia is seizures. Seizures can be associated with aphasia in children as part of the Landau–Kleffner syndrome or in adults as either an ictal or postictal Todd phenomenon. Epileptic aphasia is important to recognize, in that anticonvulsant drug therapy can prevent the episodes, and unnecessary investigation or treatment for a new lesion, such as a stroke, can be avoided. As mentioned earlier, localization of language areas in epileptic patients has contributed greatly to the knowledge of language organization in the brain. The work of Ojemann and colleagues (1989) has shown that over 15% of young epileptic patients have no Broca or no Wernicke area. In addition, a new language area, the basal temporal language area (BTLA), has been discovered through epilepsy stimulation studies, and only later confirmed in patients with spontaneous seizures (Kirshner et al., 1995).

Another transitory cause of aphasia is migraine. Wernicke aphasia may be seen in a migraine attack, usually with complete recovery over a few hours. Occasional patients may have recurrent episodes of aphasia associated with migraine (Mishra et al., 2009).

Finally, aphasia can be psychogenic, often associated with stuttering or stammering. A recent report (Binder et al., 2012) concerned three patients with stuttering or stammering, letter reversals (e.g. "low the mawn" instead of "mow the lawn"), and naming difficulty after minor head injuries. In all three, language productions were inconsistent; e.g., when a subject became angry the speech productions were much more normal. All three failed neuropsychological tests designed to detect a lack of effort (such as a digit span of only two). Patients failed to improve on easier speech production tasks such as speaking in unison, shouting, or speaking while finger-tapping. In addition, whereas developmental stutterers generally have difficulty only with the initial phoneme of a phrase, psychogenic stutterers but also some acquired cases of stuttering may hesitate on any word of a phrase.

RECOVERY AND REHABILITATION OF APHASIA

Patients with aphasia from acute disorders, such as stroke, generally show spontaneous improvement over days, weeks, and months. In general, the greatest recovery occurs during the first 3 months, but improvement may continue over a prolonged period, especially in young patients and in global aphasics (Pashek and Holland, 1988). The aphasia type often changes during recovery: global aphasia evolves into Broca aphasia, and Wernicke aphasia into conduction or anomic aphasia. Language recovery may be mediated by shifting of functions to the right hemisphere or to adjacent left hemisphere regions. As mentioned earlier, studies of language activation PET and SPECT scanning techniques are advancing our understanding of the neuroanatomy of language recovery (Heiss et al., 1999; Thompson and den Ouden, 2008; Winhuisen et al., 2007). These studies suggest that aphasia recovers best when left hemisphere areas, either in the direct language cortex or in adjacent areas, recover function. Right hemisphere activation seems to be a "second best" type of recovery.

In addition, a study of patients in the very acute phase of aphasia, with techniques of diffusion and perfusion-weighted MRI, has suggested less variability in the correlation of comprehension impairment with left temporal ischemia than has been suggested from testing of chronic aphasia, after recovery and compensation have commenced (Hillis et al., 2001).

Speech therapy, provided by speech-language pathologists, attempts to facilitate language recovery by a variety of techniques and to help the patient compensate for lost functions (see Chapter 57). Repeated practice in articulation and comprehension tasks has traditionally been used to stimulate improvement. Other techniques include melodic intonation therapy, which uses melody to involve the right hemisphere in speech production; visual action therapy, which uses gestural expression; and treatment of aphasic perseveration, which aims to reduce repetitive utterances. Two other therapeutic techniques are functional communication therapy, which takes advantage of extralinguistic communication, and cVIC or Lingraphica, a computer program originally developed for primate communication. Patients who cannot speak can learn to produce simple sentences via computer. Augmentative devices make language expression possible through use of printers or voice simulators (Kratt, 1990). Speech therapy has remained somewhat controversial, but evidence of efficacy is actually better for speech therapy than for many drugs (Kelly et al., 2010; Robey, 1998). Some studies have suggested that briefly trained volunteers can induce as much improvement as do speech-language pathologists, but large, randomized trials have clearly indicated that patients who undergo formal speech therapy recover better than untreated patients do (Robey, 1998), and more intensive, traditional therapy is likely superior to group or computer-based approaches (Kelly et al., 2010).

A new approach to language rehabilitation is the use of pharmacological agents to improve speech. Albert and colleagues (1988) first reported that the dopaminergic drug bromocriptine promotes spontaneous speech output in transcortical motor aphasia. Several other studies have supported the drug in nonfluent aphasias, although a recent controlled study showed no benefit (Ashtary et al., 2006). Stimulant drugs are also being tested in aphasia rehabilitation. As new information accumulates on the neurochemistry of cognitive functions, other pharmacologic therapies may be forthcoming.

Finally, stimulation techniques such as transcranial magnetic stimulation (Martin et al., 2009; Wong and Tsang, 2013) and direct cortical stimulation (Monti et al., 2013) are being applied to patients with aphasia. These techniques await validation by larger clinical trials. These new techniques, and their theoretical underpinnings, are discussed by Tippett et al. (2014).

REFERENCES

The complete reference list is available online at https://expertconsult .inkling.com/.

14 Dysarthria and Apraxia of Speech

Howard S. Kirshner

CHAPTER OUTLINE

MOTOR SPEECH DISORDERS
Dysarthrias
Apraxia of Speech
Oral or Buccolingual Apraxia
Aphemia
The "Foreign Accent Syndrome"
Acquired Stuttering
Opercular Syndrome

MOTOR SPEECH DISORDERS

Motor speech disorders are syndromes of abnormal articulation, the motor production of speech, without abnormalities of language. A patient with a motor speech disorder should be able to produce normal expressive language in writing and to comprehend both spoken and written language. If a listener transcribes into print or type the speech of a patient with a motor speech disorder, the text should read as normal language. Motor speech disorders include dysarthrias, disorders of speech articulation, apraxia of speech, a motor programming disorder for speech, and four rarer syndromes: aphemia, foreign accent syndrome, acquired stuttering, and the opercular syndrome. Duffy (1995), in an analysis of speech and language disorders at the Mayo Clinic, reported that 46.3% of the patients had dysarthria, 27.1% aphasia, 4.6% apraxia of speech, 9% other speech disorders (such as stuttering), and 13% other cognitive or linguistic disorders.

Dysarthrias

Dysarthrias involve the abnormal articulation of sounds or phonemes, or more precisely, abnormal neuromuscular activation of the speech muscles, affecting the speed, strength, timing, range, or accuracy of movements involving speech (Duffy, 1995). The most consistent finding in dysarthria is the distortion of consonant sounds. Dysarthria is neurogenic, related to dysfunction of the central nervous system, nerves, neuromuscular junction, or muscle, with a contribution of sensory deficits in some cases. Speech abnormalities secondary to local, structural problems of the palate, tongue, or larynx do not qualify as dysarthrias. Dysarthria can affect not only articulation, but also phonation, breathing, or prosody (emotional tone) of speech. Total loss of ability to articulate is called *anarthria*.

Like the aphasias, dysarthrias can be analyzed in terms of the specific brain lesion sites associated with specific patterns of speech impairment. Analysis of dysarthria at the bedside is useful for the localization of neurological lesions and the diagnosis of neurological disorders. An experienced examiner should be able to recognize the major types of dysarthria, rather than referring to "dysarthria" as a single disorder.

The examination of speech at the bedside should include repeating syllables, words, and sentences. Repeating consonant sounds (such as /p/, /p/, /p/) or shifting consonant sounds (/p/, /t/, /k/) can help to identify which consonants consistently cause trouble.

The Mayo Clinic classification of dysarthria (Duffy, 1995), widely used in the United States, includes six categories: (1) flaccid, (2) spastic and "unilateral upper motor neuron," (3) ataxic, (4) hypokinetic, (5) hyperkinetic, and (6) mixed dysarthria. These types of dysarthria are summarized in Table 14.1.

Flaccid dysarthria is associated with disorders involving lower motor neuron weakness of the bulbar muscles, such as polymyositis, myasthenia gravis, and bulbar poliomyelitis. The speech pattern is breathy and nasal, with indistinctly pronounced consonants. In the case of myasthenia gravis, the patient may begin reading a paragraph with normal enunciation, but by the end of the paragraph the articulation is soft, breathy, and frequently interrupted by labored respirations.

Spastic dysarthria occurs in patients with bilateral lesions of the motor cortex or corticobulbar tracts, such as bilateral strokes. The speech is harsh or "strain-strangle" in vocal quality, with reduced rate, low pitch, and consonant errors. Patients often have the features of "pseudobulbar palsy," including dysphagia, exaggerated jaw jerk and gag reflexes, and easy laughter and crying (emotional incontinence, pseudobulbar affect, or pathological laughter and crying). Another variant is the "opercular syndrome," described later in this chapter.

A milder variant of spastic dysarthria, "unilateral upper motor neuron" dysarthria, is associated with unilateral upper motor neuron lesions (Duffy, 1995). This type of dysarthria has features similar to those of spastic dysarthria, only in a less severe form. Unilateral upper motor neuron dysarthria is one of the commonest types of dysarthria, occurring in patients with unilateral strokes. Strokes, depending on their location, can also cause mixed patterns of dysarthria (see later). There is considerable evidence for the efficacy of speech therapy for post-stroke dysarthria (Mackenzie, 2011).

Ataxic dysarthria or "scanning speech," associated with cerebellar disorders, is characterized by one of two patterns: irregular breakdowns of speech with explosions of syllables interrupted by pauses, or a slow cadence of speech, with excessively equal stress on every syllable. The second pattern of ataxic dysarthria is referred to as "scanning speech." A patient with ataxic dysarthria, attempting to repeat the phoneme /p/ as rapidly as possible, produces either an irregular rhythm, resembling popcorn popping, or a very slow rhythm. Causes of ataxic dysarthria include cerebellar strokes, tumors, multiple sclerosis, and cerebellar degenerations.

Hypokinetic dysarthria, the typical speech pattern in Parkinson disease, is notable for decreased and monotonous loudness and pitch, rapid rate, and occasional consonant errors. In a study of brain activation by PET methodology (Liotti et al., 2003), premotor and supplementary motor area activations were seen in untreated patients with Parkinson disease and hypokinetic dysarthria, but not in normal subjects. Following a voice treatment protocol, these premotor and motor activations diminished, whereas right-sided basal ganglia activations increased. Hypokinetic dysarthria responds both to behavioral therapies and to pharmacologic treatment of Parkinson disease, though the efficacy of speech therapy in Parkinson disease has not been proved (Herd et al., 2012).

TABLE 14.1 Classification of the Dysarthrias

Type	Localization	Auditory signs	Diseases
Flaccid	Lower motor neuron	Breathy , nasal voice, imprecise consonants	Stroke, myasthenia gravis
Spastic	Bilateral upper motor neuron	Strain-strangle, harsh voice; slow rate; imprecise consonants	Bilateral strokes, tumors, primary lateral sclerosis
	Unilateral upper motor neuron	Consonant imprecision, slow rate, harsh voice quality	Stroke, tumor
Ataxic	Cerebellum	Irregular articulatory breakdowns, excessive and equal stress	Stroke, degenerative disease
Hypokinetic	Extrapyramidal	Rapid rate, reduced loudness, monopitch and monoloudness	Parkinson disease
Hyperkinetic	Extrapyramidal	Prolonged phonemes, variable rate, inappropriate silences, voice stoppages	Dystonia, Huntington disease
Spastic and flaccid	Hypernasality; lower motor neuron	Amyotrophic strain-strangle, harsh voice, slow rate, imprecise consonants	Upper lateral sclerosis, multiple strokes

Adapted from Duffy, J.R., 1995. Motor Speech Disorders: Substrates, Differential Diagnosis, and Management. Mosby, St. Louis; and from Kirshner, H.S., 2002. Behavioral Neurology: Practical Science of Mind and Brain. Butterworth Heinemann, Boston.

Hyperkinetic dysarthria, a pattern in some ways opposite to hypokinetic dysarthria, is characterized by marked variation in rate, loudness, and timing, with distortion of vowels, harsh voice quality, and occasional, sudden stoppages of speech. This speech pattern is seen in hyperkinetic movement disorders such as Huntington disease and dystonia musculorum deformans.

The final category, *mixed* dysarthria, involves combinations of the other five types. One common mixed dysarthria is a spastic–flaccid dysarthria seen in amyotrophic lateral sclerosis. The ALS patient has the harsh, strain-strangle voice quality of spastic dysarthria, combined with the breathy and hypernasal quality of flaccid dysarthria. Multiple sclerosis may feature a spastic–flaccid–ataxic or spastic–atraxic mixed dysarthria, in which slow rate or irregular breakdowns are added to the other characteristics seen in spastic and flaccid dysarthria. Wilson disease can involve hypokinetic, spastic, and ataxic features.

The management of dysarthria includes speech therapy techniques for strengthening muscles, training more precise articulations, slowing the rate of speech to increase intelligibility, or teaching the patient to stress specific phonemes. Devices such as pacing boards to slow articulation, palatal lifts to reduce hypernasality, amplifiers to increase voice volume, communication boards for subjects to point to pictures, and augmentative communication devices and computer techniques can be used when the patient is unable to communicate in speech. Surgical procedures such as a pharyngeal flap to reduce hypernasality or vocal fold Teflon injection or transposition surgery to increase loudness may help the patient speak more intelligibly.

Apraxia of Speech

Apraxia of speech is a disorder of the programming of articulation of sequences of phonemes, especially consonants (Ziegler et al., 2012). The motor speech system makes errors in selection of consonant phonemes, in the absence of any "weakness, slowness or incoordination" of the muscles of speech articulation (Wertz et al., 1991). The term "apraxia of speech" implies that the disorder is one of a skilled, sequential motor activity (as in other apraxias), rather than a primary motor disorder. Hillis and colleagues (2004) gave a more informal definition

of apraxia of speech, in terms of a patient who "knows what he or she wants to say and how it should sound," yet cannot articulate it properly. Consonants are frequently substituted rather than distorted, as in dysarthria. Patients have special difficulty with polysyllabic words and consonant shifts, as well as in initiating articulation of a word. Errors are inconsistent from one attempt to the next, in contrast to the consistent distortion of phonemes in dysarthria.

The four cardinal features of apraxia of speech are: (1) effortful, groping, or "trial-and error" attempts at speech, with efforts at self-correction; (2) dysprosody; (3) inconsistencies in articulation errors; and (4) difficulty with initiating utterances. Usually the patient has the most difficulty with the first phoneme of a polysyllabic utterance. The patient may make an error in attempting to produce a word on one trial, a different error the next time, and a normal utterance the third time.

Apraxia of speech is rare in isolated form, but it frequently contributes to the speech and language deficit of Broca's aphasia. A patient with apraxia of speech, in addition to aphasia, will often write better than he or she can speak, and comprehension is relatively preserved. Dronkers (1996) and colleagues have presented evidence from CT and MRI scans indicating that, although the anatomic lesions vary, patients with apraxia of speech virtually always have damage in the left hemisphere insula, whereas patients without apraxia of speech do not. This "overlapping lesion" approach to brain localization, however, can be misleading. More recent MRI correlations of apraxia of speech in acute stroke patients by Hillis and colleagues (2004), however, have pointed to the traditional Broca's area in the left frontal cortex as the site of apraxia of speech, and as the site where programming of articulation takes place. Two recent publications have drawn attention to primary progressive apraxia of speech as a variant of frontotemporal dementia (Croot et al., 2012; Duffy and Josephs, 2012). See Chapter 13 for a discussion of primary progressive aphasia and frontotemporal dementia.

Testing of patients for speech apraxia includes the repetition of sequences of phonemes (pa/ta/ka), as discussed previously under testing for dysarthria. Repetition of a polysyllabic word (e.g., "catastrophe" or "television") is especially likely to elicit apraxic errors, and having the subject repeat the same

esophagus. Involvement of pharyngeal and esophageal musculature in polymyositis and dermatomyositis is an indicator of poor prognosis and can be the source of significant morbidity. A 1-year mortality rate of 31% has been reported in individuals with inflammatory myopathy and dysphagia (Williams et al., 2003), although other investigators have reported a 1-year survival rate of 89% (Oh et al., 2007).

Dysphagia in persons with inflammatory myopathy may be due to restrictive pharyngo-esophageal abnormalities such as cricopharyngeal bar, Zenker diverticulum, and stenosis. In fact, in one study of 13 patients with inflammatory myopathy, radiographic constrictions were noted in 9 (69%) individuals, compared with 1 of 17 controls with dysphagia of neurogenic origin (Williams et al., 2003). Aspiration was also more common in the patients with myositis (61% versus 41%). The resulting dysphagia can be severe enough to require enteral feeding. Acute total obstruction by the cricopharyngeal muscle has been reported in dermatomyositis, necessitating cricopharyngeal myotomy. Other investigators have reported improvement in 50% of individuals 1 month following cricopharyngeal bar disruption; improvement was still present in 25% at 6 months (Williams et al., 2003). The reason for the formation of restrictive abnormalities in inflammatory myopathy is uncertain, but it may be that long-standing inflammation of the cricopharyngeus muscle impedes its compliance and ability to open fully (Williams et al., 2003).

Dysphagia may also develop in inclusion body myositis. It may even be the presenting symptom. In the late stages of the disorder, the frequency of dysphagia may actually exceed that seen in dermatomyositis and polymyositis. In a group of individuals in whom inclusion-body myositis mimicked and was confused with motor neuron disease, dysphagia was present in 44% (Dabby et al., 2001). In another study, dysphagia was documented in 37 of 57 (65%) patients with inclusion-body myositis (Cox et al., 2009). Abnormal function of the cricopharyngeal sphincter, probably due to inflammatory involvement of the cricopharyngeal muscle, with consequently reduced compliance, was documented in 37%. A focal inflammatory myopathy involving the pharyngeal muscles and producing isolated pharyngeal dysphagia has also been described in individuals older than age 69. It has been suggested that this is a distinct clinical entity characterized by cricopharyngeal hypertrophy, although polymyositis localized to the pharyngeal musculature has also been reported.

Dysphagia in both dermatomyositis and polymyositis may respond to corticosteroids and other immunosuppressive drugs, and these remain the mainstay of treatment. Intravenous immunoglobulin (IVIG) therapy has produced dramatic improvement in dysphagia in individuals who were unresponsive to steroids. Although inclusion-body myositis usually responds poorly to these agents, there are reports of long-lasting stabilization of dysphagia with either intravenous or subcutaneous immunoglobulin therapy (Pars et al., 2013). More often, cricopharyngeal myotomy is necessary (Oh et al., 2007).

Mitochondrial Disorders

The mitochondrial disorders are a family of diseases that develop as a consequence of dysfunction in the mitochondrial respiratory chain. Most are the result of mutations in mitochondrial deoxyribonucleic acid (DNA) genes, but nuclear DNA mutations may be responsible in some. Mitochondrial disorders are by nature multisystemic, but myopathic and neurological features often predominate, and symptoms may vary widely even between individuals within the same family.

In addition to the classic constellation of symptoms that includes progressive external ophthalmoplegia, retinitis pigmentosa, cardiac conduction defects, and ataxia, individuals with Kearns–Sayre syndrome may also develop dysphagia. Severe abnormalities of pharyngeal and upper-esophageal peristalsis have been documented in this disorder. Cricopharyngeal dysfunction is common, and impaired deglutitive coordination may also develop.

Dysphagia has also been described in other mitochondrial disorders, but descriptions are only anecdotal, and formal study has not been undertaken.

Myasthenia Gravis

Myasthenia gravis (MG) is an autoimmune disorder characterized by the production of autoantibodies directed against the α_1 subunit of the nicotinic postsynaptic acetylcholine receptors at the neuromuscular junction, with destruction of the receptors and reduction in their number. The clinical consequence of this process is the development of fatigable muscle weakness that progressively increases with repetitive muscle action and improves with rest. MG occurs more frequently in women than men; although symptoms can develop at any age, the reported mean age of onset in women is between 28 and 35, and in men, between age 42 and 49. Although myasthenic symptoms remain confined to the extraocular muscles in approximately 20% of patients, more widespread muscle weakness becomes evident in most individuals.

Involvement of bulbar musculature, with resultant dysphagia, is relatively common in MG. In approximately 6% to 30% of patients, bulbar involvement is evident from the beginning (Koopman et al., 2004); with disease progression, most eventually develop bulbar symptoms such as dysphagia and dysarthria. Dysphagia in MG can be due to dysfunction at oral, pharyngeal, or even esophageal levels, and many patients experience it at multiple levels. In a study of 20 myasthenic patients experiencing dysphagia, abnormalities in the oral preparatory phase were evident in 13 individuals (65%), oral phase dysphagia in 18 (90%), and pharyngeal phase involvement in all 20 (100%) (Koopman et al., 2004). Oral phase involvement can be due to fatigue and weakness of the tongue or masticatory muscles. In MG patients with bulbar symptoms, repetitive nerve stimulation studies of the hypoglossal nerve have demonstrated abnormalities, as have studies utilizing EMG of the masticatory muscles recorded while chewing. Pharyngeal dysfunction is also common in MG patients who have dysphagia, as demonstrated by videofluoroscopy. Aspiration, often silent, may be present in 35% or more of these individuals; in elderly patients the frequency of aspiration may be considerably higher. Bedside speech pathology assessment is not a reliable predictor of aspiration (Koopman et al., 2004). Motor dysfunction involving the striated muscle of the proximal esophagus has also been documented in MG. In one study that used testing with esophageal manometry, 96% of patients with MG demonstrated abnormalities such as decreased amplitude and prolongation of the peristaltic wave in this region. Cricopharyngeal sphincter pressure was also noted to be reduced.

It is important to remember that dysphagia can also precipitate myasthenic crisis in individuals with MG. In fact, in one study, dysphagia was considered to be a major precipitant of myasthenic crisis in 56% of patients (Koopman et al., 2004).

NEUROGENIC DYSPHAGIA

A variety of disease processes originating in the central and peripheral nervous systems can also disrupt swallowing mechanisms and produce dysphagia. Processes affecting cerebral cortex, subcortical white matter, subcortical gray matter,

OROPHARYNGEAL

Arnold–Chiari malformation
Basal ganglia disease:
  Biotin-responsive
  Corticobasal degeneration
  DLB
  HD
  Multiple system atrophy
  Neuroacanthocytosis
  PD
  PSP
  WD
Central pontine myelinolysis
Cerebral palsy
Drug related:
  Cyclosporine
  Tardive dyskinesia
  Vincristine
Infectious:
  Brainstem encephalitis
  Listeria
  Epstein–Barr virus
  Diphtheria
  Poliomyelitis
  Progressive multifocal leukoencephalopathy
  Rabies
Mass lesions:
  Abscess
  Hemorrhage
  Metastatic tumor
  Primary tumor
Motor neuron diseases:
  ALS
MS
Peripheral neuropathic processes:
  Charcot–Marie–Tooth disease
  Guillain–Barré syndrome (Miller Fisher variant)
Spinocerebellar ataxias
Stroke
Syringobulbia

ESOPHAGEAL

Achalasia
Autonomic neuropathies:
  Diabetes mellitus
  Familial dysautonomia
  Paraneoplastic syndromes
Basal ganglia disorders:
  PD
Chagas disease
Esophageal motility disorders
Scleroderma

ALS, Amyotrophic lateral sclerosis; *DLB,* dementia with Lewy bodies; *HD,* Huntington disease; *MS,* multiple sclerosis; *PD,* Parkinson disease; *PSP,* progressive supranuclear palsy; *WD,* Wilson disease.

brainstem, spinal cord, and peripheral nerves all can elicit dysphagia as a component of their clinical picture (Box 15.3).

In individuals with neurogenic dysphagia, prolonged swallow response, delayed laryngeal closure, and weak bolus propulsion combine to increase the risk of aspiration and the likelihood of malnutrition.

Stroke

Cerebrovascular disease is an extremely common neurological problem, and stroke is the third leading cause of death in the United States. It has been estimated that 500,000 to 750,000 strokes occur in the United States each year, and approximately 150,000 persons die annually following stroke. The mechanism of stroke is ischemic in 80% to 85% of cases; in the remaining 15% to 20% it is hemorrhagic. Approximately 25% of ischemic strokes are due to small-vessel disease, 50% to large-vessel disease, and 25% to a cardioembolic source. Although stroke can occur at all ages, 75% of strokes occur in individuals older than 75.

Dysphagia develops in 45% to 57% of individuals following stroke, and its presence is associated with increased likelihood of severe disability or death (Runions et al., 2004; Schaller et al., 2006). Aspiration is the most widely recognized complication of dysphagia following stroke, but undernourishment and even malnutrition occur with surprising frequency (Finestone and Greene-Finestone, 2003). Reported frequencies of nutritional deficits in patients with dysphagia following stroke range from 48% to 65%. The presence of dysphagia following stroke results in a threefold prolongation of hospital stay and increases the complication rate during hospitalization (Runions et al., 2004). It is also an independent risk factor for severe disability and death.

Finestone and Greene-Finestone (2003) have delineated a number of warning signs that can alert physicians to the presence of post-stroke dysphagia. Some are obvious, others more subtle. They include drooling, excessive tongue movement or spitting food out of the mouth, poor tongue control, pocketing of food in the mouth, facial weakness, slurred speech, coughing or choking when eating, regurgitation of food through the nose, wet or "gurgly" voice after eating, hoarse or breathy voice, complaints of food sticking in the throat, absence or delay of laryngeal elevation, prolonged chewing, prolonged time to eat or reluctance to eat, and recurrent pneumonia.

Although it is commonly perceived that the presence of dysphagia following stroke indicates a brainstem localization for the stroke, this is not necessarily so. Impaired swallowing has been documented in a significant proportion of strokes involving cortical and subcortical structures. The pharyngeal phase of swallowing is primarily impaired in brainstem infarction; in hemispheric strokes, the most striking abnormality often is a delay in initiation of voluntary swallowing. Strokes involving the right hemisphere tend to produce more impairment of pharyngeal motility, whereas left hemisphere lesions have a greater effect on oral stage function (Ickenstein et al., 2005). Dysphagia has been reported as the sole manifestation of infarction in both medulla and cerebrum.

Approximately 50% to 55% of patients with lesions in the posterior inferior cerebellar artery distribution, with consequent lateral medullary infarction (Wallenberg syndrome), develop dysphagia (Teasell et al, 2002). The fact that unilateral medullary infarction can produce bilateral disruption of the brainstem swallowing centers suggests that they function as one integrated center. Infarction in the distribution of the anterior inferior cerebellar artery can also result in dysphagia.

Following stroke within the cerebral hemispheres, dysphagia can develop by virtue of damage to either cortical or subcortical structures involved with volitional swallowing. Bilateral hemispheric damage is more likely to produce dysphagia, but it can also occur in the setting of unilateral damage. Bilateral infarction of the frontoparietal operculum may result in the anterior operculum syndrome (Foix-Chavany-Marie syndrome), which is characterized by inability to perform voluntary movements of the face, jaw, tongue, and pharynx

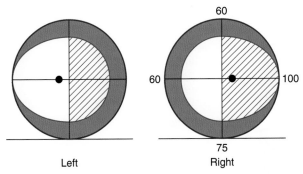

Fig. 16.1 Right homonymous hemianopia. The visual loss is often referred to the right eye, because the right temporal visual field is larger than the left nasal visual field. *Numbers* refer to the normal extent of the visual field in degrees.

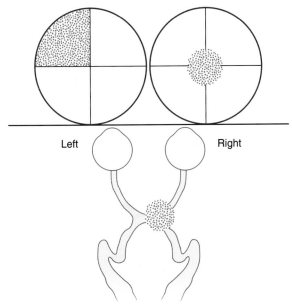

Fig. 16.2 Junctional scotoma from a lesion at the junction of the optic nerve and chiasm. The lesion affects both the right optic nerve, producing a cecocentral scotoma in the right eye, and crossing fibers in the optic chiasm, producing an upper temporal visual field defect in the left eye. The temporal visual field defect of a junctional scotoma often goes unnoticed by the patient and may only be detected with visual field testing (see Chapter 45).

BOX 16.1 Causes of Transient Monocular Visual Loss

Retinal circulation emboli
Migraine/vasospasm
Hypoperfusion (hypotension, hyperviscosity, hypercoagulability)
Ocular (optic disc edema, intermittent angle-closure glaucoma, hyphema, impending central retinal vein occlusion)
Vasculitis (e.g., giant cell arteritis)
Other (Uhthoff phenomenon, idiopathic, nonorganic)

Visual Loss in Bright Light. Some patients with reduced blood supply to the eye due to a high-grade stenosis or occlusion of the internal carotid artery report TMVL in bright light, which is likely due to impaired regeneration of photopigments secondary to ocular ischemia (Kaiboriboon et al., 2001). The TMVL can also occur following meals or with postural changes. A variety of ophthalmic abnormalities, including midperipheral retinal hemorrhages, can be present and collectively comprise the *ocular ischemic syndrome* (Chen and Miller, 2007). Other retinal diseases, such as cone dystrophies and age-related macular degeneration, can cause evanescent visual loss in bright light, also known as *hemeralopia* or *day blindness*. The visual loss in these diseases is usually bilateral, whereas it is unilateral in patients with unilateral carotid disease.

Uhthoff Phenomenon. Transient monocular visual loss with increases in body temperature is known as the Uhthoff phenomenon and most commonly occurs in patients with optic neuritis associated with demyelinating disease, but it can also occur in patients with other optic neuropathies. The phenomenon is thought to arise as a result of transient conduction block within the optic nerve. Vision returns to baseline when the body temperature returns to normal.

Transient Visual Obscurations. Transient visual obscurations are brief episodes of monocular or binocular visual loss in patients with optic disc edema. The visual loss is often precipitated by postural changes or Valsalva-like maneuvers (e.g., coughing, straining) and probably occurs secondary to transient hypoperfusion of the edematous optic nerve head. The visual loss lasts for only a few seconds, with vision rapidly returning to baseline thereafter. Similar episodes of visual loss can occur with systemic hypotension, giant cell arteritis, or retinal venous stasis. Gaze-evoked transient visual loss has been reported with orbital tumors, but can occasionally occur with optic disc edema.

Other Causes of Transient Visual Loss. Transient visual loss can also occur as a result of transient optic nerve compression by cystic lesions, such as sphenoid sinus mucoceles and craniopharyngiomas. Other ophthalmic causes of TMVL include impending central retinal vein occlusion and recurrent hyphema, although it is important to note that some causes (e.g., corneal basement membrane dystrophy, tear film dysfunction) produce visual blurring rather than actual visual loss.

Transient Binocular Visual Loss

Other than transient visual obscurations occurring in patients with bilateral optic disc edema, simultaneous complete or incomplete transient binocular visual loss is almost always due to transient dysfunction of the visual cortex. Visual migraine aura is probably the most common cause of transient binocular visual loss, especially in patients younger than 40 years (see Chapter 103). Transient binocular visual loss can also result from cerebral hypoperfusion due to vasospasm, thromboembolism, systemic hypotension, hyperviscosity, or vascular compression (Box 16.2) (Thurtell and Rucker, 2009). Transient binocular visual loss can occur in association with seizures, although they more commonly cause visual hallucinations, which can be elementary or complex, depending on the location of the seizure focus (Bien et al., 2000). Transient cortical blindness can occur in association with headache, altered mental status, and seizures in the posterior reversible encephalopathy syndrome (Hinchey et al., 1996). Transient cortical blindness can sometimes occur after head trauma, especially in children. Lastly, transient bilateral visual loss can occasionally be nonorganic in etiology, but this should remain a diagnosis of exclusion.

Sudden Monocular Visual Loss without Progression

Visual loss due to optic nerve or retinal ischemia is characteristically sudden in onset (Box 16.3) and is usually

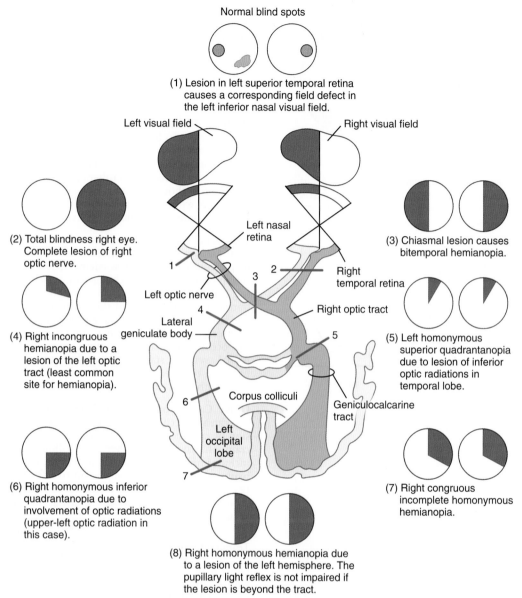

Fig. 16.3 Topographical diagnosis of visual field defects. *(Reprinted with permission from Vaughn, C., Asbury, T., Tabbara, K.F., 1989. General Ophthalmology, twelfth ed. Appleton & Lange, Norwalk, CT, p. 244.)*

BOX 16.2 Causes of Transient Binocular Visual Loss

Migraine
Cerebral hypoperfusion:
  Thromboembolism
  Systemic hypotension
  Hyperviscosity
Seizures
Posterior reversible encephalopathy syndrome
Head trauma
Optic disc edema (transient visual obscurations)

BOX 16.3 Causes of Sudden Monocular Visual Loss without Progression

Central or branch retinal artery occlusion
Anterior ischemic optic neuropathy, arteritic or nonarteritic
Posterior ischemic optic neuropathy
Branch or central retinal vein occlusion
Traumatic optic neuropathy
Central serous retinopathy
Retinal detachment
Vitreous hemorrhage
Nonorganic (functional) visual loss

---

nonprogressive, although a stuttering decline in vision may occur over several weeks in some patients with anterior ischemic optic neuropathy. *Anterior ischemic optic neuropathy* is a common cause of optic neuropathy and occurs due to loss of blood supply to the optic nerve head, resulting in optic disc edema (Rucker et al., 2004). In affected patients younger than 50 years, it is usually nonarteritic in etiology, being caused by a combination of factors that impair blood supply to the optic nerve head. In patients older than 50 years, giant cell (temporal or cranial) arteritis must be considered; urgent investigations and empirical treatment with high-dose steroids are required in these patients to prevent further devastating visual loss. Retrobulbar optic nerve infarction, also known as *posterior ischemic optic neuropathy*, is far less common, but can result from perioperative hypotension (e.g., with spinal surgery or cardiac bypass surgery) and other causes of hemodynamic shock (Rucker et al., 2004). Giant cell arteritis should be specifically considered in elderly patients with posterior ischemic optic neuropathy.

Optic nerve ischemia very rarely results from embolism or migraine. In contrast, central or branch retinal artery occlusions are caused mostly by embolic or thrombotic events. Opacification of the retinal nerve fiber layer with a cherry-red spot at the macula is the classic funduscopic appearance of acute central retinal artery occlusion (see Chapter 17). Retinal arterial occlusions can produce altitudinal, quadrantic, or complete monocular visual loss. The triad of branch retinal artery occlusions, hearing loss, and encephalopathy results from a rare microangiopathy known as *Susac syndrome* (Susac et al., 2007). A distinctive pattern of white-matter lesions with involvement of the corpus callosum is seen on magnetic resonance imaging in this disease.

Occlusion of the central retinal vein can result in sudden visual loss and an unmistakable hemorrhagic retinopathy. It usually occurs in patients with risk factors for atherosclerosis and results from venous thrombosis at the level of the lamina cribrosa of the sclera. When ischemic, it causes a dense central scotoma with sparing of peripheral vision.

Idiopathic central serous retinopathy can manifest as a positive central scotoma of sudden onset, often with symptoms of metamorphopsia or micropsia and a positive light-stress test result (see Chapter 45). It results from leakage of fluid into the subretinal space and most often occurs in young adult men with type-A personalities. The diagnosis can be difficult to make without the aid of fluorescein angiography or optical coherence tomography, as the retinal findings are subtle. Spontaneous recovery usually occurs within weeks to months, but occasionally laser photocoagulation is required to seal leaking vessels.

Traumatic optic neuropathy usually results in sudden permanent optic nerve dysfunction. The trauma can be severe or deceptively minor, causing a contusion or laceration of the optic nerve or a shearing of its nutrient vessels with subsequent infarction. Treatments, such as steroids and surgical decompression, remain controversial and mostly ineffective (Yu-Wai-Man and Griffiths, 2005, 2013).

Sudden Binocular Visual Loss without Progression

Sudden, permanent, binocular visual loss, if not caused by trauma, most commonly results from a stroke involving the retrochiasmal visual pathways and causes homonymous visual field defects (Box 16.4) (Rizzo and Barton, 2005). In patients who have no other neurological symptoms or signs, the lesion usually involves the occipital lobe. Bilateral occipital lobe infarcts can result in tubular visual field defects, checkerboard

visual field defects, or complete loss of vision in both eyes, a condition called *cortical blindness*. Cortical blindness, especially from infarction, can be accompanied by a denial of the visual loss and confabulation, a condition known as *Anton syndrome*.

Sudden binocular visual loss can result from simultaneous bilateral ischemic optic neuropathies and chiasmal compression due to *pituitary apoplexy*. Pituitary apoplexy can also cause headache, diplopia, altered mental status, and hemodynamic shock (Sibal et al., 2004), but the presentation can be subtle such that the diagnosis is missed.

Sudden Visual Loss with Progression

Sudden-onset, painful monocular visual loss that subsequently worsens is commonly due to optic nerve inflammation (optic neuritis). The visual loss typically progresses over hours to days before stabilizing and then improving. Optic neuritis is well known to be associated with multiple sclerosis and may be the first sign of the disease. The prognosis for visual recovery without treatment is excellent in most patients, although there is a poor recovery in some, such as those with optic neuritis occurring in association with neuromyelitis optica (Wingerchuk et al., 2007).

Leber hereditary optic neuropathy (LHON), a maternally transmitted disease resulting from mutations in the mitochondrial deoxyribonucleic acid (DNA) genes encoding subunits of respiratory chain complex I, can also cause sudden visual loss with subsequent progression. Primary mutations have been identified at positions 11778, 3460, and 14484 in the mitochondrial DNA. Many other mutations have been reported, but occur less frequently (Yu-Wai-Man et al., 2009). LHON produces acute or subacute painless, often permanent, central visual loss, usually in young adult men. The visual loss is initially monocular, but the other eye usually becomes affected within 6 months. Visual recovery is variable and infrequent, and depends on the mitochondrial DNA mutation. The 11778 mutation carries the worst visual prognosis, while the 14484 mutation carries the best. In the acute phase, the classic triad of ophthalmic findings includes telangiectatic vessels around the optic disc, nonedematous elevation of the optic disc, and absence of leakage from the disc on fluorescein angiography. Arteriolar narrowing can be marked, and vascular tortuosity is often a clue early in the disease. LHON can also cause loss of vision in women, but it tends to be less severe than in men.

Careful questioning of the patient with "sudden" visual loss may reveal a long-standing deficit that has suddenly been noticed (e.g., when covering the fellow eye) or that has worsened over time. In such cases, the clinician should evaluate for a slow-growing compressive lesion (Box 16.5).

Progressive Visual Loss

Progressive visual loss is the hallmark of a lesion compressing the afferent visual pathways. Common compressive lesions include pituitary tumors, aneurysms, craniopharyngiomas, and meningiomas (see Box 16.5) (Gittinger, 2005; Glaser, 1999). Granulomatous disease of the optic nerve from sarcoidosis or tuberculosis can cause chronic progressive visual loss. Optic nerve compression at the orbital apex from thyroid eye disease can occur with minimal orbital signs or ocular motility disturbance. In each of these cases, the visual loss can be so insidious as to go unnoticed until it is fortuitously discovered during a routine examination.

Hereditary or degenerative diseases of the optic nerves or retina must be included in the differential diagnosis of gradual-onset visual loss. The hereditary optic neuropathies

---

BOX 16.4 Causes of Sudden Binocular Visual Loss without Progression

Occipital lobe stroke
Bilateral ischemic optic neuropathies
Pituitary apoplexy
Head trauma
Nonorganic (functional) visual loss

BOX 16.5 Causes of Progressive Visual Loss

Anterior visual pathway inflammation:
  Optic neuritis
  Sarcoidosis
  Meningitis
Anterior visual pathway compression:
  Tumors
  Aneurysms
  Thyroid eye disease
Hereditary optic neuropathies:
  Leber hereditary optic neuropathy
  Dominant optic atrophy
Optic nerve head drusen
Glaucoma and normal-tension glaucoma
Chronic papilledema
Toxic (e.g., ethambutol) and nutritional optic neuropathies
Radiation damage to anterior visual pathways
Paraneoplastic (cancer-associated) retinopathy or optic
  neuropathy

are bilateral and are usually diagnosed during the first two decades of life (Yu-Wai-Man et al., 2009). The most common inherited optic neuropathy is the autosomal dominant variety, known as *dominant optic atrophy*. A number of mutations involving the OPA1 gene have been described in dominant optic atrophy (Yu-Wai-Man et al., 2009). The visual loss can range from mild to severe and can sometimes be asymmetrical. Characteristically, there are central or cecocentral scotomas with sparing of the peripheral fields, and temporal pallor and cupping of the optic discs. Color vision is usually abnormal. Other ophthalmic and neurological abnormalities may be present.

Drusen of the optic nerve head are extracellular deposits of plasma proteins and a variety of inorganic materials that can compress optic nerve axons near the surface of the nerve head as they enlarge (Auw-Haedrich et al., 2002). Drusen are a common cause of pseudopapilledema and can produce visual field defects including arcuate defects, blind spot enlargement, and generalized visual field constriction (Lee and Zimmerman, 2005). Loss of visual acuity is atypical, but can result from development of a secondary choroidal neovascular membrane, with subsequent hemorrhage into the macula, or anterior ischemic optic neuropathy. "Buried" drusen (i.e., those not visible with the ophthalmoscope) can also cause visual field loss; the diagnosis can be confirmed by identifying calcified deposits in the optic nerve head on ophthalmic ultrasound. Buried drusen can be seen with computed tomography if they are large enough. If central visual loss occurs in a patient with optic disc drusen and no obvious retinal lesion, a search for a retrobulbar lesion should be undertaken.

Normal-tension glaucoma (NTG) is a controversial entity that creates a diagnostic and therapeutic conundrum, since a number of conditions can give rise to a similar clinical picture (Tomsak, 1997). In true NTG, glaucomatous optic disc and visual field changes develop despite normal intraocular pressure. NTG is bilateral in 70% of patients, and the average age at diagnosis is 66 years. Women are affected approximately twice as frequently as men. NTG can be either progressive or static (Anderson et al., 2001).

Chronic papilledema from any cause of intracranial hypertension can produce progressive optic neuropathy (see Chapter 88). The optic discs often develop a milky gray color, and there is sheathing of peripapillary retinal vessels. The visual fields become constricted, with nasal defects occurring initially, followed by gradual constriction, with central vision being spared until late. Optociliary collateral vessels can develop, and sudden visual loss from ischemic optic neuropathy can rarely occur. On occasion, optic atrophy develops in the absence of papilledema or despite a decrease in intracranial pressure, possibly due to retrobulbar optic nerve compression (Thurtell et al., 2010).

Toxic and nutritional optic neuropathies are bilateral and usually progressive (Phillips, 2005; Tomsak, 1997). The nutritional variety is characterized by a history of inadequate diet, a gradual onset of painless visual loss over weeks to months, prominent dyschromatopsia, cecocentral scotomas, and development of optic atrophy late in the disease. Most cases of so-called tobacco–alcohol amblyopia are probably related to vitamin B deficiencies. Other conditions that lead to nutritional deficiency, such as bariatric surgery and ketogenic diet, can also cause bilateral optic neuropathies. Medications that are toxic to the optic nerves, including ethambutol, amiodarone, and linezolid, can cause a gradual onset of painless visual loss (Phillips, 2005). Retinal toxins, such as vigabatrin, digitalis, chloroquine, hydroxychloroquine, and phenothiazines, can also cause painless progressive binocular visual loss.

Slowly progressive visual loss from radiation damage to the anterior visual pathways, especially the retina, can result from direct radiation therapy to the eye for primary ocular tumors or metastases, or can occur after periocular irradiation for basal cell carcinomas, sinus carcinomas, and related malignancies. It can also occur after whole-brain irradiation for metastases or gliomas, or after parasellar radiation therapy for pituitary or other parasellar neoplasms (Lessell, 2004). Radiation retinopathy becomes clinically apparent after a variable latent period of months to a few years following the radiation therapy and is usually irreversible. Its incidence relates to the fraction size, total radiation dose, and use of concomitant chemotherapy. Radiation-induced retinal capillary endothelial cell damage is the initial event that triggers the retinopathy, which is usually indistinguishable from diabetic retinopathy.

Rapidly progressive bilateral visual loss can be caused by paraneoplastic processes that affect the retina or, less commonly, optic nerves (Ko et al., 2008). Small cell carcinoma of the lung is the most commonly associated tumor, but gynecological, endocrine, breast, and other tumors have been implicated. The visual loss is usually accompanied by photopsias, often precedes the diagnosis of cancer, and is associated with circulating antibodies to the tumor and retinal or optic nerve antigens (see Chapter 82). Findings similar to those of retinitis pigmentosa are present, including night blindness, constricted visual fields, and an extinguished electroretinogram. Combined treatment with chemotherapy and immunosuppression may be effective in occasional cases.

REFERENCES

The complete reference list is available online at https://expertconsult .inkling.com/.

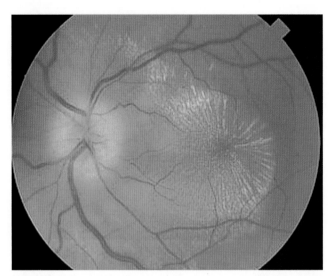

Fig. 17.14 Ophthalmoscopic appearance of idiopathic neuroretinitis in a 36-year-old woman. Fundus photograph of the patient's left eye taken 1 month after onset of visual loss shows mild residual disk edema with pallor and a robust macular star. Serologic testing for specific inflammatory diseases was unrevealing. *(With permission from Albert, D.M., Miller, J.W., Azar, D.T., et al., 2008, Neuroretinitis, in: Albert and Jakobiec's Principles and Practice of Ophthalmology. Elsevier, Saunders, pp. 1859–1863.)*

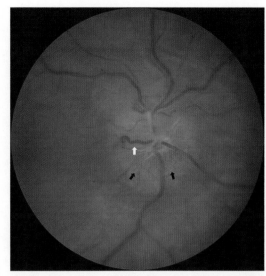

Fig. 17.15 Fundus photograph of the right eye in a patient with chronic disc swelling. Note blurred disc margins *(black arrows)* and an optociliary shunt vessel *(white arrow)*. *(Reprinted with permission from Prasad S., Volpe, N.J., Balcer, L.J., 2010. Approach to optic neuropathies: clinical update. Neurologist 16, 23–34.)*

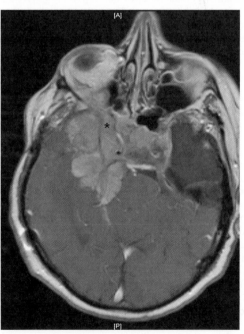

Fig. 17.16 Axial T1-weighted postcontrast MRI in a patient with an extensive sphenoid wing meningioma *(asterisk)* causing left optic nerve compression, ocular motor palsies, and proptosis. *(Reprinted with permission from Prasad S., Volpe, N.J., Balcer, L.J., 2010. Approach to optic neuropathies: clinical update. Neurologist 16, 23–34.)*

demyelinating optic neuritis (Fig. 17.14). The initial clinical presentation of these conditions may be similar, but the characteristic macular star of neuroretinitis will appear within 1 to 2 weeks, establishing the diagnosis. The distinction is critical because neuroretinitis has no association with an increased risk of MS and may be due to cat scratch disease (*Bartonella henselae*), syphilis (*Treponema pallidum*), or Lyme disease (*Borrelia burgdorferi*). In most cases, *Bartonella* infection is self-limited and does not require treatment, but in severe cases doxycycline may be effective. Other infectious causes of optic neuropathy include human immunodeficiency virus (HIV) and opportunistic infections including toxoplasmosis, cytomegalovirus, and cryptococcosis.

Paranasal sinus disease can cause a condition that mimics optic neuritis, with acute optic neuropathy and pain on eye movements, or can cause a progressive optic neuropathy resulting from compression (Rothstein et al., 1984). Optic neuropathy due to sinusitis and mucocele should be considered in patients who have clinical evidence of optic neuritis with seemingly atypical features, particularly in elderly patients with severe sinus disease, a history of fevers, ophthalmoplegia, or progression of vision loss beyond 2 weeks. Presentations after dental infection also occur.

Several compressive mass lesions cause a progressive optic neuropathy. The optic disc swells in cases of intraorbital compression, but in cases of retro-orbital compression, disc swelling typically only occurs if ICP is elevated. Chronic disc edema due to compressive lesions may be accompanied by optociliary shunt vessels and glistening white bodies on the disc surface (pseudodrusen from extruded axoplasm) (Fig. 17.15). Important causes of compressive optic neuropathy include neoplasm (including optic nerve sheath or skull base meningioma, pituitary adenoma, craniopharyngioma, dermoid and epidermoid tumors, and metastases), sinus lesions, bony processes (such as fibrous dysplasia), enlarged extraocular muscles (as in Graves disease ophthalmopathy), or aneurysms (Fig. 17.16). Meningiomas of the optic nerve sheath occur

primarily in women and can cause acuity loss associated with either disc swelling or atrophy.

Primary optic nerve neoplasms include benign juvenile pilocytic glioma in children and (rarely) malignant glioblastoma in adults (Fig. 17.17). Juvenile pilocytic astrocytoma is often associated with neurofibromatosis type 1 and may be managed conservatively with frequent ophthalmological examination through adolescence (Avery et al., 2011; Listernick et al., 2007). When clinical or radiographic progression is

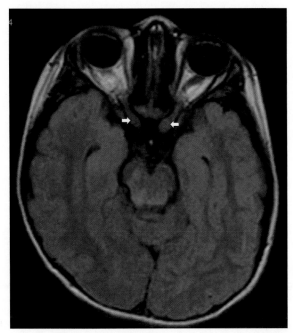

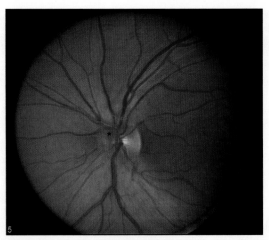

Fig. 17.18 Fundus photograph of the left eye in a patient with Leber hereditary optic neuropathy. Visual acuity was 20/200. Note hyperemia with appearance of slight nasal disc swelling *(asterisk)*. *(Reprinted with permission from Prasad S., Volpe, N.J., Balcer, L.J., 2010. Approach to optic neuropathies: clinical update. Neurologist 16, 23–34.)*

Fig. 17.17 Axial fluid-attenuated inversion recovery (FLAIR) MRI in a patient with bilateral optic nerve gliomas (juvenile pilocytic astrocytomas) *(white arrows)*. The patient had stigmata of type 1 neurofibromatosis. *(Reprinted with permission from Prasad S., Volpe, N.J., Balcer, L.J., 2010. Approach to optic neuropathies: clinical update. Neurologist 16, 23–34.)*

detected, chemotherapy should be first-line therapy, followed by radiation and rarely surgery. Malignant optic nerve glioblastoma is much rarer, affects adults, and has a considerably worse prognosis (Spoor et al., 1980). Other neoplastic conditions include lymphoma, leukemia, carcinomatous meningitis, and optic nerve metastasis. Almost any form of carcinoma can metastasize to the optic nerve; breast and lung carcinomas are the most common.

Optic neuropathy may occur as a delayed effect of radiation therapy. It can occur with or without disc edema and can sometimes be difficult to distinguish from tumor recurrence (Danesh-Meyer, 2008). Radiation optic neuropathy is suggested by exposure (typically 50-Gy dosage), characteristic 6- to 24-month time lag to symptoms, and accompanying radiation changes in proximal tissues. Progression occurs over weeks to months, and spontaneous recovery is rare. Corticosteroids may help by reducing edema in the affected optic nerve.

Visual loss in a patient with known or suspected cancer raises the possibility of a paraneoplastic optic neuropathy or retinopathy (Damek, 2005). In paraneoplastic optic neuropathy, evidence of other neurological dysfunction is common, and the antibody most commonly identified is directed toward collapsin response mediator protein 5 (CRMP5). Paraneoplastic retinopathies, on the other hand, include cancer-associated retinopathy (with antibodies to recoverin protein) and melanoma-associated retinopathy (with antibodies to rod ganglion cells).

Leber hereditary optic neuropathy (LHON) is a subacute, sequential, maternally inherited optic nerve disorder in which 80% to 90% of affected persons are males in the second or third decade of life (see Chapter 16) (Newman, 2005; Yu-Wai-Man et al., 2009). The optic disc may appear hyperemic and mildly swollen in the acute phase, although fluorescein does not demonstrate capillary leakage because true disc edema is

not present. Circumpapillary telangiectatic vessels, present in the peripapillary nerve fiber layer, are an important clue to the diagnosis (Fig. 17.18). These early funduscopic changes also may be noted in presymptomatic eyes. As the condition progresses, the discs become atrophic. Because fibers mediating the pupillary light reflex may be selectively spared, the light reflex may be preserved despite significant visual loss. Genetic diagnosis of LHON is based on the identification of related mitochondrial DNA mutations (see Chapter 93). Most patients have permanent vision loss, although a minority will experience some recovery of vision. The prognosis depends upon the specific mutation harbored; patients with mtDNA mutation T14484C are more likely to have spontaneous recovery than patients with mutations G11778A or G3460A (Newman, 2005). At present, no effective treatment for this condition is available, although idebenone has been studied and demonstrated potential benefit for preservation of vision in the unaffected eye (Chinnery and Griffiths, 2005; Klopstock et al., 2011).

Direct traumatic optic neuropathy (TON) may include nerve avulsion or transection and is easily recognized by the relevant history of injury (Sarkies, 2004) (Fig. 17.19). Fundus examination may reveal extensive intraocular hemorrhages. On the other hand, posterior indirect traumatic optic neuropathy will present with visual loss in the absence of significant fundus abnormalities; it may result from shearing forces and subsequent edema within the optic canal. Up to half of these patients may improve spontaneously (Sarkies, 2004). There is weak evidence that corticosteroid therapy may be helpful within the first 8 hours, but no other medical or surgical interventions have proven effective (Yu-Wai-Man and Griffiths, 2005, 2007).

A description of other uncommon causes of unilateral optic disc edema that occasionally can have a unilateral presentation will be discussed next.

Bilateral Optic Disc Swelling

Papilledema

The term *papilledema* refers specifically to optic disc swelling secondary to increased ICP. Disc swelling in papilledema results from blockage of axoplasmic flow in nerve fibers, increasing the volume of axoplasm in the optic disc (Hayreh, 1977). On the basis of the chronicity and fundus appearance, papilledema can be divided into four stages: early, fully developed (acute), chronic, and atrophic. The acute phase of papilledema is often suggested by a mismatch between a swollen disc and relatively spared optic nerve function, particularly central visual acuity. The most common visual field defects encountered in patients with early or acute papilledema are enlargement of the physiological blind spot, concentric constriction, and inferior nasal field loss. When acute papilledema is accompanied by decreased acuity (and often metamorphopsia), fluid typically extends within the retina to the macula itself.

In early papilledema, swelling is most prominent at the superior and inferior poles of the optic disc where the nerve fiber layer is thickest. With further development of papilledema, swelling encompasses the disc surface more uniformly,

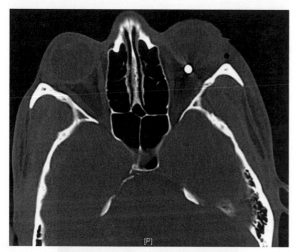

Fig. 17.19 Axial CT scan *(bone windows)* from a patient with direct left traumatic optic neuropathy due to avulsion by a BB pellet. *(Reprinted with permission from Prasad S., Volpe, N.J., Balcer, L.J., 2010. Approach to optic neuropathies: clinical update. Neurologist 16, 23–34.)*

and the degree of disc elevation increases (Fig. 17.20). The retinal veins may distend slightly, and the disc may appear mildly hyperemic. These vascular changes result from nerve fiber swelling causing compression of capillaries and venules, leading to venous stasis and dilation, formation of microaneurysms, and finally disc and peripapillary splinter hemorrhages (see Fig. 17.20). Retinal cotton-wool spots may occur secondary to ischemia in the nerve fiber layer that is normally transparent. Spontaneous venous pulsations usually are absent once the ICP exceeds 18 cm H_2O. Although papilledema typically is bilateral, it can be asymmetrical because of differences in transmitted pressure related to anatomical variation in the meningeal covering of the intracranial and intracanalicular optic nerves (Killer et al., 2003).

Fluorescein angiography in the setting of acute papilledema may reveal absent fluorescence during the retinal arterial phase as a result of delayed circulation caused by disc swelling. Dilated capillaries, microaneurysms, and flame-shaped hemorrhages may appear in the arteriovenous phase. Fluorescein may leak from dilated capillaries in the venous phase.

The disc appearance changes as papilledema becomes chronic, usually after weeks to months. The nerve fiber layer may appear pale and take on a gliotic appearance as a result of optic atrophy and astrocytic proliferation (Fig. 17.21). Hemorrhages are less prominent (and often have resolved completely). The disc takes on a "champagne cork" appearance in which small, glistening white bodies (pseudodrusen) are present owing to extruded axoplasm after prolonged stasis. Shunt vessels due to compensatory dilation of preexisting communications between the retinal and ciliary circulation may appear.

If increased ICP and papilledema persist, optic nerve axons become damaged, and visual field loss develops. At this stage, optic disc swelling lessens, and pallor develops (atrophic papilledema). Finally, patients with end-stage papilledema exhibit secondary optic nerve atrophy (disc pallor) without evidence of swelling. Chronic atrophic papilledema, unlike the acute phase, is often characterized by loss of visual acuity with severely constricted visual fields.

Papilledema can be the consequence of numerous disease processes that elevate the intracranial pressure. An expanding mass lesion such as a brain tumor, cerebral edema due to stroke, or intracranial hemorrhage will increase ICP, particularly in a younger patient without age-related brain atrophy.

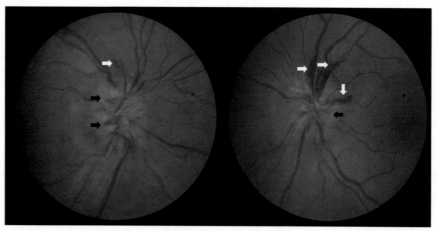

Fig. 17.20 Fundus photographs in a patient with acute papilledema. Note that swelling of the peripapillary nerve fiber layer causes an obscured view of underlying retinal vessels *(black arrows)*. Splinter hemorrhages, which also suggest true papilledema rather than pseudopapilledema, are seen *(white arrows)*. *(Reprinted with permission from Prasad S., Volpe, N.J., Balcer, L.J., 2010. Approach to optic neuropathies: clinical update. Neurologist 16, 23–34.)*

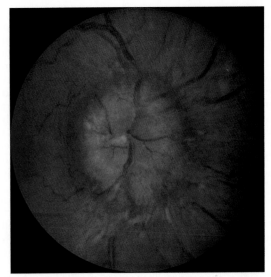

Fig. 17.21 Fundus photograph of the right eye of a patient with chronic papilledema. Note pale, gliotic "champagne-cork" disc appearance, without retinal hemorrhages. *(Reprinted with permission from Prasad S., Volpe, N.J., Balcer, L.J., 2010. Approach to optic neuropathies: clinical update. Neurologist 16, 23–34.)*

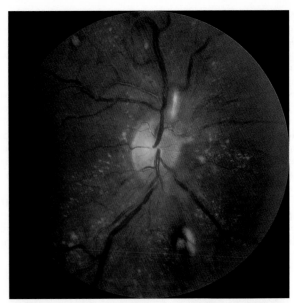

Fig 17.22 Disc edema, cotton wool spots, and retinal hemorrhages from malignant hypertension.

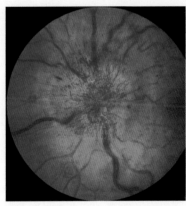

Fig. 17.23 Diabetic papillopathy in a patient with type 1 diabetes. Note the telangiectatic vessels on the disc surface. *(With permission from Kanski, J.J., 2009. Clinical Ophthalmology: A Synopsis. Neuro-ophthalmology, 2nd edn. Butterworth Heinemann, Oxford.)*

Compression of the ventricular system in the posterior fossa is particularly likely to cause papilledema. Venous sinus thrombosis is another common cause, especially in pregnancy and other states of hypercoagulability. Cryptococcal meningitis is the infectious disorder most commonly associated with significant papilledema.

Pseudotumor cerebri, or idiopathic intracranial hypertension, can lead to disc swelling and progressive visual loss. The condition is most common in obese women, but modest weight gain (by 5%–15%) even in nonobese women is a risk factor for disease. Additional risk factors are the use of tetracycline derivatives or vitamin A, and if these agents are being taken they should be discontinued. Weight loss can be imperative in the management of pseudotumor cerebri. In the short term, treatment with acetazolamide can improve symptoms and reduce optic disc swelling. In refractory cases, optic nerve sheath fenestration or cerebrospinal fluid (CSF) shunting may be indicated to reduce the possibility of progressive, permanent visual loss.

Malignant Hypertension

A marked elevation in blood pressure may produce bilateral optic disc swelling indistinguishable from papilledema (Hayreh, 1977). Peripapillary cotton-wool spots and retinal microhemorrhages are other prominent features in patients with malignant hypertension (Fig. 17.22). Encephalopathy owing to posterior reversible encephalopathy syndrome (PRES) is common but not always present. The changes associated with malignant hypertension can occur at lower blood pressures in patients with renal failure.

Diabetic Papillopathy

Diabetic papillopathy is a rare cause of bilateral (or sometimes unilateral) disc swelling in patients with type 1 diabetes (Barbera et al., 1996). This entity is distinct from typical NAION in that there is often bilateral, simultaneous optic nerve involvement. Often visual loss is minimal, with the exception of an enlarged physiological blind spot. Disc edema may be accompanied by marked capillary telangiectasias overlying the disc surface (Fig. 17.23). Neuroimaging and lumbar puncture may be necessary to distinguish this condition from papilledema. The pathogenesis is unclear but may relate to a mild impairment of blood flow causing disc swelling without infarction of the optic nerve head (as in the case of premonitory NAION). In many cases, the optic disc edema resolves without residual visual deficit.

Other Causes

Leber's hereditary optic neuropathy, as discussed earlier, can frequently present with simultaneous bilateral visual loss and disc swelling. Anemia, hyperviscosity syndromes, pickwickian syndrome, hypotension, and severe blood loss are other uncommon causes of bilateral optic disc swelling. The clinical setting generally provides clues to the diagnosis. In addition, any of the entities described under unilateral optic disc edema, particularly the infiltrative disorders, rarely can cause bilateral disc swelling. In children, optic neuritis commonly is bilateral and often is associated with bilateral papillitis (disc swelling).

Bilateral ischemic optic neuropathies should prompt immediate evaluation for giant cell (temporal) arteritis in patients older than 55 years. Although most toxic optic neuropathies manifest with normal-appearing optic discs, disc edema is characteristic of methanol poisoning.

Pseudopapilledema

In patients with pseudopapilledema, visible optic disc drusen (hyaline bodies) may be present. Even when disc drusen are not apparent, the distinction between true disc swelling and pseudopapilledema can frequently be made on the basis of fundus examination findings (Table 17.1). The most important distinguishing feature is the clarity of the peripapillary nerve fiber layer. In patients with true disc edema, the nerve fiber layer is hazy, obscuring the underlying retinal vessels,

whereas in pseudopapilledema, this layer can remain distinct. In addition, the presence of spontaneous venous pulsations (SVPs) supports the diagnosis of pseudopapilledema, although SVP can be absent in pseudopapilledema as well. Although subretinal hemorrhages may be present in patients with pseudopapilledema (particularly in the setting of optic disc drusen), splinter hemorrhages are characteristic of true papilledema. When buried drusen are present under the disc surface, the clinical distinction between papilledema and pseudopapilledema can be challenging, and ocular ultrasonography can help demonstrate hyperechoic signals consistent with drusen. Finally, fluorescein angiography will show leakage in papilledema but not pseudopapilledema (Lam et al., 2008).

Optic Disc Drusen

Optic disc drusen, which constitute a common cause of pseudopapilledema, refers to calcium deposits within the optic nerve head. Although their etiology is unclear, drusen may result from axonal degeneration owing to altered axoplasmic flow, particularly in the setting of a small optic canal (Lam et al., 2008). In children, disc drusen tend to be buried, whereas in adults, they often are visible on the disc surface (Figs. 17.24 and 17.25). The progression from buried to surface drusen in individual patients has been well documented. The prevalence of optic disc drusen is approximately 2% within the general population, and they can be bilateral in two-thirds of cases. Optic disc drusen are much more common in Caucasian patients than in African Americans and may be genetic, inherited in an autosomal dominant pattern with incomplete penetrance.

Patients with optic disc drusen generally do not complain of visual symptoms, although rarely a patient may experience transitory visual obscurations similar to those described by patients with true papilledema. Although patients may be unaware of a visual field defect, such deficits are common, occurring in approximately 70% of eyes with visible disc drusen and in 35% of those with pseudopapilledema but no visible drusen (Lam et al., 2008). These deficits can slowly progress and probably result from nerve fiber layer thinning and axonal dysfunction caused by the drusen. The visual field defects, therefore, generally follow a nerve fiber bundle distribution, most commonly affecting the inferior nasal visual

TABLE 17.1 Differentiation of Early Papilledema and Pseudopapilledema

Feature	Papilledema	Pseudopapilledema
Disc color	Hyperemic	Pink, yellowish pink
Disc margins	Indistinct early at superior and inferior poles, later entire margin	Irregularly blurred, may be lumpy
Vessels	Normal distribution, slight fullness; spontaneous venous pulsations absent	Emanate from center, frequent anomalous pattern, ± spontaneous venous pulsations
Nerve fiber layer	Dull as a result of edema, which may obscure blood vessels	No edema; may glisten with circumpapillary halo of feathery light reflections
Hemorrhages	Splinter	Subretinal, retinal, vitreous

Reprinted with permission from Beck, R.W., Smith, C.H., 1988. Neuro-Ophthalmology: A Problem-Oriented Approach. Little, Brown, Boston.

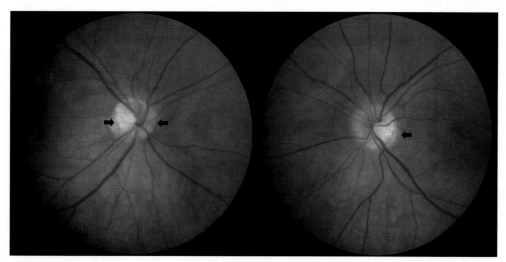

Fig. 17.24 Fundus photographs in a patient with pseudopapilledema. There is a "lumpy-bumpy" disc appearance due to visible disc drusen *(black arrows)*. Note that retinal vessels are not obscured by nerve fiber layer edema. Spontaneous venous pulsations may also indicate pseudopapilledema. *(Reprinted with permission from Prasad S., Volpe, N.J., Balcer, L.J., 2010. Approach to optic neuropathies: clinical update. Neurologist 16, 23–34.)*

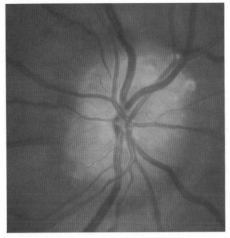

Fig. 17.25 Optic disc drusen. Visible excrusences on the disc surface represent optic disc drusen, which are one example of pseudopapilledema. *(With permission from Gili, P., Flores-Rodríguez, P., Yangüela, J., et al., 2013. Using autofluorescence to detect optic nerve head drusen in children. J AAPOS 17(6), 568–571.)*

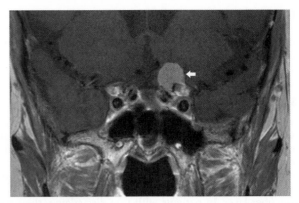

Fig 17.26 Left optic nerve compression due to meningioma of the planum sphenoidale.

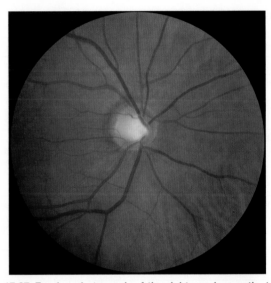

Fig. 17.27 Fundus photograph of the right eye in a patient with glaucoma. The cup-to-disc ratio has increased to approximately 0.7. The intraocular pressure was 29 mm Hg before treatment. *(Reprinted with permission from Prasad S., Volpe, N.J., Balcer, L.J., 2010. Approach to optic neuropathies: clinical update. Neurologist 16, 23–34.)*

field. Enlargement of the blind spot and generalized field constriction also may occur. In addition, visual field loss in the setting of optic disc drusen can occur secondary to superimposed ischemic optic neuropathy or an associated retinal degeneration.

OPTIC NEUROPATHIES WITH NORMAL-APPEARING OPTIC DISCS

Many optic neuropathies manifest initially with a completely normal disc appearance; these are classified as retrobulbar optic neuropathies. The disc appearance is normal because the pathological process is posterior to the lamina cribrosa. As with the swollen disc, the differential diagnosis depends on whether optic nerve involvement is unilateral or bilateral.

Unilateral Presentations

The most common causes of unilateral retrobulbar optic neuropathy are optic neuritis and compressive lesions. The time course of vision loss usually is helpful in distinguishing between these two entities. No definite way exists to differentiate these disorders on examination, but the detection of a superior temporal field defect in the fellow eye (a junctional scotoma) is highly suggestive of a compressive lesion affecting the anterior optic chiasm and the posterior optic nerve, involving the decussating fibers (termed *Willebrand knee* or *genu*) (Fig. 17.26). Posterior (retrobulbar) ischemic optic neuropathy (PION) may occur in patients with giant cell arteritis, other vasculitides, or severe blood loss (Chang and Miller, 2005; Hayreh, 2004). For practical purposes, no retrobulbar correlate to NAION exists.

Bilateral Presentations

Bilateral optic neuropathies in which the optic discs appear normal include nutritional optic neuropathy (including tobacco–alcohol amblyopia), vitamin B_{12} or folate deficiencies, toxic optic neuropathy (from heavy metals), drug-related optic neuropathy (due to ethambutol, chloramphenicol, isoniazid, and others), and inherited optic neuropathies. When these conditions are chronic, optic atrophy may ensue. Other diagnostic considerations in this category include bilateral compressive lesions and bilateral retrobulbar optic neuritis. Finally, posterior indirect traumatic optic neuropathy can result from shearing forces and subsequent edema within the optic canal.

OPTIC NEUROPATHIES WITH OPTIC ATROPHY

Any optic neuropathy that produces damage to the optic nerve may result in optic atrophy. Compressive lesions characteristically will cause progressive visual loss and optic atrophy. The presence of gliotic changes suggests that the disc was previously swollen.

Glaucoma is the most common type of optic neuropathy and it is typically identified by elevated intraocular pressure and optic disc cupping (Fig. 17.27) (Jonas and Budde, 2000). However, angle closure glaucoma may present with painful acute visual loss, resembling the features of optic neuritis. Distinguishing characteristics include the severity of pain (which can be excruciating) and a red eye with an enlarged, nonreactive pupil. Normal-tension glaucoma is more difficult to recognize but will present with optic disc cupping and

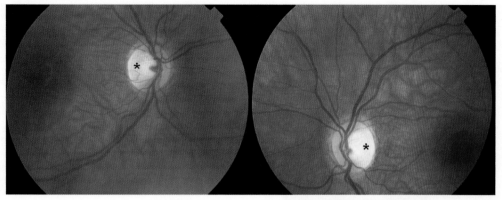

Fig. 17.28 Fundus photographs in a patient with dominant optic atrophy. Note extreme temporal pallor, with excavated appearance *(asterisks). (Reprinted with permission from Prasad S., Volpe, N.J., Balcer, L.J., 2010. Approach to optic neuropathies: clinical update. Neurologist 16, 23–34.)*

progressive field constriction, despite normal intraocular pressures (Anderson et al., 2001).

Dominantly inherited optic atrophy typically presents with insidious asymmetrical visual loss in childhood (Newman, 2005). These patients often have a striking disc appearance, with pallor and excavation of the temporal portion of the disc (Fig. 17.28). The disorder is due to mutations of the OPA1 gene, with autosomal inheritance and variable penetrance. The OPA gene product is believed to target the mitochondria and support membrane stability. Because over 90 different pathogenic OPA1 mutations have been described, available genetic tests are less sensitive compared to those for LHON.

Optic atrophy also occurs as a consequence of disorders of the retina, optic chiasm, and optic tract. Patients with lesions of the optic chiasm or tract can demonstrate bow-tie atrophy, with pallor of the nasal and temporal portions of the disc in the setting of temporal field loss. Acquired geniculocalcarine lesions (posterior to the optic tract) do not produce disc pallor, although congenital lesions may lead to optic atrophy through trans-synaptic degeneration.

CONGENITAL OPTIC DISC ANOMALIES

Congenital optic nerve anomalies (in addition to optic disc drusen, as discussed earlier in this chapter) include a tilted optic disc and optic nerve dysplasia. Visual loss associated with a congenital disc anomaly can range from total blindness to minimal dysfunction.

Tilted Optic Disc

A tilted optic disc usually is easily recognizable on fundus examination. The disc may appear foreshortened on one side, and one portion may appear elevated, with the opposite end depressed (Fig. 17.29). Often the retinal vessels run in an oblique direction. Tilted optic discs are of neurological importance in that they usually are bilateral and may be associated with temporal field loss, thus mimicking a chiasmal syndrome. However, differentiation from chiasmal disease generally is possible because visual field defects in patients with tilted discs typically do not respect the vertical meridian.

Optic Nerve Dysplasia

Of the several types of optic nerve dysplasia, optic nerve hypoplasia is the most common (Taylor, 2007). In this condition, the optic disc appears small and surrounded by choroid

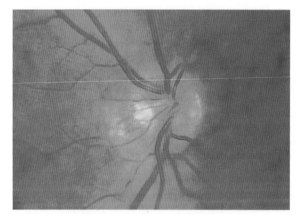

Fig. 17.29 Tilted optic disc. The disc in the fellow eye had a similar appearance.

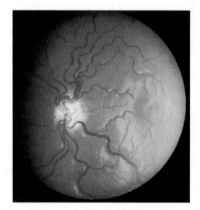

Fig. 17.30 Optic nerve hypoplasia (ONH) with some pallor. The disc is the inner circle of the two seen on the photograph; hence the term double-ring of ONH. Note the relatively large size of the blood vessels at the surface of the disc. *(With permission from Richard B. Goldbloom, Color Plate in Pediatric Clinical Skills, pp. 1–4, fourth edition, Copyright © 2011, 2003, 1997, 1992 by Saunders, an imprint of Elsevier Inc.)*

and retinal pigment changes that resemble a double ring (Fig. 17.30). The abnormality may be unilateral or bilateral. In most cases, no specific cause is identifiable. The frequency of optic nerve hypoplasia appears to be increased in children of mothers who had diabetes mellitus or ingested antiepileptic

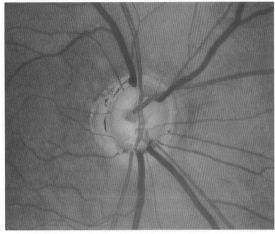

Fig. 17.31 Optic disc coloboma. *(With permission from Trobe, Jonathan D., MD, Congenital Optic Nerve Disorders, in Rapid Diagnosis in Ophthalmology: Neuro-Ophthalmology. January 1, 2008, pp. 11–21. © 2008.)*

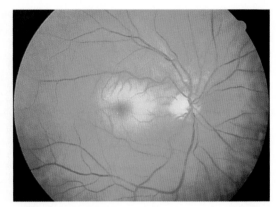

Fig. 17.32 Central retinal artery occlusion. Note the cherry-red spot in the center of the macula, with surrounding whitening of the retina.

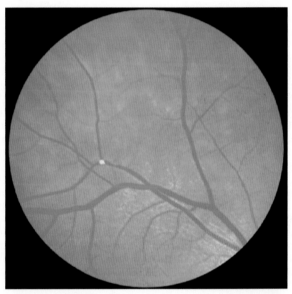

Fig. 17.33 Hollenhorst plaque. Note the bright yellow cholesterol embolus lodged at the retinal artery bifurcation. *(With permission from Dunlap, A.B., Kosmorsky, G.S., Kashyap, V.S., 2007, The fate of patients with retinal artery occlusion and Hollenhorst plaque. J Vasc Surg 46(6), 1125–1129.)*

drugs, quinine, or lysergic acid diethylamide (LSD) during pregnancy. De Morsier syndrome (septo-optic dysplasia) is characterized by developmental abnormalities of structures sharing an embryological forebrain derivation, including bilateral optic nerve hypoplasia, absent septum pellucidum, and pituitary gland dysfunction (Taylor, 2007). Optic nerve aplasia, or complete absence of the optic discs, is extremely rare.

Optic nerve coloboma is more common than optic nerve hypoplasia and results from incomplete closure of the fetal fissure (Fig. 17.31). It may occur as an isolated finding or as part of a congenital syndrome including Aicardi syndrome and trisomy 13. Another type of congenital anomaly, the optic pit, is manifested as a small grayish area, usually located in the inferior temporal portion of the optic disc. In some optic nerve dysplasias, the disc appears enlarged. This is true of the so-called morning glory disc in which a large whitish concavity is surrounded by pigmentation that resembles a morning glory flower. This appearance occurs because defective closure of the embryonic fissure is followed by growth of glial tissue and vascular remnants.

RETINAL DISORDERS
Retinal Arterial Disease

Retinal arterial disease can manifest as a central retinal artery occlusion, branch retinal artery occlusion (CRAO/BRAO), or amaurosis fugax (transient monocular visual loss). Carotid artery atherosclerotic disease is the most common cause, but cardiac valvular disease must also be considered. Evaluation and treatment for retinal arterial disease are similar to those for stroke and cerebrovascular disease in general because the annual risk of stroke or death in patients with visible retinal emboli can be increased 10-fold to 8.5% compared with controls. Acute retinal artery occlusion (CRAO/BRAO) is characterized by retinal whitening (edema) secondary to infarction. In CRAO, these findings usually are more prominent in the posterior pole than they are in the periphery (Fig. 17.32). A marked narrowing of the retinal arterioles often is noted. Because the fovea (the center of the macula) receives the majority of its blood supply from the choroid and there are no overlying retinal ganglion cells, this area retains its normal reddish-orange color, producing the characteristic cherry-red

spot. The retinal edema usually subsides fairly rapidly over days to weeks. After resolution, the retinal appearance typically returns to normal, although the prognosis for visual recovery generally is poor.

When present, retinal emboli most often are located at arteriolar bifurcations (Fig. 17.33). Visualization of retinal emboli is more common in BRAO than in CRAO. They take on a glistening or whitish or yellowish appearance and may be located on or near the optic disc or in the retinal periphery. The three major types of retinal emboli are (1) cholesterol (Hollenhorst plaques, most commonly from the carotid artery), (2) platelet-fibrin (most commonly from the cardiac valves), and (3) calcific (from either a carotid or cardiac source). It is difficult to accurately distinguish among these on the basis of fundus examination alone. With impaired blood flow after a CRAO, a portion of a retinal arteriole may take on a whitish appearance. This represents not an embolus, but rather stagnant lipid in the blood or changes in the arteriole wall.

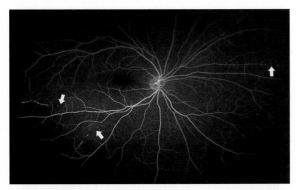

Fig. 17.34 Fluoroscein angiogram demonstrating branch retinal arteriolar occlusions in a patient with Susac's syndrome.

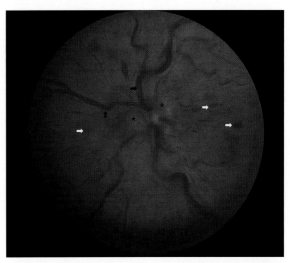

Fig. 17.35 Fundus photograph of the left eye in a patient with central retinal vein occlusion. Note mild disc swelling and hyperemia *(asterisks)*, engorgement of retinal veins *(black arrows)*, and intraretinal dot-and-blot hemorrhages *(white arrows)*. *(Reprinted with permission from Prasad, S., Volpe, N.J., Balcer, L.J., 2010. Approach to optic neuropathies: clinical update. Neurologist 16, 23–34.)*

Branch Retinal Artery Occlusions and Encephalopathy (Susac Syndrome)

Branch retinal artery occlusions and encephalopathy (Susac syndrome) is a rare disorder characterized by multiple branch retinal artery occlusions and neurological dysfunction (Gross and Eliashar, 2005; Susac, 2004). Susac syndrome most commonly affects women between the ages of 20 and 40 years. A viral syndrome may precede the development of ocular and neurological signs. The most prominent neurological manifestations are impaired mentation, sensorineural hearing loss, and visual deficits relating to BRAOs, although the full triad of these symptoms is rarely present initially. Cerebrospinal fluid in patients with Susac syndrome shows a mild lymphocytic pleocytosis and elevated protein. Antinuclear antibody (ANA) testing and cerebral arteriography are generally normal, but brain MRI most often demonstrates multiple areas of high signal intensity that resemble demyelinating plaques on T2-weighted images. Fluoroscein angiography can be very helpful to demonstrate characteristic areas of vascular permeability and arteriolar blockage (Fig. 17.34).

Ocular Ischemic Syndrome

Generalized ocular ischemia indicates involvement of both retinal and ciliary circulations in the eye. Signs of optic nerve and retinal ischemia may be present, as well as ophthalmoplegia and evidence of anterior segment ischemia (iris atrophy, loss of pupil reactivity, cataract formation, rubeosis iridis). Carotid artery occlusion or dissection and giant cell arteritis are the primary considerations in patients with ocular ischemia.

Retinal Vein Occlusion

Central or branch retinal vein occlusions rarely occur in patients younger than 50 years. The diagnosis is established clinically by the presence of characteristic retinal hemorrhages in the setting of acute vision loss. These occur diffusely in central retinal vein occlusion and focally in branch retinal vein occlusion (Fig. 17.35). Disc edema often is present and in some cases is the predominant fundus feature. In ischemic occlusion, treatment with panretinal photocoagulation can improve prognosis. No direct associations between retinal vein occlusion and carotid artery atherosclerotic disease are recognized. Patients require evaluation for vascular risk factors but generally do not require carotid imaging or ultrasound examination. In cases of bilateral retinal vein occlusion, patients should be evaluated for hyperviscosity syndromes or hypercoagulable states.

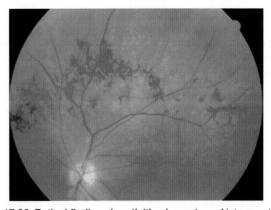

Fig. 17.36 Retinal findings in retinitis pigmentosa. Note prominent bony spicule changes in the retinal midperiphery.

Retinal Degenerations

Among the many diseases of retinal degeneration, several are associated with neurological disease. The cause of retinitis pigmentosa (RP) is degeneration of the retinal rods and cones. Rods are predominantly affected early in the course of RP, impairing night vision. Visual field loss occurs first in the midperiphery and progresses to severe field constriction. Pigmentary retinal changes that look like bony spicules are the hallmark of RP (Fig. 17.36). In some cases, however, pigment changes are not prominent, and the visual field loss may be mistaken for a neurological disorder. Even without the characteristic bony spicule-type changes, the diagnosis of RP can be made on the basis of the retinal thinning, narrowing of retinal arterioles, and waxy optic disc pallor. RP may be associated with Kearns–Sayre syndrome, Cockayne syndrome, Refsum syndrome, Batten disease, inherited vitamin E deficiency, and spinocerebellar ataxia type 7.

Retinal photoreceptor degenerations also can occur as a remote effect of cancer (the paraneoplastic retinopathies). These include cancer-associated retinopathy (CAR), which affects primarily rods and manifests with night blindness;

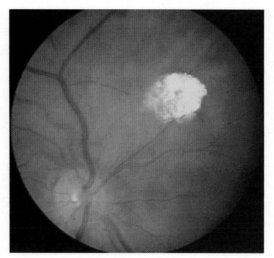

Fig. 17.37 Astrocytic hamartoma in a patient with tuberous sclerosis.

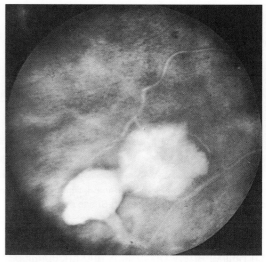

Fig. 17.38 Retinal angioma in a patient with von Hippel–Lindau disease.

cancer-associated cone dysfunction, which manifests as dyschromotopsia; melanoma-associated retinopathy, which has a relatively better prognosis; and others. Visual acuity in these conditions initially can range from normal to significantly impaired, typically with a rapid rate of deterioration. Arteriolar narrowing is a consistent finding, and pigmentary changes in the retina are variable. Electroretinography is markedly abnormal (showing reduced to extinguished rod and cone components). Antiphotoreceptor antibodies often can be identified in the serum, although the specificity of these tests remains imperfect. Treatment of the underlying malignancy typically does not improve vision, but immunosuppression with steroids can be effective.

Progressive cone dystrophies are retinal degenerations that commonly demonstrate autosomal dominant inheritance. Typically, vision loss develops in both eyes, beginning in adolescence and worsening over several years. Early in the course of cone dystrophy, the fundus may appear normal; with time, however, pigmentary changes develop in the macula, and electroretinography demonstrates characteristic reductions of the photopic response.

Phakomatoses

Retinal findings are common in phakomatoses that affect the nervous system, particularly tuberous sclerosis and von Hippel–Lindau disease. Neurological features of phakomatoses are described in Chapter 100. In tuberous sclerosis, retinal astrocytic hamartomas are characteristic (Fig. 17.37). These usually are multiple and may appear either as a fullness in the retinal nerve fiber layer or as a nodular refractile lesion (mulberry type). Von Hippel–Lindau disease is characterized by the presence of one or more retinal angiomas that appear as reddish masses with a feeding artery and a draining vein

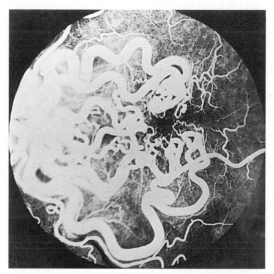

Fig. 17.39 Fluorescein angiogram of a racemose arteriovenous malformation in the retina in a patient with Wyburn–Mason disease.

(Fig. 17.38). Treatment with photocoagulation or cryotherapy may be necessary. Wyburn–Mason disease is characterized by racemose arteriovenous malformations in the retina (Fig. 17.39).

REFERENCES

The complete reference list is available online at https://expertconsult .inkling.com.

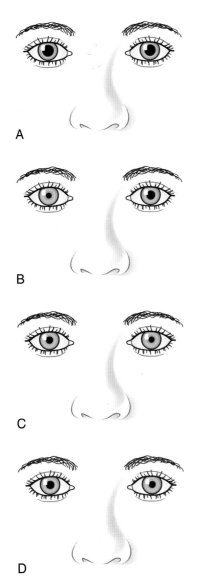

Fig. 18.4 Left tonic pupil. A, In darkness, anisocoria is minimal because the normal right pupil is dilated. **B,** In bright light, anisocoria is enhanced because the normal right pupil constricts, while the tonic pupil does not. **C,** A near stimulus results in constriction of the tonic pupil, giving light-near dissociation. **D,** A few seconds after return of gaze to a distant target, the normal right pupil has redilated, but the tonic pupil remains small.

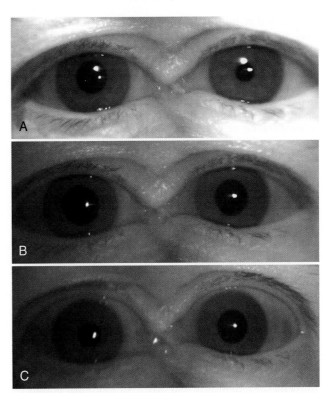

Fig. 18.5 Right tonic pupil. A, When viewed in bright light, there is anisocoria with a larger right pupil. **B,** When viewed in dim light, the anisocoria is less prominent due to dilation of the normal left pupil. **C,** Thirty minutes after instillation of dilute pilocarpine, the right pupil is constricted due to the presence of cholinergic supersensitivity.

pupil at the initial presentation of head trauma, stroke, or an intracranial mass lesion is associated with 75% mortality (Clusmann et al., 2001). Although dilute pilocarpine has been reported to produce constriction of the pupil in this situation, it should definitely constrict after administration of 1% pilocarpine (see Table 18.1). This may help in differentiating isolated pupillary enlargement from oculomotor palsy from pharmacological pupillary enlargement, because a pharmacological pupil should not constrict with pilocarpine. See Chapter 104 for a complete discussion of oculomotor nerve anatomy and clinical lesions; Fig. 104.3 shows an example of oculomotor palsy.

Iris Sphincter Injury and Ischemia. Blunt trauma to the eye can damage the iris sphincter, causing mydriasis (pupillary enlargement) with poor pupillary constriction to both light

and near stimuli. Tears at the pupillary margin may be evident. The pupil may be smaller than normal (spastic miosis) immediately after the injury, but it becomes dilated and poorly reactive after a few minutes. This course of events may simulate those of uncal herniation. Iris ischemia may cause mydriasis, poor pupillary reactivity, and iris transillumination defects. Iris ischemia may occur with acute angle closure glaucoma and ocular ischemic syndrome, both of which are usually accompanied by poor vision and pain. Additional signs of acute angle closure glaucoma include corneal edema and ocular injection. The ocular ischemic syndrome can occur in patients with severe stenosis of an internal carotid artery or stenoses of the internal and external carotid arteries on one side. Associated eye findings include neovascularization of the retina, optic disc, or iris (rubeosis iridis), anterior uveitis (iritis), and ocular hypotony. Some forms of iris degeneration, such as iris atrophy, may cause pupillary dilation, often with irregularity of the pupillary outline.

Pharmacological Mydriasis. Pharmacological mydriasis usually occurs after accidental or intentional instillation of anticholinergic agents such as atropine. Accidental mydriasis usually occurs with hand-to-eye contact in individuals who have contact with dilating agents; examples include following application of a scopolamine skin patch for motion sickness, administration of eye drops to a family member with eye disease, or exposure to plants with parasympathetic blocking activity such as angel's trumpet or Jimson weed (Andreola et al., 2008; Spina and Taddei, 2007). Inadvertent administration of nebulized ipratropium into the eye via an ill-fitting face mask in a critically ill patient may result in unilateral mydriasis that mimics isolated pupillary involvement from oculomotor nerve compression due to intracranial hypertension with uncal herniation (Eustace et al., 2004). However, pharmacologically dilated pupils tend to be larger than the dilated pupil of oculomotor nerve palsy. Sympathomimetic agents, such as phenylephrine, give mydriasis that is less marked and prolonged than that caused by anticholinergic agents. Pharmacologically dilated pupils do not constrict after administration of 1% pilocarpine (see Table 18.1).

Anisocoria Greater in the Dark

Horner Syndrome. The classic Horner syndrome triad of sympathetic dysfunction consists of ipsilateral ptosis, miosis, and facial anhidrosis. The lesion may be anywhere along the three-neuron sympathetic pathway (described in Pupil Anatomy and Neural Control). Anhidrosis is only present with lesions of the first- or second-order (preganglionic) neurons because the fibers serving facial sweating take a pathway distinct from those destined for the dilator muscle after synapsing in the superior cervical ganglion. The ptosis results from impaired innervation of the Müller muscle, which contributes only slightly to maintenance of lid opening. As a result, only mild ptosis will be evident with sympathetic dysfunction. Apparent enophthalmos (an illusion of a "sunken" eye) due to palpebral fissure narrowing from involvement of the Müller muscle in combination with subtle elevation of the lower lid ("reverse" or "upside down" ptosis) from involvement of lower lid smooth muscle may occur. An additional finding on examination is dilation lag, the delayed dilation of the Horner pupil in darkness (Pilley and Thompson, 1975) (Fig. 18.6).

The differential diagnosis for Horner syndrome varies for a preganglionic lesion (first- or second-order neuron) versus a postganglionic (third-order neuron) lesion; differentiation between the two will dictate the diagnostic approach. Localization of a preganglionic versus a postganglionic lesion can be made with pupillary diagnostic eye drops (Mughal and Longmuir, 2009). Hydroxyamphetamine (1%) is used for this purpose. However, some prefer to confirm the presence of

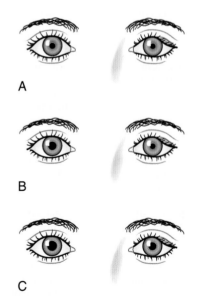

Fig. 18.6 Left Horner syndrome. A, Mild upper lid ptosis and miosis in room light. **B,** Anisocoria is increased at 5 seconds after the lights are dimmed, due to dilation lag of left pupil. **C,** Fifteen seconds after the lights are dimmed, left pupil exhibits increased dilation compared to the image in **B.**

Horner syndrome using cocaine or apraclonidine eye drop testing rather than proceeding directly to localization testing. Administration of diagnostic and localizing drops cannot be done on the same day; at least 24 hours must separate the eye drop tests. From a practical standpoint, cocaine and hydroxyamphetamine are difficult to obtain. Cocaine is a controlled substance, must be kept under lock and key, and results in positive urine toxicology for 2 days after ocular administration (Jacobson et al., 2001). Hydroxyamphetamine eye drops can be obtained from compounding pharmacies. Cocaine inhibits reuptake of norepinephrine at the sympathetic terminus. The result is dilation of a normal pupil but impaired dilation of the sympathetically denervated pupil, with a resultant increase in the anisocoria. Lack of dilation after cocaine administration occurs with both preganglionic and postganglionic lesions. Hydroxyamphetamine induces the third-order neuron to release any stored norepinephrine. It will dilate a normal pupil and a pupil with an intact third-order sympathetic neuron. Therefore, if pupillary dilation occurs in a Horner pupil, the lesion is localized to the preganglionic first- or second-order neurons. If pupillary dilation fails to occur, a third-order neuron lesion is likely (Fig. 18.7, A-B).

Apraclonidine, in a 0.5% solution, is a recent addition to the diagnostic armamentarium for Horner syndrome (Koc et al., 2005). It is an α-adrenergic agonist approved for lowering of intraocular pressure. After bilateral instillation of apraclonidine in a patient with Horner syndrome, there is reversal of the anisocoria caused by dilation of the Horner pupil and either constriction of or no change in the normal pupil (Fig. 18.8). This occurs because apraclonidine is a weak α-1 agonist; the Horner pupil dilates due to denervation supersensitivity. In addition, the Horner-induced ptosis resolves; however, this alone cannot be used to confirm diagnosis, because elevation of the eyelid may be seen in normal eyes. Apraclonidine as a replacement for cocaine in the diagnosis of Horner syndrome is promising, but further study is needed; it remains unclear how much time is needed for denervation supersensitivity to develop (Kardon, 2005). A positive apraclonidine test has been reported within 3 hours of lesion onset; however, a false-negative result has been reported up to 16 days after carotid dissection (Cooper-Knick et al., 2011; Dewan et al., 2009; Lebas et al., 2010).

Any lesion along the course of the three-neuron sympathetic pathway may cause Horner syndrome. Two conditions deserve detailed description, owing to their clinical importance and potential ominous prognosis if left undetected; these are carotid dissection, with presentation as an isolated painful Horner syndrome, and Pancoast tumor. Acute onset of a painful Horner syndrome, especially after neck trauma or manipulation (e.g., chiropractic manipulation), should lead to suspicion for a carotid dissection. The intracranial precavernous portion of the carotid artery can be affected and it is not uncommon for a dissection in this portion to be missed on magnetic resonance angiography (MRA) and detected only by careful examination of non–contrast-enhanced fat-saturated axial T1-weighted magnetic resonance imaging (MRI) through the base of the skull, looking for a crescent of hyperintense T1 signal surrounding the carotid artery flow void (see **Fig. 18.7,** C, D). Treatment typically consists of antiplatelet therapy with aspirin to minimize the risk of emboli from the dissected artery (Giorgiadis et al., 2009). A preganglionic Horner syndrome, particularly in a patient with a history of tobacco use, should prompt a search for a pulmonary apical neoplasm or Pancoast tumor. Outside of these two settings, the workup for Horner syndrome consists of neuroimaging of the affected portion of the sympathetic pathway: brain and spine (the entire cervical and first two thoracic segments) MRI with contrast for a preganglionic lesion, and brain MRI with contrast

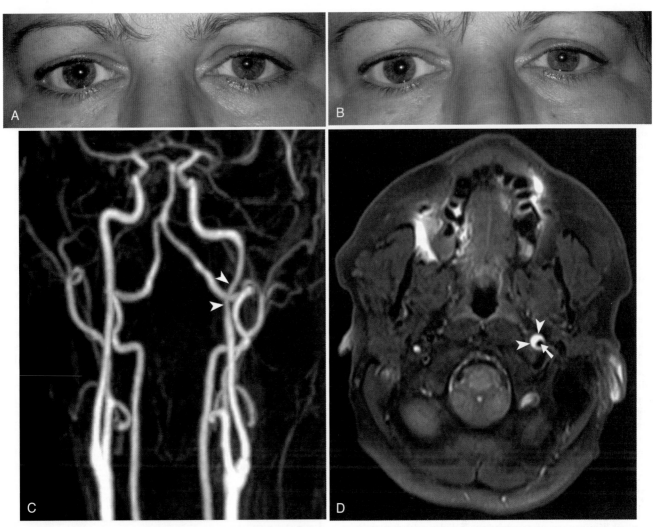

Fig. 18.7 Acute, painful, left postganglionic (third-order neuron) Horner syndrome secondary to a left internal carotid artery dissection. **A,** Left miosis and slight ptosis. **B,** Failure of left pupil to dilate after 1% hydroxyamphetamine instillation, confirming the postganglionic location of the lesion. **C,** Magnetic resonance angiography, showing subtle focal narrowing of the left internal carotid artery (*arrowheads*). **D,** T1-weighted axial magnetic resonance image without contrast, showing a left internal carotid artery dissection with a crescent of hyperintense blood in the wall of the artery (*arrowheads*) causing narrowing of the artery lumen (*white arrow*).

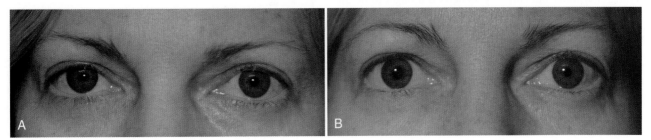

Fig. 18.8 A, Right Horner syndrome with mild right ptosis and anisocoria with a small right pupil. **B,** Forty minutes after administration of 0.5% apraclonidine. Note reversal of anisocoria secondary to dilation of the Horner pupil and resolution of the ptosis.

and MRA for a postganglionic lesion (Almog et al., 2010; Davagnanam et al., 2013). In children, the majority of Horner syndromes are congenital; however, birth trauma, vascular malformations, carotid dissection, and neoplasm (neuroblastoma) are possible causes. The recommended evaluation in children includes neuroimaging and urinary catecholamine testing to screen for neuroblastoma (Smith et al., 2010).

Anterior Uveitis (Iris Inflammation). Acute inflammatory disease involving the iris (anterior uveitis or iritis) may cause pupillary constriction. If inflammation persists, adhesions between the iris and lens (posterior synechiae) may lead to pupillary irregularity and immobility. Usually the inflamed eye is red and the patient reports pain and photophobia. However, some chronic forms of anterior uveitis can cause iris adhesions without these manifestations. Syphilis most commonly causes Argyll–Robertson pupils but may cause focal iris inflammation and degeneration. Infiltration of the iris by tumor or amyloid can also cause irregular pupils.

Episodic Anisocoria

Anisocoria may be intermittent. Physiological anisocoria can vary from week to week and occasionally from hour to hour. A rare condition known as *tadpole pupil* results from intermittent spasms of segments of the dilator muscle; often, these patients have an underlying Horner syndrome (Thompson et al., 1983). A related phenomenon is oculo-sympathetic spasm associated with lesions of the cervical spinal cord.

Benign episodic unilateral mydriasis is a diagnosis of exclusion in which episodes of pupillary dilation last from minutes to a few days (Jacobson, 1995). Some patients have migraine or a trigeminal autonomic cephalgia, but many patients have isolated monocular visual blurring or are asymptomatic during episodes (Antonaci et al., 2010). The frequency of episodes varies from several per week to one every few years. Some patients have asymmetrical parasympathetic insufficiency as a cause of the episodes, while others have asymmetrical sympathetic hyperactivity. Cyclical oculomotor palsy is a rare condition in which periodic oculomotor spasms occur in a patient with oculomotor nerve palsy. During the spasms, the eyelid rises, the exotropic eye moves to the midline, and the pupil constricts. In some cases, the spasms involve only the pupil. Intermittent spasm of portions of the pupillary sphincter may occur in traumatic oculomotor nerve paralysis and with aberrant regeneration. Unilateral pupillary dilation and other pupillary signs can also occur during seizures, and rhythmic pupillary oscillations have been reported with Creutzfeld–Jakob disease (Nagasaka et al., 2010).

Pupillary Light-Near Dissociation

The term *light-near dissociation* refers to pupils that have marked diminution of constriction to light, with better constriction to near stimuli. The differential diagnosis includes tonic pupil, Argyll–Robertson pupil, the dorsal midbrain syndrome, and severe bilateral optic neuropathy (Han et al., 2010). Tonic pupils were described earlier (Anisocoria Greater in the Light). Argyll–Robertson pupils are small and irregular. In the past, this condition was most commonly seen in the setting of syphilis, but currently diabetes is thought to be the most common cause, although the pupils are not miotic. Localization of the underlying lesion is unclear, but possibilities include the ciliary ganglion and the dorsal midbrain (Thompson and Kardon, 2006). The dorsal midbrain or Parinaud syndrome (see Chapter 21) consists of impaired vertical gaze, convergence-retraction nystagmus, and lid retraction (Collier sign), in addition to pupillary light-near dissociation. It is often due to pineal gland lesions, hydrocephalus, or stroke. Light-near dissociation in this syndrome may be due to destruction of the dorsally located olivary pretectal nuclei involved in the pupillary light reflex (see Pupil Anatomy and Neural Control), with relative sparing of the fibers serving the pupillary near response, which arise from a more ventral pathway.

EYELID ABNORMALITIES
Eyelid Anatomy and Neural Control

The width of the palpebral fissure is determined by the balance of action of the orbicularis oculi muscle, the levator palpebrae superioris muscle, smooth Müller muscle, and the periorbital and eyelid connective tissues. The orbicularis oculi is innervated by the facial nerve, the levator palpebrae superioris by the oculomotor nerve, and the Müller muscle by the sympathetic nervous system. Activation of the orbicularis oculi results in eye closure. The levator palpebrae and, to a lesser extent, Müller muscle are responsible for maintaining eye opening. See Chapter 104 for a complete discussion of the anatomy of the facial and oculomotor nerves.

Pathological Conditions of the Eyelids
Clinical Presentation and Examination

Patients with abnormal eyelids may present complaining of a change in the physical appearance of one or both eyelids, or they may complain of symptoms related to impaired eyelid function such as eye pain or blurred vision from exposure keratopathy due to excessive eyelid opening or incomplete eyelid closure. In contrast, patients may be unaware of a problem but have had an asymmetrical eye appearance brought to their attention by an acquaintance or family member. Patients will often indicate that they have a "droopy eye" even if the side with the smaller palpebral fissure is the normal side and the side with the widened palpebral fissure is abnormal. It is up to the examiner to determine which side is abnormal. Familiarity with the resting position of the eyelids is therefore essential for determining whether a pathological state exists.

Steps in the examination of the eyelids are summarized in Box 18.1. The normal palpebral fissure is between 12 and 15 mm wide. At rest, the upper eyelid normally covers the upper 1 to 2 mm of the iris, and the margin of the lower eyelid just touches the lower border of the iris (Fig. 18.9). In an eye with upper lid retraction, the lid touches the upper border of the iris or sclera is visible between the iris and the upper lid

---

BOX 18.1 Clinical Examination of the Eyelids

Observe for at least 1 minute, looking for the following:
  Palpebral fissure asymmetry
  The resting position of each upper and lower eyelid relative to the iris edge
  Upper or lower lid retraction and scleral show
  Ptosis
  Proptosis (protruding eye) or enophthalmos (inward or "sunken" eye)
  Eyelid edema or scarring
  Blink rate (normal is roughly 18 times per minute)
Assess lid position in different gaze directions
If ptosis is present, assess for worsening with prolonged upgaze
Observe gentle and forced lid closure
Examine for pupillary abnormalities, ocular motor abnormalities, and facial weakness

---

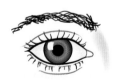 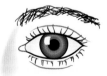

Fig. 18.9 Normal eyelid position. Upper lid covers the upper 1 to 2 mm of the iris. Lower lid just touches the lower edge of the iris.

familiarity, and is involved in odor learning and memory (Gottfried et al., 2002). The entorhinal cortex preprocesses information entering the hippocampus, whereas the amygdala seems to respond to the intensity of emotionally significant odors. The orbitofrontal cortex combines input from taste, texture, and smell and plays a vital role in flavor perception and hedonics (Rolls and Grabenhorst, 2008).

Gustation

Taste is critical for identifying substances in foods and beverages, such as sugars and poisonous alkaloids, that promote or disrupt homeostasis. In addition to being located within the oral cavity, bitter and sweet taste-related receptors are found in the alimentary and respiratory tracts, where they are involved in metabolism and bacterial defense. In the oral cavity, the taste receptor cells are located within taste buds, small flask-like structures on the surface of the oral epithelium, mostly on protuberances called papillae (Figs. 19.3 and 19.4). Like olfactory receptor cells, taste receptor cells periodically die and become replaced.

Humans possess approximately 7,500 oral taste buds. The buds on the *fungiform papillae*, as well as those on the *anterior folliate papillae* and *soft palate*, are innnervated by CN VII. Those on the *posterior folliate papillae* and *circumvalate papillae* are innervated by CN IX. Taste buds within the oral pharynx are supplied by the vagus (CN X) nerve.

A small family of three G-protein-coupled receptors (GPCRs) termed T1R1, T1R2, and T1R3, encode sweet and umami (monosodium glutamate-like) sensations. Bitter is mediated by the T2R receptors, a family of ~30 GPCRs expressed on cells different from those that express sweet and umami receptors. Salty sensations arise from the entrance of Na^+ ions into the cells via specialized membrane channels, such as the amiloride-sensitive Na^+ channel. Although sour taste has been suggested to depend upon a range of receptors, PKD2L1 is likely the primary sour taste receptor. The nerves innervating the taste buds converge centrally into the nucleus of the solitary tract of the brainstem. From there fibers project to centers within the upper regions of the ventral posterior nuclei of the thalamus via the medial lemniscus. Information is then sent to the amygdala and several cortical regions, including the primary somatosensory cortex and the anterior insular cortex. Neurons within these regions respond to taste, touch, and in some cases odors.

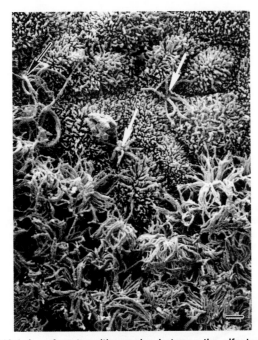

Fig. 19.1 A surface transition region between the olfactory and respiratory epithelia. The bottom half displays olfactory epithelium, the top half respiratory epithelium. Arrows identify olfactory receptor cell dendritic endings with cilia. Bar = 5 μm. *With permission from Menco, B. P. M., Morrison, E. E., 2003, Morphology of the mammalian olfactory epithelium: form, fine structure, function, and pathology, in: Doty, R. L. (Ed.), Handbook of Olfaction and Gustation, 2nd edn. Marcel Dekker, New York, pp. 17–49.*

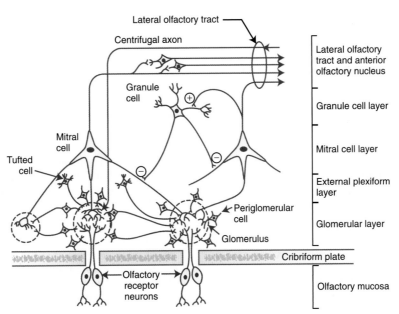

Fig. 19.2 Schematic of olfactory bulb structures, neurons, and layers. *With permission from Alloway, K.D., Pritchard, T.C., 2007, Medical Neuroscience, 2nd edn. Hayes Barton, Raleigh, NC.*

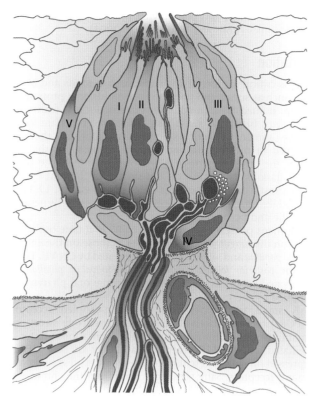

Fig. 19.3 Idealized drawing of longitudinal section of mammalian taste bud. Cells of types I, II, and III are elongated and form the sensory epithelium of the bud. These cells have different types of microvillae within the taste pit and may reach the taste pore. Type IV cells are basal cells and type V are marginal cells. Synapses are most apparent at the bases of type III cells. The connecting taste nerves have myelin sheaths. *With permission from Witt, M., Reutter, K., 2015. Anatomy of the tongue and taste buds., in: Doty, R.L. (Ed.), Handbook of Olfaction and Gustation, 3rd edn. Wiley-Liss, New York, pp. 639–665. Copyright © 2015 Richard L. Doty.*

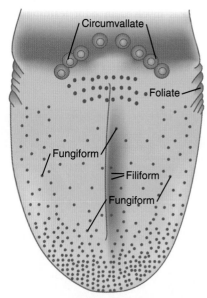

Fig. 19.4 Schematic representation of the tongue demonstrating the relative distribution of the four main classes of taste papillae. Note that the fungiform papillae can vary considerable in size, and that they are more dense on the anterior and lateral regions of the tongue. *Copyright © 2006 Richard L. Doty*

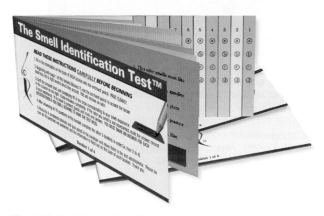

Fig. 19.5 Booklets of the University of Pennsylvania Smell Identification Test (UPSIT). The test comprises 4 booklets, each containing 10 microencapsulated scratch and sniff odorants that are released by a pencil tip. Associated with each odorant is a multiple-choice question about which of four possibilities is correct. Forced-choice answers are recorded on the last page of each booklet and assessed with a simple scoring key. *Copyright © 2004 Sensonics, Inc., Haddon Heights, NJ. Reprinted with permission.*

The "taste code" interpreted by the brain depends on the specific neurons that are activated and the patterns of firing that occur both within and between these nerves. As with odors, the brain must remember what a particular tastant tastes like (e.g., sweet) and a matching or comparison of information coming from the taste pathways must be made at some point in the CNS. Much of the "integration" of gustatory information with other sensory input occurs at the level of the orbitofrontal cortex. Secondary connections through anterior limbic structures are involved in emotion, reward valuation, and reward-related decision-making (Rolls, 2013).

CHEMOSENSORY TESTING

The most widely used olfactory tests are psychophysical tests of odor identification and detection (Doty, 2007). In identification tests, a subject is typically asked to identify, usually from a list of alternatives, the quality of the sensation experienced when sniffing or tasting a stimulus. A response is required even if no sensation is perceived, a procedure called forced-choice responding. For example, the most popular odor identification test—the 40-item "scratch and sniff" University of Pennsylvania Smell Identification Test or UPSIT—requires a subject to identify the name of each odor from a list of four alternatives (Fig. 19.5) (Doty et al., 1984b). The

number of correct answers determines the degree of deficit and allows for both an overall absolute classification of function (i.e., normosmia, mild microsmia, moderate microsmia, severe microsmia, anosmia) and a relative classification based upon percentiles from age- and sex-related norms. Malingering can be discerned from improbable responses in the forced-choice situation.

In an odor detection threshold test, a subject is typically presented with an odor and one or more blanks in random fashion and asked to identify which of the stimuli is stronger or otherwise discernable from the other stimuli. A common procedure is to present stronger stimuli when a miss occurs and weaker stimuli when a hit occurs following a defined algorithm. This is termed a "staircase procedure" and the

6. damage to taste-related central nervous system structures from disorders such as multiple sclerosis, tumors, epilepsy, and stroke.

Lesions caudal to the pons produce ipsilateral deficits, whereas lesions within the pons proper can produce ipsilateral, contralateral, or bilateral deficits. Both ipsilateral and contralateral taste deficits have been noted in patients with lesions of the insular cortex, reflecting the bilateral representation of taste function at this level (Pritchard et al., 1999). Unlike CN VII, CN IX is relatively protected along its path, although iatrogenic interventions can result in CN IX injury (e.g., from tonsillectomy, bronchoscopy, laryngoscopy, and radiation therapy), and this nerve is not immune to damage from tumors, vascular lesions, and infection. On rare occasion epilepsy or migraine is associated with a gustatory prodrome or aura, and some tastes may actually trigger seizures or migraine attacks.

A number of medications have been implicated in taste dysfunction, including antineoplastic agents, antirheumatic drugs, antibiotics, and blood pressure medications (Doty et al., 2008). Terbinafine, a popular antifungal, can produce long-lasting loss of sweet, sour, bitter, and salty taste perception (Doty and Haxel, 2005). A double-blind study found that eszopiclone, a widely used sleep medication, induces a bitter dysgeusia in approxiately two-thirds of individuals tested (Doty et al., 2009). This sensation was related to the time since drug administration, was stronger for women than for men, and correlated with both saliva and blood levels of the drug.

Alterations in chemosensory function are well-established as a consequence of radiation and chemotherapy for cancer patients. Taste thresholds can increase during chemotherapy and qualitative changes, such as the development of a metallic taste, are frequently reported (Gamper et al., 2012). In one study of nasopharyngeal cancer patients receiving radiotherapy who developed impairment in olfactory function, decreased olfactory bulb volume was noted (Veyseller et al., 2014).

CLINICAL EVALUATION OF TASTE AND SMELL

Etiology can usually be established from a clinical history that explores symptom nature, onset, duration, pattern of fluctuations, and potential precipitating events, such as upper respiratory infections that occurred prior to symptom onset. Information regarding head trauma, smoking habits, drug and alcohol abuse (e.g., intranasal cocaine, chronic alcoholism in the context of Wernicke and Korsakoff syndromes), exposures to pesticides and other toxic agents, and medical interventions are informative. The possibility of multiple or cumulative effects cannot be discounted. A determination of all the medications that the patient was taking before and at the time of symptom onset is important, as are comorbid medical conditions potentially associated with taste and smell impairment, such as renal failure, liver disease, hypothyroidism, diabetes, and dementia. Delayed puberty in association with anosmia (with or without midline craniofacial abnormalities, deafness, and renal anomalies) suggests the possibility of Kallmann syndrome. Recollection of epistaxis, discharge (clear, purulent or bloody), nasal obstruction, allergies, and somatic symptoms, including headache or irritation, have potential localizing value. Questions related to memory, parkinsonian signs, and seizure activity (e.g., automatisms, occurrence of blackouts, auras, and déjà vu) should be posed. The possibility of malingering should be considered, particularly if litigation is involved. Intermittent smell loss usually implies an obstructive disorder, such as from rhinosinusitis or

other inflammatory problem. Sudden smell loss alerts the practitioner to head trauma, ischemia, infection, or a psychiatric condition. Gradual smell loss can be a marker for the development of a progressive obstructive lesion, cumulative drug effects, or simply presbyosmia or presbygeusia. While losses secondary to head trauma are most commonly abrupt, in some cases the loss appears over time or only becomes apparent to the patient after a long interval. In addition to quantitative sensory evaluation, which is key in defining the dysfunction, neurological and otorhinolaryngological (ORL) examinations, along with appropriate brain and nasosinus imaging, aid in the evaluation of patients with olfactory or gustatory complaints. Blood serum tests may be helpful in identifying conditions such as diabetes, infection, heavy metal exposure, nutritional deficiency (e.g., B_6, B_{12}), allergy, and thyroid, liver, and kidney disease.

TREATMENT AND MANAGEMENT

Management of chemosensory disorders is condition specific. Medical or surgical interventions are available for most patients with obstructive or inflammatory disorders (e.g., allergic rhinitis, glossitis, polyposis, intranasal or intraoral neoplasms). For example, in cases of rhinosinusitis, an oral taper of prednisone can initially be used to quell general inflammation followed by topical administration of the nasal spray or drops in the inverted head position, such as the Moffett position (Canciani and Mastella, 1988). Candidiasis or other oral infections can be quelled with topical antifungal and antibiotic treatments. Some salty or bitter dysgeusias respond to chlorohexidine mouth wash, possibly as a result of its strong positive charge (Wang et al., 2009). Patients with excessive oral dryness, including dryness due to medications, often benefit from the use of mints, lozenges, or sugarless gum, as well as oral pilocarpine or artificial saliva.

Medications that induce distortions of smell or taste can often be discontinued and other types of medications or modes of therapy substituted, although reversal of the dysfunction may take months (Doty et al., 2008). Antioxidants, such as alpha-lipoic acid, may be effectual in some cases of hyposmia, hypogeusia, dysosmia, dysgeusia, and burning mouth syndrome (Hummel et al., 2002), although strong scientific evidence for such efficacy is lacking. Despite being widely mentioned in the medical literature, zinc and vitamin A therapies unlikely benefit olfactory disturbances except when frank deficiencies are present, although both of these agents may improve taste dysfunction secondary to hepatic deficiencies (Deems et al., 1991b). Studies reporting positive effects of theophylline, acupuncture, and transcranial magnetic stimulation are not convincing and generally lack appropriate control groups. There are reports that some antiepileptics and antidepressants (e.g., amitriptyline) may be of value in treating some chemosensory disturbances, particularly following head trauma. Donepezil (an acetylcholinesterase inhibitor) has been reported to improve both cognitive and odor identification scores in patients with Alzheimer disease (Velayudhan and Lovestone, 2009).

It is of interest that repeated exposure to odorants may, in fact, increase sensitivity to them in both animals and humans, providing a rationale for therapies in which multiple odors are smelled before and after going to bed (Hummel et al., 2009). In one study, patients with post-infectious and post-traumatic olfactory impairment were put through 16 weeks of "training" of smelling four separate odorants, which resulted in an increase in function for both groups (Konstantinidis et al., 2013). Importantly, spontaneous recovery over time occurs in some instances, providing hope to at least some patients. In a longitudinal study of 542 patients with smell loss from a variety of causes, modest improvement occurred over an average time period of 4 years in about half of the participants (London, et al., 2008). However, normal age-related function returned in only 11% of the anosmic and 23% of the hyposmic patients. The amount of dysfunction present at the time of presentation, not etiology, was the best predictor of prognosis.

An important but overlooked element of therapy comes from chemosensory testing itself. Confirmation or lack of conformation of loss is beneficial to patients, particularly ones who come to believe they may be "crazy" as a result of unsupportive medical providers or family members. Quantitative testing places the patient's problem into overall perspective and if considerable function is present, patients can be informed of a more positive prognosis. It is extremely therapeutic for an older person to become aware that, while his or her smell function is not what it used to be, it still falls above the average of his or her peer group. It is unfortunate that many such patients are simply told by their physician they are getting old and nothing can be done for them, often exacerbating or leading to depression and decreased self-esteem.

REFERENCES

The complete reference list is available online at https://expertconsult .inkling.com/.

20 Cranial and Facial Pain

J. D. Bartleson, David F. Black, Jerry W. Swanson

CHAPTER OUTLINE

HISTORY
  Types of Headaches
  Onset of Headaches
  Frequency and Periodicity of Episodic Headaches
  Temporal Profile
  Time of Day and Precipitating Factors
  Location
  Quality and Severity
  Premonitory Symptoms, Aura, and Accompanying
    Symptoms
  Aggravating and Mitigating Factors
  Family History of Headaches
  Prior Evaluation
  Prior Treatment
  Disability
  Patient Concerns and Reasons for Seeking Help
  Other Medical or Neurological Problems

EXAMINATION

DIAGNOSTIC TESTING
  Neuroimaging and Other Imaging Studies
  Cerebrospinal Fluid Tests
  Electrophysiological Testing
  General Medical Tests
  Special Examinations and Consultations

FURTHER OBSERVATION

Headache is an exceedingly common symptom that affects virtually everyone at some time in their life. It is estimated that nearly half of the world's adult population has an active headache disorder (Robbins and Lipton, 2010). Headache is one of the most common reasons for outpatient healthcare visits in the United States. Patients with head and/or face pain typically present for medical attention because the discomfort is severe, interferes with work and/or leisure activities, or raises the patient's or family's concern about a serious underlying cause.

Headache disorders are classified as primary or secondary (Box 20.1) (IHS, 2013). The primary headache disorders do not have an underlying structural cause, but all the primary headache disorders can be stimulated by secondary conditions. The diagnosis of head and face pain depends on three elements: the history, neurological and general examinations, and appropriate investigations, if needed. Treatment of headaches is discussed in Chapter 103.

HISTORY

The gold standard for diagnosis and management of headache is a careful interview and neurological and general medical examinations (De Luca and Bartleson, 2010). In the vast majority of patients with headache, the neurological and general examinations will be normal, and the diagnosis is based entirely on the history. Therefore, clinicians are well advised to spend most of their time interviewing the patient.

History-taking for head and face pain is similar to that for other presenting complaints, but several specific aspects should be addressed. The questions listed in Box 20.2 are useful, and the discussion that follows illustrates some responses and their implications. Usually one begins by asking the patient to describe their symptoms or, alternatively, simply by asking how they can be helped. This approach allows patients to relax and say what they had planned to say. Usually the patient will speak for less than 2 minutes if not interrupted. Once the patient has had an opportunity to speak, directed but open-ended questions (see Box 20.2) can be asked.

Types of Headaches

Many individuals have more than one type of headache. It is valuable to establish this information at the beginning of the interview so each type of pain can be carefully delineated. A change in an established headache pattern can indicate a new condition.

Onset of Headaches

A stable headache disorder of many years' duration is almost always of benign origin. Migraine headaches often begin in childhood, adolescence, or early adulthood. A headache of recent onset obviously has many possible causes, including the new onset of either a benign or serious condition. "Recent onset" has been defined differently by various authors; the typical range is from 1 to 12 months. In general, the more recent the onset of headache, the more worrisome the possible cause. The "worst ever" headache, an increasingly severe headache, or change for the worse in an existing headache pattern all raise the possibility of an intracranial lesion. Headaches of instantaneous onset suggest an intracranial hemorrhage, usually in the subarachnoid space, but also can be caused by intracerebral hemorrhage, cerebral venous thrombosis, intra- and extracranial arterial dissection, pituitary apoplexy, spontaneous intracranial hypotension, reversible cerebral vasoconstriction syndrome (RCVS), acute hypertensive crisis, and other conditions that must be excluded with the first occurrence of so-called "thunderclap headache" (Ju and Schwedt, 2010). If no underlying cause is discovered despite expedited, thorough investigation, a diagnosis of primary thunderclap headache can be considered. Onset of a new headache in patients older than 50 years raises suspicion of an intracranial lesion (e.g., subdural hematoma) or giant cell (temporal or cranial) arteritis (GCA). A history of antecedent head or neck injury should be sought; even a relatively minor injury can be associated with subsequent development of epidural, subdural, subarachnoid, or intraparenchymal hemorrhage and post-traumatic dissection of the carotid or vertebral arteries (Debette and Leys, 2009). However, post-traumatic headaches can occur following head injury in the absence of any demonstrable pathology.

BOX 20.1 Headache Classification

THE PRIMARY HEADACHES

Migraine and its subtypes
Tension-type headache and its subtypes
Trigeminal autonomic cephalalgias
    Cluster headache
    Paroxysmal hemicrania
    Short-lasting unilateral neuralgiform headache attacks
    Hemicrania continua
Other primary headache disorders
    Primary cough headache
    Primary exercise headache
    Primary headache associated with sexual activity
    Primary thunderclap headache
    Cold-stimulus headache
    External-pressure headache
    Primary stabbing headache
    Nummular headache
    Hypnic headache
    New daily persistent headache

THE SECONDARY HEADACHES

Headache attributed to trauma or injury to the head and/or neck
Headache attributed to cranial or cervical vascular disorder
Headache attributed to nonvascular intracranial disorder
Headache attributed to a substance or its withdrawal
Headache attributed to infection
Headache attributed to disorder of homeostasis
Headache or facial pain attributed to disorder of the cranium, neck, eyes, ears, nose, sinuses, teeth, mouth, or other facial or cervical structure
Headache attributed to psychiatric disorder

PAINFUL CRANIAL NEUROPATHIES, OTHER FACIAL PAINS, AND OTHER HEADACHES

Painful cranial neuropathies and other facial pains
Other headache disorders

From The International Classification of Headache Disorders, 3rd edition (beta version), 2013.

BOX 20.2 Useful Questions to Ask the Patient with Headache

- How many types of headache do you have?
- When and how did each type begin?
- If the headaches are episodic, what is the frequency and duration?
- How long does it take for your headaches to reach maximal intensity?
- How long do your headaches last?
- When do the headaches tend to occur, and what factors trigger your headaches?
- Where does your pain start, and how does it evolve?
- What is the quality of your pain?
- How severe is your pain?
- Is the pain steady or pulsating (throbbing), or both?
- Are there symptoms that herald the onset of your headache?
- What are they, when do they begin, and how long do they last?
- Are there symptoms that accompany your headaches?
- Do you get nauseated with your headaches?
- Does light and/or noise bother you a lot more when you have a headache than when you don't?
- Do your headaches limit your ability to work, study, or do what you need to do for at least 1 day?
- Does anything aggravate your pain (e.g., exertion)?
- Are your headaches getting better or worse, or are they about the same?
- What treatments have been used to treat the headaches, both acutely and preventively?
- What helps your pain?
- Is there a family history of headaches?
- What prior testing have you had?
- Do you have other medical or neurological problems?
- What do you think might be causing your headaches?
- How disabling are your headaches?
- Why are you seeking help now?

---

exclusion of aneurysmal subarachnoid hemorrhage (Ducros, 2012; IHS, 2013).

Frequency and Periodicity of Episodic Headaches

Migraine may be episodic or chronic. Chronic migraine is defined as headache occurring on ≥ 15 days per month for 3 ≥ months which has the features of migraine headache on ≥ 8 days per month. Chronic migraine usually develops in individuals with a history of episodic migraine headaches. Chronic migraine may occur with or without medication overuse. Some patients with apparent medication overuse do not improve after drug withdrawal.

Episodic cluster headaches typically occur daily for several weeks or months and are followed by a lengthy headache-free interval. Chronic cluster headaches occur at least every other day for more than 1 year or with remissions lasting < 1 month. If there is no regular periodicity, it is useful to inquire about the longest and shortest periods of freedom between headaches. Having the patient monitor headache frequency, duration, intensity, triggers, and medication use on a headache calendar or in a diary is helpful in diagnosis and measuring response to treatment. Tension-type headaches can be infrequently (< 12 days per year) or frequently episodic (≥ 12 and < 180 days per year).

Thunderclap headache recurring over a few days or weeks raises the possibility of RCVS, a diagnosis that requires

Temporal Profile

A chronic daily headache without migrainous or autonomic features is likely to be a chronic tension-type headache. Untreated migraine pain usually peaks within 1 to 2 hours of onset and lasts 4 to 72 hours. Cluster headache is typically maximal immediately (if the patient awakens with the headache in progress) or peaks within minutes (if it begins while awake). Cluster headaches are more common in men and are infrequently inherited. Cluster headaches can last 15 to 180 minutes (usually 45 to 120 minutes). Headaches similar to cluster but lasting only 2 to 30 minutes and occurring several or many times a day are typical of episodic or chronic paroxysmal hemicrania, both of which are more common in women and are prevented by indomethacin (Goadsby, 2012). Primary stabbing headaches ("ice-pick pains") are momentary, typically lasting seconds. Stabbing headaches are more common in patients with migraine and tend to vary in location. Tension-type headaches commonly build up over hours and last hours to days to years. Headache that is daily and unremitting from onset, usually in patients without prior headaches, is classified as new daily persistent headache and may have features suggestive of migraine or tension-type headache. A chronic, continuous, unilateral headache of moderate severity with superimposed attacks of more intense pain, associated with autonomic features, suggests the diagnosis of hemicrania continua, an indomethacin-responsive syndrome. Occipital neuralgia and trigeminal neuralgia manifest as brief shocklike pains, often triggered by stimulation in the territory served by the affected nerve. Occasionally a dull pain in the same nerve distribution persists longer, often after a series of brief, sharp pains. Short-lasting *u*nilateral *n*euralgiform headache with *c*onjunctival injection and *t*earing (SUNCT) is a rare syndrome consisting of paroxysms of first-division trigeminal nerve pain, lasting 5 to 240 seconds but occurring 3 to 200 times per day with the associated autonomic symptoms for which it is named (Goadsby, 2012).

Time of Day and Precipitating Factors

Cluster headaches often awaken patients from a sound sleep and may occur at the same time each day in an individual person. Hypnic headaches usually begin after age 50 years and regularly awaken the patient at a particular time of night. Unlike cluster headaches, they are usually bilateral and not associated with autonomic phenomena (Holle et al., 2013). Migraine headaches can occur at any time but often begin in the morning. A headache of recent onset that disturbs sleep or is worse on waking may be caused by increased intracranial pressure. Tension-type headaches typically are present during much of the day and often are more severe later in the day. Obstructive sleep apnea may be accompanied by the frequent occurrence of headache on awakening, as might medication overuse headache ("rebound headache") and headache due to caffeine withdrawal. If headache begins while the patient is asleep, it is impossible to tell whether the onset was gradual or abrupt.

Patients with chronic recurrent headaches often recognize factors that trigger an attack. Migraine headaches may be precipitated by bright light, menstruation, weather changes, caffeine withdrawal, fasting, alcohol (particularly beer and wine), sleeping more or less than usual, stress and release from stress, certain foods and food additives, perfume and smoke, and others. Alcohol can trigger a cluster headache within minutes of ingestion. If bending, lifting, coughing, or Valsalva maneuver brings on a headache, an intracranial lesion, especially one involving the posterior fossa, must be considered. Exertional headache and headache associated with sexual activity are both worrisome. Although either can occur as a primary headache disorder unassociated with structural disease or can be associated with migraine, both types can also be due to subarachnoid hemorrhage, arterial dissection, and RCVS, which must be excluded with the first occurrence of such headaches. Intermittent headaches that are worsened by sitting or standing and improved by lying down are characteristic of a cerebrospinal fluid (CSF) leak. If there is no history of lumbar puncture, head trauma, or neurosurgical intervention, a spontaneous CSF leak may be the cause (Mokri, 2013). Lancinating face pain triggered by facial or intraoral stimuli occurs with trigeminal neuralgia. Glossopharyngeal neuralgia typically is triggered by chewing, swallowing, or talking, although cutaneous trigger zones in and about the ear are occasionally present.

Location

Asking the patient to outline the location of his or her pain with their finger can be very helpful. Trigeminal neuralgia is confined to one or more branches of the trigeminal nerve. The patient may be able to localize one or more trigger points on the face or in the mouth and then show how the pain spreads. Pain in the throat may be due to a local process or to glossopharyngeal neuralgia. Carotid artery dissection commonly presents with unilateral neck, face, and head pain, is frequently associated with an ipsilateral Horner syndrome, and often follows head or neck trauma.

Migraine is commonly unilateral, can be confined to the front or back of the head, and can affect the neck. Migraine pain can start on one side and spread to the other or be bilateral from onset. Cluster headaches are unilateral during an attack and typically are centered in, behind, or around one eye. Some patients' cluster headaches switch sides with different cluster periods, and a smaller number experience side shifts within a cluster period. The typical tension-type headache is generalized, although it may begin in the neck muscles and affect chiefly the occipital region or predominate frontally. When pain is localized to the eye, mouth, or ear, local processes involving these structures must be considered. Otalgia may be caused by a process involving the tonsil and posterior tongue. With chronic unilateral facial pain, an underlying lesion often cannot be identified. Occasionally, however, facial pain may be a symptom of nonmetastatic lung cancer (Pembroke et al., 2013).

Quality and Severity

The character and quality of the patient's pain can have significance. In most cases, the type of pain can be designated as sharp, aching, or burning. Headaches may be steady or throbbing (pulsating) in character. It may be helpful to ask the patient to grade the severity of pain on a scale of 1 to 10. Patients who report their pain level is 20 are hurting but may be prone to exaggerate. Migraine pain often has a pulsating quality that may be superimposed on a more continuous pain. The pain of cluster headache is characteristically severe, boring, and steady and often described as a "hot poker." SUNCT produces moderately severe pain in the orbital or temporal region and may be described as sharp and stabbing or (rarely) pulsatile. Tension-type headaches usually are described as a steady feeling of fullness, tightness, or pressure, or like a cap, band, or vise. Headaches caused by meningeal irritation, whether related to infectious meningitis or blood, are typically severe. Trigeminal neuralgia pain is severe, brief, sharp, electric shocklike, or stabbing; pains can occur up to several times per minute, and a milder ache may persist between paroxysms of pain. Glossopharyngeal neuralgia pain is similar in character to that of trigeminal neuralgia.

Premonitory Symptoms, Aura, and Accompanying Symptoms

Some patients have premonitory symptoms that precede a migraine headache by hours. These can include psychological changes (e.g., depression, euphoria, irritability) or somatic symptoms (e.g., constipation, diarrhea, abnormal hunger, fluid retention, increased urination). The term aura refers to focal cerebral symptoms associated with a migraine attack. These symptoms can last 5 to 60 minutes but usually last 10 to 30 minutes. Aura symptoms typically precede the headache but can continue into the headache phase or begin during the headache. Visual symptoms are most common and may consist of either positive (scintillating lights, spots, or zig-zag lines) or negative (scotomas or visual field loss) phenomena, or both. The visual symptoms characteristically affect both eyes simultaneously but can, rarely, affect one eye alone. Less common hemispheric symptoms, such as unilateral somatosensory disturbances (tingling and/or numbness) or dysphasic language disturbance, may occur with or without visual symptoms. Aura symptoms usually have a gradual onset and offset; they typically increase and decrease over minutes. If more than one symptom occurs (e.g., visual plus somatosensory), the onsets usually are staggered and not simultaneous. Patients can experience migraine aura without an associated headache. Positive symptoms, the slow spread of symptoms, and staggered onsets help differentiate migraine aura from focal symptoms caused by cerebrovascular disease.

Symptoms originating from the brainstem or both cerebral hemispheres simultaneously, such as vertigo, dysarthria, ataxia, auditory symptoms, diplopia, bilateral visual symptoms in both eyes, bilateral paresthesias, and decreased level of consciousness, may accompany migraine with brainstem aura (formerly called basilar-type migraine) (IHS, 2013). Vertigo without other brainstem signs can also accompany migraine headaches. Migraine with aura that includes motor weakness can be due to familial hemiplegic migraine if there is a family history in at least one first- or second-degree relative, or due to sporadic hemiplegic migraine if there is no family history. It can be difficult for the patient to differentiate sensory loss from true weakness. Nausea, vomiting, photophobia, phonophobia, and osmophobia characteristically accompany migraine attacks. In addition, lacrimation, rhinorrhea, and nasal congestion can accompany migraine headache and mimic headache of sinus origin (Cady et al., 2005). Ipsilateral miosis, ptosis, lacrimation, conjunctival injection, and nasal stuffiness commonly accompany cluster headache; sweating and facial flushing on the side of the pain are much less common. Similar autonomic features also accompany episodic and chronic paroxysmal hemicrania and hemicrania continua. Very short attacks (5–240 seconds) with ipsilateral conjunctival injection and tearing suggest SUNCT (Goadsby, 2012). Horner syndrome is common in carotid artery dissection. In the setting of acute transient or persistent monocular visual loss, GCA and carotid dissection and stenosis should be considered. Temporomandibular joint dysfunction includes jaw pain precipitated or aggravated by movement of the jaw or clenching of the teeth and is associated with reduced range of jaw movement, joint clicking, and tenderness over the joint. Headache accompanied by fever suggests an infection. Headache associated with persistent or progressive diffuse or focal CNS symptoms, including seizures, implies a structural cause. Purulent or bloody nasal discharge suggests an acute sinus cause for the headache. Likewise, a red eye raises the possibility of an ocular process such as infection or acute glaucoma. A history of polymyalgia rheumatica, jaw claudication, or tenderness of the scalp arteries in an older person strongly suggests GCA. Transient visual obscurations upon standing, usually pulsatile tinnitus, diplopia (especially for objects in the distance), and papilledema may be associated with increased intracranial pressure from any cause, including idiopathic intracranial hypertension (pseudotumor cerebri).

Aggravating and Mitigating Factors

Worsening of headache as a result of a cough or physical jolt suggests an intracranial component to the pain. Sufferers of cluster headache tend to endure their pain in an agitated state, pacing and moving about, while patients with migraine prefer to lie still. Precipitation or marked worsening of headache in the upright position and/or relief with recumbency suggests intracranial hypotension. Routine physical activity, light, sound, and smells typically aggravate migraine headaches. Rest, especially sleep, and avoidance of light and noise and application of cold tend to benefit the migraineur. Massage, ice, or heat may reduce the pain associated with a tension-type headache. Local application of pressure over the affected eye or ipsilateral temporal artery, the local application of heat or cold, and (rarely) brief intense physical activity may alleviate the pain of cluster headache.

Family History of Headaches

Migraine often is an inherited disorder, and a family history of migraine (sometimes referred to as "sick headaches") is present in about two-thirds of patients. Tension-type headaches also can be familial. Cluster headache is inherited in about 5% of sufferers. Familial hemiplegic migraine is a rare autosomal dominant variant of migraine with aura, wherein the aura includes hemiparesis lasting minutes to 24 hours.

Prior Evaluation

The patient should be asked about prior consultations and testing. If appropriate, the records and actual imaging studies can be obtained for review.

Prior Treatment

Response to treatment should be sought, including agents used to treat individual headache attacks acutely and those used prophylactically. The dose, frequency, and duration of each treatment should be reviewed. This information provides an opportunity to determine whether acute medications have been overused and whether prophylactic medications were optimized. A history of the use of caffeine-containing substances also should be elicited because they may cause or aggravate headaches through rebound withdrawal.

Disability

Baseline and follow-up assessment of headache-related disability is helpful in judging the effects of treatment and guiding headache therapy. The Migraine Disability Assessment Scale (MIDAS) is one useful validated clinical tool (Andrasik et al., 2005).

Patient Concerns and Reasons for Seeking Help

Headache pain can produce significant fear and anxiety regarding serious disease. The patient should be encouraged to express any concerns so that each can be appropriately addressed.

The question of why the patient is seeking help may be obvious if the problem is of recent onset. If the problem is chronic, however, it can be useful to inquire why the patient has come for aid at this time. Red and yellow flags (see Box 20.3) help identify which patients are more likely to have a secondary cause of their pain.

Other Medical or Neurological Problems

A history of past and current medical and neurological conditions, injuries, operations, and medication allergies should be obtained. A list of all current medications and dietary supplements should be recorded. A number of medications can cause headache, including hormonal, cardiovascular, and gastrointestinal agents (De Luca and Bartleson, 2010).

EXAMINATION

The examination begins the moment the physician encounters the patient. Careful observation helps determine whether the patient appears ill, anxious, or depressed, and whether the history is reliable. The patient who is unable to give a reasonably coherent history should be suspected of having an abnormal mental status. Although typically the physical examination of the headache patient shows no abnormalities, findings on examination may yield important clues about the underlying cause.

Vital signs, especially blood pressure and pulse, should be assessed. Extremely high blood pressure can cause headache.

BOX 20.3 Headache Warning Flags

RED FLAGS FOR WORRISOME HEADACHES

- Head or neck injury
- New onset or new type or worsening pattern of existing headache
- New level of pain (e.g., worst ever)
- Abrupt or split-second onset
- Triggered by Valsalva maneuver or cough
- Triggered by exertion
- Triggered by sexual activity
- Headache during pregnancy or puerperium
- Age > 50 years
- Neurological signs or symptoms
  - Seizures
  - Confusion
  - Impaired alertness
  - Weakness
  - Papilledema
- Systemic illness
  - Fever
  - Nuchal rigidity
  - Weight loss
  - Scalp artery tenderness
- Secondary risk factors
  - Cancer
  - Immunocompromised host
    - Human immunodeficiency virus (HIV)
    - On immunosuppressants
- Recent travel
  - Domestic
  - Foreign

YELLOW FLAGS FOR WORRISOME HEADACHES

- Wakes patient from sleep at night
- New onset side-locked headaches
- Postural headaches

From De Luca, G.C., Bartleson, J.D., 2010. When and how to investigate the patient with headache. Semin Neurol 30, 133–134. Used with permission.

If there is a question of fever, temperature can be measured. The body habitus should be noted. Patients with pseudotumor cerebri, typically young women, are usually obese. The general examination can include auscultation of the heart and lungs, palpation of the abdomen, and examination of the skin. A neurological examination, including assessment of the mental status, gait, cranial nerves, reflexes, and motor and sensory systems, is essential. The skull and cervical spine should be examined. The skull should be palpated for lumps and local tenderness. The area over an infected sinus may be tender. Thickened, tender, irregular temporal arteries with a reduced pulse suggest GCA. In both migraine and tension-type headaches, the scalp may be tender. A short neck or low hairline suggests basilar invagination or a Chiari malformation. In an infant, bulging of the fontanelles suggests increased intracranial pressure, most commonly caused by hydrocephalus. Measuring head circumference is important in a child. The cervical spine also should be tested for tenderness and mobility. Nuchal rigidity on passive neck flexion and Kernig sign indicate meningeal irritation.

DIAGNOSTIC TESTING

In most cases, the history, together with the neurological and physical examinations, is all that is needed to make a diagnosis, especially in the patient with long-standing headaches. Migraine, tension-type headaches, and cluster headaches usually can be diagnosed with a high degree of certainty, and it is often possible to proceed directly to management.

In some situations, the diagnosis is uncertain, and additional diagnostic testing should be considered. The worrisome headache "warning flags" that increase the likelihood of a serious underlying intracranial process and often lead to additional testing are listed in Box 20.3. Red flags are more worrisome than yellow flags. Investigation of the patient with headache includes almost all tests used in neurology and neurosurgery, as well as various medical studies. Selection of appropriate tests depends on the diagnostic formulation after the history and examination; indiscriminate use of batteries of tests is unwarranted.

Neuroimaging and Other Imaging Studies

Computed Tomography and Magnetic Resonance Imaging

Computed tomography (CT) and magnetic resonance imaging (MRI) are extremely useful tests in evaluating patients with headache. CT is best utilized when investigating for acute intracranial hemorrhage, assessing bony anatomy, or evaluating for sinusitis. While CT can detect intracranial processes such as tumors, hematomas, cerebral infarctions, abscesses, hydrocephalus, and meningeal processes, MRI provides higher sensitivity and specificity, and is therefore the preferred diagnostic study for these entities. Advantages of CT over MRI include lower cost, a faster scan for those patients who either cannot remain still or are claustrophobic, compatibility with pacemakers and other retained metal objects, and widespread availability. The iodinated contrast used in CT has been associated with allergic reactions and contrast-induced nephropathy. The contrast agent used in MRI is less likely to produce allergic reactions or renal damage, but it has been associated with nephrogenic systemic fibrosis, typically in patients with pre-existing renal impairment. The imaging modality of choice to investigate various causes of headache is shown in Box 20.4.

CT can detect acute subarachnoid hemorrhage in at least 95% of patients if sufficient bleeding has occurred and the patient is scanned promptly. If findings on the CT scan are normal and the history is suggestive of recent subarachnoid hemorrhage, a lumbar puncture should be performed to assess for red blood cells and xanthochromia. Evidence of bleeding (i.e., red blood cells and xanthochromia) can last for up to 1-2 weeks after a subarachnoid hemorrhage.

CT can be helpful for evaluating abnormalities of the skull, orbit, sinuses, facial bones, and the bony cervical spine. Changes associated with intracranial hypotension are best shown with MRI and include enhancement of the pachymeninges, sagging of the brain, engorged veins, and subdural fluid collections (Mokri, 2013). The cervical spinal cord and exiting nerve roots are much better shown with MRI than with plain CT. Myelography with CT can be used to image the spine as an alternative to MRI. Magnetic resonance angiography is a noninvasive method that can demonstrate intracranial and extracranial vascular occlusive disease including large-vessel dissection, intracranial arteriovenous malformations, and aneurysms. CT angiography also can show arterial disease although arterial calcifications may confound accurate luminal diameter measurements. Intracranial venous sinus thrombosis is best shown with gadolinium-enhanced magnetic resonance venography, but CT venography techniques continue to improve. For headache that is acute in onset or follows trauma, CT is the preferred imaging study to look for subarachnoid and other intracranial bleeding. For evaluation of patients

BOX 20.4 Imaging Modality of Choice to Investigate Causes of Headache

MRI PREFERRED

Vascular Disease:

Cerebral infarction
Venous infarction

Neoplastic Disease:

Primary and secondary brain tumors (especially in posterior fossa)
Skull base tumors
Meningeal carcinomatosis and lymphomatosis
Pituitary tumors

Infections:

Cerebritis and brain abscess
Meningitis
Encephalitis

Other:

Chiari malformation
Cerebrospinal fluid hypotension with pachymeningeal enhancement and brain sag
Foramen magnum and upper cervical spine lesions
Pituitary apoplexy
Rare encephalopathies and headache (CADASIL*, MELAS†, SMART‡)

CT PREFERRED

Fractures (Calvarium)

Acute Hemorrhage (Subarachnoid, Intracerebral)

Paranasal Sinus and Mastoid Air Cell Disease

MRI AND CT EQUAL

MR Angiography/CT Angiography:

Vasculitis (large and medium sized vessels)
Intracranial aneurysms
Carotid and vertebral artery dissections
Reversible cerebral vasoconstriction syndrome

MR Venography/CT Venography:

Cerebral venous thrombosis

*CADASIL—cerebral autosomal dominant arteriopathy with subcortical infarcts and leukoencephalopathy.
†MELAS—mitochondrial encephalomyopathy, lactic acidosis, and strokelike episodes.
‡SMART—strokelike migraine attacks after radiation therapy.
CT, computed tomography; MRI, magnetic resonance imaging.
Copyrighted and used with permission of Mayo Foundation for Medical Education and Research.

with subacute and chronic headache, MRI is recommended (Sandrini et al., 2004). MRI can reveal more than CT, but many of the abnormalities will be incidental, including asymptomatic cerebral infarctions, small aneurysms, and benign brain tumors (Vernooij et al., 2007).

Plain Radiographs and Other Imaging of the Skull, Sinuses, and Cervical Spine

Plain radiographs of the skull are unnecessary in the routine evaluation of patients with headache, but they can infrequently be useful in patients with an unusual bony abnormality found on physical examination or in the pediatric population where radiographs may answer the clinical questions without exposing the child to higher doses of radiation used with CT. Although plain radiographs of the sinuses can show infection, hemorrhage, fracture, or tumor, CT provides much greater definition and has become the test of choice for these conditions. Occipitonuchal pain may result from degenerative disk and joint disease of the mid- and upper cervical spine. Rheumatoid arthritis and ankylosing spondylitis can lead to craniocervical junction instability and pain. Fat-saturated post-gadolinium T1-weighted MR images as well as inversion recovery sequences can be very helpful in demonstrating marrow edema and joint fluid abnormalities seen in many spondyloarthropathies (Lacout et al., 2008). Tomographic images or CT may be needed to show bony changes in the upper cervical spine and craniocervical junction. Flexion and extension, odontoid, and pillar views of the cervical spine can help exclude ligamentous damage and fractures in patients with a history of head and neck injury. MRI is the imaging study of choice for spinal cord and nerve root pathology.

Temporomandibular Joint/Dental Imaging Studies

Panoramic X-ray examination, MRI, or CT of the temporomandibular joints may be helpful in selected patients. The presence of temporomandibular joint disease should not be taken as proof that the patient's headaches are related. Dental radiographs are useful if a dental origin for the pain is suspected.

Cerebral Angiography

Cerebral angiography is rarely needed in the initial investigation of headache. It can be helpful in confirming vascular disease including arterial dissections, arteriovenous malformations, intracranial aneurysms, RCVS, and CNS vasculitis.

Myelography with Computed Tomography and Radioisotope Studies for Detection of Cerebrospinal Fluid Leaks

In addition to MRI of the brain and spine, myelography with CT and isotope cisternography (typically with indium-111) can be helpful in determining the presence and location of a spontaneous, post-traumatic, or postoperative CSF leak.

Cerebrospinal Fluid Tests

CSF examination can diagnose or exclude meningitis, encephalitis, subarachnoid hemorrhage, and leptomeningeal cancer and lymphoma. It can also document increased or decreased intracranial pressure and confirm the diagnosis of headache and neurological deficits with CSF lymphocytosis (HaNDL) (Gomez-Aranda et al., 1997). Measurement of the opening CSF pressure should always be performed.

Electrophysiological Testing

Electroencephalography is not useful in the investigation of headache unless the patient also has a history of seizures, syncope, or episodes of altered awareness, and there is no indication for use of evoked potentials (Sandrini et al., 2004).

General Medical Tests

A few blood tests are important in the investigation of headache. Elevation of the erythrocyte sedimentation rate (ESR), often to 100 mm per hour or higher, is frequently seen in GCA. A normal ESR does not exclude the condition, because 4% of patients with positive findings on temporal artery biopsy have a normal ESR (Smetana and Shmerling, 2002).

examiner's nose in the middle. More sophistication can be brought to the clinical examination by looking at the vestibulo-ocular reflex, with the patient in a rotary chair and looking at an object that moves with the chair. A rotating striped drum is used to examine for optokinetic nystagmus (OKN), and Frenzel goggles can be used to remove fixation.

Disorders of Pursuit. Pursuit movements include fixation (pursuit at 0 degrees velocity). Small, 0.1- to 0.3-degree square-wave movements of the eyes are often seen even in normal individuals during fixation. *Square-wave jerks* are so named because in eye-movement recordings they appear as two saccades in opposite directions separated by a short period of no movement, giving a square appearance to the recording. Square-wave jerks exceeding 10 per minute are indicative of central nervous system disease, but they are not as specific for cerebellar ataxia as large-amplitude square-wave jerks. Square-wave jerks larger than 10 degrees in amplitude are called *macro–square-wave jerks*. Cerebellar disease also slows down pursuit movements, requiring catch-up saccades to keep up with a moving target. Such saccadic intrusions and intrusions of square-wave jerks give a "ratchety" appearance to pursuit movement.

Disorders of Saccades. Saccade velocity is normal in cerebellar disease, but its accuracy is impaired so that both hypometric and hypermetric saccades are seen. Such saccades are followed by a corrective saccade in the appropriate direction (Munoz, 2002). The dorsal oculomotor vermis (OMV) composed of lobules V–VII and related fastigial nuclear cells play a role in saccade amplitude and accuracy; bilateral OMV lesions cause hypometric saccades and in contrast bilateral lesions of the fastigial nucleus result in hypermetric saccades (Kheradmand and Zee, 2011).

Other Saccadic Intrusions. *Ocular flutter* differs from square-wave jerks in that the back-and-forth horizontal saccades are not separated by an intersaccade interval. *Opsoclonus* is characterized by continuous saccades in all directions in a chaotic fashion. Both ocular flutter and opsoclonus are associated with cerebellar disease, especially paraneoplastic or postinfectious syndromes.

Nystagmus. Gaze-evoked nystagmus is elicited when eccentric gaze is maintained at about 30 degrees from the midline. There are repetitive drifts of the eyes toward the midline, followed by saccades to the eccentric position. The fast phase of the nystagmus is always to the side of the eccentric gaze. This nystagmus is usually seen in cerebellar disease. When typical gaze-evoked nystagmus fatigues and reverses direction after a few seconds, it is called *rebound nystagmus*. Rebound nystagmus may also appear as a transient nystagmus in the opposite direction when the eye is returned to midline. Rebound nystagmus is also seen in cerebellar disease. *Downbeat nystagmus* is characterized by a rapid phase in the down direction in primary position of the eyes. Such downbeat nystagmus becomes more prominent with downgaze or gaze to the side. Downbeat nystagmus is typically seen in craniovertebral junction abnormalities such as Arnold-Chiari malformation, but it can also occur in some degenerative ataxias such as spinocerebellar ataxia type 6. Finally, upbeat primary position nystagmus can be seen in lesions of the anterior vermis.

Vestibulo-Ocular Reflex. In a rotary chair, normal individuals can suppress the vestibular-ocular reflex (VOR) and keep their eyes on an object moving slowly with the chair. Patients with cerebellar disease cannot inhibit the VOR, so the eyes drift away from the object and make catch-up saccades as the chair is rotated.

Speech and Bulbar Function

Speech is evaluated by listening to patients' spoken words and asking them to speak standard phrases. Speech in cerebellar disease is characterized by slowness, slurring of the words, and a general inability to control the process of articulation, leading to unnecessary hesitations and stops, omissions of pauses when needed, and an accentuation of syllables when not needed. Also, there is a moment-to-moment variability in the volume and pitch of words and inappropriate control of the breathing needed for speech, causing a scanning dysarthria. Both speech execution and the motor programming of speech may be defective in cerebellar disease (Spencer and Slocomb, 2007). Mild dysphagia is not uncommon in cerebellar disease. In children, a form of "cerebellar mutism" has been described after posterior fossa surgery. This is transient and followed by more typical cerebellar dysarthria.

Cognitive-Affective Features

A number of studies have suggested that cerebellar lesions can be accompanied by changes in cognitive and behavioral functions. Such changes have included defective executive function (often noted on the Wisconsin card sorting test) and defective visual and verbal memory and verbal fluency tasks. Acute cerebellar lesions may be accompanied by subtle language deficits, and a syndrome of cerebellar mutism has been noted in children with acute cerebellar lesions.

Neurological Signs in Patients with Sensory Ataxia

For patients with sensory ataxia, the major basis of ataxia is defective proprioception. Patients can be shown to have impaired position and vibration sense, and the deep tendon reflexes are often lost because of afferent fiber pathology. The Romberg test is positive. Many degenerative ataxic syndromes combine features of cerebellar and proprioceptive deficits in variable proportion.

DIAGNOSTIC APPROACH TO ATAXIA

Recognizing an ataxic basis for the patient's coordination problems and gait is usually easy. Other neural disorders that can give rise to similar problems with gait and dexterity—nerve and muscle disorders, spinal cord diseases, and basal ganglia diseases, for example—can usually be distinguished on the basis of physical signs alone.

Some patients with bilateral frontal lobe lesions may have a gait disorder superficially resembling ataxia (Brun ataxia or frontal ataxia). However, limb and eye-movement signs of cerebellar disease are absent, and the gait abnormalities are out of proportion to the limb signs. Often the patient may experience a sense of being glued to the ground ("magnetic" gait). Other gait disorders associated with dystonia or chorea may also be occasionally mistaken for cerebellar ataxia.

Neurological examination also determines whether the ataxia is primarily cerebellar, primarily sensory, or a combination of both. This led Greenfield to classify ataxic disorders as spinal, cerebellar, or spinocerebellar in nature. Further diagnostic considerations and avenues for investigation are aimed at making a specific diagnosis (Box 22.1), and management is dependent on the diagnosis. This can be a daunting task, especially when the disease appears to be "degenerative" in nature (i.e., associated with cerebellar atrophy). As an example, the Online Mendelian Inheritance in Man website lists more than 800 genetic disorders alone in which ataxia can occur. In the appropriate clinical setting when the initial diagnostic process (e.g., imaging studies) has been unfruitful, it may be important to educate the patient about the possibility of not being able to come to a specific diagnosis before embarking on an expensive process of laboratory studies. In patients with ataxia, many additional pieces of information may be useful in arriving at a diagnosis. These include age at onset (Table 22.1); the tempo of disease (Table 22.2); whether the ataxia is predominantly spinal, spinocerebellar, cerebellar, or associated with spasticity (Box 22.2); the presence or absence of noncerebellar neurological signs (Table 22.3); and the occurrence of any distinctive systemic features (Table 22.4).

BOX 22.1 Acquired and Genetic Causes of Ataxia

ACQUIRED CAUSES OF ATAXIA

Congenital: "ataxic" cerebral palsy, other early insults
Vascular: ischemic stroke, hemorrhagic stroke, AVMs
Infectious/transmittable: acute cerebellitis, postinfectious encephalomyelitis, cerebellar abscess, Whipple disease, HIV, CJD
Toxic: alcohol, anticonvulsants, mercury, 5FU, cytosine arabinoside, lithium
Neoplastic/compressive: gliomas, ependymomas, meningiomas, basal meningeal carcinomatosis, craniovertebral junction abnormalities
Immune: MS, paraneoplastic syndromes, anti-GAD, gluten ataxia
Deficiency: hypothyroidism, vitamin B_1 and B_{12}, vitamin E

GENETIC CAUSES OF ATAXIA

Autosomal recessive: FA, AT, AVED, AOA 1, AOA 2, MIRAS, ARSACS, other newly defined autosomal recessive ataxias
Ataxia in other genetic diseases not traditionally classified as an "ataxia"
Autosomal dominant: SCA types 1 through 31, episodic ataxias (types 1, 2, others)
X-linked, including fragile X tremor-ataxia syndrome (FXTAS)
Mitochondrial: NARP, MELAS, MERRF, others including Kearns-Sayre syndrome

AOA, Ataxia with oculomotor apraxia; *ARSACS*, autosomal recessive spastic ataxia of Charlevoix-Saguenay; *AT*, ataxia telangiectasia; *AVED*, ataxia with vitamin E deficiency; *AVMs*, arteriovenous malformations; *CJD*, Creutzfeldt–Jakob disease; *FA*, Friedreich ataxia; *5FU*, 5 fluorouracil; *GAD*, glutamic acid decarboxylase; *HIV*, human immunodeficiency virus; *MELAS*, mitochondrial encephalopathy, lactic acidosis, stroke-like episodes; *MERRF*, myoclonus epilepsy with ragged red fibers; *MIRAS*, mitochondrial recessive ataxic syndrome; *MS*, multiple sclerosis; *NARP*, neuropathy, ataxia, and retinitis pigmentosa; *SCA*, spinocerebellar ataxia.

TABLE 22.1 Causes of Ataxia Related to Age at Onset

Age at onset	Acquired	Genetic
Infancy	Ataxic cerebral palsy, other intrauterine insults	Inherited congenital ataxias (Joubert, Gillespie)
Childhood	Acute cerebellitis; cerebellar abscess; posterior fossa tumors such as ependymomas, gliomas; AVM; congenital anomalies such as Arnold–Chiari malformation; toxic such as due to anticonvulsants; immune related to neoplasms (opsoclonus-myoclonus)	FA; other recessive ataxias; ataxia associated with other genetic-metabolic diseases; EA syndromes; mitochondrial disorders; SCAs such as SCA 2, SCA 7, SCA 13, DRPLA
Young adult	Abscesses; HIV; mass lesions such as meningiomas, gliomas, AVM; immune such as MS; Arnold–Chiari malformation; hypothyroidism; toxic such as alcohol and anticonvulsants	FA; SCAs, inherited tumor syndromes like von Hippel–Lindau syndrome, ataxias associated with other genetic-metabolic diseases
Older adult	Same as above plus "idiopathic" ataxia, immune related such as anti-GAD and gluten ataxia	More benign SCAs such as SCA 6

AVM, Arteriovenous malformation; *DRPLA*, dentate-rubral-pallidoluysian atrophy; *EA*, episodic ataxia; *FA*, Friedreich ataxia; *HIV*, human immunodeficiency virus; *MS*, multiple sclerosis; *SCA*, spinocerebellar ataxia (*note*: SCA indicates a dominantly inherited ataxic disease).

TABLE 22.2 Causes of Ataxia Based on Onset and Course

Tempo	Acquired diseases	Genetic diseases
Episodic		Many inborn errors of metabolism; EA syndromes
Acute (hours/days)	Strokes, ischemic and hemorrhagic; MS; infections; parainfectious syndromes; toxic disorders	
Subacute (weeks/months)	Mass lesions in the posterior fossa; meningeal infiltrates; infections such as HIV; CJD; deficiency syndromes such B_1 and B_{12}; hypothyroidism; immune disorders such as paraneoplastic, gluten, and anti-GAD ataxia; alcohol	
Chronic	Mass lesions such as meningiomas; craniovertebral junction anomalies; alcoholic; idiopathic/sporadic cerebellar ataxia; MSA	Most genetic disorders such as FA, AT, and other AR ataxias; SCAs

AR, Autosomal recessive; *AT*, ataxia telangiectasia; *CJD*, Creutzfeldt-Jakob disease; *EA*, episodic ataxia; *FA*, Friedreich ataxia; *GAD*, glutamic acid decarboxylase; *HIV*, human immunodeficiency virus; *MS*, multiple sclerosis; *MSA*, multiple system atrophy; *SCA*, spinocerebellar ataxia (dominantly inherited).

BOX 23.1 Classification of Parkinsonism

I. Parkinson disease
 Parkinson disease—sporadic
 Parkinson disease—hereditary (see Table 23.1)
II. Multisystem degenerations ("parkinsonism plus")
 Progressive supranuclear palsy
 Multiple system atrophy (Shy-Drager syndrome):
  MSA-P striatonigral degeneration)
  MSA-C (olivopontocerebellar atrophy)
 Lytico-Bodig disease, or amyotrophic lateral sclerosis and
  parkinsonism-dementia complex of Guam
 Corticobasal degeneration
 Progressive pallidal atrophy
 Parkinsonism-dementia complex
 Pallidopyramidal disease
III. Heredodegenerative parkinsonism
 Dopa-responsive dystonia
 Huntington disease
 Wilson disease
 Hereditary ceruloplasmin deficiency
 Neurodegeneration with brain iron accumulation (pantothenate
  kinase-associated neurodegeneration, also known as
  Hallervorden–Spatz disease)
 Olivopontocerebellar and spinocerebellar atrophies, including
  Machado–Joseph disease
 Frontotemporal dementia with parkinsonism (FTDP)
 Gerstmann–Sträussler–Scheinker syndrome
 Familial progressive subcortical gliosis

 Lubag (X-linked dystonia-parkinsonism)
 Familial basal ganglia calcification
 Mitochondrial cytopathies with striatal necrosis
 Ceroid lipofuscinosis
 Familial parkinsonism with peripheral neuropathy
 Parkinsonian-pyramidal syndrome
 Neuroacanthocytosis
 Hereditary hemochromatosis
 Neuroferritinopathy
 Aceruloplasminemia
IV. Secondary (acquired, symptomatic) parkinsonism
 Infectious: postencephalitic, acquired immunodeficiency
  syndrome, subacute sclerosing panencephalitis, Creutzfeldt–
  Jakob disease, prion diseases
 Drugs: dopamine receptor blocking drugs (antipsychotic,
  antiemetic drugs), reserpine, tetrabenazine, methyldopa,
  lithium, flunarizine, cinnarizine
 Toxins: MPTP, carbon monoxide, manganese, mercury, carbon
  disulfide, cyanide, methanol, ethanol
 Vascular: multi-infarct disease
 Trauma: pugilistic encephalopathy disease
 Other: parathyroid abnormalities, hypothyroidism,
  hepatocerebral degeneration, brain tumor, paraneoplastic,
  normal-pressure hydrocephalus, noncommunicating
  hydrocephalus, syringomesencephalia, hemiatrophy-
  hemiparkinsonism, peripherally induced tremor and
  parkinsonism, psychogenic

---

causative genetic mutation, clinicians must learn about these genetic forms of parkinsonism not only to understand the pathogenic mechanisms but also to learn how to interpret and use the increasingly available gene tests, including whole exome and whole genome sequencing, for genetic counseling (MacArthur et al., 2014). There is growing appreciation for different subtypes of PD and the need to develop diagnostic criteria based on clinical, genetic, and pathological features (Thenganatt and Jankovic, 2015). Besides genetic causes, there are many other causes of parkinsonism and of parkinsonism combined with other neurological deficits (atypical parkinsonism or parkinsonism-plus syndromes) (Box 23.1).

Motor Abnormalities

Early in the course of the disease, many patients with parkinsonism are unaware of any motor deficit. Often the patient's spouse comments on a reduction in facial expression (often misinterpreted as depression), a reduction in arm swing while walking, and a slowing of activities of daily living, most notably dressing, feeding, and walking. The patient may then become aware of a reduction in manual dexterity, with slowness and clumsiness interfering with activities. PD is typically asymmetrical, especially early in the course. A painful shoulder is one of the most common early symptoms of PD, possibly related to decreased arm swing and secondary joint changes or shoulder muscle rigidity, often misdiagnosed as bursitis, arthritis, or a rotator cuff disorder. Besides shoulder pain as one example of a sensory symptom related to underlying motor abnormality, painful dystonia and other etiologies can contribute to pain and discomfort associated with PD (Ha and Jankovic, 2012). Handwriting often becomes slower and smaller (micrographia), with speed and size decreasing as the task continues. Eventually the writing may become illegible. Dressing tasks such as fastening small buttons or getting arms

into sleeves are often difficult. Hygiene becomes impaired. As with most other tasks, disability is greater if the dominant arm is more affected; shaving, brushing teeth, and other repetitive movements usually are affected the most. Use of eating utensils becomes difficult, chewing is laborious, and choking while swallowing may occur. If the latter is an early and prominent complaint, one must consider bulbar involvement in one of the parkinsonism-plus syndromes, such as progressive supranuclear palsy (PSP) and multiple system atrophy (MSA) (Jellinger, 2014; Low et al, 2015) (Table 23.2).

Speech becomes slurred and loses its volume (hypophonia), and as a result, patients often must repeat themselves. Like gait, speech may be *festinating*; that is, it gets faster and faster (tachyphemia). A large number of additional speech disturbances may occur, including stuttering and *palilalia*, an involuntary repetition of a phrase with increasing rapidity. Early and pronounced voice changes often indicate a diagnosis other than PD (e.g., palilalia is more commonly a feature of PSP and MSA). A harsher, nasal quality of the voice, which is quite distinctive from the hypophonic monotone of PD, also suggests the diagnosis of PSP. A higher-pitched quivering, "whiny" voice may suggest MSA, especially if it is associated with frequent sighing, respiratory gasps, laryngeal stridor, and other respiratory problems (Mehanna and Jankovic, 2010).

Another problem related to impairment of bulbar function is excessive salivation and drooling. Initially this may occur only at night, but later it can be present throughout the day, at times necessitating the constant use of a tissue or handkerchief.

Getting in and out of a chair or car and climbing in and out of the bathtub may cause problems and most patients switch to showering instead of bathing. Many patients misinterpret these difficulties as resulting from "weakness." Generalized loss of energy and easy fatigability are also common complaints. Walking becomes slowed and shuffling, with

TABLE 23.2 Parkinsonian Syndromes: Differential Diagnosis

	PD	PSP	MSA-P	MSA-C	CBD	DLB	PDACG
Bradykinesia	+	+	+	±	+	±	+
Rigidity	+	+	+	+	+	±	+
Gait disturbance	+	+	+	+	+	±	+
Tremor	+	−	±	±	±	−	+
Ataxia	−	−	−	+	−	−	±
Dysautonomia	±	±	+	+	−	±	±
Dementia	±	+	±	−	±	+	+
Dysarthria or dysphagia	±	+	+	+	+	±	+
Dystonia	±	±	±	−	+	−	−
Eyelid apraxia	±	+	±	−	±	−	±
Limb apraxia	−	±	−	−	+	±	−
Motor neuron disease	−	−	±	−	−	−	+
Myoclonus	±	−	±	±	+	±	−
Neuropathy	−	−	−	±	−	−	−
Oculomotor deficit	−	+	−	+	+	±	±
Sleep impairment	±	±	±	±	−	±	
Asymmetrical findings	+	±	±	−	+	−	
L-dopa response	+	−	±	±	−	−	
L-dopa dyskinesia	+	−	±	−	−	−	
Family history	±	−	−	−	−	−	
Putaminal T2 hypointensity	−	±	+	+	−	−	−
Lewy bodies	+	−	±	±	±	+	−

CBD, Corticobasal degeneration; *DLB*, dementia with Lewy bodies; *MSA-C*, multiple system atrophy, cerebellar type; *MSA-P*, multiple system atrophy, parkinsonian type; *PD*, Parkinson disease; *PDACG*, amyotrophic lateral sclerosis and parkinsonism-dementia complex of Guam; *PSP*, progressive supranuclear palsy.

flexion of the knees and a narrow base. When involvement is asymmetrical, one leg may drag behind the other. Stride then shortens, and turns include multiple steps (turning en bloc). Later, patients may note a tendency to advance more and more rapidly with shorter and shorter steps (festination), at times seemingly propelled forward with a secondary inadequate attempt to maintain the center of gravity over the legs. When this occurs, a nearby wall or an unobstructed fall may be the only method of stopping. Alternatively, the feet may seem glued to the floor, the so-called freezing phenomenon, or motor block. Early on, this is appreciated when the patient initiates walking (start hesitation), is turning (especially in an enclosed space), or attempts to walk through an enclosed area or a narrow passage such as a doorway or walking in or out of an elevator. When combined with poor postural stability, prominent freezing results in the tendency to fall forward or to the side while turning. Later, impaired postural reflexes may cause falls without a propulsive or freezing precipitant. The early occurrence of falls suggests a diagnosis of PSP or other parkinsonian disorder rather than PD. Turning over in bed and adjusting the bedclothes often become difficult. Patients may have to sit up first and then turn, and later the spouse may have to help roll the person over or adjust position for comfort.

Cognitive, Autonomic, and Sensory Abnormalities

The complaints of patients with parkinsonism are not limited to the motor system, and a large variety of nonmotor symptoms, many of which are probably not directly related to dopaminergic deficiency, often emerge as the disease progresses. In many cases, they become more disabling than the classic motor problems (Lim et al., 2009) (see Table 23.2). Dementia occurs in a variety of parkinsonian syndromes (see Chapters 95 and 97). Depression is also a common problem, and patients often lose their assertiveness and become withdrawn, more passive, and less motivated to socialize. The term *bradyphrenia* describes the slowness of thought processes and inattentiveness often seen.

Complaints related to autonomic dysfunction are also common. In all parkinsonian syndromes, constipation is a common complaint and may become severe. However, fecal incontinence does not occur in PD unless the motor disability is such that the patient cannot maneuver to the bathroom, dementia is superimposed, or impaction has led to overflow incontinence. Bladder complaints such as frequency, nocturia, and the sensation of incomplete bladder emptying may occur. Urinary incontinence is especially suggestive of MSA. A mild to moderate degree of orthostatic hypotension is common in parkinsonian disorders, and antiparkinsonian drugs often aggravate the problem (see Chapter 96). If the autonomic features, particularly erectile dysfunction, sphincter problems, and orthostatic lightheadedness, occur early or become the dominant feature, one must consider the possibility of MSA (see Chapter 95). Impotence with early loss of nocturnal or morning erections and inability to maintain erection during intercourse is suggestive of MSA. The other symptom that may precede the onset of motor problems associated with several parkinsonian disorders, particularly PD, MSA, or dementia with Lewy bodies, is rapid eye movement (REM) sleep behavior disorder. One characteristic nonmotor feature of PD is excessive greasiness of the skin and seborrheic dermatitis, characteristically seen over the forehead, eyebrows, and malar area.

In addition to pain, there are many other sensory symptoms associated with PD (Patel et al., 2014). Visual complaints are usually not a prominent feature, with the following specific exceptions. In PD (and many other parkinsonian disorders), diplopia may occur during reading secondary to impaired convergence. Visual complaints sometimes occur in other parkinsonian disorders, particularly PSP (see Chapter 96). Oculogyric crises, which are sudden episodes of involuntary ocular deviation (most often up and to the side) in the absence of neuroleptic drug exposure, are virtually pathognomonic of parkinsonism after encephalitis lethargica, although they may occur in rare neurometabolic disorders as well. Sensory loss is not part of parkinsonism, although patients with PD may have poorly explained positive sensory complaints such as numbness and tingling, aching, and painful sensations that are sometimes quite disabling. Peripheral neuropathy suggests another disorder or an unrelated problem (e.g., diabetes mellitus), although a higher-than-expected incidence of peripheral neuropathy, possibly related to levodopa treatment and elevated methylmalonic acid levels, has been suggested (Toth et al., 2010).

Although a variety of neurophysiological and computer-based methods for quantitating the severity of the various parkinsonian symptoms and signs have been proposed, most studies rely on clinical rating scales. Non-demented patients can reliably self-administer and complete the historical section of the UPDRS, now available in a revised version referred to as the *Movement Disorder Society (MDS)-UPDRS* (http://www.movementdisorders.org). The revision clarifies some ambiguities and more adequately assesses the nonmotor features of PD, which are among the most disabling symptoms, particularly in more advanced stages of the disease (Goetz et al., 2010). Some clinical research studies supplement the UPDRS by a more objective timed test such as the Purdue Pegboard Test and movement and reaction times. Many scales, such as the Parkinson's Disease Questionnaire-39 (PDQ-39) and the Parkinson's Disease Quality of Life Questionnaire (PDQL), attempt to assess the overall quality of life (Jankovic, 2008).

Onset and Course

As in other movement disorders, the age at onset of a parkinsonian syndrome is clearly important in considering a differential diagnosis. Although the majority of patients are adults, parkinsonism does occur in childhood (see Box 23.1). PD, particularly the tremor-dominant subtype, usually has a slow onset and very gradual progression, although the "postural instability gait difficulty" (PIGD) subtype is more rapidly progressive with less favorable prognosis (Thenganatt and Jankovic, 2014a). Generally, patients with early-onset PD and those with a tremor-dominant form tend to progress at a slower rate and are less likely to have an associated cognitive decline than those with postural instability and the gait difficulty form of PD. Other disorders (e.g., those due to toxins, cerebral anoxia, infarction) may present abruptly or progress more rapidly (resulting in so-called malignant parkinsonism) or may even improve spontaneously (e.g., those due to drugs, certain forms of encephalitis).

Examination and Clinical Signs

The diagnosis of parkinsonism often is immediately apparent on first contact with the patient. The facial expression, low-volume voice, tremor, poverty of movement, shuffling gait, and stooped posture provide an immediate and irrevocable first impression of parkinsonism. However, the physician must perform a detailed assessment, searching for any atypical features in attempting to distinguish between PD and other parkinsonian disorders (Morris and Jankovic, 2012). Loss of facial expression (*hypomimia*) often is an early sign of PD. But occasional patients have a wide-eyed, anxious, worried expression due to furrowing of the brow ("procerus sign") and deep facial folds, which strongly suggests PSP. Blink frequency usually is reduced, although *blepharoclonus* (repetitive spasms of the lids on gentle eye closure) and reflex blepharospasm (e.g., precipitated by shining a light into the eyes or manipulating the lids) also may be seen. Spontaneous blepharospasm and apraxia of lid opening occur less often. Patients with apraxia of lid opening (not a true apraxia) are not able to open their eyes after spontaneous or voluntary closure and often must use their fingers to forcefully open their eyes, and once the eyes are fixated on an object, the eyelids remain open. Primitive reflexes, including the inability to inhibit blinking in response to tapping over the glabella (Myerson sign) and palmomental reflexes, are nonspecific and are commonly present in many parkinsonian disorders (Brodsky et al., 2004).

Various types of tremor, most notably rest and postural varieties, often accompany parkinsonian disorders. Patients should be observed with hands resting on their laps or thighs, and they should be instructed to hold their arms in an outstretched position or in a horizontal position with shoulders abducted, elbows flexed, and hands palms-down in front of their faces in the so-called "wing-beating position". Rest tremor often re-emerges after a period of quiescence in a new position (*re-emergent tremor*) (Jankovic, 2008). This re-emergent tremor, which is often the most troublesome parkinsonian tremor because it interferes with holding objects steadily against gravity, may be wrongly attributed to postural tremor and lead to misdiagnosis as essential tremor. A true kinetic (intention) tremor, elicited by the finger-to-nose maneuver, is much less common in patients with PD and other parkinsonian disorders and usually indicates involvement of cerebellar connections. A jerky (myoclonic) postural tremor is suggestive of a diagnosis of MSA rather than PD. Head tremor (*titubation*) suggests a diagnosis other than PD, such as essential tremor, dystonic neck tremor, or a cerebellar tremor associated with the cerebellar form of MSA (MSA-C), spinocerebellar atrophy, or multiple sclerosis (MS).

Rigidity is an increase in muscle tone, usually equal in flexors and extensors and present throughout the passive range of movement. This contrasts with the distribution and velocity-dependent nature of spasticity (the clasp-knife phenomenon). Paratonia (or Gegenhalten), on the other hand, increases with repetitive passive movement and attempts to get the patient to relax. It may be difficult to distinguish between milder forms of paratonia and rigidity, especially in the legs. Characteristically, the performance of voluntary movements in the opposite limb (e.g., opening and closing the fist or abduction-adduction of the shoulder) brings out rigidity, a phenomenon known as *activated rigidity* (Froment sign). Superimposed on the rigidity may be a tremor or cogwheel phenomenon. This, like the milder forms of rigidity, is better appreciated by placing one hand over the muscles being tested (e.g., placing the left thumb over the biceps and the remaining fingers over the triceps while flexing and extending the elbow with the right hand). The distribution of the rigidity sometimes is helpful in differential diagnosis. For example, pronounced nuchal rigidity with much less hypertonicity in the limbs suggests the diagnosis of PSP, whereas an extreme degree of unilateral arm rigidity or paratonia suggests *corticobasal degeneration* (CBD) or *corticobasal syndrome* (CBS). The latter term is suggested for cases diagnosed clinically, as only a minority of patients with clinical features of CBS have pathologically proven CBD (Ling et al., 2014).

Akinesia and bradykinesia are appreciable on examination in several ways. Automatic movements normally expressed in conversation, such as gesturing with hands while speaking, crossing and uncrossing the legs, and repositioning the body in the chair diminish or are absent. The performance of rapid, repetitive, and alternating movements such as finger tapping, opening and closing the fist, pronation-supination of the forearm, and foot tapping is slow, with a gradual reduction in amplitude and eventual cessation of movement (*freezing*). In addition to fatiguing, there may be hesitation in initiating movement and arrests in ongoing movement. The severely afflicted patient may be barely able to perform the task. There is a tendency for rapid repetitive movements to take on the frequency of an accompanying tremor. In such cases, instruct the patient to slow the movement and attempt to complete it voluntarily. In contrast to PD, PSP patients have small amplitude of finger separation (often at a rapid rate) without progressive decrement on repetitive finger tapping (Ling et al., 2012). Watching the patient write is an important part of the examination. Observation may reveal great slowness and effort, even in someone with minimal change in the size of the script. In addition to micrographia, writing and drawing show a tendency to fatigue, with a further reduction in size as the task proceeds and a concomitant action tremor. This is in contrast to handwriting in patients with ET, which tends to be larger and tremulous.

Postural disturbances are common in parkinsonian disorders. The head usually tilts forward and the body becomes stooped, often with pronounced kyphosis and varying degrees of scoliosis, typically away from the side of the onset of parkinsonian signs, such as rest tremor (Ashour and Jankovic, 2006). The arms become flexed at the elbows and wrists, with varying postural deformities in the hands, the most common being flexion at the metacarpophalangeal joints and extension at the interphalangeal joints, with adduction of all the fingers and opposition of the thumb to the index finger (*striatal hand*) (Fig. 23.2, *A*). Flexion also occurs in the joints of the legs. Variable foot deformities occur, the most common being hammer toe-like disturbances in most of the toes, occasionally with extension of the great toe (*striatal foot*) (Fig. 23.2, *B*), which may be misinterpreted as an extensor plantar response. Initially, abnormal foot posturing may be induced by action, occurring only during walking or weight bearing. The flexed or simian posture sometimes is extreme, with severe flexion at the waist (*camptocormia*) (Jankovic, 2010) (Fig. 23.2, *C*). Some patients, particularly those with MSA, exhibit scoliosis or tilted posture (*Pisa sign*) (Fig. 23.2, *D*). Despite the truncal flexion, the position of the hands in patients with PD often remains above the beltline because of flexion of the elbows. Occasional patients remain upright or even demonstrate a hyperextended posture. Hyperextension of the neck is particularly suggestive of PSP, whereas extreme flexion of the neck (head drop or bent spine) suggests MSA (Fig. 23.2, *D*) but also PD.

Postural instability is characteristic of parkinsonian disorders, particularly the postural instability and gait difficulty forms of PD, PSP, and MSA. As patients rise from a sitting position, poor postural stability, slowness, narrow base, and not repositioning the feet often combine to cause them to fall back into the chair "in a lump." PSP patients may "rocket" out of the chair inappropriately quickly, failing to recognize their inability to maintain stability on their feet. The PD patient may require several attempts, push off the arms of the chair, or need to be pulled up by an assistant. Gait disturbances in typical parkinsonism include lack of arm swing, shortened and later shuffling stride, freezing in the course of walking (especially when initiating gait and when approaching a door frame or a potential obstruction or a chair). Patients with PD turn en bloc, whereas patients with PSP tend to pivot when they turn. In more severe cases of PD or PSP, propulsion and retropulsion may occur spontaneously, resulting in falls (Jankovic, 2008). In addition, walking often brings out or exacerbates a rest tremor in patients with PD. To assess postural instability, the physician performs the pull test. Standing behind the patient, the examiner pulls the patient backward by the shoulders, carefully remaining close behind to prevent a fall (Morris and Jankovic, 2012). Once postural reflexes are impaired, there may be retropulsion or multiple backward steps in response to the postural perturbation. Later there is a tendency to fall en bloc without retropulsion or even normal attempts to recover or to cushion the fall.

In PD, the base of the gait is usually narrow, and tandem gait is performed well. When the gait is wide-based, a superimposed ataxia is a consideration, as is seen in MSA-C, although some of the spinocerebellar atrophies may present with parkinsonism and ataxia (see Chapter 97). Toe walking (*cock-walk*) is seen in some parkinsonian disorders (e.g., due to manganese poisoning), and a peculiar loping gait may indicate the rare patient with akinesia in the absence of rigidity, which may be one phenotype of PSP. The so-called magnetic foot, or marche à petits pas, of senility (also seen in vascular parkinsonism due to multiple infarctions, Binswanger disease, and normal pressure hydrocephalus) more commonly results in a lower-body parkinsonism, typically associated with cerebrovascular disorders such as lacunar strokes (Mehanna and Jankovic, 2013). A striking discrepancy of involvement between the lower body and the upper limbs, with normal or even excessive arm swing, is an important clue to the diagnosis of vascular parkinsonism.

Differential Diagnosis

Although dementia commonly occurs in PD, this feature, particularly when present relatively early in the course, must alert the physician to other possible diagnoses (see Chapter 95), including dementia with Lewy bodies, particularly if the cognitive deficit is accompanied by visual hallucinations, or the coincidental association of unrelated causes of cognitive decline, such as Alzheimer's disease (Svenningsson et al., 2012). Prominent eye movement disturbances are found in a number of conditions, including PSP, MSA-C, postencephalitic parkinsonism, CBD, and Machado–Joseph disease (SCA3). It is important to assess not only horizontal and vertical gaze (typically impaired in PSP) but also optokinetic nystagmus to note whether vertical saccadic eye movements (particularly as the optokinetic tape moves in upward direction) are impaired, as in PSP. The oculocephalic (doll's eye) maneuver must be performed when ocular excursions are limited, seeking supportive evidence of supranuclear gaze palsy. Patients with PSP typically have trouble making eye contact because of disturbed visual refixation. As a result of persistence of visual fixation when PSP patients turn, their head turn lags behind their body turn. Obvious pyramidal tract dysfunction usually suggests diagnoses other than PD. An exaggerated grasp response indicates disturbance of the frontal lobes and the possibility of a concomitant dementing process. Occasionally a pronounced flexed posture in the hand may be confused with a grasp reflex, and the examiner must be convinced that there is active contraction in response to stroking of the palm. The abnormalities of rapid, repetitive, and alternating movements described earlier can be confused with the clumsy awkward performance of limb-kinetic apraxia (Zadikoff and Lang, 2005). More importantly, the

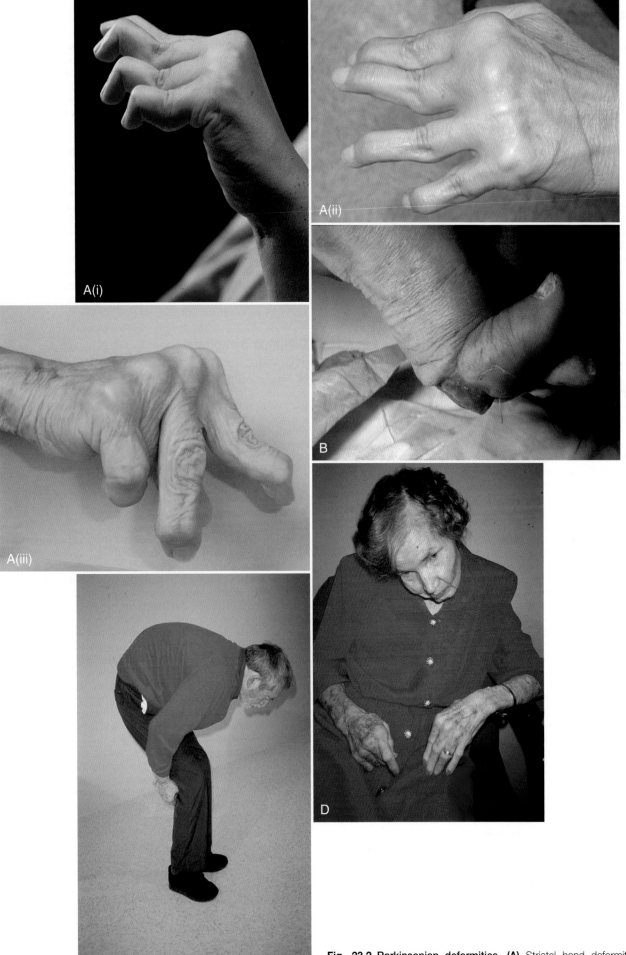

Fig. 23.2 Parkinsonian deformities. (A) Striatal hand deformities; **(B)** Striatal foot deformity; **(C)** Camptocormia in a patient with PD; **(D)** Pisa sign and anterior neck flexion in a patient with MSA.

abnormalities in performance of repetitive movement must not be confused with the disruption of rate, rhythm, and force typical of the dysdiadochokinesia of cerebellar disease. A helpful maneuver in testing for the presence of associated cerebellar dysfunction is to have the patient tap with the index finger on a hard surface. Watching and, in particular, listening to the tapping often allows a distinction to be made between the slowness and decrementing response of parkinsonism and the irregular rate and force of cerebellar ataxia. Testing for ideomotor apraxia, as seen in CBS, should also be performed by asking the patient to mimic certain hand gestures (intransitive tasks) such as the "victory sign" or the University of Texas "hook 'em horns sign" (extension of the second and fifth finger and flexion of the third and fourth finger) or to simulate certain activities (transitive tasks [using a tool or utensil]) such as brushing teeth and combing hair. However, in the later stages of many parkinsonian disorders, rigidity and other motor disturbances may make results of these tests difficult to interpret. In PD or MSA, the less affected limb may show mirror movements as the patient attempts to perform rapid repetitive or alternating movements with the most affected limb (Espay et al., 2005). On the other hand, in CBS, the most affected limb may mirror movements performed in the less affected limb. Some patients with parkinsonism and frontal lobe involvement exhibit signs of perseveration such as the *applause sign*, manifested by persistence of clapping after instructing the patient to clap consecutively three times as quickly as possible. Although initially thought to be characteristic of PSP, it is also present in some patients with other parkinsonian disorders (Wu et al., 2008).

The presence of other abnormal movements in an untreated patient may indicate a diagnosis other than PD. Seek evidence of stimulus-sensitive myoclonus by producing sudden loud noise or using light touch or pinprick in the digits and the proximal palm or the sole of the foot. Easily elicited and nonfatiguing myoclonic jerks in response to these stimuli may be seen not only in patients with CBS and MSA but also in some patients with PD and dementia.

Despite a variety of sensory complaints, patients with PD do not show prominent abnormalities on the sensory examination, aside from the normal increase in vibration threshold that occurs with age (Patel et al., 2014). Cortical sensory disturbances suggest a diagnosis of CBS. Wasting and muscle weakness are not characteristic of PD, although later in the course of the disease, severely disabled patients show disuse atrophy and severe problems in initiating and maintaining muscle activation that are often difficult to separate from true weakness. Combinations of upper and lower motor neuron weakness occur in several other parkinsonian disorders (see Table 23.2).

Assessing autonomic function is important not only in patients suspected of having MSA, but also in patients with PD, many of whom have dysautonomia. At the bedside, this includes an evaluation of orthostatic changes in blood pressure and pulse (in supine position and at least 3 minutes after standing) and, in appropriate circumstances, the patient's response to the Valsalva maneuver, mental arithmetic, and the cold pressor test, among others. Finally, perform sequential examinations over time, carefully searching for the development of additional findings that may provide a clue to the diagnosis. Several parkinsonian syndromes present initially as pure parkinsonism; only later with disease progression do other signs develop.

TREMOR

Tremor is rhythmic oscillation of a body part, produced by either alternating or synchronous contractions of reciprocally innervated antagonistic muscles. Tremors usually have a fixed frequency, although the rate may appear irregular. The amplitude of the tremor can vary widely, depending on both physiological and psychological factors. The basis of further categorization is the position, posture, and motor performance necessary to elicit it. A *rest tremor* occurs with the body part in complete repose, although when a patient totally relaxes or sleeps this tremor usually disappears. Maintenance of a posture, such as extending the arms parallel to the floor, reveals a *postural tremor*; moving the body part to and from a target brings out an *intention tremor*. The use of other descriptive categories has caused some confusion in tremor terminology. *Action tremor* has been used for both postural and kinetic (also known as *intention*) tremors. Whereas a *kinetic tremor* is present throughout goal-directed movement, the term *terminal tremor* applies to the component of kinetic tremor that exaggerates when approaching the target. *Ataxic tremor* refers to a combination of kinetic tremor plus limb ataxia. Box 23.2 provides a list of differential diagnoses for the three major categories of tremor and other rhythmic movements that occasionally are confused with tremor.

Common Symptoms

A description of symptoms occurs under the various categories of tremor. All people have a normal or physiological tremor demonstrable with sensitive recording devices. Two common pathological tremor disorders that are often confused are parkinsonian rest tremor and essential tremor. Although Chapter 96 discusses both conditions in detail, we discuss helpful distinguishing points here in view of the frequency of misdiagnosis.

Rest Tremor

A rest tremor occurs with the body part in complete repose and often dampens or subsides entirely with action. For this reason, patients with pure rest tremor experience greater social embarrassment than functional disability, unless, as noted earlier, the rest tremor re-emerges during postural holding. Indeed, in some cases it is a family member or friend who first observes the tremor, which is noticeable to the patient only later. Alternatively, some patients complain of the sensation of trembling inside long before a rest tremor becomes overt. Early on, rest tremor may be intermittent and often precipitated only by anxiety or stress. The onset of most types of tremor is in the arms, often beginning asymmetrically. In the face, rest tremor usually affects the lips and jaw, and the patient may note a rhythmic clicking of the teeth. In the limbs, the tremor usually is most distally in the fingers (pill rolling) or may manifest by flexion-extension or a supination-pronation, oscillatory movement of the wrist and forearm, and flexion-extension movement of the ankle. In severe forms, it may be present more proximally, causing the entire body to shake. The presence of head tremor (titubation) should raise the possibility of essential tremor or of dystonic tremor associated with cervical dystonia or cerebellar outflow tremor, as is seen in patients with MS or posterior fossa disorders. Tremor in the legs, and especially in the feet while sitting, is usually caused by parkinsonian rest tremor. A history of progression from unilateral arm tremor to additional involvement of the ipsilateral leg suggests parkinsonism rather than essential tremor. Once the tremor has become noticeable to the patient, a variety of methods are used to conceal the movement, such as holding one hand with the other, sitting on the affected hand, or crossing the legs to dampen a tremulous lower limb. Many patients find that they can briefly abort the tremor.

BOX 23.2 Classification and Differential Diagnosis of Tremor

RESTING TREMORS

PD
Other parkinsonian syndromes (less common)
Midbrain (rubral) tremor (Holmes tremor): rest < postural < intention
WD (also acquired hepatocerebral degeneration)
Essential tremor

POSTURAL TREMORS

Physiological tremor
Exaggerated physiological tremor; these factors can also aggravate other forms of tremor:
  Stress, fatigue, anxiety, emotion
  Endocrine: hypoglycemia, thyrotoxicosis, pheochromocytoma
  Drugs and toxins: adrenocorticosteroids, β-agonists, dopamine agonists, amphetamines, lithium, tricyclic antidepressants, neuroleptics, theophylline, caffeine, valproic acid, alcohol withdrawal, mercury ("hatter's shakes"), lead, arsenic, others
Essential tremor (familial or sporadic)
Primary writing tremor and other task-specific tremors
Orthostatic tremor
With other CNS disorders:
  PD (postural tremor, re-emergent tremor, associated essential tremor)
  Other akinetic-rigid syndromes
  Idiopathic dystonia, including focal dystonias

With peripheral neuropathy:
  Charcot-Marie-Tooth disease (called the *Roussy-Levy syndrome*)
  Other peripheral neuropathies
Cerebellar tremor

INTENTION TREMORS

Diseases of cerebellar outflow (dentate nuclei, interpositus nuclei, or both, and superior cerebellar peduncle):
  MS, trauma, tumor, vascular disease, WD, acquired hepatocerebral degeneration, drugs, toxins (e.g., mercury), others

MISCELLANEOUS RHYTHMIC MOVEMENT DISORDERS

Psychogenic tremor
Rhythmic movements in dystonia (dystonic tremor, myorrhythmia)
Rhythmic myoclonus (segmental myoclonus, e.g., palatal or branchial myoclonus, spinal myoclonus), myorrhythmia
Oscillatory myoclonus
Asterixis
Clonus
Epilepsia partialis continua
Hereditary chin quivering
Spasmus nutans
Head bobbing with third ventricular cysts
Nystagmus

CNS, Central nervous system; *MS,* multiple sclerosis; *PD,* Parkinson disease; *WD,* Wilson disease.

Postural Tremor

In contrast to a pure rest tremor, postural tremors, especially with pronounced terminal accentuation, can result in significant disability. Many such patients are mistaken as having "bad nerves." People who perform delicate work with their hands (e.g., jewelers, surgeons) become aware of this form of tremor earlier than most. The average person usually first appreciates tremor in the acts of feeding and writing. Carrying a cup of liquid, pouring, or eating with a spoon often brings out the tremor. Writing is tremulous and sloppy, questioning the patient's signature on a check. The voice may be involved in essential tremor. Again, anxiety and stress worsen the tremor, and patients often notice that their symptoms are especially bad in public. The most common cause of postural tremor seen in movement disorders clinics is essential tremor (Jankovic, 2009).

Patients often adopt compensatory mechanisms to lessen the disability caused by tremor. Many give up certain tasks such as serving drinks and eating specific foods (e.g., soup), especially in public. When the tremor is very asymmetrical, patients often switch to using the less-affected hand for many tasks, including writing. Bringing a cup to the mouth becomes difficult; later, a straw is required. When writing, patients may use the other hand to steady the paper or the writing hand itself. Patients often switch from cursive to print, and the use of heavier or thicker writing instruments sometimes makes the script more legible. In some patients with parkinsonian disorders and severe rest tremor, the tremor may also be present while the patient holds an outstretched or wing-beating posture. This tremor usually occurs after a latency of several seconds, hence the term *re-emergent tremor* (Jankovic, 2008); in contrast, in essential tremor the tremor is evident immediately on taking up a new posture. Some patients with essential tremor also have rest tremor and develop other parkinsonian

features. There is also evidence that some patients with essential tremor have an increased risk for developing PD (Fekete and Jankovic, 2011).

Other Types of Tremor

Various types of writing disturbances may combine with tremor. Primary writing tremor is one form of task-specific tremor that affects the writing act in isolation, with little or no associated postural or terminal tremor interfering with other acts. Dystonic writer's cramp can involve additional tremulousness on writing. Distinction is required from the voluntary excessive squeezing of the pen or pressing onto the page often seen in patients with essential tremor or primary writing tremor, which is attributable to their attempts to lessen the effect of tremor on writing. In addition, patients with postural tremor may consciously slow their writing to improve accuracy, but this is a voluntary compensatory mechanism not associated with the micrographia and fatigue that accompany parkinsonism.

Tremor in the head and neck, or titubation, occurs in isolation or combined with a postural tremor elsewhere, especially in the arms, as is seen in patients with essential tremor. When the head tremor is irregular and is associated with abnormal head posture and uneven contractions or hypertrophy of the neck muscles, the possibility of cervical dystonia requires consideration (dystonic tremor). Head tremor is rarely a source of physical disability but may create social embarrassment. Patients occasionally complain of a similar tremor of the voice. This is particularly noticeable to others who are listening to the patient on the telephone, and many ask the patient whether they are sad or have been crying.

Less often, patients with postural tremors note a similar tremor in the legs and trunk. The awareness of this form of tremor clearly depends on the activity performed. One form of postural tremor, orthostatic tremor, characteristically presents not as tremor but rather difficulty and insecurity on standing. It is associated with a 14- to 16-Hz tremor in the legs and trunk (Yaltho and Ondo, 2014). This tremor typically subsides if the patient walks about, leans against something, or sits down.

Other Clues in the History

Although patients with several different types of tremor may indicate that alcohol transiently reduces their shaking, a striking response to small amounts of alcohol is particularly characteristic of essential tremor (Mostile and Jankovic, 2010). Clues to the possible presence of factors aggravating the normal physiological tremor (see Box 23.2) require further inquiry.

Examination

In addition to clinical examination, various physiological, accelerometric, and other computer-based techniques can be employed to assess tremor, but a clinical rating scale usually is most practical, particularly in clinical trials. The Tremor Research Group (TRG) has developed a rating scale that can be used to quantitatively assess all types of tremor, particularly essential tremor, the most common type encountered in clinical practice (Box 23.3). The TRG Essential Tremor Rating Scale (TETRAS) is currently being validated and has been found to correlate well with quantitative computer-based systems (Mostile et al., 2010). Besides rest tremor, postural tremor, and kinetic limb tremor, examine patients for tremor of the head. With the patient seated or standing, head tremor may be evident as vertical ("yes-yes") nodding (*tremblement affirmatif*) or side-to-side ("no-no") horizontal shaking (*tremblement negatif*). There may be combinations of the two, with rotatory movements. Subtle head tremors may only be appreciated when the examiner holds the patient's cranium while testing with the other hand for extreme lateral eye movements. Head tremors usually range from 1.5 to 5 Hz and are most commonly associated with essential tremor or cervical dystonia and with diseases of the cerebellum and its outflow pathways.

BOX 23.3 Tremor Research Group Rating Scale

INSTRUCTIONS FOR COMPLETING THE OBSERVER TREMOR PORTION

1. Head tremor: Subject is seated upright. The head is observed for 10 seconds in midposition and for 5 seconds each during several provocative maneuvers. First the subject is asked to rotate his or her head to the maximum lateral positions slowly in each direction. The subject is then asked to deviate his or her eyes to the maximum lateral positions while the examiner gently touches the subject's chin.
   0 = No tremor.
   1 = Tremor seen or felt during provocative maneuvers.
   2 = Mild tremor seen at midposition or moderate tremor seen with provocative maneuvers.
   3 = Moderate tremor seen at midposition or severe tremor seen with provocative maneuvers.
   4 = Severe tremor seen at midposition.
2a. Face tremor: Subject is seated upright and asked to smile and pucker his or her lips, each for 5 seconds. Tremor is specifically assessed for the lower facial muscles (excluding jaw and tongue) and upper face (eye closure).
   0 = No tremor.
   1 = Mild tremor seen only with active muscle contraction.
   2 = Mild tremor seen at rest or moderate tremor seen with active muscle contraction.
   3 = Moderate tremor seen at rest or severe tremor seen with muscle contraction.
   4 = Severe tremor seen at rest.
2b. Tongue tremor: Subject is seated upright and asked to open his or her mouth for 5 seconds and then stick out his or her tongue for 5 seconds.
   0 = No tremor.
   1 = Mild tremor seen only with active muscle contraction.
   2 = Mild tremor seen at rest or moderate tremor seen with active muscle contraction.
   3 = Moderate tremor seen at rest or severe tremor seen with active muscle contraction.
   4 = Severe tremor seen at rest.
2c. Jaw tremor: Subject is seated upright and asked to maximally open his or her mouth and clench the jaw for 5 seconds.
   0 = No tremor.
   1 = Mild tremor seen only with active muscle contraction.

2 = Mild tremor seen at rest or moderate tremor seen with active muscle contraction.
3 = Moderate tremor seen at rest or severe tremor seen with active muscle contraction.
4 = Severe tremor seen at rest.

3. Voice tremor: First assess speech during normal conversation; then ask subject to produce an extended "aaa" sound and "eee" sound for 5 seconds each.
   0 = No tremor.
   1 = Barely perceptible tremor only during provocative maneuver.
   2 = Mild but clear tremor present with speaking.
   3 = Moderate tremor (no voice breaks).
   4 = Severe tremor (with voice breaks or unintelligible speech).
4. Arm tremor: Subject is seated upright. Tremor is assessed during four arm maneuvers (rest, forward horizontal reach posture, lateral "wing-beating" posture, and kinesis) for 5 seconds in each posture. Left and right arms may be assessed simultaneously. Amplitude assessment should be estimated using the maximally displaced point of the hand at the point of greatest displacement along any single plane. For example, the amplitude of a pure supination-pronation tremor, pivoting around the wrist, would be assessed at either the thumb or fifth digit.
   a. Rest tremor. The subject should have his or her elbows on the arm rests. (If this is the previous assessment, no specific instructions should be given if the subject did not naturally assume an acceptable arm position for elbows on the arm rests, with hands resting freely.) Begin the second assessment only after the subject appears relaxed in the new position.
   b. Forward outstretched postural tremor. Subject should bring his or her arms forward, slightly lateral to midline and parallel to the ground. The wrists should also be straight and the fingers slightly and comfortably abducted so that they do not touch each other.
   c. Lateral "wing-beating postural" tremor. Subject abducts his or her arms parallel to the ground and flexes the elbows so that the two hands do not quite touch each other. The fingers are slightly and comfortably abducted so that they do not touch each other, with the pointer finger at shoulder height.

BOX 23.3 Tremor Research Group Rating Scale (Continued)

d. Kinetic tremor. Subject extends only his or her pointer finger, then touches a set object located at the same height (parallel to the ground) and slightly lateral to the midline. The subject then touches his or her own nose or chin and repeats this back-and-forth motion five times. Only the position along the trajectory of greatest tremor amplitude is assessed. This will typically be either at the nose or chin or at the point of full extent.

e. Tremor while walking: Have the patient walk a minimum of 6 m at a normal pace to and from the examiner, and observe his or her hands.

Rest Tremor:
0 = No tremor.
1 = Tremor is barely visible or present only with mental provocation or reinforcement.
1.5 = Tremor is visible, but is < 1 cm amplitude.
2 = Tremor is 1–3 cm amplitude.
2.5 = Tremor is 3–5 cm amplitude.
3 = Tremor is 5–10 cm amplitude.
3.5 = Tremor is 10–20 cm amplitude.
4 = Tremor is > 20 cm amplitude.

Postural Tremor:
0 = No tremor.
1 = Tremor is barely visible.
1.5 = Tremor is visible, but is < 1 cm amplitude.
2 = Tremor is 1–3 cm amplitude.
2.5 = Tremor is 3–5 cm amplitude.
3 = Tremor is 5–10 cm amplitude.
3.5 = Tremor is 10–20 cm amplitude.
4 = Tremor is > 20 cm amplitude.

Kinetic Tremor:
0 = No tremor.
1 = Tremor is barely visible.
1.5 = Tremor is visible, but is < 1 cm amplitude.
2 = Tremor is 1–3 cm amplitude.
2.5 = Tremor is 3–5 cm amplitude.
3 = Tremor is 5–10 cm amplitude.
3.5 = Tremor is 10–20 cm amplitude.
4 = Tremor is > 20 cm amplitude.

Tremor While Walking:
0 = No tremor.
1 = Tremor is barely visible.
1.5 = Tremor is visible, but is < 1 cm amplitude.
2 = Tremor is 1–3 cm amplitude.
2.5 = Tremor is 3–5 cm amplitude.
3 = Tremor is 5–10 cm amplitude.
3.5 = Tremor is 10–20 cm amplitude.
4 = Tremor is > 20 cm amplitude.

5. Trunk tremor: Subject is comfortably seated in a chair and asked to flex both legs at the hips 30 degrees above parallel to the ground for 5 seconds. The knees are passively bent so that the lower leg is perpendicular to the ground. The legs are not allowed to touch. Tremor is evaluated around the hip joints and the abdominal muscles.
0 = No tremor.
1 = Tremor present only with hip flexion.
2 = Obvious but mild tremor.
3 = Moderate tremor.
4 = Severe tremor.

6. Leg tremor action: Subject is comfortably seated and asked to raise his or her legs parallel to the ground with knees extended for 5 seconds. The legs are slightly abducted so they do not touch. Tremor amplitude is assessed at the end of the feet.
0 = No tremor.
1 = Barely perceptible tremor.
2 = Obvious but mild tremor.
3 = Moderate tremor; < 5 cm amplitude at any point.
4 = Severe tremor; > 5 cm amplitude.

7. Leg tremor rest: Subject is comfortably seated with knees flexed and feet resting on the ground. Tremor amplitude is assessed at the point of maximal displacement.
0 = No tremor.
1 = Barely perceptible tremor.
2 = Obvious but mild tremor.
3 = Moderate tremor; < 5 cm amplitude at any point.
4 = Severe tremor; > 5 cm amplitude.

8. Standing tremor: Subject is standing, unaided if possible. The internal malleoli are 5 cm apart. Arms are down at the sides. Tremor is assessed at any point on the legs or trunk.
0 = No tremor.
1 = Barely perceptible tremor.
2 = Obvious but mild tremor.
3 = Moderate tremor.
4 = Severe tremor.

9. Spiral drawings: Ask the subject to draw the requested figures. Test each hand without leaving the hand or arm on the table. Use only a ballpoint pen.
0 = Normal.
1 = Slightly tremulous. May cross lines occasionally.
2 = Moderately tremulous or crosses lines frequently.
3 = Accomplishes the task with great difficulty. Figure still recognizable.
4 = Unable to complete drawing. Figure not recognizable.

10. Handwriting: Have patient write "Today is a nice day."
0 = Normal.
1 = Mildly abnormal. Slightly untidy, tremulous.
2 = Moderately abnormal. Legible, but with considerable tremor.
3 = Markedly abnormal. Illegible.
4 = Severely abnormal. Unable to keep pencil or pen on paper without holding down with the other hand.

11. Hold pencil approximately 1 mm above a point on a piece of paper for 10 seconds.
0 = No tremor.
1 = Tremor is barely visible.
1.5 = Tremor is visible, but is < 1 cm amplitude.
2 = Tremor is 1–3 cm amplitude.
2.5 = Tremor is 3–5 cm amplitude.
3 = Tremor is 5–10 cm amplitude.
3.5 = Tremor is 10–20 cm amplitude.
4 = Tremor is > 20 cm amplitude.

12. Pour water from one glass into another, using styrofoam coffee cups filled 1 cm from top. Rated separately for right and left hands.
0 = Absolutely no visible tremor.
1 = More careful than a person without tremor. No water is spilled.
2 = Spills a small amount (<10%).
3 = Spills large amount (10%–50%).
4 = Unable to pour without spilling most.

A parkinsonian rest tremor may involve the jaw and lips. A similar tremor of the perioral and nasal muscles, the *rabbit syndrome*, has been associated with antipsychotic drug therapy but also occurs in PD. In many disorders, voluntary contraction of the facial muscles induces an action tremor. In addition, a postural tremor of the tongue often is present on tongue protrusion. In the case of tremors of head and neck structures, it is important to observe the palate at rest for the slower rhythmic movements of palatal myoclonus (also called *palatal tremor*). Occasionally, tremor spares the palate, with similar movements affecting other branchial structures. Demonstration of a voice tremor requires asking the patient to hold a note as long as possible. Superimposed on the vocal tremulousness may be a harsh, strained quality or abrupt cessation of airflow during the course of maintaining the note, which suggests a superimposed dystonia of the larynx (*spasmodic dysphonia*).

A parkinsonian rest tremor characteristically has a frequency in the range 4 to 6 Hz. The frequency of postural arm tremors varies depending on cause and severity; essential tremor usually is in the range of 5 to 10 Hz, with the greater-amplitude tremors tending to be slower. Exaggerated physiological tremor has a frequency of 8 to 12 Hz. Many patients with parkinsonism demonstrate a combination of slower resting and faster postural tremors. Some patients with slower, larger-amplitude forms of essential tremor have a definite resting component.

A rest tremor in the limbs occurs even with the muscles in complete repose. Even a small amount of muscle activity, as may occur if the patient is somewhat anxious or the limb is not completely at rest, may bring out a higher-frequency action postural tremor. It is sometimes impossible to abate this postural tremor during a stressful office interview. Stress and concentration may bring out an occult rest tremor, such as the performance of serial sevens. Although a rest tremor characteristically subsides when the patient maintains a posture (e.g., holding the arms outstretched parallel to the floor), it may recur after a few seconds. As noted earlier, the re-emergent tremor that occurs after a latency of a few seconds (and sometimes as long as 1 minute) suggests an underlying parkinsonian disorder (Jankovic, 2008). Carrying out goal-directed movements, such as finger-to-nose testing, usually causes the tremor to dampen further or subside completely. On the other hand, a typical postural tremor associated with essential tremor usually occurs without latency after the initiation of a posture and may worsen further at the endpoints of goal-directed movement (*terminal tremor*). The slower kinetic tremor of cerebellar disease occurs throughout the movement but also worsens upon reaching the target. Occasionally, pronounced bursts of muscle activity in a patient with terminal tremor cause individual separate jerks, which give the impression of superimposed myoclonus. *Essential myoclonus* is an autosomal dominant disorder, and affected patients and their relatives have both jerk-like myoclonus and postural tremor phenomenologically identical to essential tremor. Most patients previously diagnosed with *essential myoclonus* probably have myoclonus-dystonia syndrome, many due to mutations in the gene coding for ε-sarcoglycan (*SGCE*).

Having the patient point the index fingers at each other under the nose (without touching the fingers together or touching the face) with the arms abducted at the sides and the elbows flexed can demonstrate both distal tremor in the hands and proximal tremors. An example of proximal tremor is the slower wing-beating tremor of cerebellar outflow pathway disease, as may be seen in WD. Tremor during the course of slowly pronating and supinating the forearms with the arms outstretched or with forceful abduction of the fingers occurs in patients with primary writing tremor. Holding a full cup of water with the arm outstretched often amplifies a postural tremor, and picking up the full cup, bringing it to the mouth, and tipping it to drink enhances the terminal tremor, often causing spillage. In addition to writing, one should have the patient draw with both hands separately. Useful drawing tasks include an Archimedes spiral, a wavy line from one side of the page to the other (Fig. 23.3), and an attempt to carefully draw a line or spiral between two well-defined, closely opposed borders. Another useful test designed to bring out position-specific tremor is the dot approximation test, in which the patient is instructed to be seated at the desk with elbow elevated and to hold the tip of the pen or pencil (for at least 10 seconds) as close as possible to a dot drawn on a sheet of paper without touching it. Many patients with action tremors note marked exacerbation of their tremor during this specific task.

In the legs, in addition to the standard heel-to-shin testing which brings out kinetic and terminal tremors, it may be possible to demonstrate a postural tremor by having the patient hold the leg off the bed and attempt to touch the examiner's finger with the great toe. With the legs flexed at the knees and abducted at the hips and the feet held flat on the bed, synchronous rhythmic 3-Hz abductions of the thighs may occur in patients with atrophy of the anterior vermis, as seen in alcoholic cerebellar degeneration.

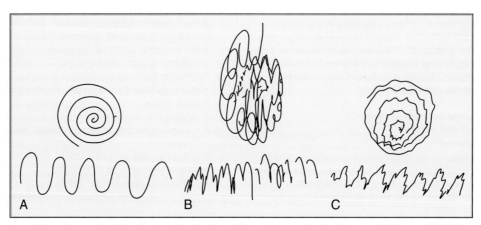

Fig. 23.3 Archimedes spiral and wavy-line drawings by the examiner **(A)** and by a patient with essential tremor **(B, C)**, in whom the tremor is asymmetrical and more evident in the right hand **(B)** than in the left hand **(C)**.

On standing unsupported, patients with orthostatic tremor develop rapid, rhythmic contractions of leg muscles, causing the kneecaps to bob up and down. This dampens or subsides on walking. In contrast, cerebellar disease results in slower titubation of axial structures and the head, seen in the upright position. Often, observing the gait helps differentiate between upper-limb rest tremor and postural tremor that persists at rest as a result of stress. The former usually is clearly evident during walking, whereas the latter usually subsides. Obviously, observing additional features of the gait is helpful in making these distinctions as well.

Certain tremors persist in all positions. Disease in the midbrain involving the superior cerebellar peduncle near the red nucleus (possibly also involving the nigrostriatal fibers) results in the so-called midbrain, or rubral, tremor (*Holmes tremor*). Characteristically, this form of tremor combines features of the three tremor classes. It is often present at rest, increases with postural maintenance, and increases still further, sometimes to extreme degrees, with goal-directed movement. Another form of rest tremor is myorhythmia, defined as repetitive, rhythmic, slow (1–4 Hz) tremor affecting chiefly cranial and limb muscles. It is typically usually associated with lesions involving the brainstem, thalamus, or other diencephalic structures, some with potentially treatable etiologies.

Tremor also may be a feature of psychiatric disease, representing a conversion reaction or even malingering. Usually, certain features are atypical or incongruous. This psychogenic tremor differs from most organic tremors in that the frequency is often quite variable, and concentration and distraction often abate the tremor instead of increasing it (Thenganatt and Jankovic, 2014b).

DYSTONIA

Dystonia is a disorder dominated by sustained muscle contractions, which often cause twisting and repetitive movements or abnormal postures (Albanese et al., 2013). The term *dystonia* is used in three major contexts: (1) to describe the specific form of involuntary movement (i.e., a physical sign), (2) to refer to a syndrome caused by a large number of different disease states, or (3) to refer to the idiopathic form of dystonia, in which these movements usually occur in isolation without additional neurological abnormalities (Box 23.4).

Dystonic movements may be slow and twisting or quite rapid, resembling the shock-like jerks of myoclonus. There may be additional rhythmic movements, especially when the patient actively attempts to resist the involuntary movement. If the patient relaxes, allowing the limb to move as it pleases, the abnormal dystonic posturing usually becomes evident, and the rhythmic dystonic tremor lessens. This position in which dystonic tremor ceases is the *null point*. A faster distal postural tremor similar to essential tremor is a common associated feature. The varied nature of these movements often causes the misdiagnosis of dystonia as some other type of movement disorder.

Another common error in diagnosis is the mislabeling of dystonia as hysteria. Stress and anxiety aggravate the movements, and rest and even hypnosis alleviate the movements. Patients often discover a variety of peculiar maneuvers (sensory tricks) that they can use to lessen or even completely abate the dystonic movements and postures (discussed in this chapter and in Chapter 96). The abnormal movements and postures may occur only during the performance of certain acts and not others that use the same muscles. An example of this action, *task-specific dystonia*, is involvement of the hand only in writing (writer's cramp or graphospasm) or playing a musical instrument, but not with other manual tasks such as using utensils. Dystonia of the oromandibular region only on speaking or

eating is another example of task-specific dystonia, as is dystonia in legs and trunk that occurs only on walking forward but not on walking backward, climbing stairs, or running. On the other hand, some dystonias occur only during running (Wu and Jankovic, 2006). A final source of possible confusion with hysteria is the occurrence of dystonia after injury to the affected limb or after prolonged immobilization such as casting. Such peripherally induced dystonia, which is usually fixed rather than mobile, may be associated with a complex regional pain syndrome (previously referred to as *reflex sympathetic dystrophy*), depression, and personality changes and may occur on a background of secondary gain or litigation and other features of psychogenic dystonia (Thenganatt and Jankovic, 2014c; van Rooijen et al., 2011).

Common Symptoms

Dystonia can affect almost all striated muscle groups. Common symptoms include forced eyelid closure (*blepharospasm*); jaw clenching, forced jaw opening, or involuntary tongue protrusion (oromandibular or lingual dystonia); a harsh, strained, or breathy voice (laryngeal dystonia or spasmodic dysphonia); and involuntary deviation of the neck in any plane or combination of planes (cervical dystonia or spasmodic torticollis) (Albanese et al., 2013). Other symptoms are spasms of the trunk in any direction, which variably interfere with lying, sitting, standing, or walking (axial dystonia); interference with manual tasks (often only specific tasks in isolation: the occupational cramps); and involvement of the leg, usually with inversion and plantar flexion of the foot, causing the patient to walk on the toes. All these disorders may slowly progress to the point of complete loss of voluntary function of the affected part. On the other hand, only certain actions may be impaired, and the disorder may remain focal in distribution. Chapter 96 deals with each of these forms of dystonia in more detail.

The age at onset and distribution of dystonia often are helpful in determining the possible cause. Box 23.4 details the many causes of inherited and acquired dystonias (dystonia due to a known specific cause) (Albanese et al., 2013). Whereas some patients with dystonia have "pure dystonia" without any other neurological deficit (*isolated dystonia*), others have additional clinical features such as parkinsonism, spasticity, weakness, myoclonus, dementia, seizures, and ataxia (*combined dystonia*). Typically, childhood-onset primary dystonia (e.g., classic, Oppenheim, or DYT1 dystonia) begins in distal parts of the body (e.g., graphospasm, foot inversion) and spreads to a generalized dystonia. On the other hand, dystonia beginning in adult life usually is limited to one or a small number of contiguous regions such as the face and neck, remains focal or segmental, and rarely becomes generalized. Generalized involvement or onset in the legs in an adult usually implies the possibility of a secondary cause such as PD or some other parkinsonian disorder. Involvement of one side of the body (*hemidystonia*) is strong evidence of a lesion in the contralateral basal ganglia, particularly the putamen (Wijemanne and Jankovic, 2009). Most primary dystonias start as action dystonia occurring during some activity such as writing and walking or running, but consider peripheral or central trauma and psychogenic dystonia when the dystonia occurs at rest and consists of a fixed posture (Thenganatt and Jankovic, 2014c). A fixed posture maintained during sleep or anesthesia implies superimposed contractures or a musculoskeletal disturbance mimicking the postures of dystonia. Although rest and sleep lessen dystonia in many, some note a striking diurnal variation. The diurnal variation manifests with little or no dystonia on rising in the morning, followed by the progressive development of

---

BOX 23.4 Etiological Classification of Dystonia

I. Inherited or Acquired
  A. Inherited (isolated)
  B. Inherited (combined)
II. Acquired dystonia (dystonia due to a known specific cause)
  Parkinson disease
  Progressive supranuclear palsy
  Multiple system atrophy
  Corticobasal degeneration
  Alternating hemiplegia of childhood
  Biopterin-deficient diseases
  Aromatic amino acid decarboxylase deficiency (dopamine
    agonist-responsive dystonia)
  Pelizaeus–Merzbacher disease
  Lesch–Nyhan syndrome
  Dystonia deafness
  Huntington disease
  Spinocerebellar degenerations
  Dentatorubral-pallidoluysian atrophy
  Hereditary spastic paraplegia with dystonia
  Thalamo-olivary degeneration with encephalopathy
  Wilson disease
  Neurodegeneration with brain iron accumulation
  Hypoprebetalipoproteinemia, acanthocytosis, retinitis
    pigmentosa, and pallidal degeneration
  Ataxia-telangiectasia
  Ataxia oculomotor apraxia
  Neuroacanthocytosis
  Rett syndrome
  Intraneuronal inclusion disease
  Infantile bilateral striatal necrosis
  Familial basal ganglia calcifications
  Hereditary spastic paraplegia with dystonia
  Associated with metabolic disorders:
    1. Amino acid disorders
      Glutaricacidemia
      Methylmalonicacidemia
      Homocystinuria
      Hartnup disease
      Tyrosinemia
      Glucose transporter-1 (GLUT-1) deficiency
    2. Lipid disorders
      Metachromatic leukodystrophy
      Ceroid lipofuscinosis
      Niemann-Pick disease type C (dystonic lipidosis,
        histiocytosis); defect in cholesterol esterification; caused
        by mutation in NPC1 gene 18q11) and HE1 gene
        (14q24.3)
      Gangliosidoses (GM1, GM2 variants)
      Hexosaminidase A and B deficiency
    3. Other metabolic disorders
      Biopterin-deficient diseases
      Triosephosphate isomerase deficiency
      Aromatic amino acid decarboxylase deficiency (dopamine
        agonist-responsive dystonia)
      Biotin-responsive basal ganglia disease
      Leigh disease
      Leber disease

  Perinatal cerebral injury and kernicterus: athetoid cerebral
    palsy, delayed-onset dystonia
  Infection: viral encephalitis, encephalitis lethargica,
    Reye syndrome, subacute sclerosing panencephalitis,
    Creutzfeldt–Jakob disease, human immunodeficiency
    virus
  Other: tuberculosis, syphilis, acute infectious torticollis
  Drugs: L-dopa and dopamine agonists, dopamine receptor-
    blocking drugs, fenfluramine, anticonvulsants, flecainide,
    ergots, certain calcium channel blockers
  Toxins: magnesium, carbon monoxide, carbon disulfide,
    cyanide, methanol, disulfiram, 3-nitroproprionic acid, wasp
    sting
  Metabolic: hypoparathyroidism
  Paraneoplastic brainstem encephalitis
  Vitamin E deficiency
  Primary antiphospholipid syndrome
  Cerebrovascular or ischemic injury, Sjögren syndrome
  Multiple sclerosis
  Central pontine (and extrapontine) myelinolysis
  Brainstem lesions
  Spinal cord lesions
  Syringomyelia
  Brain tumor
  Arteriovenous malformation
  Head trauma and brain surgery (thalamotomy)
  Lumbar stenosis
  Peripheral trauma (with causalgia)
  Electrical injury
III. Other hyperkinetic syndromes associated with dystonia
  A. Tic disorders with dystonic tics
  B. Paroxysmal dyskinesias
    1. Paroxysmal kinesigenic dyskinesia
      (16p11.2–q12.1)
    2. Paroxysmal nonkinesigenic dyskinesia (2q33–35)
    3. Paroxysmal exertion-induced dyskinesia
      (16p12–q12)
    4. Paroxysmal hypnogenic dyskinesia (largely a frontal
      lobe seizure disorder with a gene localized to
      20q13.2–13.3)
IV. Psychogenic
V. Pseudodystonia
  Atlanto-axial subluxation
  Syringomyelia
  Arnold–Chiari malformation
  Trochlear nerve palsy
  Vestibular torticollis
  Posterior fossa mass
  Soft-tissue neck mass
  Congenital postural torticollis
  Congenital Klippel–Feil syndrome
  Isaacs syndrome
  Satoyoshi syndrome
  Stiff person syndrome
  Dupuytren contractures
  Trigger digits
  Ventral hernia

---

problems as the day goes on, sometimes to the point of becoming unable to walk late in the day. This diurnal variability strongly suggests a diagnosis of dopa-responsive dystonia, although this feature is present in only about half of the patients (Wijemanne and Jankovic, 2015). Important clues to the cause of dystonia are (1) the nature of symptom onset

(sudden versus slow) and (2) its course, whether rapid or slow progression or episodes of spontaneous remission.

The family history must be reviewed in detail with the awareness that affected relatives may have limited or distinctly different involvement from that of the patient. The categorization of genetic dystonias according to loci is somewhat arbitrary (Lohmann and Klein, 2013; Moghimi et al., 2014). Obtaining a birth and developmental history is critical in view of the frequency of dystonia after birth trauma, birth anoxia, and kernicterus. As with the other dyskinesias, seek a history of such features as previous encephalitis, drug use, and head trauma. There is also increasing support for the ability of peripheral trauma to precipitate various forms of dystonia, and occasionally this is combined with a complex regional pain syndrome, also called *reflex sympathetic dystrophy* (van Rooijen et al., 2011).

Examination

Action dystonia is commonly the earliest manifestation of primary (idiopathic) dystonia. It is important to observe patients performing the acts that are most affected. Later, other tasks precipitate similar problems, the use of other parts of the body causes the dystonia to become evident in the originally affected site, and the dystonia may overflow to other sites. Still later, dystonia is periodically evident at rest, and even later the posturing may be persistent and difficult to correct passively, especially when secondary joint contractures develop. A significant deviation from this progression, particularly with the early appearance of dystonia at rest, should encourage the physician to search carefully for a secondary cause (see Box 23.4).

It is important to recognize the natural variability of dystonia, especially the effects of stress and anxiety. This is exemplified by blepharospasm, in which stress often increases the eylid closure but increased concentration associated with talking such as occurs during a conversation or a visit to the doctor often reduces the severity of the problem. If only placing reliance on the degree of disability seen in the office, the physician may underestimate the severity of the blepharospasm and may misdiagnose the problem as hysterical.

Depending on the cause of the dystonia, several other neurological abnormalities may be associated. Consider WD in any patient with onset of dystonia before age 60 (Mak and Lam, 2008). Many secondary dystonic disorders (listed in Box 23.4 and discussed in Chapter 96) result in additional psychiatric or cognitive disturbances, seizures, or pyramidal tract or cerebellar dysfunction. Ocular motor abnormalities suggest a diagnosis of Leigh disease, dystonic lipidosis, ataxia-telangiectasia, ataxia-oculomotor apraxia syndrome, HD, Machado–Joseph disease (SCA3), or other spinocerebellar atrophies. Optic nerve or retinal disease raises the possibility of Leigh disease, other mitochondrial cytopathies, GM2 gangliosidosis, ceroid lipofuscinosis, and neurodegeneration with brain iron accumulation (NBIA) (McNeill et al., 2008; Schneider et al., 2013). One of the most common causes of NBIA is pantothenate kinase–associated neurodegeneration, previously called *Hallervorden-Spatz disease* (Schneider et al., 2013). Other causes include neuroferritinopathy, infantile neuroaxonal dystrophy, aceruloplasminemia, and PLA2G6-associated neurodegeneration. Lower motor neuron and peripheral nerve dysfunction occur with neuroacanthocytosis, ataxia-telangiectasia, ataxia-oculomotor apraxia syndrome, metachromatic leukodystrophy, Machado–Joseph disease (SCA3), and other multisystem degenerations. Occasionally, prominent dystonic postures or pseudoathetosis occurs secondary to profound proprioceptive loss due to peripheral nerve, spinal cord, or brain lesions. The dystonia itself may cause additional neurological problems such as spinal cord or cervical root compression from long-standing torticollis, and peripheral nerve entrapment from limb dystonia. Also, independent of the cause, long-standing dystonic muscle spasms often result in hypertrophy of affected muscles (e.g., the sternocleidomastoid muscle in cervical dystonia).

Although the general medical examination must be thorough, the diagnosis is largely based on the history and observed phenomenology of the movement disorder (Morris and Jankovic, 2012). As always, carefully seek the ophthalmological and systemic signs of WD. Abdominal organomegaly also may indicate a storage disease. Minor tongue and lip mutilation is seen in neuroacanthocytosis, in which orolingual action dystonia may be prominent (Walker et al., 2006). Oculocutaneous telangiectasia and evidence of recurrent sinopulmonary infections suggest ataxia-telangiectasia. Musculoskeletal abnormalities may simulate dystonia; rarely, dysmorphic features may serve as a clue to a mucopolysaccharidosis.

CHOREA

The term *chorea* derives from the Greek *choreia*, meaning "a dance." This hyperkinetic movement disorder consists of irregular, unpredictable, brief, jerky movements that flow randomly from one part of the body to another (Jankovic and Roos, 2014). The term *choreoathetosis* describes slow chorea, typically seen in patients with cerebral palsy. Besides these disorders, there are numerous other causes of chorea (Jankovic, 2009), most of which are listed in Box 23.5.

Common Symptoms

Initially, patients, particularly those with HD, often are unaware of the presence of involuntary movements, and the family may simply interpret the chorea as normal fidgetiness (Jankovic and Roos, 2014). The earliest patient complaints usually are those of clumsiness and incoordination, such as dropping or bumping into things. The limbs occasionally strike closely placed objects. In moderate to severe cases, patients may complain of abnormal involuntary jumping or jerking of the limbs and trunk. However, even when movements are overt, many patients deny their presence or only admit to being minimally aware of them. This discrepancy is particularly striking in the case of *tardive dyskinesia*, in which the patient often appears completely unaware of or indifferent to constant and severe movements of the mouth and tongue (Waln and Jankovic, 2013). In contrast to chorea associated with HD, which often predominantly involves the upper face (Jankovic and Roos, 2014), patients with *tardive dyskinesia* have repetitive, coordinated (stereotypic), rather than random movements, of their tongue and mouth. Although the involuntary movements associated with *tardive dyskinesia* may superficially seem choreic, the muscle contractions are more predictable and repetitive, and the movements are more coordinated, often resembling seemingly purposeful motor acts such as chewing. Patients with orofacial chorea or stereotypy often have difficulties keeping their dentures in place and they may grind their teeth (bruxism) or cause biting of the tongue or inner cheek. *Stereotypies* are continuous, repetitive movements, which represent the most common phenomenology of tardive dyskinesia (Edwards et al., 2012). Other causes of stereotypies, besides tardive dyskinesia, include autistic disorders and schizophrenia.

Other features often associated with chorea, particularly HD, include motor impersistence manifested by inability to maintain tongue protrusion (*trombone tongue*) and pendular reflexes, probably caused by motor hypotonia (Jankovic and Roos, 2014). Speech may be slurred, halting, and periodically interrupted, especially in HD, in which speech disturbances are severe and often do not correlate with the severity of chorea. Here, in addition to dysarthria, there is usually a reduction in the spontaneity and quantity of speech output. Problems with feeding result from a combination of limb chorea, which causes sloppiness, and swallowing difficulties,

Developmental and aging choreas
  Physiological chorea of infancy
  Cerebral palsy (anoxic), kernicterus
  Buccal-oral-lingual dyskinesia and edentulous orodyskinesia
  In older adults, senile chorea (probably several causes)
Hereditary choreas
  Huntington disease
  Benign hereditary chorea (TITF1 gene mutations)
  Neuroacanthocytosis
  Other central nervous system degenerations:
    olivopontocerebellar atrophy, Machado–Joseph disease and
    other spinocerebellar atrophies, ataxia-telangiectasia, ataxia
    oculomotor apraxia types 1 and 2, tuberous sclerosis of
    basal ganglia, pantothenate kinase-associated
    neurodegeneration, neurodegeneration with brain iron
    accumulation (Hallervorden–Spatz disease),
    neuroferritinopathy, "Huntington disease-like" disorders (e.g.,
    PRNP, junctophilin or JPH3 mutations, SCA2, SCA17)
  Neurometabolic disorders: Wilson disease, Lesch-Nyhan
    syndrome, lysosomal storage disorders, amino acid
    disorders, Leigh disease, porphyria
Drugs: neuroleptics (tardive dyskinesia), antiparkinsonian drugs,
  amphetamines, cocaine, tricyclic antidepressants, oral
  contraceptives
Toxins: alcohol intoxication and withdrawal, anoxia, carbon
  monoxide, manganese, mercury, thallium, toluene
Metabolic
  Hyperthyroidism
  Hypoparathyroidism (various types)
  Pregnancy (chorea gravidarum)
  Hypernatremia and hyponatremia, hypomagnesemia,
    hypocalcemia
  Hypoglycemia and hyperglycemia (the latter may cause
    hemichorea, hemiballism)
  Acquired hepatocerebral degeneration
  Nutritional (e.g., beriberi, pellagra, vitamin B12 deficiency in
    infants)
Infectious and postinfectious
  Sydenham chorea
  Encephalitis lethargica
  Various other infectious and postinfectious encephalitis,
    Creutzfeldt–Jakob disease
Immunological
  Systemic lupus erythematosus
  Henoch–Schönlein purpura
  Others (rarely): sarcoidosis, multiple sclerosis, Behçet disease,
    polyarteritis nodosa
Vascular (often hemichorea)
  Infarction or hemorrhage
  Arteriovenous malformation, moyamoya disease
  Polycythemia rubra vera
  Migraine
  Following cardiac surgery with hypothermia and extracorporeal
    circulation in children
Tumors
Trauma, including subdural and epidural hematoma
Miscellaneous, including paroxysmal choreoathetosis

which can result in choking and aspiration. Eating is particularly difficult for patients with *neuroacanthocytosis* (previously termed *chorea-acanthocytosis*), in which severe orolingual dystonia (eating dystonia) can cause the tongue to push the food out of the mouth almost as quickly as the patient puts it in. Patients with this dystonia often place food at the back of the tongue and throw the head back to initiate swallowing. This lingual movement may resemble the orolingual stereotypy typically observed in patients with tardive dyskinesia or tardive dystonia. One form of choreic movement in patients with neuroacanthocytosis is continuous truncal bending and extending movements, giving the appearance of a "rubber man," most apparent while the patient is standing or walking. Disturbances of stance and gait can be an early complaint in patients with chorea. The patient may note a tendency to sway and jerk while standing and an unsteady, uneven gait often likened to a drunken stagger. Later still, added postural instability in HD results in falls. Respiratory dyskinesias may cause the patient to feel short of breath or unable to obtain enough air (Mehanna and Jankovic, 2010). Patients with involvement of the pelvic region may complain bitterly of thrusting and rocking movements in the lower trunk and pelvis. Respiratory and pelvic involvements are sources of complaint more often in tardive dyskinesia than in other choreic movement disorders.

Other Clues in the History

It is obvious from a review of Box 23.5 that it is impractical to discuss additional historical clues for every cause of chorea. We therefore limit discussion here to a few practical and important points.

Age at onset and manner of progression vary depending on the cause. A helpful distinction made here is between benign hereditary chorea, associated with *NKX2-1* (formerly called *TITF1*) gene (14q13.1–q21.1) mutation, and HD (Patel and Jankovic, 2014). In the former, chorea typically begins in childhood with a slow progression and little cognitive change, whereas HD presenting in childhood is more often of the akinetic-rigid variety, with severe mental changes and rapid progression.

In most cases, the onset of chorea is slow and insidious. An abrupt or subacute onset is more typical of many of the symptomatic causes of chorea, such as Sydenham chorea, hyperthyroidism, cerebral infarcts, and neuroleptic drug withdrawal (withdrawal emergent syndrome) (Mejia and Jankovic, 2010), systemic lupus erythematosus (SLE), and other autoimmune choreas (Baizabal-Carvallo and Jankovic, 2012; Baizabal-Carvallo et al., 2013a). A pattern of remissions and exacerbations suggests the possibility of drugs, SLE, and rheumatic fever, whereas brief (minutes to hours) bouts of involuntary movement indicate a paroxysmal dyskinesia (Waln and Jankovic, 2015).

A recent history of streptococcal throat infection and musculoskeletal or cardiovascular problems in a child suggests a diagnosis of rheumatic (Sydenham) chorea. Rheumatic chorea tends to occur every 5 to 10 years in a community when a new population of children becomes susceptible to *Streptococcus* infection. One may obtain a previous history of rheumatic fever, particularly in women who develop chorea during pregnancy or while taking birth control pills. Chorea gravidarum may be more common in women with prior history of rheumatic chorea. The individual contractions in Sydenham disease are slightly longer (>100 msec) than those in HD (50 to 100 msec), and there are often associated features such as dysarthria, oculogyric deviations, "milkmaid's grip," obsessive-compulsive behavior, and other features, including the prior history of streptococcal infection, that support the diagnosis of Sydenham disease.

In women, chorea during pregnancy or a history of previous fetal loss suggests the possibility of SLE with anticardiolipin antibodies, even in the absence of other features of collagen vascular disease. Symptoms isolated to one side of the body suggest a structural lesion in the contralateral basal ganglia. However, many patients who complain of unilateral involvement have abnormalities of both sides on examination.

A careful family history is crucial. The most common cause of inherited chorea is HD, which has fully penetrant autosomal dominant transmission (Frank and Jankovic, 2010; Jankovic and Roos, 2014). The family history can be misleading, however, because the clinical features of the disease in other family members may have been mainly behavioral, and psychiatric disturbances and the chorea hardly noticed.

Examination

The range of choreiform movements is quite broad, including eyebrow lifting or depression, lid winking, lip pouting or pursing, cheek puffing, lateral or forward jaw movements, tongue rolling or protruding, head jerking in any plane (a common pattern is a sudden backward jerk followed by a rotatory sweep forward), shoulder shrugging, trunk jerking or arching, pelvic rocking, and flitting movements of the fingers, wrists, toes, and ankles. Patients incorporate choreic jerks into voluntary movements, perhaps in part to mask the presence of the dyskinesia (so-called parakinesis).

Chorea often alters the performance of various tasks such as finger-to-nose testing and rapid alternating movements, causing a jerky, interrupted performance. Standing and walking often aggravate the chorea. Particularly in HD, the gait is irregular and lurching and has bizarre characteristics, not simply explained by increased chorea. The gait usually is wide-based despite the absence of typical ataxia. Patients may deviate from side to side in a zigzag fashion with lateral swaying and additional spontaneous flexion. In addition, the stride may be irregularly longer or shorter and the speed slowed, with some features similar to those of a parkinsonian gait, such as loss of arm swing, festination, propulsion, and retropulsion. One or both arms may be flexed at the elbow as if holding a purse over the forearm.

Respiratory irregularities are common, especially in tardive dyskinesia, but are also present in other movement disorders (Mehanna and Jankovic, 2010). Periodic grunting, respiratory gulps, humming, and sniffing may be present in this and other choreic disorders, including HD. Other movement disorders often combine with chorea. Dystonic features probably are the most common and are seen in many conditions. Less common but well recognized are parkinsonism (e.g., with juvenile HD, neuroacanthocytosis, and WD), tics (e.g., in neuroacanthocytosis), myoclonus (e.g., in juvenile HD), tremor (e.g., in WD and HD), and ataxia (e.g., in juvenile HD and some spinocerebellar ataxias). Tone usually is normal to low. Muscle bulk is typically preserved, although weight loss and generalized wasting are common in HD. When distal weakness and amyotrophy are present, one must consider accompanying anterior horn cell or peripheral nerve disease, as in neuroacanthocytosis, ataxia-telangiectasia, Machado–Joseph disease, and spinocerebellar ataxias (see Chapter 97). Reduced tendon reflexes occur. On the other hand, chorea often results in hung-up and pendular reflexes, probably caused by the occurrence of a choreic jerk after the usual reflex muscle contraction.

Depending on the cause (see Box 23.5), several other neurological disturbances may be associated with chorea. In HD, for example, cognitive changes, motor impersistence (e.g., difficulty maintaining eyelid closure, tongue protrusion, constant handgrip), apraxias (especially orolingual), and oculomotor dysfunction are all quite common (see Chapter 96). *Milkmaid's grip*, appreciated as an alternating squeeze and release when the patient is asked to maintain a constant, firm grip of the examiner's fingers, probably is caused by a combination of chorea and motor impersistence.

TABLE 23.3 Neuroleptic-Induced Movement Disorders

Acute, transient	Chronic, persistent
Dystonic reaction	Tardive stereotypy
Parkinsonism	Tardive chorea
Akathisia	Tardive dystonia
Neuroleptic malignant syndrome	Tardive akathisia Tardive tics Tardive myoclonus Tardive tremor Persistent parkinsonism Tardive sensory syndrome

Modified from Jankovic, J., 1995. Tardive syndromes and other drug-induced movement disorders. Clin Neuropharmacol 18, 197–214.

TARDIVE DYSKINESIA

In contrast to the random and unpredictable flowing nature of chorea, tardive dyskinesia usually demonstrates repetitive stereotypical movements, which are most pronounced in the orolingual region (Mejia and Jankovic, 2010; Waln and Jankovic, 2013). These include chewing and smacking of the mouth and lips, rolling of the tongue in the mouth or pushing against the inside of the cheek (*bon-bon sign*), and periodic protrusion or flycatcher movements of the tongue. The speed and amplitude of these movements can increase markedly when the patient is concentrating on performing rapid alternating movements in the hands. Patients often have a striking degree of voluntary control over the movements and may be able to suppress them for a prolonged period when asked to do so. On distraction, however, the movements return immediately. Despite severe facial movements, voluntary protrusion of the tongue is rarely limited, and this act often dampens or completely inhibits the ongoing facial movements. This contrasts with the pronounced impersistence of tongue protrusion seen in HD, which is far out of proportion to the degree of choreic involvement of the tongue. In addition to stereotypies, many other movement disorders are associated with the use of dopamine receptor blockers (Table 23.3).

Besides the impersistence typically seen in HD, several other clinical factors help distinguish between HD and tardive dyskinesia. Involuntary movements in tardive dyskinesia typically localize to the lower face, whereas in HD, irregular contractions of the frontalis muscles and associated elevation of the eyebrows is common (Jankovic and Roos, 2014). Despite the rocking movements of the pelvis, tapping of the feet, and shifting of the weight from side to side while standing (some of which may be caused by akathisia), the gait often is normal in patients with tardive dyskinesia, although a bizarre ducklike gait can be seen. This contrasts with the strikingly abnormal, irregular, dance-like, gait in many choreic disorders, especially in HD.

Tardive dyskinesia caused by neuroleptic drugs such as the antipsychotics and other dopamine receptor blockers, particularly metoclopramide, is not the only cause of orobucco-linguo-masticatory stereotypic movements (Mejia and Jankovic, 2010; Waln and Jankovic, 2013). Other drugs, particularly dopamine agonists in PD, anticholinergics, and antihistamines, cause a similar form of dyskinesia. Multiple infarctions in the basal ganglia and possibly lesions in the cerebellar vermis result in similar movements. Older adults, especially the edentulous, often have a form of stereotypic orofacial movement, usually with minimal lingual involvement. Here, as in tardive dyskinesia, inserting dentures in the mouth may dampen the movements, and placing a finger to the lips can also suppress them. Another important diagnostic consideration and source of clinical confusion is idiopathic oromandibular dystonia. Orofacial and limb stereotypies, often preceded by psychiatric symptoms, may also be seen in women with ovarian teratomas, less frequently in males with testicular tumors, and in children as part of anti-N-methyl-D-aspartate receptor (NMDAR) encephalitis (Baizabal-Carvallo and Jankovic, 2012; Baizabal-Carvallo et al., 2013b).

BALLISM

Ballism, or ballismus, is the least common of the well-defined dyskinesias (Jankovic, 2009). The name derives from the Greek word for "to throw," and the movements of ballism are high in amplitude, violent, and flinging or flailing in nature. As in chorea, they are rapid and nonpatterned. The prominent involvement of more proximal muscles of the limbs usually accounts for the throwing or flinging nature. Lower-amplitude distal movements also may be seen, and occasionally there is even intermittent prolonged dystonic posturing. Some authors emphasize the greater proximal involvement and the persistent or ceaseless nature of ballism in contrast to chorea. However, it is more likely that ballism and chorea represent a continuum rather than distinct entities. The coexistence of distal choreic movements, the discontinuous nature in less-severe cases, and the common evolution of ballism to typical chorea during the natural course of the disorder or with treatment all support this theory. Ballism usually confines to one side of the body, called *hemiballismus*. Occasionally, only one limb is involved (*monoballism*); rarely, both sides are affected (*biballism*) or both legs (*paraballism*). Box 23.6 lists the various causes of hemiballism.

The flinging movements of ballism often are extremely disabling to patients, who drop things from their hands or damage closely placed objects. Self-injury is common, and examination often reveals multiple bruises and abrasions. Additional signs and symptoms depend on the cause, location, and extent of the lesion, which is usually in the contralateral subthalamic nucleus or striatum (see Chapter 96).

TICS

Tics are the most varied of all movement disorders. Patients with Tourette syndrome, the most common cause of tics, manifest motor or phonic tics and a wide variety of associated symptoms (Jankovic and Kurlan, 2011). Tics are brief and intermittent movements (*motor tics*) or sounds (*phonic tics*). Motor tics typically consist of sudden, abrupt, transitory, often repetitive, and coordinated (stereotypical) movements that may resemble gestures and mimic fragments of normal behavior, vary in intensity, and are repeated at irregular intervals. The movements are most often brief and jerky (clonic); however, slower, more prolonged movements (tonic or dystonic tics) also occur. Several other characteristic features are helpful in distinguishing this movement disorder from other dyskinesias. Patients usually experience an inner urge or local premonitory sensations before making the movement, which is temporarily relieved by its performance. Tics are voluntarily suppressible for variable periods, but this occurs at the expense of mounting inner tension and the need to allow the tic to occur. Indeed, a large proportion of people with tics, when questioned carefully, admit that they intentionally produce the movements or sounds that comprise their tics (in contrast to most other dyskinesias) in response to the uncontrollable inner urge or a premonitory sensation. Box 23.7 provides examples of the various types of tics. Motor and phonic tics are divisible further as simple or complex. Simple motor tics are random, brief, irregular muscle twitches of isolated body segments, particularly the eyelids and other facial muscles, the neck, and the shoulders. In contrast, complex motor tics are coordinated, patterned movements involving a number of muscles in their normal synergistic relationships. A wide variety of other behavioral disturbances may be associated with tic disorders, and it is sometimes difficult to separate complex tics from some of these comorbid disorders. These comorbid disturbances include attention deficit with or without hyperactivity, obsessive-compulsive behavior, impulsive behavior, and externally directed and self-destructive behavior, including self-mutilation (Jankovic and Kurlan, 2011). In some cases, the self-injurious behavior can be quite serious and even life threatening ("malignant Tourette"). Some Tourette syndrome patients also manifest sudden and transitory cessation of all motor activity (*blocking tics*), including speech, without alteration of consciousness. These blocking tics are caused by either prolonged tonic or dystonic tics that interrupt ongoing motor activity such as speech (*intrusions*), or by a sudden inhibition of ongoing motor activity (*negative tic*).

BOX 23.6 Causes of Ballism

Infarction or ischemia, including transient ischemic attacks; usually lacunar disease, hypertension, diabetes, atherosclerosis, vasculitis, polycythemia, thrombocytosis, other causes
Hemorrhage
Tumor
 Metastatic
 Primary
Other focal lesions (e.g., abscess, arteriovenous malformation, tuberculoma, toxoplasmosis, multiple sclerosis plaque, encephalitis, subdural hematoma)
Hyperglycemia (nonketotic hyperosmolar state)
Drugs (phenytoin, dopamine agonists in Parkinson disease)

BOX 23.7 Phenomenological Classification of Tics

SIMPLE MOTOR TICS

Eye blinking; eyebrow raising; nose flaring; grimacing; mouth opening; tongue protrusion; platysma contractions; head jerking; shoulder shrugging, abduction, or rotation; neck stretching; arm jerks; fist clenching; abdominal tensing; pelvic thrusting; buttock or sphincter tightening; hip flexion or abduction; kicking; knee and foot extension; toe curling

SIMPLE PHONIC TICS

Sniffing, grunting, throat clearing, shrieking, yelping, barking, growling, squealing, snorting, coughing, clicking, hissing, humming, moaning

COMPLEX MOTOR TICS

Head shaking, teeth gnashing, hand shaking, finger cracking, touching, hitting, jumping, skipping, stamping, squatting, kicking, smelling hands or objects, rubbing, finger twiddling, echopraxia, copropraxia, spitting, exaggerated startle

COMPLEX PHONIC TICS

Coprolalia (wide variety, including shortened words), unintelligible words, whistling, panting, belching, hiccupping, stuttering, stammering, echolalia, palilalia (also mental coprolalia and palilalia)

Simple and complex phonic tics comprise a wide variety of sounds, noises, or formed words (see Box 23.7). The term *vocal tic* usually applies to these noises. However, because many of these sounds do not use the vocal cords, we prefer the term *phonic tic*. Although the presence of phonic tics is required for the diagnosis of definite Tourette syndrome, this criteria is artificial because phonic tics are essentially motor tics that result in abnormal sounds. Possibly the best-known (although not the most common) example of complex phonic tic is *coprolalia*, the utterance of obscenities or profanities. These are often slurred or shortened or may intrude into the patient's thoughts but not become verbalized (mental coprolalia) (Freeman et al., 2009). In addition, patients with Tourette syndrome often exhibit copropraxia (obscene gestures) and echopraxia (mimicked gestures).

Like most dyskinesias, tics usually increase with stress. In contrast to other dyskinesias, however, relaxation (e.g., watching television at home) often results in an increase in the tics, probably because the patient does not feel the need to suppress them voluntarily. Distraction or concentration usually diminishes tics, which also differs from most other types of dyskinesia. Many patients with idiopathic tics note spontaneous waxing and waning in their nature and severity over weeks to months, and periods of complete remission are possible. Many people with tics are only mildly affected, and many are even unaware that they demonstrate clinical features. This must be kept in mind when reviewing the family history and planning treatment. Finally, tics are one of the few movement disorders that can persist during all stages of sleep, although they usually subside in sleep.

There is no diagnostic test for Tourette syndrome; the diagnosis is based on clinical criteria according to the DSM-V (American Psychiatric Association, 2013) which appears in Box 23.8.

Common Symptoms

Box 23.9 lists causes of tic disorders. Most are primary or idiopathic, and within this group, the onset almost always occurs in childhood or adolescence (Tourette syndrome). The male-to-female ratio in patients with Tourette syndrome is approximately 3 : 1. Idiopathic tics occur on a spectrum from a mild, transitory, single, simple motor tic to chronic, multiple, simple, and complex motor and phonic tics.

Patients and their families complain of a wide variety of symptoms (see Box 23.7). They may have seen numerous other specialists (e.g., allergists for repetitive sniffing, otolaryngologists for throat clearing, ophthalmologists for excessive eye blinking or eye rolling, and psychologists and psychiatrists for various neurobehavioral abnormalities). Often, someone close to the patient or a teacher suggests the diagnosis of Tourette syndrome to the family after learning about it in the media. Children may verbalize few complaints or feel reluctant to speak of the problem, especially if they have been subject to ridicule by others. Even young children, when questioned carefully, can provide the history of urge to perform the movement that gradually culminates in the release of a tic and the ability to control the tic voluntarily at the expense of mounting inner tension. Children may be able to control the tics for prolonged periods but often complain of difficulty concentrating on other tasks while doing so. Some give a history of requesting to leave the schoolroom and then releasing the tics in private (e.g., in the washroom). Peers and siblings often chastise or ridicule the patient, and parents or teachers, not recognizing the nature of the disorder, may scold or punish the child for what are thought to be voluntary bad habits (indeed, an older term for tics is *habit spasms*).

The history may include an exposure to stimulants for hyperactivity. Review the family history for the wide range of associated symptoms such as obsessive-compulsive behavior and attention deficit disorder. Additional neurological complaints, including other dyskinesias, suggest the possibility of a secondary cause of the tics. Although tics may sometimes appear as highly unusual and bizarre movements and sounds, tics are rarely of psychogenic origin (Baizabal-Carvallo and Jankovic, 2014).

BOX 23.8 DSM-5 Diagnostic Criteria: Tourettes Disorder (307.23 (F95.2))

1. Both multiple motor and one or more vocal tics have been present at some time during the illness, although not necessarily concurrently.
2. The tics may wax and wane in frequency but have persisted for more than 1 year since first tic onset.
3. Onset is before age 18 years.
4. The disturbance is not attributable to the physiological effects of a substance (e.g., cocaine) or another medical condition (e.g., Huntington's disease, postviral encephalitis).

Reprinted with permission from the Diagnostic and Statistical Manual of Mental Disorders, Fifth Edition, (© 2013). American Psychiatric Association.

BOX 23.9 Etiological Classification of Tics

I. Physiological tics
   A. Mannerisms
II. Pathological tics
   A. Primary
      Sporadic:
      1. Transient motor or phonic tics (<1 year)
      2. Chronic motor or phonic tics (>1 year)
      3. Adult-onset (recurrent) tics
      4. Tourette syndrome
      Inherited:
      1. Tourette syndrome
      2. Huntington disease
      3. Primary dystonia
      4. Neuroacanthocytosis
   B. Secondary ("tourettism")
      1. Infections: encephalitis, Creutzfeldt–Jakob disease, Sydenham chorea
      2. Drugs: stimulants, L-dopa, carbamazepine, phenytoin, phenobarbital, antipsychotics
      3. Toxins: carbon monoxide
      4. Developmental: static encephalopathy, mental thoughts but retardation, chromosomal abnormalities
      5. Other: head trauma, stroke, neurocutaneous syndromes, chromosomal abnormalities, schizophrenia, neuroacanthocytosis, degenerative disorders
III. Related disorders
   A. Stereotypies
   B. Self-injurious behaviors
   C. Hyperactivity syndrome
   D. Compulsions
   E. Excessive startle
   F. Jumping disease, latah, myriachit

Modified from Jankovic, J., 2001. Tourette's syndrome. N Engl J Med 345, 1184–1192.

Examination

In most patients with tics, the neurological examination is entirely normal. In patients with primary tic disorders, the presence of other neurological, cognitive, behavioral, and neuropsychological disturbances may simply relate to extension of the underlying cerebral dysfunction beyond the core that accounts for pure tic phenomena. Patients with secondary forms of tics (e.g., neuroacanthocytosis, tardive tics) may demonstrate other involuntary movements such as chorea, dystonia, and other neurological deficits (see Box 23.7). Careful interview stressing the subjective features that precede or accompany tics usually allows the distinction between true dystonia or myoclonus, and dystonic or clonic tics.

Despite bitter complaints by the family, it is common for patients to show little or no evidence of a movement disorder during an office appointment. Aware of this, the physician must attempt to observe the patient at a time when he or she is less likely to be exerting voluntary control, such as in the waiting room. If no movements have been witnessed during the interview, the physician should seemingly direct attention elsewhere (e.g., to the parents) while observing the patient out of the corner of the eye. The patient often releases the tics while changing in the examining room, particularly after suppressing tics during the interview. The physician should attempt to view the patient at this time or at least listen for the occurrence of phonic tics. If all else fails, ask the patient voluntarily to mimic the movements. This, in combination with associated symptoms such as urge, voluntary release, control, and the often varied and complex nature of the movements, usually is enough to provide the diagnosis, even if the physician never witnesses spontaneous tics in the office. Finally, ask the parents to provide home videos of the patient. Although tics usually start in childhood, some adults may present with tics and other features of Tourette syndrome. In most of these adults with tics one can find evidence of childhood onset of tics which spontaneously remitted after adolescence and recurred later during adulthood (Jankovic and Kurlan, 2011).

MYOCLONUS

Myoclonus is a sudden, brief, shock-like involuntary movement possibly caused by active muscle contraction (*positive myoclonus*) or inhibition of ongoing muscle activity (*negative myoclonus*). The differential diagnosis of myoclonus is broader than that of any other movement disorder (Box 23.10). To exclude muscle twitches, such as fasciculations caused by lower motor neuron lesions, some authors have insisted that an origin in the CNS be a component of the definition. Although the majority of cases of myoclonus originate in the CNS, occasional cases of brief shock-like movements clinically indistinguishable from CNS myoclonus occur with spinal cord or peripheral nerve or root disorders.

The clinical patterns of myoclonus vary widely. The frequency varies from single, rare jerks to constant, repetitive contractions. The amplitude may range from a small contraction that cannot move a joint to a very large jerk that moves the entire body. The distribution ranges from focal involvement of one body part, to segmental (involving two or more contiguous regions), to multifocal, to generalized. When the jerks occur bilaterally, they may be symmetrical or asymmetrical. When they occur in more than one region, they may be synchronous in two body parts (within milliseconds) or asynchronous. Myoclonus usually is arrhythmic and irregular, but in some patients it is very regular (rhythmic), and in others there may be jerky oscillations that last for a few seconds and then fade away (oscillatory). Myoclonic jerks may occur spontaneously without a clear precipitant or in response to a wide variety of stimuli, including sudden noise, light, visual threat, pinprick, touch, and muscle stretch. Attempted movement (or even the intention to move) may initiate the muscle jerks (action or intention myoclonus). *Palatal myoclonus* is a form of segmental myoclonus manifested by rhythmic contractions of the soft palate. The rhythmicity has led to the alternative designation of *palatal tremor*. Symptomatic palatal myoclonus/tremor, usually manifested by contractions of the levator palatini, may persist during sleep; this form of palatal myoclonus usually is associated with some brainstem disorder. In contrast, essential palatal myoclonus/tremor consists of rhythmic contractions of the tensor palatini, often associated with a clicking sound in the ear, and disappears with sleep. Symptomatic but not essential palatal myoclonus often is associated with hypertrophy of the inferior olive. Another term proposed for essential palatal tremor is *isolated palatal tremor*, with several different subtypes or causes possible, including tics, psychogenic (probably accounting for a large proportion of these cases), and volitional (Dijk and Tijssen, 2010; Zadikoff et al., 2006).

Common Symptoms

As may be seen from the foregoing description and the long list of possible causes of myoclonus, the symptoms in these patients are quite varied. For simplification, we briefly review the possible symptoms with respect to four major etiological subcategories in Box 23.10.

Physiological forms of myoclonus occurring in normal subjects vary depending on the precipitant. Probably the most common form is the jerking most of us have experienced on falling asleep (*hypnagogic myoclonus*, or *jactitation*). This very familiar phenomenon is rarely a source of concern. Occasionally, anxiety- or exercise-induced myoclonus causes concern. The history usually is clear, and there is little to find (including abnormal movements) when the patient is seen.

In the *essential myoclonus* group, patients usually complain of isolated muscle jerking in the absence of other neurological deficits (with the possible exception of tremor and dystonia). The movements may begin at any time from early childhood to late adult life and may remain static or progress slowly over many years. The family history may be positive, and some patients note a striking beneficial effect of alcohol (Mostile and Jankovic, 2010). Associated dystonia, present in some patients, also may respond to ethanol. Essential myoclonus and myoclonus dystonia are probably the same disorder.

Myoclonus occurring as one component of a wide range of seizure types is *epileptic myoclonus*. Many of these patients give a clear history of seizures as the dominant feature. Myoclonic jerks may be infrequent and barely noticeable to the patient or may occur frequently and cause pronounced disability. Myoclonus on waking in the morning or an increasing frequency of the myoclonic jerks may forewarn of a seizure soon to come. The clinical pattern of myoclonus in this instance also varies widely. Sensitivity to photic stimuli and other sensory input may be prominent. Occasional patients demonstrate isolated myoclonic jerks in the absence of additional seizure activity. In these cases, the family history may be positive for seizures, and the electroencephalogram (EEG) often demonstrates a typical centrencephalic seizure pattern that is otherwise asymptomatic (such as a 3-Hz spike-and-wave pattern). In others, myoclonus and seizures are equally prominent (the myoclonic epilepsies). These may or may not be associated with an apparent progressive encephalopathy (most often with cognitive dysfunction and ataxia) in the absence of a definable, underlying, symptomatic cause.

TABLE 23.5 Investigation of Movement Disorders

Movement disorder investigation	A	C	B	D	T	M
Routine hematology (including sedimentation rate)	+	+	+	+	–	+
Routine biochemistry (including Ca2+, uric acid, liver function tests)	+	+	+	+	+	+
Serum copper, ceruloplasmin (with or without 24-hour urine Cu, liver biopsy, radiolabeled Cu studies)	++	++	–	++	+	+
Slit-lamp examination	++	++	–	++	+	+
Thyroid function	+	++	–	+	–	+
Antistreptolysin O test, anti-DNase B, antihyaluronidase	–	+	–	+	+	–
Antinuclear factor, LE cells, other immunological studies, anticardiolipin antibodies, venereal disease research laboratories test	+	++	+	+	–	+
Blood acanthocytes	+	+	–	+	+	+
Lysosomal enzymes	+	+	–	+	+	+
Urine organic and amino acids	+	+	–	+	–	+
Urine oligosaccharides and mucopolysaccharides	+	+	–	+	–	+
Serum lactate and pyruvate	+	+	–	+	–	+
DNA tests for gene mutations	+	+	–	+	–	+
Bone marrow for storage cells (including electron microscopy)	+	+	–	+	–	+
Electron microscopy of leukocytes; biopsy of liver, skin, and conjunctiva	+	+	–	+	–	+
Nerve or muscle biopsy	+	+	–	+	–	+
Oligoclonal bands	+	+	+	+	–	+
Computed tomography or magnetic resonance imaging	++	++	++	++	+	++
Electroencephalography	+	+	–	+	+	++
Electromyography and nerve conduction studies	+	+	–	+	+	+
Evoked potentials	+	+	–	+	–	++
Electroretinogram	+	+	–	+	–	+
Neuropsychological testing	+	+	–	–	+	–

Note: The extent of investigation depends on factors such as age of onset, nature of progression, and presence of historical or clinical atypical features suggesting a secondary cause of the movement disorder in question.

++, Very important or often useful; +, sometimes helpful; +, questionably helpful; – rarely or never helpful. A, Akinetic rigid syndrome; B, hemiballism; C, chorea; D, dystonia; M, myoclonus; T, tics.

TABLE 23.6A Etiological Classification of Dystonia-Inherited (Isolated)

Classification	Chromosome gene mutation gene product	Pattern of inheritance	Onset	Distribution, additional features	Origin/comment
DYT1	9q34, GAG deletion, TOR1A/TorsinA	AD	C	Distal limbs, generalized	Penetrance: 30% AJ, 70% NJ
DYT2	NM	AR			Spanish gypsies, Iranian Jews
DYT6	8q21-22 THAP1	AD	A, C	Cervical, cranial, brachial	German-American Mennonite-Amish
DYT7	18p	AD	A	Cervical, cranial, spasmodic dysphonia, hand tremor	German
DYT13	1p36.13-32	AD	A, C	Cranial-cervical and upper limb	Italian
DYT17	20p11.22-q13.12	AR	C	Cervical dystonia, dysphonia, segmental, generalized	Lebanese
DYT21	2q14.3-q21.3	AD	A	Late onset	Sweden
DYT23	9q34.11, CIZ1	AD	A	Cervical	Caucasians
DYT24	3, ANO3	AD	A	Cranial-cervical-laryngeal, tremor, myoclonus	European
DYT25	18p, GNAL	AD	A	Cervical>cranial>arm	European

TABLE 23.6B Etiological Classification of Dystonia-Inherited (Combined)

Classification	Chromosome gene mutation gene product	Pattern of inheritance	Onset	Distribution, additional features	Origin/comment
DYT3	Xq *TAF1*	XR	A	Parkinsonism	Filipinos (Lubag) mosaic striatal gliosis
DYT4	19p13.3-p13.2 *TUBB4 (β-tubulin 4a)*	AD	C,A	Whispering dysphonia, cranial, cervical, limb, gait disorder, facial atrophy, ptosis, edentulous	Australian
DYT5a	14q22.1 *GCH1*/GTP cyclohydrolase I	AD	C	Gait disorder, parkinsonism, myoclonus, spasticity	Dopa-responsive dystonia, diurnal fluctuation
DYT5b	11p15.5 tyrosine hydroxylase	AR	C	Gait disorder, parkinsonism, myoclonus, spasticity	Dopa-responsive dystonia, diurnal fluctuation
DYT 8/20	10q22 *KCNMA1* α-subunit of a Ca-sensitive K channel	AD	C	Paroxysmal nonkinesigenic dyskinesia, epilepsy	European origin
DYT 9/18	1p35-p31 *SLC2A1* glucose transporter type 1 (GLUT1)	AD	C (infancy)	Paroxysmal exercise induced dyskinesia (dystonia or chorea) with or without epilepsy and hemiplegic migraine	Delayed development, microcephaly, ataxia, hypoglychorrhachia
DYT 10/19	16p11.2-q12.1 *PRRT2* proline-rich transmembrane protein 2	AD	C	Paroxysmal kinesigenic dyskinesia, epilepsy	migraines, episodic ataxia

the putamen). The cause of hemiballism or hemichorea is usually a structural lesion in the contralateral subthalamic nucleus or striatum. The cause is commonly a small lacunar infarction, so MRI typically is more successful than CT in localizing the lesion. A pattern of high signal in the striatum (especially the putamen) on T1 imaging is characteristic of hemiballism due to hyperosmolar nonketotic hyperglycemia. In patients with parkinsonism, imaging must assess the possibility of hydrocephalus (either obstructive or communicating), midbrain atrophy (as in PSP), and cerebellar and brainstem atrophy (as in olivopontocerebellar atrophy). MRI clearly is much more effective in demonstrating these posterior fossa abnormalities than is CT. Atrophy of the head of the caudate nucleus occurs in HD, but it is not specific for this disorder and does not correlate with the presence or severity of chorea. Multiple infarctions, intracerebral calcification (better seen on CT), mass lesions (e.g., tumors, arteriovenous malformations), and basal ganglia lucencies (as seen in various disorders) may be found in patients with several movement disorders such as parkinsonism, chorea, and dystonia. In patients with striatonigral degeneration (one subcategory of MSA with prominent parkinsonism), T2-weighted and proton-density MRI scans often demonstrate a combination of striatal atrophy and hypointensity, with linear hyperintensity in the posterolateral putamen. T2-weighted gradient echo MRI often demonstrates hypointense putaminal changes (Brooks et al., 2009). The "hot cross bun" sign in the pons and hyperintensity in the middle cerebellar peduncles on fluid-attenuated inversion recovery (FLAIR) imaging also suggest MSA-C. The latter feature as well as additional supratentorial white-matter changes and atrophy also occur in the fragile X tremor ataxia syndrome (FXTAS). Sagittal-view MRI in patients with PSP can show atrophy of the rostral midbrain tegmentum; the most rostral midbrain, the midbrain tegmentum, the pontine base, and the cerebellum appear to correspond to the bill, head, body, and wing, respectively, to form a "hummingbird" or "penguin" sign (although this is a rather

late imaging feature). Further developments in MRI promise to improve our ability to differentiate between various degenerative disorders, especially if they are associated with characteristic pathological features. Examples are deposition of pigments or heavy metals. T1-weighted hyperintensity in the basal ganglia occurs in hyperglycemia, manganese toxicity, hepatocerebral disease, WD, abnormal calcium metabolism, neurofibromatosis, hypoxia, and hemorrhage. Striatal T1-weighted hypointensity and T2-weighted hyperintensity suggest mitochondrial disorders. Striatal T2-weighted hypointensity, with hyperintensity of the mesencephalon sparing the red nucleus and the lateral aspect of the substantia nigra, gives the appearance of "face of the giant panda" sign, the typical MRI appearance of WD. T2-weighted MRI in PKAN typically shows hypointensity in the globus pallidus surrounding an area of hyperintensity, the "eye of the tiger" sign (McNeill et al., 2008; Schneider et al., 2013).

Magnetic resonance spectroscopy also holds promise for differentiating disorders with various neurodegenerative patterns or neurometabolic disturbances. Positron emission tomography (PET) using fluorodeoxyglucose, fluorodopa, and other radiolabeled compounds (e.g., demonstrating labeling of dopamine receptors) has shown reproducible changes in such conditions as HD and parkinsonian disorders. For example, F-dopa PET scans show reduced uptake in both the putamen and caudate in patients with atypical parkinsonism (e.g., PSP, MSA), whereas the caudate usually is preserved in patients with PD. The patterns of abnormalities seen may predict the underlying pathological changes and thus may be useful in differential diagnosis. Developments in single-photon emission computed tomography (SPECT) suggest that this will probably become a useful diagnostic tool in evaluating and diagnosing certain movement disorders. For example, SPECT study of the dopamine transporter (DAT) helps differentiate PD (and other parkinsonian disorders with degeneration of the substantia nigra) from other tremor disorders such as essential tremor. Finally, recent studies suggest that

TABLE 24.2 Summary of Clinical Features Differentiating Parkinson Disease from Symptomatic Parkinsonism in Patients with an Akinetic-Rigid Gait Syndrome

Feature	Parkinson disease	Symptomatic parkinsonism
Posture	Stooped (trunk flexion)	Stooped or upright (trunk flexion/ extension)
Stance	Narrow	Often wide-based
Initiation of walking	Start hesitation	Start hesitation, magnetic feet
Steps	Small, shuffling	Small, shuffling
Stride length	Short	Short
Freezing	Common	Common
Leg movement	Stiff, rigid	Stiff, rigid
Speed	Slow	Slow
Festination	Common	Rare
Arm swing	Minimal or absent	Reduced or excessive
Heel-to-toe walking	Normal	Poor (truncal ataxia)
Postural reflexes	Preserved in early stages	Absent at early stage
Falls	Late (forward, tripping)	Early and severe (backward, tripping, or without apparent reason)

most common of which are multiple system atrophy, corticobasal degeneration, and progressive supranuclear palsy (Jankovic, 2015). A number of clinical signs help distinguish among these conditions (Table 24.2). In progressive supranuclear palsy, the typical neck posture is one of extension, with axial and nuchal rigidity rather than neck and trunk flexion as in PD. A stooped posture with exaggerated neck flexion is sometimes a feature of multiple system atrophy. A distinguishing feature of progressive supranuclear palsy and multiple system atrophy is the early appearance of falls due to loss of postural and righting responses, in comparison to the preservation of these reactions in PD until later stages of the illness. There also may be an element of ataxia in these akinetic-rigid syndromes that is not evident in PD. The disturbance of postural control in progressive supranuclear palsy is coupled with impulsivity due to frontal executive dysfunction leading to reckless lurching movements during postural changes when sitting or arising, and toppling falls. Falls occur in 80% of patients with progressive supranuclear palsy and can be dramatic, leading to injury. Accordingly, the patient who presents with falls and an akinetic-rigid syndrome is more likely to have one of these conditions rather than PD. Finally, the dramatic response to levodopa that is typical of PD does not occur in these other akinetic rigid syndromes, although some cases of multiple system atrophy respond partially for a short period.

In addition to the hypokinetic disorders discussed previously, diseases of the frontal lobe including tumors (glioma or meningioma), anterior cerebral artery infarction, obstructive or communicating hydrocephalus (especially normal-pressure hydrocephalus), and diffuse small vessel cerebrovascular disease (multiple lacunar infarcts and Binswanger disease) also produce disturbance of gait and balance. These pathologies interrupt connections among the frontal lobes, other cortical areas, and subcortical structures especially the striatum. The clinical appearance of the gait in frontal lobe lesions varies from a predominantly wide-based unsteady ataxic gait to an akinetic-rigid gait with slow, short steps and a tendency to shuffle. It is common for a patient to present with a combination of these features. In the early stages, the stance base is wide, with an upright posture of the trunk and shuffling when starting to walk or turning corners. There may be episodes of freezing. Arm swing is normal or even exaggerated, giving the appearance of a "military two-step" gait. The normal fluidity of trunk and limb motion is lost. In contrast, voluntary upper limb and hand movements are normal and there is a lively facial expression. This "lower half parkinsonism" is commonly seen in diffuse small vessel cerebrovascular disease. The marche à petits pas of Dejerine and Critchley's atherosclerotic parkinsonism refers to a similar clinical picture. Patients with this clinical syndrome commonly are misdiagnosed as having PD. The normal motor function of the upper limbs, retained arm swing during walking, upright truncal posture, wide-based stance, upper motor neuron signs including pseudobulbar palsy, and the absence of a resting tremor distinguish this syndrome from PD. In addition, the lower half parkinsonism of diffuse cerebrovascular disease generally does not respond to levodopa treatment (see Box 24.4). Walking speed in subcortical arteriosclerotic encephalopathy is slower than in cerebellar gait ataxia or PD (Ebersbach et al., 1999). Slowness of movement and the lack of heel-to-shin ataxia distinguish the wide-based stance of this syndrome from that of cerebellar gait ataxia (see Table 24.1).

As the underlying condition progresses, the unsteadiness and slowness of movement become more pronounced. There may be great difficulty initiating a step (start hesitation, "slipping clutch") as if the feet were glued to the floor ("magnetic feet"). Attempts to take a step require assistance and the patient seeks support from nearby objects or persons. There may be excessive upper body movement as the patient tries to free the feet to initiate walking. Once walking is underway, steps may be better, but small, shuffling, ineffective steps (freezing) re-emerge when attempting to turn. Such patients rarely exhibit the festination of PD, but a few steps of propulsion or retropulsion may be taken. Postural and righting reactions are impaired and eventually lost. Falls are common and follow the slightest perturbation. In contrast, these patients are often able to make stepping, walking, or bicycling leg movements with the legs when seated or lying supine but cannot step or walk when standing. This discrepancy may reflect poor control of truncal motion and dysequilibrium when standing, making stepping impossible without falling (Thompson, 2007). The inability to stand from sitting or lying and difficulty turning over in bed are other signs of impaired truncal movement in the higher level gait disorder of frontal lobe disease. Frontal signs such as paratonic rigidity (gegenhalten) of the arms and legs, grasp reflexes in the fingers and toes, and brisk tendon reflexes with extensor plantar responses are common. Urinary incontinence and dementia frequently occur. Brain imaging with MRI reveals the majority of conditions causing this syndrome, such as diffuse cerebrovascular disease, cortical atrophy, or hydrocephalus.

Some patients display fragments of this clinical picture. Those with the syndrome of gait ignition or gait initiation failure exhibit profound start hesitation and freezing, but step size and rhythm are normal once walking is underway. Sensory cues may facilitate stepping. Balance while standing or walking is normal. These findings are similar to those seen with walking in PD, but speech and upper limb function are normal, and there is no response to levodopa. Brain imaging results are normal. This syndrome has also been described as "pure akinesia" and "primary progressive freezing of gait."

Some cases develop stuttering speech and hypokinetic handwriting. The slowly progressive evolution of symptoms suggests a degenerative condition. Follow-up studies indicate this may be one expression of progressive supranuclear palsy (Riley et al., 1994) or other neurodegenerations (Factor et al., 2006). Occasionally, isolated episodic festination with truncal flexion is encountered. Others complain of a loss of the normal fluency of stepping when walking and a conscious effort is required to maintain a normal stepping rhythm and step size. These symptoms may be associated with subtle dysequilibrium, manifesting as a few brief staggering steps to one side or a few steps of retropulsion after standing up, turning quickly, or making other rapid changes in body position. Finally, some elderly patients experience severe walking difficulties that resemble those described in frontal lobe disease. The history in these syndromes is one of gradual onset, without stroke-like episodes or identifiable structural or vascular lesions of the frontal lobes or cerebral white matter on imaging. The criteria for normal pressure hydrocephalus are not fulfilled, there are no signs of parkinsonism, and levodopa is ineffective. There is no evidence of more generalized cerebral dysfunction, as occurs in Alzheimer disease. Indeed, it is rare for patients with Alzheimer disease to develop difficulty walking until the later stages of the disease. The cause of these syndromes is unknown although it is increasingly recognized that subcortical white-matter pathology may exist without apparent MRI lesions (Jokinen et al., 2013).

ELDERLY GAIT PATTERNS, CAUTIOUS GAITS, AND FEAR OF FALLING

Healthy, neurologically normal elderly people tend to walk at slower speeds than their younger counterparts. The slower speed of walking is related to shorter and shallower steps with reduced excursion at lower limb joints. In addition, stance width may be slightly wider than normal, and synergistic associated arm and trunk movements are less vigorous. The rhythmicity of stepping is preserved. These changes give the normal elderly gait a cautious or guarded appearance. Factors contributing to a general decline in mobility of the elderly include degenerative joint disease, reducing range of limb movement, and decreased cardiovascular fitness, limiting exercise capacity. These changes in the elderly gait pattern provide a more secure base to compensate for a subtle age-related deterioration in balance.

In unselected elderly populations, a more pronounced deterioration in gait and postural control may be seen. Walking speed is slower, steps are shorter, stride length is reduced, stance phase of walking is increased, and variability in stride time is increased. These changes are most marked in those who fall.

Elderly patients with an insecure gait characterized by slow short steps, en bloc turns, and falls often have signs of multiple neurological deficits, such as (1) mild proximal weakness of neuromuscular origin, (2) subtle sensory loss (mild distal light touch and proprioceptive loss, blunted vestibular or visual function), (3) mild spastic paraparesis due to cervical myelopathy, and (4) impaired truncal control as discussed earlier without any one lesion being severe enough to explain the walking difficulty. The cumulative effect of these multiple deficits may account for perceived instability and dysequilibrium. Musculoskeletal disorders, postural hypotension, and loss of confidence (especially after falls) are further factors contributing to a cautious gait pattern. In this situation, brain imaging is valuable to look for frontal and periventricular white-matter ischemic lesions that correlate with imbalance, increased body sway, falls, and cognitive decline (Baezner et al., 2008).

Falls lead to a marked loss of confidence when walking and a cautious or protected gait. A cautious gait is a normal response to the perception of impaired or threatened balance and a fear of falling. Such patients adopt a crouched posture and take short shallow steps. They may be unable to walk without support, holding onto furniture, leaning on walls, and avoiding crowded or open spaces because of a fear of falling. The gait improves dramatically when support is provided. Accordingly, a cautious gait should be interpreted as compensatory and not specific for any level of the gait classification. A formal program of gait retraining may help restore confidence and improve the ability to walk.

PERCEPTIONS OF INSTABILITY AND ILLUSIONS OF MOVEMENT

A number of syndromes have been described in which middle-aged individuals complain of unsteadiness and imbalance associated with "dizziness," sensations or illusions of semi-continuous body motion, sudden brief body displacements, or body tilt. These sensation symptoms develop in open spaces where there are no visible supports (space phobia) or in particular situations such as on bridges, stairs, and escalators or in crowded rooms. Such symptoms are associated with the development of phobic avoidance behavior and the syndrome of phobic postural vertigo (Brandt, 1996). Prolonged illusory swaying and unsteadiness after sea or air travel is referred to as the mal de débarquement syndrome. Past episodes of a vestibulopathy may suggest a subtle semicircular canal or otolith disturbance, but a disorder of vestibular function is rarely confirmed in these syndromes. Fear of falling and anxiety are common accompaniments. These symptoms must be distinguished from the physiological "vertigo" and unsteadiness accompanying visual-vestibular mismatch or conflict when observing moving objects, focusing on distant objects in a large panorama, or looking upward at a moving object.

RECKLESS GAIT PATTERNS

Reckless gaits are seen in patients with impaired postural responses and poor truncal control who do not recognize their instability and take risks that result in falls and injuries. Such patients make inappropriate movements of the feet and trunk when sitting or standing without due caution or monitoring of body posture. The most striking examples occur in frontal dementias such as progressive supranuclear palsy and frontotemporal dementias in which impulsivity and a failure to adapt to the precarious balance are part of the cognitive decline.

HYSTERICAL AND PSYCHOGENIC GAIT DISORDERS

A gait disorder is one of the commoner manifestations of a psychogenic, functional or hysterical movement disorder. The typical gait patterns encountered include:

1. transient fluctuations in posture while walking,
2. knee buckling without falls,
3. excessive slowness and hesitancy,
4. a crouched, stooped or other abnormal posture of the trunk,
5. complex postural adjustments with each step,
6. exaggerated body sway or excessive body motion especially brought out by tandem walking, and
7. trembling, weak legs (Hayes et al., 1999).

The more acrobatic hysterical disorders of gait indicate the extent to which the nervous system is functioning normally and capable of high-level coordinated motor skills and postural control to perform complex maneuvers. Suggestibility, variability, improvement with distraction, and a history of sudden onset or a rapid, dramatic, and complete recovery are common features of psychogenic gait (and movement) disorders in general. A classical discrepancy is illustrated by the Hoover sign in the patient with an apparently paralyzed leg when examined supine. As the patient lifts the normal leg, the examiner places a hand under the "paralyzed" leg and feels the presence (and strength) of synergistic hip extension. The general neurological exam often reveals a variety of other signs suggestive of psychogenic origin such as "give way weakness" and nonphysiological sensory disturbances. One must be cautious in accepting a diagnosis of hysteria, however, because a bizarre gait may be a presenting feature of primary torsion dystonia, and unusual truncal and leg postures may be encountered in truncal and leg tremors. Finally, higher level gait disorders often have a disconnect between the standard neurological exam and the gait pattern.

MUSCULOSKELETAL DISORDERS AND ANTALGIC GAIT
Skeletal Deformity and Joint Disease

Degenerative osteoarthritis of the hip may produce leg shortening in addition to mechanical limitation of leg movement at the hip, giving rise to a waddling gait or a limp. Leg shortening with limping in childhood may be the presenting feature of hemiatrophy due to a cerebral or spinal lesion or spinal dysraphism. Examination of the legs may reveal lower motor neuron signs, sensory loss with trophic ulcers of the feet, and occasionally, upper motor neuron signs such as a brisk knee reflex. Lumbosacral vertebral abnormalities (spina bifida), bony foot deformities, and a cutaneous hairy patch over the lumbosacral region are clues to the diagnosis. In adult life, spinal dysraphism (diastematomyelia with a tethered cord) may first become symptomatic after a back injury, with the development of walking difficulties, leg and lower back pain, neurogenic bladder disturbances, and sensory loss in a leg. Imaging of the spinal canal reveals the abnormality.

Painful (Antalgic) Gaits

Most people at one time or another experience a limp caused by a painful or an injured leg. Limps and gait difficulties due to joint disease, bone injury, or soft-tissue injury are not usually accompanied by muscle weakness, reflex change, or sensory loss. Limitation of the range of joint movement at the hip, knee, or ankle to reduce pain leads to short steps with a fixed leg posture. Hip disease causes a variety of gait adjustments; it is important to examine the range of hip movements (while supine) and any associated pain during passive movements of the hip in a patient with a gait disorder. Pain due to intermittent claudication of the cauda equina is most commonly caused by lumbar spondylosis and, rarely, by a spinal tumor. Diagnosis is confirmed by spinal imaging. It may be difficult to distinguish this syndrome from calf muscle claudication secondary to peripheral vascular disease. Examination after exercise may resolve the issue by revealing a depressed ankle jerk or radicular sensory loss, with preservation of arterial pulses in the leg. Other painful conditions affecting the spine, lower limbs, and soft tissue, such as plantar fasciitis, can affect gait.

REFERENCES

The complete reference list is available online at https://expertconsult .inkling.com/.

25 Hemiplegia and Monoplegia

Karl E. Misulis, E. Lee Murray

CHAPTER OUTLINE

ANATOMY AND PHYSIOLOGY
   Motor System Anatomy
   Localization of Motor Deficits
HEMIPLEGIA
   Cerebral Lesions
   Brainstem Lesions
   Spinal Lesions
   Peripheral Lesions
   Psychogenic Hemiplegia
MONOPLEGIA
   Cerebral Lesions
   Brainstem Lesions
   Spinal Lesions
   Peripheral Lesions
PITFALLS IN THE DIFFERENTIAL DIAGNOSIS OF HEMIPLEGIA AND MONOPLEGIA

Hemiplegia and monoplegia are more likely to be due to discrete focal lesions than diffuse lesions, so these presentations are especially suited to clinical-anatomic localization. Similarly, imaging studies are likely to be revealing with hemiplegia or monoplegia but the focus of imaging must be directed by clinical suspicion.

Hemiplegia and monoplegia are motor symptoms and signs, but associated sensory abnormalities are essential to localization, so these are discussed when appropriate. Sensory deficit syndromes are discussed in more depth in Chapter 30. Motor power begins with volition, the conscious effort to initiate movement. Lack of volition does not produce weakness but rather results in akinesia. Projections from the premotor regions of the frontal lobes to the motor strip result in activation of corticospinal tract (CST) neurons, which then have a descending pathway which is detailed later.

Localization begins with identification of weakness. Differentiation is made among the following distributions:

- Generalized weakness
- Monoplegia
- Hemiplegia
- Paraplegia.

Only hemiplegia and monoplegia are discussed in this chapter.

ANATOMY AND PHYSIOLOGY
Motor System Anatomy

Anatomic localization begins with a good understanding of anatomy and physiology. Focal deficits such as hemiplegia and monoplegia are more likely to be due to a focal structural lesion than diffuse disorders so anatomy is of prime importance.

The neuroanatomical locus of motor initiative is unknown and likely diffuse but motor planning likely begins in the premotor cortex. Integrating sensory information into the planning stage, neurons of the premotor cortex project widely to targets including motor cortex, prefrontal cortex, parietal cortex, supplementary motor cortex area, basal ganglia, thalamus, and spinal cord. Output from the primary motor cortex descends through the internal capsule to the brainstem and spinal cord as the pyramidal tract.

Pyramidal Tract

Pyramidal tract axons become the corticobulbar and corticospinal tracts. Most of the descending axons cross in the brainstem to activate contralateral cranial nerve nuclei or descend into the spinal cord in the lateral corticospinal tract. These neurons generally supply limb muscles. A minority of the motor axons descend in the spinal cord uncrossed in the anterior corticospinal tract where some of these axons cross before they supply contralateral motoneurons. Some of descending neurons which are uncrossed supply ipsilateral axial muscles.

The premotor cortex is divided into divisions which have cytoarchitectural foundations and some functional implications, but real topographic organization develops in the primary motor cortex where mapping of the body areas served by regions of the cortex produces a distorted representation of the body—the homunculus (Fig. 25.1).

Descending corticospinal pathways through the internal capsule are topographically organized though not as precisely as in the motor cortex. Within the internal capsule, the corticospinal tracts are generally in the posterior limb, with the face and arm axons anteriorly and the leg axons posteriorly.

As the corticospinal axons descend through the spinal cord, the presence of crossed and uncrossed axons makes for complex effects of lesions on motor function. In addition, whereas there is some topographic organization to the corticospinal tracts, this is not as clinically relevant as that of the motor cortex or even internal capsule (Morecraft et al., 2002).

Basal Ganglia

The basal ganglia likely modulate motor activity rather than directly activate it. They seem to play a role in control of initiation of movement by the pre-motor and motor cortical regions. In addition to the role of the basal ganglia in motor function, they are implicated in other functions, including memory.

Afferents to the basal ganglia are from the cerebral cortex and thalamus to the striatum. Efferents from the striatum are largely to the globus pallidus and substantia nigra. The globus pallidus projects in turn to the thalamus.

Cerebellum

The cerebellum monitors and modulates motor activities, responding to motor commands and inputs from sensory receptors from joints, muscles, and vestibular system. The cerebellum is somewhat topographically organized with gait and axial musculature represented at and near the midline and limb motor activity served laterally in the cerebellar hemispheres.

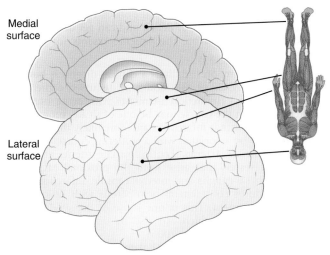

Fig. 25.1 Representation of the body on the motor cortex. Face and arms are represented laterally, and legs are represented medially, with cortical representation of the distal legs bordering on the central sulcus.

TABLE 25.1 Cerebral Lesions

Lesion location	Symptoms	Signs
Motor cortex	Weakness and poor control of the affected extremity, which may involve face, arm, and leg to different degrees	Incoordination and weakness that depends on the location of the lesion within the cortical homunculus; often associated with neglect, apraxia, aphasia, or other signs of cortical dysfunction
Internal capsule	Weakness that usually affects the face, arm, and leg almost equally	Often associated with sensory impairment in same distribution
Basal ganglia	Weakness and incoordination on the contralateral side	Weakness, often without sensory loss; no neglect or aphasia
Thalamus	Sensory loss	Sensory loss with little or no weakness

Localization of Motor Deficits

Lesions of the cerebral cortex produce weakness depending on location and size. Lesions of the motor cortex will affect primarily the muscles represented by that area, as visualized by the homunculus. If the lesion is small and localized to the motor cortex then the deficit can be purely or solely motor. If the lesion is larger and involves sensory afferents then a sensory deficit is expected.

Lesions of the internal capsule can potentially involve just motor axons but because of proximity of adjacent structures, some sensory involvement is more common. Lesions producing limited motor involvement of one limb are not common from internal capsule lesions.

Lesions of the descending corticospinal tracts in the brainstem produce hemiplegia typically with other brainstem signs, such as crossed sensory symptoms, cranial nerve deficits, or ataxia not explained by weakness.

Lesions of the corticospinal tract in the spinal cord usually produce upper motoneuron deficits below the level of the lesions but also often produce lower motoneuron deficits at the level of the lesion. Lesions so restricted in the cord as to produce hemiparesis or the Brown–Sequard syndrome are rare.

Lesions and disorders of the basal ganglia commonly produce contralateral motor dysfunction, although more likely manifest as difficulty with motor control than hemiplegia or monoplegia. Disorders with focal motor symptoms from basal ganglia dysfunction include Parkinson disease, dystonia, hemiballismus, and Huntington disease.

Lesions of the cerebellum do not produce hemiplegia or monoplegia but rather ipsilateral limb ataxia if a lateral lesion, and gait ataxia if a midline lesion.

HEMIPLEGIA
Cerebral Lesions

Cerebral lesions constitute the most common cause of hemiplegia. Lesions in either cortical or subcortical structures may be responsible for the weakness (Table 25.1).

Cortical Lesions

Cortical lesions produce weakness that is more focal than the weakness seen with subcortical lesions. Figure 25.1 is a diagrammatic representation of the surface of the brain, showing how the body is mapped onto the surface of the motor-sensory cortex: the homunculus. The face and arm are laterally represented on the hemisphere, whereas the leg is draped over the top of the hemisphere and into the interhemispheric fissure.

Small lesions of the cortex can produce prominent focal weakness of one area, such as the leg or the face and hand, but hemiplegia—paralysis of both the leg and arm on the same side of the body—is not expected from a cortical lesion unless the damage is extensive. The most likely cause of cortical hemiplegia would be a stroke involving the entire territory of the internal carotid artery.

Infarction. Both cortical and subcortical infarctions can produce weakness, but cortical infarctions are more likely than subcortical infarctions to be associated with sensory deficits. Also, many cortical infarctions are associated with cortical signs—neglect with nondominant hemisphere lesions and aphasia with dominant hemisphere lesions. Unfortunately, this distinction is not absolute because subcortical lesions also occasionally can produce these signs.

Initial diagnosis of infarction usually is made on clinical grounds. The abrupt onset of the deficit is typical. Weakness that progresses over several days is unlikely to be caused by infarction, although some infarcts can show worsening for a few days after onset. Progression over days suggests demyelinating disease or infection. Progression over weeks suggests a mass lesion such as tumor. Progression over seconds to minutes in a marching fashion suggests either epilepsy or migraine; not all migraine-associated deficits are associated with concurrent or subsequent headache.

Computed tomography (CT) scans often do not show infarction for up to 3 days after the event but are performed emergently to rule out mass lesion or hemorrhage. Small infarctions may never be seen on CT. Magnetic resonance imaging (MRI) is superior in showing both old and new infarctions; diffusion-weighted imaging (DWI) in conjunction with *apparent diffusion coefficient* (ADC) on MRI distinguishes recent infarction from old lesions.

Middle Cerebral Artery. The middle cerebral artery (MCA) supplies the lateral aspect of the motor sensory cortex, which controls the face and arm. On the dominant side, speech centers also are supplied—the Broca area (expression) in the posterior frontal region and the Wernicke area (reception) on the superior aspect of the temporal lobe.

Cortical infarction in the territory of the MCA produces contralateral hemiparesis, usually associated with other signs of cortical dysfunction such as aphasia with left hemisphere lesions or neglect with right hemisphere lesions. Weakness is much more prominent in the arm, hand, and face than in the leg. Hemianopia sometimes is seen, especially with large MCA infarctions, as a result of infarction of the optic radiations. MCA infarction is suspected with hemiparesis plus cortical signs of aphasia or neglect. Confirmation is with imaging.

Anterior Cerebral Artery. The anterior cerebral artery (ACA) supplies the inferior frontal and parasagittal regions of the frontal and anterior parietal lobes. This region is responsible for leg movement and is important for bowel and bladder control. Infarction in the ACA distribution produces contralateral leg weakness. The arm may be slightly affected, especially the proximal arm, with sparing of hand and face. In some patients, both ACAs arise from the same trunk, so infarction produces bilateral leg weakness; this deficit can be mistaken clinically for myelopathy and is in the differential diagnosis for suspected cord infarction or other acute myelopathy.

ACA infarction is suggested by a clinical presentation of unilateral or bilateral leg weakness and CST signs. Confirmation is with MRI.

Posterior Cerebral Artery. The posterior cerebral arteries (PCAs) are the terminal branches of the basilar artery. They supply most of the occipital lobes and the medial aspect of the temporal lobes. PCA infarction is not expected to produce weakness but produces contralateral hemianopia, often with memory deficits due to bilateral hippocampal infarction.

The clinical diagnosis of PCA infarction may be missed because an examiner may not look for hemianopia in a patient who otherwise presents only with confusion. Visual complaints may be vague or nonexistent.

PCA infarction is suggested by a clinical presentation of acute confusion or visual disturbance, or both. A finding of hemianopia is supportive evidence. Imaging can show not only the area of infarction but also the location of the vascular defect—unilateral or bilateral PCA or basilar artery.

Mass Lesion. While infarction presents with deficits with localization dependent on vascular anatomy, mass lesions are not so constrained. Lesions may affect motor and sensory systems with complex symptomatology. The etiology of these non-vascular cortical lesions is usually trauma, tumor, or infection. Diagnosis of acute trauma is typically easy but identification of the remote effects of trauma may be difficult, especially when limited history is available.

Hemiplegia from mass lesion can be produced by large lesion of the cerebral hemisphere, at which point nonmotor symptoms would be evident, including cortical signs, sensory abnormalities, and/or visual field abnormalities. Subcortical mass lesions are seldom as restricted to internal capsule/basal ganglia as infarction.

Subcortical Lesions

Subcortical lesions are more likely to produce equal weakness of the contralateral face, arm, and leg than cortical lesions because of the convergence of the descending axons in the internal capsule. The internal capsule is a particularly common location for lacunar infarctions and also can be affected by hemorrhage in the adjacent basal ganglia or thalamus. Weakness of sudden onset is most likely to be the result of infarction, with hemorrhage in a minority of cases. Demyelinating

disease is characterized by a subacute onset. Tumors are associated with a slower onset of deficit and can get quite large in subcortical regions before the patient presents for medical attention.

Infarction. Infarction usually is a clinical diagnosis but can be confirmed by CT or MRI scans, as discussed earlier (see Cortical Lesions). Infarction manifests with acute onset of deficit, although the course may be one of steady progression or stuttering. Lacunar infarctions are more likely than cortical infarctions to be associated with a stuttering course.

Lenticulostriate Arteries. Lenticulostriate arteries are small penetrating vessels that arise from the proximal MCA and supply the basal ganglia and internal capsule. Infarction commonly produces contralateral hemiparesis with little or no sensory involvement. This is one cause of the syndrome of pure motor stroke, which can also be due to a brainstem lacunar infarction (Lastilla, 2006).

Thalamoperforate Arteries. Thalamoperforate arteries are small penetrating vessels that arise from the PCAs and supply mainly the thalamus. Infarction in this distribution produces contralateral sensory disturbance but also can cause movement disorders such as choreoathetosis or hemiballismus; hemiparesis is not expected.

Demyelinating Disease. Demyelinating disease comprises a group of conditions whose pathophysiology implicates the immune system.

Multiple Sclerosis. Multiple sclerosis (MS) manifests with any combination of white-matter dysfunction. Hemiparesis can develop, especially if large plaques affect the CST fibers in the hemispheres. Hemiparesis is even more likely with brainstem or spinal demyelinating lesions, because small lesions can produce more profound deficits in these areas. The diagnosis is suggested by the progression over days plus a prior history of episodes of relapsing and remitting neurological deficits. Episodes of weakness that last for only minutes are likely not to be due to demyelinating disease but rather to transient ischemic attack (TIA) or migraine equivalent.

Diagnosis is based on clinical grounds for most patients, but the finding of areas of increased signal intensity on MRI T2-weighted images is suggestive for MS. Active demyelinating lesions often show enhancement on gadolinium-enhanced T1-weighted images. Cerebrospinal fluid (CSF) examination usually is performed and can give normal findings or show elevated protein, a mild lymphocytic pleocytosis, or oligoclonal bands of immunoglobulin G (IgG) in the CSF.

Acute Disseminated Encephalomyelitis. Acute disseminated encephalomyelitis (ADEM) is a demyelinating illness that is monophasic but in other respects manifests like a first attack of MS (Wingerchuk, 2006). This entity sometimes is called *parainfectious encephalomyelitis,* although the association with infection is not always certain. Symptoms and signs at all levels of the central nervous system (CNS) are common, including hemiparesis, paraplegia, ataxia, and brainstem signs. Diagnosis is based on clinical grounds, because MRI cannot definitively distinguish between MS and ADEM. CSF examination may show a mononuclear pleocytosis and elevation in protein, but these findings are neither always present nor specific. Even the presence or absence of oligoclonal IgG in the CSF cannot differentiate between ADEM and MS. Patients who present clinically with ADEM should be warned of the possibility of having recurrent events indicative of MS.

Progressive Multifocal Leukoencephalopathy. Progressive multifocal leukoencephalopathy (PML) is a demyelinating disease caused by reactivation of the JC virus, usually seen in immunodeficient patients. Predisposed patients include those with acquired immunodeficiency syndrome (AIDS), leukemia, lymphoma, tuberculosis, and sarcoidosis. Patients receiving immunosuppressive therapies, such as natalizumab, rituximab, cyclophosphamide, or cyclosporine for various autoimmune diseases, are also at risk. Visual loss is the most common presenting symptom and weakness the second. MRI scan shows multiple white-matter lesions. CSF examination either reveals no abnormality or shows a lymphocytic pleocytosis or elevated protein, or both. Brain biopsy is required for specific diagnosis, although JC virus deoxyribonucleic acid (DNA) can be detected in the CSF by polymerase chain reaction (PCR) assay in most patients. PML is suggested when a patient with immunodeficiency presents with subacute to chronic onset of neurological deficits and multifocal white-matter lesions on MRI.

Although there are no proven treatments, general principles can be applied, namely improving immunological status by treatment of underlying disease and the removal of immunosuppressive therapies. Caution should be taken when reinstating the immune system as it can lead to IRIS (immune reconstitution inflammatory syndrome), which can lead to worsening neurological status. IRIS can be managed with a short course of high dose IV corticosteroids. Natalizumab-induced PML can be managed by plasma exchange.

Migraine. Migraine can be divided into many subdivisions, including the following:

- Common migraine
- Classic migraine
- Basilar migraine
- Complicated migraine
- Hemiplegic migraine
- Migraine equivalent.

All but common migraine can cause hemiplegia (Black, 2006). *Common migraine* is episodic headache without aura; by definition, there should be no deficit. *Classic migraine* is episodic headache with aura, most commonly visual. *Basilar migraine* is episodic headache with brainstem signs including vertigo and ataxia; this variant is a disorder mainly of childhood. *Complicated migraine* is that in which the aura lasts for hours or days beyond the duration of the headache. *Hemiplegic migraine*, as its name suggests, is characterized by paralysis of one side of the body, typically with onset before the headache; this variant often is familial. *Migraine equivalent* is characterized by the presence of episodic neurological symptoms without headache.

Migrainous infarction features sustained deficit plus MRI evidence of infarction that had developed from the migraine. Definitive diagnosis is problematic because patients with migraine have a higher incidence of stroke not associated with a migraine attack.

The diagnosis of migraine is suggested by the combination of young age of the patient with few risk factors, and a marching deficit that can be conceptualized as migration of spreading electrical depression across the cerebral cortex. Imaging often is necessary to rule out hemorrhage, infarction, and demyelinating disease.

Seizures. Postictal contralateral hemiplegia or hemiparesis can occur in patients with a unilateral hemispheric seizure disorder. This situation is identified by history and slowing on the electroencephalogram (EEG) contralateral to the side of weakness.

Tumors. Tumors affecting the cerebral hemispheres commonly present with progressive deficits including hemiparesis. Coordination deficit usually develops before the weakness. Cortical dysfunction is commonly present, such as aphasia with dominant hemisphere lesions and neglect. Other signs of expanding tumors may include headache, seizures, confusion, and visual field defects.

Tumor should be suspected in a patient with progressive motor deficit over weeks, especially with coexistent seizures or headache. MRI with contrast enhancement is more sensitive than CT for identification of tumors.

Infections. Infections can present as hemiplegia, usually with a subacute onset. Bacterial abscess of the brain can present with subacute progression of hemiparesis. This can occur in isolation, from dental or other source, or in the bed of an infarction, such as in a patient with bacterial endocarditis (Mori et al., 2003; Okubo et al., 1998). With acute onset of weakness and then progressive worsening, embolic infarction and then abscess in the region of the infarction has to be considered.

Viral infections such as encephalitis can present with hemiplegia but usually are associated with other symptoms. Hemiparesis from HSV encephalitis would be expected to be associated with fever, mental status changes, headache, and/or seizures (Ahmed et al., 2013).

Alternating Hemiplegia of Childhood. Alternating hemiplegia of childhood is a rare condition characterized by attacks of unilateral weakness, often with signs of other motor deficits (e.g., dyskinesias, stiffness) and oculomotor abnormalities (e.g., nystagmus) (Zhang et al., 2003). Attacks begin in young childhood, usually before age 18 months; they last hours, and deficits accumulate over years. Initially, patients are normal, but with time, persistent neurological deficits become obvious. A benign form can occur on awakening in patients who are otherwise normal and do not develop progressive deficits; this entity is related to migraine. Diagnostic studies are often performed, including MRI, electroencephalography, and angiography, but these usually show no abnormalities. Alternating hemiplegia is suggested when a young child presents with episodes of hemiparesis, especially on awakening, not associated with headache.

Hemiconvulsion–Hemiplegia–Epilepsy Syndrome. In young children with the rare condition called hemiconvulsion–hemiplegia–epilepsy syndrome, unilateral weakness develops after the sudden onset of focal seizures. The seizures are often incompletely controlled. Neurological deficits are not confined to the motor system and may include cognitive, language, and visual deficits. Unlike alternating hemiplegia, the seizures and motor deficits are consistently unilateral, although eventually the unilateral seizures may become generalized. Imaging findings may be normal initially, but eventually atrophy of the affected hemisphere is seen (Freeman et al., 2002). CSF analysis is not specific, but a mild mononuclear pleocytosis may develop because of the CNS damage and seizures. Rasmussen encephalitis is a cause of this syndrome.

Brainstem Lesions

Brainstem lesions producing hemiplegia are among the easiest to localize because associated signs of cranial nerve and brainstem dysfunction are almost always present.

Brainstem Motor Organization

Figure 25.2 shows the anatomical organization of the motor systems of the brainstem. Motor pathways descend through the CST to the pyramidal decussation in the medulla, where they cross to innervate the contralateral body. Lesions of the pons and midbrain above this level produce contralateral hemiparesis, which may involve the contralateral face. Rostral lesions of the medulla produce contralateral weakness, whereas more caudal medullary lesions produce ipsilateral cranial

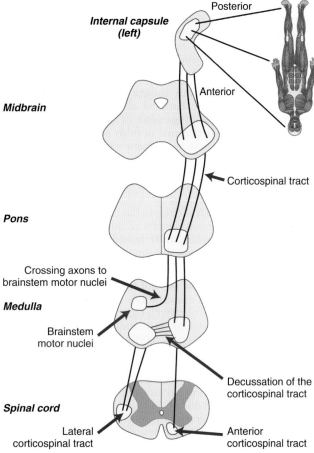

Fig. 25.2 Brainstem motor organization, beginning with internal capsule. Corticospinal tract remains topographically organized throughout brainstem and spinal cord, although isolated lesions below cerebral cortex are unlikely to produce topographically specific damage.

nerve signs with a contralateral hemiparesis and sensory deficit.

Sensory pathways from the nucleus gracilis and nucleus cuneatus cross at about the same level as the motor fibers of the CST, so deficits in light touch and position sense tend to parallel the distribution of the motor deficit. By contrast, the spinothalamic tracts have already crossed in the spinal cord and ascend laterally in the brainstem. Accordingly, lesions of the lower medulla may produce contralateral loss of pain and temperature sensation and ipsilateral loss of touch and position sense. Lesions above the mid-medulla produce a contralateral sensory defect of all modalities similar to that from cerebral lesions, yet the clues to brainstem localization can include the following:

- Ipsilateral facial sensory deficit from a trigeminal lesion
- Ipsilateral hemiataxia from damage to the cerebellar hemispheres or nuclei
- Ocular motor weakness from any of multiple lesion locations
- Ipsilateral Horner syndrome from damage of the descending sympathetic tracts.

Common Lesions

Table 25.2 shows some of the important lesions of the brainstem and their associated motor deficits. Brainstem lesions

usually are due to damage to the penetrating branches of the basilar artery. Patients present with contralateral weakness along with other deficits that help localize the lesion. Hemiataxia often develops and can be mistaken for hemiparesis, so careful examination is essential.

Spinal Lesions

Spinal lesions can produce hemiplegia sparing the face, although they mostly will cause bilateral deficits typical of myelopathy. A spinal cord lesion should be suspected in a patient with bilateral weakness, bowel or bladder control deficits, and back pain.

Spinal Hemisection (Brown–Séquard Syndrome)

Spinal hemisection is seldom seen in clinical practice. This entity is usually associated with intradural tumors, trauma, inflammatory conditions such as demyelinating disease, and occasionally spinal infarction. Spondylotic myelopathy, disk disease, and most extradural tumors typically produce symmetrical deficits. Patients with the spinal hemisection syndrome present with weakness ipsilateral to and below the lesion. In addition, segmental motor loss may be seen with involvement of the motoneurons at the level of the lesion. Sensory abnormalities include loss of pain and temperature contralateral to and below the lesion. Position sense may be affected ipsilateral to the lesion.

Transverse Myelitis

Transverse myelitis is an acute myelopathic process that is presumed to be autoimmune in origin. Patients present with motor and sensory deficits below the lesion, usually in the form of a paraplegia. The abnormalities typically are bilateral but may be asymmetrical. MRI may show increased signal on T2 images, enlargement of the cord, and/or enhancement in the spinal cord, which has an appearance that differs subtly from that in involvement in MS.

Transverse myelitis is a clinical diagnosis. The primary differential diagnosis is between MS and neuromyelitis optica (NMO).

Spinal Cord Compression

Spinal cord compression usually is due to disk protrusion, spondylosis, or acute trauma, but neoplastic and infectious causes should always be considered (Shedid and Benzel, 2007). Disk disease and spondylosis typically are in the midline, so bilateral findings are expected. Extradural tumors also usually produce bilateral findings. Intradural tumors may produce unilateral deficits and occasionally can manifest as Brown–Séquard syndrome.

Lesions below the cervical spinal cord would produce not hemiplegia but rather monoplegia of a lower limb or paraplegia. Spondylosis with cord compression produces lower motoneuron (LMN) weakness at the level of the lesion and CST signs below the level of the lesion. Spinal cord compression resulting in paralysis should be evaluated as quickly as possible with MRI. Myelography should be considered if MRI is not urgently available.

Spinal Cord Infarction

Anterior spinal artery infarction usually causes paraparesis and spinothalamic sensory loss below the level of the lesion; dorsal column function is preserved. Rarely, one segmental branch of the anterior spinal artery can be involved with unilateral spinal cord damage and monoparesis or hemiparesis.

TABLE 25.2 Brainstem syndromes

Named disorder	Lesion location	Signs
Midbrain		
Weber syndrome	CN III, ventral midbrain, CST	Contralateral hemiparesis, CN III palsy
Benedikt syndrome	CN III, ventral midbrain, CST, red nucleus	Contralateral hemiparesis, third nerve palsy, intention tremor, cerebellar ataxia
Top-of-the-basilar syndrome	Occipital lobes, midbrain oculomotor nuclei, cerebral peduncle, medial and temporal lobe, thalamus	Contralateral hemiparesis, cortical blindness, oculomotor deficits, memory difficulty, contralateral sensory deficit
Pons		
Millard–Gubler syndrome	CN VI, CN VII, ventral pons	Contralateral hemiparesis, CN VI and CN VII palsies
Clumsy hand syndrome	CST	Contralateral hemiparesis, dysarthria, often with facial weakness
Pure motor hemiparesis (due to pons lesion)	Ventral pons	Contralateral hemiparesis with corticospinal tract signs
Ataxic hemiparesis (due to pons lesion)	CST, cerebellar tracts	Contralateral hemiparesis with impaired coordination
Foville syndrome	CN VII, ventral pons, paramedian pontine reticular formation	Ipsilateral CN VII palsy, contralateral hemiparesis, gaze palsy to the side of the lesion
Medulla		
Medial medullary syndrome	CST, medial lemniscus, hypoglossal nerve	Contralateral hemiparesis, loss of position and vibratory sensation, ipsilateral tongue paresis
Lateral medullary syndrome	Spinothalamic tract, trigeminal nucleus, cerebellum and inferior cerebellar peduncle, vestibular nuclei, nucleus ambiguus	No hemiparesis usually produced, but hemiataxia may be mistaken for hemiparesis; dysphagia, hemisensory loss, face weakness, Horner syndrome are common

CN, cranial nerve; *CST*, corticospinal tract.

Spinal cord infarction is suggested when a patient presents with paraparesis or paraplegia of acute onset, and MRI of the spine does not show cord compression nor does MRI of the brain show bilateral ACA infarction.

Peripheral Lesions

Peripheral lesions are not expected to produce hemiplegia. A pair of peripheral lesions affecting an arm and leg on the same side, however, may occasionally masquerade as hemiplegia. Differentiation depends on identification of the individual lesions as being within the distribution of one nerve, nerve root, or plexus division. The tendon reflexes are likely to be depressed in patients with peripheral lesions, rather than increased as with CST lesions.

Amyotrophic lateral sclerosis can produce weakness of one limb, followed by weakness of the other limb on the same side, with progression over months or even years. Usually the combined presence of upper motoneuron (UMN) and LMN involvement without sensory changes and lack of bowel/bladder involvement supports the diagnosis. If the predominant involvement is UMN in type, the picture can look like that of a progressive hemiparesis.

Mononeuropathy multiplex can manifest as separate lesions affecting individual limbs; involvement of an arm and leg on the same side can give the impression of hemiparesis. Diabetes is the most common cause, but other causes include leprosy, vasculitis, and predisposition to pressure palsies. Diagnosis is by electromyography (EMG), which can differentiate mononeuropathies from polyneuropathy (Misulis, 2003).

Psychogenic Hemiplegia

Psychogenic or *functional* weakness includes both conversion reaction and malingering. In conversion reaction, the patient is not conscious of the nonorganic nature of the deficit, whereas in malingering, the patient makes a conscious effort to fool the examiner. Some secondary gain for the patient, either psychological or economic, is a factor with both types. In malingering, the secondary gain usually is more obvious and may be disability payments, litigation, family attention, or avoidance of stressors or tasks. Clues to functional weakness include the following:

- Improvement in strength with coaching
- Give-way weakness
- Inconsistencies in examination—for example, inability to extend the foot but able to walk on toes
- Hoover sign (when the patient lies supine on the bed and lifts one leg at a time, the examiner should feel effort to press down with the opposite heel if the tested leg is truly paralyzed; failure to do so constitutes the Hoover sign)
- Paralysis in the absence of other signs of motor system dysfunction, including tone and reflex changes.

Diagnosis of functional weakness is based on inconsistencies on examination and elimination of the possibility of organic disease. Functional weakness should be diagnosed with caution. It is easy to dismiss the patient's complaints after an inconsistent feature is seen, especially if some secondary gain is obvious. Unfortunately, a patient with organic problems may have a functional overlay, which may exaggerate otherwise subtle clinical findings.

If functional weakness is suspected, some diagnostic testing often is required to rule out neurological disease, although such investigations should be kept to a minimum.

MONOPLEGIA
Cerebral Lesions

Cerebral lesions more commonly produce hemiplegia than monoplegia, but isolated limb involvement can occasionally occur, especially with cortical involvement. The arm segment of the motor–sensory cortex lies on the lateral aspect of the hemisphere adjacent to the sylvian fissure. Subcortical lesions are less likely than cortical lesions to produce monoplegia because of the dense packing of the fibers of the CST in the internal capsule.

Infarction

The arm region of the motor cortex is supplied by the MCA. Infarction of a branch of the MCA can produce isolated arm weakness, although facial involvement and cortical signs are expected (Paciaroni et al., 2005). With more extensive lesions, visual fields can be abnormal because of infarction of the optic radiations. Mild leg weakness also can occur with medial cortical involvement of the infarct. The leg segment of the cortex lies in the parasagittal region and is supplied by the ACA. ACA infarction produces weakness of the contralateral leg.

Transient Ischemic Attack

Episodic paralysis of one limb sometimes is due to TIA. The main considerations in the differential diagnosis are migraine and seizure. Abrupt onset and absence of positive (muscle activating) motor symptoms argue in favor of TIA.

Migraine

Migraine can produce sensation that marches along one limb, usually the arm. This marching pattern differs from the abrupt onset of stroke. Involvement of only the leg is unusual. The headache phase typically begins as the neurological deficit is resolving. Weakness can develop as part of the migraine aura, but this is much less likely than sensory disturbance. Not all migrainous weakness is followed by headache.

Seizure

Seizure classically produces positive motor symptoms with jerking or stiffness. Focal seizures rarely can produce negative motor symptoms including paralysis. In such cases, the seizure can be impossible to diagnose without EEG, so EEG may be indicated in selected patients with unexplained focal weakness. Ictal paralysis can have abrupt onset and offset and can even resemble negative myoclonus.

Focal seizure activity may be suggested by subtle twitching or disturbance of consciousness associated with the episodes. In comparison with TIAs, seizures usually are more frequent and have a shorter duration. Lastly, postictal weakness of one limb can occur.

Multiple Sclerosis

Multiple Sclerosis can produce monoplegia secondary to a discrete white-matter plaque in the cerebral hemisphere, but because it is a subcortical disease, hemiparesis is more common. The corticospinal tracts are somatotopically organized, so monoparesis is theoretically possible but uncommon. Onset of symptoms is subacute.

Tumors

Tumors deep to the cortex rarely produce monoplegia because the involvement is not sufficiently discrete to affect only one limb. Cortical involvement makes single-limb involvement more likely. Parasagittal lesions often produce leg involvement, which initially can be unilateral. Meningiomas often arise from one side of the falx, so they predominantly affect the opposite leg, initially with weakness, incoordination, and CST signs. With progression, bilateral symptoms develop.

Bilateral leg weakness with CST signs can be due to either cerebral or spinal lesions, although single leg deficit is only rarely due to a spinal cause. Metastatic tumors often are found at the gray/white junction; in this location, they can produce focal cortical damage. Early on, the lesion may be too small to produce other neurological symptoms, but with increasing growth, it is more likely to produce focal seizures. Tumor is suspected with insidious progression of focal deficit, especially if combined with headache or seizures.

Infections

Infections are an uncommon cause of monoplegia but this presentation is possible. Brain abscess in the region of the motor strip can produce weakness largely confined to one extremity, arm more than leg. Viral encephalitis produces different patterns of involvement depending on whether it is herpes simplex virus (HSV). Non-HSV encephalitis commonly produces an encephalopathy, with focal motor deficit being unlikely. HSV encephalitis with often temporal lobe involvement can produce arm and face weakness but hemiparesis, seizures and language defect are more common (Mekan et al., 2005). Involvement of brain outside of the temporal lobes is seen in a small but important group of patients and can produce symptoms appropriate to the lesion, e.g., frontal or occipital. Brainstem can rarely be affected with no evident hemispheric involvement (Jereb et al., 2005).

Brainstem Lesions

Brainstem lesions seldom produce monoplegia because of the tight packing of the fibers of the CSTs in the brainstem. Unilateral cerebellar hemisphere lesions may produce appendicular ataxia, which is most obvious in the arm, although this should be distinguished from monoparesis by the absence of weakness or CST signs.

Spinal Lesions

Spinal lesions can produce weakness from segmental damage to nerve roots or CSTs. Weakness at the level of the lesion is in a radicular distribution and may be associated with muscle atrophy and loss of segmental reflexes. Weakness below the lesion can be unilateral or bilateral and is associated with CST signs.

Peripheral Lesions

Peripheral lesions usually produce monoparetic weakness in the distribution of a single nerve, nerve root, or plexus. A few conditions, such as amyotrophic lateral sclerosis and focal spinal muscular atrophy, may produce weakness in a monomelic (monoplegic) distribution.

Pressure Palsies

Intermittent compression of a peripheral nerve can produce transient paresis of part of a limb. The patient may think the entire limb is paralyzed, but detailed examination shows that

TABLE 25.3 Peripheral Nerve Lesions of the Arm

Lesion	Clinical findings	Electromyography findings
Median neuropathy		
Carpal tunnel syndrome	Weakness and wasting of abductor pollicis brevis if severe; sensory loss on palmar aspect of first through third digits	Slow median motor and sensory NCV through the carpal tunnel; denervation of abductor pollicis brevis if severe
Anterior interosseous syndrome	Weakness of flexor digitorum profundus, pronator quadratus, flexor pollicis longus	Denervation in flexor digitorum profundus, flexor pollicis longus, pronator quadratus
Pronator teres syndrome	Weakness of distal median-innervated muscles; tenderness of pronator teres	Slow median motor NCV through proximal forearm denervation of distal median-innervated muscles
Compression at the ligament of Struthers	Weakness of distal median-innervated muscles	As for pronator teres syndrome, with the addition of denervation of pronator teres
Ulnar neuropathy		
Palmar branch damage	Weakness of dorsal interossei; no sensory loss	Normal ulnar NCV; denervation of first dorsal interosseus but not abductor digiti minimi
Entrapment at Guyon canal	Weakness of ulnar intrinsic muscles; numbness over fourth and fifth digits	Slow ulnar motor and sensory NCV through wrist
Entrapment at or near the elbow	Weakness of ulnar intrinsic muscles; numbness over fourth and fifth digits	Slow ulnar motor NCV across elbow, denervation in first dorsal interosseus, abductor digiti minimi, and ulnar half of flexor digitorum profundus
Radial neuropathy		
Posterior interosseus syndrome	Weakness of finger and wrist extensors; no sensory loss	Denervation in wrist and finger extensors; sparing of the supinator and extensor carpi radialis
Compression at the spiral groove	Weakness of finger and wrist extensors; triceps usually spared; sensory loss on dorsal aspects of first digit	Slow radial motor NCV across spiral groove; denervation in distal radial-innervated muscles; triceps may be affected with proximal lesions

NCV, nerve conduction velocity.

the paresis is limited to a nerve distribution. Recovery from the weakness usually occurs so rapidly that examination often is not possible before the improvement. Predisposition to pressure palsies can be seen in two main circumstances: on a hereditary basis and in the presence of peripheral polyneuropathy.

Hereditary Neuropathy with Predisposition to Pressure Palsies. Hereditary neuropathy with predisposition to pressure palsies is associated with episodic weakness and sensory loss associated with compression of isolated nerves. This disorder is inherited as an autosomal dominant condition with a deletion or mutation in the gene for peripheral myelin protein 22 (PMP-22). Nerve conduction studies will show slowing commonly across the compression area (carpal tunnel, cubital tunnel, and femoral head). NCVs also may be reduced in asymptomatic gene carriers (Chance, 2006).

Pressure Palsies in Polyneuropathy. Patients with polyneuropathy may have an increased susceptibility to pressure palsies. Areas of demyelination are more likely to have a depolarizing block produced by even mild pressure.

Mononeuropathies

Table 25.3 shows some important peripheral nerve lesions of the arm. Table 25.4 shows some important peripheral nerve lesions of the leg.

Median Nerve. The most common median neuropathy is carpal tunnel syndrome, but other important anatomical lesions, including anterior interosseus syndrome and pronator teres syndrome, have been described.

Carpal Tunnel Syndrome. Carpal tunnel syndrome is the most common mononeuropathy. The median nerve is compressed as it passes under the flexor retinaculum at the wrist.

TABLE 25.4 Peripheral Nerve Lesions of the Leg

Lesion	Clinical findings	Electromyography findings
Sciatic neuropathy	Weakness of tibial- and peroneal-innervated muscles, with sensory loss on posterior leg and foot	Denervation distally in tibial- and peroneal-innervated muscles
Peroneal neuropathy	Weakness of foot extension and eversion and toe extension	Denervation in tibialis anterior; NCV across fibular neck may be slowed
Tibial neuropathy	Weakness of foot plantar flexion	Denervation of gastrocnemius
Femoral neuropathy	Weakness of knee extension; weakness of hip flexion if psoas involved	Denervation in quadriceps, sometimes psoas

NCV, nerve conduction velocity.

Patients present with numbness on the palmar aspect of the first through the third digits. Forced flexion or extension of the wrist commonly exacerbates the sensory symptoms. Weakness of the abductor pollicis brevis may develop in advanced cases.

This condition would not normally be considered in the differential diagnosis for monoparesis, but because the patient can complain of weakness that is more extensive than the actual deficit, it is considered here. Clinical diagnosis can be confirmed by EMG.

Anterior Interosseus Syndrome. The anterior interosseous nerve is a branch of the median nerve in the forearm that supplies some of the forearm muscles. Damage can occur distal to the elbow, producing a syndrome that essentially is purely motor. Weakness of finger flexion is prominent. Affected muscles include the flexor digitorum profundus to the second and third digits (the portion to the fourth and fifth digits is innervated by the ulnar nerve). The distal median nerve entering the hand is unaffected because the anterior interosseous nerve arises from the main trunk of the median nerve.

Diagnosis is suspected by weakness of the median nerve–innervated finger flexors, with sparing of the abductor pollicis brevis and ulnar nerve–innervated flexors. EMG can confirm the diagnosis.

Pronator Teres Syndrome. The median nerve distal to the elbow can be damaged as it passes through the pronator teres muscle. All median-innervated muscles of the arm are affected except for the pronator teres itself. The clinical picture is that of an anterior interosseous syndrome plus distal median neuropathy. The pronator teres may be tender, and palpation may exacerbate some of the distal pain.

Ulnar Nerve. Ulnar entrapment is most common near the elbow and at the wrist. Entrapment at the elbow produces weakness of the ulnar-innervated intrinsic muscles. Weakness of long flexors of the fourth and fifth digits also can develop. When the entrapment is at the wrist, the weakness is isolated to the intrinsic muscles of the hand, and more proximal muscles are unaffected. Although most of the intrinsic muscles of the hand are ulnar innervated, a few are median innervated and are unaffected in ulnar neuropathy.

The diagnosis of ulnar neuropathy is suggested when a patient complains of pain or numbness on the ulnar aspect of the hand. Additional findings that support this diagnosis include weakness and wasting of the intrinsic muscles of the hand, which is especially easy to see in the first dorsal interosseous.

Radial Nerve Palsy. Radial neuropathy is most commonly seen above the elbow, such that wrist and finger extensors are mainly affected. The triceps also can be affected. Radial nerve palsy is most commonly due to a pressure palsy in alcoholic intoxication. Peripheral neuropathy makes the development of pressure neuropathy of the radial nerve more likely.

Femoral Neuropathy. Femoral neuropathy can occur at the level of the lumbar plexus secondary to compression by intra-abdominal contents (fetus or neoplasm), but we also have seen it from damage incurred during angiography or surgery. Patients present with pain in the thigh and weakness of knee extension. They usually report that the leg "gives out" during walking or that they cannot get out of a chair without using their arms. Examination may show quadriceps weakness, but this muscle group is so strong that the examiner may not be able to detect the deficit. Lower leg muscles must be examined to ensure that muscles in the sciatic distribution are normal. Diagnosis is confirmed by EMG showing denervation confined to the femoral nerve distribution. Unfortunately, electrical signs of denervation may not be obvious for up to 4 weeks after the injury. CT scan imaging of the abdomen and pelvis should be considered to evaluate for possible mass compression of the femoral nerve.

Sciatic Neuropathy. Sciatic neuropathy can have multiple causes, including acute trauma and chronic compressive lesions. The term *sciatica* describes pain in the distribution of the sciatic nerve in the back of the leg. It usually is due to radiculopathy (see Radiculopathies, later). An intramuscular injection into the sciatic nerve rather than the gluteus muscle is an occasional cause of sciatic neuropathy, which is characterized by initial severe pain followed by a lesser degree of pain and weakness.

Piriformis syndrome is a condition in which the sciatic nerve is compressed by the piriformis muscle. This is a difficult diagnosis to make, requiring demonstration of increased pain on tensing the piriformis muscle by flexing and adducting the hip. Piriformis syndrome should be considered in patients presenting with symptoms and signs referable to the sciatic nerve but with no evident cause seen on imaging of the lumbar spine and plexus.

Diagnosis of sciatic neuropathy is considered when a patient presents with pain or weakness of the lower leg muscles. EMG can confirm the distribution of denervation. NCS is usually normal.

Peroneal (Fibular) Neuropathy. The *peroneal nerve* is appropriately designated as the *fibular nerve* in many modern scientific publications and texts because of the proximity to the fibula and to distinguish it from *perineal nerves*. While this may become standard, we will continue to use the term *peroneal* for this discussion. Peroneal neuropathy can develop from a lesion at the fibular neck, the popliteal fossa, or even the sciatic nerve in the thigh. The peroneal division of the sciatic nerve is more susceptible to injury than the tibial division, so incomplete sciatic injury affects predominantly the peroneal innervated muscles—tibialis anterior, extensor digitorum brevis, and peroneus. In addition, the peroneal division innervates the short head of the biceps femoris. This is an important muscle to remember because distal peroneal neuropathy spares this muscle, whereas a proximal sciatic neuropathy, a peroneal division lesion, or a radiculopathy is expected to cause denervation not only in the tibialis anterior but also the short head of the biceps femoris (Marciniak et al., 2005).

Radiculopathies

Radiculopathy produces weakness of one portion of a limb. Common radiculopathies are summarized in Table 25.5. Complete paralysis of all of the muscles of an arm or leg is not caused by radiculopathy, other than in traumatic avulsion of multiple nerve roots. Roots serving arm power include

TABLE 25.5 Radiculopathies

Level	Motor deficit	Sensory deficit
Cervical radiculopathy		
C5	Deltoid, biceps	Lateral upper arm
C6	Biceps, brachioradialis	Radial forearm and first and second digits
C7	Wrist extensors, triceps	Third and fourth digits
C8	Intrinsic hand muscles	Fifth digit and ulnar forearm
T1	Intrinsic muscles of the hand, especially APB	Axilla
Lumbar radiculopathy		
L2	Psoas, quadriceps	Lateral and anterior thigh
L3	Psoas, quadriceps	Lower medial thigh
L4	Tibialis anterior, quadriceps	Medial lower leg
L5	Peroneus longus, gluteus medius, tibialis anterior, extensor hallucis longus	Lateral lower leg
S1	Gastrocnemius, gluteus maximus	Lateral foot and fourth and fifth digits

APB, abductor pollicis brevis.

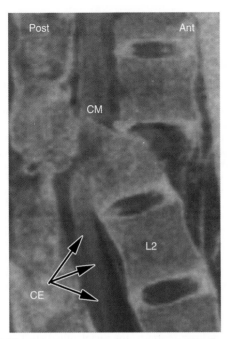

Fig. 26.3 Magnetic resonance imaging demonstrating the effects of trauma to the thoracolumbar portion of the spine with a crush injury of the cauda equina (CE) and conus medullaris (CM) portion of the spinal cord. Note T12/L1-level spine fracture and dislocation.

a third of these patients suffer considerable central pain. Affected limb and pelvic floor muscles develop flaccid weakness, and electromyography shows denervation after either a conus medullaris or cauda equina injury, especially following anatomically complete lesions.

Both conus medullaris and cauda equina injuries are associated with bladder, bowel, and sexual dysfunction. Urodynamic evaluations typically demonstrate detrusor areflexia, and a rectal exam identifies a flaccid anal sphincter. In addition, the bulbocavernosus reflex is typically absent or diminished, and reflexogenic erection in males is commonly lost.

Imaging studies (e.g., plain radiographs, CT, MRI) identify structural pathology. Burst fractures and fracture dislocations are common injuries to the spinal column that result in neurological deficits, suggesting a conus medullaris or cauda equina involvement. Following trauma to the thoracolumbar spine, imaging studies can be used to assess spinal stability and identify detailed aspects of spine fractures, including the presence and location of bone fragments, spinal canal encroachment, epidural hematomas, and herniated disks. A variety of treatment options exist (e.g., surgical stabilization of the spine, decompression of the conus medullaris and nerve roots).

A lumbar spinal stenosis due to a congenitally small-diameter spinal canal or central disk and spondylotic narrowing one or more levels below L1 may present with a subtle course. Over months to years, lower extremity numbness or pain, usually in an L3–S1 single or multiradicular pattern, accompanies standing and walking, often gradually progressing to limit walking distance. Pain is commonly accompanied by weakness, but patients may not be aware of their deficit. Clinical insight into this diagnosis and the upper level of cauda compression is gained by a manual muscle examination after a few minutes of being supine, followed by having the subject walk for about 500 feet, and then immediately retesting strength. Transient paresis or greater paresis in the affected

root distribution often is found immediately after the walk and resolves within a minute or two.

PAIN AND AUTONOMIC DYSFUNCTION

In addition to motor and sensory impairments, pain and dysfunction in the autonomic nervous system can aid localization of spinal cord syndromes. Pain is frequently associated with spinal cord injuries, along with autonomic impairments that may affect blood pressure and heart rate, bladder, bowel, sexual, and cardiorespiratory functions. The type and severity of autonomic dysfunction depends on the location of pathology and severity of the spinal cord injury. International spinal cord injury societies recommend a systematic approach to document remaining autonomic function after a spinal cord injury (Alexander et al., 2009).

Pain Syndromes

Distinct pain syndromes may develop as a result of compression, inflammation, or injury to the vertebral column, ligaments, the dura mater, nerve roots, dorsal horn, and ascending spinal cord sensory tracts. Neuropathic pain may take the form of *paresthesia* (abnormal but not unpleasant sensation that is either spontaneous or evoked), *dysesthesia* (an abnormal, unpleasant sensation that is spontaneous or evoked), *allodynia* (pain evoked by ordinary stimuli such as touch or rubbing), and *hyperalgesia* (an augmented response to a stimulus that is usually painful).

Local Pain

Localized neck or back pain may result from irritation or injury to innervated spine structures including ligaments, periosteum, and dura. The pain is typically deep and aching, may vary with a change in position, and often becomes worse from increased load or weight bearing on affected structures. Percussion or palpation over the spine may in some patients worsen the local pain. When the injured or diseased spine structures are irritated, secondary symptoms may develop and include muscle spasm and a more diffusely located pain. Musculoligamentous sources of pain often persist for more than a week post spine surgery and develop with compensatory overuse of joints and muscles. Such pain must be distinguished from central neurogenic pain, but can amplify it.

Projected Pain

A pathological process involving the facet joints may be experienced as focal or radiating pain in an upper or lower extremity. When a nerve root is irritated or injured, the projected pain is radicular.

Radicular pain commonly has a sharp, stabbing quality or causes dysesthesia. It may be exacerbated by activities that stretch the affected nerve root (e.g., straight leg raising or flexion of the neck). Straining or coughing may also increase the intensity and severity of radicular pain. Nerve root irritation may also result in sensory and motor deficits following the same dermatome and myotome distribution as the affected nerve root. This helps localize the level of spinal cord injury that is causing paraplegia.

Central Neurogenic Pain

Paresthesia, dysesthesia, allodynia, and *hyperalgesia* accompany injury to the spinal cord in at least half of patients, as well as after thalamocortical stroke. Regardless of segmental level or completeness of injury, most patients with a traumatic spinal cord injury develop a clinically significant pain syndrome at some post-lesion time point (Waxman and Hains, 2006). Neuropathic pain after spinal cord injury may affect different locations. At-level pain is primarily derived from local cellular and neuroplastic changes in the dorsal horn and sensory roots at the segments of injury. Below-level pain is located in body segments receiving innervation from the spinal cord caudal to the lesioned segments. Above-level neurogenic pain is less common.

Pain developing after a spinal cord injury is commonly described as burning, pricking, or aching in quality. It can be experienced as deep or superficial. Some patients develop a severe and excruciating pain syndrome after cord or cauda trauma that is at-level and below-level even in the absence of any cutaneous or proprioceptive sensation, which requires centrally acting medications to control. The most recently FDA-approved medication for spinal pain is pregabaline. The mechanisms for such painful phantom phenomena are not well understood but include structural and molecular dorsal horn, thalamic, and cortical adaptations to ordinary and noxious inputs.

Autonomic Dysreflexia

Injuries to the spinal cord that result in paraplegia from a lesion above T6 may also impair autonomic control and result in episodes of severe hypertension or hypotension. Autonomic dysreflexia represents an acute syndrome characterized by excessive and uncontrolled sympathetic output from the spinal cord. As a result, the blood pressure is suddenly and markedly elevated. Associated symptoms include headache; malaise; blurring of vision; flushed, sweaty skin above the level of injury; and pale, cool skin below it. An episode of autonomic dysreflexia can be triggered by any noxious stimulation below the segmental level of injury. Common triggers include bladder distension, constipation, rectal fissures, joint injury, and urinary tract infection. Autonomic dysreflexia may present soon after the initial injury but more commonly becomes symptomatic several months after the spinal cord injury. Prevention is the best approach. Treatment of acute symptoms targets removal of noxious stimuli and cautious lowering of the blood pressure (see Chapter 63).

Bowel and Bladder Dysfunction

Normal bladder and bowel control depend on segmental reflexes involving both autonomic and somatic motor neurons, as well as descending and ascending tracts of the spinal cord (Fowler et al., 2008). As a result, bladder and bowel function may be impaired after an injury to any segmental level of the spinal cord. Different clinical syndromes develop depending on whether the injury or disease process affects the sacral spinal cord directly or higher segmental levels. Traumatic spinal cord injuries with paraplegia taking place above the T12 vertebra will interrupt spinal cord long-tract connections between supraspinal micturition centers in the brainstem and cerebral cortex and the sacral spinal cord. An upper motoneuron syndrome follows, with detrusor–sphincter dyssynergia caused by impaired coordination of autonomic and somatic motor control of the bladder detrusor and external urethral sphincter, respectively. Incomplete bladder emptying results. In addition, the upper motoneuron syndrome also includes detrusor hyper-reflexia with increased pressure within the bladder. In contrast, injury to the T12 vertebra and below results in a direct lesion to the sacral spinal cord and associated nerve roots. A direct lesion to preganglionic parasympathetic neurons and somatic motoneurons of the Onuf nucleus located within the S2–S4 spinal cord segments results in denervation of pelvic targets. Injuries to both the conus medullaris and cauda equina present as a lower motoneuron syndrome characterized by weak or flaccid detrusor function. Urinary retention follows, with risk of overflow incontinence. The goal for all bladder care is to avoid retrograde urine flow, urinary tract infections, and renal failure. Management of both upper and lower motoneuron bladder impairment commonly includes clean intermittent bladder catheterizations. Chapter 47 discusses evaluation and treatment.

REFERENCES

The complete reference list is available online at https://expertconsult .inkling.com/.

27 Proximal, Distal, and Generalized Weakness

David C. Preston, Barbara E. Shapiro

CHAPTER OUTLINE

CLINICAL PRESENTATION BY AFFECTED REGION
General Considerations
Ocular Muscles
Facial and Bulbar Muscles
Neck, Diaphragm, and Axial Muscles
Proximal Upper Extremity
Distal Upper Extremity
Proximal Lower Extremity
Distal Lower Extremity

BEDSIDE EXAMINATION OF THE WEAK PATIENT
Observation
Muscle Bulk and Deformities
Muscle Palpation, Percussion, and Range of Motion
Muscle Tone
Strength
Fatigue
Reflexes
Sensory Disturbances
Peripheral Nerve Enlargement
Fasciculations, Cramps, and Other Abnormal
  Muscle Movements

FUNCTIONAL EVALUATION OF THE WEAK PATIENT
Walking
Arising from the Floor
Stepping Onto a Stool
Psychogenic Weakness

CLINICAL INVESTIGATIONS IN MUSCULAR WEAKNESS
Serum Creatine Kinase
Electromyography
Muscle Biopsy
Genetic Testing
Exercise Testing

DIFFERENTIAL DIAGNOSIS BY AFFECTED REGION AND OTHER MANIFESTATIONS OF WEAKNESS
Disorders with Prominent Ocular Weakness
Disorders with Distinctive Facial or Bulbar Weakness
Disorders with Prominent Respiratory Weakness
Disorders with Distinctive Shoulder-Girdle or
  Arm Weakness
Disorders with Prominent Hip-Girdle or Leg Weakness
Disorders with Fluctuating Weakness
Disorders Exacerbated by Exercise
Disorders with Constant Weakness
Acquired Disorders Causing Weakness
Lifelong Disorders
Other Conditions

Muscle weakness may be due to disorders of the central nervous system (CNS) or peripheral nervous system (PNS). The PNS includes the primary sensory neurons in the dorsal root ganglia, nerve roots, peripheral nerves, neuromuscular junctions, and muscles. Although not strictly peripheral, the primary motor neurons (anterior horn cells) in the brainstem and spinal cord are also conventionally included as part of the PNS. The neurological examination allows separation of the causes of weakness arising at these different locations. If the pattern of weakness is characteristic of upper motor neuron (UMN) dysfunction (i.e., weakness of upper-limb extensors and lower-limb flexors) together with hyper-reflexia and extensor plantar responses, the weakness clearly is of CNS origin. Weakness with sensory loss may occur in both CNS disorders and disorders of the nerve roots and peripheral nerves. Weakness without sensory loss may also occur from CNS disorders, but in the PNS this pattern of weakness occurs in disorders of the anterior horn cell, neuromuscular junction, or muscle. Rarely in the PNS, peripheral motor fibers are the site of pathology (e.g., as occurs in multifocal motor neuropathy with conduction block). Although fatigue often accompanies most disorders of weakness, marked fatigue, especially when involving the extraocular, bulbar, and proximal upper limb muscles, often indicates a disorder of the neuromuscular junction.

The motor unit is the primary building block of the PNS and includes the anterior horn cell, its motor nerve, terminal nerve fibers, and all their accompanying neuromuscular junctions and muscle fibers. This chapter concentrates on disorders of the motor unit and disorders that may also involve the peripheral sensory nerves. The pattern of weakness often localizes the pathological process to the primary neurons, nerve roots, peripheral nerves, neuromuscular junctions, or muscles. Muscle weakness changes functional abilities that are more or less specific to the muscle groups affected. Recognizable patterns of symptoms and signs often allow a reasonable estimation of the anatomical involvement. Identifying these patterns is the first step in the differential diagnosis of weakness, as certain disorders affect specific muscle groups. This chapter begins with a review of the symptoms and signs of muscular weakness with respect to the muscle groups affected. A discussion follows of the bedside examinations, functional examinations, and laboratory tests often used in evaluating patients with muscle weakness. The chapter concludes with an approach to the differential diagnosis of muscle weakness based on which muscle groups are weak, whether the muscle weakness is constant or fluctuating, and whether the disorder is genetic or acquired.

CLINICAL PRESENTATION BY AFFECTED REGION
General Considerations

As muscles begin to weaken, the associated clinical features depend more on which muscles are involved than on the cause of involvement. A complicating factor in evaluating weakness is the patient's interpretation of the term *weak*. Although physicians use this term to denote a loss of muscle power, patients tend to apply it more loosely in describing their symptoms. Even more confusing, many people use the words *numb* and *weak* interchangeably, so the clinician should not accept a complaint of weakness at face value; the patient should be questioned further until it is clear that weakness means loss of muscle strength.

If the patient has no objective weakness when examined, the clinician must rely on the history. In patients with weak muscles, a fairly stereotypical set of symptoms emerges according to which muscle groups are weak (discussed later in this section). The patient whose weakness is caused by depression or malingering has vague symptoms, avoids answering leading questions, and the stereotypical symptoms of weakness are seldom volunteered. Instead, these patients make such statements as "I just can't do (the task)," or "I can't climb the stairs because I get so tired and have to rest." When pressed regarding these symptoms, it becomes apparent that specific details are lacking. Patients who cannot get out of a low chair because of real weakness explain exactly how they have to maneuver themselves into an upright position (e.g., pushing on the chair arms, leaning forward in the seat, and bracing their hands against the furniture). The examiner should avoid providing patients with clinical details they appear to be searching for. Asking whether pushing on the arms of the chair is required to stand up provides the patient with key information that may later be used in response to the questions of baffled successive examiners. In addition, it often is difficult to differentiate true muscle weakness from apparent weakness that accompanies tendon or joint contractures or is secondary to pain. For example, patients with primary orthopedic conditions often complain of weakness. In these patients, however, pain with passive or active motion often is a prominent part of the symptoms.

In evaluating weakness, the first key task is to discern which muscle groups are affected. In this regard, it is helpful to consider the involvement of specific body regions: ocular; facial and bulbar; neck, diaphragm, and axial; proximal upper extremity; distal upper extremity; proximal lower extremity; and distal lower extremity.

Ocular Muscles

Extraocular muscle weakness results in ptosis or diplopia. When looking in the mirror, the patient may notice drooping of the eyelids, or family and friends may point it out. It is important to keep in mind that ptosis occasionally develops in older patients as a consequence of aging (i.e., partial dehiscence of the levator muscles) or a sequela of ocular surgery (e.g., lens implantation for cataracts). To differentiate between acute and chronic ptosis, it helps to look at prior photographs. Because the ocular myopathies often are familial, examination of family members is useful. Bilateral ptosis may result in compensatory backward tilting of the neck to look ahead or upward. Rarely, this postural adaptation may lead to neck pain and fatigue as the prominent symptoms. In addition, true ptosis often results in compensatory contraction of the frontalis muscles to lessen the ptosis, resulting in a characteristic pattern of a droopy eyelid with prominent forehead furrowing produced by contraction of the frontalis muscle. Weakness of extraocular muscles may result in diplopia. Mild diplopia, however, may cause only blurring of vision, sending the patient to the ophthalmologist for new eyeglasses. It also is worth asking the patient whether closing one eye corrects the diplopia, because neuromuscular weakness is not among the causes of monocular diplopia.

Facial and Bulbar Muscles

Patients experience facial weakness as a feeling of stiffness or sometimes as a twisting or altered perception in the face (note

that patients often use the word *numbness* in describing facial weakness). Drinking through a straw, whistling, and blowing up balloons are all particularly difficult tasks for these patients and may be sensitive tests for facial weakness, particularly when such weakness dates from childhood. Acquaintances may notice that the patient's expression is somehow changed. A pleasant smile may turn into a snarl because of weakness of the levator anguli oris muscles. In lower facial weakness, patients may notice drooling and difficulty retaining their saliva, often requiring them to carry a tissue in the hand—the so-called napkin sign—which often accompanies bulbar involvement in amyotrophic lateral sclerosis (ALS). A common observation in mild long-standing facial weakness, as in patients with facioscapulohumeral (FSH) muscular dystrophy, is a tendency for the patient to sleep with the eyes open from weakness of the orbicularis oculi. Weakness of masticatory muscles may result in difficulty chewing, sometimes with a sensation of fatigue and discomfort, as may occur with myasthenia gravis (MG). Pharyngeal, palatal, and tongue weakness disturbs speech and swallowing. A flaccid palate is associated with nasal regurgitation, choking spells, and aspiration of liquids. Speech may become slurred or acquire a nasal or hoarse quality. In contrast with central lesions, no problem with fluency or language function is observed.

Neck, Diaphragm, and Axial Muscles

Neck muscle weakness becomes apparent when the patient must stabilize the head. Riding as a passenger in a car that brakes or accelerates, particularly in emergencies, may be disconcerting for the patient with neck weakness, because the head rocks forward or backward. Similarly, when the patient is stooping or bending forward, weakness of the posterior neck muscles may cause the chin to fall on the chest. A patient with neck-flexion weakness often notices difficulty lifting the head off the pillow in the morning. As neck weakness progresses, patients may develop the *dropped head syndrome*, in which they no longer can extend the neck, and the chin rests against the chest (Fig. 27.1). This posture leads to several secondary difficulties, especially with vision and swallowing.

Shortness of breath often develops when diaphragm muscles weaken, especially when individuals lie flat or must exert themselves. These symptoms can be mistakenly attributed to lung or heart disease. Severe diaphragmatic weakness leads to hypoventilation and carbon dioxide retention. This may first be manifested as morning headaches or vivid nightmares. Later, hypercapnia results in sedation and a depressed mental state. Rarely, axial and trunk muscles can be involved early in the course of a neuromuscular disorder. Weakness of the abdominal muscles may make sit-ups impossible. Focal weakness of the lower abdominal muscles results in an obvious protuberance that superficially mimics an abdominal hernia. Patients with weakness of the paraspinal muscles are unable to maintain a straight posture when sitting or standing, although they can do so when lying on the bed (so-called *bent spine syndrome*).

Proximal Upper Extremity

A feeling of tiredness often is the first expression of shoulder weakness. The weight of the arms is sufficient to cause fatigue. Early on, the patient experiences fatigue while performing sustained tasks with the hands held up, especially over the head. The most problematic activities include painting the ceiling, shampooing or combing the hair, shaving, and simply trying to lift an object off a high shelf.

the thumb distal to the wrist, and the peroneal nerve at the fibular head at the knee.

Fasciculations, Cramps, and Other Abnormal Muscle Movements

All limbs are examined to determine the presence or absence of fasciculations. A *fasciculation* is a brief twitch caused by the spontaneous firing of one motor unit. Fasciculations may be difficult or impossible to see in infants or obese patients. They can be present in normal people, so their presence in the absence of wasting or weakness is of no significance (*benign fasciculations*). Fasciculations that are widespread and seen on every examination may indicate denervating disease, particularly anterior horn cell disease. Mental or physical fatigue, caffeine, cigarette smoking, or drugs such as amphetamines exacerbate fasciculations.

In some patients who have been careful to avoid exposure to exacerbating factors, disease-related fasciculations may be absent or appear benign. This should be kept in mind during the evaluation. Abundant fasciculations may be difficult to differentiate from *myokymia*, which is a more writhing, bag of worms–like motion of muscle. Myokymia results from repetitive bursting of a motor unit (i.e., grouped fasciculations) and characteristically is associated with certain neuromuscular conditions (e.g., radiation injury, Guillain–Barré syndrome).

Similar to fasciculations, cramps may be benign or accompany several neuropathic conditions. A *cramp* is a painful involuntary muscle contraction. Cramps occur when a muscle is contracting in a shortened position. During a cramp, the muscle becomes hard and well defined. Stretching the muscle relieves the cramp. Superficially, a muscle contracture that occurs in a metabolic myopathy may resemble a cramp, although these two entities are completely different on electrophysiological testing. During a contracture, electrical silence is characteristic, whereas numerous motor units fire at high frequencies during a cramp.

FUNCTIONAL EVALUATION OF THE WEAK PATIENT
Walking

Alteration of gait may occur with weakness of the muscles of the hip and back, leg, and shoulder. In normal walking, when the heel hits the ground, the action of the hip abductors, which stabilize the pelvis, serves to counteract the shock. Thus in a sense, the hip abductors act as shock absorbers. Weakness of these muscles disturbs the normal fluid movement of the pelvis during walking, so when the heel hits the ground, the pelvis dips to the other side; bilateral weakness produces a waddle. Additionally, weakness of the hip extensors and back extensors makes it difficult for the patient to maintain a normal posture. Ordinarily the body is carried so that the center of gravity is slightly forward of the hip joint. To maintain an erect posture, the hip and back extensors are in continual activity. If these muscles become weak, the patient often throws the shoulders back so that the weight of the body falls behind the hip joints. This postural adjustment accentuates the lumbar lordosis. Alternatively, with pronounced weakness of the quadriceps muscles, the patient stabilizes the knee by throwing it backward. When the knee is hyperextended, it locks, deriving its stability from the anatomy of the joint rather than from muscular support. Finally, weakness of the muscles of the lower leg may result in a *steppage gait*, in which a short throw at the ankle midswing affects dorsiflexion of the foot. The foot then rapidly comes to the ground before the toes fall back into plantar flexion. Shoulder weakness may be observed

as the patient walks; the arms hang loosely by the sides and tend to swing in a pendular fashion rather than with a normal controlled swing.

Arising from the Floor

The normal method for arising from the floor depends on the age of the patient. The young child can spring rapidly to the feet without the average observer being able to dissect the movements. The elderly patient may turn to one side, place a hand on the floor, and rise to a standing position with a deliberate slowness. Despite such variability, abnormalities caused by muscle weakness are easily detectable. The patient with hip muscle weakness will turn to one side or the other to put the hand on the floor for support. The degree of turning is proportional to the severity of the weakness. Some patients must turn all the way around until they are in a prone position before they draw their feet under them to begin the standing process. Most people arise to a standing position from a squatting position, but the patient with hip extensor and quadriceps muscle weakness finds it easier to keep the hands on the floor and raise the hips high in the air. This has been termed the *butt-first maneuver*; the patient forms a triangle with the hips at the apex and the base of support provided by both hands and feet on the floor, and then laboriously rises from this position, usually by pushing on the thighs with both hands to brace the body upward. The progress of recovery or progression of weakness can be documented by noting whether the initial turn is greater than 90 degrees, whether unilateral or bilateral hand support is used on the floor and thighs, whether this support is sustained or transitory, and whether a butt-first maneuver is used. The entire process is known as the *Gower maneuver*, but it is useful to break it up into its component parts (Fig. 27.5).

Stepping onto a Stool

For a patient with hip and leg weakness, stepping onto an 8-inch-high footstool is equivalent in difficulty to a normal person's stepping up onto a coffee table. This analogy is apt because the required maneuvers are similar in both cases.

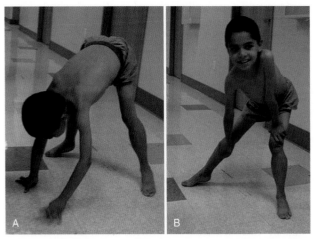

Fig. 27.5 Gower sign in a 7-year-old boy with Duchenne muscular dystrophy. **A,** Butt-first maneuver as hips are hoisted in the air. **B,** Hand support on the thighs. *(From McDonald, C.M., 2012. Clinical approach to the diagnostic evaluation of hereditary and acquired neuromuscular diseases. Phy Med Rehabil Clin N Am 23(3), 495–563. Copyright © 2012 Elsevier Inc.)*

Whereas the patient with normal strength readily approaches a footstool and easily steps onto it, the patient with weakness often hesitates in front of the stool while contemplating the task. A curious little maneuver occurs, known colloquially as the *fast-foot maneuver*. Normal persons can easily take the weight of the body on one leg, straightening out the knee as they stand on the footstool. Patients with weakness feel unsafe. They like to get both feet under them before straightening the knees and rising to their full height. To accomplish this, they place one foot on the footstool. While the knee of this leg is still bent, they quickly transfer the other foot from the floor to the footstool and then straighten the knees. This gives the impression of a hurried transfer of the trailing foot from floor to footstool, hence the term *fast foot*. As the weakness increases, the pelvis may dip toward the floor as the leading leg takes up the strain and the patient's weight transfers from the foot on the floor to the foot on the stool, the so-called *hip dip*. Finally, if the weakness is severe, patients may either use hand support on the thighs or appear to gather themselves in and throw the body onto the footstool. Analysis of the various components—the hesitation, fast foot, hip dip, and throw—together with the presence or absence of hand support may provide a sensitive measure of changes in the disease state.

Psychogenic Weakness

An experienced examiner should be able to differentiate real weakness from psychogenic weakness. The primary characteristic of psychogenic weakness is that it is unpredictable and fluctuating. Muscle strength may suddenly give out when a limb is being evaluated. The patient has difficulty knowing the exact muscle strength expected and cannot adequately counter the examiner's resistance. This gives rise to a wavering, collapsing force. Tricks are useful to bring out the discrepancy in muscle performance. For example, if the weak thigh cannot lift off the chair in a seated position, then the legs should not swing up onto the mattress when being seated on the examining table. When the examiner suspects that weakness of shoulder abduction is feigned, the patient's arm is placed in abduction. With the examiner's hand on the elbows, the examiner can instruct the patient to push toward the ceiling. At first, the downward pressure is very light, and the patient is unable to move the examiner's hand toward the ceiling. However, the arm does not fall down either, and as the downward pressure is gradually increased, continued exhortation to push the examiner's hand upward results in increasing resistance to the downward pressure. The examiner ends up putting maximum weight on the outstretched arm, which remains in abduction. The logical conclusion is that the strength is normal. Patients do not realize this because they believe that because they did not move the examiner's hand upward, they must be weak.

CLINICAL INVESTIGATIONS IN MUSCULAR WEAKNESS

In the investigation of diseases of the motor unit, the most helpful tests are measurement of the serum concentration of creatine kinase (CK), electrodiagnosis, and muscle biopsy. These are available to all physicians. Genetic testing increasingly provides definitive diagnosis. In addition, if facilities are available, exercise testing can provide useful information.

Serum Creatine Kinase

The usefulness of measuring the serum CK concentration in the diagnosis of neuromuscular diseases is in differentiating between neurogenic disease, in which normal or mild to moderate elevations of CK may be seen, and myopathies, in which the CK concentration often is markedly increased. Notable exceptions exist. CK concentrations rarely may be elevated as high as *10 times normal in patients with spinal muscular atrophy*, and occasionally in those with ALS (see Chapter 98). Measurements of serial CK concentrations generally follow the progress of the disease. However, problems have been recognized with both of these uses. Foremost is the determination of the normal level. Race, gender, age, and activity level are important in determining normal values. All studies on CK concentration show that gender and race affect values. In a survey of 1500 hospital employees, using carefully standardized methods, it was possible to detect three populations, each with characteristic CK values. The upper limits of normal (97.5th percentile) were as follows:

- Black men only: 520 U/liter
- Black women, nonblack men: 345 U/liter
- Nonblack women: 145 U/liter

The nonblack population included Hispanics, Asians, and Caucasians. Because expression of the upper limit is as a percentile of the mean, by definition, 2.5% of the normal population will have levels above the upper limit of normal. Although this does not seem like a large proportion, in a town of 100,000, 2,500 people would have abnormal levels. The point is that the upper limit of normal CK concentration is not rigid and requires intelligent interpretation. Although the serum CK concentration can be useful in determining the course of an illness, judgment is required because changes in CK values do not always mirror the clinical condition. In treating inflammatory myopathies with immunosuppressive drugs or corticosteroids, a steadily declining CK concentration is reassuring, whereas concentrations that are creeping back up when the patient is presumably in remission may be concerning.

Serum CK concentrations are also useful for determining whether an illness is monophasic. A bout of myoglobinuria is usually associated with very high concentrations of CK. The concentration then declines steadily by approximately 50% every 2 days. This pattern indicates that a single episode of muscle damage has occurred. Patients with CK concentrations that do not decline in this fashion or that vary from high to low on random days have an ongoing illness. Finally, exercise may cause a marked elevation in CK, which usually peaks 12 to 18 hours after the activity but may occur days later. CK concentrations are more likely to increase in people who are sedentary and then undertake unaccustomed exercise than in a trained individual.

Electromyography

The EMG study is an operator-sensitive study, and an experienced electromyographer is essential to perform and interpret an EMG correctly. Chapter 35 discusses the principles of EMG. The EMG study may provide much useful information. An initial step in the assessment of the weak patient is to localize the abnormality in the motor unit: neuropathic, myopathic, or neuromuscular junction. Nerve conduction studies and needle electrode examination are particularly useful for identifying neuropathic disorders and localizing the abnormality to anterior horn cells, roots, plexus, or peripheral nerve territories (see Chapters 98, 106, and 107). Repetitive nerve stimulation and single-fiber EMG can aid in elucidating disorders of the neuromuscular junction. Needle electrode examination may help distinguish between the presence of abnormal muscle versus nerve activity, depending on the presence of acute and chronic denervation, myotonia, neuromyotonia, fasciculations, cramps, and myokymia.

inheritance. Acute infantile SMA (*Werdnig–Hoffmann disease*) is a severe and usually fatal illness characterized by marked weakness of the limbs and respiratory muscles. Children with the intermediate form of SMA (chronic Werdnig–Hoffmann disease or spinal muscular atrophy type 2) also have severe weakness, rarely maintaining the ability to walk for more than a few years. The progression of the illness is not steady. The condition may plateau for some years, with periods of more rapid deterioration. Scoliosis is common. A fine tremor of the outstretched hands is characteristic. The chronic juvenile form of SMA (*Kugelberg–Welander syndrome*) begins sometime during the first decade of life, and patients walk well into the second decade or even into early adult life. Scoliosis is less common than in the infantile form. This condition is consistent with a normal lifespan. Finally, adult-onset SMA leads to slowly progressive proximal muscle weakness after the age of 20 years.

The inherited muscular dystrophies cause progressive, nonfluctuating weakness. Aside from the inherited distal muscular dystrophies discussed earlier in the chapter, other muscular dystrophies manifest with proximal muscle weakness. *Duchenne muscular dystrophy*, inherited as an X-linked recessive trait caused by mutations in the *DMD* gene, is associated with an absence of dystrophin. Clinically, the combination of proximal weakness in a male child with hypertrophic calf muscles and contractures of the Achilles tendons gives the clue to the diagnosis. The serum CK concentration is markedly elevated. Although muscle biopsy is diagnostic, genetic testing is now preferred to confirm the diagnosis (see Chapter 50). The clinical features of *Becker muscular dystrophy* are identical except for later onset and slower progression. Cardiomyopathy also is a feature. Female carriers of the gene usually are free of symptoms but may present with limb–girdle distribution weakness or cardiomyopathy.

The limb–girdle dystrophies constitute a well-accepted diagnostic classification despite their clinical and genetic heterogeneity. Weakness begins in the hips, shoulders, or both and spreads gradually to involve the rest of the limbs and the trunk. The genetics of these disorders is constantly expanding (see Chapter 50), and genetic testing is now available for many limb–girdle dystrophies.

Severe early-onset limb–girdle dystrophy similar in phenotype to Duchenne muscular dystrophy, including calf hypertrophy, occurs in the *sarcoglycanopathies*. The cause is a deficiency in one of the dystrophin-associated glycoproteins (sarcoglycans α, β, γ, and δ). The inheritance pattern in these disorders is autosomal recessive, not X-linked, and the sarcoglycanopathies affect both genders equally. Cardiac involvement is rare, and mental retardation is not part of the phenotype. Another cause of a severe Duchenne-like phenotype is mutation of the *FKRP* gene, also inherited in an autosomal recessive manner.

With less severe limb–girdle phenotypes, several genetic causes have been recognized, and inheritance is both autosomal recessive and autosomal dominant. In general, the phenotype in the autosomal recessive group is clinically more severe, with earlier onset of weakness and more rapid progression.

Diagnostic evaluation of limb–girdle muscular dystrophies is rapidly evolving and covered in greater depth in Chapter 110. Genetic testing for dystrophin, sarcoglycans, and other genes may be appropriate before performance of muscle biopsy. If the appropriate genetic tests are uninformative, then muscle biopsy is indicated. The biopsy specimen will show dystrophic changes, separating limb–girdle dystrophy from other (inflammatory) myopathies and from denervating diseases such as SMA. Immunohistochemical analysis of dystrophic muscle may provide a specific diagnosis, but not in all cases. Unfortunately, many patients with limb–girdle muscular dystrophies do not receive a specific diagnosis.

With the exception of Welander myopathy, predominantly lower-extremity weakness is the usual presentation of hereditary distal myopathies. Among these disorders are the Markesbery–Griggs–Udd, Nonaka, and Laing myopathies, which affect anterior compartment muscles in the leg, and Miyoshi myopathy, which affects predominantly the posterior calf muscles.

In patients with inclusion-body myositis, the quadriceps and forearm finger flexor muscles often are preferentially involved. In some patients, this involvement may be asymmetrical at the onset. The other inflammatory myopathies—polymyositis and dermatomyositis—affect proximal, predominantly hip–girdle muscles in a symmetrical fashion. Although rare, the Lambert–Eaton myasthenic syndrome manifests with proximal lower-extremity weakness in more than half of patients, similar to a myopathy. Hyporeflexia and autonomic and sensory symptoms may suggest the diagnosis. EMG often is diagnostic.

Ascending weakness of subacute onset with hyporeflexia, usually with numbness, is the hallmark of Guillain–Barré syndrome. The examiner should take care to look for a spinal sensory level and UMN signs, because a spinal cord lesion can mimic this presentation. When present, bulbar weakness is helpful in the diagnosis. Respiratory weakness may result. As discussed earlier, multiple neuromuscular causes of weakness of subacute onset with respiratory failure are recognized.

Distal muscle weakness and atrophy are the hallmarks of neurogenic disorders. In both the demyelinating and axonal forms of Charcot–Marie–Tooth disease, the problem in the legs antedates that in the hands. In ALS, the weakness often is asymmetrical and may combine with UMN signs.

Disorders with Fluctuating Weakness

An important consideration in the differential diagnosis is whether the weakness is constant or fluctuating. Even constant weakness may vary somewhat in degree, depending on how the patient feels. It is well recognized that an individual's physical performance is better on days when they feel energetic and cheerful and is less optimal on days when they feel depressed or are sick. Such factors can also be expected to affect the patient with neuromuscular weakness. The examiner should make specific inquiries to determine how much variability exists. Does the strength fluctuation relate to exercise or time of day? Symptoms and signs provoked by exercise imply a disorder in the physiological or biochemical mechanisms governing muscle contraction. Pain, contractures, and weakness after exercise often are characteristic of abnormalities in the biochemistry of muscle contraction. Pathological fatigue is the hallmark of neuromuscular junction abnormalities.

Factors other than exercise may result in worsening or improvement of the disease. Some patients notice that fasting, carbohydrate loading, or other dietary manipulations make a difference in their symptoms. Such details may provide a clue to underlying metabolic problems. Patients with a defect in lipid-based energy metabolism are weaker in the fasting state and may carry a candy bar or sugar with them. The patient with hypokalemic periodic paralysis may notice that inactivity after a high-carbohydrate meal precipitates an attack.

The usual cause of weakness that fluctuates markedly on a day-to-day basis or within a space of several hours is a defect in neuromuscular transmission, metabolic abnormality, or channel disorder (e.g., periodic paralysis), rather than one of the muscular dystrophies. Most neurologists recognize that the cardinal features of MG are ptosis, ophthalmoparesis, dysarthria, dysphagia, and proximal weakness (see Chapter 109). On clinical examination, the hallmark of MG is pathological muscle fatigue. Normal muscles fatigue if exercised sufficiently, but in MG, fatigue occurs with little effort. Failure of neuromuscular transmission may prevent holding the arms in an outstretched position for more than a few seconds or maintenance of sustained upgaze. Frequently the patient is relatively normal in the office, making the diagnosis of myasthenia more difficult; the history and ancillary studies (assay for acetylcholine receptor antibodies, anti-MuSK antibodies, and EMG with repetitive stimulation or single-fiber EMG) must be relied on to establish the diagnosis.

In the Lambert-Eaton myasthenic syndrome, fluctuating weakness also may occur, but the fluctuating character is less marked than in MG. Weakness of the shoulder and especially the hip girdle predominates, with the bulbar, ocular, and respiratory muscles relatively spared. Exceptions to this latter rule are recognized, and some presentations of Lambert-Eaton myasthenic syndrome mimic MG. Typically, reflexes are reduced or absent at rest. After a brief period of exercise, weakness and reflexes often are improved (facilitation), which is the opposite of the situation in MG. The electrophysiological correlate of this phenomenon is the demonstration of a marked incremental response to rapid, repetitive nerve stimulation or brief exercise. The underlying pathophysiology of Lambert-Eaton myasthenic syndrome is an autoimmune or paraneoplastic process mediated by anti–voltage-gated calcium channel antibodies; commercial testing for these antibodies is available.

Patients with periodic paralysis note attacks of weakness, typically provoked by rest after exercise (see Chapter 109). Inheritance of the primary periodic paralyses is as an autosomal dominant trait secondary to a sodium or calcium channel defect (see Chapter 99). In the hyperkalemic (sodium channel) form, patients experience weakness that may last from minutes to days; beginning in infancy to early childhood, the provocation is by rest after exercise or potassium ingestion. Potassium levels generally are high during an attack. In the hypokalemic (calcium channel) form, weakness may last hours to days, is quite severe beginning in the early teens, manifests more in males than in females, and the provocation is by rest after exercise or carbohydrate ingestion. Potassium levels generally are low during an attack.

Secondary hypokalemic periodic paralysis occurs in a subset of patients with thyrotoxicosis. The syndrome is clinically identical to primary hypokalemic periodic paralysis, except for the age at presentation, which usually is in adulthood. In both types of primary periodic paralysis, paralysis may be total, but with sparing of bulbofacial muscles. Respiratory muscle paralysis is rare in hypokalemic periodic paralysis. Patients with paramyotonia congenita also may experience attacks of weakness, especially in the cold. EMG with special protocols for exercise and cooling may be diagnostic; genetic testing also is available for these disorders.

Disorders Exacerbated by Exercise

Fatigue and muscle pain provoked by exercise, the most common complaints in patients presenting to the muscle clinic, often are unexplained. Diagnoses such as fibromyalgia (see Chapter 28) may confound the examination. Biochemical defects are being detected in an increasing number of patients with exercise-induced fatigue and myalgia. The metabolic abnormalities that impede exercise are disorders of carbohydrate metabolism, lipid metabolism, and mitochondrial function (see Chapter 110). The patient's history may give some clue to the type of defect.

Fatty acids provide the main source of energy for resting muscle. Initiation of vigorous exercise requires the use of intracellular stores of energy because blood-borne metabolites initially are inadequate. It takes time for the cardiac output to increase, for capillaries to dilate, and for the blood supply to muscle to be increased, and an even longer time to mobilize fat stores in the body in order to increase the level of fatty acids in the blood. Because muscle must use its glycogen stores for energy in this initial phase of heavy exercise, defects of glycogen metabolism cause fatigue and muscle pain in the first few minutes of exercise. As exercise continues, the blood supply increases, resulting in an increased supply of oxygen, glucose, and fatty acids. After 10 to 15 minutes, the muscle begins to use a mixture of fat and carbohydrate. The use of carbohydrate is not tolerated for long periods, however, because it would deplete the body's glycogen stores, potentially resulting in hypoglycemia. After 30 to 40 minutes of continued endurance exercise, the muscle is using chiefly fatty acids as an energy source. Patients with defective fatty acid metabolism easily tolerate the initial phase of exercise. With endurance exercise lasting 30 to 60 minutes, however, they may become incapacitated. Similarly, in the fasting state, the body is more dependent on fatty acids, which it uses to conserve glucose. Thus, the patient with a disorder of fatty acid metabolism may complain of increased symptoms when exercising in the fasting state. Ingestion of a candy bar may give some relief because this quickly boosts the blood glucose level. Patients with fatty acid metabolism defects often have well-developed muscles, because they prefer relatively intense, brief, power exercise such as weight lifting.

Disorders of mitochondrial metabolism vary in presentation. In some types, recurrent encephalopathic episodes occur, often noted in early childhood and resembling Reye disease (see Chapter 93). In other types, particular weakness of the extraocular and skeletal muscles is a presenting feature. In still other types, usually affecting young adults, the symptoms are predominantly of exercise intolerance. Defects occur in the electron transport system or cytochrome chain that uncouples oxygen consumption from the useful production of adenosine triphosphate (ATP). The resulting limit on available ATP causes metabolic pathways to operate at their maximum with even a light exercise load. Resting tachycardia, high lactic acid levels in the blood, excessive sweating, and other indications of hypermetabolism may be noted. This clinical picture may lead to an erroneous diagnosis of hyperthyroidism. It is essential always to measure the serum lactic acid concentration when a mitochondrial myopathy is suspected, even though the level is normal in some patients. In addition to lactate, ammonia and hypoxanthine concentrations also may be elevated.

Patients with suspected metabolic defects should undergo forearm exercise testing. A blood pressure cuff should not be used for the ischemic portion of the test, because this may be hazardous in patients with defects in the glycolytic pathway.

Disorders with Constant Weakness

With disorders characterized by constant weakness, the course is one of stability or steady deterioration. Without treatment, periods of sustained objective improvement or major differences in strength on a day-to-day basis are lacking. The division of this group of disorders into subacute and chronic also needs clarification. *Subacute* means that weakness appeared over weeks to months in a previously healthy person. In contrast, *chronic* implies a much less definite onset and prolonged course. Although the patient may say that the weakness came on suddenly, a careful history elicits symptoms that go back many years. This division is not absolute. Patients with polymyositis, usually a subacute disease, may have a slow course mimicking a muscular dystrophy. Patients with a muscular dystrophy may have a slow decrease in strength but suddenly lose a specific function such as standing from a chair or climbing stairs and believe their deterioration to be acute in onset.

Acquired Disorders Causing Weakness

The usual acquired disorders that produce weakness are motor neuron diseases; inflammatory, toxic, or endocrine disorders of muscle; neuromuscular transmission disorders; and peripheral neuropathies with predominantly motor involvement. The first task is to determine whether the weakness is neuropathic, myopathic, or secondary to a neuromuscular transmission defect. In some instances this is straightforward, and in others it is very difficult. For instance, some cases of motor neuron disease with predominantly LMN dysfunction may mimic inclusion-body myositis, and Lambert–Eaton myasthenic syndrome may mimic polymyositis. If fasciculations are present, the disorder must be neuropathic. If reflexes are absent and muscle bulk is preserved, suspect a demyelinating neuropathy, although presynaptic neuromuscular junction disorders (e.g., Lambert–Eaton myasthenic syndrome) also show hyporeflexia with normal muscle bulk. The presence of sensory signs or symptoms, even if mild, may indicate a peripheral neuropathy or involvement of the CNS. Often, separating these conditions requires serum CK testing, EMG, and muscle biopsy.

ALS is the most common acquired motor neuron disease. Although peak age at onset is from 65 to 70 years, the disorder can occur at any adult age. It often follows a relatively rapid course preceded by cramps and fasciculations. Examination shows muscle atrophy and often widely distributed fasciculations. If the bulbar muscles are involved, difficulties with swallowing and speaking also are present. The diagnosis is relatively simple if unequivocal evidence of UMN dysfunction accompanies muscle atrophy and fasciculations. UMN signs include slowness of movement, hyper-reflexia, Babinski sign, and spasticity. A weak, atrophic muscle associated with an abnormally brisk reflex is almost pathognomonic for ALS. The finding of widespread denervation on needle electrode examination in the absence of any sensory abnormalities or demyelinating features on nerve conduction testing supports the diagnosis. In all patients without bulbar involvement, it is important to rule out spinal pathology, because the combination of cervical and lumbar stenosis occasionally may mimic ALS with respect to clinical and electrophysiological findings.

In patients with only LMN dysfunction, it is essential to exclude the rare diagnosis of *multifocal motor neuropathy with conduction block*, a condition usually treatable with intravenous gamma globulin. Patients with multifocal motor neuropathy with conduction block usually have no bulbar features or UMN signs, and a characteristic finding includes demyelination (i.e., conduction block) on motor nerve conduction testing. Because the underlying pathophysiological process is conduction block, weakness usually is more severe than expected for the observed degree of atrophy. However, atrophy occurs, especially when the condition is of long duration.

Although most adults with motor neuron disease have ALS or one of its variants, sporadic forms of adult-onset SMA and especially X-linked spinobulbar muscular atrophy (Kennedy's Disease) can occur as well. In these cases, the progression of weakness is much slower, and UMN involvement is absent. Of importance, these latter cases, especially Kennedy disease, often have elevated CK levels in the range of 500 to 1500 U/liter.

If the patient has a myopathy, acquired and inherited causes should be considered. A discussion of the presentation of inherited myopathic disorders appears earlier in the chapter. Causes of acquired myopathies include inflammatory conditions and a large number of toxic, drug-induced, and endocrine disorders. Inflammatory myopathies include polymyositis, dermatomyositis, and inclusion-body myositis and often run a steadily progressive course, although some fluctuations occur, particularly in children. Onset of weakness in polymyositis and dermatomyositis is subacute, weakness is proximal, and serum CK levels usually are increased. If an associated rash is present, little doubt exists about the diagnosis of dermatomyositis. If a rash is absent, polymyositis may be difficult to differentiate clinically from any of the other causes of proximal weakness. Sometimes the illness occurs as part of an overlap syndrome in which fragments of other autoimmune diseases (e.g., scleroderma, lupus, rheumatoid arthritis) are involved. Polymyositis sometimes is difficult to differentiate from a muscular dystrophy, even after muscle biopsy; some inflammatory changes occur in muscular dystrophies, most notably in FSH muscular dystrophy. Other signs of systemic involvement such as malaise, transitory aching pains, mood changes, and loss of appetite are more common in polymyositis than in limb–girdle dystrophy.

Inclusion-body myopathy typically has a chronic, insidious onset. It occasionally mimics polymyositis but more often mimics ALS associated with LMN dysfunction. Clues to the diagnosis are male gender, onset after the age of 50 years in most patients, slower progression, and characteristic involvement of the quadriceps and long finger flexors. Some patients may have proximal muscle weakness, as in polymyositis, whereas others may have predominantly distal weakness mimicking that of ALS and other neuropathic conditions. Serum CK generally is elevated but occasionally may be normal. As with other chronic inflammatory myopathies, interpreting the EMG study may be difficult and requires an experienced examiner, because inclusion-body myopathy often shows a combination of myopathic and neuropathic features. Inclusion-body myopathy, unlike polymyositis, often is unresponsive to immunosuppressive therapy. Pathological features include rimmed vacuoles and intracytoplasmic and intranuclear filamentous inclusions.

Toxic, drug-induced, and endocrine disorders are always considerations in the differential diagnosis of acquired myopathies. Among toxins, alcohol is still one of the most common and may produce both an acute and a chronic myopathic syndrome. Several prescription medicines are associated with myopathies. Most prominent are corticosteroids, cholesterol-lowering agents (i.e., statins), and colchicine.

Although neuromuscular transmission disorders are always diagnostic considerations in patients with fluctuating symptoms, the Lambert–Eaton myasthenic syndrome may be an exception. It often manifests with progressive proximal lower-extremity weakness without fluctuations. Clues to the diagnosis include a history of cancer, especially small-cell lung cancer (although in many patients the myasthenic syndrome may predate the discovery of the cancer), hyporeflexia, facilitation of strength and reflexes after brief exercise, and coexistent autonomic symptoms, especially urinary and sexual dysfunction in men.

Sensory features separate peripheral neuropathies from disorders of the motor unit. The notable exception is multifocal motor neuropathy with conduction block, discussed earlier. Other neuropathies also may manifest with predominantly motor symptoms. Among these are toxic neuropathies (from dapsone, vincristine, or lead, or an acute alcohol-related neuropathy) and some variants of Guillain–Barré syndrome (especially the acute motor axonal neuropathy syndrome).

Lifelong Disorders

Most patients presenting to the neuromuscular clinic will have lifelong or at least very chronic, presumably inherited, disorders. These include inherited disorders of muscle (e.g., dystrophies, congenital myopathies), anterior horn cell (e.g., spinal muscular atrophies), peripheral nerves (e.g., Charcot–Marie–Tooth polyneuropathy), or very rarely, neuromuscular transmission (e.g., congenital myasthenic syndromes). In some of these disorders, the responsible genetic abnormality has been identified. An important point in the differential diagnosis is to determine whether the weakness is truly progressive. The examiner should ask questions until the progressive or nonprogressive nature of the disease is ascertained. The severity of the disease is not proof of progression. It is difficult to imagine that a 16-year-old girl confined to her wheelchair with spinal muscular atrophy and scoliosis and having difficulty breathing has a relatively nonprogressive disorder, but careful questioning may reveal no loss of function for several years. Furthermore, it is not sufficient to ask the patient in vague and general terms whether the illness is progressive. Questioning should be specific; for example, "Are there tasks you cannot perform now that you could perform last week (month, year)?" The examiner also must be alert for denial, which is common in young patients with increasing weakness. The 18-year-old boy with limb–girdle dystrophy may claim to be the same now as in years gone by, but questioning may reveal that he was able to climb stairs well when he was in high school, whereas he now needs assistance in college.

Lifelong Nonprogressive Disorders

Some patients complain of lifelong weakness that has been relatively unchanged over many years. Almost by definition, such disorders have to start in early childhood. Nonprogression of weakness does not preclude severe weakness. Later-life progression of such weakness may occur as the normal aging process further weakens muscles that have little functional reserve. One major group of such illnesses is the congenital nonprogressive myopathies, including central core disease, nemaline myopathy, and congenital fiber-type disproportion. The typical clinical picture in these diseases is that of a slender dysmorphic patient with diffuse weakness (Fig. 27.10). Other features may include skeletal abnormalities such as high-arched palate, pes cavus, and scoliosis, which are supportive of the presence of weakness in early life. Deep tendon reflexes are depressed or absent. Though unusual, severe respiratory involvement may occur in all these diseases. The less severe (non-X-linked) form of myotubular (centronuclear) myopathy is suggested by findings of ptosis, extraocular muscle weakness, and facial diplegia. Muscle biopsy usually provides a specific morphological diagnosis in the congenital myopathies; specific genetic testing is now available for many of the congenital myopathies. Several varieties of congenital muscular dystrophy (CMD) are recognized. The weakness in CMD manifests in the newborn period, with the affected child presenting as a floppy baby. Skeletal deformities and contractures may be present. CNS abnormalities, including cognitive impairment, seizures, and structural brain or eye abnormalities may be present. The classification is based on the involved protein function and causative gene mutation. The main CMD subtypes, grouped by the involved protein function and gene in which causative mutations occur, include defects in structural proteins, glycosylation, proteins of the endoplasmic reticulum and nuclear envelope, and mitochondrial membrane proteins. The disorders with CNS structural abnormalities are very severe; for example, characteristics of Fukuyama CMD include microcephaly, mental retardation, and seizures

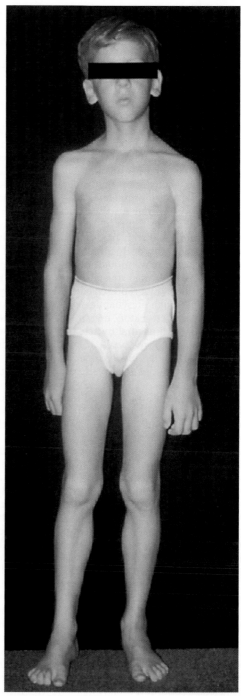

Fig. 27.10 The patient with a congenital myopathy is slender, without focal atrophy. Shoulder–girdle weakness is apparent from the horizontal set of the clavicles.

with severe disability. The serum CK concentration may be markedly elevated in CMDs. The muscle biopsy specimen shows dystrophic changes, and immunohistochemistry often provides a specific diagnosis. Tests for some of the gene mutations are commercially available.

Lifelong Disorders Characterized by Progressive Weakness

Most diseases in the category of lifelong disorders characterized by progressive weakness are inherited progressive disorders of anterior horn cells, peripheral motor nerve, or muscle.

Among these are the spinal muscular atrophies, Charcot–Marie–Tooth polyneuropathies, and muscular dystrophies. Mild day-to-day fluctuations in strength may occur in these disorders, but the overall progression is steady (i.e., the disorder is slowly progressive from the start and remains that way); it will not suddenly change course and become rapidly progressive. As mentioned earlier, patients may experience long periods of stability when their disease is seemingly nonprogressive.

Traditional attempts to categorize disorders are based on whether the disorder is caused by anterior horn cell, peripheral motor nerve, or muscle disease, along with a specific pattern of muscle weakness. Certain characteristic patterns of weakness often suggest specific diagnoses. For example, the names of FSH and oculopharyngeal muscular dystrophies reflect their selective involvement of muscles. Today, all disorders are redefined and categorized in accordance with their specific genetic abnormality.

Other Conditions

No scheme of analysis is perfect in clinical medicine, and many exceptions to the guidelines provided earlier exist. Most notable are disorders restricted to various parts of the body. The etiology for such localized illness is often unclear, but may represent a form fruste of a disorder with a specific gene defect. Examples include branchial myopathy and quadriceps myopathy, as well as the focal forms of motor neuron disease such as benign monomelic amyotrophy. These diseases often are "benign" in that they do not shorten life. The weakness may cause disability, although it is usually mild.

REFERENCES

The complete reference list is available online at http://expertconsult .inkling.com.

28 Muscle Pain and Cramps

Leo H. Wang, Glenn Lopate, Alan Pestronk

CHAPTER OUTLINE

GENERAL FEATURES OF PAIN

MUSCLE PAIN: BASIC CONCEPTS
  Nociceptor Terminal Stimulation and Sensitization
  Nociceptive Axons

CLINICAL FEATURES OF MUSCLE PAIN
  General Features of Muscle Pain
  Evaluation of Muscle Discomfort

MUSCLE DISCOMFORT: SPECIFIC CAUSES
  Myopathies with Muscle Pain
  Muscle Cramps
  Other Involuntary Muscle Contraction Syndromes
  Myalgia Syndromes without Chronic Myopathy

GENERAL FEATURES OF PAIN

Pain is an uncomfortable sensation with sensory and emotional components. Short episodes of pain or discomfort localized to muscle are a near universal experience. Common causes of short-term muscle discomfort are unaccustomed exercise, trauma, cramps, and systemic infections. Chronic muscle discomfort is also relatively common. In the population of the United States aged 25 to 74 years, 10% to 14% have chronic pain related to the joints and musculoskeletal system. Pain localized to muscle may be due to noxious stimuli in muscle or referral from other structures including skin, nerves, connective tissue, joints, and bone. Common syndromes with pain localized to muscle but no histological muscle pathology include fibromyalgia and small-fiber neuropathies. The referral of pain from other structures to muscle may involve stimulation of central neural pathways or secondary noxious contraction of muscle.

The best categorization of pain in muscle and other tissues is by temporal and qualitative features. Cutaneous pain is thought to be subjectively experienced as two phases: the first phase perceived as sharp, well-localized, and lasting as long as the stimulus. A delayed second phase of pain is experienced as dull, aching or burning, and more diffuse. In contrast to cutaneous pain, visceral, muscular, or chronic pain is more likely experienced subjectively similar to the second phase of cutaneous pain, and has more sensory and affective components. Pain from stimulation of diseased tissue is often associated with *hyperalgesia*, in which a noxious stimulus produces an exaggerated pain sensation, or with *allodynia*, pain induced by a normally innocuous stimulus.

Sensitization is the reduction of the pain threshold and can be the result of changes in molecular composition, cellular interactions, and network connectivity throughout the pain system. Neuropathic pain, localized to muscle or other tissues, is associated with increased afferent axon activity and occurs spontaneously or after peripheral stimuli. It may be related to central or peripheral sensitization.

MUSCLE PAIN: BASIC CONCEPTS

Generation of pain localized to muscle involves activation of afferent axons, conduction of pain signals through the peripheral and central nervous systems (PNS and CNS), and central processing of properties of the afferent signals.

Nociceptor Terminal Stimulation and Sensitization

Stimuli of afferent axons can be mechanical or chemical (for review see Mense, 2009). Mechanosensory transduction is mediated by mechanosensitive ion channels such as the transient receptor potential vanilloid 4 (TRPV4) channel or members of the degenerin/epithelial sodium channel (DEG/ENaC) family. Endogenous chemical stimuli of muscle nociceptors include protons (H^+) and adenosine triphosphate (ATP), which are increased in muscle with damage. In humans, injection of acidic buffered solution into muscle elicits pain. Acid-sensing ion channels (ASICs) are a subfamily of the DEG/ENaC superfamily. ASIC1 and ASIC3 are expressed on sensory axons innervating skeletal and cardiac muscles. ASIC3 may initiate the anginal pain associated with myocardial ischemia. The heat and capsaicin receptor TRPV1 can also be activated under strong acidic conditions.

The second important chemical cause of muscle pain is ATP. ATP is present in increased levels in muscle interstitium during ischemic muscle contraction. Injection of ATP also elicits pain. Many peripheral nociceptors express ATP purinergic receptors. In muscle, ATP primarily activates the $P2X_2$ and $P2X_3$ receptors. $P2X_3/P2X_{2/3}$ receptor antagonists can reverse mechanical hyperalgesia that occurs with inflammation.

Other chemical substances (bradykinin, serotonin, prostaglandin E2 (PGE2), and NGF) that most likely do not activate pain afferents at physiological levels can induce pain at supraphysiological levels, or can sensitize peripheral nociceptive afferents. Sensitization of nociceptive axon terminals is reduction of the threshold for their stimulation into the innocuous range. Sensitization of nociceptor terminals can have two effects on axons: (1) an increase in the frequency of action potentials in normally active nociceptors or (2) induction of new action potentials in a population of normally silent small axons.

Bradykinin, serotonin, and prostaglandins are normally sequestered in normal tissue and increase in damaged tissue. Bradykinin is the protease product of the plasma protein kallidin. In damaged tissue, kallidin is exposed to and cleaved by tissue kallikreins forming bradykinin. Serotonin is normally stored in platelets and is released when the platelets are in damaged tissue. Bradykinin and serotonin are only mildly painful when injected into human muscle. Bradykinin produces more pain after the injection of PGE2 or serotonin.

PGE2 is present in delayed onset muscle soreness (DOMS). PGE2 is released from endothelial and other tissue cells. The depression of muscle nociceptor activity by aspirin may reflect inhibition of the effects of PGE2.

Endogenous substances proposed to play roles in activating or sensitizing peripheral nociceptive afferents include neurotransmitters (serotonin, histamine, glutamate, nitric oxide, adrenaline), neuropeptides (substance P, neurokinin 1, brady-kinin, nerve growth factor (NGF), calcitonin gene-related peptide), and inflammatory mediators (prostaglandins, cytokines). In humans, intramuscular injection of glutamate, capsaicin, levoascorbic acid, acromelic acid-A (a kainoid mushroom toxin), hypertonic saline (sodium chloride 5%–6%), and potassium chloride causes pain. Glutamate is an important neurotransmitter in the CNS pain pathway, and peripherally, is probably more important in sensitizing muscle afferents. Increased levels of glutamate in muscle correlate temporally with the appearance of pain after exercise or experimental injections of hypertonic saline. There are no specific membrane receptors for hypertonic saline (sodium chloride 5%–6%) and potassium chloride; they activate muscle nociceptors through changing membrane equilibrium potential.

Lactate, an anaerobic metabolite, probably does not play a primary role in directly stimulating muscle pain. Patients with myophosphorylase deficiency do not produce lactate under ischemia yet experience pain. Lactate may potentiate the effects of H^+ ions on ASIC3 channels in activating pain-related axons.

Many receptors that respond to chemical stimuli are also activated by changes in temperature: TRPA1 (ankyrin-repeat transient receptor potential) receptors are activated by cold temperatures, TRPV1 and TRPV3 by warm temperatures. Gain-of-function TRPA1 mutations are associated with familial episodic pain syndromes (Kremeyer et al., 2010).

No matter what the stimuli, the propagation of generated pain signal is dependent on sodium channels. Important sodium channels expressed in muscle nociceptive afferents include the tetrodotoxin-sensitive sodium channel (Na_v) 1.7 (*SCN9A*) and the tetrodotoxin-resistant sodium channels $Na_v1.8$ and 1.9 (*SCN10A* and *SCN11A*, respectively). Mutations in genes for these channels may cause loss or increase of pain (Waxman and Zamponi, 2014).

Nociceptive Axons

Many of the afferent axons that transmit painful stimuli from muscle (nociceptors) have free nerve endings (see excellent review by Mense and Gerwin, 2010). These free nerve endings do not have corpuscular receptive structures such as pacinian or paciniform corpuscles. They appear as a "string of beads," thin stretches of axon (with diameters of 0.5–1.0 µm) with intervening varicosities. Most free nerve endings are ensheathed by a single layer of Schwann cells that leave bare some of the axon membranes, where only the basal membrane of the Schwann cell separates the axon membrane from the interstitial fluid. A single fiber has several branches that extend over a broad area. These terminal axons (nerve endings) end near the perimysium, adventitia of arterioles, venules, and lymphatic vessels, but do not contact muscle fibers (see Fig. 28.1, *A*). It is not clear whether nociceptive afferents can have both cutaneous and muscle branches. The varicosities in the free terminals contain granular or dense core vesicles containing glutamate and neuropeptides such as substance P (SP), vasoactive intestinal peptide (VIP), calcitonin gene-related peptide (CGRP), and somatostatin. When the afferents are activated, neuropeptides are released into the interstitial tissue and may activate other nearby muscle nociceptors.

Action potentials arising in nociceptor terminals induce or potentiate pain by two mechanisms: *centripetal conduction* to central branches of afferent axons brings nociceptive signals directly to the CNS. *Centrifugal conduction* of action potentials along peripheral axon branches causes indirect effects by activating other unstimulated nerve terminals of the same nerve and causing release of glutamate and neuropeptides into the extracellular medium. These chemical substances can stimulate or sensitize terminals on other nociceptive axons. This is the basis for the axon reflex and the wheal and flare around a cutaneous lesion.

Group III (class Aδ cutaneous afferent) thinly myelinated and group IV (class C cutaneous afferent) unmyelinated afferent axons conduct the pain-inducing stimuli from muscle to the CNS. Group III nociceptive axons are thinly myelinated and conduct impulses at moderately slow velocities (3–13 m/sec). Group III fibers can end in free nerve terminals (possibly for mediating a more spontaneous pain) or other receptors such as paciniform corpuscles. Group IV fibers are unmyelinated, conduct impulses at very slow velocities (0.6–1.2 m/sec), end as free nerve endings, and are the main mediators of the diffuse, dull, or burning muscle pain.

Group II axons are large and myelinated, and conduct impulses at rapid velocities, mainly from muscle spindles. They normally mediate innocuous stimuli, and stimulation may reduce the perception of pain (by acting on the nociceptive afferents in the spinal cord). Inflammation or repetitive stimulation can sensitize group II afferents (phenotypic switch), which then mediate mechanical allodynia in some tissues.

The cell bodies of all afferents are located in the dorsal root ganglion; the central process enters the CNS through the dorsal root (Fig. 28.2). Central terminals of nociceptive axons from muscle end in lamina I of the superficial dorsal horn and laminae IV–VI of the neck of the dorsal horn of the spinal cord. Cutaneous afferents end in the same areas, but in addition can also terminate in lamina II. Dorsal horn neurons have convergent inputs from afferents from both muscle and skin, and therefore activation of cutaneous afferents may be experienced as muscle pain.

Glutamate is the main neurotransmitter of pain in the CNS and binds NMDA and AMPA receptors. With short-lasting or low-frequency discharges, glutamate is only able to activate AMPA receptors, causing short-lasting and ineffective depolarization of the dorsal horn neuron. Additional inhibitory signals are also present to suppress the conductance of the pain signal: (1) inhibitory signal from the group II myelinated peripheral afferent; and (2) the inhibitory descending pain tracts which contact the central process of the peripheral afferent using glycine and GABA as inhibitory neurotransmitters. With long-lasting and high-frequency discharges, persistent glutamate signal activates NMDA receptors which have been shown to be critically important in the development of chronic nociceptive hypersensitivity. In addition, SP, when released, activates NK1 receptors which lead to increased NMDA receptor conductivity and de novo expression of NMDA receptors. Functional changes in AMPA/NMDA receptor activity are one mechanism resulting in central sensitization. Other mechanisms include metabolic changes in neurons and surrounding glia, and changes in synaptic structure.

Dorsal horn neurons convey pain signals primarily through the contralateral lateral spinothalamic tract, with minor projections through the spinoreticular and spinomesencephalic tracts. The spinothalamic tract terminates in the lateral thalamic nuclei and then relays to the primary and secondary somatosensory cortex, prefrontal cortex (for cognitive and affective pain), anterior cingulate cortex, and insular cortex.

The spinoreticular tract relays information to the medial nuclei of the thalamus, and mediates the autonomic component of pain sensations. The spinomesencephalic tract projects to the amygdala (which processes the emotional and memory aspect of pain).

Afferents conveying muscle pain have different midbrain and thalamic relays than do cutaneous afferents and activate different cortical areas. In addition, interneurons and descending CNS pathways modulate muscle afferents differently than

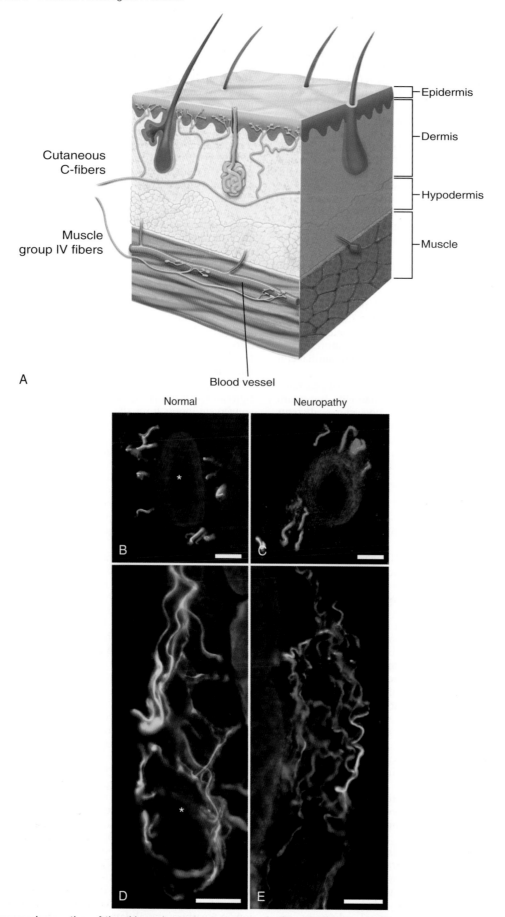

Fig. 28.1 Sensory innervation of the skin and muscle. A, C-fiber and group IV fiber innervation of the skin and muscle. **B–E,** Double label staining (yellow) of nonmyelinating Schwann cell cytoplasm by NCAM (red) and unmyelinated axons by peripherin (green) is much more abundant in the blood vessels (labeled with *) of normal muscle compared to muscle from a patient with small fiber neuropathy where the majority of Schwann cell processes are devoid of axons (bar = 20 μm). *(Courtesy of Amir Dori, Glenn Lopate, and Alan Pestronk.)*

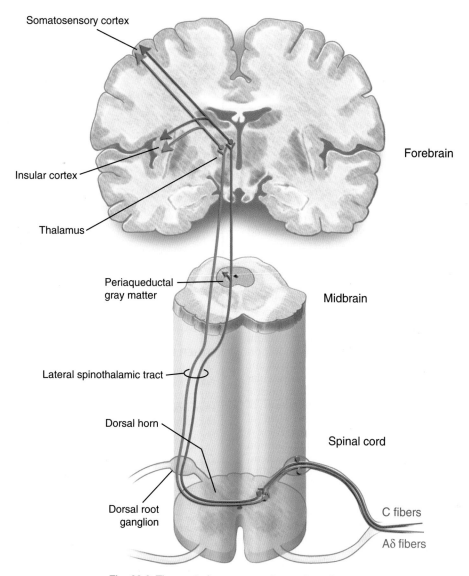

Somatosensory cortex

Forebrain

Insular cortex

Thalamus

Periaqueductal
gray matter

Midbrain

Lateral spinothalamic tract

Dorsal horn

Spinal cord

Dorsal root
ganglion

C fibers

Aδ fibers

Fig. 28.2 The central nervous system pain pathway.

cutaneous afferents. For example, descending antinociceptive pathways that originate in the mesencephalon with connections in the medulla and spinal cord are an important modulator of pain and may be stronger for muscle afferents.

CLINICAL FEATURES OF MUSCLE PAIN
General Features of Muscle Pain

In the clinical setting, patients describe muscle discomfort using a variety of terms: pain, soreness, aching, fatigue, cramps, or spasms. Pain with muscle cramps has an acute onset and short duration. Cramp pain is associated with palpable muscle contraction, and stretching the muscle provides immediate relief. Pain originating from fascia and periosteum has relatively precise localization. Cutaneous pain differs from muscle pain by its distinct localization and sharp, pricking, stabbing, or burning nature. Pain with small-fiber neuropathies is often present outside length-dependent distributions and may be located in proximal as well as distal regions. In fibromyalgia syndromes, it is common for patients to complain that fatigue accompanies their muscle discomfort. Depression is more common in patients with chronic

musculoskeletal pain (18%) than in a population without chronic pain (8%).

Evaluation of Muscle Discomfort

The basis for the classification of disorders underlying muscle discomfort can be anatomical, temporal in relation to exercise, muscle pathology, and the presence or absence of active muscle contraction during the discomfort (Pestronk, 2014). Evaluation of muscle discomfort typically begins with a history that includes the type, localization, inducing factors, and evolution of the pain; drug use; and mood disorders. The physical examination requires special attention to the localization of any tenderness or weakness. The pain may produce the appearance of weakness by preventing full effort. Typical of this type of "weakness" on examination is sudden reduction in the apparent level of effort, rather than smooth movement through the range of motion expected with true muscle weakness. The sensory examination is important because small-fiber neuropathies commonly cause discomfort with apparent localization in muscle. A general examination is needed to evaluate the possibility that pain may be arising from other tissues such as joints. Blood studies may include creatine kinase (CK), aldolase, complete blood cell count, sedimentation rate, potassium, magnesium, calcium, phosphate, lactate, thyroid functions, and evaluation for systemic immune disorders. CK values of African Americans are higher than those of other races (up to three times higher than Caucasian Americans) (Kenney et al., 2012). Evaluate urine myoglobin in patients with a high CK and severe myalgias, especially when they relate to exercise. Electromyography (EMG) may suggest myopathy or if normal may indicate that muscle pain is arising from anatomical loci other than muscle. Nerve conduction studies may detect an underlying neuropathy, but objective documentation of small-fiber neuropathies can require quantitative sensory testing or skin biopsy with staining of intraepidermal nerves. We have recently developed a novel staining technique of small nerve fibers that quantitates perivascular innervation, and shows there is reduced innervation of blood vessels within muscle in patients with small-fiber neuropathy (see Fig. 28.1, *B–E*) (Dori et al., 2015).

Magnetic resonance imaging could show increased muscle signal on fast spin echo T2 fat-saturated or short-tau inversion recovery (STIR) sequences. Muscle ultrasound can be a useful and noninvasive method of localizing and defining types of muscle pathology. Muscle biopsy is most often useful in the presence of another abnormal test result such as a high serum CK, aldolase, lactate, or an abnormal EMG. However, important clues to treatable disorders such as fasciitis or systemic immune disorders (connective tissue pathology, perivascular inflammation, or granulomas) may be present in muscle in the absence of other positive testing. Examination of both muscle and connective tissue increases the yield of muscle biopsy in syndromes with muscle discomfort. There is increased diagnostic yield from muscle biopsies if in addition to routine morphological analysis and processing, histochemical analysis includes staining for acid phosphatase, alkaline phosphatase, esterase, mitochondrial enzymes, glycolytic enzymes, C_{5b-9} complement, and MHC Class I. Measurement of oxidative enzyme activities can reveal evidence of mitochondrial disease as a cause of muscle discomfort or fatigue, even in disorders with no histopathological abnormalities. While disorders of glycogen and lipid metabolism often result in abnormal muscle histochemistry, deficiencies in some enzymes (e.g., phosphoglycerate kinase or carnitine palmitoyltransferase (CPT) II deficiencies) may not cause muscle pathology and diagnosis is best made by genetic testing. Ultrastructural examination of muscle rarely provides additional information in muscle pain syndromes.

MUSCLE DISCOMFORT: SPECIFIC CAUSES

Muscle pain is broadly divisible into groups depending on its origin and relation to the time of muscle contraction. Myopathies may be associated with muscle pain without associated muscle contraction (myalgias) (Boxes 28.1 and 28.2). Muscle pain during muscle activity (Box 28.3; also see Box 28.2) may occur with muscle injury, myopathy, cramps, or tonic (relatively long-term) contraction. Some pain syndromes perceived as arising from muscle originate in other tissues, such as connective tissue, nerve, or bone, or have no clear morphological explanation for the pain (Box 28.4).

Myopathies with Muscle Pain

Myopathies that produce muscle pain (see Box 28.1) are usually associated with weakness, a high serum CK or aldolase, or an abnormal EMG (Pestronk, 2014). Immune-mediated or inflammatory myopathies may produce muscle pain or tenderness, especially with an associated systemic connective

---

BOX 28.1 Myopathic Pain Syndromes*

INFLAMMATORY

Inflammatory and immune myopathies:
  Systemic connective tissue disease
  Perimysial pathology: tRNA synthetase antibodies
  Fasciitis
  Childhood dermatomyositis
Muscle infections:
  Viral myositis
  Pyomyositis
  Toxoplasmosis
  Trichinosis

RHABDOMYOLYSIS ± METABOLIC DISORDER

Glycogen storage disease type V (Myophosphorylase deficiency): McArdle disease
Glycogen storage disease type VII (Phosphofructokinase deficiency)
Carnitine palmitoyltransferase II
Mitochondrial myopathies
Malignant hyperthermia syndromes
Familial Recurrent Rhabdomyolysis (Myoglobinuria) in Childhood (LPIN1 mutations)

OTHER MYOPATHIES WITH PAIN OR DISCOMFORT

Myopathy with tubular aggregates ± cylindrical spirals
Adult-onset nemaline rod myopathy
Multicore disease
Fiber-type disproportion myopathy
Myopathy with deficiency of iron-sulfur clusters
Myopathy with tubulin-reactive crystalline inclusions
Myopathy with hexagonally cross-linked crystalloid inclusions
Myoadenylate deaminase deficiency
Neuromyopathy with internalized capillaries
Myotonias: myotonic dystrophy 2; dominant myotonia congenita (occasional)
Muscular dystrophies (occasional): Duchenne, Becker, limb-girdle dystrophy types 1A, 1C, 2C, 2D, 2E, 2H, 2I, 2L; ANO5-deficient myopathy
Selenium deficiency
Vitamin D deficiency
Toxic myopathy: eosinophilia myalgia, rhabdomyolysis
Hypothyroid myopathy
Mitochondrial disorders (fatigue or myalgias with exercise)
Camurati-Engelmann syndrome (bone pain)

DRUGS AND TOXINS

*Usual associated features: weakness, abnormal electromyogram.

---

tissue disease or pathological involvement of connective tissue (including myopathies with anti-tRNA synthetase antibodies). Pain is common in childhood dermatomyositis, immune myopathies associated with systemic disorders, eosinophilia-myalgia syndromes, focal myositis, and infections. Myopathies due to direct infections (e.g., bacterial, viral, toxoplasmosis, trichinosis) are usually painful. Metabolic myopathies, including myophosphorylase and CPT II deficiencies, typically produce muscle discomfort or fatigue with exercise and less prominently at rest. As a rule, disorders of carbohydrate utilization (e.g., myophosphorylase deficiency) produce pain and fatigue after short, intense exercise, whereas lipid disorders (e.g., CPT II deficiency) cause muscle discomfort with sustained exercise. Myophosphorylase deficiency causes exercise intolerance with myalgias, weakness, and painful contractures.

BOX 28.2 Muscle Discomfort Associated with Drugs and Toxins

INFLAMMATORY MYOPATHY

Definite:
  Hydralazine
  Penicillamine
  Procainamide
  1,1'-Ethylidinebis[tryptophan]
  Toxic oil syndrome
Possible:
  Cimetidine
  Imatinib mesylate
  Interferon-α
  Ipecac
  Lansoprazole
  Leuprolide
  Levodopa
  Penicillin
  Phenytoin
  Propylthiouracil
  Sulfonamide

RHABDOMYOLYSIS ± CHRONIC MYOPATHY

Alcohol
ε-Amino caproic acid
Amphetamines
Cocaine
Cyclosporine
Daptomycin
Hypokalemia
Isoniazid
Lipid-lowering agents*:
  Bezafibrate
  Clofibrate
  Fenofibrate
  Gemfibrozil
  Lovastatin
  Simvastatin
  Pravastatin
  Fluvastatin
  Atorvastatin
  Cerivastatin
  Nicotinic acid
  Red yeast rice
Labetalol
Lithium
Organophosphates
Propofol
Snake venom
Tacrolimus
Zidovudine

PAINFUL MYOPATHY ± RHABDOMYOLYSIS

Colchicine
Emetine
Fenoverine
Germanium
Hypervitaminosis E

Taxenes
Zidovudine

MYALGIA ± MYOPATHY

All-trans-retinoic acid
Amiodarone
Amphotericin
Azathioprine
Beta-blockers (rare)
Bryostatin 1
Bumetanide
Calcium channel blockers
Captopril
Cholesterol-lowering agents
Ciguatoxin
Corticosteroid withdrawal
Cytotoxics
Danazol
Enalapril
Estrogen
Gemcitabine
Gold
Interferon-α: 2a and 2b
Isotretinoin
Ketorolac
Laxatives
Methotrexate[†]
Mercury (organic)
Metolazone
Mushrooms (Orellanine/Psilocybe)
Mycophenolate mofetil
Nitrofurantoin
Oral contraceptives
Paclitaxel
Retinoids
Quinolone derivatives
Rifampin
Spanish toxic oil
Suxamethonium (succinylcholine)
Vinca alkaloids
Zimeldine

CRAMPS

Albuterol
Anticholinesterase
Bergamot (bergapten)
Caffeine
Clofibrate
Cyclosporine
Diuretics (chronic, excessive use)
Lithium
Nifedipine
Terbutaline
Tetanus
Theophylline
Vitamin A

*Especially with concurrent cyclosporine A, danazol, erythromycin, gemfibrozil, niacin, colchicine.
†With concurrent pantoprazole.

BOX 28.3 Cramps* and Other Involuntary Muscle Contraction Syndromes

CRAMP SYNDROMES

Ordinary:
  Common in normal individuals, especially gastrocnemius muscle, older age
  Pregnancy
Systemic disorders:
  Dehydration: hidrosis, diuretics, hemodialysis
  Metabolic: low Na^+, Mg^{2+}, Ca^{2+}, glucose, uremia, cirrhosis
  Endocrine: thyroid (hyper- or hypothyroid), hypoadrenal, hyperparathyroid
Ischemia
Drug-induced
Denervation, partial: motor neuron disease, spinal stenosis, radiculopathy, neuropathy (including small-fiber neuropathy)
Syndromes: cramp-fasciculation, Satoyoshi syndrome

OTHER CONTRACTION SYNDROMES

Central disorders: stiff person syndrome, spasticity, tetanus, dystonia
Peripheral nerve disorders: neuromyotonia, tetany, myokymia, partial denervation
Muscle: contractures, myotonia, myoedema

FAMILIAL MUSCLE CONTRACTION SYNDROMES

Muscular dystrophy: Becker; LGMD 1C
Myotonia: myotonia congenita, myotonia fluctuans, acetalozamide-responsive myotonia, myotonic dystrophy
Contractures:
  Brody syndrome: ATP2A1
  Glycogen disorders: myophosphorylase deficiency
  Rippling muscle syndrome: Caveolin-3
  HANAC: COL4A1
  Neuropathic
Cramps: autosomal dominant:
  Schwartz–Jampel: Perlecan, LIFR
  Neuromyotonia and myokymia: KCNQ2; KCNA1
  Geniospasm
  Crisponi: CRLF1
  Myofibrillar myopathy

POSSIBLE TREATMENTS FOR CRAMPS AND OTHER MUSCLE SPASMS

Normalize metabolic abnormalities
Quinine sulfate, 260 mg qhs or bid
Carbamazepine, 200 mg bid or tid
Phenytoin, 300 mg daily
Gabapentin, 300 mg qhs
Tocainide, 200–400 mg bid
Verapamil, 120 mg daily
Amitriptyline, 25–100 mg qhs
Vitamin E, 400 International Units daily
Riboflavin, 100 mg daily
Diphenhydramine, 50 mg daily
Calcium, 0.5–1 g elemental Ca^{++} daily

bid, Twice daily; *qhs,* daily at bedtime; *tid,* three times daily.
*Usual features: sudden involuntary painful muscle contractions (usually involve single muscles, especially gastrocnemius); local cramps in other muscles often associated with neuromuscular disease. Precipitants: muscle contraction, occasionally during sleep. Relief: passive muscle stretch, local massage.

BOX 28.4 Pain Syndromes without Chronic Myopathy*

PAIN OF UNCERTAIN ORIGIN

Polymyalgia rheumatica
Fibromyalgia
Chronic fatigue syndrome
Infections:
  Viral and postviral syndromes
  Brucellosis
Endocrine
  Thyroid: increased or decreased
  Parathyroid: increased or decreased
Familial Mediterranean fever

PAIN WITH DEFINED ORIGIN

Connective tissue disorders:
  Systemic
  Fasciitis
Joint disease
Bone: osteomalacia, fracture, neoplasm
Vascular: ischemia, thrombophlebitis
Polyneuropathy:
  Small-fiber polyneuropathies
  Guillain–Barré
Radiculoneuropathy
Central nervous system: restless legs syndrome, dystonias (focal)

PAIN OF MUSCLE ORIGIN WITHOUT CHRONIC MYOPATHY

Muscle ischemia: atherosclerosis, calciphylaxis
Muscle overuse syndromes:
  Delayed-onset muscle soreness (DOMS)
  Cramps
Drugs, toxins
Muscle injury (strain)

*Usual features: muscle pain; may interfere with effort but no true weakness; present at rest, may increase with movement; muscle morphology and serum creatine kinase normal.

The pain is proportional to the amount of exercise. Rhabdomyolysis is usually associated with muscle pain and tenderness that can persist for days after the initial event. It may occur with a defined metabolic or toxic myopathy or sporadically in the setting of unaccustomed exercise, especially in hot weather. Rhabdomyolysis may produce renal failure—a life-threatening complication and therefore the etiology and any precipitants should be aggressively pursued. Normal physiological responses to strenuous exercise (such as basic training) can result in CK up to 50 times the upper limit of normal (Kenney et al., 2012). These patients experience muscle soreness but not weakness or swelling. They have no myoglobinuria, renal failure, or electrolyte disturbances and the condition is probably benign. Medications, such as cholesterol-lowering agents, may produce a painful myopathy with prominent muscle fiber necrosis and a very high serum CK. Rhabdomyolysis can occur, especially at high doses. However, more commonly, cholesterol-lowering agents produce a myalgia syndrome with no defined muscle pathology.

Muscular dystrophy and mitochondrial disorders are usually painless. Occasional patients with mild Becker muscular dystrophy or mitochondrial syndromes with minimal or no weakness may experience a sense of discomfort such as myalgias, fatigue, or cramps, especially after exercise. Hereditary myopathies with occasional reports of muscle discomfort or spasms in patients (or carriers) include certain limb–girdle muscular dystrophies, facioscapulohumeral dystrophy, myotonic dystrophy type 2, and some mild congenital myopathies. Pain in hereditary myopathies is often due to musculoskeletal problems secondary to the weakness. Several myopathies defined by specific morphological changes in muscle but whose cause is unknown commonly have myalgias or exercise-related discomfort. These syndromes include tubular aggregates with or without cylindrical spirals, focal depletion of mitochondria, internalized capillaries, and adult-onset rod myopathies.

Muscle Cramps

Muscle cramps (see Box 28.3) are localized, typically uncomfortable muscle contractions (Miller and Layzer, 2005). Characteristic features include a sudden involuntary onset in a single muscle or muscle group, with durations of seconds to minutes and a palpable region of contraction. Occasionally there is distortion of posture. Fasciculations often occur before and after the cramp. Muscle cramps are thought to originate in motor axons or nerve terminals. EMG during cramps demonstrates rapid, repetitive motor unit action potentials ("cramp discharges") at rates from 40 to 150 per second that increase and then decrease during the course of the cramp. CNS influences on cramps are minor and probably involve modulation of cramp thresholds. The EMG can distinguish cramps from other types of muscle contraction (e.g., contracture and myoedema are electrically silent).

Cramps usually arise during sleep or exercise and are more likely to occur when muscle contracts. Pain syndromes associated with cramps include discomfort during a muscle contraction and soreness after the contraction due to muscle injury. Cramps, especially those in the calf or foot muscles, are common in normal people of any age. They may be more common in the elderly (up to 50%), at the onset of exercise, at night, during pregnancy, and with fasciculations. These types of cramps are usually idiopathic and benign. In up to 60% of patients with cramps, small-fiber neuropathy may be the only underlying disease discovered after routine evaluation (Lopate et al., 2013).

Cramps that occur frequently in muscles other than the gastrocnemius often herald an underlying neuromuscular disorder. The presence of fasciculations with mild cramps but no weakness usually represents benign fasciculation syndrome. When the muscle cramps are more disabling, the condition is often called cramp-fasciculation syndrome. EMG is normal except for the presence of fasciculations. Repetitive nerve stimulation at 10 Hz provokes after-discharges of motor unit action potentials.

While neurogenic disorders that produce partial denervation of muscles (e.g., amyotrophic lateral sclerosis, radiculopathies, polyneuropathies) are a common cause of cramps, other etiologies (see Boxes 28.2 and 28.3) include drugs and metabolic, neuropathic, and inherited disorders.

When EMG shows neuropathy, myokymia, and/or neuromyotonia, the diagnosis is Isaac syndrome. Patients with the more severe Morvan syndrome also have limbic encephalitis and autonomic disturbances. Antibodies to the voltage-gated potassium channel complex are common in Isaac and Morvan syndromes, but also occur less commonly in patients with the cramp-fasciculation syndrome or in patients with neuropathic pain.

Treatment of cramp syndromes involves management of the underlying disorder and/or symptomatic trials of medications. Stretching affected muscles can relieve cramps. Active stretching, by contracting the antagonist, may be especially effective treatment because it evokes reciprocal inhibition. There is no clear benefit of prophylactic stretching on the frequency of cramps. Symptomatic treatment can reduce abnormal muscle contractions or the discomfort produced by the contractions. Quinine, tonic water, and related drugs can be effective in treating nocturnal muscle cramps, but side effects may outweigh benefits. Increased salt intake and magnesium lactate or citrate may help treat leg cramps during pregnancy.

Other Involuntary Muscle Contraction Syndromes

Diffuse muscle contraction syndromes, usually arising from the PNS or CNS (dystonias), often show widespread and continuous spontaneous motor unit fiber discharges. They may produce considerable discomfort. Causes are hereditary syndromes, CNS disorders, drugs, or toxins (see Boxes 28.2 and 28.3). Tetany, typically associated with hypocalcemia or alkalosis, causes spontaneous repetitive discharges often at very high rates. Myokymia can often be seen on the skin as vermicular or spontaneous rippling. EMG shows rhythmic or semi-rhythmic bursts of normal-appearing motor units at 30 to 80 Hz. Malignant hyperthermia and neuroleptic malignant syndrome both cause diffuse muscle rigidity and, if severe, rhabdomyolysis, as well as dysautonomia. They are usually triggered after drug exposure, immediately after halothane or depolarizing muscle relaxant in malignant hyperthermia and days to weeks after exposure to a variety of dopamine antagonists for neuroleptic malignant syndrome.

Muscle contractions originating from muscle include electrically active forms due to myotonia and electrically silent contractures. *Myotonia* is repetitive firing of muscle fibers at rates of 20 to 80 Hz, with waxing and waning of the amplitude and frequency. Triggering the action potentials may be mechanical or electrical stimulation. Myotonic contractions are usually not painful, except for exercise-induced muscle cramps in myotonia fluctuans or acetalozamide-responsive myotonia (both a result of mutations in *SCN4A*). Mexiletine helps the stiffness and improves quality of life. Patients with recessive myotonia congenita often note fatigue. *Muscle contractures* are active, painful muscle contractions in the absence of electrical activity. (The term is also used to describe fixed resistance to stretch of a shortened muscle due to fibrous connective tissue changes or loss of sarcomeres in the muscle.) Contractures differ clinically from cramps, having a more prolonged time course, no resolution by muscle stretch, and occurrence only in an exercised muscle. Electrically silent muscle contractures occur in myopathies including myophosphorylase deficiency and other glycolytic disorders, Brody syndrome, rippling muscle disease, and hypothyroidism (myoedema).

Myalgia Syndromes without Chronic Myopathy

Pain originating from muscle, often acute, may occur in the absence of a chronic myopathy (see Box 28.4). Muscle ischemia causes a squeezing pain in the affected muscles during exercise. Ischemia produces pain that develops especially rapidly (within minutes) if muscle is forced to contract at the same time; the pain subsides quickly with rest. Cramps and overuse syndromes are associated with pain during or immediately after muscle use. DOMS occurs 12 to 48 hours after exercise and lasts for hours to days. Muscle contraction or palpation exacerbates discomfort. Serum CK is often increased and STIR MRI changes may be present. DOMS is most commonly precipitated by eccentric muscle contraction (contraction during muscle stretching) or unaccustomed exercise and may be associated with repetitive overstretching of elastic noncontractile tissues. Muscle fatigue after exercise may occur via separate excitation/contraction coupling pathways than those that cause DOMS (Iguchi and Shields, 2010).

Exercise training and gentle stretching typically protects against DOMS.

Polymyalgia syndromes have pain localized to muscle and other structures. Polymyalgia pain is often present at rest and variably affected by movement. Serum CK and EMG are normal. No major pathological change in muscle occurs unless the discomfort produces disuse and atrophy of type II muscle fibers. Muscle biopsies may also show changes associated with systemic immune disorders, including inflammation around blood vessels or in connective tissue. Polymyalgia syndromes can have identified causes including systemic immune disease, drug toxicity, and small-fiber polyneuropathies.

A series of clinical criteria define some syndromes of unknown pathophysiology associated with muscle discomfort (polymyalgia rheumatica, fibromyalgia, and chronic fatigue syndrome). *Polymyalgia rheumatica* usually occurs after age 50 years and manifests with pain and stiffness in joints and muscles, weight loss, and low-grade fever. The pain is symmetrical, involving the shoulder, neck, and hip girdle, and is greatest after inactivity and sleeping. Polymyalgia rheumatica can be associated with temporal arteritis and an elevated sedimentation rate (>40 mm/h). Pain improves within a few days after treatment with corticosteroids (prednisone, 20 mg/day). The diagnosis of *chronic fatigue syndrome* requires symptoms of persistent and unexplained fatigue. Four or more symptoms must occur for the 6 months after the onset of fatigue, including impaired memory or concentration, sore throat, tender cervical or axillary lymph nodes, muscle pain, pain in multiple joints, new headaches, unrefreshing sleep, or malaise after exertion. Rest does not alleviate fatigue, which substantially compromises daily function. Chronic fatigue syndrome may improve spontaneously over time.

Fibromyalgia is diagnosed when there is a history of at least 3 months of widespread musculoskeletal pain, most commonly around the neck and shoulders, and examination findings of excessive tenderness in predefined anatomical sites on the trunk and extremities. Patients may also note fatigue and disturbed sleep, headache, cognitive difficulty, and aggravation of symptoms by exercise, anxiety, or stress. The etiology of fibromyalgia is unknown. While CNS sensitization has been proposed to explain widespread hyperalgesia, more recently peripheral nerve abnormalities have been documented. The loss of cutaneous C-fibers, and possibly muscle nociceptor abnormalities, may underlie the pathophysiology of fibromyalgia. Several studies have shown impaired small-fiber function as demonstrated by abnormalities in intraepidermal nerve fiber density, quantitative sensory testing, and pain-related evoked potentials (Oaklander et al., 2013; Üçeyler et al., 2013). Dysfunction of autonomic nerves is found in some patients. In addition, there are consistent abnormalities on questionnaires and rating scales designed to evaluate patients with neuropathy.

Decreasing the central sensitization to pain is the focus of the pharmacological treatment of fibromyalgia and chronic pain. Medications include tricyclic antidepressants, selective serotonin and norepinephrine reuptake inhibitors, gabapentin, and pregabalin. No clear evidence exists for the superiority of any one medication. Low-impact aerobic exercise training may reduce pain and pressure thresholds over tender points. Cognitive behavioral therapy may be useful.

Pain or discomfort localized to muscle may arise in other structures. For example, hip disease can suggest the misdiagnosis of a painful proximal myopathy with apparent leg weakness. In this situation, external or internal rotation of the thigh commonly evokes proximal pain. Radiological studies can confirm the diagnosis. Disorders of bone and joints, connective tissue, endocrine systems, vascular supply, peripheral nerves and roots, and the CNS may also present with discomfort localized to muscle.

REFERENCES

The complete reference list is available online at https://expertconsult .inkling.com/.

29 Hypotonic (Floppy) Infant

W. Bryan Burnette

CHAPTER OUTLINE

APPROACH TO DIAGNOSIS
History
Physical Examination
Diagnostic Studies
SPECIFIC DISORDERS ASSOCIATED WITH HYPOTONIA IN INFANCY
Cerebral Disorders
Combined Cerebral and Motor Unit Disorders
Spinal Cord Disorders
Peripheral Nerve Disorders
Neuromuscular Junction Disorders
Muscle Disorders
SUMMARY

Floppy, or hypotonic, infant is a common scenario encountered in the clinical practice of child neurology. It can present significant challenges in terms of localization and is associated with an extensive differential diagnosis (Box 29.1). As with any clinical problem in neurology, attention to certain key aspects of the history and examination allows correct localization within the neuraxis and narrows the list of possible diagnoses. Further narrowing of the differential is achievable with selected testing based on the aforementioned findings. Understanding the anatomical and etiological aspects of hypotonia in infancy necessarily begins with an understanding of the concept of tone. *Tone* is the resistance of muscle to stretch. Categorization of tone differs among authors, but assessment is performed with the patient at rest and all parts of the body fully supported; examination involves tonic or phasic stretching of a muscle or the effect of gravity. Tone is an involuntary function and therefore separate and distinct from strength or power, which is the maximum force generated by voluntary contraction of a muscle. Function at every level of the neuraxis influences tone, and disease processes affecting any level of the neuraxis may reduce tone. Although a comprehensive review of conditions associated with hypotonia in infancy is beyond the scope of a single chapter, this chapter considers the basic approach to evaluating the floppy infant and considers several key disorders.

APPROACH TO DIAGNOSIS

History

Several features of the history may point to a specific diagnosis or category of diagnoses leading to hypotonia, or may permit distinguishing disorders present during fetal development from disorders acquired during the perinatal period. Thoroughly investigate a family history of disorders known to be associated with neonatal hypotonia, especially in the mother or in older siblings. Certain dominantly inherited genetic disorders (e.g., myotonic dystrophy) are associated with *anticipation* (earlier or more severe expression of a disease in successive generations). Such disorders may be milder and therefore undiagnosed in the mother. A maternal history of spontaneous abortion, fetal demise, or other offspring who died in infancy may also provide clues to possible diagnoses. A history of reduced fetal movement is a common feature of disorders associated with hypotonia, and may indicate a peripheral cause (Vasta et al., 2005). A history of maternal fever late in pregnancy suggests in utero infection, while a history of a long and difficult delivery followed by perinatal distress suggests hypoxic-ischemic encephalopathy with or without accompanying myelopathy. Among the many potential causes of neonatal hypotonia, acquired perinatal injury is far more common than inherited disorders and is rarely overlooked. However, also consider the possibility of a motor unit disorder leading to perinatal distress and hypoxic-ischemic encephalopathy.

Physical Examination
General Features of Hypotonia

Assessing tone in an infant involves both observation of the patient at rest and application of certain examination maneuvers designed to evaluate both axial and appendicular musculature. Beginning with observation, a normal infant lying supine on an examination table will demonstrate flexion of the hips and knees so that the lower extremities are clear of the examination table, flexion of the upper extremities at the elbows, and internal rotation at the shoulders (Fig. 29.1). A hypotonic infant lies with the lower extremities in external rotation, the lateral aspects of the thighs and knees touching the examination table, and the upper extremities either extended down by the sides of the trunk or abducted with slight flexion at the elbows, also lying against the examination table. Evaluation of the *traction response* is done with the infant in supine position; the hands are grasped and the infant pulled toward a sitting position. A normal response includes flexion at the elbows, knees, and ankles, and movement of the head in line with the trunk after no more than a brief head lag. The head should then remain erect in the midline for at least a few seconds. An infant with axial hypotonia demonstrates excessive head lag with this maneuver (Fig. 29.2, A), and once upright, the head may continue to lag or may fall forward relatively quickly. Absence of flexion of the limbs may also be seen and indicates either appendicular hypotonia or weakness. The traction response is normally present after 33 weeks postconceptional age. Vertical suspension is performed by placing hands under the infant's axillae and lifting the infant without grasping the thorax. A normal infant has enough power in the shoulder muscles to remain suspended without falling through, with the head upright in the midline and the hips and knees flexed. In contrast, a hypotonic infant held in this manner slips through the examiner's hands (see Fig. 29.2, B), often with the head falling forward and the legs extended at the knees. Infants with axial hypotonia related to brain injury may also demonstrate crossing, or *scissoring*, of the legs in this position, which is an early manifestation of appendicular hypertonia. In *horizontal suspension*, the infant is held prone with the abdomen and chest against the palm of the examiner's hand (see Fig. 29.2, C). A normal infant maintains the head above horizontal with the limbs flexed, while

---

BOX 29.1 Differential Diagnosis of the Floppy Infant

CEREBRAL HYPOTONIA

Chromosomal disorders:
   Prader-Willi Syndrome
Chronic nonprogressive encephalopathy
Chronic progressive encephalopathy
Benign congenital hypotonia

COMBINED CEREBRAL AND MOTOR UNIT DISORDERS

Acid maltase deficiency
Congenital myotonic dystrophy
Syndromic congenital muscular dystrophies
Congenital disorders of glycosylation
Lysosomal disorders
Infantile neuroaxonal dystrophy

SPINAL CORD DISORDERS

Acquired spinal cord lesions
Spinal muscular atrophy
Infantile spinal muscular atrophy with respiratory distress
X-linked spinal muscular atrophy

PERIPHERAL NERVE DISORDERS

Congenital hypomyelinating neuropathy/Dejerine-Sottas
   disease

NEUROMUSCULAR JUNCTION DISORDERS

Juvenile myasthenia gravis
Neonatal myasthenia gravis
Congenital myasthenic syndromes
Infant botulism

MUSCLE DISORDERS

Congenital myopathies:
   Centronuclear myopathy
   Nemaline myopathy
   Central core disease
Nonsyndromic congenital muscular dystrophies:
   Merosin-deficient congenital muscular dystrophy
   Ullrich congenital muscular dystrophy
Other muscular dystrophies:
   Infantile facioscapulohumeral dystrophy

---

a hypotonic infant drapes over the examiner's hand with the head and limbs hanging limply. Other examination findings in hypotonic infants include various deformities of the cranium, face, limbs, and thorax. Infants with reduced tone may develop occipital flattening, or *positional plagiocephaly*, as the result of prolonged periods of lying supine and motionless.

Localization

Once the presence of hypotonia in an infant is established, the next step in determining causation is localization of the abnormality to the brain, spinal cord, motor unit, or multiple sites. A *motor unit* is a single spinal motor neuron and all the muscle fibers it innervates and includes the motor neuron with its cell body, axon, and myelin covering; the neuromuscular junction; and muscle. The major "branch point" at this stage of the assessment is whether the lesion is likely to be in the brain, at a more distal site, or at multiple sites. Review of the recent literature suggests that 60%–80% of cases of hypotonia in infancy are due to central causes, while 15%–30% are due to peripheral abnormalities (Peredo and Hannibal, 2009).

The key features of disorders of cerebral function, particularly the cerebral cortex, are encephalopathy and seizures. Encephalopathy manifesting as decreased level of consciousness may be difficult to ascertain, given the large proportion

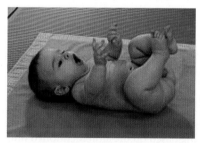

Fig. 29.1 **Normal infant lying supine with legs flexed and arms adducted.** *(With permission from Kobesova, A., and Kolar, P., 2014, Developmental kinesiology: three levels of motor control in the assessment and treatment of the motor system, J Bodyw Mov Ther 18(1), 23–33, Elsevier.)*

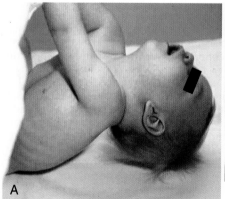
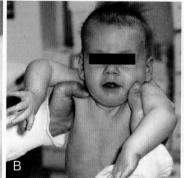
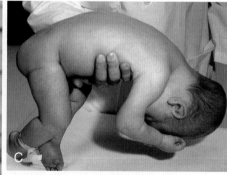

Fig. 29.2 **A,** Hypotonic infant demonstrating abnormal traction response with excessive head lag. **B,** Ventral suspension in a hypotonic infant, with elevation of shoulders and arms (slip-through). **C,** Horizontal suspension with the head and limbs hanging limply. *(With permission from Bodensteiner, J. B., 2008, The evaluation of the hypotonic infant, Semin Pediatr Neurol 15(1), 10–20, Elsevier.)*

of time normal infants spend sleeping. However, full-term or near-term infants with normal brain function spend at least some portion of the day awake with eyes open, particularly with feeding. Encephalopathy also manifests with excessive irritability or poor feeding, although the latter problem is rarely the sole feature of cerebral hemispheric dysfunction and may occur with disorders at more distal sites. Infants with centrally mediated hypotonia of many different etiologies frequently have relatively normal power despite a hypotonic appearance. Power may not be observable under normal conditions because of a paucity of spontaneous movement, but it may be observable with application of a noxious stimulus such as a blood draw or placement of a peripheral intravenous catheter. Other indicators of central rather than peripheral dysfunction include *fisting* (trapping of the thumbs in closed hands), normal or brisk tendon reflexes, and normal or exaggerated primitive reflexes. Tendon reflexes should be tested with the infant's head in the midline and the limbs symmetrically positioned; deviations from this technique often result in spuriously asymmetrical reflexes. *Primitive reflexes* are involuntary responses to certain stimuli that normally appear in late fetal development and are supplanted within the first few months of life by voluntary movements. Abnormalities of these reflexes include absent or asymmetrical responses, obligatory responses (persistence of the reflex with continued application of the stimulus), or persistence of the reflexes beyond the normal age range. Two of the most sensitive primitive reflexes are the Moro and asymmetrical tonic neck reflexes. The *Moro reflex* is a startle response present from 28 weeks after conception to 6 months postnatal age (Gingold et al., 1998). Quickly dropping the infant's head below the level of the body while holding the infant supine with the head supported in one hand and the body supported in the other readily elicits this reflex. The normal response consists of initial abduction and extension of the arms with opening of the hands, followed quickly by adduction and flexion with closure of the hands. The *tonic neck reflex* is a vestibular response and is present from term until approximately 3 months of age. The response is elicited by rotating the head to one side while the infant is lying supine. The normal response is extension of the ipsilateral limbs while the contralateral limbs remain flexed. Central disorders resulting in hypotonia may also be associated with dysmorphism of the face or limbs, or malformations of other organs. Various defects in O-linked glycosylation of α-dystroglycan, a protein associated with the dystrophin glycoprotein complex that stabilizes the sarcolemma, result in structural defects of the brain, eye, and skeletal muscle.

Disorders of the spinal cord leading to neonatal hypotonia are usually secondary to perinatal injury. Spinal cord injury may occur in the setting of a prolonged, difficult vaginal delivery with breech presentation, resulting in trauma to the spinal cord, or may result from hypoxic-ischemic injury to the cord concurrently with encephalopathy. In the latter case, hypotonia may initially be attributable to the encephalopathy. In cases of hypotonia resulting from spinal cord injury, diminished responsiveness to painful stimuli, sphincter dysfunction with continuous leakage of urine and abdominal distension, and priapism may provide clues to localization of the lesion.

The hallmark of disorders of the motor unit is weakness. Tendon reflexes are absent or reduced. Tendon reflexes reduced out of proportion to weakness usually indicate a neuropathy, often a demyelinating neuropathy, whereas tendon reflexes reduced in proportion to weakness are more likely to result from myopathy or axonal neuropathy. The motor unit is the final common pathway for all reflexes, and for this reason, primitive reflexes are depressed or absent in motor unit disorders. This phenomenon may hinder detection of central nervous system (CNS) abnormalities when lesions at both levels coexist. Other abnormalities related to motor unit disorders in infants include underdevelopment of the jaw (micrognathia), a high arched palate, and chest wall deformities, in particular pectus excavatum. Muscle atrophy may also occur but also occurs in cerebral disorders. Sensory function is not assessable in detail in a neonate or young infant, particularly in the presence of encephalopathy, although reduced responsiveness to pinprick may provide clues to the presence of a polyneuropathy or spinal cord lesion in the setting of normal mental status. Some motor unit disorders may result in perinatal distress due to weakness and may result in a superimposed encephalopathy that confounds the localization of hypotonia.

Hypotonic infants may have reduced movement during fetal development, leading to fibrosis of muscles or of structures associated with joints, as well as foreshortening of ligaments. This results in restricted joint range of motion, or *contractures.* The term *arthrogryposis* refers to joint contractures that develop prenatally. The most common form of arthrogryposis is unilateral or bilateral clubfoot. The most severe end of this clinical spectrum is *arthrogryposis multiplex congenita*, or multiple joint contractures. The causes of this condition may be abnormalities of the intrauterine environment, motor unit disorders, or disorders of the CNS. Hypotonia in utero may also result in congenital hip dysplasia.

Diagnostic Studies

Selective laboratory testing allows confirmation of the clinical localization of hypotonia, and in many cases leads to identification of a specific diagnosis. In all cases, ancillary testing guided by historical features and examination findings has the greatest chance of yielding a diagnosis. Available modalities include various forms of neuroimaging; electrophysiological techniques including electroencephalography (EEG), nerve conduction studies (NCS), electromyography (EMG), and repetitive nerve stimulation; muscle and nerve biopsy; and other laboratory studies such as serum creatine kinase (CK), metabolic studies, and genetic studies.

Neuroimaging

Neuroimaging studies, in particular magnetic resonance imaging (MRI), are most useful when suspecting structural abnormalities of the CNS. T1-weighted images most readily detect congenital malformations of the brain and spinal cord, while T2-weighted images and various T2-based sequences reveal abnormalities of white matter and show evidence of ischemic injury. Specialized techniques such as MR spectroscopy may show evidence of mitochondrial disease (Matthews et al., 1993) or disorders of cerebral creatine metabolism (Frahm et al., 1994). When performing neuroimaging studies that require sedation on hypotonic infants, give particular consideration to airway management and other safety issues.

Electroencephalography

Electroencephalography may be informative when seizures are suspected as either a cause of unexplained encephalopathy or a result of a more global disturbance of brain function. EEG may also reveal evidence of underlying structural abnormalities and thus increase the pretest probability of a diagnostic finding on neuroimaging.

Creatine Kinase

Creatine kinase catalyzes the conversion of creatine to phosphocreatine, which serves as a reservoir for the buffering and regeneration of adenosine triphosphate (ATP). It expresses in many human tissues, in particular smooth muscle, cardiac muscle, and skeletal muscle. The concentration of CK detectable in serum increases in any condition in which tissues expressing high levels of the enzyme undergo breakdown. Serum CK concentration may be elevated in congenital myopathies, congenital muscular dystrophies, or spinal muscular atrophy, but levels may also be elevated transiently following normal vaginal deliveries or with perinatal distress. Conversely, serum CK is normal in some congenital myopathies and inherited neuropathies.

Metabolic Studies

Removal of low-molecular-weight toxic metabolites across the placenta typically prevents inborn errors of metabolism (e.g., amino acidopathies, organic acidurias, urea cycle defects, fatty acid oxidation defects, mitochondrial disorders) from causing in utero injury. More commonly, these disorders manifest in a previously healthy newborn who develops hypotonia, encephalopathy, or seizures within the first 24 to 72 hours after birth, after oral feeding begins and toxic intermediates begin to accumulate in the blood. Although detection of many disorders is by state-mandated newborn screens, these results may not be available before an affected infant becomes symptomatic. For this reason, newborns who develop hypotonia and encephalopathy after an unremarkable first few days of life should have enteral feedings held until metabolic studies such as blood ammonia level, plasma amino acid, acylcarnitine profile, and urine organic acids have definitively excluded an inborn error of metabolism. Because neonatal sepsis has a similar presentation, undertake investigation for infection with cultures of blood, urine, and cerebrospinal fluid in such cases; empirical antimicrobial therapy should be initiated while diagnostic studies are pending.

Nerve Conduction Studies and Electromyography

Nerve conduction studies and EMG are the studies of choice in a suspected motor unit disorder when other available clinical information does not suggest a specific diagnosis. The two techniques are complementary and always performed together. They allow distinction between primary disorders of muscle and peripheral nerve disorders when the two are indistinguishable on clinical grounds. Repetitive nerve stimulation (RNS) studies evaluate the integrity of the neuromuscular junction, abnormalities of which are not detectable with routine nerve conduction studies or EMG. The most commonly observed abnormality on low-rate (2–3 Hz) RNS studies of patients with various forms of myasthenia is a significant decrement, usually defined as 10% or greater, in the amplitude of the compound motor action potential (CMAP) between the first and fourth or fifth stimuli of a series. Single-fiber EMG (SFEMG) is a highly specialized technique that evaluates the delay in depolarization between adjacent muscle fibers within a single motor unit, referred to as *jitter*. This modality is highly sensitive for neuromuscular junction abnormalities but has a low specificity and requires a cooperative patient. SFEMG with stimulation of the appropriate nerve has been described in pediatric patients (Tidwell and Pitt, 2007), but experience with this technique in infants is limited to a small number of centers. The utility of these neurophysiology studies is dependent on the skill and experience of the clinician performing the tests, as well as the precision of the question posed.

Muscle Biopsy

Muscle biopsy is integral to the diagnosis of certain inherited muscle disorders such as congenital myopathies, congenital muscular dystrophies, and metabolic myopathies and may also aid in the distinction between myopathies and motor neuron disorders. Give careful consideration to the site chosen for biopsy. Ideally, a muscle should be chosen that is moderately but not severely weak and that has not undergone needle EMG. Another important consideration is the quantity of tissue obtained. Obtain a sufficient quantity of tissue to rapidly freeze a portion for routine histochemical stains, submit additional tissue for specialized studies such as biochemical assays, electron microscopy, or genetic studies, and have additional tissue available to be stored for possible future studies. In practical terms, this usually entails obtaining at least three separate specimens weighing 1 to 1.5 g each. Although needle biopsy may procure an adequate sample in some cases, open biopsy is more likely to yield an appropriate amount of tissue, thereby avoiding the need for a second surgical procedure and its attendant risks. The value of muscle biopsy, as with neurophysiology studies, depends on the experience of the interpreting laboratory and the focus of the question asked by the referring clinician. In addition to these factors, proper handling of the tissue between the operating room and the receiving laboratory is a critical link in the chain of custody. This step is often the most difficult to control, but it requires attention equal to the other steps in the process in order to maximize the probability of obtaining a diagnostic sample and minimize the risk of subjecting the patient to a second procedure.

Nerve Biopsy

Nerve biopsy plays a more limited role in the diagnosis of hypotonia in infancy. It is nevertheless appropriate when a peripheral neuropathy is suspected on clinical grounds, but available testing fails to yield a diagnosis. The sural nerve is usually chosen because of its accessibility and the relatively minor deficit produced by its removal. Sural nerve biopsy is most likely to be informative in the setting of an abnormal response on nerve conduction studies. The limited choice of peripheral nerves available for biopsy confines use of this procedure to centers with considerable experience. Submit portions of the nerve for routine histochemical stains, paraffin-embedded sections, and thin plastic sections, the latter processed for light microscopy or electron microscopy.

Genetic Testing

In some cases of hypotonia in infancy, the combination of clinical history, examination, and ancillary testing points toward a specific genetic diagnosis. Genetic testing is commercially available for many conditions, and the number continues to expand rapidly. Consult one or more of the accessible resources such as the Internet-based Online Mendelian Inheritance in Man or GeneTests.org for the most current information on testing for specific disorders. When a chromosomal disorder is suspected, consider array comparative genomic hybridization (aCGH), a technique that has an increased diagnostic yield by 5%–17% over traditional karyotyping (Prasad and Prasad, 2011). The newer technique of whole exome sequencing will likely further increase the diagnostic yield of the genetic evaluation of hypotonia, but its application to this clinical problem has been limited to date.

Serology

In cases of a suspected neuromuscular junction disorder such as myasthenia gravis, assays of antibodies directed against the sarcolemmal nicotinic acetylcholine receptor or muscle-specific kinase are commercially available. Autoimmune myasthenia gravis is rare in infancy, but absence of the antibodies is required for the diagnosis of a congenital myasthenic syndrome. Several forms of myasthenia gravis occur in infancy and are discussed in greater detail later in this chapter.

SPECIFIC DISORDERS ASSOCIATED WITH HYPOTONIA IN INFANCY
Cerebral Disorders

Regardless of etiology, hypotonia is a common feature of disturbed function of the cerebral hemispheres in neonates and infants and, as previously noted, is frequently characterized by diminished tone that is disproportionate to the degree of weakness. Disorders of cerebral function in infancy are also frequently associated with concurrent axial hypotonia and appendicular hypertonia. Overall, central disorders are a far more common cause of hypotonia than motor unit diseases. Although a comprehensive listing of all such disorders is beyond the scope of a single chapter, a number of important categories of cerebral causes of hypotonia are considered here.

Chromosomal Disorders

Hypotonia is a prominent feature of many disorders associated with large- or small-scale chromosomal abnormalities. Such disorders also are frequently associated with a dysmorphic appearance of the face and hands. Among the most common of these disorders is *Prader–Willi syndrome*, which is caused by various abnormalities resulting in absence of paternally expressed genes within the PWS/Angelman syndrome region on chromosome 15 (Kim et al., 2012). Pathogenic defects in this region include paternal deletion, uniparental disomy, or an imprinting defect. Affected individuals often have profound hypotonia and poor feeding in infancy, suggesting a disorder of the motor unit or a combined cerebral and motor unit disorder. However, serum CK, EMG, muscle biopsy, and brain MRI are normal. The commonly recognized morphological features of almond-shaped eyes, narrow biparietal diameter, and relatively small hands and feet may not be readily apparent in early infancy. DNA methylation analysis is the only technique that will diagnose PWS in all three molecular classes and differentiate PWS from Angelman syndrome (AS) in deletion cases (Glenn et al., 1996, 1997; Kubota et al., 1996). A DNA methylation analysis consistent with PWS is sufficient for clinical diagnosis, though not for genetic counseling purposes. Parental DNA samples are not required to differentiate the maternal and paternal alleles. The most robust and widely used assay targets the 5′ CpG island of the SNURF-SNRPN (typically referred to as SNRPN) locus, and will correctly diagnose PWS in more than 99% of cases (Glenn et al., 1996; Kubota et al., 1997). The promoter, exon 1, and intron 1 regions of SNRPN are unmethylated on the paternally expressed allele and methylated on the maternally repressed allele. Normal individuals have both a methylated and an unmethylated SNRPN allele, while individuals with PWS have only the maternally methylated allele. Methylation-specific multiplex-ligation probe amplification (MS-MLPA) can also determine the parental origin in this region (Kim et al., 2012).

Failure to thrive in infancy gives way in early childhood to hyperphagia and a characteristic pattern of behavioral abnormalities, intellectual disability, and hypogonadism.

Chronic Nonprogressive Encephalopathy

Chronic nonprogressive encephalopathy describes a clinical syndrome with many potential causes, including cerebral dysgenesis related to a genetic disorder, in utero infection, toxic exposure, inborn error of metabolism, or vascular insult. Perinatal brain injury resulting in a chronic encephalopathy is readily diagnosable and typically associated with a reduced level of consciousness and seizures. Hypoxic-ischemic brain injury in the newborn manifests with low Apgar scores, and lactic acidosis along with other indicators of injury to other vital organs is often present. Hypotonia related to ischemic brain injury usually gives way to spasticity. In cases of remote in utero injury or cerebral dysgenesis, hypotonia may be the only manifestation of the problem in the perinatal period. Clues to the presence of cerebral dysgenesis include malformations of other organs and abnormalities of head size or shape. In such cases, obtain an MRI of the brain, and a chromosomal anomaly should be sought with karyotype and chromosomal microarray analysis. The onset of hypotonia in a previously healthy neonate or infant is almost always cerebral in origin and may also relate to infection, vascular injury, or an inborn error of metabolism.

Chronic Progressive Encephalopathy

Chronic progressive encephalopathy more commonly presents with developmental regression than with hypotonia. Inborn errors of metabolism involving small molecules may cause this clinical presentation, but more frequently the cause is a disorder of lysosomal or peroxisomal metabolism leading to progressive accumulation of storage material in various tissues. These disorders frequently manifest with progressive facial dysmorphism, organomegaly, or skeletal dysplasia in addition to neurological decline. Among disorders causing chronic progressive encephalopathy, various autosomal recessive defects of peroxisome biogenesis in the Zellweger syndrome spectrum (ZSS) are most commonly associated with profound hypotonia in infancy. The most severely affected individuals present with neonatal hypotonia, poor feeding, encephalopathy, seizures, and craniofacial dysmorphism (Steinberg et al., 2006). Stippling of the patellae and other long bones (chondrodysplasia punctata) may be seen on skeletal survey, and affected individuals may have evidence of hepatic dysfunction as well as hepatic cysts on abdominal imaging. Measurement of plasma very-long-chain fatty acid (VLCFA) concentrations identifies elevated levels of C26:0 and C26:1, and ratios of C24/C22 and C26/C22 indicate a defect in peroxisomal fatty acid metabolism. Abnormalities in 12 different PEX genes, all of which encode peroxins (proteins required for peroxisome assembly), have been identified in ZSS, with two-thirds having pathogenic mutations in the PEX1 gene (Collin and Gould, 1999; Maxwell et al., 2002; Walter et al., 2001). Management is supportive, and the most severely affected infants do not survive beyond the first year of life.

Benign Congenital Hypotonia

Benign congenital hypotonia refers to infants with early hypotonia who later develop normal tone. It is a diagnosis made only in retrospect and has become less common in the era of high-resolution neuroimaging and genetic testing. Nevertheless, there remains a subset of children, often with a family history of a similarly affected parent or sibling who was undiagnosed. Intellectual disability of varying degrees frequently becomes apparent in later life.

Combined Cerebral and Motor Unit Disorders

Several genetic diseases manifest with abnormalities of both the brain and the motor unit. These conditions can present considerable diagnostic challenges.

Acid Maltase Deficiency

Acid maltase deficiency, an autosomal recessive deficiency of the lysosomal enzyme acid α-1,4-glucosidase, presents with a severe skeletal myopathy and cardiomyopathy and may also be associated with encephalopathy. Routine histochemical stains show accumulation of glycogen in lysosomal vacuoles and within the sarcoplasm. The diagnosis is confirmed with biochemical assay of enzyme activity in muscle or in cultured skin fibroblasts. Recombinant human enzyme is approved by the U.S. Food and Drug Administration (FDA) for replacement therapy, which can prolong survival (Kishnani et al., 2006).

Congenital Myotonic Dystrophy

Congenital myotonic dystrophy is an autosomal dominant disorder that typically presents in adolescence or early adulthood, but in some instances may be associated with profound hypotonia and weakness of the face and limbs in infancy. Approximately 25% of infants born to mothers with myotonic dystrophy are affected in this way, although the diagnosis in the mother may be unrecognized (Rakocevic-Stojanovic et al., 2005). Survivors of perinatal distress often have global developmental delay, with both intellectual impairment and motor disability throughout childhood, then develop myotonia and other characteristic symptoms of the muscular dystrophy as they approach puberty. To date, only myotonic dystrophy type 1, caused by abnormal expansion of a trinucleotide repeat within the gene DMPK, has been associated with a congenital presentation. Genetic testing is commercially available.

Infantile Facioscapulohumeral Dystrophy

Facioscapulohumeral dystrophy (FSHD) is another dominantly inherited muscular dystrophy presenting most frequently in early adulthood, but which may have a congenital presentation. The genetic abnormality is contraction of a 3.3-kb repeat array at the D4Z4 locus. Those with the smallest integral number of repeats may have diffuse hypotonia and weakness in infancy and account for less than 5% of cases (Klinge et al., 2006). Affected infants may have cognitive impairment, epilepsy, and progressive sensorineural hearing loss. Serum CK is normal or mildly elevated. Family history may include a mildly affected parent, although cases also result from de novo mutations. Genetic testing is commercially available.

Syndromic Congenital Muscular Dystrophies

A group of congenital muscular dystrophies due to defects of O-linked glycosylation of dystroglycan, a component of the dystrophin–glycoprotein complex spanning the plasma membrane of skeletal myocytes, are associated with severe myopathy, a cerebral cortical malformation referred to as *cobblestone lissencephaly*, and ocular defects such as retinal dysplasia. In addition to profound hypotonia and weakness, affected infants often have intractable epilepsy. These diagnoses are suspected based on the characteristic constellation of abnormalities and have been clinically categorized as *Fukuyama congenital muscular dystrophy*, *Walker–Warburg syndrome*, and *muscle-eye-brain disease*. Thus far, eight different causative genes have been identified (Godfrey et al., 2011), and there appears to be a far greater degree of phenotypic overlap among the different genotypes than was previously appreciated.

Congenital Disorders of Glycosylation

Congenital disorders of glycosylation are a group of recessively inherited defects in 21 different enzymes that modify N-linked oligosaccharides (Jaeken et al., 2009). Many forms present with hypotonia in infancy. The most common form, type Ia, results from a deficiency of the phosphomannomutase enzyme. In addition to hypotonia, affected infants may have hyporeflexia, global developmental delay, failure to thrive, seizures, and evidence of hepatic dysfunction, coagulopathy, and elevated thyroid-stimulating hormone (TSH). Characteristic examination findings include inverted nipples and an abnormal distribution of subcutaneous fat. Facial dysmorphism occurs but is not present in all cases. Brain MRI shows cerebellar hypoplasia. Analysis of transferrin isoforms in serum by isoelectric focusing reveals a characteristic pattern indicative of a defect in the early steps of the N-linked oligosaccharide synthetic pathway. Commercially available genetic testing identifies pathogenic sequence variants in 95% of affected individuals. Although cerebral dysfunction dominates the early clinical picture, some patients develop a demyelinating peripheral neuropathy in the first or second decade of life (Gruenwald, 2009).

Lysosomal Disorders

Certain defects of lysosomal hydrolases, in particular *Krabbe disease* and *metachromatic leukodystrophy*, result in progressive degeneration of both central and peripheral myelin (Korn-Lubetzki et al., 2003), producing both an encephalopathy and motor unit dysfunction (Cameron et al., 2004). Both disorders are associated with characteristic white matter abnormalities on brain MRI, and biochemical assays on peripheral blood of β-galactocerebrosidase in the case of Krabbe, and of arylsulfatase A in the case of metachromatic leukodystrophy confirm the diagnosis.

Infantile Neuroaxonal Dystrophy

Neuroaxonal dystrophy is a rare autosomal recessive disorder caused by mutations in the PLA2G6 gene, which encodes a calcium-independent phospholipase (Gregory et al., 2008). The classic form may present as early as 6 months of age with hypotonia, although psychomotor regression is more common, and progressive spastic tetraparesis and optic atrophy with visual impairment follow. Brain MRI shows bilateral T2 hypointensity of the globus pallidus, indicative of progressive iron accumulation, as well as thinning of the corpus callosum and cerebellar cortical hyperintensities. Nerve conduction studies show evidence of an axonal sensorimotor polyneuropathy with active denervation on EMG. The characteristic pathological finding is of enlarged and dystrophic-appearing axons on biopsy of skin, peripheral nerve, or other tissue-containing peripheral nerve. Commercially available genetic testing identifies abnormalities in approximately 95% of children with early symptom onset.

Spinal Cord Disorders

Disorders of the spinal cord leading to generalized hypotonia in infancy usually involve the cervical spine at a minimum but may involve the entire cord. They include both acquired processes and genetic syndromes.

Acquired Spinal Cord Lesions

Acquired spinal cord lesions relate to trauma sustained during delivery or occur as a part of the spectrum of hypoxic-ischemic encephalopathy. As previously noted, the highest risk of spinal cord injury occurs in vaginal deliveries with breech presentation, particularly when the head is hyperextended in utero. Herniation of the brainstem through the foramen magnum, as well as injury to the cerebellum, may also occur. Cervical spine injury may also occur in cephalic presentations with midforceps delivery, especially in cases of prolonged rupture of membranes. In both traction injury and hypoxic-ischemic injury, encephalopathy often dominates the early clinical picture and may obscure the extent of spinal cord dysfunction. Potential indicators in the acute phase include bladder distention with dribbling of urine and impaired sweating below the level of the lesion. Signs of spasticity gradually supplant early flaccid paraparesis. As mental status improves, the level and extent of motor impairment becomes apparent. MRI of the spine in the acute stage may show cord edema or hemorrhage, whereas imaging obtained later in the course may reveal cord atrophy.

Spinal Muscular Atrophy

Spinal muscular atrophy (SMA) is the most common inherited disorder of the spinal cord resulting in hypotonia in infancy, occurring with an incidence of approximately 1 in 10,000 live births per year (Sugarman et al., 2012). It is an autosomal recessive disorder in which the molecular defect leads to impaired regulation of programmed cell death in anterior horn cells and in motor nuclei of lower cranial nerves. Both populations of motor neurons are progressively lost, producing hypotonia and weakness of limb and truncal musculature, as well as bulbar dysfunction. In approximately 95% of cases, the genetic defect is homozygous deletion of the survival motor neuron 1 (SMN1) gene, which is located on the telomeric region of chromosome 5q13 (Ogino and Wilson, 2002). A virtually identical centromeric gene on 5q13, referred to as *SMN2*, encodes a similar but less biologically active product (Swoboda et al., 2005). While no more than two copies of SMN1 are present in the human genome, variable numbers of SMN2 copies are present. The protein product of SMN2 appears to partially rescue the SMA phenotype such that a larger SMN2 copy number generally results in a milder presentation and disease course.

Historically, SMA patients have been categorized into different phenotypes or syndromes based on age of presentation and maximum motor ability achieved. The disease results from a common genetic abnormality with a spectrum of phenotypic severity contingent upon modifying factors that include SMN2 copy number and other loci not yet identified. The classification of the most severely affected patients, with weakness and hypotonia evident at birth, is SMA type 0. These infants may have arthrogryposis multiplex congenita in addition to diffuse weakness of limb and trunk muscles, but facial weakness is usually mild if present. Perinatal respiratory failure causes death in early infancy. SMA type 1, also referred to as *Werdnig–Hoffmann disease*, is a designation given to infants who develop weakness within the first 6 months of life. These infants may appear normal at birth or may appear hypotonic. Facial expression is usually normal, and arthrogryposis is usually absent. Weakness is worse in proximal than in distal muscles and worse in the lower extremities, which may lead to suspicion of a congenital myopathy or muscular dystrophy. Further confounding the diagnosis is the presence of an elevated serum CK in a substantial portion of patients (Rudnick-Schoneborn et al., 1998), although CK rarely rises above 1000 U/L. In addition to limb weakness, affected infants demonstrate abdominal breathing due to relative preservation of diaphragm function as compared to abdominal and chest wall musculature. Needle EMG shows evidence of both acute and chronic denervation in the limbs and serves to distinguish this disorder from myopathies with a similar presentation.

Genetic testing is commercially available for SMN-related SMA. Among the 5% of patients without homozygous deletion of SMN1, most are compound heterozygotes with the characteristic deletion on one allele and a point mutation on the other. Parents of affected children are heterozygotes for deletion of SMN1 in a majority of cases, although a 2% rate of de novo mutations is reported in SMA patients (Wirth et al., 1997). The natural history of SMA is unique among anterior horn cell disorders in that the progression of weakness is most rapid early in the disease course and subsequently slows. Nevertheless, in the absence of supportive measures, median survival is 8 months, with death due to respiratory failure. Survivors have normal cognitive development. Although no effective treatment exists, therapeutic strategies aimed at increasing the biological activity of SMN2 are the subjects of ongoing clinical trials (Arnold and Burghes, 2013).

Infantile Spinal Muscular Atrophy with Respiratory Distress Type 1

Infantile spinal muscular atrophy with respiratory distress type 1 (SMARD1), previously classified as a variant of SMA type 1, is a rare and distinct autosomal recessive anterior horn cell disorder. Unlike SMN-related SMA, affected infants develop early diaphragmatic paralysis and distal limb weakness that progresses to complete paralysis. Many have intrauterine growth restriction and are born with ankle contractures. Approximately one-third are born prematurely. Similar to SMN-related SMA, EMG and muscle biopsy reveal evidence of chronic active denervation. The causative gene encodes the immunoglobulin μ-binding protein 2 (IGHMBP2), for which testing is commercially available (Grohmann et al., 2001).

X-linked Spinal Muscular Atrophy

This rare X-linked anterior horn cell degenerative disorder shares a considerable degree of phenotypic overlap with SMN-related SMA. Distinctive features include polyhydramnios secondary to impaired fetal swallowing, arthrogryposis, and axonal sensory and motor abnormalities on nerve conduction studies (Dlamini et al., 2013). Consider the diagnosis in any simplex case of a male infant with an SMA phenotype and normal SMN1 copy number. The only known causative gene encodes the ubiquitin-like modifier activating enzyme 1 (UBA1, formerly UBE1), for which commercial testing is available.

Peripheral Nerve Disorders

Polyneuropathies, both inherited and acquired, are a rare cause of infantile hypotonia. The two most common clinical designations for infantile polyneuropathies are *congenital hypomyelinating neuropathy* (CHN) and *Dejerine-Sottas disease* (DSD). In recent years, mounting evidence reveals that neither entity is a monogenic disorder, nor are they clearly distinct from one another. Clinical features include hypotonia, distal or diffuse weakness, absent tendon reflexes, and evidence on nerve conduction studies of a demyelinating polyneuropathy. Traditionally, DSD was classified as hereditary motor and sensory neuropathy (HSMN) type III, but at least four genes associated with various demyelinating HMSN subtypes have been linked to the DSD and CHN phenotypes, including PMP22, MPZ, EGR2, and PRX (Plante-Bordenueve and Said, 2002). In general, patients with an infantile presentation are homozygotes or compound heterozygotes for mutations in the causative genes. The most common acquired autoimmune peripheral neuropathies, Guillain–Barré syndrome and chronic inflammatory demyelinating polyneuropathy (CIDP), occur rarely in the first year of life and typically present with weakness and hypotonia in a previously normal infant.

Neuromuscular Junction Disorders

Disorders of neuromuscular transmission resulting in hypotonia in infancy also feature varying degrees of weakness or fatigability. Appreciation of the latter is by fluctuating ptosis, weak suck, or premature discontinuation of oral feedings. Neuromuscular junction disorders presenting with hypotonia in infancy include juvenile myasthenia gravis, neonatal myasthenia gravis resulting from placental transmission of maternal antibodies against the fetal postsynaptic acetylcholine receptor, congenital myasthenic syndromes, and infant botulism.

Juvenile Myasthenia Gravis

Approximately 10% to 15% of cases of autoimmune myasthenia gravis due to endogenous production of antibodies directed against sarcolemmal nicotinic acetylcholine receptors or muscle-specific kinase occur in individuals younger than 16 years of age. The disorder is particularly rare in the first year of life (Andrews, 2004). The small number of infantile cases reported in the literature limits the conclusions drawn with respect to the occurrence of measurable antibody titers, treatment, and outcomes in this age group.

Neonatal Myasthenia

In approximately 15% of infants born to mothers with autoimmune myasthenia gravis, transitory symptoms of myasthenia occur in the neonatal period related to transfer of acetylcholine receptor antibodies across the placenta. Because the fetal nicotinic acetylcholine receptor is different from the adult form, the expression of myasthenic symptoms in newborns depends on the maternal production of antibodies against the fetal receptor (Gardnerova et al., 1997). These antibodies are not active against the adult form of the receptor and therefore do not contribute to maternal symptoms. Likewise, antibodies against the fetal receptor are not detectable by commercially available assays. For these reasons, neither maternal symptom severity nor the maternal antibody titer predicts the likelihood or severity of neonatal myasthenic symptoms. As with juvenile myasthenia gravis, the predominant symptoms are ocular or bulbar, although generalized hypotonia or weakness may occur. Rarely, affected infants have arthrogryposis due to prenatal exposure to fetal antibodies, leading to prolonged immobility in utero. Affected infants may require respiratory support temporarily or symptomatic therapy with subcutaneous neostigmine prior to oral feeds to prevent fatigue and premature discontinuation of feeding. In a majority of cases, the symptoms resolve within the first month of life (Papazian, 1992).

Congenital Myasthenic Syndromes

Several genetic disorders of neuromuscular transmission have been identified as causing hypotonia; fluctuating or persistent weakness of ocular, bulbar, or limb muscles; or arthrogryposis in infancy. The basis of one widely used classification scheme of congenital myasthenic syndromes (CMS) is whether the abnormality occurs in the presynaptic motor nerve terminal, the synaptic cleft, or the postsynaptic sarcolemma. The cause of the presynaptic disorder is a defect in the enzyme choline acetyltransferase, which synthesizes the neurotransmitter, whereas the synaptic defect results from deficiency of the end-plate cholinesterase. The causes of the postsynaptic disorders are various abnormalities of the structure, localization, or kinetics of the acetylcholine receptor. Inheritance of most CMS is autosomal recessive, except for the slow channel syndrome, which is autosomal dominant. The clinical presentation is similar to other forms of myasthenia occurring in

infancy, although deficiencies of the presynaptic enzyme choline acetyltransferase and of the postsynaptic acetylcholine receptor-associated protein rapsyn are also associated with sudden episodes of apnea (Hantai et al., 2004). Infants with CMS have negative antibody studies and demonstrate a decremental response on RNS. Specialized electrophysiological testing on fresh muscle biopsy specimens has been useful as a diagnostic tool but is not widely available. Of the 16 different genes currently known to be associated with CMS (Finlayson et al., 2013), testing is commercially available for 12, while testing of the others is available on a research basis only. Most forms of CMS are treated with cholinesterase inhibitors and/or the potassium channel inhibitor, 3,4-diaminopyridine. However, cholinesterase inhibitors may exacerbate end-plate cholinesterase deficiency, defects in the postsynaptic DOK-7 protein, and slow-channel syndrome. The latter form of the disorder may respond to fluoxetine (Harper et al., 2003), while improvement with oral ephedrine (Lashley et al., 2010) or salbutamol (Lorenzoni et al., 2013) has been reported in patients with defects in the DOK-7 gene. The natural history of CMS is highly variable even among patients with the same genotype.

Infant Botulism

Spores of the Gram-positive anaerobe *Clostridium botulinum*, an organism found in soil and in some cases in contaminated foods, produce an exotoxin that prevents anchoring of acetylcholine-containing vesicles to the presynaptic nerve terminal of the neuromuscular junction, disrupting neuromuscular transmission and resulting in flaccid weakness. In adults, the cause of botulism is ingestion of the preformed toxin; the organism itself cannot survive in the acidic environment of the adult digestive tract. By contrast, infants who ingest spores may be colonized and develop botulism from in situ production of the toxin. Affected infants may present any time after 2 weeks of age and may have relatively greater involvement of bulbar than appendicular muscles. The characteristic finding on RNS is an increment in the CMAP with high-rate (50 Hz) stimulation (Cornblath et al., 1983). Diagnostic confirmation is obtained by testing a stool or enema specimen with a bioassay in mice inoculated against different strains of toxin. Aside from supportive measures, early administration of botulinum immune globulin shortens the course of the disease (Arnon et al., 2006). In most cases, treatment should be initiated based on the clinical suspicion and should not be delayed while awaiting results of the bioassay.

Muscle Disorders

Subsets of disorders that cause hypotonia in infancy relate to developmental or structural defects of myocytes and do not affect cerebral function. The *congenital myopathies* are developmental muscle disorders with distinctive features on muscle histology. Most are autosomal recessive or X-linked, although some are allelic with dominantly inherited conditions with later symptom onset. Common features include diffuse weakness and hypotonia with normal or mildly elevated serum CK, nonspecific myopathic abnormalities on EMG, and predominance of type I fibers on muscle histology. The diagnosis is contingent upon biopsy findings and in some cases can be confirmed with commercially available genetic testing. A recommended diagnostic approach based upon clinical features and skeletal muscle pathology is outlined in a recent review by North et al. (2014). Cognition is usually normal, and there are no abnormalities of other organs. Weakness may be severe but is typically static or slowly progressive, and some affected infants show improved strength through the early childhood

TABLE 30.5 Common Sensory Syndromes

Syndrome	Localization	Sensory features	Associated findings
Acute inflammatory demyelinating polyneuropathy	Demyelinating lesion of peripheral nerves and roots	Dysesthesias and paresthesias that may be painful, along with sensory loss	Areflexia common early in the course; motor findings predominant
Sensory neuropathy	Axonal or neuronal damage involving predominantly sensory axons	Burning pain, often with superimposed dysesthesias and paresthesias	Reflexes often suppressed distally early in the course
Carpal tunnel syndrome	Compression of the median nerve at the wrist	Numbness on the thumb and index and middle fingers	Weakness and wasting of the abductor pollicis brevis may occur in severe cases
Ulnar neuropathy	Ulnar nerve compression, most likely near the elbow and at the wrist	Loss of sensation on the fourth and fifth digits	Weakness of the interossei often evident with advanced cases
Syringomyelia	Fluid-filled cavity that expands the spinal cord, damaging segmental neurons and white matter tracts	Loss of pain and temperature at the levels of the lesion (capelike distribution; suspended sensory loss); dissociated sensory loss (i.e., affecting spinothalamic sensation and sparing posterior column sensation)	Weakness at the levels of the lesion can develop with motoneuron damage; spasticity below the lesion can develop in severe cases
Thalamic infarction	Infarction of the territory of the thalamoperforate arteries	Sensory loss and sensory ataxia involving the contralateral body	Weakness may develop; aphasia or neglect suggesting cortical damage can rarely develop with involvement of thalamocortical connections
Thalamic pain syndrome	Previous sensory stroke in the thalamus produces neuropathic pain of central origin	Burning dysesthetic pain in the contralateral body, especially distally in the limbs	Other signs of the thalamic damage are typical, including sensory loss
Trigeminal neuralgia	Dysfunction of the trigeminal nerve root	Paroxysms of lancinating electric shock-like neuropathic pain are seen; no other cranial nerve abnormality and no weakness are seen	No sensory loss or motor findings

sensory loss on the ipsilateral face (from trigeminal involvement) plus loss of pain and temperature sensation on the contralateral body (from damage to the ascending spinothalamic tract). With this syndrome, however, the motor findings eclipse the sensory findings; these include ipsilateral cerebellar ataxia, bulbar weakness resulting in dysarthria and dysphagia, and Horner syndrome.

Medial medullary syndrome typically results from occlusion of a branch of the vertebral artery and is less common than lateral medullary syndrome. Patients have loss of contralateral position and vibration sensation, but again, the motor findings predominate, including contralateral hemiparesis and ipsilateral paresis of the tongue.

Ascending damage in the brainstem from vascular and other causes also can produce contralateral sensory loss, but as with the aforementioned syndromes, the sensory findings are trivial compared with the motor findings.

Cerebral Sensory Lesions

Thalamic Lesions. Pure sensory deficit of cerebral origin usually arises from damage to the thalamus. The thalamus receives vascular supply from the thalamoperforate arteries, which are branches of the posterior cerebral arteries, often with some contribution from the posterior communicating arteries. In some patients, both thalami are supplied by one posterior cerebral artery, so bilateral thalamic infarction can develop from unilateral arterial occlusion. Thalamic pain syndrome is an occasional sequela of a thalamic sensory stroke and is characterized by spontaneous pain localized to the distal arm and leg, exacerbated by contact and stress.

Cortical Lesions. Lesions of the postcentral gyrus produce more sensory symptoms than motor symptoms. Infarction of this region involving a branch of the middle cerebral artery can produce sensory loss with little or no motor loss. More posterior lesions may spare the primary modalities of sensation (pain, temperature, touch, joint position) but instead impair higher sensory function, with manifestations such as graphesthesia, two-point discrimination, and the perception of double simultaneous stimuli.

COMMON SENSORY SYNDROMES

Some common sensory syndromes are outlined in Table 30.5. Many of these are associated with motor deficits as well.

Peripheral Syndromes
Sensory Polyneuropathy

The most common presenting complaint among patients with distal symmetrical peripheral polyneuropathy is sensory disturbance. The disturbance can be negative (decreased discrimination and increased threshold) or positive (neuropathic pain, paresthesias, dysesthesias), or both. Most neuropathies involve motor and sensory fibers, although the initial symptoms usually are sensory.

Nerve conduction studies can evaluate the status of the myelin sheath, thereby identifying patients with predominantly demyelinating polyneuropathies, including acute inflammatory demyelinating polyneuropathy (AIDP) and chronic inflammatory demyelinating polyneuropathy (CIDP). Electromyography (EMG) can demonstrate denervation and hence axonal damage, thereby identifying the motor involvement of many neuropathies with predominantly axonal features (Misulis and Head, 2002).

Cerebrospinal fluid (CSF) analysis can be helpful for identifying some immune-mediated and inflammatory neuropathies. Nerve biopsy can help with diagnosis of a variety of neuropathies.

Diabetic Neuropathies

Diabetic sensory neuropathy affects mainly small myelinated and unmyelinated axons, thereby producing disordered pain and temperature sensation. The findings often appear to be a paradox to the affected patient: loss of sensation yet with burning pain. Pathophysiologically, this makes perfect sense. The damaged axons cannot carry the patterns of action potentials, which accounts for the loss of sensation, yet spontaneous action potentials from damaged nerve endings, plus increased susceptibility to discharge from mechanical stimuli, cause the perceived neuropathic pain.

Small Fiber Neuropathy

Small fiber neuropathies (SFN) typically present as a progressive burning pain, commonly seen first in the feet. Lancinating pain, numbness, and paresthesias along with symptoms of autonomic dysfunction are commonly seen. Examination demonstrates abnormalities of pinprick and temperature sensation in most patients. Vibratory perception is often affected. Reflexes commonly are normal. Conventional electrodiagnostic studies are normal, as they only access large fiber nerves. Since sweat glands are innervated by small fiber nerves, quantitative sudomotor axon reflex test (QSART) exams are highly specific and sensitive. Improvements in pathology techniques have made skin biopsies an effective and safe method for diagnosing SFN.

Common etiologies include diabetes mellitus, autoimmune/paraneoplastic, vitamin deficiencies/toxicities, toxic exposure to alcohol, heavy metals, and medications. Amyloidosis should also be considered, especially when accompanied by profound autonomic dysfunction.

Acquired Immunodeficiency Syndrome-Associated Neuropathies

Human immunodeficiency virus type 1 (HIV-1) infection can produce a variety of neuropathic presentations. One of the most common is a painful, predominantly sensory polyneuropathy (Robinson-Papp and Simpson, 2009). The diagnosis can be confirmed by nerve conduction studies, EMG, and the appropriate clinical findings. CSF analysis and biopsy usually are not necessary unless an HIV-1-associated vasculitis or infection (such as cytomegalovirus) is present.

Toxic Neuropathies

Some toxic neuropathies can be predominantly sensory. Such presentations most commonly are seen in patients with chemotherapy-induced peripheral neuropathy (Gutiérrez-Gutiérrez et al., 2010). Although motor abnormalities do occur, the sensory symptoms eclipse the motor symptoms for most patients. Development of dysesthesias, burning, and loss of sensation is the characteristic presentation. The neuropathy can be severe enough to be dose limiting for some patients and may continue to progress for months after cessation of chemotherapy administration.

Patients with neuropathy that develops during chemotherapy can be presumed to have toxic neuropathy. If the association is not clear, however, other possibilities should be considered, including paraneoplastic and nutritional causes. Atypical features of chemotherapy-induced neuropathy include appearance of symptoms after completion of the chemotherapy regimen and development of prominent neuropathy with administration of agents that are seldom neurotoxic.

Among the uncommon toxic neuropathies is B6/pyridoxine. Excess supplementation can cause a painful sensory neuropathy, associated with degeneration of the dorsal root ganglia (Perry et al., 2004). With further excessive doses, motor involvement can occur but this is far less common.

Amyloid Neuropathy

Primary amyloidosis can produce a predominantly sensory neuropathy in approximately one-third of affected patients (Simmons and Specht, 2010). Familial amyloid polyneuropathy is a dominantly inherited condition. Patients present with painful dysesthesias plus loss of pain and temperature sensation. Weakness develops later. Autonomic dysfunction is typical. Eventually the sensory loss can be severe enough to make the affected extremities virtually anesthetic. The diagnosis can be suspected on clinical grounds, and confirmation requires positive results on either DNA genetic testing or nerve biopsy.

Proximal Sensory Loss

Proximal sensory loss involving the trunk and upper aspects of the arms and legs is uncommon but can be seen in patients with porphyria or diabetes and in some patients with proximal plexopathies with a restricted distribution. Other rare causes of proximal sensory loss include Tangier disease, Sjögren syndrome, and paraneoplastic syndrome (Rudnicki and Dalmau, 2005). These neuropathic processes can be associated with pain in addition to the sensory loss. Motor deficit also is common, with weakness in a proximal distribution.

Patients with thoracic sensory loss also should be evaluated for thoracic spinal cord lesion, which may not always be associated with corticospinal tract signs.

Temperature-Dependent Sensory Loss

Leprosy can produce sensory deficits that predominantly affect cooler regions of the skin including the fingers, toes, nose, and ears (Wilder-Smith and Van Brakel, 2008). Temperature sensation initially is impaired, with subsequent involvement of pain and touch sensation in the cooler skin regions. The deficit gradually ascends to warmer areas, typically in a stocking-glove distribution, with frequent trigeminal and ulnar nerve involvement.

Acute Inflammatory Demyelinating Polyradiculoneuropathy

Acute inflammatory demyelinating polyradiculoneuropathy (AIDP), or Guillain-Barré syndrome, is an autoimmune process characterized by rapid progression of inflammatory demyelination of the nerve roots and peripheral nerves. Patients present with generalized weakness that may spread from the legs upwards or occasionally from cranial motor nerves downwards. Sensory symptoms generally are overshadowed by the motor loss. Tendon reflexes are lost as the weakness progresses (Hughes and Cornblath, 2005).

The diagnosis of AIDP is suspected in a patient who presents with progressive weakness with areflexia. Nerve conduction studies can confirm slowing, especially proximally (F-waves are particularly affected). CSF analysis shows increased protein level without a prominent cellular response (albuminocytological dissociation).

Mononeuropathy

Of the many recognized mononeuropathies, the most common is carpal tunnel syndrome, with ulnar neuropathy a close second. Although not classically considered a mononeuropathy, radiculopathy can be considered to fall into this category because one peripheral nerve unit is affected.

Carpal Tunnel Syndrome. Compression of the median nerve at the wrist produces sensory loss on the palmar aspects of the first through the third digits. Motor symptoms and signs can develop with increasing severity of the mononeuropathy, but the sensory symptoms predominate, especially early in the course (Bland, 2005).

Nerve conduction studies usually show slowing of sensory and motor conduction of the median nerve through the carpal tunnel at the wrist. The slowing is present when conduction elsewhere is normal or at least when the distal slowing is far out of proportion to the slowing from neuropathy elsewhere. The EMG findings usually are normal, but denervation in the abductor pollicis brevis may develop with severe disease.

Ulnar Neuropathy. Ulnar neuropathy is commonly due to compression in the region of the ulnar groove. Patients present with numbness in the ulnar two fingers (fourth and fifth digits). Weakness of the interossei develops with advanced ulnar neuropathy in any location, but sensory symptoms predominate, especially early in the course (Cut, 2007).

Motor nerve conduction studies show slowing of conduction across the elbow or wrist—the two common sites for ulnar nerve entrapment. Findings on sensory nerve conduction studies also will be abnormal if the lesion is at the wrist. EMG can show denervation in the ulnar-innervated intrinsic muscles of the hand.

Radial Neuropathy. Radial neuropathy is often due to compression of the nerve in the spiral groove. Prototypically, this is seen in patients with alcohol intoxication, although cases are not confined to this association. Damage to the radial nerve in the spiral groove results in damage to muscles innervated distally to the triceps. Patients typically present with wrist drop, and sensory symptoms are minimal. Compression of the radial nerve distally in the forearm near the wrist can produce sensory loss and dysesthesias on the radial side of the dorsum of the hand, and in this case there is no motor loss.

Diagnosis is suspected clinically from the wrist drop in the absence of weakness of muscles of the arm innervated by other nerves; note that examination of median and ulnar-innervated muscles can be difficult if the radial deficit is severe. Sensory findings, when present, are typical. Sensory findings in a radial nerve distribution without motor involvement suggest distal radial sensory nerve damage (e.g., from pressure, handcuffs, intravenous catheter insertion, or other local trauma).

Radiculopathy

Radiculopathy commonly produces pain or sensory loss, or both, in the distribution of one or more nerve roots. Motor symptoms and signs develop with increasing severity, but sensory symptoms (usually pain) may be present for years without motor symptoms. Reflex abnormalities are common in radiculopathy.

Table 30.6 presents clinical features of common radiculopathies. Although cervical and lumbar radiculopathies are

TABLE 30.6 Radiculopathies

Nerve root	Sensory loss	Motor loss	Reflex abnormality
C5	Radial forearm	Deltoid, biceps	None
C6	Digits 1 and 2	Biceps, brachioradialis	Biceps
C7	Digits 3 and 4	Wrist extensors, triceps	Triceps
C8	Digit 5	Intrinsic hand muscles	None
L2	Lateral and anterior upper thigh	Psoas, quadriceps	None
L3	Lower medial thigh	Psoas, quadriceps	Patellar (knee)
L4	Medial lower leg	Tibialis anterior, quadriceps	Patellar (knee)
L5	Lateral lower leg	Peronei, gluteus medius, tibialis anterior, toe extension	None
S1	Lateral foot, digits 4 and 5, outside of sole	Gastrocnemii, gluteus maximus	Achilles tendon (ankle)

discussed here, any level can be affected. Diabetic radiculopathy and herpes zoster commonly affect thoracic dermatomes, as well as cervical and thoracic dermatomes usually unaffected by spondylosis or disk disease.

Radiculopathy is best investigated using MRI. In patients younger than 45 years of age, the most common etiological disorder is disk disease. In older patients, spondylosis and osteophyte formation predominate. The latter is slower to progress and less likely to be associated with spontaneous remissions and exacerbations. EMG can be helpful to identify any axonal damage from radiculopathy, which may help determine the need, location, and timing of decompressive surgery.

Spinal Syndromes

Myelopathy

Myelopathy typically produces sensory loss, although the motor and reflex findings eclipse the sensory findings in most patients. Nevertheless, when a patient presents with back pain with or without leg weakness, a sensory level should be sought.

Some basic "pearls" regarding sensory testing in patients with suspected myelopathy follow:

- A defined line-like level is not expected.
- The sensory mapping is not as precise as that shown on dermatome charts.
- The sensory loss is seldom complete, which makes precise localization even more difficult.
- The sensory level may not be at the same level on the two sides of the body—a discrepancy of up to several levels can be seen.
- Look for dissociated sensory loss due to crossed projections of pain/temperature versus uncrossed touch/proprioception projections.
- Discrepancy in sensory level between posterior column and spinothalamic levels can occur because of intersegmental projections of the axons of the posterolateral (Lissauer) tract.

- The sensory level may be much higher than might be expected from motor examination or pain. This is because the lesion may be much higher than indicated by the levels of clinical findings, reinforcing the basic precept that the examiner must start from the level of the symptoms and consider higher levels.

Syringomyelia

Syringomyelia is the presence of a syrinx, or fluid-filled space, in the spinal cord that extends over several to many segments. This is most commonly associated with a Chiari malformation (Koyanagi and Houkin, 2010). The mass effect of the syrinx produces damage to the fibers crossing in the anterior commissure that are destined for the spinothalamic tract, which conveys pain and temperature sensation. With more severe enlargement of the syrinx, damage to the surrounding ascending tracts may occur, affecting sensation below the level of the lesion. By the time this develops, segmental motoneuron damage and descending corticospinal tract damage are almost always present, and clinical signs of these changes can be seen.

Spinal Hemisection

The spinal hemisection syndrome (Brown–Séquard syndrome) is classically described as the result of surgical or traumatic hemisection of the cord, but this presentation is rarely if ever encountered in clinical practice. Below the level of the lesion, ipsilateral deficits in vibration and proprioception from dysfunction of the dorsal columns, as well as contralateral deficits in pain and temperature from damage to the spinothalamic tracts, are the characteristic findings. Ipsilateral weakness also is seen from damage to the corticospinal tracts.

The diagnosis is suggested by the clinical presentation. This is a condition that can easily be missed unless the examiner assesses individual sensory modalities. MRI usually is performed to look for inflammatory or structural causes of the condition.

Tabes Dorsalis and Related Disorders

Tabes dorsalis is due to involvement of the dorsal roots by late neurosyphilis. Patients present with sensory ataxia, lightning pains, and often a slapping gait. Tendon reflexes are depressed (Marra, 2009).

Syphilitic myelitis is a rare complication of neurosyphilis, characterized by progressive weakness and spasticity. Motor symptoms dominate in this condition, with lesser sensory symptoms than with tabes dorsalis. MRI of the spine must be performed to look for other structural causes of myelopathy.

Brain Syndromes
Thalamic Infarction and Hemorrhage

Thalamic infarction typically produces contralateral hemisensory loss and is the main cause of a pure sensory stroke. All modalities are affected to variable degrees. The thalamus and its vascular supply are not organized so that specific portions of the sensory system are affected without dysfunction of other sensory systems and regions. MRI is most sensitive for visualization of acute thalamic lesions but CT is performed when MRI is unavailable or contraindicated.

Thalamic Pain Syndrome (Central Post-Stroke Pain)

Thalamic pain syndrome is an occasional sequela to thalamic infarction that usually affects the entire contralateral body, from face through arm, trunk, and leg. The pain, mainly distal in the limbs, is present at rest but is exacerbated by sensory stimulation. The distribution of the pain may shift so that the pain is poorly localized (Nicholson, 2004). Sensory detection thresholds are increased. Involvement of the posterior ventrobasal region is thought to be necessary for production of thalamic pain.

In a patient with a known history of thalamic infarction, additional study usually is not needed when thalamic pain occurs. If the pain develops long after the infarction, however, repeated scanning to look for a new pathological process such as recurrent infarction, hemorrhage, or (less likely) tumor is warranted.

The term *central post-stroke pain syndrome* is increasingly used, since not all post-stroke pain syndromes are due to primary thalamic damage, although the thalamus is still felt to be an important part of the pathophysiology (Klit, Finnerup, and Jensen, 2009).

Trigeminal Neuralgia

Trigeminal neuralgia is a painful condition that produces lancinating pain in the distribution of part of the trigeminal nerve. This is prototypical neuropathic pain. Patients have paroxysms of pain that usually last for seconds. Sensory loss does not occur, so its presence encourages further search for other diagnoses. Imaging studies commonly are performed in the evaluation of trigeminal neuralgia but seldom are revealing.

Mental Neuropathy (Numb Chin Syndrome)

While development of isolated numbness and/or pain in the chin region may seem insignificant, it is often an ominous finding suggestive of an underlying and possibly undiagnosed malignancy. The diagnosis of a mental neuropathy warrants an aggressive malignancy evaluation. Nonmalignant etiologies include trauma and other jaw pathologies, multiple sclerosis, infections, connective tissue diseases, vasculitis and sickle cell crisis, in both adult and pediatric patients (Hamdoun et al., 2012; Laurencet et al, 2000).

Cortical Infarction

Infarction of the sensory cortex serving the face and arm is due to thromboembolism of branches of the middle cerebral artery. Infarction in the anterior cerebral artery territory produces sensory loss affecting the leg. Motor symptoms and signs are usually present, as are sensory abnormalities; however, if the region of infarction is limited, the sensory findings may be much more prominent than the motor findings.

Deficits of Higher Sensory Perception

Multiple disorders have been described as producing defects in higher sensory processing. These include, in part, neonatal insult, autism, early developmental disorders, stroke, Alzheimer disease, head injury, and post-traumatic stress disorder. The total scope and features of these disorders are not completely understood, and since they are less able to be localized than more elemental sensory deficits, they are studied less often. Most of the clinical descriptions are anecdotal, with few control comparisons.

Sensory processing disorder is a term which has not yet been incorporated into standard diagnostic terminology, but there is increasing indication that this is likely a family of disorders with a variety of substrates and features (Koziol et al., 2011). The anatomical structures which serve higher sensory processing and integration are as broad as the brain itself and include cerebral cortex, basal ganglia, cerebellum, and the thalamus.

The disorder can manifest as difficulty with processing sensory data into complex meaning, and difficulty with attention to or interpretation of sensory stimuli and even electrophysiological responses from the brain. Sensory processing disorder crosses the border between sensory perception and attention, hence the multitude of studies examining sensory perception in autism spectrum disorder (Cygan et al., 2014).

The *sensory profile* is an assessment tool in the form of a long questionnaire which addresses, in part, some of the higher sensory processing, and without making a definitive diagnosis, can be helpful for identifying patients who may have difficulty with sensory processing (Brown et al., 2001; Dunn, 1994). While initially developed for use in children, an adult sensory profile assessment is now in use.

Infants with low birth weight and with neonatal insult appear to be at increased risk for sensory processing disorder (Gill et al., 2013; Wickremasinghe et al., 2013). Not surprisingly, children with autism also exhibit increased risk for this (Puts et al., 2014). Presently, sensory processing is not routinely assessed in clinical practice, but the clinician should be aware of the concept and the potential manifestations of related disorders.

Clinical manifestations of sensory processing disorders can include misinterpretation of sensory data resulting in poorly organized motor output and impaired incorporation of sensory stimuli in learning. This can affect not just responses to audio and visual stimuli but to almost any modality, cause deficiency or excess cognitive response to sensory stimulation, or even accentuate a drive to get sensory inputs.

Functional (or Psychogenic) Sensory Loss

Functional sensory loss is less common than other positive functional neurological symptoms such as seizures or paralysis. In fact, it is easy to mistakenly ascribe a pattern of sensory loss to a nonanatomical cause when in fact true disease is present. Such misdiagnosis is particularly common with thalamic infarction and plexus dysfunction. Of note, embellished sensory or motor loss, although obvious to the examiner, may be superimposed on a real neurological deficit. The patient may be unintentionally helping the examiner yet essentially ruining the credibility of the report.

Cautionary notes should be borne in mind. In general, however, clinical presentations suggesting functional sensory loss include:

- Sensory loss exactly splitting the midline, with a minimal transition zone
- Circumferential sensory loss around the body or an extremity
- Failure to perceive vibration with a precise demarcation
- Loss of vision or hearing on the same side of the body as for the cutaneous sensory deficit
- Total anesthesia.

The discrepancies in total anesthesia can be failure to perceive any sensory stimulus on an extremity that moves perfectly well. This degree of sensory loss would be expected to produce sensory ataxia. Another trap for a patient with psychogenic anesthesia of a limb involves tapping the limb while the patient's eyes are closed; consequent movement of the limb confirms the functional nature of the deficit. Third, if the anesthetic limb is an arm, examining for sensory abnormality while the arms are folded across the chest can be confusing for the malingering patient, especially if performed quickly.

PITFALLS

Additional text available at http://expertconsult.inkling.com.

REFERENCES

The complete reference list is available online at https://expertconsult .inkling.com/.

31 Arm and Neck Pain

Michael Ronthal

CHAPTER OUTLINE

CLINICAL ASSESSMENT
History
Examination
PATHOLOGY AND CLINICAL SYNDROMES
Spinal Cord Syndromes
Radiculitis
Brachial Plexopathy
Thoracic Outlet Syndrome
Suprascapular Nerve Entrapment
Carpal Tunnel Syndrome
Ulnar Entrapment at the Elbow
Radial Nerve–Posterior Interosseus Nerve Syndrome
Complex Regional Pain Syndrome
"In-Between" Neurogenic and Non-Neurogenic Pain
    Syndrome—Whiplash Injury
Rheumatoid Arthritis of the Spine
Non-Neurological Neck/Arm Pain Syndromes

Evaluation of the patient with arm and/or neck pain is based on a careful history and clinical examination. Diagnosis of the common causes and a treatment plan can almost always be accomplished in the office before laboratory investigation, but further study may be required if the patient fails to improve or has other specific indications for imaging or electrical studies.

A useful approach is to consider the diagnosis in terms of pain-sensitive structures in the neck and upper limbs. These structures may be part of the nervous system or may involve joints, muscles, and tendons. Neurological causes should be considered based on the innervation of the neck and arm, and non-neurological causes are based on dysfunction of the other anatomical structures of the arm or neck. Because nerve root irritation generates neck muscle spasm, this type of pain is usually lumped into the "neurological" category. Some essentially non-neurological conditions have neurological complications and are grouped in this chapter as "in-between" disorders.

CLINICAL ASSESSMENT
History

Neurological Causes of Pain: Sites That Can Trigger Pain

Muscle Spasm. Posterior cervical muscles in spasm trigger local pain that is aggravated by neck movement, and the diagnosis is supported by the finding of palpable spasm and tenderness. The pain may radiate upward to the occipital region and over the top of the head to the bifrontal area. It is usually described as constant, aching, or bursting, or as a tight band or pressure sensation on top of the head. Pain with similar characteristics can be triggered by abnormalities of the facet joints, cervical vertebrae, and even intervertebral disk pathology, which is also instrumental in the genesis of neck muscle spasm.

Neck mobility is best assessed by testing for movement in each of the main planes of movement, flexion and extension, lateral flexion to the right and left, and rotation to the right and left. Normally in flexion, the chin can touch the sternum, and in rotation the chin can approximate the point of the shoulder.

Central Pain. Dysfunction affecting the ascending sensory tracts in the spinal cord may generate pain or paresthesias in the arm(s) or down the trunk and lower limbs. An electric shock-like sensation provoked by neck flexion and spreading to the arms, down the spine, and even into the legs is thought to originate in the posterior columns of the cervical spinal cord (Lhermitte sign). Although the symptom is frequent in patients with multiple sclerosis (MS), it is nonspecific and simply indicates a pathological process in the cervical cord. Sharp, superficial, burning pain or itching points to dysfunction in the spinothalamic system, whereas deep, aching, boring pain with paresthesias of tightness, squeezing, or a feeling of swelling suggests dysfunction in the posterior column system. The sensory symptoms indicate the dysfunctional tract but are poor segmental localizers.

Nerve Root Pain. If the pathology involves a nerve root, it is referred into the upper limb in a dermatome distribution. Brachialgia (arm pain) aggravated by neck movement, coughing, or sneezing suggests radiculopathy and when these trigger features are present one can be fairly certain that the pain is radicular in character. Nerve root pain is typically lancinating in character, but it can present as a dull ache in the arm.

Repetitive sudden shooting pains radiating from the occipital region to the temporal areas or vertex suggest the diagnosis of occipital neuralgia. There may be local tenderness over the greater or lesser occipital nerve, and a local injection of corticosteroid plus local anesthetic is both diagnostic and therapeutic. Failure to respond suggests that the craniovertebral junction area should be imaged.

Ulnar Nerve Pain. Ulnar nerve entrapment causes numbness or pain radiating down the medial aspect of the arm to the little and ring fingers. Symptoms are often worse at night when the patient sleeps with a flexed elbow, and they may interrupt sleep. Ulnar paresthesias are also triggered by pressure on the nerve when resting the elbow on the arm of a chair or desk. Tapping on the nerve in the ulnar groove at the elbow may evoke a tingly electrical sensation in the little and ring fingers—Tinel sign.

Median Nerve Pain. Median nerve entrapment in the carpal tunnel classically awakens the patient from sleep with numbness and tingling in the thumb, index, and middle fingers, which is relieved by "shaking out" the hand. Pain generated in the median nerve can be sharp and lancinating and radiates to the thumb, index, and middle fingers. While entrapment in the carpal tunnel is common, occasionally the site of entrapment is at the elbow as the nerve passes under the pronator muscle.

Plexus Pain. Infiltrative or inflammatory lesions of the brachial plexus produce severe brachialgia radiating down the

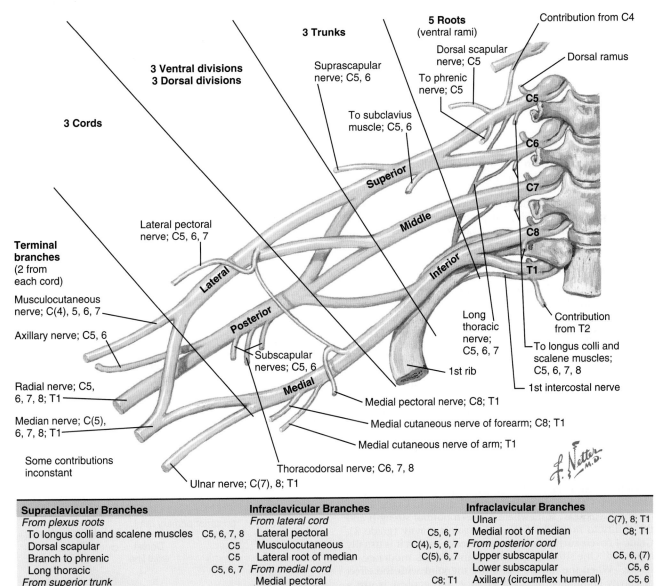

3 Trunks

5 Roots
(ventral rami)

Contribution from C4

3 Ventral divisions
3 Dorsal divisions

Suprascapular
nerve; C5, 6

Dorsal scapular
nerve; C5

Dorsal ramus

To phrenic
nerve; C5

3 Cords

To subclavius
muscle; C5, 6

C5

Superior

C6

C7

Middle

**Terminal
branches**
(2 from
each cord)

Lateral pectoral
nerve; C5, 6, 7

C8

Lateral

Inferior

T1

Musculocutaneous
nerve; C(4), 5, 6, 7

Contribution
from T2

Posterior

Axillary nerve; C5, 6

Long
thoracic
nerve;
C5, 6, 7

To longus colli and
scalene muscles;
C5, 6, 7, 8

Subscapular
nerves; C5, 6

Radial nerve; C5,
6, 7, 8; T1

Medial

1st rib

1st intercostal nerve

Medial pectoral nerve; C8; T1

Median nerve; C(5),
6, 7, 8; T1

Medial cutaneous nerve of forearm; C8; T1

Medial cutaneous nerve of arm; T1

Some contributions
inconstant

Thoracodorsal nerve; C6, 7, 8

Ulnar nerve; C(7), 8; T1

Supraclavicular Branches		Infraclavicular Branches		Infraclavicular Branches	
From plexus roots		*From lateral cord*		Ulnar	C(7), 8; T1
To longus colli and scalene muscles	C5, 6, 7, 8	Lateral pectoral	C5, 6, 7	Medial root of median	C8; T1
Dorsal scapular	C5	Musculocutaneous	C(4), 5, 6, 7	*From posterior cord*	
Branch to phrenic	C5	Lateral root of median	C(5), 6, 7	Upper subscapular	C5, 6, (7)
Long thoracic	C5, 6, 7	*From medial cord*		Lower subscapular	C5, 6
From superior trunk		Medial pectoral	C8; T1	Axillary (circumflex humeral)	C5, 6
Suprascapular	C5, 6	Medial cutaneous nerve of arm	T1	Thoracodorsal	C5, 6
To subclavius muscle	C5, 6	Medial cutaneous nerve of forearm	C8; T1	Radial	C5, 6, 7, 8

Fig. 31.1 Brachial plexus: schema. *(Netter illustration from* www.netterimages.com *© Elsevier Inc. All rights reserved.)*

upper limb and also spreading to the shoulder region. Radiation to the ulnar two fingers suggests that the origin is in the lower brachial plexus, and radiation to the upper arm, forearm, and thumb suggests an upper plexopathy. Patients with thoracic outlet syndrome complain of brachialgia and numbness or tingling in the upper limb or hand when working with objects above the head. The thoracic outlet syndrome is an overdiagnosed condition, but certainly exists, and maneuvers are designed to test for compromise of the neurovascular structures passing through the thoracic outlet. The arm is extended at the elbow, abducted at the shoulder, and then rotated posteriorly. The examiner palpates the radial pulse while listening with a stethoscope over the brachial plexus in the supraclavicular fossa. The patient takes a deep inspiration and turns the head to one or the other side. Many normal individuals lose their radial pulse, but the emergence of a bruit does suggest at the least vascular entrapment (Adson test). The patient then exercises the hands held above the head with extended elbows—numbness, pain, or paresthesias, often

with pallor of the hand, supports the diagnosis (Roos test) (Fig. 31.1).

Non-Neurological Causes of Neck Pain and Brachialgia

Pain arising in muscle is deep, aching, and boring. In the cervical region, it is localized to the shoulders and sometimes radiates down the arm. If the patient is over 50 years of age, a sedimentation rate should be checked; if it is markedly elevated, the diagnosis of polymyalgia rheumatica should be considered. Patients with fibromyalgia may have pain in the neck, shoulders, and arms, with trigger spots or nodules that are exquisitely tender even to light pressure.

If pain is triggered or aggravated by joint movement of the upper limb, arthritis or tendonitis is the likely cause. Particular attention should be paid to these characteristics: pain on shoulder abduction is usually tendinitis, rotator cuff pathology, or pericapsulitis related. The tendons anteriorly and at the lateral point of the shoulder may be tender to pressure. More diffuse tenderness anterior to the shoulder joint indicates bursitis. Tenderness over the medial or lateral epicondyle at the elbow indicates local inflammation, and pain on active or passive wrist or finger joint movement suggests tendonitis or arthritis of the fingers. The pain of epicondylitis may radiate down the forearm in a pseudoneuralgic fashion, but precipitation by active wrist extension or grip indicates a rheumatological cause.

Examination

The physical examination is designed to localize a neurological deficit which may be related to spinal cord, nerve roots, or peripheral nerves. Evaluation for non-neurological pathology is also required because rheumatological problems often complicate a primarily neurological problem. A detailed knowledge of motor and sensory neuroanatomy is required for accurate localization.

Motor Signs—Atrophy and Weakness

The examination begins with inspection. Particular attention is paid to atrophy of muscles of the shoulders, arms, and the small muscles of the hands. Fasciculations are often due to anterior horn cell disease, but they may be part of the neurology of cervical spondylosis and radiculopathy. Significant sensory signs would argue against anterior horn cell degeneration.

Muscles in the various myotomes must be tested individually. When there is unilateral weakness, the contralateral side can act as a control, but some standard measure of strength is necessary for accurate evaluation when bilateral weakness is present. If one can overcome the action of a muscle by resisting or opposing its action close to the joint it moves, using an equivalent equipotent muscle of the examiner (fingers test fingers, whole arm tests biceps), then that muscle is by definition, weak. The degree of weakness can be graded, and the 5-point (Medical Research Council [MRC]) grading scale is often used. Grade 5 represents normal strength. Grade 4 represents "weakness" somewhere between normal strength and the ability to move the limb only against gravity (grade 3). Grade 4 covers such a wide range of weakness that it is usually expanded. One simple expansion is into "mild, moderate, or severe." When the muscle can move the joint with the effect of gravity eliminated, it is graded at 2, and grade 1 is just a flicker of movement. Even when the patient complains primarily of symptoms in the upper limbs, the lower limbs must be examined for signs of myelopathy.

The finding of hypertonia, weakness, sensory loss, increased tendon reflexes, and/or extensor plantar reflexes indicates cord dysfunction. These signs, when combined with radicular signs in the upper limbs, indicate a spinal cord lesion in the neck. The distribution of weakness is all important in localizing the problem to nerve root, plexus, peripheral nerve, muscle, or even upper motor neuron (central weakness). It is useful to use a simplified schema of radicular anatomical localization when evaluating nerve root weakness because overlap of segmental innervation of muscles can complicate the analysis (Table 31.1).

A distribution of weakness that does not conform to a clearly defined anatomical distribution of cervical roots or a single peripheral nerve in the upper limb suggests plexopathy. Upper plexus lesions cause mainly shoulder abduction weakness, and lower plexus lesions will affect the small muscles of the hand.

Sensory Signs

Skin sensation is tested in a standardized manner starting with pinprick appreciation at the back of the head (C2), followed

TABLE 31.1 Segmental Innervation Scheme for Anatomical Localization of Nerve Root Lesions

Segment level	Muscle(s)	Action
C4	Supraspinatus	First 10 degrees of shoulder abduction
C5	Deltoid Biceps/brachialis/ brachioradialis	Shoulder abduction Elbow flexion
C6	Extensor carpi radialis longus	Radial wrist extension
C7	Triceps	Elbow extension
C7	Extensor digitorum	Finger extension
C8	Flexor digitorum	Finger flexion
T1	Interossei	Finger abduction and adduction
	Abductor digiti minimi	Little finger abduction

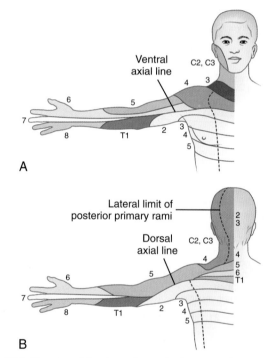

Fig. 31.2 Diagram of the dermatomes in the upper limbs. A, Anterior aspect. Although variability and overlap across the interrupted lines are evident, little or no overlap occurs across the continuous lines (i.e., dorsal and ventral axial lines). The examiner should routinely choose one spot in the "middle" of a dermatome and test at that point in all patients. C4 usually terminates at the point of the shoulder, T3 is almost always in the axilla, and T4 spreads across the chest so that C4 abuts T4 approximately at the nipple line. **B,** Posterior aspect.

by sequentially testing sensation in the cervical dermatomes, down the shoulder, over the deltoid, down the lateral aspect of the arm to the lateral fingers, and then proceeding to the medial fingers and up the medial aspect of the arm (Fig. 31.2). The procedure is repeated with a wisp of cotton to test touch sensation and test tubes filled with cold and warm water to test temperature sensation. Position sense in the distal phalanx of a finger is tested by immobilizing the proximal joint and supporting the distal phalanx on its medial and lateral sides and then moving it up or down in small increments. The patient, with eyes closed, reports the sensation of movement and its direction. Loss of position sense in the fingers usually indicates a very high cervical cord lesion.

Tendon Reflexes

Examination of the tendon reflexes helps localize segmental nerve root levels, but in cervical spondylosis, which is by far the most common underlying pathology, the reflexes are often preserved or even increased despite radiculopathy, because of an associated myelopathy. An absent or decreased biceps reflex localizes the root level to C5, and an absent triceps reflex localizes the level to C6 or C7. An absent biceps reflex but with spread so that triceps or finger flexors contract is called an *inverted biceps jerk* and is strong evidence for C5 radiculopathy.

PATHOLOGY AND CLINICAL SYNDROMES
Spinal Cord Syndromes

Intramedullary Lesions

Primary intramedullary lesions may be neoplastic, inflammatory, or developmental. The most common presenting symptom of spinal cord tumor is pain, which is present in about two-thirds of patients, usually radicular in distribution, often aggravated by coughing or straining, and worse at night.

Dissociated sensory signs (segmental loss of pinprick and temperature sensation with preserved light touch, vibration, and position sense) in the upper limbs suggests central cord pathology. Long-tract signs in the lower limbs will, ultimately, develop in progressive acquired lesions. Magnetic resonance imaging (MRI) reveals swelling of the spinal cord. The most common tumors are glioma, lymphoma, and ependymoma.

Cervical myelitis presents with rapid onset of radicular and long-tract symptoms and signs and may be due to MS, postinfectious encephalomyelitis, or neuromyelitis optica, or it may be without an obvious cause (idiopathic).

Syringomyelia, a cystic intramedullary lesion of variable and unpredictable progression, may present with deep aching or boring pain in the upper limb, often characteristically referred to the ear. Asymmetrical lower motor neuron signs (radiculopathic) in the upper limbs, with dissociated suspended sensory loss (i.e., has an upper and lower border to the impairment of pinprick and temperature sensation), is suggestive of a syrinx. However, the most common cause of intramedullary cord dysfunction is extrinsic spinal cord compression.

Extramedullary Lesions

Extramedullary lesions, whatever the pathology, may result in any combination of root, central cord, and long-tract signs and symptoms. The most common cause of cervical nerve root and spinal cord compression is cervical spondylosis. This is a degenerative disorder of the cervical spine characterized by disk degeneration with disk space narrowing, bone overgrowth producing spurs and ridges, and hypertrophy of the facet joints, all of which can compress the cord or nerve roots. Hypertrophy of the spinal ligaments, with or without calcification, may contribute to compression. Hypertrophic osteophytes are present in approximately 30% of the population, and the incidence increases with age. The presence of such degenerative changes does not indicate that the patient has symptoms due to these changes; other pathology can also be present. Furthermore, the degree of bony change does not always correlate with the severity of the signs and symptoms

it produces. This chronic degenerative process is sometimes referred to as *hard disk* as opposed to an acute disk herniation or *soft disk* in which the onset is acute with severe neck pain and brachialgia. Patients with cervical spondylosis often awake in the morning with a painful stiff neck and diffuse nonpulsatile headache that resolves in a few hours. The lesion is most commonly at C5/6 and/or C6/7 and the focal signs are likely to reflect root dysfunction at those levels. Wasting and weakness of the small muscles of the hands, but particularly weakness of abduction of the little finger is often present. This sign localizes to lower segmental levels but there may be no observable anatomical change at those levels and it is labeled as a false localizer.

Restricted neck movement is always present with significant cervical spondylosis. Bladder dysfunction with frequency, urgency, and urgency incontinence or the finding of long-tract signs indicates the need for imaging of the cervical spine both to exclude pathology other than cervical spondylosis and also to define the severity of the spinal cord compression. Immobilization in a cervical collar often helps with the symptoms and signs of cervical spondylosis. The role of surgery as treatment is discussed in Chapter 106.

Other Cord Compression Syndromes

Extramedullary cord compression by pathology in the epidural space may be due to a primary or metastatic tumor. A Schwannoma or nerve sheath tumor produces signs and symptoms related to the nerve root on which it arises, and as it enlarges, progressive myelopathic dysfunction occurs. Plain radiographs of the cervical spine may demonstrate an enlarged intervertebral foramen and the MRI is diagnostic. A meningioma may present in a similar fashion and is more frequent in the thoracic region.

The initial presenting symptom of epidural spinal cord compression due to metastatic malignancy is pain in over 90% of patients. Malignant bone pain is usually localized to the vertebra involved and percussion tenderness over the vertebral spine is a good localizing sign. As the pathology spreads to the epidural space radicular pain occurs. Plain radiographs of the cervical spine may show bony pathology with the preservation of disk spaces but the imaging modality of choice is MRI. The whole spinal column should be scanned because the pathology is often at multiple sites, some of which may be subclinical. Spinal cord compression due to metastatic disease is a neurological emergency requiring treatment with immediate high-dose steroids and either local irradiation or surgical decompression.

Epidural infection may be either acute and pyogenic, or chronic when the organism is likely to be mycobacterial or fungal. Pyogenic epidural abscess may present acutely with fever, severe pain localized to a rigid neck, radicular pain, and rapidly progressive root and myelopathic signs, but at times the presentation is more subacute with less systemic evidence of infection. Imaging reveals early loss of the disk space which enhances with contrast material, and the infection spreads into the epidural space and then into the bone with vertebral collapse. Optimal therapy is surgical decompression and evacuation combined with 6–12 weeks of appropriate antimicrobial therapy for pyogenic infections and more prolonged treatment for tuberculosis.

The differential diagnosis of a rapidly progressive, painful, epidural lesion also includes spinal subarachnoid, subdural, or epidural hemorrhage. Bleeding is usually associated with some form of coagulopathy or anticoagulant therapy but sometimes occurs with vascular anomalies. The sudden onset of severe pain in the neck with or without radicular pain may be due to a local hemorrhage and after reversal of the coagulation deficit, if there is cord compression, surgical decompression.

Radiculitis

Herpes zoster may infect cervical sensory root ganglia. The pain is typically radicular, and the diagnosis becomes clear when, after 2 to 10 days, the typical vesicular rash appears. Motor involvement occasionally occurs, and when it does, it has a predilection for C5/6 segments. Myelitis with long-tract signs is seen in less than 1% of patients. If the pain lasts longer than 3 months after crusting of the skin lesions, postherpetic neuralgia has developed. The pain is described as constant, nagging, burning, aching, tearing, and itching, upon which are superimposed electric shocks and jabs. Treatment of postherpetic neuralgia pain is discussed in Chapters 103 and 106.

Brachial Plexopathy

Brachialgia and physical signs not respecting a single nerve root, associated with tenderness to palpation in the supraclavicular notch, should arouse suspicion of a brachial plexopathy.

Brachial Neuritis (Neuralgic Amyotrophy, Parsonage-Turner Syndrome)

Brachial neuritis is characterized by the abrupt onset of severe unilateral constant unrelenting pain in the shoulder and arm, worse at night, and rarely bilateral. The syndrome afflicts mainly young adult men. Within a week or so, muscle weakness, atrophy, and fasciculations are evident, mainly in the shoulder girdle but occasionally more distally, and distributed in more than one myotome. Despite the pain, there is usually little or no sensory loss. Pathogenesis is thought to be autoimmune/inflammatory, and a number of antecedent inciting events have been described, including immunization, infections, and trauma. The syndrome is also associated with autoimmune diseases and Hodgkin disease. There is no proven specific treatment, but a short course of corticosteroids is usually given. In general, treatment is supportive, and the pain mostly runs its course in 6 to 8 weeks. In some patients, recovery from paralysis can take up to a year, and occasionally there is some permanent mild weakness.

A subset of patients with a familial history has recurrent attacks. Hereditary neuralgic amyotrophy is autosomal dominant, and many have deletions of the PMP-22 gene in a portion of the distal long arm of chromosome 17.

Brachial Plexopathy in Cancer Patients

Plexopathy in patients with cancer, particularly those with breast cancer or lymphoma who have been irradiated, poses a problem: is this radiation plexopathy or malignant infiltration of the brachial plexus? Malignant infiltration is more likely to be extremely painful, and is more likely to involve the lower plexus. There may be an associated Horner syndrome. Radiation plexitis is less likely to cause severe pain and often involves the upper plexus. Both syndromes are slowly progressive but radiation plexitis is likely to be of longer duration. Neurophysiological studies with EMG can be helpful and myokymia and fasciculations support the diagnosis of radiation plexitis. Imaging with MRI to detect tumor infiltration has a sensitivity of 96%, specificity of 95%, and a positive predictive value of 95%. Occasionally locally malignant, relentless, and recurrent schwannoma occurs in a plexus that has been irradiated many years before.

Thoracic Outlet Syndrome

Entrapment may involve the brachial plexus, the subclavian artery, or both. Sagging musculature with postural abnormalities including droopy shoulders and a long neck contribute to the predisposition for thoracic outlet syndrome.

A supernumerary cervical rib or simply an elevated transverse process of the seventh cervical vertebra may be seen on plain radiographs. The rib may articulate with the superior aspect of the first rib, or a fibrous band may extend from its tip to the tip of the abnormal transverse process and connect to the first rib. The abnormal structure compresses the plexus particularly when the upper limb is elevated above head level. Pain and paresthesias radiate to the ulnar side of the hand and fingers and there is weakness of the intrinsic muscles of the hand secondary to lower plexus compression. The thoracic outlet maneuvers (Adson and Roos tests) described previously are generally considered to be unreliable but do raise suspicion. The neurological examination may be normal or there may be weakness of abductor digiti minimi with hypothenar sensory loss. Occasionally the abductor pollicis brevis muscle is particularly atrophic and weak, mimicking carpal tunnel syndrome.

The diagnosis is usually one of exclusion: imaging of the cervical spine is normal, and nerve conduction studies below the clavicle are also normal. Venous and arterial anatomy can be studied by catheter angiography, Doppler, or MR angiography and venography. Electrophysiological studies that show partial denervation of the small muscles of the hand and a decreased sensory nerve action potential amplitude from the little finger are compatible with the diagnosis of thoracic outlet syndrome.

In all cases a conservative approach should be tried initially. Postural exercises and thoracic outlet muscle strengthening exercises with instructions for ergodynamics at work and correction of unusual sleep posture may provide relief in 50–90% of patients, usually within 6 weeks. Failure of conservative treatment and ongoing symptoms prompts consideration of a surgical opinion.

Suprascapular Nerve Entrapment

The suprascapular nerve may be entrapped or injured as it passes through the suprascapular notch (see Chapter 107). It is occasionally cut in the process of lymph node biopsy. The branch to the infraspinatus muscle can be entrapped at the spinoglenoid notch by a hypertrophied inferior transverse scapular ligament. The patient complains of deep pain at the upper border of the scapula, aggravated by shoulder movement, and there may be atrophy and weakness of the supra- and more commonly the infraspinatus muscles. The supraspinatus muscle accounts for the first 10 degrees of shoulder abduction, and the infraspinatus muscle externally rotates the arm.

Carpal Tunnel Syndrome

Carpal tunnel syndrome, the most common entrapment neuropathy, is more frequent in women and may present in pregnancy. It is now accepted as an occupational hazard secondary to repetitive stress as in, for example, typing, and occasionally it is the presenting symptom of underlying systemic disease. The nerve is entrapped in the bony confines of the carpal tunnel, which is roofed by the transverse carpal ligament.

Pregnancy, diabetes, rheumatoid arthritis, hypothyroidism, sarcoidosis, acromegaly, and amyloid infiltration of the ligament are possible underlying causes, and appropriate screening blood studies should be performed on all patients with carpal tunnel syndrome.

Numbness or pain radiates to the thumb, index, and middle fingers and often wakes the patient at night. At times there is diffuse brachialgia. Atrophy and weakness of the abductor pollicis brevis muscle may be marked, but the motor deficit itself is rarely the cause of disability. Significant sensory loss in median nerve distribution can be a handicap when using the hand out of sight.

Examination reveals atrophy of the abductor pollicis brevis muscle, which produces a longitudinal furrow in the thenar eminence. There is weakness of thumb abduction. In theory there should also be weakness of the opponens pollicis, but patients recruit the long flexor tendons when testing opposition, so weakness is hard to identify. The palmar cutaneous nerve branch leaves the median nerve proximal to the flexor retinaculum and supplies the skin over the thenar eminence and proximal palm on the radial aspect of the hand.

Hence, sensory loss secondary to dysfunction of the median nerve in the carpal tunnel involves the distal thumb, index, and middle fingers but not the thenar eminence itself, a useful diagnostic point.

The Phalen test is performed by holding the wrist in complete flexion, and the test is considered positive when numbness or tingling in a median nerve distribution is seen within 20 seconds, but the latency before the sensory symptoms occur can be up to a minute. Sensitivity is about 74% and the false-positive rate is about 25%. The Tinel sign may be elicited by tapping the median nerve at the wrist.

Confirmation of the diagnosis is provided by nerve conduction studies and electromyography (EMG): distal motor and sensory latencies are prolonged, and polyphasic reinnervation potentials are seen in the abductor pollicis brevis muscle. More extensive and expensive investigations are usually not warranted, but sonography and MRI have been utilized in difficult cases. Initial relief of the sensory symptoms can be obtained with the use of wrist splints, but patients with unremitting pain or significant motor and sensory signs, together with confirmatory nerve conduction studies, should be offered decompressive surgery. This is usually curative. The surgeon should always send the excised flexor retinaculum for histopathological examination to exclude amyloid deposition.

Occasionally, carpal tunnel syndrome may be mimicked by entrapment of the median nerve more proximally at the elbow. Here it passes beneath the thick fascial band between the biceps tendon and the forearm fascia and then between the two heads of the pronator teres muscle. As the nerve passes between the heads of the pronator teres, it supplies that muscle as well as the flexor carpi radialis (which flexes and abducts the hand at the wrist) and the flexor digitorum superficialis (which flexes the fingers at the interphalangeal joints with the proximal phalanx fixed). After it passes between the two heads of the pronator teres muscle, it supplies the flexor pollicis longus muscle (which flexes the distal phalanx of the thumb with the proximal phalanx fixed), the flexor digitorum profundus muscle to the first and second digits (which flexes the distal phalanx with the middle phalanx fixed), and the pronator quadratus muscle (which pronates the forearm with the elbow completely flexed). Nerve conduction studies may localize the site of pathology, and the EMG precisely defines which muscles are involved.

Ulnar Entrapment at the Elbow

The ulnar nerve can be entrapped proximal to the epicondylar notch or as it passes through the cubital tunnel at the elbow, where a fibro-osseous canal is formed by the medial condyle, ulnar collateral ligament, and the flexor carpi ulnaris muscle.

Structural narrowing of the canal aggravated by occupational stress and a sustained flexion posture, especially when sleeping, and repetitive flexion/extension movements aggravate entrapment. Although numbness and tingling are more common than pain, both are referred to the hypothenar eminence and the little and ring fingers. A positive Tinel sign at the elbow over the ulnar nerve helps localize the site. There is wasting and weakness of the small muscles of the hand (excluding the abductor pollicis brevis and opponens muscles, which are median innervated). There is decreased sensation over the palmar aspect of the ring and little fingers, and there may be decreased sensation on the medial and dorsal aspect of the hand and ulnar two fingers in the distribution of the dorsal branch of the ulnar nerve. In severe chronic cases, clawing of the fourth and fifth digits results from weakness of the third and fourth lumbrical muscles. Nerve conduction studies localize the area of entrapment. If the symptoms do not resolve by avoiding prolonged elbow flexion, and the physical signs are significant, surgical decompression should be considered (see Chapter 107).

Radial Nerve–Posterior Interosseus Nerve Syndrome

Having passed through the spiral groove of the humerus, the radial nerve pierces the lateral intermuscular septum to lie in front of the lateral condyle of the humerus between the brachialis and brachioradialis muscles. There it bifurcates to form the superficial branch, which provides sensory innervation to the lateral dorsal hand and the deep branch, referred to as the *posterior interosseus nerve*. This branch supplies the finger and thumb extensors and the extensor carpi radialis brevis muscle, which is of lesser importance for radial wrist extension (extensor carpi radialis longus is dominant, and its nerve supply comes off slightly more proximally, so radial wrist extension is spared in lesions of the posterior interosseus nerve). The deep branch passes through the fibrous edge of the extensor carpi radialis muscle through a slit in the supinator muscle (arcade of Frohse). Entrapment of the posterior interosseous nerve here produces symptoms similar to those of lateral epicondylitis—lateral arm pain or a dull ache in the deep extensor muscle area, which radiates proximally and distally and is increased with resisted active supination of the forearm. Extension of the elbow, wrist, and middle fingers against resistance increases the lateral elbow pain. Tenderness may be elicited over the posterior interosseous nerve just distal and medial to the radial head. Posterior interosseous entrapment pain is typically seen in manual laborers and occasionally in typists. The site of pathology is easily localized by EMG and nerve conduction studies, and surgical decompression is usually successful. Occasionally a neoplasm of the nerve causes the same symptoms, and some surgeons prefer MRI prior to surgery.

Complex Regional Pain Syndrome

The complex regional pain syndrome (CRPS) encompasses syndromes previously called reflex sympathetic dystrophy (RSD), causalgia, shoulder–hand syndrome, Sudeck atrophy, transient osteoporosis, and acute atrophy of bone (see Chapters 54, 107, and 108). By consensus, the syndrome requires the presence of regional pain and sensory changes following a noxious event. The pain is of a severity greater than that expected from the inciting injury and is associated with abnormal skin color or temperature change, abnormal sudomotor activity, or edema. *Type I CRPS* refers to patients with RSD without a definable nerve lesion, and *type II CRPS* refers to cases where a definable nerve lesion is present (formerly called *causalgia*). A soft tissue injury is the inciting event in about 40% of patients, a fracture in 25%, and myocardial infarction in 12%.

The pathophysiology is unclear, but because many patients respond to sympathetic block and because autonomic features are prominent it has been suggested that there is an abnormal reflex arc that follows the route of the sympathetic nervous system and is modulated by cortical centers. There is decreased sympathetic outflow to the affected limb and autonomic manifestations previously ascribed to sympathetic overactivity are now thought to be due to catecholamine hypersensitivity. Significant emotional disturbance at the time of onset is present in many patients and stress may be a precipitating factor.

Three stages of progression have been described:

* Stage I: sensations of diffuse burning, sometimes throbbing, aching, sensitivity to touch or cold, with localized edema. Vasomotor disturbances produce altered skin color and temperature.
* Stage II: progression of soft-tissue edema, with thickening of skin and articular soft tissues and muscle wasting. This may last 3 to 6 months.
* Stage III: progression to limitation of movement, often with a frozen shoulder, contractures of the digits, waxy trophic skin changes, and brittle ridged nails. Plain radiographs show severe demineralization of adjacent bones.

Motor impairment is not necessary to make the diagnosis, but weakness, tremor, or dystonia is sometimes present.

The diagnosis is essentially clinical. Diffuse, severe, nonsegmental pain with cyanosis or mottling, increased sweating and shiny skin, swollen nonarticular tissue, and coldness to touch are characteristic. Hypersensitivity to pinprick may preclude precise sensory testing. There may be associated myofascial trigger points and tendonitis about the shoulder.

Autonomic testing may help with the diagnosis; the resting sweat output and quantitative sudomotor axon reflex test used together are 94% sensitive and 98% specific and are excellent predictors of a response to sympathetic block. Bony changes including osteoporosis and joint destruction may be seen. Bone scintigraphy is most sensitive in stage I and less useful in later stages. A stellate ganglion block may be useful both therapeutically and diagnostically (see Chapter 107).

These patients require a good deal of psychological support as well as trials of symptomatic medication. Drugs that sometimes work are prazosin, propranolol, nifedipine or verapamil, guanethidine or phenoxybenzamine, and antidepressants. Biophosphonates may prevent bone resorption and are also helpful with pain control. A trial of stellate ganglion block, which can be repeated if successful, is worthwhile. Sympathectomy has been used for progressive disease in patients who have previously responded to sympathetic block.

"In-Between" Neurogenic and Non-Neurogenic Pain Syndrome—Whiplash Injury

"Whiplash is an acceleration-deceleration mechanism of energy transfer to the neck. It may result from rear-end or side impact motor vehicle collisions but can also occur during diving or other mishaps. The impact may result in bony or soft tissue injuries (whiplash injury), which in turn may lead to a variety of clinical manifestations (whiplash-associated disorders)."

—**Quebec Task Force on Whiplash Associated Disorders**(Spitzer et al., 1995)

Rear-end motor vehicle collisions are responsible for 85% of whiplash injuries, and about 1 million such injuries occur in the United States every year. Severe injuries can cause rupture of ligaments, avulsion of vertebral endplates, fractures, and disk herniations, often associated with cervical nerve root or spinal cord damage. The severity of injury can be graded:

* Grade I injuries: pain, stiffness, and tenderness in the neck—no physical signs
* Grade II injuries: grade I symptoms together with physical signs of decreased range of movement and point tenderness
* Grade III injuries: neurological signs are present—weakness, sensory loss, absent reflex or long-tract signs.

The prognosis is related to the severity of injury:

* Neck pain longer than 6 months after injury: grade I, 44%; grade II, 81%; grade III, up to 90%
* Headache longer than 6 months after injury: grade I, 37%; grade II, 37%; grade III, 70%
* In general, about 40% of patients report complete recovery at 2 years, and about 45% continue to have major complaints 2 years after the injury.

The cause of persistent symptoms in patients with minor injuries is unknown, and little evidence exists for a structural basis for chronic whiplash pain in this group. The difference between a trivial injury and one of more significance should be based on the presence or absence of neurological signs.

About 20% of patients complain of cognitive symptoms after whiplash; cognitive dysfunction is likely to be functional or malingering.

The influence of compensation and legal action in whiplash-associated disorders remains controversial. Two studies from Lithuania, where only a minority of car drivers are insured for personal injury, demonstrated both retrospectively and prospectively significantly less symptomatology than for similar accidents in the United States; in Lithuania, at 1 year, no significant difference existed between collision and control groups. The Quebec Task Force emphasizes that whiplash is essentially a benign condition, with the majority of patients recovering, but it is the refractory minority that accounts for an inordinate proportion of the costs. Support, physical therapy, muscle relaxants, and antidepressants are the main therapeutic options, but if neurological signs are present, imaging of the cervical spine with MRI is indicated. Persistence of pain for more than 6 weeks should indicate referral to a more specialized service; often a multidisciplinary team approach is best.

Rheumatoid Arthritis of the Spine

Rheumatoid arthritis in the cervical spine involves all the synovial joints, but it is particularly problematic when it involves the atlantoaxial articulation. Local inflammation and pannus formation cause pain on neck movement and there may be rupture of the transverse ligament that holds the odontoid process in place to cause atlantoaxial subluxation. Pain is referred to the neck below the ear lobe, and there may be a high myelopathy. Instability can cause sudden death. Spine radiographs show excessive space between the anterior arch of the atlas and the odontoid process.

Non-Neurological Neck/Arm Pain Syndromes

Patients with non-neurological causes for acute, subacute, or chronic neck and arm pain are frequently referred for neurological opinion. They may have no focal deficits or have minor nerve root or peripheral nerve signs that are incidental to their main complaint. Usually the clue to diagnosis is to be found in the history: a good story of movement aggravating or triggering the pain signposts the cause.

Fibromyalgia and Myofascial Syndrome

Within the group of rheumatological disorders, fibromyalgia is considered to be the most common cause of generalized musculoskeletal pain in women between the ages of 20 and 55 years; its prevalence is approximately 2%. The pain may initially be localized to the neck and shoulders but can spread diffusely over the body. It may follow an episode of physical or emotional trauma or a flu-like illness and be associated with depression and fatigue, which are present in more than 90% of cases. Many patients may have a true sleep disorder. The only physical sign is muscle tenderness and the finding of "trigger spots," multiple tender palpable nodules in the muscles. The diagnostic criteria are widespread musculoskeletal pain and excess tenderness in at least 11 of 18 predefined anatomic sites.

Myofascial pain is considered to be a localized form of fibromyalgia, with pain in one anatomic region such as the neck and shoulder with local tenderness. The cause and pathology of the condition are unknown and there is no specific treatment. Most patients are tried on muscle relaxants and antidepressants with physical therapy and exercise. Failure to respond warrants a trial of trigger point injections of corticosteroid in local anesthetic.

Polymyalgia Rheumatica

Polymyalgia rheumatica, more common in patients over the age of 50, presents with severe aching, pain, and tenderness in the neck and shoulder girdle muscles in association with a markedly elevated erythrocyte sedimentation rate. The condition responds dramatically to small doses of oral steroid. Some cases are associated with temporal arteritis. If there is weakness, one should consider the diagnosis of polymyositis, and the serum creatine kinase should be measured.

Tendonitis, Bursitis, and Arthritis

Shoulder. Pain triggered by shoulder joint movement suggests tendonitis, capsulitis, or an internal derangement of the joint. Flexion and elevation of the shoulder that evokes pain is often called the *impingement sign*. Patients with a painful arc syndrome often respond to local corticosteroid injections into the tender tendons. Tenderness anterior to the shoulder joint suggests bursitis, which also usually responds to local corticosteroid injection. Weakness of extreme shoulder abduction indicates a rotator cuff tear, but pain on movement makes evaluation difficult, and MRI of the shoulder may be needed to establish the diagnosis. Acromioclavicular joint arthritis causes a more diffuse shoulder pain aggravated by arm elevation, and the diagnosis rests on radiographs of the shoulder joint. Nonsteroidal anti-inflammatory medications help.

In patients with marked limitation of shoulder joint movement such that the scapula moves *en bloc* with the arm and is associated with movement-evoked pain, a diagnosis of "frozen shoulder" or adhesive capsulitis is made. Treatment for adhesive capsulitis is not all that satisfactory. Analgesics and physical therapy help in a limited way; the course is likely to consist of many months of discomfort but, in the end, with resolution.

Elbow

Epicondylitis. Pain in the elbow region triggered by clenching the fist (which tenses the extensor muscles and irritates their points of origin), or pain that increases with resisted finger and/or wrist extension and flexion suggests the diagnosis of epicondylitis. Local tenderness will be found medially or laterally over the distal end of the humerus. Lateral epicondylitis is known as "tennis elbow" and medial epicondylitis as "golfer's elbow." Treatment with a velcro rubber band support over the tender area at the elbow supplemented by local corticosteroid injections is usually helpful. Occasionally, these patients require surgery.

Olecranon Bursitis. Local tenderness and swelling at the point of the elbow (Popeye joint) makes the diagnosis of olecranon bursitis. The condition may follow local irritation but can be a manifestation of gout and occasionally represents a pyogenic infection. The bursa should be aspirated for diagnosis.

Wrist

Tendonitis. Wrist tendonitis is diagnosed by finding local tendon tenderness over the tendons which are also tender when stretched. De Quervain tenosynovitis is diagnosed by the presence of tenderness over the radial aspect of the wrist and evoking pain by ulnar flexion, with the thumb held in the closed fist (Finklestein test). Splinting or casting and the use of local steroids usually resolves the process.

Hands. In addition to the complaint of pain on finger joint movement, there may be swelling of the joints and joint inflammation, as indicated by rubor. Pain in the fingers, worse in the morning, aggravated by movement and not associated with numbness (as in carpal tunnel), suggests rheumatoid arthritis. Spindling of the fingers or other joint deformity occurs.

Distal signs in the terminal interphalangeal joints suggest osteoarthritis or psoriatic arthropathy. Bony swelling of the terminal phalanges (Heberden nodes) is likely to be due to osteoarthritis, which can cause local pain and tenderness. Red, hot, painful, hypersensitive extremities, especially hypersensitive to heat, suggest the diagnosis of erythromelalgia. This may represent abnormal sensitization of thermal receptors or abnormal platelet function and is sometimes associated with blood dyscrasias. Erythromelalgia usually responds to aspirin.

REFERENCES

The complete reference list is available online at https://expertconsult .inkling.com/.

32 Lower Back and Lower Limb Pain

Karl E. Misulis, E. Lee Murray

CHAPTER OUTLINE

ANATOMY AND PHYSIOLOGY
APPROACH TO DIAGNOSIS OF LOW BACK AND LEG PAIN
  History and Examination
  Differential Diagnosis of Lower Back and Leg Pain
  Evaluation
CLINICAL SYNDROMES
  Lower Back and Leg Pain
  Leg Pain without Lower Back Pain
  Lower Back Pain without Leg Pain
PITFALLS

Lower back pain is one of the most common reasons for neurological and neurosurgical consultation. In many of the patients who present with lower back pain, the pain either developed or was exacerbated as a result of occupational activity. Lower limb pain is a common accompaniment to lower back pain but can occur independently.

The list of considerations in the differential diagnosis of lower back and lower leg pain is extensive and includes neural, bone, and non-neurological disorders. Although lower back pain usually is thought of as either neuropathic (specifically, radiculopathy-associated) or mechanical in origin, other possible sources of pain, including urolithiasis, tumors, infections, vascular disease, and other intra-abdominal processes, must be considered in the differential diagnosis.

ANATOMY AND PHYSIOLOGY

The lumbosacral spinal cord terminates in the conus medullaris at the level of the body of the L1 vertebra (Fig. 32.1). The motor and sensory nerve roots from the lumbosacral cord form the cauda equina. From there, the motor and sensory nerve roots unite at the dorsal root ganglion to form the individual spinal nerves. These anastomose in the lumbosacral plexus (Fig. 32.2), from which run the major nerves supplying the leg (Table 32.1).

Pain in the lower back can have many origins. A good beginning for the differential diagnosis is determining whether the leg also has pain.

A complicating factor in this consideration is that local spine pain can be referred—that is, felt at a distance—because of the common nerve root innervation of the proximal spinal nerves and peripheral nerves supplying distal parts of the leg.

Causes of lower back pain without leg pain include:

- Ligamentous strain
- Muscle strain
- Facet pain
- Bony destruction
- Inflammation

Causes of lower back plus lower limb pain include:

- Radiculopathy
- Plexopathy

Important causes of leg pain without low back pain include:

- Sciatic neuropathy
- Femoral neuropathy
- Peroneal neuropathy
- Meralgia paresthetica
- Peripheral polyneuropathies

Isolated tibial neuropathy is uncommon. Individual peripheral nerve lesions usually are caused by local trauma, entrapment by connective tissue, or involvement with mass lesions.

Lower back pain occasionally is caused by non-neurological and nonskeletal lesions. Some of the most important causes are:

- Urolithiasis
- Ovarian cysts and carcinoma
- Endometriosis
- Bladder or kidney infection
- Abdominal aortic aneurysm
- Visceral ischemia or other aortic ischemic disease.

APPROACH TO DIAGNOSIS OF LOW BACK AND LEG PAIN

The first step in diagnosis is localization of the causative lesion. History and examination usually allow differentiation among mechanical, neuropathic, and non-neurological pain.

History and Examination

The history should focus first on features of the back and leg pain:

- Mode of onset
- Character
- Distribution
- Associated motor and sensory symptoms
- Bladder and bowel control
- Exacerbating and remitting factors
- History of predisposing factors (e.g., trauma, cancer, osteoporosis)

For example, the acute onset of lower back pain radiating down the leg suggests a lumbosacral radiculopathy. Onset with exertion suggests a herniated disk as a cause of the radiculopathy. Progressive symptom development can be from any expanding lesion, such as a tumor, infection, or expanding disk extrusion.

Patients with lower back and leg pain usually have more symptoms than signs of neurological dysfunction. Therefore, if examination shows sensory and motor signs in a specific radicular or neural distribution, a detectable structural lesion is more likely.

The neurological examination is targeted to determine whether the symptoms are accompanied by abnormal neurological signs. General examination of the lower limb is important. Muscle groups that can be tested include:

- Hip–girdle muscles:
  - Hip flexors (psoas, sartorius)
  - Hip extensors (gluteus maximus, semitendinosus, semimembranosus, biceps femoris)

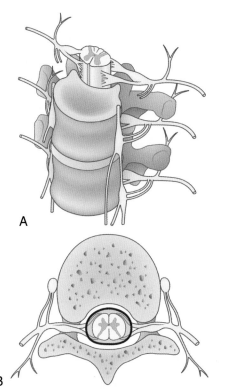

A

B

Fig. 32.1 Oblique **(A)** and axial **(B)** views of the spine showing anatomical relationships between neural and bone elements.

- Hip adductors (adductor group: longus, brevis, magnus)
- Hip abductors (gluteus medius, gluteus minimus, piriformis)
- Knee muscles:
  - Knee extension (quadriceps)
  - Knee flexion (semitendinosus, semimembranosus, biceps femoris)
- Ankle and foot muscles:
  - Foot plantar flexion (gastrocnemius)
  - Foot dorsiflexion (tibialis anterior)
  - Foot everters (peronei)
  - Foot inverters (tibialis posterior)
  - Toe extension (extensor digitorum)
  - Great toe extension (extensor hallucis longus)
  - Toe plantar flexion (flexor digitorum longus)
  - Great toe flexion (flexor hallucis longus)

Sensory examination should include the important nerve roots and peripheral nerve distributions: the femoral, peroneal, tibial, and lateral femoral cutaneous, lumbar roots L2–L5, and sacral root S1. Reflexes to be studied include the Achilles, patellar, and plantar reflexes.

Exacerbation of pain with some maneuvers also can be revealing. Stretch of damaged nerves results in increased pain by deforming the axon membrane, thereby increasing membrane conductance, depolarizing the nerve, and producing repetitive action potentials. Straight leg raising augments pain in a lumbosacral radiculopathy. Hip extension exacerbates pain of upper lumbar radiculopathy or that due to damage to the upper parts of the lumbar plexus, such as from carcinomatous infiltration or inflammation.

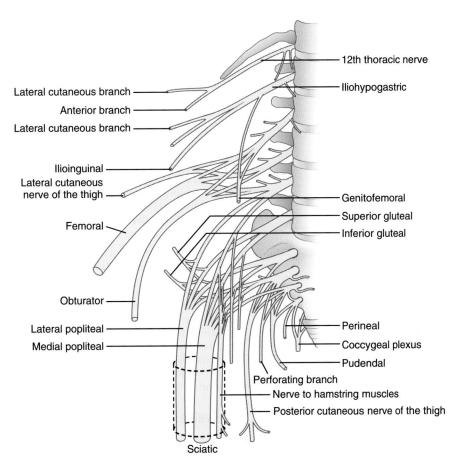

Lateral cutaneous branch
Anterior branch
Lateral cutaneous branch
Ilioinguinal
Lateral cutaneous nerve of the thigh
Femoral
Obturator
Lateral popliteal
Medial popliteal

12th thoracic nerve
Iliohypogastric
Genitofemoral
Superior gluteal
Inferior gluteal
Perineal
Coccygeal plexus
Pudendal
Perforating branch
Nerve to hamstring muscles
Posterior cutaneous nerve of the thigh
Sciatic

Fig. 32.2 Anatomy of the lumbosacral plexus. *(Reprinted with permission from Bradley, W.G., 1974. Disorders of the Peripheral Nerves. Blackwell, Oxford, p. 29.)*

TABLE 32.1 Motor and Sensory Function of Lumbosacral Nerves

Nerve	Origin	Motor function	Sensory function
Femoral	Lumbar plexus, L2–L4	Extension of knee, flexion of thigh	Anterior thigh
Saphenous	Distal sensory branch of femoral nerve	None	Inside aspect of lower leg
Lateral femoral cutaneous	Branch of lumbar plexus, L2–L3	None	Lateral thigh
Obturator	Lumbar plexus, L2–L4	Adduction of thigh	Medial aspect of upper thigh
Sciatic	Combined roots from lumbosacral plexus, partially separated into tibial and peroneal divisions	Foot plantar (tibial division) and dorsiflexion (peroneal division), foot inversion (tibial) and eversion (peroneal)	Lateral, anterior, and posterior aspects of lower leg and foot
Tibial	Lumbosacral plexus, L4–S3	Plantar flexion and inversion of foot	Posterior lower leg and sole of foot
Peroneal	Lumbosacral plexus, L5–S2	Dorsiflexion and eversion of foot	Dorsum of foot and lateral lower leg
Superficial peroneal	Distal sensory branch of peroneal nerve	None	Dorsum of foot
Sural	Cutaneous branches of peroneal and tibial nerves	None	Lateral foot to sole

TABLE 32.2 Classification of Lower Back and Lower Limb Pain

Type	Examples
Mechanical pain	Facet pain Bony destruction Sacroiliac joint inflammation Osteomyelitis Diskitis Lumbar spondylosis
Neuropathic pain	Polyneuropathy Radiculopathy from disk disease, zoster, and diabetes Mononeuropathy including sciatic, femoral, lateral femoral cutaneous, and peroneal neuropathies Plexopathy from cancer, abscess, hematoma, and autoimmune processes
Non-neurologic pain	Urolithiasis Retroperitoneal mass Ovarian cyst or carcinoma Endometriosis

Armed with the abnormalities recognized from this history and examination, the neurologist may come to a conclusion about the localization of the lesion. This knowledge narrows the differential diagnosis substantially.

Differential Diagnosis of Lower Back and Leg Pain

The differential diagnosis of lower back and leg pain can be addressed as shown in Tables 32.2 through 32.5. Classification into mechanical and neuropathic categories is useful for narrowing the scope of diagnostic considerations. The possibility of non-neurological causes should always be kept in mind.

Some basic guidelines for the differential diagnosis of lower back and leg pain are as follows:

- Pain confined to the lower back generally is caused by a low back disorder.
- Pain confined to the leg usually is caused by a leg disorder, although neuropathic pain from lumbar spine disease can radiate down the leg without back pain in a minority of patients.
- Pain in both the low back and the leg usually is caused by lumbar radiculopathy or, less commonly, lumbosacral plexopathy.
- Clinical abnormalities confined to one nerve root distribution usually are caused by intervertebral disk disease or lumbosacral spondylosis producing radiculopathy.
- Clinical abnormalities that involve several nerve distributions usually are caused by plexus lesions, with cauda equina lesions being the alternative diagnosis.
- Bilateral lesions suggest proximal damage in the spinal canal affecting the roots of the cauda equina.
- Impairment of bladder control indicates either a cauda equina lesion or, less commonly, a bilateral sacral plexopathy.
- Non-neurological causes of lower back pain are possible and particularly include urolithiasis, abdominal aortic aneurysm, ischemia, and other intra-abdominal pathological processes.
- Multiple lesions can make the differential diagnosis more difficult. For example, radiculopathies at two or more levels may look like a plexopathy or peripheral neuropathic process.

Non-neurological causes of lower back pain include urolithiasis, ovarian cysts, endometriosis, pelvic carcinoma, bladder infection, and other retroperitoneal lesions including tumor, abscess, abdominal aortic aneurysm, visceral ischemia, and hematoma. These conditions produce pain that does not radiate unless neural structures are involved. Neural involvement in the abdomen and pelvis can produce radiating pain that can be clinically differentiated from radiculopathy only if multiple nerve roots are involved. Early involvement of bowel or bladder function together with abdominal pain suggests one of these non-neurological conditions.

Evaluation

Diagnostic evaluation of lower back and lower leg pain begins with proper clinical localization and classification of the complaint. Diagnostic tests are summarized in Table 32.6 (Russo, 2006). The tests used depend on the clinical

SECTION A   General Principles

33   Laboratory Investigations in Diagnosis and Management of Neurological Disease

Robert B. Daroff, Joseph Jankovic, John C. Mazziotta, Scott L. Pomeroy

CHAPTER OUTLINE

DIAGNOSTIC YIELD OF LABORATORY TESTS

INTERPRETATION OF RESULTS OF LABORATORY INVESTIGATIONS

RISK AND COST OF INVESTIGATIONS
Risk-to-Benefit Analysis
Cost-to-Benefit Analysis

PRIORITIZATION OF TESTS

RELIABILITY OF LABORATORY INVESTIGATIONS

DECISION ANALYSIS

RESEARCH INVESTIGATIONS AND TEACHING HOSPITALS

PATIENT CONFIDENTIALITY

ROLE OF LABORATORY INVESTIGATIONS IN NEUROLOGICAL DISEASE MANAGEMENT

The history and examination are key to making the diagnosis in a patient with neurological disease (see Chapter 1). Laboratory investigations are becoming increasingly important in diagnosis and management, however, and are discussed in some detail in later chapters on the specific disorders. A test may be diagnostic (e.g., the finding of cryptococci in the cerebrospinal fluid [CSF] of a patient with a subacute meningitis, a low vitamin E level in a patient with ataxia and tremor, a low serum vitamin B_{12} level in a patient with a combined myelopathy and neuropathy).

Laboratory tests should be directed to prove or disprove the hypothesis that a certain disease is responsible for the condition in the patient. They should not be used as a "fishing expedition." Sometimes, a physician who cannot formulate a differential diagnosis from the clinical history and examination is tempted to order a wide range of tests to see what is abnormal. In addition to the high costs involved, this approach is likely to add to the confusion because "abnormalities" may be found that have no relevance to the patient's complaints. For instance, many patients are referred to neurologists to determine whether they have multiple sclerosis (MS) because their physicians requested magnetic resonance imaging (MRI) of the brain for some other purpose such as the investigation of headaches. If the MRI shows small T2-weighted abnormalities in the centrum semiovale (changes that are seen in a proportion of normal older adults and in those with hypertension and diabetes), the neuroradiologist will report that the differential diagnosis includes MS, despite the fact that the patient has no MS symptoms.

Moreover, neuroimaging modalities have expanded remarkably in the past decade, and the neurologist ordering these tests should be familiar with each one, so that appropriate sequences and methods are used to address the particular question presented by the patient's history. Also, because of the increasing use of pacemakers, deep brain stimulators, and other devices, the neurologist should be aware that certain precautions must be taken before MRI scans are ordered; in many instances, computed tomography (CT) scans or alternative investigations must be used to avoid potential danger to the patient.

Results of laboratory tests can be used to determine response to treatment. For instance, the high erythrocyte sedimentation rate (ESR) typical with cranial arteritis falls with corticosteroid treatment and control of the condition. A rising ESR as the corticosteroid dosage is reduced indicates that the condition is no longer adequately controlled and that headaches and the risk of loss of vision will soon return.

It is important to use laboratory tests judiciously and to understand their sensitivity, specificity, risks, and costs. The physician must understand how to interpret the hematological, biochemical, and bacteriological studies and the specific neurodiagnostic investigations. The latter studies include clinical neurophysiology, neuroimaging, and the pathological study of biopsy tissue. Knowledge of the various DNA tests available and their interpretation is critical before they are ordered; their results may have far-reaching implications not only for the patient but for all other family members. The neurologist also must have a working knowledge of several related disciplines that provide specific investigations to aid in neurological diagnosis. These include neuropsychology, neuro-ophthalmology, neuro-otology, uroneurology, neuroepidemiology, clinical neurogenetics, neuroimmunology and neurovirology, and neuroendocrinology. Chapters 43 through 52 describe these disciplines and the investigations they offer.

Biopsy of skeletal muscle or peripheral nerve may be needed to diagnose neuromuscular diseases. A brain biopsy may be needed to diagnose a tumor, infection, vasculitis, or (rarely) degenerative disease of the nervous system.

The investigations used to diagnose neurological disease change rapidly. Genetic studies of DNA mutations in the blood now allow the diagnosis of Huntington disease (HD), a growing number of spinocerebellar ataxias and parkinsonian disorders, a form of autosomal dominant dystonia (DYT1), Duchenne and other muscular dystrophies, many forms of Charcot–Marie–Tooth (CMT) disease, Rett syndrome, fragile X premutation, and a variety of other neurogenetic disorders (see http://www.ncbi.nlm.nih.gov/gtr; http://www.genetests .org; http://www.geneclinics.org; http://www.ncbi.nlm.nih .gov/omim). For genetic disorders with a very large number of causative mutations, such as CMT, step-wise evaluations are preferred to avoid unnecessary testing and excessive cost. Mutations of over 30 different genes have been found to be causative of CMT, but mutations in only four genes, PMP22 (duplication), MPZ, GJB1, and MFN2, account for 95% of cases. It is judicious to first test for mutations in these four genes before extending to the broader panel. Whole exome sequencing is increasingly utilized as a diagnostic approach for the identification when genetic disorder is suspected in cases with unusual phenotype.

Blood tests for human immunodeficiency virus infection (HIV), Lyme disease, and other infections and for various paraneoplastic syndromes affecting the nervous system also can be diagnostic. For example, three types of anti-Purkinje cell antibodies are recognized: anti-Yo (PCA-1), seen with tumors of breast, ovary, and adnexa; atypical anti-cytoplasmic antibody (anti-Tr or PCA-Tr), seen with Hodgkin disease and tumors of the lung and colon; and PCA-2, identified mostly with lung tumors. In addition, three antineuronal antibodies can be detected: anti-Hu (ANNA-1), seen in conjunction with encephalomyelitis, small cell lung tumor, and tumors of breast, prostate, and neuroblastoma; anti-Ri (ANNA-2), found with tumors of breast and ovary; and atypical anti-Hu, seen with tumors of lung, colon, adenocarcinoma, and lymphoma. Anti-CV2 (CRMP) antibody, expressed by oligodendrocytes, is associated with a syndrome of ataxia and optic neuritis and has been seen with small cell lung carcinoma. Anti-NMDA antibodies are associated with progressive psychiatric disturbances, memory impairment, dyskinesias, and decreased responsiveness together with hypoventilation and autonomic instability. Anti-NMDA encephalitis in many cases is associated with ovarian teratomas; symptoms may substantially improve with removal of the tumor and immunomodulation, so prompt diagnosis and treatment is important.

Antibodies directed to a serum protein, Ma (anti-Ma1 and anti-Ma2), have been seen in patients with limbic encephalitis associated with testicular and other tumors. Antibodies directed to amphiphysin have been detected in patients with a cerebellar syndrome and small cell lung carcinoma. Antibodies against a glutamate receptor are seen in rare patients with a pure cerebellar syndrome associated with cancer and a variety of autoimmune diseases. Antibodies against glutamic acid decarboxylase (anti-GAD) have been seen in patients with the stiff person syndrome and in patients with ataxia in a setting of an autoimmune disease such as diabetes, thyroid disease, or vitiligo. Antigliadin antibodies are helpful in evaluating patients with unexplained ataxia. As a result of advances in laboratory technology, genetic, immunological, and other blood tests are expanding the ability of clinicians to confirm the diagnosis of an increasing number of neurological disorders, obviating more invasive studies.

MRI has replaced CT for most conditions, and MR angiography and venography have largely replaced conventional catheter-based blood vessel imaging studies. In general, older, more invasive tests are now used for therapy rather than diagnostics. For example, the diagnosis and cause of an acute stroke may be determined by MRI, but catheter angiography is used to deliver intra-arterial tissue plasminogen activator (tPA) or perform embolectomies. The neurologist must know enough about each laboratory test to request it appropriately and to interpret the results intelligently. As a rule, it is inappropriate to order a laboratory test if the result will not influence diagnosis or management. Tests should be used to diagnose and treat disease, not to protect against litigation. When used judiciously, laboratory investigations serve both purposes; when ordered indiscriminately, they serve neither.

DIAGNOSTIC YIELD OF LABORATORY TESTS

When choosing tests, the neurologist must decide what information will help distinguish between the diseases on the differential diagnostic list. A test is justified if the result will confirm or rule out a certain disease or alter patient management, provided that it is not too risky or painful. A lumbar puncture (LP) is justified if the clinical picture is that of meningitis, when the test may both confirm the diagnosis and reveal the responsible organism. Culture and sensitivity testing should not be ordered on every sample of CSF sent to the laboratory, however, if meningitis is not in the differential diagnosis. Because the LP is invasive, with potential complications, it is not justified unless an abnormal finding will aid in the diagnosis. No test is justified unless the finding will influence the diagnostic process.

The physician should provide full clinical information and highlight the questions for which answers are being sought from the investigations. The electrophysiologist will look more carefully for evidence of denervation in a certain myotome if the patient has a syndrome suggesting herniation of that disk. The neuroradiologist will obtain additional views to search for evidence of a posterior communicating artery aneurysm if the neurologist reports a third nerve palsy in a patient with subarachnoid hemorrhage.

INTERPRETATION OF RESULTS OF LABORATORY INVESTIGATIONS

Every biological measurement in a population varies over a normal range, which usually is defined as plus or minus 2 or 3 standard deviations (SDs) from the mean value; 2 SDs encompass 96%, and 3 SDs encompass 99% of the measurements from a normal population. Even with 3 SDs, one normal person in 100 has a value outside the normal range. Therefore, an abnormal result may not indicate the presence of a disease. It also is important to know the characteristics of the normal population used to standardize a laboratory test. Ranges that were normalized using adults are almost never correct for newborns and children. Ranges normalized using a hospitalized population may not be accurate for ambulatory people.

An abnormal test result may not be caused by the disorder under investigation. For example, an elevated serum creatine kinase (CK) concentration can result from recent exercise, electromyography (EMG) or intramuscular injection, liver disease, or myocardial infarction (MI), as well as from a primary muscle disease. A common problematic finding for pediatric neurologists is centrotemporal spikes on the electroencephalogram (EEG) in a child with headache or learning disability who has never had a seizure. The EEG should not have been ordered in the first place, and to give such a patient antiepileptic drugs would compound poor judgment in diagnosis with worse judgment in management.

The neurologist should personally review test results that are ordered. In most instances, the actual imaging studies should be reviewed in addition to the report, and when appropriate, the neuroradiologist should participate. Similarly, for neurologists experienced in pathology, biopsy findings may be reviewed with the neuropathologist. The neurologist who knows the patient may be of great help in interpreting imaging or pathological studies.

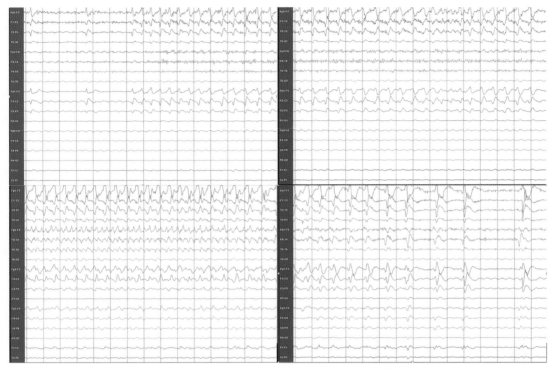

Fig. 34.18 Nonconvulsive seizure (arising from left hemisphere, spreading to right hemisphere).

a cEEG monitoring appears to predict a lower seizure risk (Shafi et al., 2012).

Electrographic Identification of Nonconvulsive Seizures

Figure 34.18 depicts an unequivocal nonconvulsive seizure. The discharge lasts >10 seconds, and has the classic electrographic features of a seizure, with clear evolution in frequency, amplitude, morphology, and spatial extent. However, not all nonconvulsive seizures are as clear-cut, and the lack of concordant clinical signs can make some nonconvulsive seizures difficult to identify. Box 34.2 lists proposed criteria for NCS (Chong and Hirsch, 2005). Some cEEG patterns resemble electrographic seizures, but fail to meet all of these criteria. When the EEG pattern is equivocal, a therapeutic trial of benzodiazepines can be helpful. However, the interpretation of the benzodiazepine trial may itself be difficult, because clinical improvement may be delayed, and because electrographic and clinical improvement may require loading doses of other anticonvulsant medications.

The "Ictal-Interictal Continuum"

In the ICU setting, the distinction between recurrent interictal epileptiform discharges and ictal discharges can be challenging. Electrographic patterns often wax and wane, evolving from patterns that are clearly ictal to those that are clearly interictal and vice versa. This can frustrate consistent EEG reporting, and more importantly, can present challenges to clinicians who must decide which EEG patterns warrant treatment, and how aggressively they should be treated. Most experts recommend treating unequivocal nonconvulsive seizures and equivocal patterns with a clear clinical correlate. There is less consensus on treatment of equivocal patterns without clinical correlate. Chong and Hirsch have proposed a conceptual framework termed the "ictal-interictal continuum" (Chong and Hirsch, 2005) (Fig. 34.19), in which various electrographic patterns are plotted according to their likelihood

---

BOX 34.2 Criteria for Nonconvulsive Seizures

Any pattern lasting at least 10 seconds satisfying any one of the following 3 primary criteria:

PRIMARY CRITERIA:

1. Repetitive generalized or focal spikes, sharp waves, spike-and-wave, or sharp-and-slow wave complexes at ≥3/sec.
2. Repetitive generalized or focal spikes, sharp waves, spike-and-wave, or sharp-and-slow wave complexes at <3/sec and the secondary criterion.
3. Sequential rhythmic, periodic, or quasi-periodic waves at ≥1/sec and unequivocal evolution in frequency (gradually increasing or decreasing by at least 1/sec, e.g., from 2 to 3/sec), morphology, or location (gradual spread into or out of a region involving at least 2 electrodes). Evolution in amplitude alone is not sufficient. Change in sharpness without other change in morphology is not adequate to satisfy evolution in morphology.

SECONDARY CRITERION:

Significant improvement in clinical state or appearance of previously absent normal EEG patterns (such as a posterior dominant rhythm) temporally coupled to acute administration of a rapidly acting AED. Resolution of the "epileptiform" discharges, leaving diffuse slowing without clinical improvement and without appearance of previously absent normal EEG patterns, would not satisfy the secondary criterion.

Reprinted with permission from Chong, D.J., Hirsch, L.J., 2005, Which EEG patterns warrant treatment in the critically ill? Reviewing the evidence for treatment of periodic epileptiform discharges and related patterns. J Clin Neurophysiol 22(2), 79–91.

to represent an ictal phenomenon and their potential to cause secondary neuronal injury. Standardized terminology for rhythmic and periodic EEG patterns occurring during critical care EEG recordings has recently been developed by a committee of the American Clinical Neurophysiology Society (Hirsch et al., 2013).

Periodic Discharges

Periodic discharges (PDs) are characterized by spikes, sharp waves, or sharply contoured slow waves that recur periodically or pseudo-periodically, usually every 1–2 seconds. Periodic discharges may be generalized (GPDs: generalized periodic discharges, formerly called GPEDs; Fig. 34.20), unilateral

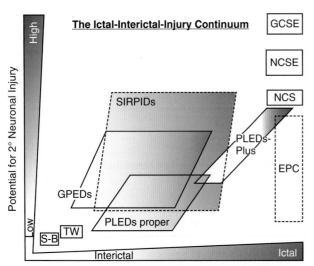

Fig. 34.19 The ictal-interictal continuum. *(Reprinted with permission from Chong, D.J., Hirsch, L.J., 2005, Which EEG patterns warrant treatment in the critically ill? Reviewing the evidence for treatment of periodic epileptiform discharges and related patterns. J Clin Neurophysiol 22(2), 79–91.)*

(LPDs: lateralized periodic discharges, formerly called PLEDs), or bilaterally independent (BIPDs: bilateral independent periodic discharges, formerly called BIPLEDs; Fig. 34.21). PDs are frequently associated with focal brain injury such as ischemia, hemorrhage, or infection. By definition, they do not meet the formal criteria for a seizure. However, they frequently occur following prolonged seizures. There is controversy about the meaning of PDs, their potential contribution to secondary brain injury, and consequently the need for their treatment. They may simply be markers of encephalopathy or focal brain injury, rather than a pathologic entity that requires treatment. However, PDs have been associated with poor outcome following status epilepticus (Jaitly et al., 1997; Nei et al., 1999).

Stimulus-Induced Rhythmic, Periodic, or Ictal Discharges

The periodic epileptiform discharges described earlier generally occur spontaneously and do not change in response to arousal or external stimulation. However, occasionally electrographic patterns consistently occur following stimulation or arousal of a comatose patient (Fig. 34.22). These stimulus-sensitive EEG patterns have been termed stimulus-induced rhythmic, periodic, or ictal discharges, or SIRPIDs (Hirsch et al., 2004). It is often unclear whether SIRPIDs represent ictal phenomena such as reflex seizures or interictal phenomena such as an abnormal arousal pattern. There is debate about how aggressively these patterns should be treated. Most SIRPIDs are not accompanied by clinical signs, although occasionally they may correlate with focal motor seizures, in which case the case for treatment may be more compelling (Hirsch et al., 2008).

Quantitative EEG

Increasing awareness and concern about nonconvulsive seizures has led to a growing demand for continuous EEG monitoring in intensive care units, generating large volumes of data that can be overwhelming to interpret using conventional reviewing techniques that display 10–20 seconds of raw EEG data per screen. To address this challenge and facilitate

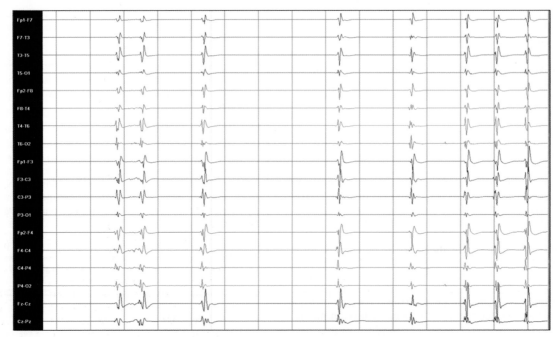

Fig. 34.20 Generalized periodic discharges (GPDs).

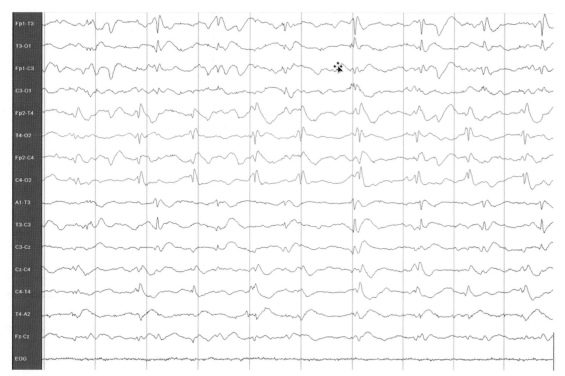

Fig. 34.21 Bilateral independent periodic discharges (BIPDs).

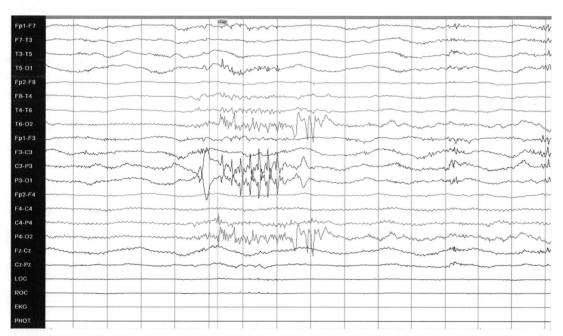

Fig. 34.22 Stimulus-induced rhythmic, periodic, or ictal discharges (SIRPIDs) in response to noise.

interpretation of prolonged EEG recordings, several quantitative EEG (QEEG) display tools have been developed to provide insight into trends in the EEG over time and to highlight significant electrographic events. However, it is important to emphasize that QEEG tools should not replace careful review of the underlying raw EEG. Table 34.1 lists QEEG display tools commonly available from various manufacturers and their primary clinical applications. One of the most appealing applications of quantitative EEG displays is their potential use as a screening tool for seizures. Figures 34.23, A and B illustrate the typical appearance of seizures on amplitude-integrated

EEG (aEEG) and color density spectral array (CDSA) displays, respectively. aEEG is a technique that displays time-compressed and rectified EEG amplitude on a semi-logarithmic scale. The top and bottom margins of the aEEG tracing reflect the maximum and minimum EEG amplitudes at a given time. CDSA is a technique that applies fast-Fourier transformation (FFT) to convert raw EEG signals into a time-compressed and color-coded display, also termed a color spectrogram. Frequency-specific EEG power is depicted on the y-axis, with varying degrees of EEG power (power = amplitude^2) depicted using a color-coded scale. The sensitivity of QEEG displays for

TABLE 34.1 Overview of Commonly Available Quantitative EEG Display Tools

Quantitative EEG display tool	Primary clinical applications
Amplitude-integrated EEG (aEEG)	Background assessment, Seizure-identification
Envelope trend	Seizure-identification
Color spectrogram (CDSA, CSA, DSA)	Seizure-identification
Total Power	Seizure-identification
Rhythmicity detector (i.e. R2D2)	Seizure-identification
Alpha-delta ratio	Background assessment, ischemia detection
Alpha variability	Background assessment, ischemia detection
Asymmetry indices	Background assessment, ischemia detection
Burst-suppression index	Background assessment

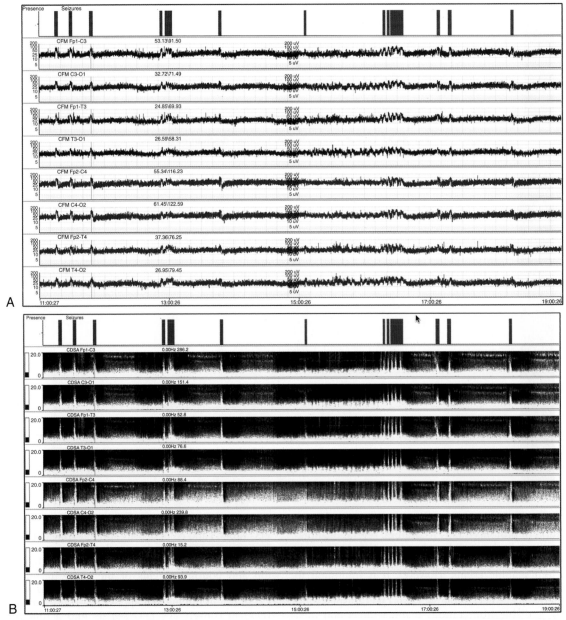

Fig. 34.23 A, Recurrent seizures depicted on an 8-hour aEEG display. **B,** Recurrent seizures depicted on an 8-hour CDSA display. Electrographic seizures identified on the raw EEG are indicated by the blue bars at the top of each figure. An 8-channel double-distance longitudinal bipolar montage. On the aEEG display **(A)**, seizures are associated with a rise in both the bottom and top margin of the aEEG tracing. On the CDSA display **(B)**, seizures are associated with bright bands of color, indicating higher power EEG activity across a wider range of frequencies.

TABLE 36.2 Changes in TMS Measurements in Various Neurological Disorders

	MT	MEP/RC	SP	LICI	SICI	ICF	SAI	SI	CBI
Movement disorders									
Parkinson disease	—		↓	↑	↓	—	—	↓	—
Dystonia	—	↑	↓	↓/↑	↓	—	—	↓	
Huntington disease			↑		↓	↑			
PKD	—	—	—	↓	—/↓	—			
Other degenerative disorders									
Alzheimer disease	↓/—	↑			↓	—	↓		
Cerebellar degeneration	↑		↑/—	↑	—	↓			↓
Amyotrophic lateral sclerosis	↓/↑	↑	↓	↓	↓	↑			—
Generalized Epilepsy	↓/—		↑/—	↓/—	↓	—			
Migraine	↑/—		↑/—	↓	—/↓	↑/—			

PKD, paroxysmal kinesigenic dyskinesia; MT, motor threshold; MEP, motor-evoked potential; RC, recruitment curve; SP, silent period; LICI, long-interval intracortical inhibition; SICI, short-interval intracortical inhibition; ICF, intracortical facilitation; SAI, short-latency afferent inhibition; SI, surround inhibition; CBI, cerebellar inhibition; ↑, increased; ↓, reduced; —, unchanged.

TABLE 36.3 Acute Effects of Neurological Drugs on TMS Measurements

Drugs	MT	MEP/RC	CSP	LICI	SICI	ICF	SICF	SAI
Na+ channel blockers	↑↑	=/↓	=		=/↓	=/↓	=	
GABA_A agonists	=	↓↓	—/↑		↓↓/—	↓/—	↓	
GABA_B agonists	—		↓	↓	↑	↓	—	
Glutamate (NMDA) antagonists	=	=	=		↑	↓	—	
Levodopa / dopamine agonists	=	=/↓	↑↑/—		↑↑/—	=	↓	
Dopamine antagonists	=	↑	=		=/↓	—/↑		
Norepinephrine agonists	=	↑	—		=/↓	↑↑		
Serotonin reuptake inhibitor	=	↑	—		↓	↔		
Anticholinergics	—/↓	—/↑	=	↑	—/↓	—/↑		↓
Other drugs								
Ethanol	—	—	↑		↑		↓	
Gabapentine	=		↑↑		↑↑		↓↓	
Levetiracetam	—/↑	↓	—/↑		=		=	
Topiramate	—		—		↑			
Piracetam							↓	

MT, motor threshold; MEP, motor-evoked potential; RC, recruitment curve; SP, silent period; LICI, long-interval intracortical inhibition; SICI, short-interval intracortical inhibition; ICF, intracortical facilitation; SICF, short-interval intracortical facilitation; SAI, short-latency afferent inhibition; ↑, increased; ↓, reduced; —, unchanged; ↑↑, ↓↓, =, consistent observations in two or more studies.

which is not affected by dopaminergic medications. SI is reduced or absent in the asymptomatic side of patients with unilateral Parkinson disease (Shin et al., 2007). Dopaminergic drugs enhance SICI and prolong SP, whereas dopamine-blocking agents reduce SICI and increase ICF. These observations suggest that motor cortex excitability depends on the balance between different inhibitory mechanisms, some of which are under basal ganglia control. Several studies measured changes in TMS parameters after subthalamic nucleus deep brain stimulation (DBS). SP is lengthened and ICF is enhanced after DBS, but no SP change was observed in another study. Reduced SAI presumably associated with dopaminergic medications and reduced LAI were restored by DBS.

Dystonia

In patients with focal dystonia, reduced SICI is not site-specific and was also observed in unaffected sides in patients with upper limb dystonia, and in hand muscles in patients with cervical and facial dystonia. In patients with dystonia, shorten-ing of SP is observed, but only in dystonic muscles. In writer's cramp, decrease in LICI was observed in the symptomatic hand during muscle activation. Both SICI and LICI were found to be abnormal in psychogenic dystonia, which limits the value of these measures in differentiating organic from psychogenic disorders (Espay et al., 2006; Quartarone et al., 2009). SICI is normal in dopa-responsive dystonia (DYT5) (Hanajima et al., 2007). Recruitment curve, SP, SICI, LICI, ICF, and SICF were all normal in patients with myoclonus-dystonia (DYT15) (Li et al., 2008; van der Salm et al., 2009). In patients with focal dystonia, LAI is diminished or absent, but SAI is normal. SI is reduced or absent in patients with focal hand dystonia (Sohn and Hallett, 2004b), but may be extended in patients with paroxysmal kinesigenic dyskinesia (Shin et al., 2010). In patients with focal dystonia, PAS-induced plasticity is abnormally enhanced with loss of topographic specificity, even in nondystonic parts of the body (Quartarone et al., 2008; Weise et al., 2011). This abnormal enhancement is not observed in patients with psychogenic dystonia (Quartarone et al., 2009). Abnormally enhanced PAS-induced plasticity may also be helpful for distinguishing PD-like patients showing normal dopamine transporter scans (SWEDDs: scans without evidence of dopaminergic deficit) from PD patients (Schwingenschuh et al., 2010).

Huntington Disease

Patients with Huntington disease have shown prolonged SP, which correlates with the severity of chorea. However, preclinical and early-stage patients with Huntington disease showed normal SP, normal or increased motor threshold, normal SICI with slightly higher SICI threshold, enhanced ICF, and reduced SAI (Nardone et al., 2007; Schippling et al., 2009).

Other Neurodegenerative Disorders
Dementia and Mild Cognitive Impairment

In Alzheimer disease, motor cortical hyperexcitability was demonstrated by TMS, which included reduced MT, enhanced MEP, and reduced SICI. However, intracortical facilitation appeared normal, as measured by ICF and SICF. Reduced MT was significantly correlated with the severity of cognitive impairments. SAI, representing cholinergic system function, is reduced in patients with Alzheimer disease, and is reversed by the oral administration of cholinesterase inhibitors. Abnormal SAI in combination with a large increase in SAI after a single dose of anticholinesterase inhibitor may indicate a favorable response to these drugs. SAI was also found to be abnormal in patients with Lewy body dementia, but is usually normal in frontotemporal dementia (Di Lazzaro et al., 2006). SAI is usually normal in patients with MCI, but found to be reduced in amnestic MCI with multiple domain impairments, suggesting that this type of MCI might be a phenotype of incipient AD (Nardone et al., 2012).

Amyotrophic Lateral Sclerosis

In amyotrophic lateral sclerosis (ALS), abnormalities in MT are inconsistent, presumably due to heterogeneity of the ALS phenotype and the stage of the disease at time of testing (Vucic et al., 2013). While some studies found an increased MT or even an absence of MEPs, others have reported either normal or reduced MT. Longitudinal studies have shown a reduction of MTs early in the disease course, increasing to the point of cortical inexcitability with disease progression (Vucic et al., 2013). Increases in MEP amplitudes along with reduced MT have been documented particularly in the early stage of ALS, suggesting that cortical hyperexcitability is an early feature of ALS (Vucic et al., 2011). Absence or reduction in CSP has been reported in ALS, most prominently in early stages of the disease, which appears to be specific for ALS among various neuromuscular disorders (Vucic et al., 2013). Decreased SICI with increase in ICF has also been demonstrated in ALS, but not observed in ALS mimic disorders (Vucic et al., 2011). Central motor conduction time (CMCT) is typically modestly prolonged in ALS, probably reflecting axonal degeneration of the upper motor neurons.

Cerebellar Disorders

In patients with various types of cerebellar degeneration, MT, CSP and LICI are often increased. ICF is reduced without change in SICI, and CBI is usually reduced or absent. However, these changes are different among the various types of cerebellar degeneration (Schwenkreis et al., 2002). In patients with inherited cerebellar ataxia, reduced ICF can be more specific for spinocerebellar ataxia (SCA) 2 and 3, while prolonged CCT was found in patients with Friedreich ataxia and SCA 1, 2 and 6.

Epilepsy and Antiepileptic Drugs

There are several different mechanisms for the genesis of epileptic seizures and for the modes of action of antiepileptic drugs (AEDs). TMS can be used to give information about these mechanisms by measuring cortical excitability. For example, motor threshold is decreased in untreated patients with idiopathic generalized epilepsy. On the other hand, in progressive myoclonic epilepsy, threshold is normal, but there is loss of cortical inhibition demonstrated with paired pulses at 100–150 milliseconds and an increase in facilitation at 50 milliseconds. Prolonged SP was found in idiopathic generalized epilepsy and also in partial motor seizure. Within 48 hours after a generalized tonic-clonic seizure, ICF is reduced while SICI is normal, presumably representing a protective mechanism against spreading or recurrence of seizures. Increased motor cortical excitability including reduced motor threshold, increased ICF, and reduced SICI and LICI, was observed in the 24 hours before a seizure, while the opposite changes in motor cortical excitability measures were seen in the 24 hours after a seizure (Badawy et al., 2009). SICI is reduced but ICF is normal in progressive or juvenile myoclonic epilepsy. LICI is also reduced in progressive myoclonic epilepsy and also in idiopathic generalized epilepsy. Weaker SICI and ICF in the hemisphere ipsilateral to seizure onset were found to have a predictive value for seizure attacks in the subsequent 48 hours in temporal lobe epilepsy patients with acute drug withdrawal (Wright et al., 2006). A long-term follow-up study in drug-naïve patients with generalized or partial epilepsy demonstrated that a decrease in cortical excitability such as increased motor threshold and increased SICI and LICI after medication predicted a high probability of being seizure-free after one year of treatment (Badawy et al., 2010).

Specific effects can be seen with various AEDs in normal subjects (Kimiskidis et al., 2014). AEDs which enhance the action of GABA, such as vigabatrin, gabapentin, and lorazepam, increase SICI, but have no effect on MT. In contrast, the AEDs blocking voltage-gated sodium or calcium channels, phenytoin, carbamazepine, and lamotrigine, increase MT without significant effects on SICI (Ziemann et al., 1996). In addition to elucidating these mechanisms, TMS can potentially be used to quantify physiological effects in individual patients, and this may be more valuable in some circumstances than monitoring blood levels of AEDs.

Stroke

Several studies have attempted to correlate clinical recovery from stroke to the characteristics of MEPs. MEPs are often absent in severely affected stroke patients. In mildly affected patients, MEPs are usually of longer latency, smaller amplitude, and higher motor threshold. The presence of MEPs in the early stage of stroke is associated with a good functional recovery (Hendricks et al., 2002). Conversely, absence of MEPs in paretic limb with concomitantly increased MEP amplitudes in the unaffected limb predicts poor recovery. In addition, the presence of ipsilateral MEPs in the paretic limb in response to the stimulation of the unaffected hemisphere is also associated with poor recovery. The recovery of MEP latency is highly correlated with return of hand function. A motor threshold higher than normal is often associated with the signs of spasticity. Noninvasive mapping of the motor cortex can be carried out with TMS using the figure-of-eight-shaped coil. This technique has been used to evaluate cortical reorganization in various conditions. In stroke patients, it has been demonstrated that cortical reorganization of the motor output still occurs up to several months after insult. There is progressive enlargement of the motor maps of the recovering affected part. SICI is reduced in the affected hemisphere in the acute phase of a motor cortical stroke, and remains reduced regardless of functional recovery. SICI also tends to be reduced in the unaffected hemisphere, but returns to be normal subsequently or can be greater than that in the affected hemisphere in patients showing good recovery. Enhanced SICI may lead to reduced activity in the unaffected hemisphere, which enhances activity of the affected hemisphere and promotes recovery.

Multiple Sclerosis (MS)

CCT measurement has been applied in the evaluation of patients with multiple sclerosis, where there is frequent involvement of the corticospinal tract. Typically there is either a unilateral or bilateral prolongation of CCT consistent with demyelinating lesions in the corticospinal tract (Schlaeger et al., 2013; Schmierer et al., 2002). Prolonged CCT is more pronounced in progressive MS than in relapsing-remitting MS. Similar to other evoked potential studies, MEPs vary considerably in latency, amplitude, and shape in patients with multiple sclerosis when they are measured consecutively. An increased motor threshold is also frequently observed in patients with multiple sclerosis.

Migraine

Several studies have shown an increased MT in patients with migraine, but some studies also showed normal MT. CSP is usually normal, but in some studies shortened CSP was found in the hand as well as facial muscles. SICI was normal in one study, but reduced in another study. ICF was normal in one study, but increased in another. Because of the high prevalence of visual symptoms, many studies have investigated the cortical excitability of the occipital cortex, and have found a reduced phosphene threshold for occipital TMS (similar to MT for motor cortical TMS) in patients with migraine with aura (Badawy et al., 2012).

Cervical Myelopathy and Other Spinal Cord Lesions

TMS is a useful tool for detection of cervical myelopathy, along with somatosensory evoked potential. In patients with cervical myelopathy, MEPs as well as the ratio of MEP/CMAP (compound muscle action potential) are usually reduced. CCT is prolonged, and their interside difference is increased. Simultaneous recordings from muscles innervated by different myelomers can help define the spinal level where the lesion involves. Prolonged CCT often correlates with the clinical severity and the degree of cord compression observed in MRI. In a study recruiting large number of patients with cervical myelopathy (Lo et al., 2004), the sensitivity of TMS in differentiating the presence and absence of MRI cord abnormality was 100% and the specificity was around 85%. CCT measures of the muscles innervated by cranial nerves such as the trapezius or the tongue may help differentiate ALS from cervical myelopathy. Abnormal CCT to these muscles indicates high probability of ALS.

THERAPEUTIC APPLICATIONS
Rationale for rTMS

The rationale of repetitive TMS for the therapy of neurological and psychiatric disorders draws from the concept that stimulation can alter brain activity and physiology. The idea is to compensate or even to reverse functional abnormalities thought to cause clinical deficits, assuming that normal functioning can be restored. This assumption remains to be proven. Promising randomized controlled therapeutic studies may provide a proof of concept, and the clinical use of rTMS for the treatment of depression has been approved in the USA and in some European countries.

Currently the best evidence in support of this concept comes from deep brain stimulation, although with DBS the effect is contemporaneous with the stimulation, while with rTMS the desired effect is after the stimulation. DBS above all in Parkinson disease (PD) improves motor deficits, and modulates brain activity and motor cortex physiology. Although the causality has yet to be proven, these studies point to widespread effects of DBS across the motor circuit that connects motor cortex, basal ganglia, and thalamus. This raises hope that stimulating elsewhere within this circuit could achieve similar effects. Particular interest lies in the motor cortex due to its accessibility to rTMS. Functional imaging demonstrates widespread activation of the motor circuit by rTMS targeting the primary motor cortex (M1) (Okabe et al., 2003) and the dorsal pre-motor cortex (dPMC) (Bestmann et al., 2005) supporting this concept. Further support comes from rTMS of M1 and the prefrontal cortex releasing dopamine in the caudate and putamen corresponding to their cortico-striatal projections (Strafella et al., 2001, 2003).

Basic Principles of rTMS

In addition to single and paired pulse stimulation, TMS can be applied repetitively (rTMS), inducing effects which persist beyond the stimulation. This persistence implies functional and structural changes in synaptic strength, which constitutes the basic mechanism in plasticity.

Plasticity is the ability of the brain for change and underlies normal brain functions such as motor learning or adaptation to an environmental change. Plasticity is also responsible for spontaneous recovery after brain injury, such as stroke. rTMS and other means of brain stimulation can make plastic changes, and diverse patterns of stimulation will produce different effects.

Generally, early plastic changes are alterations in synaptic strength and later changes will include anatomical changes such as sprouting and alterations of dendritic spines. By analogy to basic synaptic physiology, strengthening of synaptic strength is called long-term potentiation (LTP) and reducing synaptic strength is called long-term depression (LTD). Changes induced by rTMS are considered LTP-like or LTD-like, depending on whether excitability is increased or decreased (Quartarone et al., 2006; Quartarone and Hallett, 2013). Plastic changes can occur only within a certain range, which is referred to as homeostatic plasticity (Abraham and Tate, 1997; Bienenstock et al., 1982; Turrigiano and Nelson, 2004). The stimulation protocol defines the polarity of effects which can be excitatory or inhibitory. High-frequency or rapid rTMS ≥ 5 Hz, generally increases excitability, whereas low-frequency or slow rTMS, usually 1 Hz, induces a decrease (inhibition). There are patterned stimulation protocols and some derive their rationale from studies in brain physiology. A promising stimulation protocol, theta-burst stimulation (TBS), is thought to simulate normal firing patterns in the hippocampus by coupling gamma-frequency bursts (50 Hz) with theta-rhythm (5 Hz). TBS given continuously (cTBS) leads to depression, whereas if the TBS is given in periodic short trains, there is an increase of excitability (Huang et al., 2006). Quadripulse TMS is the delivery of clusters of four pulses at different intervals given every 5 seconds. Short intervals in the cluster of about 5 milliseconds will lead to facilitation, whereas longer intervals of about 50–100 milliseconds will lead to depression (Hamada et al., 2008). These are all methods of homosynaptic plasticity where activity of a synapse will lead to its own change. Heterosynaptic plasticity involves two inputs into the same synapse; as described earlier, this can be done with the TMS technique called paired-associative stimulation (PAS), which combines a peripheral nerve and subsequent motor cortex stimulation by TMS (Stefan et al., 2000), but this has not yet been applied in therapy. These stimulation effects have been explored principally in the motor cortex in the healthy young and may not directly be extrapolated to effects in brain disorders and in nonmotor areas. The efficacy of intermittent rTMS is contingent on its ability to induce effects which persist minutes to hours beyond the stimulation period (Chen et al., 1997; Gangitano et al., 2002; Maeda et al., 2000). Plasticity has been probed in various brain disorders and appears preserved, for instance, in PD (Benninger, 2013).

There are safety concerns with rTMS and these have been summarized by an international committee (Rossi et al., 2009). Seizures are the most serious acute adverse effect of rTMS, although extremely rare, and primarily result from excitatory stimulation protocols exceeding safety limits. Particular precaution is warranted in vulnerable patients with disease conditions or drugs which potentially lower the seizure threshold. There are no reports of irreversible stimulation effects.

Current Concepts of Therapeutic Application of rTMS

A rapidly growing number of randomized controlled studies have probed the therapeutic potential of rTMS in various brain disorders. Therapeutic applications include rTMS as an adjunct to conventional therapy, in treatment-refractory cases, and as a first line therapy. rTMS promotes learning during repetitive practice (Ackerley et al., 2010), and combining rTMS with rehabilitative and other types of interventions may enhance the therapeutic benefit. The rationale of rTMS is to promote plasticity. rTMS may offer an alternative to invasive procedures including DBS and epidural cortex stimulation, and may simulate the condition after electrode implantation to determine the eligibility of candidates in a pre-surgical evaluation and contribute to validating a cortical target. rTMS probes plasticity and has advanced our knowledge of the pathophysiology of various brain disorders. rTMS could provide a diagnostic test such as in differentiating organic dystonia with altered plasticity in the PAS paradigm from intact plasticity in psychogenic dystonia (Quartarone et al., 2009).

An extensive review of current concepts and guidelines for the potential therapeutic use of rTMS in various brain disorders has been recently published (Lefaucheur et al., 2014). This review focuses on approved applications and discusses selected therapeutic approaches to illustrate the diversity of rationales and possibilities.

Depression

Currently the strongest evidence for rTMS is found for the treatment of depression, and this indication is now clinically approved in the USA and in some countries in Europe (George et al., 2013). A large, multicenter randomized controlled trial (RCT) found significant reduction in depression scores with HF (10 Hz) rTMS to the left dorsolateral prefrontal cortex (DLPFC) compared to placebo in the acute treatment of major depression (O'Reardon et al., 2007). This led to the FDA approval despite a negative multicenter RCT published in the same year (Herwig et al., 2007). There has been a discussion about this discrepancy which some had attributed to the methodological differences. A subsequent RCT supported the

antidepressant efficacy of rapid rTMS of the left DLPFC (George et al., 2010), and a current meta-analysis provides further support (Berlim et al., 2013a).

Electroconvulsive therapy provided the initial rationale for rTMS with the intent to modulate brain networks involved in the pathophysiology of depression. The targets had been derived from neurophysiological and imaging research in patients with depression pointing to functionally opposite changes in the prefrontal cortices. This concept of disbalance has found support in therapeutic trials demonstrating similar efficacy of both the approved excitatory rapid rTMS of the left DLPFC and the inhibitory slow rTMS aimed at the hyperactivity of the right DLPFC (Chen et al., 2013). Interestingly, there are nonresponders to either protocol who have benefited from side switching, but no predictor of therapeutic success has been identified which could guide individual therapy. The few controlled studies found no superiority of bilateral over unilateral stimulation of either side (Berlim et al., 2013b).

In conclusion, rapid rTMS of the left DLPFC offers a therapeutic option in medication–refractory major depression. The therapeutic effect increases with repeated interventions and may be stronger in younger patients and depression of recent onset (George et al., 2011).

Auditory Hallucinations and Negative Symptoms in Schizophrenia

The increased pathological activity in the primary and associative auditory areas in the left temporoparietal cortex presumed to underlie auditory hallucinations provides the rationale for inhibitory rTMS protocols. The results are ambiguous with both positive and negative studies (both of Class II and III), though a few meta-analyses point to a possible therapeutic efficacy of inhibitory rTMS. Larger studies are needed.

Negative symptoms in schizophrenia may result from functional disturbance in the prefrontal cortex. Various stimulation protocols have targeted frontal areas, but only facilitatory rapid rTMS to the left dorsolateral prefrontal cortex (DLPFC) has been promising.

Parkinson Disease

The success of DBS in Parkinson disease has raised interest in rTMS as an alternative therapy. PD may offer a model to investigate whether rTMS can improve symptoms and reverse functional changes in the motor network. The motor system affected in PD lends itself ideally for cause–effect exploration.

The current disease model suggests that dysfunction of the cortico-striato-thalamo-cortical circuit results in a deficient thalamo-cortical drive and impaired facilitation of the motor cortex to cause motor symptoms (Mink, 1996; Wichmann et al., 2011). Decreased cortical activation and excitability during planning and performance of voluntary activity may represent a neurophysiological correlate of bradykinesia (Chen et al., 2001). The rationale of rapid rTMS is to increase motor cortex activation and excitability. Though pilot studies were promising and meta-analyses concluded modest efficacy of rTMS in improving motor function (Elahi et al., 2009; Fregni et al., 2005), the results of therapeutic trials remain ambiguous, including two recent Class I RCTs applying more powerful stimulation parameters failing to confirm efficacy (Benninger et al., 2011, 2012). Larger RCTs of different stimulation protocols are needed. A promising therapeutic concept arises from the postulated role of oscillatory activity in normal brain physiology and in the pathogenesis of brain disorders. In PD, presumed pathological oscillatory beta-activity in the motor cortex and basal ganglia characterizes bradykinesia, and

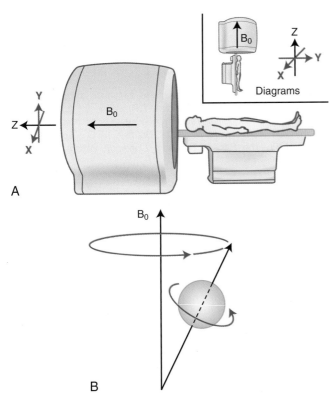

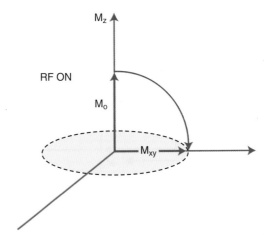

Fig. 39.4 Flipping the net magnetization vector. When a 90-degree radiofrequency (RF) pulse is applied, the net magnetization vector of the protons (M_o) is flipped from the vertical (z) plane to the horizontal (xy) plane. *(Reprinted with permission from Hashemi, R.H., Bradley, W.G., Lasanti, C.J., 2004. MRI—The Basics. 2nd edn. Lippincott Williams & Wilkins, Philadelphia.)*

Fig. 39.3 A, Magnetization in a magnetic resonance imaging scanner. Direction of external magnetic field is in the head–foot direction in the scanner. However, in diagrams that follow, the frame of reference is turned, so that the *z* direction is up *(inset).* **B,** Precession. In an external magnetic field (B_o), protons spin around their own axis and "wobble" about the axis of the magnetic field. This phenomenon is called *precession.* (**A** *from Higgins, D., 2010. ReviseMRI. Available at* http://www.revisemri.com/questions/basicphysics/precession; **B** *Reprinted with permission from Hashemi, R.H., Bradley, W.G., Lasanti, C.J., 2004. MRI—The Basics. 2nd edn. Lippincott Williams & Wilkins, Philadelphia.)*

commercial production today produce magnetic fields at strengths of 1.5 or 3.0 tesla (T).

When the patient is placed in the MRI scanner, the magnetic dipoles in the tissues line up relative to the external magnetic field. Some dipoles will point in the direction of the external field ("north"), some will point in the opposite direction ("south"), but the net magnetization vector of the dipoles (the sum of individual spins) will point in the direction of the external field ("north"), and this will be the tissue's acquired net magnetization. At this point, a small proportion of the protons (and therefore the net magnetization vector of the tissue) is aligned along the external field (longitudinal magnetization), and the protons precess with a certain frequency. The term *precession* describes a proton spinning about its own axis and its simultaneous wobbling about the axis of the external field (see Fig. 39.3, *B*). The frequency of precession is directly proportional to the strength of the applied external magnetic field.

As a next step in obtaining an image, a radiofrequency pulse is applied to the part of the body being imaged. This is an electromagnetic wave and, if its frequency matches the precession frequency of the protons, *resonance* occurs. Resonance is a very efficient way to give or receive energy. In this process, the protons receive the energy of the applied radiofrequency pulse. As a result, the protons flip, and the net

magnetization vector of the tissue ceases transiently to be aligned with that of the external field but flips into another plane, thereby *transverse magnetization* is produced. One example of this is the 90-degree radiofrequency pulse that flips the entire net magnetization vector by 90 degrees to the transverse (horizontal) plane (Fig. 39.4). What we detect in MRI is this transverse magnetization, and its degree will determine the *signal intensity*. Through the process of electromagnetic induction, rotating transverse magnetization in the tissue induces electrical currents in *receiver coils*, thus accomplishing signal detection. Several cycles of excitation pulses by the scanner with detection of the resulting electromagnetic signal from the imaged subject are repeated per imaged slice. This occurs while varying two additional magnetic field gradients along the *x* and *y* axes for each cycle. Varying the magnetic field gradient along these two additional axes, known as *phase* and *frequency encoding*, is necessary to obtain sufficient information to decode the spatial coordinates of the signal emitted by each tissue voxel. This is accomplished using a mathematical algorithm known as a *Fourier transform*. The final image is produced by applying a gray scale to the intensity values calculated by the Fourier transform for each voxel within the imaging plane, corresponding to the *signal intensity* of individual tissue elements.

T1 and T2 Relaxation Times

During the process of resonance, the applied 90-degree radiofrequency pulse flips the net magnetization vectors of the imaged tissues to the transverse (horizontal) plane by transmitting electromagnetic energy to the protons. The radiofrequency pulse is brief, and after it is turned off the magnitude of the net magnetization vector starts to decrease along the transverse or horizontal plane and return ("recover or relax") toward its original position, in which it is aligned parallel to the external magnetic field. The relaxation process, therefore, changes the magnitude and orientation of the tissue's net magnetization vector. There is a decrease along the horizontal or transverse plane and an increase (recovery) along the longitudinal or vertical plane (Fig. 39.5).

To understand the meaning of T1 and T2 relaxation times, the decrease in the magnitude of the horizontal component of the net magnetization vector and its simultaneous increase

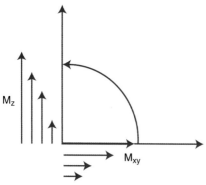

Fig. 39.5 T1 and T2 relaxation. When the radiofrequency (RF) pulse is turned off, two processes begin simultaneously: gradual recovery of the longitudinal magnetization (M_z) and gradual decay of the horizontal magnetization component (M_{xy}). These processes are referred to as *T1* and *T2 relaxation*, respectively. *(Reprinted with permission from Hashemi, R.H., Bradley, W.G., Lasanti, C.J., 2004. MRI—The Basics. 2nd edn. Lippincott Williams & Wilkins, Philadelphia.)*

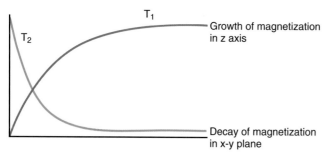

Fig. 39.6 This diagram illustrates the simultaneous recovery of longitudinal magnetization (T1 relaxation) and decay of horizontal magnetization (T2 relaxation) after the RF pulse is turned off. *(Reprinted with permission from Hashemi, R.H., Bradley, W.G., Lasanti, C.J., 2004. MRI—The Basics. 2nd edn. Lippincott Williams & Wilkins, Philadelphia.)*

in magnitude along the vertical plane should be analyzed independently. These processes are in fact independent and occur at two different rates, T2 relaxation always occurring more rapidly than T1 relaxation (Fig. 39.6). The *T1 relaxation time* refers to the time required by protons within a given tissue to recover 63% of their original net magnetization vector along the vertical or longitudinal plane immediately after completion of the 90-degree radiofrequency pulse. As an example, a T1 time of 2 seconds means that 2 seconds after the 90-degree pulse is turned off, the given tissue's net magnetization vector has recovered 63% of its original magnitude along the vertical (longitudinal) plane. Different tissues may have quite different T1 time values (T1 recovery or relaxation times). T1 relaxation is also known as *spin-lattice relaxation*.

While T1 relaxation relates to the longitudinal plane, *T2 relaxation* refers to the decrease of the transverse or horizontal magnetization vector. When the 90-degree pulse is applied, the entire net magnetization vector is flipped in the horizontal or transverse plane. When the pulse is turned off, the transverse magnetization vector starts to decrease. The T2 relaxation time is the time it takes for the tissue to lose 63% of its original transverse or horizontal magnetization. As an example, a T2 time of 200 ms means that 200 ms after the 90-degree pulse has been turned off, the tissue will have lost 63% of its transverse or horizontal magnetization. The decrease of the net

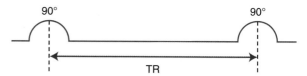

Fig. 39.7 Repetition time. This pulse sequence diagram demonstrates the concept of repetition time (TR), which is the time interval between two sequential radio frequency pulses. *(Reprinted with permission from Hashemi, R.H., Bradley, W.G., Lasanti, C.J., 2004. MRI—The Basics. 2nd edn. Lippincott Williams & Wilkins, Philadelphia.)*

magnetization vector in the horizontal plane is due to dephasing of the individual proton spins as they precess at slightly different rates owing to local inhomogeneities of the magnetic field. This dephasing of the individual proton magnetic dipole vectors causes a decrease of the transverse component of the net magnetization vector and loss of signal. T2 relaxation is also known as *spin-spin relaxation*. Just like the T1 values, the T2 time values of different tissues may also be quite different. Tissue abnormalities may alter a given tissue's T1 and T2 time values, ultimately resulting in the signal changes seen on the patient's MR images.

Repetition Time and Time to Echo

As mentioned earlier, the amount of the signal detected by the receiver coils depends on the magnitude of the net magnetization vector along the transverse or horizontal plane. Using certain operator-dependent parameters, it is possible to influence how much net magnetization strength (in other words, vector length) will be present in the transverse plane for the imaged tissues at the time of signal acquisition. During the imaging process, the initial 90-degree pulse flips the entire vertical or longitudinal magnetization vector into the horizontal plane. When this initial pulse is turned off, recovery along the longitudinal plane begins (T1 relaxation). Subsequent application of a second radiofrequency pulse at a given time after the first pulse will flip the net magnetization vector that recovered so far along the longitudinal plane back to the transverse plane. As a result, we can measure the magnitude of the net longitudinal magnetization that had recovered within each voxel at the time of application of the second pulse, provided that signal acquisition is begun immediately afterwards. The time between these radiofrequency pulses is referred to as *repetition time*, or TR (Fig. 39.7). It is important to realize that contrary to the T1 and T2 times, which are properties of the given tissue, the repetition time is a controllable parameter. By selecting a longer TR, for instance, we allow more time for the net magnetization vector to recover before we flip it back to the transverse plane for measurement. A longer TR, because it increases the amount of signal that can potentially be detected, will also result in a higher signal-to-noise ratio, with higher image quality.

As described earlier, the other process that begins after the initial radiofrequency pulse is turned off is the decrease of net horizontal or transverse magnetization, owing to dephasing of the proton spins (T2 relaxation). *Time to echo* (TE) refers to the time we wait until we measure the magnitude of the remaining transverse magnetization. TE, just like TR, is a parameter controlled by the operator. If we use a longer TE, tissues with significantly different T2 values (i.e., different rates of loss of transverse magnetization component) will show more difference in the measured signal intensity (transverse magnetization vector size) when the signals are collected. However, there is a tradeoff. If the TE is set too high,

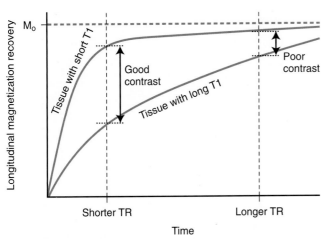

Fig. 39.8 T1-weighting. When imaging tissues with different T1 relaxation times, selecting a short TR will increase T1 weighting, as the magnitudes of their recovered longitudinal magnetizations will be different. By selecting a longer TR, longitudinal magnetization of both tissues will recover significantly, and there will be a smaller difference between the magnitudes of their recovered magnetization vectors; therefore, the T1 weighting will be less.

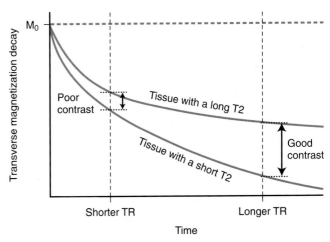

Fig. 39.9 T2-weighting. In tissues with different T2 relaxation times, selecting a short TE will not result in much T2 weighting, because there is no major difference *yet* between the loss of their transverse magnetizations. However, by selecting a longer TE, we allow a significant difference to develop between the amount of transverse magnetization of the two tissues, so more T2 weighting is added to the image.

the signal-to-noise ratio of the resulting image will drop to a level that is too low, resulting in poor image quality.

Tissue Contrast (T1, T2, and Proton Density Weighting)

By using various TR and TE values, it is possible to increase (or decrease) the contrast between different tissues in an MR image. Achieving this contrast may be based on either the T1 or the T2 properties of the tissues in conjunction with their proton density. Selecting a long TR value reduces the T1 contrast between tissues (Fig. 39.8). Thus, if we wait long enough before applying the second 90-degree pulse, we allow enough time for all tissues to recover most of their longitudinal or vertical magnetization. Because T1 is relatively short, even for tissues with the longest T1, this is possible without resulting in excessively long scan times. Since after a long TR, the longitudinally oriented net magnetization vectors of separate tissue types are all of similar magnitudes prior to being flipped into the transverse plane by the second pulse, a long TR will result in little T1 tissue contrast. Conversely, by selecting a short TR value, there will be significant variation in the extent to which tissues with different T1 relaxation times will have recovered their longitudinal magnetization prior to being flipped by the second 90-degree pulse (see Fig. 39.8). Therefore, with a short TR, the second pulse will flip magnetization vectors of different magnitudes into the transverse plane for measurement, resulting in more T1 contrast between the tissues.

During T2 relaxation in the transverse plane, selecting a short TE will give higher measured signal intensities (as a short TE will not allow enough time for significant dephasing, i.e., transverse magnetization loss), but tissues with different T2 relaxation times will not show much contrast (Fig. 39.9). This is because by selecting a short time until measurement (short TE) we do not allow significant T2-related magnitude differences to develop. If we select longer TE values, tissues with different T2 relaxation times will have time to lose different amounts of transverse magnetization, and therefore by the time of signal measurement, different signal intensities will be

measured from these different tissues (see Fig. 39.9). This is referred to as *T2 contrast*.

Based on the described considerations, selecting TR and TE values that are both short will increase the T1 contrast between tissues, referred to as *T1 weighting*. Selecting long TR and long TE values will cause increased T2 contrast between tissues, referred to as *T2 weighting*.

On T1-weighted images, substances with a longer T1 relaxation time (such as water) will be darker. This is because the short TR does not allow as much longitudinal magnetization to recover, so the vector flipped to the transverse plane by the second 90-degree pulse will be smaller with a lower resulting signal strength. Conversely, tissues with shorter T1 relaxation times (such as fat or some mucinous materials) will be brighter on T1-weighted images, as they recover more longitudinal magnetization prior to their proton spins being flipped into the transverse plane by the second 90-degree pulse (Fig. 39.10). Among many other applications of T1-weighted images, they allow for evaluation of BBB breakdown: areas with abnormally permeable BBB show increased signal after the intravenous administration of gadolinium. Gadolinium administration is contraindicated in pregnancy. Breastfeeding immediately after receiving gadolinium is generally regarded to be safe (Chen et al., 2008). Renally impaired patients are susceptible to an uncommon but serious adverse reaction to gadolinium, *nephrogenic systemic fibrosis* (Marckmann et al., 2006).

On T2-weighted images, substances with longer T2 relaxation times (e.g., water) will be brighter because they will not have lost as much transverse magnetization magnitude by the time the signal is measured (Fig. 39.11). The T1 and T2 signal characteristics of various tissues or substances found in neuroimaging are listed in Table 39.1.

What happens if we select long TR and short TE values? With the longer TR, the T1 differences between the tissues diminish, whereas the short TE does not allow much T2 contrast to develop. The signal intensity obtained from the various tissues, therefore, will mostly depend on their relative proton densities. Tissues having more proton density, and thereby larger net magnetization vectors, will have greater signal intensity. This set of imaging parameters is referred to as *proton density (PD) weighting*.

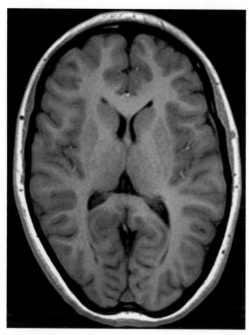

Fig. 39.10 Axial T1-weighted image of a normal subject, obtained with a 3-T scanner.

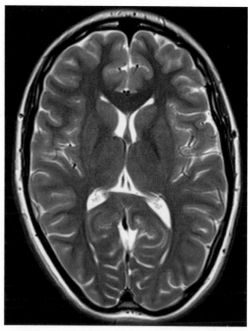

Fig. 39.11 Axial T2-weighted image of a normal subject, obtained with a 3-T scanner.

TABLE 39.1 MRI Signal Intensity of Some Substances Found in Neuroimaging

	T1-weighted image	T2-weighted image
Air	↓↓↓↓	↓↓↓↓
Free water/CSF	↓↓↓	↑↑↑
Fat	↑↑↑	↑
Cortical bone	↓↓↓	↓↓↓
Bone marrow (fat)	↑↑	↑
Edema	↓	↑↑
Calcification	↓ (Heavy amounts of Ca^{++}) ↑ (Little Ca^{++}, some Fe^{+++})	↓
Mucinous material	↑	↓
Gray matter	Lower than in T2-WI	
White matter	Higher than in T2-WI	
Muscle	Similar to gray matter	Similar to gray matter
Blood products:		
• Oxyhemoglobin	Similar to background	↑
• Deoxyhemoglobin	↓	↓
• Intracellular methemoglobin	↑↑	↓
• Extracellular methemoglobin	↑↑	↑↑
• Hemosiderin	↓	↓↓↓

CSF, Cerebrospinal fluid; *MRI*, magnetic resonance imaging; *T2-WI*, T2-weighted image.

Magnetic Resonance Image Reconstruction

To construct an MR image, a slice of the imaged body part is selected, then the signal coming from each of the voxels making up the given slice is measured. Slice selection is achieved by setting the external magnetic field to vary linearly along one of the three principal axes perpendicular to the axial, sagittal, and coronal planes of the subject being imaged. As a result, protons within the slice to be imaged will precess at a Larmor frequency different from the Larmor frequency within all other imaging planes perpendicular to the axis along which the magnetic field gradient is applied. The *Larmor frequency* is the natural precession frequency of protons within a magnetic field of a given strength and is calculated simply as the product of the magnetic field, B_0, and the gyromagnetic ratio, gamma. The precession frequency of a hydrogen proton is therefore directly proportional to the strength of the applied magnetic field. The gyromagnetic ratio for any given nucleus is a constant, with a value for hydrogen protons of 42.58 MHz/T. In slices at lower magnetic strengths of the gradient, the protons precess more slowly, whereas in slices at higher magnetic field strengths, the protons precess more quickly. Based on the property of nuclear magnetic resonance, the applied radiofrequency pulse (which flips the magnetization vector to the transverse plane) will stimulate only those protons with a precession frequency that matches the frequency of the applied radiofrequency pulse. By selecting the frequency of the stimulating radiofrequency pulse during the application of the slice selection gradient, we can choose which protons (those with a specific Larmor frequency) to stimulate ("make resonate"), and thereby we can select which slice of the body to image (Fig. 39.12).

After excitation of the slice to be imaged, using the slice selection gradient, the spatial coordinates of each voxel within the slice must be encoded to determine how much signal is coming from each voxel of that slice. This is achieved by means of two additional gradients that are orthogonal to each other within the imaging plane, known as the *frequency encoding gradient* and the *phase encoding gradient*. The phase

images, with associated hyperintensity in the surrounding white matter representing vasogenic edema. Foci of hemorrhage may be present but not too commonly. There is moderate mass effect associated with the lesions, and with contrast, a variable degree and pattern of enhancement is noted (diffuse or ringlike). This tumor is highly infiltrative, usually cannot be fully removed by surgery, and the median survival is 3 to 4 years.

Oligodendroglioma. Oligodendroglioma accounts for 5% to 10% of all gliomas. It arises from the oligodendroglia that form the myelin sheath of the central nervous system (CNS) pathways. Oligodendroglioma occurs most commonly in young and middle-aged adults, with a median age of onset within the fourth to fifth decades and a male predominance of up to 2 : 1. Seizure is often the presenting symptom. The most common location is the supratentorial hemispheric white matter, and it also involves the cortical mantle. The tumor often has cystic components and at least microscopically, in 90% of cases also shows calcification. Hemorrhage and necrosis are rare, and the mass effect is not impressive. On MRI (Koeller and Rushing, 2005) the appearance is heterogeneous, and the tumor is hypo- and isointense on T1 and hyperintense on T2. With gadolinium, the enhancement is variable, usually patchy, and the periphery of the lesion tends to enhance more intensely. Oligodendrogliomas are hypercellular and have been noted to appear hyperintense on diffusion-weighted images (Fig. 39.19).

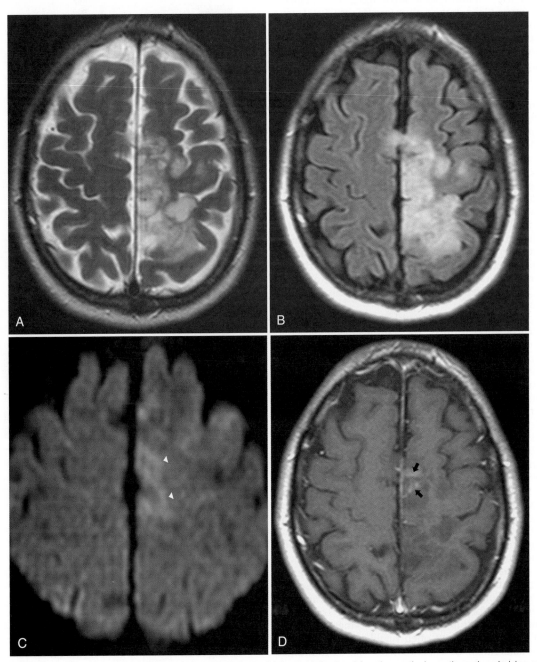

Fig. 39.19 Oligodendroglioma. A mass lesion is seen in the left medial frontal lobe, involving the cortical mantle and underlying white matter. **A, B,** On T2 and FLAIR images, the tumor is hyperintense. **C,** On diffusion-weighted image, faint hyperintensity due to the hypercellular nature of this tumor is noted *(arrowheads)*. **D,** With contrast, a few areas of enhancement are seen that tend to involve periphery of lesion *(arrows)*.

Gliomatosis Cerebri. Gliomatosis cerebri, a rare glial neoplasm, usually presents in the third decade of life. The glial tumor cells are disseminated throughout the parenchyma and infiltrate large portions of the neuraxis. Macroscopically it appears homogeneous and is seen as enlargement/expansion of the parenchyma; the gray/white matter interface may become blurred, but the architecture is otherwise not altered. The hemispheric white matter is involved first, then the pathology spreads to the corpus callosum, followed by both hemispheres. Later, the deep gray matter (basal ganglia, thalamus, massa intermedia) may be affected as well. Diffuse tumor infiltration often extends into the brainstem, cerebellum, and even the spinal cord. Histologically, most cases of gliomatosis cerebri are WHO grade III.

The MRI appearance is iso- to hypointense on T1 and hyperintense on T2. Hemorrhage is uncommon, and enhancement is also rare, at least in the early stages (Fig. 39.20). Later, multiple foci of enhancement may appear, signaling more malignant transformation. The imaging appearance is similar to that of encephalitis, lymphoma, or subacute sclerosing panencephalitis, but in these disorders, clinical findings are more pronounced.

Glioblastoma Multiforme. Glioblastoma multiforme is a highly malignant tumor classified as grade IV by the WHO. It is most common in older adults, usually appearing in the fifth and sixth decades. GBM is the most common primary brain neoplasm, representing 40% to 50% of all primary neoplasms and up to 20% of all intracranial tumors. It forms a heterogeneous mass exhibiting cystic and necrotic areas and often a hemorrhagic component as well. The most common locations are the frontal and temporal lobes. The tumor is highly infiltrative and has a tendency to spread along larger pathways such as the corpus callosum and invade the other hemisphere, resulting in a characteristic "butterfly" appearance. GBM has also been described to spread along the ventricular surface in the subarachnoid space and may also invade the meninges. There are reported cases of extracranial glioblastoma metastases.

Structural neuroimaging distinguishes between multifocal and multicentric glioblastomas. The term *multifocal glioblastoma* refers to multiple tumor islands in the brain that arose from a common source via continuous parenchymal spread or meningeal/CSF seeding; therefore, they are all connected, at least microscopically. *Multicentric glioblastoma* refers to multiple tumors that are present independently, and physical connection between them cannot be proven, implying they are separate de novo occurrences. This is less common, having been noted in 6% of cases.

On MRI (Fig. 39.21) glioblastomas usually exhibit mixed signal intensities on T1- and T2-weighted images. Cystic and necrotic areas are present, appearing as markedly decreased signal on T1-weighted and hyperintensity on T2-weighted images. Mixed hypo- and hyperintense signal changes due to hemorrhage are also seen. The hemorrhagic component can also be well demonstrated by gradient echo sequences or by SWI. The core of the lesion is surrounded by prominent edema, which appears hypointense on T1-weighted and hyperintense on T2-weighted images. Besides edema, the signal changes around the core of the tumor reflect the presence of infiltrating tumor cells and, in treated cases, postsurgical reactive gliosis and/or post-irradiation changes. Following administration of gadolinium, intense enhancement is noted, which is inhomogeneous and often ringlike, also including multiple nodular areas of enhancement. The surrounding edema and ringlike enhancement at times makes it difficult to distinguish glioblastoma from cerebral abscess. DWI is helpful in these cases; glioblastomas are hypointense with this

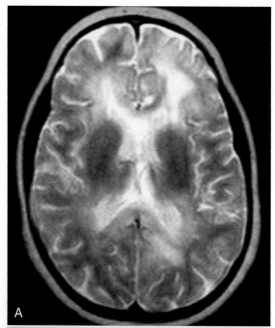

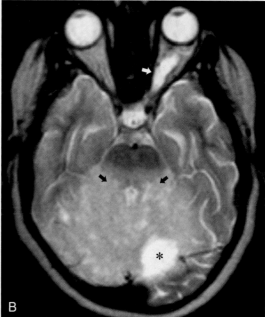

Fig. 39.20 Gliomatosis cerebri. A, Axial T2-weighted magnetic resonance (MR) image of brain shows bilateral patchy areas of increased signal intensity in periventricular white matter. **B,** Axial T2-weighted MR image of brain obtained at the level of the upper pons shows diffuse thickening and hyperintensity of left optic nerve *(white arrow)* and increased signal intensity in posterior aspect of pons and in cerebellum *(black arrows).* A focus of very high signal intensity is present in posterior left cerebellar hemisphere (*). *(From Yip, M., Fisch, C., Lamarche, J.B., 2003. AFIP archives: gliomatosis cerebri affecting the entire neuraxis. Radiographics 23, 247–253.)*

technique, whereas abscesses exhibit remarkable hyperintensity on diffusion-weighted images.

Owing to its aggressive growth (the tumor size may double every 10 days) and infiltrative nature, the prognosis for patients with glioblastoma is very poor. Despite surgery, irradiation, and chemotherapy the median survival is 1 year.

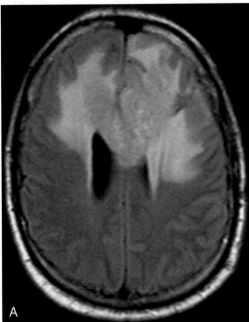

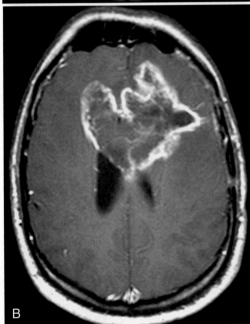

Fig. 39.21 Glioblastoma multiforme. A, Axial FLAIR image demonstrates a mass lesion spreading across the corpus callosum to involve both frontal lobes in a symmetrical fashion ("butterfly" appearance). Tumor is isointense, exerts mass effect on the sulci and the lateral ventricles, and is surrounded by vasogenic edema. **B,** On axial T1 postcontrast imaging, tumor exhibits heterogeneous irregular enhancement, most marked at its periphery.

Ependymoma. Although ependymomas are primarily extra-axial tumors (within the fourth ventricle), intraparenchymal ependymomas arising from ependymal cell remnants of the hemispheric parenchyma are also well known, so this tumor type is discussed here. Ependymomas comprise 5% to 6% of all primary brain tumors; 70% of cases occur in childhood and the first and second decades, and ependymoma is the third most common posterior fossa tumor in children. Ependymomas arise from differentiated ependymal cells, and the most common location (70%) is the fourth ventricle. The

tumor is usually well demarcated and is separated from the vermis by a CSF interface. The tumor may be cystic and may contain calcification and hemorrhage but these features are more common in supratentorial ependymomas. It may extrude from the cavity of the fourth ventricle through the foramina of Luschka and Magendie. Spreading via CSF to the spinal canal (drop-metastases) may occur, but on spine imaging ependymoma is more commonly noted to arise from the ependymal lining of the central canal, presenting as an intramedullary spinal cord tumor. A subtype, myxopapillary ependymoma, is almost always restricted to the filum terminale.

Ependymomas are hypo- to isointense on T1-weighted, and iso- to hyperintense on T2-weighted images. With gadolinium, intense enhancement is seen, mostly involving the solid components of the tumor, whereas the cystic components tend to exhibit rim enhancement. The differential diagnosis for infratentorial ependymoma includes medulloblastoma, pilocytic astrocytoma, and choroid plexus papilloma.

Lymphoma. Primary CNS lymphoma (PCNSL) is a non-Hodgkin lymphoma, which in 98% of cases is a B-cell lymphoma. It once accounted for only 1% to 2% of all primary brain tumors, but this percentage has been increasing, mostly because of the growing acquired immunodeficiency syndrome (AIDS) population. The peak age of onset is 60 in the immunocompetent population and age 30 in immunocompromised patients. Lesions may occur anywhere within the neuraxis, including the cerebral hemispheres, brainstem, cerebellum, and spinal cord, although the most common location (90% of cases) is supratentorial. PCNSL lesions are highly infiltrative and exhibit a predilection for sites that contact subarachnoid and ependymal surfaces as well as the deep gray nuclei.

The imaging appearance of PCNSL depends on the patient's immune status. The tumor is hypo- to isointense on T1-weighted and hypo- to slightly hyperintense on T2-weighted images. Contrast enhancement is usually intense. In immunocompetent patients (Zhang et al., 2010) the lesion is often single, tends to abut the ventricular border (Costa et al., 2006), and ring enhancement is uncommon (Fig. 39.22). In immunocompromised patients, usually multiple, often ring-enhancing lesions are seen, which are most commonly located in the periventricular white matter and the gray/white junction of the lobes of the hemispheres, but the deep central gray matter structures and the posterior fossa may be involved as well. Overall, the imaging appearance appears more malignant in the immunocompromised cases and may be difficult to differentiate from toxoplasmosis. Other components of the differential diagnosis in patients with multiple PCNSL lesions include demyelination, abscesses, neurosarcoidosis, and metastatic disease.

Extra-axial Primary Brain Tumors

Descriptions of schwannomas and the more rare extra-axial primary brain tumor types—esthesioneuroblastoma, central neurocytoma, and subependymoma—are available in the online version of this chapter (http://www.expertconsult.com).

Meningiomas. Meningiomas are the most common primary brain tumors of nonglial origin and make up 15% of all intracranial tumors. The peak age of onset is the fifth decade, and there is a striking female predominance that may be related to the fact that some meningiomas contain estrogen and progesterone receptors. These tumors arise from meningothelial cells. In 1% to 9% of cases, multiple tumors are seen. The most common locations are the falx (25%), convexity (20%), sphenoid wing, petrous ridge (15% to 20%), olfactory

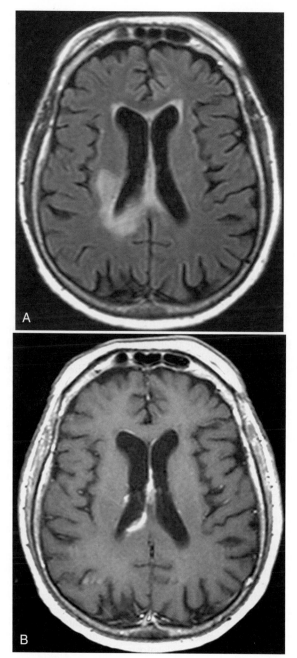

Fig. 39.22 CNS lymphoma in an immunocompetent individual.
A, FLAIR sequence depicts a single hyperintense lesion with spread along the ventricular border. **B,** After contrast administration, multiple areas of enhancement are seen within the lesion, without a ring-like enhancement pattern.

On T1-weighted images, meningiomas are usually iso- to slightly hypointense. The appearance on T2 can be iso-, hypo-, or hyperintense to the gray matter. Although MRI does not reveal the histological subtypes of meningiomas with absolute certainty, there have been observations according to which fibroblastic and transitional meningiomas tend to be iso- to hypointense on T2-weighted images, whereas the meningothelial or angioblastic type is iso- or more hyperintense. Not uncommonly, the skull adjacent to a meningioma will exhibit subtle thickening, a useful diagnostic clue in some cases.

After gadolinium administration, meningiomas typically exhibit intense homogeneous enhancement. A quite typical imaging finding on postcontrast images is the *dural tail sign*, which refers to the linear extension of enhancement along the dura, beyond the segment on which the tumor is based. Earlier this had been attributed to en plaque extension of the meningioma along these dural segments and was thought to be specific for this type of tumor. However, recently it has been recognized that this imaging appearance is not specific to this situation and may be seen in other tumors, secondary to increased vascularity/hyperperfusion or congestion of the dural vessels after irradiation and as a postsurgical change.

Primitive Neuroectodermal Tumor. *Primitive neuroectodermal tumor* (PNET) is a collective term that includes several tumors arising from cells that are derived from the neuroectoderm and are in an undifferentiated state. The main tumors that belong to the PNET group are medulloblastomas, esthesioneuroblastomas, and pinealoblastomas. The tumors belonging to the PNET group are fast growing and highly malignant. The most common mode of metastatic spread for PNETs is via CSF pathways, an indication for imaging surveillance of the entire neuraxis when these tumors are suspected.

Medulloblastoma. Medulloblastomas arise from the undifferentiated neuroectodermal cells of the roof of the fourth ventricle (superior or inferior medullary velum, vermis). They represent 25% of all cerebral tumors in children, usually presenting in the first and second decade. The tumor fills the fourth ventricle, extending rostrally toward the aqueduct and caudally to the cisterna magna, frequently resulting in obstructive hydrocephalus. Leptomeningeal and CSF spread may also occur, resulting in spinal drop metastases. Cystic components and necrosis may be present. Calcification is possible. On CT, medulloblastoma typically appears as a heterogeneous, generally hyperdense midline tumor occupying the fourth ventricle, with mass effect and variable contrast enhancement. The MRI signal (Koeller and Rushing, 2003) is heterogeneous; the tumor is iso- or hypointense on T1 and hypo-, iso-, or hyperintense on T2. Contrast administration induces heterogeneous enhancement (Fig. 39.24). Restricted diffusion may be seen on DWI/ADC (Gauvain et al., 2001). Consistent with its site of origin, indistinct borders between the tumor and the roof of the fourth ventricle may be observed, aiding in the differential diagnosis, which in children includes atypical, rhabdoid-teratoid tumor, brainstem glioma, pilocytic astrocytoma, choroid plexus papilloma, and ependymoma. The adult differential diagnosis includes the latter two entities in addition to metastasis and hemangioblastoma. Medulloblastoma does not tend to extrude via the foramina outside of the fourth ventricle, facilitating differentiation from ependymoma. In children, choroid plexus papilloma is more likely to occur within the lateral ventricle.

Pineoblastoma. Pineoblastomas are highly cellular tumors that are similar in MRI appearance to pineocytomas. However, they tend to be larger (>3 cm), more heterogeneous, frequently cause hydrocephalus, and also may spread via the CSF.

groove (5% to 10%), parasellar region (5% to 10%), and the posterior fossa (10%). Rarely, an intraventricular location has been reported. Meningiomas often appear as smooth hemispherical or lobular dural-based masses (Fig. 39.23). Calcification is common, seen in at least 20% of these tumors. Meningiomas also often exhibit vascularity. The extra-axial location of the tumor is usually well appreciated owing to a visible CSF interface between tumor and adjacent brain parenchyma. Meningiomas may become malignant, invading the brain and eroding the skull. In such cases, prominent edema may be present in the brain parenchyma, to the extent that the extra-axial nature of the tumor is no longer obvious.

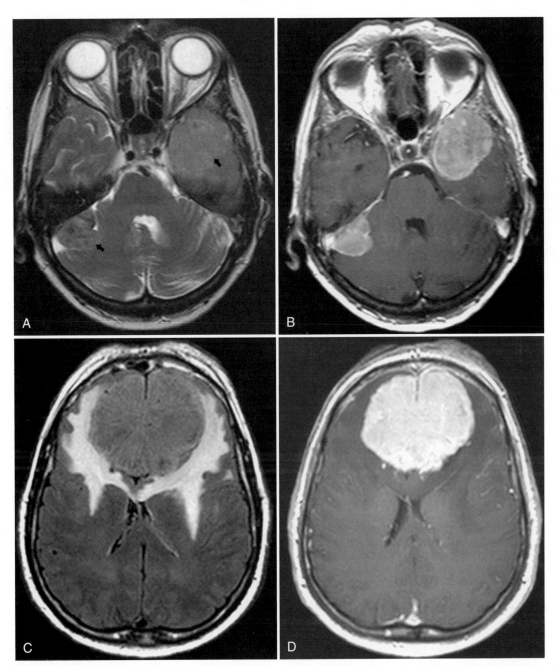

Fig. 39.23 Two cases of meningioma. In the first **(A, B)** two extra-axial mass lesions are seen, one arising from the tentorium and the other from the sphenoid wing in the left middle cranial fossa *(arrows)*. These compress the right cerebellar hemisphere and the left temporal lobe, respectively. **A,** On T2-weighted image, the masses are mostly isointense with foci of hypointensity. **B,** After gadolinium administration, the masses enhance homogeneously. Note the small dural tail along the tentorium. In the second case **(C, D)** a large olfactory groove meningioma that exerts significant mass effect on the frontal lobes, corpus callosum, and lateral ventricles is presented. **C,** On FLAIR image, hyperintense vasogenic edema is seen in the compressed brain parenchyma. **D,** Tumor enhances homogeneously with gadolinium.

This tumor is isointense to gray matter on T1, with moderate heterogeneous enhancement following administration of gadolinium. Like other PNETs, the hypercellularity of pineoblastoma results in T2-weighted signal that tends to be iso- or hypointense relative to gray matter, and restricted diffusion may also be seen. Cysts within the tumor may appear markedly hyperintense on T2, peripheral edema less so. In cases accompanied by hydrocephalus, FLAIR imaging may reveal uniform hyperintensity in a planar distribution along the margins of the lateral ventricles due to transependymal flow of CSF. Peripheral calcifications or intratumoral hemorrhage

will exhibit markedly hypointense signal with blooming artifact on T2* (pronounced *T2-star*) images. Differential diagnostic considerations include germ cell tumor, pineocytoma, and (uncommonly) metastases.

Other Pineal Region Tumors. Besides pineoblastomas, which histologically belong to the group of primitive neuroectodermal tumors, the pineal gland may also develop tumors of pinealocyte origin (pineocytoma) and germ cell tumors.

Pineocytoma. Pineocytomas are homogeneous masses containing more solid components, but cysts may also be present.

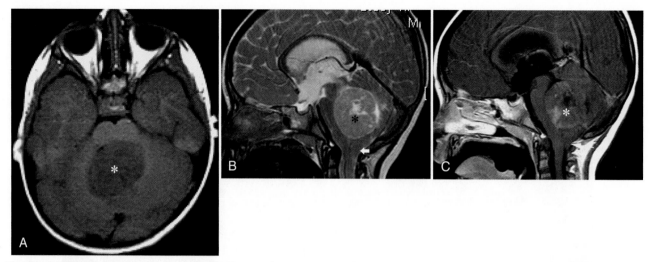

Fig. 39.24 Medulloblastoma. A large mass lesion is seen (*) filling and expanding the fourth ventricle. **A,** On T1-weighted image, tumor is partially iso- but mostly hypointense. **B,** On T2-weighted image, tumor shows iso- and hyperintense signal change; it compresses/displaces the brainstem and cerebellum. On sagittal images, note the secondary Chiari malformation (caudal displacement of cerebellar tonsils) due to mass effect *(arrow)*. **C,** On T1 postcontrast image, there is a heterogeneous enhancement pattern.

These tumors have a round, well-defined, noninvasive appearance. Calcification is commonly seen, but hemorrhage is uncommon. These tumors may be hypointense on T2 and exhibit a variable (central, nodular) pattern of intense enhancement after gadolinium administration (Fakhran and Escott, 2008).

Germ Cell Tumors (Germinoma). Masses in the pineal region are most often germ cell tumors, usually germinomas. Less common types include teratoma, choriocarcinoma, and embryonal carcinoma. Germinomas are well-circumscribed round or lobulated lesions. Hemorrhage and calcification are rare. Metastases may spread via CSF, so the entire neuraxis should be imaged if these tumors are suspected. MRI signal characteristics are variable, with iso- to hyperintense signal relative to gray matter on both T1 and T2. With gadolinium, intense contrast enhancement is seen.

Subependymal Giant Cell Astrocytoma. Subependymal giant cell astrocytoma, a WHO grade I tumor, arises from astrocytes in the subependymal zone of the lateral ventricles and develops into an intraventricular tumor in the region of the foramen of Monro. It is seen almost exclusively in patients with tuberous sclerosis. Just like central neurocytoma, this tumor is also prone to cause obstructive hydrocephalus. The tumor is heterogeneously hypo- to isointense on T1 and heterogeneously hyperintense on T2-weighted images, with possible foci of hypointensity due to calcification. On FLAIR, an isointense to hyperintense solid tumor background may be punctuated by hyperintense cysts. FLAIR is also useful to assess for the possible presence of hyperintense cortical tubers, which if present aid in the differential diagnosis. With gadolinium, intense enhancement is seen.

Choroid Plexus Papilloma. Choroid plexus papilloma is a well-circumscribed, highly vascular, intraventricular WHO grade I tumor derived from choroid plexus epithelium. In children it is usually seen in the lateral ventricle, while in adults it tends to involve the fourth ventricle. General imaging characteristics include a villiform or bosselated "cauliflower-like" appearance. Hemorrhage and calcification are noted occasionally in the tumor bed. The tumor's location frequently causes obstructive hydrocephalus. On MRI, the appearance is hypo- or isointense to normal brain on T1 and iso- to hyperintense on T2-weighted images. The latter

may also show punctate or linear/serpiginous signal flow voids within the tumor. Calcification (25%) or hemorrhage manifest as a markedly hypointense blooming artifact on T2* gradient echo images. With gadolinium, intense enhancement is seen. Choroid plexus carcinomas are malignant tumors that may invade the brain parenchyma and may also spread via CSF.

Tumors in the Sellar and Parasellar Region

The sellar and parasellar group of extra-axial masses include pituitary micro- and macroadenomas and craniopharyngiomas. Meningiomas, arachnoid cysts, dermoid and epidermoid cysts, optic pathway gliomas, hamartomas, metastases, and aneurysms are also encountered in the para- and suprasellar region.

Pituitary Adenomas. The distinction between micro- and macroadenomas is based on their size: tumors less than 10 mm are microadenomas, the larger tumors are macroadenomas. These tumors may arise from hormone-producing cells, such as prolactinomas or growth hormone–producing adenomas, resulting in characteristic clinical syndromes. Pituitary adenomas are typically hypointense on T1-weighted and hyperintense on T2-weighted images, relative to the surrounding parenchyma. This signal change, however, is not always conspicuous, especially in the case of small microadenomas. Gadolinium administration helps in these cases, when the microadenoma is visualized as relative hypointensity against the background of the normally enhancing gland (Fig. 39.26). Following a delay, this difference in enhancement is often no longer apparent, and if the postcontrast images are obtained in a later phase, a reversal of contrast may be noted. The adenoma takes up contrast in a delayed fashion and is seen as hyperintense against the more hypointense gland from where the contrast has washed out. Sometimes when the signal characteristics are not conspicuous, only alteration of the size and shape of the pituitary gland or shifting of the infundibulum may indicate the presence of a microadenoma. Because of this, it is important to be familiar with the normal range of pituitary gland sizes, which depend on age and gender. In adults, a gland height of more than 9 mm is worrisome. In the younger population, however, different normal values have

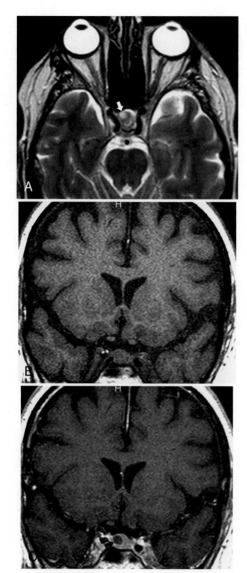

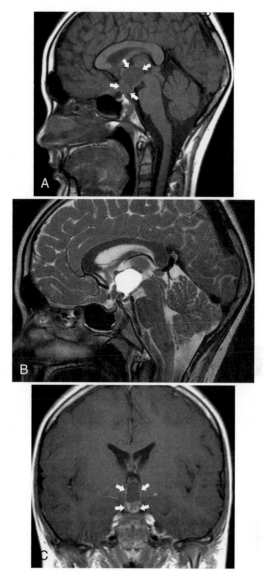

Fig. 39.26 Pituitary microadenoma. A, Axial T2-weighted image demonstrates a round area of hyperintensity on right side of pituitary gland *(arrow)*. **B,** On coronal noncontrast T1-weighted image, the gland has an upward convex morphology, and there is a vague hypointensity in its right side *(arrow)*. **C,** On coronal T1-weighted postcontrast image, the microadenoma is well seen as an area of hypointensity *(arrow)* against the background of the normally enhancing gland parenchyma.

Fig. 39.28 Craniopharyngioma. A, On sagittal T1-weighted image, a suprasellar mass lesion has a prominent T1 hypointense cystic component *(arrows)*. **B,** On sagittal T2-weighted image, the cyst is hyperintense. **C,** With gadolinium, both the rim of the cyst and the solid portion of the mass exhibit enhancement *(arrows)*.

been established. Before puberty, the normal height is 3 to 5 mm. At puberty in girls, the gland height may be 10 to 11 mm and may exhibit an upward convex morphology. In boys at puberty, the height is 6 to 8 mm, and the upward convex morphology can be normal. The size and shape of the gland may also change during pregnancy: convex morphology may appear, and a gland height of 10 mm is considered normal.

While microadenomas are localized to the sellar region, macroadenomas may become invasive and extend to the suprasellar region and may displace/compress the optic chiasm or even the hypothalamus. Extension to the cavernous sinus is also possible (see eFig. 39.27).

Craniopharyngioma. Craniopharyngiomas are believed to originate from the epithelial remnants of the Rathke pouch.

This WHO grade I tumor may be encountered in children, and a second peak incidence is in the fifth decade (Eldevik et al., 1996). The most common location is the suprasellar cistern (Fig. 39.28), but intrasellar tumors are also possible. The tumor may cause expansion of the sella or erosion of the dorsum sellae. In the suprasellar region, displacement of the chiasm, the anterior cerebral arteries, or even the hypothalamus is possible. Craniopharyngiomas have both solid and cystic components. Histologically, the more common adamantinomatous and the less common papillary forms are distinguished. The adamantinomatous type frequently exhibits calcification. The MRI signal is heterogeneous. Solid portions are iso- or hypointense on T1, whereas cystic components exhibit variable signal characteristics depending on the amount of protein or the presence of blood products. On T2, the solid and cystic components are sometimes hard to distinguish, as they are both usually hyperintense. Areas of calcification may appear hypointense on T2. With contrast, the solid portions of the tumor exhibit intense enhancement.

Metastatic Tumors

Intracranial metastases are detected in approximately 25% of patients who die of cancer. Cerebral metastases comprise over half of brain tumors (Vogelbaum and Suh, 2006) and are the most common type of brain tumor in adults (Klos and O'Neill, 2004). Most (80%) metastases involve the cerebral hemispheres, and 20% are seen in the posterior fossa. Pelvic and colon cancer have a tendency to involve the posterior fossa. Intracranial metastases, depending on the type of tumor, may involve the skull and the dura, the brain, and also the meninges in the form of meningeal carcinomatosis. Among all tumors that metastasize to the bone, breast and prostate cancer and multiple myeloma are especially prone to spread to the skull and dura. Most often, carcinomas involve the brain and get there by hematogenous spread. Systemic tumors with the greatest tendency to metastasize to brain are lung (as many as 30% of lung cancers give rise to brain metastases), breast (Fig. 39.29), and melanoma (Fig. 39.30). Cancers of the gastrointestinal tract (especially colon and rectum) and the kidney are the next most common sources. Other possibilities include gallbladder, liver, thyroid gland, pancreas, ovary, and testicles. Tumors of the prostate, esophagus, and skin (other than melanoma) hardly ever form brain parenchymal metastases.

It is important to highlight the potential imaging differences between primary and metastatic brain tumors, since a significant percentage of patients found to have brain metastasis have no prior diagnosis of cancer. Cerebral parenchymal metastases can be single (usually with kidney, breast, thyroid, and lung adenocarcinoma) or (more commonly) multiple (in small cell carcinomas and melanoma) and tend to involve the gray/white matter junction. Seeing multiple tumors at the corticomedullary junction favors the diagnosis of metastatic lesions over a primary brain tumor. The size of metastatic lesions is variable, and the mass effect and peritumoral edema is usually prominent and, contrary to that seen with primary brain tumors, frequently out of proportion to the size of the tumor itself. The edema is vasogenic, persistent, and involves the white matter, highlighting the intact cortical sulci as characteristic fingerlike projections. It is hypointense on T1 and hyperintense on T2 and FLAIR. The tumor itself exhibits variable, often heterogeneous signal intensity, especially if the metastasis is hemorrhagic (15% of brain metastases). Tumors that tend to cause hemorrhagic metastases include melanoma; choriocarcinoma; and lung, thyroid, and kidney cancer. The tumor signal characteristic can be unique in mucin-producing colon adenocarcinoma metastases, where the mucin and protein content cause a hyperintense signal on T1-weighted images.

Detection of intracerebral metastases is facilitated by administration of gadolinium, and every patient with neurological symptoms and a history of cancer needs to have a gadolinium-enhanced MRI study. The enhancement pattern of metastatic tumors can be solid or ringlike. To improve the diagnostic yield, triple-dose gadolinium or magnetization transfer techniques have been used, which improve detection of smaller metastases that are not so conspicuous with single-dose contrast administration. A triple dose of gadolinium improves metastasis detection by as much as 43% (van Dijk et al., 1997). Meningeal carcinomatosis can also be detected by contrast administration, which can reveal thickening of the meninges and/or meningeal deposits of the metastatic tumor.

For demonstration of the role of advanced structural neuroimaging in brain tumor surgery planning, please see the online version of this chapter, available at http://www.expertconsult.com.

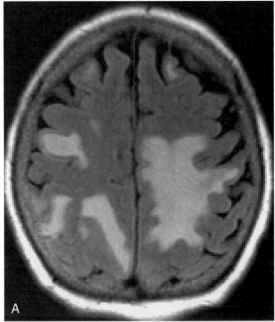

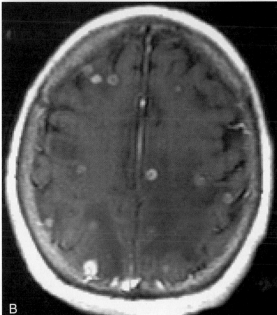

Fig. 39.29 Brain metastases from breast cancer. A, On axial FLAIR image, multiple areas of vasogenic edema extend into subcortical white matter with fingerlike projections. **B,** On axial T1-weighted postcontrast image, numerous small enhancing mass lesions are scattered in both hemispheres at the gray/white junction. Both homogeneous and ringlike enhancement patterns are present.

Ischemic Stroke

Acute Ischemic Stroke. With the introduction of thrombolytic therapy in the treatment of acute ischemic stroke, timely diagnosis of an ischemic lesion, determining its location and extent, and demonstrating the amount of tissue at risk has become essential (see Chapters 65 and 68). CT imaging remains of great value in the evaluation of acute stroke; it is readily available, and newer CT modalities including CT angiography and CT perfusion imaging are coming into greater use. The applicability of CT to acute stroke continues to be

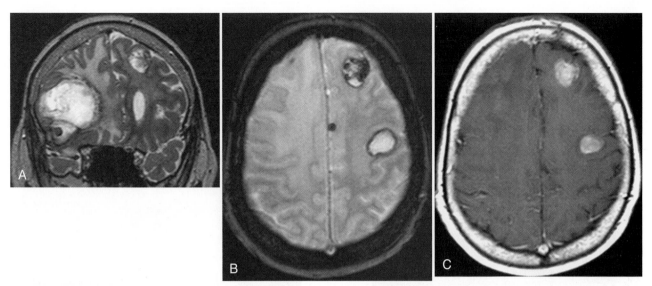

Fig. 39.30 Hemorrhagic melanoma metastases. A, Coronal T2-weighted image demonstrates a large hyperintense mass in the right frontal lobe, with associated hyperintense vasogenic edema and mass effect. A smaller mass lesion with similar signal characteristics is present at the gray/white junction in the left frontal lobe. Note surrounding rim of hypointensity, indicating hemosiderin deposition within these hemorrhagic metastases. **B,** On gradient echo, hypointense blood degradation products are well seen within the metastases. **C,** Following gadolinium administration, intense enhancement is noted.

enhanced by the ever-increasing rapidity with which scans can be acquired, allowing for greater coverage of tissues with thinner slices. The technological advances allowing for rapid acquisition of data have led to 4D imaging, where complete 3D data sets of the brain are serially obtained over very short time intervals, allowing for higher temporal and spatial resolutions in brain perfusion studies of acute ischemic stroke patients.

CT is very useful in detecting hyperdense hemorrhagic lesions as the cause of stroke. Early ischemic stroke, however, may not cause any change on unenhanced CT, making it difficult to determine the extent of the ischemic lesion and the amount of tissue at risk. CT is especially limited in evaluating ischemia in the posterior fossa, owing to streak artifacts at the skull base. Despite these limitations, early signs of acute ischemia on unenhanced CT may be helpful in the first few hours after stroke. CT signs of acute ischemia include blurring of the gray/white junction and effacement of the sulci due to ischemic swelling of the tissues. Blurring of the contours of the deep gray matter structures is of similar significance. In cases of internal carotid artery occlusion, middle cerebral artery main segment (M1) occlusion, or more distal occlusions, intraluminal clot may be seen as a focal hyperdensity, sometimes referred to as a *hyperdense MCA*, or *hyperdense dot sign* (Fig. 39.32).

Several MRI modalities as well as CT perfusion studies are capable of providing data regarding cerebral ischemia and perfusion to assist in the evaluation for possible thrombolytic therapy very early after symptom onset. DWI with ADC mapping is considered to be the most sensitive method for imaging acute ischemia (Figs. 39.33 to 39.36). In humans, the hyperintense signal indicating restriction of diffusion is detected within minutes after onset (Hossmann and Hoehn-Berlage, 1995).

Temporal Evolution of Ischemic Stroke on Magnetic Resonance Imaging

Acute Stroke. Initially, the hyperintense signal on DWI is caused by decreased water diffusivity due to swelling of the ischemic nerve cells (for the first 5 to 7 days), then it

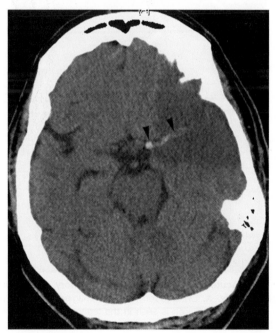

Fig. 39.32 Evolving ischemic stroke in the territory of the left middle cerebral artery. On this noncontrast CT scan, a hyperdense signal is seen in the distal left internal carotid artery and in the M1 segment of the left middle cerebral artery, indicating presence of a blood clot *(arrowheads)*. There is hypodensity in the corresponding area of the left hemisphere, demonstrating the evolving ischemic infarct.

increasingly results from the abnormal T2 properties of the infarcted tissue (T2 shine-through). For this reason, a reliable estimation of the age of the ischemic lesion is not possible by looking at DWI images alone. Imaging protocols for acute ischemic stroke usually include T1- and T2-weighted fast spin echo images, FLAIR sequences, and DWI with ADC maps.

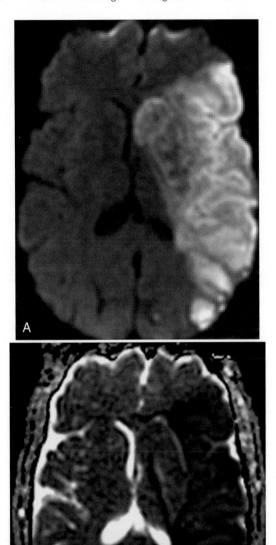

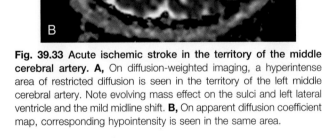

Fig. 39.33 Acute ischemic stroke in the territory of the middle cerebral artery. A, On diffusion-weighted imaging, a hyperintense area of restricted diffusion is seen in the territory of the left middle cerebral artery. Note evolving mass effect on the sulci and left lateral ventricle and the mild midline shift. **B,** On apparent diffusion coefficient map, corresponding hypointensity is seen in the same area.

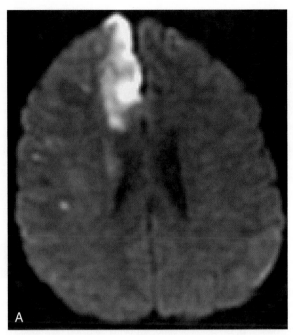

Fig. 39.34 Acute ischemic stroke in the territory of the anterior cerebral artery. A, On diffusion-weighted imaging, a hyperintense area of restricted diffusion is seen in the right medial frontal lobe, involving the territory of the anterior cerebral artery.

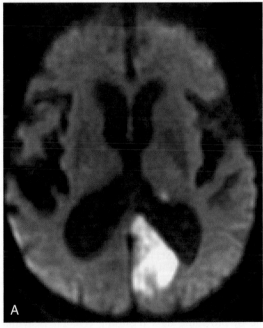

Fig. 39.35 Acute ischemic stroke in the territory of the posterior cerebral artery. A, On diffusion-weighted imaging, a hyperintense area of restricted diffusion is seen in the left medial occipital lobe, involving the territory of the posterior cerebral artery.

These sequences together confirm the diagnosis of ischemia, determine its extent, and allow for an approximate estimation of the time of onset (Srinivasan et al., 2006). On ADC maps, the values decrease initially after the onset of ischemia (i.e., the signal from the affected area becomes progressively more hypointense). This reaches a nadir at 3 to 5 days but remains significantly low until the seventh day after onset. After this time, the values increase (the signal gets more and more hyperintense) and return to the baseline values in 1 to 4 weeks (usually in 7 to 10 days). Therefore, ADC maps are quite useful for the estimation of the age of the lesion: if the signal of the area is hypointense on an ADC map, the lesion is likely less than 7 to 10 days old. If the area is isointense or hyperintense on the ADC map, the onset was likely more than 7 to 10 days ago. As already noted, although these signal changes take place on ADC maps, the DWI images remain hyperintense, without noticeable changes of intensity by visual inspection.

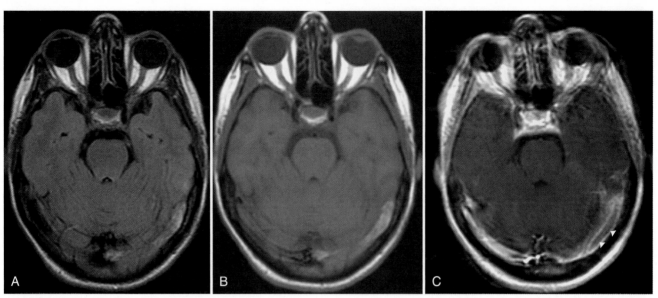

Fig. 39.46 Left transverse and sigmoid sinus thrombosis with a small left temporal lobe area of venous ischemia. This 48-year-old patient presented with a new-onset seizure and right visual field deficit that resolved later. **A,** Axial FLAIR image reveals abnormal hyperintense signal in the left transverse and sigmoid sinus, indicating thrombosis. Compare to the right transverse sinus, with the normal hypointense flow void. This FLAIR image also shows a small but noticeable area of hyperintensity due to venous ischemia in the left temporal lobe. **B,** Noncontrast T1-weighted image also reveals abnormal hyperintense signal in the involved venous sinuses. Again, compare with the contralateral sinus. **C,** Postcontrast T1-weighted image reveals normal filling in the sinus on the right, but there is no filling along the visualized segment of the left transverse sinus *(arrowheads).*

a false assumption of thrombosis. Gadolinium-enhanced images help in these cases, demonstrating contrast filling/enhancement in the sinuses and confirming the absence of thrombosis. A normal variant of venous sinus hypoplasia/aplasia may result in decreased/absent flow signal on MRV, falsely interpreted as thrombosis. T1- and T2-weighted images, however, are usually able to demonstrate the absence of thrombus in the sinus. These examples highlight the importance of reviewing all necessary image modalities (MRV, T2-weighted images, T1-weighted images with and without contrast) to make or reject a diagnosis of venous sinus thrombosis.

Hemorrhagic Cerebrovascular Disease

Structural neuroimaging is crucial in the evaluation of hemorrhagic cerebrovascular disease. Besides detection of the hematoma itself, its location can provide useful information regarding its etiology. Lobar hematomas, especially along with small, scattered, parenchymal microbleeds, raise the possibility of cerebral amyloid angiopathy, whereas putaminal, thalamic, or cerebellar hemorrhages are more likely to be of hypertensive origin. Other underlying lesions such as brain tumors causing hemorrhages can be detected by structural imaging. This section discusses hemorrhagic cerebrovascular disease and cerebral intraparenchymal hematoma, whereas other causes of hemorrhage such as trauma or malignancy are discussed in other sections. Please also refer to Chapters 66 and 67 for a clinical neurological review of intracerebral hemorrhages.

For decades, noncontrast CT scanning has been (and in most emergency settings still is) the essential tool for initial evaluation of intracerebral hemorrhage. In hyperacute (<12 hours after onset) and acute hemorrhage (12 to 48 hours), the patient's hematocrit largely determines the lesion's degree of density on CT. With a normal hematocrit, both retracted and unretracted clots exhibit hyperdensity that contrasts sufficiently with the isodense background of brain parenchyma to

be easily detectable. In cases of anemia, however, small hemorrhagic lesions may potentially be overlooked owing to their lower CT density and may even be isodense to brain. The following sections describing the appearance of hemorrhage on CT and MRI studies all assume a normal hematocrit.

In the acute stage, the hematoma is seen as an area of hyperdensity on CT. The associated mass effect depends on the size and location. Effacement of the ventricles, cortical sulci, or basal cisterns is often seen. Various degrees of midline shift or subtypes of herniation (transtentorial, subfalcine, etc.) may occur. The surrounding edema is seen as hypodensity and tends to appear irregular with varying thickness depending on the degree of involvement of adjacent white matter tracts, which are preferentially affected. The initially distinct border of the hematoma changes within days to a few weeks after onset and becomes irregular and "moth-eaten" due to the phagocytic activity of macrophages. Small hematomas may disappear on CT within 1 week; in the case of larger hematomas, the process may take more than a month. Small hemorrhages may resolve without any residual change, while those that are larger are gradually replaced by an encephalomalacic cavity of decreased density and ex vacuo enlargement of the adjacent CSF spaces.

The appearance of hemorrhagic cerebrovascular disease on MRI is very complex regarding both signal heterogeneity on individual scans and subsequent changes in appearance over successive imaging studies. Signal characteristics of hemorrhage vary widely across different pulse sequences (T1, T2, T2* gradient echo) depending on the age of the hemorrhage; presence of oxyhemoglobin, deoxyhemoglobin, methemoglobin, and hemosiderin; changing water content within the clot; and integrity of erythrocyte membranes. Understanding the typical MRI appearance of each stage in the evolution of a hemorrhage allows one to estimate its age, because biochemical and structural changes characteristic of each stage (macroscopic and microscopic) occur along a predictable time line. In addition to conventional (T1- and T2-weighted) images, the gradient echo technique has been used to detect even small intracerebral hemorrhages, given its sensitivity to the paramagnetic properties (magnetic field distorting effects) of various blood products. More recently introduced into clinical practice, the technique of SWI offers the greatest sensitivity for chronic hemorrhage to date and is particularly useful in evaluating punctate hemorrhages in patients with diffuse shear injury secondary to prior head trauma.

A discussion of the MR imaging features of hemorrhage is best organized according to the stages of hemorrhage evolution as follows.

Hyperacute Hemorrhage (0 to 24 Hours). In the early (hyperacute) phase of intraparenchymal hemorrhage (<24 hours) the red blood cells are intact, and a mixture of oxy- and deoxyhemoglobin is present (Bakshi et al., 1998). In this stage, the signal on T1-weighted images is isointense to the brain, so even larger hematomas may be missed on this pulse sequence. On T2-weighted images, the oxyhemoglobin portion is hyperintense and deoxyhemoglobin is hypointense, resulting in the gradual appearance of a hypointense rim and gradually increasing hypointense foci within the hematoma as the amount of deoxyhemoglobin increases from the periphery. Such hypointense foci are also seen on FLAIR. Between the clot and the deoxyhemoglobin-containing rim, thin intervening clefts of fluid-like T2 hyperintensity may be seen as an initial manifestation of clot retraction. On gradient echo images, hyperacute hemorrhage will exhibit heterogeneously isointense to markedly hypointense signal, the latter corresponding to deoxyhemoglobin content in more peripheral portions of the clot. The amount of edema is mild in this stage, usually seen as a thin rim that is hyperintense on T2 and FLAIR images and hypointense on T1-weighted images (Atlas and Thulborn, 1998).

Acute Hemorrhage (1 to 3 Days). During this stage, hemoglobin is transformed to deoxyhemoglobin, but the membranes of the erythrocytes are still intact (Bakshi et al., 1998). The hematoma becomes slightly hypointense on T1 and strikingly hypointense on T2-weighted images (Fig. 39.47). On GRE, proton spins in the presence of paramagnetic deoxyhemoglobin dephase rapidly during TE, resulting in signal loss and, therefore, hypointensity of the hematoma on this pulse sequence. The surrounding edema, which is more extensive during this stage, is hypointense on T1 and hyperintense on T2.

Early Subacute Hemorrhage (3 Days to 1 Week). As blood degradation evolves, deoxyhemoglobin is converted to methemoglobin. At this stage, the blood degradation products are still intracellular (Bakshi et al., 1998). Intracellular methemoglobin is hyperintense on T1 and hypointense on T2-weighted images. T1 shortening is primarily the result of dipole-dipole interactions between heme iron and adjacent water protons, facilitated by a conformational change that occurs when deoxyhemoglobin is converted to methemoglobin.

Signal changes on T2 occur via a different mechanism. Sequestration of methemoglobin within the intact red blood cell membrane results in a locally paramagnetic environment adjacent to the diamagnetic, methemoglobin-free extracellular compartment. These differences in the local magnetic fields, present at a microscopic level, cause rapid dephasing of proton spins and signal loss during TE as water molecules diffuse rapidly through this heterogeneous environment. Therefore, on T2-weighted images the presence of intracellular methemoglobin results in hypointensity of the hemorrhage. These signal changes start from the periphery of the hematoma where the deoxyhemoglobin-to-methemoglobin transformation first occurs. During this stage, the amount of edema starts to decrease.

Late Subacute Hemorrhage (1 to 4 Weeks). In the late subacute phase, the membranes of the red blood cells disintegrate, and methemoglobin becomes extracellular (Bakshi et al., 1998). Extracellular methemoglobin contains Fe^{3+}, which has five unpaired electrons. This leads to a dipole-dipole interaction which, contrary to intracellular methemoglobin, causes hyperintense signal change on both T1- and T2-weighted images (Fig. 39.48).

During this stage (usually 2 weeks after the hemorrhage) hemosiderin deposition begins, typically at the periphery of the hematoma where macrophages reside. A dark peripheral rim appears on GRE and T2-weighted images, initially thin, then progressively thicker. The amount of edema around the hematoma continues to decrease gradually.

Chronic Hemorrhage (>4 Weeks). In the chronic stage (Bakshi et al., 1998), the core of larger hematomas turns into a slitlike or linear cavity with CSF signal characteristics, being hypointense on T1 and FLAIR and hyperintense on T2-weighted images. At the periphery of the lesion, macrophages continue to remove iron from the extracellular methemoglobin; hemosiderin and ferritin are deposited in their lysosomes, resulting in a rim of hypointense signal on T2-weighted and GRE images. This hypointense rim becomes progressively more prominent during the transition from the late subacute to chronic stage (Fig. 39.49).

If the hemorrhage is small, eventually its entire area will be occupied by hemosiderin deposition. Smaller hemorrhages or microbleeds, such as those seen in amyloid angiopathy or after head trauma, are visualized as multiple uniformly hypointense foci on GRE images. Susceptibility-weighted images are even more sensitive to magnetic filed distortion due to blood products and can reveal microbleeds that are missed even by conventional gradient echo images. It is important to keep in mind that because of magnetic field distortion, the area of hypointensity on GRE or susceptibility-weighted images is larger than the actual size of the bleed. GRE or, ideally, SWI should be part of every MRI protocol for brain trauma.

Hemorrhage, like many other lesions to the brain, provokes reactive gliosis. In the chronic stage, surrounding gliosis is seen as mildly hyperintense signal on T2 and FLAIR images.

Superficial siderosis, a chronic sequela of bleeding into the subarachnoid space, and cerebral amyloid angiopathy, a hemorrhage-prone condition, are discussed in the online version of this chapter, available at http://www.expertconsult.com.

Infection

Structural neuroimaging can provide useful information for evaluating infectious diseases of the CNS. The imaging modality of choice is MRI, which is able to demonstrate even subtle parenchymal abnormalities and inflammatory involvement of the meninges. Please visit http://www.expertconsult.com to view this section. For a review of the etiology, clinical presentation, and treatment of infections of the nervous system, see Chapters 77–79.

Noninfectious Encephalitis

Multiple Sclerosis and Other White Matter Diseases

Inflammatory and noninflammatory lesions of the corpus callosum, leukodystrophy (Krabbe disease, metachromatic leukodystrophy, adrenoleukodystrophy), radiation leukoencephalopathy, posterior reversible encephalopathy syndrome, and central pontine myelinolysis are discussed in the online version of this chapter, available at http://www.expertconsult.com.

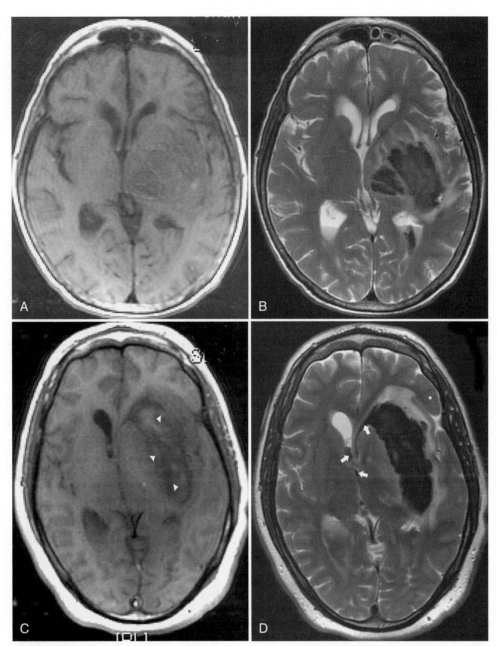

Fig. 39.47 Two cases of acute parenchymal hemorrhage. A, B, Large acute left basal ganglia hemorrhage. On noncontrast T1-weighted image **(A)** only faint hypointensity is noted. On axial T2-weighted image **(B)** the hematoma appears as a striking hypointensity with developing hyperintense edema in surrounding parenchyma. Note associated mass effect. **C–D,** In this case, the basal ganglia hematoma is in a more advanced stage. On T1-weighted image **(C)** the area is still mostly hypointense, but its center is now turning hyperintense because of intracellular methemoglobin *(arrowheads)*. On corresponding T2-weighted image **(D)** the hematoma is still hypointense (as intracellular methemoglobin is also hypointense on T2), but the surrounding hyperintense edema is more prominent, and the mass effect is increased as well. Note that hemorrhage is also present within the ventricle, making the prognosis worse *(arrows)*.

Multiple Sclerosis. Multiple sclerosis is a demyelinating disease with autoimmune inflammatory reaction against the myelin sheath of CNS pathways (see Chapter 80). MRI is essential for the diagnosis of MS by demonstrating the typical inflammatory demyelinating lesions disseminated in time and space (Fig. 39.59). It is also used for disease monitoring and assessment of response to therapy.

MS white matter lesions may occur supratentorially or infratentorially, as well as within the spinal cord (imaging of spinal cord MS lesions is described later). Best evaluated on

T2-weighted images, infratentorial lesions may be seen within the medulla, pons, midbrain, or cerebellum. Characteristic locations include the pontine tegmentum, periaqueductal region, cerebral peduncles, middle and superior cerebellar peduncles, and the white matter of the cerebellar hemispheres. Punctate or small lesions that are present directly adjacent to the fourth ventricle or cisterns are sometimes difficult to detect on T2-weighted images but are not uncommon. Infratentorial lesions are generally smaller than supratentorial lesions and are also less frequently hypointense on conventional

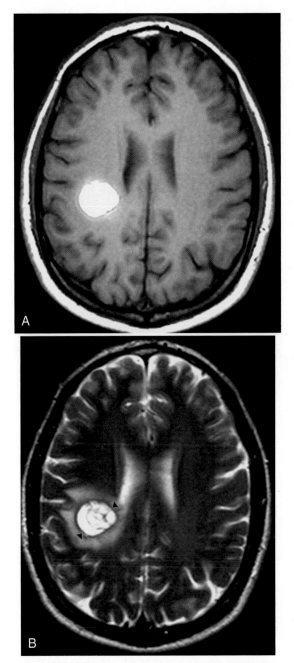

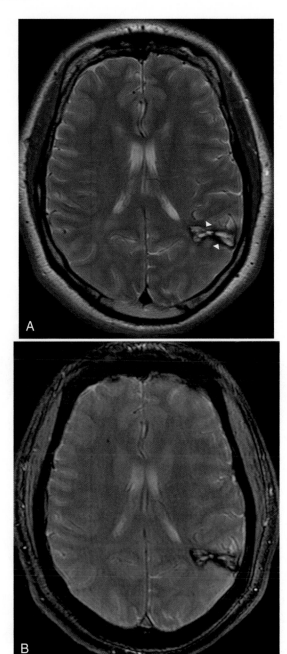

Fig. 39.48 Late subacute parenchymal hemorrhage. A, On noncontrast T1-weighted image, there is a hematoma in the right corona radiata. This exhibits homogeneous hyperintense signal. **B,** On T2-weighted image, the hematoma also appears as homogeneous hyperintensity. Signal characteristics are typical for the presence of extracellular methemoglobin in a late subacute hematoma. Note beginning of hypointense hemosiderin deposition at the rim of the hematoma on T2-weighted image *(arrowheads)*.

Fig. 39.49 Chronic parenchymal hemorrhage. A, Axial T2-weighted image reveals a slitlike cavitary lesion in the left parietal lobe. Its center has CSF-like hyperintense signal, but there is a rim of hypointensity due to hemosiderin deposition along its border *(arrowheads)*. **B,** Axial gradient echo image reveals markedly hypointense hemosiderin deposition along the border of the chronic hemorrhage.

T1-weighted images; they commonly appear hypointense on T1-weighted 3D spoiled gradient echo pulse sequences.

Supratentorial white matter lesions are usually best appreciated using the FLAIR pulse sequence, which nulls out CSF signal that may obscure periventricular abnormalities on conventional T2-weighted images. Periventricular (PV) and subcortical white matter lesions typically are small in size and morphologically are generally ovoid or round on axial images. On sagittal views, PV lesions often exhibit a thin linear or

fingerlike morphology (Dawson fingers), with the long axis of the lesion oriented perpendicularly to the wall of the lateral ventricle in a PV distribution. The PV distribution of many MS lesions is well demonstrated on SWI imaging, which reveals a single tiny, profoundly hypointense dot or thin linearity at the center of a significant proportion of demyelinating lesions. It represents a venule and is visible because of the magnetic susceptibility effects of deoxygenated venous blood, to which SWI is particularly sensitive.

Although the distribution of white matter lesions in MS has a somewhat random appearance, the hemispheres

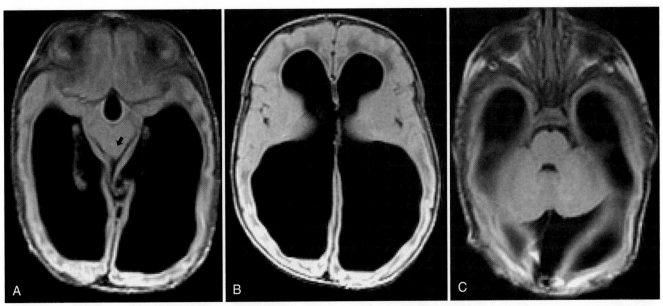

Fig. 39.95 Obstructive hydrocephalus. A–C, In this case of congenital obstructive hydrocephalus, the cerebral aqueduct appears stenotic *(small arrow)*. There is extreme dilatation of the third and lateral ventricles, with the cerebral tissue being extremely thinned. The fourth ventricle is normal in size.

Vascular Malformations

The various vascular malformations (arteriovenous malformations, cavernous malformations, developmental venous anomaly, and capillary telangiectasia) are discussed in the online version of this chapter, available at http://www.expertconsult.com. Please also see Chapters 66 and 67 for review.

Cerebrospinal Fluid Circulation Disorders

Abnormalities in CSF and intraspinal cord flow cause changes in the brain or spinal cord that are readily identifiable by CT or MRI. Hydrocephalus is an abnormal intracranial accumulation of CSF that interferes with normal brain function (see Chapter 88). It should be distinguished from dilation of the ventricles and subarachnoid space due to decreased brain volume, which can be normal or pathological and has been called *hydrocephalus ex vacuo*. We will avoid using this term, because true hydrocephalus often requires treatment by shunting. Hydrocephalus may follow increased CSF production or impaired resorption. Resorption occurs not only via the pacchionian granulations in the venous sinuses but through the brain lymphatic system as well. Traditionally, two main types of hydrocephalus are distinguished: obstructive and nonobstructive. Nonobstructive hydrocephalus is due to increased CSF production, as with choroid plexus papillomas in children. Depending on whether CSF flow from the ventricular system to the subarachnoid space is intact or impeded, we can distinguish between communicating and noncommunicating types of obstructive hydrocephalus. Some processes increase CSF ICP but not the volume of intracranial CSF, causing the syndrome of idiopathic intracranial hypertension (known as *pseudotumor cerebri*). Interruption of CSF circulation can also happen at the craniocervical junction, where pathologies that interfere with the return of CSF from the spinal subarachnoid space to the intracranial compartment, as happens in the Chiari malformations, can arise. Finally, CSF intracranial volume may be abnormally reduced, causing the syndrome of intracranial hypotension.

Obstructive, Noncommunicating Hydrocephalus. Depending on the site of obstruction, various segments of the ventricular system will enlarge. Obstruction at the foramen of Monro causes unilateral or bilateral enlargement of the lateral ventricles. Aqueductal stenosis, which may be congenital, leads to enlargement of the third and lateral ventricles, but the fourth ventricle is normal in size (Fig. 39.95). Obstruction of the foramina of Luschka and Magendie results in enlargement of the third, fourth, and lateral ventricles. Other possible imaging findings include thinning and upward bowing of the corpus callosum. In third ventricle enlargement, the optic and infundibular recesses are widened. When the evolution of the hydrocephalus is rapid, transependymal CSF flow induces a T2 hyperintense signal (best seen on FLAIR sequences) along the walls of the involved ventricular segments, and in the case of the lateral ventricles, most pronounced at the frontal horns.

Normal-Pressure Hydrocephalus. In this type of hydrocephalus, there is enlargement of the ventricles, most pronounced for the third and lateral ventricles (Fig. 39.96). The subarachnoid spaces at the top of the convexity are typically compressed, but the larger sulci, such as the interhemispheric sulcus and the sylvian fissure, may be dilated as well as the ventricles (Kitagaki et al., 1998). In this case, the cross-sections of the dilated sulci often have the appearance of a "U" rather than the appearance of a "V" characteristic of atrophy. These morphologic findings are more helpful than flow studies. Increased CSF flow in the cerebral aqueduct may cause a hypointense "jet-flow" sign on all sequences. Quantitative CSF flow studies (cine phase-contrast MR imaging) are frequently used for evaluation of patients with suspected normal-pressure hydrocephalus. However, the distinction between using MRI to diagnose normal-pressure hydrocephalus versus determining the probability of clinical improvement from shunt placement should be kept in mind, as studies seem to show that MRI may be better at the former than the latter. Although CSF flow studies had been thought to help to predict shunt responsiveness (Bradley et al., 1996), later studies have challenged

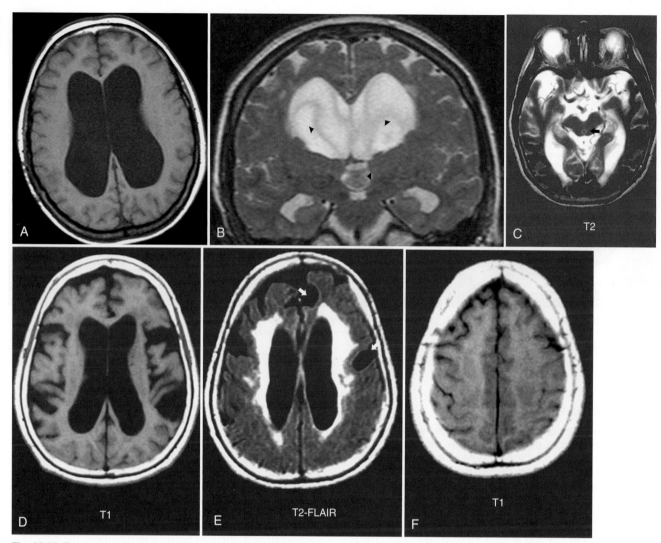

Fig. 39.96 Two cases of normal-pressure hydrocephalus. In the first case **(A)** axial noncontrast T1-weighted images demonstrate significant enlargement of the ventricles, which is clearly out of proportion to the size of the superficial CSF spaces. The parietal sulci appear somewhat effaced. **B,** Coronal T2-weighted image also exhibits prominent ventricular enlargement. Note intraventricular artifact due to CSF pulsation *(arrowheads)*, indicating hyperdynamic flow. The second case demonstrates communicating hydrocephalus. Images **C–F** are axial sections of the MRI from a 71-year-old woman with progressive gait and cognitive impairment, as well as urinary incontinence. Note the low signal in the sylvian aqueduct, owing to a flow void from high-velocity CSF flow through this structure **(C,** *arrow*). Although basal cisterns **(C)** and interhemispheric and sylvian fissures **(D, E)** are dilated, sulci in the high convexity **(F)** are compressed. Trans-ependymal reabsorption of CSF, suggested by the homogeneous high signal in the periventricular white matter **(E),** need not occur in all cases of symptomatic hydrocephalus. In addition to the compressed sulci in the convexity, the U shape of some of the dilated sulci **(E,** *white arrows*) is helpful to make the diagnosis.

this view (Dixon et al., 2002; Kahlon et al., 2007). Traditionally it has been hypothesized that in this condition there is a problem with CSF absorption at the level of the arachnoid granulations, since normal-pressure hydrocephalus has been observed as a late complication after meningitis or subarachnoid hemorrhage that caused meningeal involvement/scarring. But this syndrome, often associated with vascular disease in older people, may also be the result of decreased superficial venous compliance and a reduction in the blood flow returning via the sagittal sinus (Bateman, 2008). The term *normal pressure* is a misnomer because long-term monitoring of ventricular pressure has shown recurrent episodes of transient pressure elevation.

Chiari Malformation. Depending on associated structural abnormalities, different types of Chiari malformation are

distinguished. In the most common, type 1 Chiari, there is caudal displacement of the tip of the cerebellar tonsils 5 mm or more below the level of the foramen magnum. Most often this malformation is accompanied by a congenitally small posterior fossa. However, acquired forms of tonsillar descent also exist, either due to space occupying intracranial pathology or to a low-pressure environment in the spinal canal, such as after lumboperitoneal shunt placement. In typical Chiari 1, the ectopic cerebellar tonsils are frequently peg shaped, but otherwise the cerebellum is of normal morphology. There is usually crowding of the structures at the level of the foramen magnum. The 5-mm diagnostic cutoff value has been selected in adults, as this condition tends to be symptomatic and clinically significant at this or higher measured values. If the tonsils are caudal to the level of the foramen magnum by less than 5 mm, the term *low-lying cerebellar tonsils* is used; this is

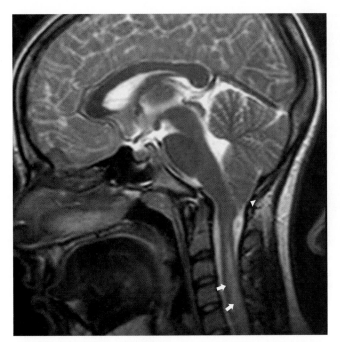

Fig. 39.97 Chiari type 1 malformation. Sagittal T2-weighted image demonstrates caudal displacement of the cerebellar tonsil through the foramen magnum into the cervical spinal canal (arrowhead). The tonsil is characteristically peg-shaped. There is a prominent longitudinal hyperintense cavity in the visualized cervical spinal cord segment, consistent with a syrinx (arrows).

frequently an asymptomatic incidental finding. When evaluating younger patients or children, it is to be remembered that the considered "normal" position of the cerebellar tonsils is different in the various age groups. In the first decade, 6 mm below the foramen magnum is considered the upper limit of normal, and with increasing age, there is an "ascent" of the tonsils, with a 5-mm cutoff value in the second and third decades, 4 mm up to the eighth decade, and 3 mm in the ninth decade of life (for review see Nash et al., 2002). Tonsillar ectopia and crowding at the foramen magnum interfere with return of CSF from the spinal to the intracranial subarachnoid space. This may lead, by still-disputed mechanisms, to syrinx formation in the spinal cord (see Fig. 39.97). If there is imaging evidence of a Chiari malformation on brain MRI, it is essential to image the cervical and thoracic cord to rule out a syrinx.

In Chiari type 2 malformation, there is a developmental abnormality of the hindbrain and caudal displacement not only of the cerebellar tonsils but also the cerebellum, medulla, and fourth ventricle. The cervical spinal nerve roots are stretched/compressed, and there is often a spinal cord syrinx present. Other abnormalities include lumbar or thoracic myelomeningocele; hydrocephalus is often present as well. Chiari type 3 malformation is an even more severe developmental abnormality, with cervical myelomeningocele or encephalocele.

🚫 For a description of idiopathic intracranial hypertension (pseudotumor cerebri) and of the imaging sequelae of intracranial hypotension please see the online version of this chapter at http://www.expertconsult.com.

Orbital Lesions

🚫 The structural neuroimaging of orbital lesions is discussed online at http://www.expertconsult.com.

Spinal Diseases
Spinal Tumors

Tumors affecting the spinal region can be classified according to their predominant location, intrinsic to the vertebral column itself or within the spinal canal. Spinal canal tumors may be intramedullary or extramedullary. Intramedullary tumors involve the spinal cord parenchyma, whereas extramedullary tumors are outside the spinal cord but within the spinal canal. Depending on their relation to the dura, extramedullary tumors may be classified as intradural or extradural. As tumors grow, they can spread to other compartments. For example, metastases in the vertebral bodies often extend to the epidural space and cause spinal cord compression. Tumors in pre- and paravertebral locations may also extend to the extradural space, either through the vertebral bodies, as happens with metastatic lung cancer, or through the neural foramina, as in lymphoma.

Vertebral Metastases, Extradural Tumors. In the majority of cases, tumors involving the vertebrae are metastatic in origin. Half of all vertebral metastatic tumors are from lung, breast (Fig. 39.102), and prostate cancer. Kidney and gastrointestinal tumors, melanoma, and those arising from the female reproductive organs are other common sources. Of all structural neuroimaging techniques, MRI is the imaging modality of choice to evaluate vertebral metastases, with sensitivity equal to and specificity better than bone scan (Mechtler and Cohen, 2000). MR imaging protocols for the evaluation of vertebral metastases typically include T1-weighted images with and without gadolinium, T2-weighted images, and STIR sequences. Typically, osteolytic metastases appear as hypointense foci on noncontrast T1-weighted images, hyperintense signal on T2 and STIR sequences, and enhance on postcontrast images. The enhancement may render the previously T1 hypointense metastatic foci isointense, interfering with their detection. Therefore, precontrast T1-weighted images should always be obtained as well. Osteoblastic metastases, such as seen in prostate cancer, are hypointense on T2-weighted images. Besides the vertebral bodies, metastases preferentially involve the pedicles. With marked involvement, the vertebral body may collapse.

Extradural tumors most commonly result from spread of metastatic tumors to the epidural space, directly from the vertebral body or from the prevertebral/paravertebral space. These mass lesions in the epidural space initially indent the thecal sac, and as they grow, they displace and eventually compress the spinal cord or cauda equina. If spinal cord compression is long-standing and severe enough, T2 hyperintense signal change may appear in the involved cord segment as a result of edema and/or ischemia secondary to compromised local circulation. An example of tumor spread from a paravertebral focus is lymphoma, which may extend into the spinal canal through the neural foramen. When intraspinal extension is suspected in a patient with lymphoma, MRI is the study of choice (Fig. 39.103). In cases of epithelial tumors, by the time of presentation, plain radiographs reveal the intraspinal extension with more than 80% sensitivity, but in patients with lymphoma, plain radiographs are still normal in almost 70% of cases (Mechtler and Cohen, 2000).

In the smaller group of extradural primary spinal tumors, multiple myeloma is the most common in adults. Involvement of the vertebral bone marrow may occur in multiple small foci, but diffuse involvement of an entire vertebral body is also possible. Myelomatous lesions are hypointense on T1, hyperintense on T2-weighted images, and highly hyperintense on STIR sequences. There is marked enhancement after gadolinium administration.

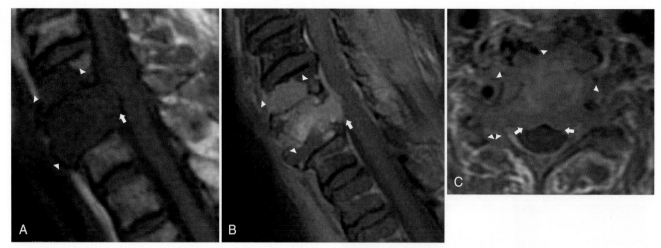

Fig. 39.102 Spinal metastasis. MRI from a 52-year-old woman with breast cancer. **A,** Sagittal T1-weighted image reveals hypointense signal in two adjacent vertebral bodies *(arrowheads)*. Metastatic mass extends beyond the vertebral bodies into the epidural space *(arrow)*. **B,** Sagittal T1-weighted, fat-suppressed postcontrast image better delineates the extent of the tumor. **C,** Axial postcontrast image demonstrates tumor spread toward the pre- and paravertebral space *(arrowheads)*, into the epidural space *(small arrows)* and into the pedicle *(double arrowheads)*.

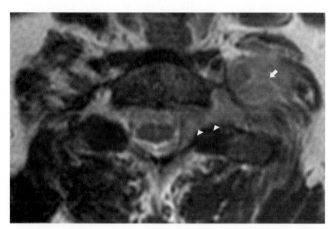

Fig. 39.103 Lymphoma. A left paravertebral tumor *(arrow)* extends through the left neural foramen into the cervical spinal canal *(arrowheads)*.

Extramedullary Intradural Spinal Tumors. This group of tumors includes leptomeningeal metastases, meningiomas, nerve sheath tumors, embryonal tumors (teratoma), congenital cysts (epidermoid, dermoid), and lipoma.

Leptomeningeal Metastases. Leptomeningeal metastases result from tumor cell infiltration of the leptomeningeal layers (pia and arachnoid). NonHodgkin lymphoma, leukemia, breast and lung cancer, melanoma, and gastrointestinal cancers are the most common sources of metastases. Leptomeningeal seeding also occurs from primary CNS tumors such as malignant gliomas, ependymoma, and neuroblastomas. The optimal imaging modality to detect leptomeningeal seeding is gadolinium-enhanced MRI, which reveals linear or multifocal nodular enhancing lesions along the surface of the spinal cord or nerve roots. The diagnostic yield can be improved by using higher doses of gadolinium.

Spinal Meningiomas. Most (90%) spinal meningiomas are intradural, but extradural extension also occurs. The tumors displace/compress the spinal cord or nerve roots. MRI signal characteristics can be variable: they often exhibit isointense

signal to the spinal cord on both T1- and T2-weighted images, but T2 hypointensity may also be seen. Similar to intracranial meningiomas, these tumors enhance in an intense homogeneous fashion (Fig. 39.104). In patients with neurofibromatosis type 2, the entire spine should be imaged because multiple meningiomas may be present.

Nerve sheath tumors and embryonal tumors that belong to this group of spinal tumors are described in the online version of this chapter, available at http://www.expertconsult.com.

Intramedullary Tumors. The most common primary spinal cord tumors are astrocytomas and ependymomas, representing 80% to 90% of all primary malignancies. For best structural assessment of intramedullary tumors (primary and metastatic), MR imaging with and without gadolinium should be obtained.

Ependymoma. Ependymomas are more common in males and in about 50% of cases involve the lower spinal cord in the region of the conus medullaris and cauda equina. The myxopapillary type arises from the ependymal remnants of the filum terminale. Ependymomas are usually well demarcated and may exhibit a T1 and T2 hypointense pseudocapsule. This is important from a surgical standpoint, because these tumors may usually be removed with minimal injury to the surrounding cord parenchyma. The involved cord is expanded. On T1-weighted images, ependymomas are usually isointense to the spinal cord or, rarely, hypointense. On T2-weighted images, they are usually hyperintense relative to the spinal cord. The tumor may have a hemorrhagic component as well, in which case the signal characteristic is usually heterogeneous, depending on the stage of the hemorrhage. Ependymomas are often associated with a rostral or caudal cyst, which is hypointense on T1 and hyperintense on T2-weighted images. With gadolinium, intense homogeneous enhancement is seen within the solid portion of the tumor.

Astrocytoma. Astrocytomas occur in both the pediatric and adult populations. Their peak incidence is in the third to fifth decades of life. They have a preference for the thoracic cord segments. Up to three-quarters are low grade. They exhibit T1 hypointensity and appear hyperintense on T2-weighted images. Although the tumor margin is usually poorly defined, subtotal resection is often possible. A cyst or syringomyelic

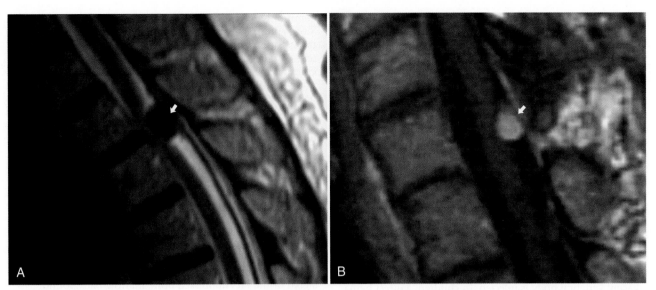

Fig. 39.104 Two cases of meningioma. A, Sagittal T2-weighted image demonstrates a hypointense extramedullary dural-based mass lesion that causes marked spinal cord compression *(arrow)*. **B,** Sagittal T1-weighted postcontrast image reveals an extramedullary dural-based mass lesion in a similar location. The mass enhances homogeneously *(arrow)*.

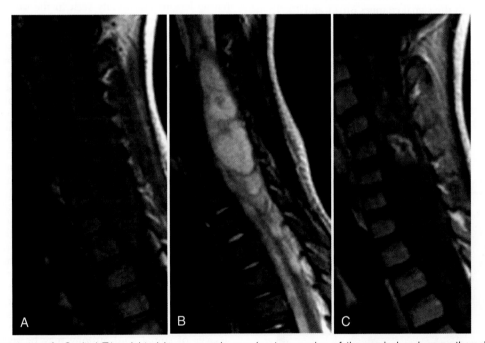

Fig. 39.106 Astrocytoma. A, Sagittal T1-weighted image reveals prominent expansion of the cervical and upper thoracic cord due to a T1-hypointense intramedullary tumor. **B,** Sagittal T2-weighted image demonstrates the hyperintense mass. **C,** Sagittal T1-weighted postcontrast image reveals a patchy heterogeneous pattern of enhancement.

cavity is associated with spinal cord astrocytoma in up to 50% of cases. Contrary to intracranial low-grade gliomas, spinal astrocytomas typically enhance, often in a heterogeneous fashion (Fig. 39.106).

Intramedullary Metastases. Lung and breast cancer are the most common sources of intramedullary metastases, but lymphoma, colorectal cancer, and renal cell cancer may also metastasize to the cord. Metastases have some preference for the conus medullaris but may be multiple in 10% of cases and involve other cord segments as well. Their signal intensity varies; mucus-containing breast or colon cancer metastases can be hyperintense on noncontrast T1-weighted images. On postcontrast images, intense enhancement is seen, which may be homogeneous or ringlike. Associated edema is frequently seen as surrounding T1 hypointensity and T2 hyperintensity. The cord may be expanded to variable degrees.

Vascular Disease

This section is available online at http://www.expertconsult.com. Please also refer to Chapter 69.

Infection

Infections of the spine may involve the disk spaces as well as the vertebral bodies. Neurological emergency occurs when the infection proceeds to the epidural space, leading to abscess formation that can result in spinal cord compression.

Discitis and Osteomyelitis. The most common pathogen responsible for discitis and osteomyelitis is *Staphylococcus aureus*. The most common route of transmission is hematogenous, and in these cases the lumbar spine is involved most frequently, usually at the L3/4 or L4/5 levels. Contiguous spread of infection may also occur, and postoperative causes (such as after instrumentation) have been documented as well. In adults the discitis/osteomyelitis complex generally begins with infection of the subchondral bone marrow inferior to the cartilage endplate. Infection of the subchondral region of a vertebral body results in subsequent perforation of the vertebral endplate, leading to infection of the intervertebral disc, or discitis. The infected disk decreases in height and in conjunction with spread of infection through the disk, the adjacent vertebral body is infected. In children, a direct hematogenous route to the disk can cause discitis to occur before the development of osteomyelitis. Discitis and osteomyelitis are typically hypointense relative to normal disks and vertebrae on T1-weighted images and hyperintense on T2-weighted images, indicating edema. On STIR, markedly hyperintense signal correlates with the signal changes on T1 and T2. There is destruction of the endplates and, therefore, the endplate/disk margin is poorly seen. With gadolinium, there is enhancement of the infected marrow and irregular peripheral enhancement at the periphery of the involved disk (Fig. 39.108). Pathological fractures of the infected vertebrae may also be seen.

Epidural Abscess, Paravertebral Phlegmon. The pathologies of epidural abscess and paravertebral phlegmon are most commonly seen as complications of discitis and osteomyelitis. Since epidural abscess and resultant spinal cord compression represent a neurological emergency, besides the affected vertebral bodies and disks, it is important to always evaluate the epidural space for abscess and the paraspinal tissues for phlegmon (purulent inflammation and diffuse infiltration of soft or connective tissue) if discitis and/or osteomyelitis are seen. Epidural abscess may be missed on conventional T1- and T2-weighted images because its signal characteristics may blend in with its surroundings. The central portion of the abscess may exhibit hyperintensity similar to CSF on T2-weighted images while exhibiting iso- to hypointense signal relative to the spinal cord on T1-weighted images. With gadolinium administration, however, intense enhancement is noted (Fig. 39.109). Just as may occur with compression due to epidural tumors, the compressed spinal cord segment may exhibit T2 hyperintense signal alteration. Phlegmon in the paravertebral tissues also enhances peripherally with gadolinium. This paravertebral infectious process is also well seen on STIR sequences as hyperintensity against the hypointense signal of the fat-suppressed bone marrow background.

Noninfectious Inflammatory Disorders

Multiple Sclerosis. Multiple sclerosis (see Chapter 80) commonly affects the spinal cord. Simultaneous cerebral demyelinating lesions are usually seen in the same patient but less frequently in cases of Devic disease (neuromyelitis optica), which is associated with anti-aquoporin-4 antibodies (Matsushita et al., 2010). On MRI studies of the spinal cord in MS patients, the cervical segments are most commonly involved (Fig. 39.110). The lesions are hyperintense on T2-weighted images and are seen even more conspicuously on sagittal STIR sequences. The lower signal-to-noise ratio of STIR makes this sequence less specific than T2-weighted images for cord lesions, but it is more sensitive. STIR is generally useful only in the sagittal plane, and findings on this sequence should always be correlated with T2 images. Lesional signal changes with either technique are patchy and segmental, often discretely overlapping with the dorsal, anterior, or lateral columns of the spinal cord. The lateral and dorsal columns are affected most frequently. The signal changes are usually in the peripheral regions of the cord, but individual lesions may intersect with the central cord gray matter as well. In MS, the lesions typically do not span more than two vertebral lengths rostrocaudally and tend to involve less than half of the cross-section of the cord. Following administration of gadolinium, active cord lesions may exhibit homogeneous or open-ring enhancement. Large active MS lesions may cause swelling, with local expansion of the cord. In patients with a severe clinical picture or a long-standing history of MS, varying degrees of spinal cord atrophy may be seen. In less severe cases, volumetric analysis may reveal atrophy not detectable by visual inspection.

Acute Disseminated Encephalomyelitis. The widespread demyelinating lesions in this condition commonly involve the spinal cord as well. Diffuse or multifocal T2 hyperintense signal changes with variable degrees of cord swelling may be seen (Fig. 39.111). There is a variable amount of enhancement after gadolinium administration.

Transverse Myelitis. Transverse myelitis is an inflammatory disorder of the spinal cord that involves the gray as well as the white matter. The inflammation involves one or more (typically 3 to 4) cord segments and usually more than two-thirds of the cross-sectional area of the cord (Fig. 39.112). Transverse myelitis etiologies include viral infection, postviral or post-vaccine autoimmune reactions, vasculitis, mycoplasma

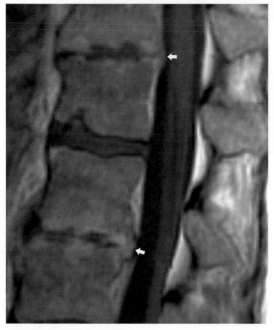

Fig. 39.108 Discitis and osteomyelitis. Two levels are involved *(arrows)*. Sagittal T1-weighted postcontrast image demonstrates decreased disk height and destruction of the adjacent endplates. With gadolinium, there is irregular enhancement of the infected marrow.

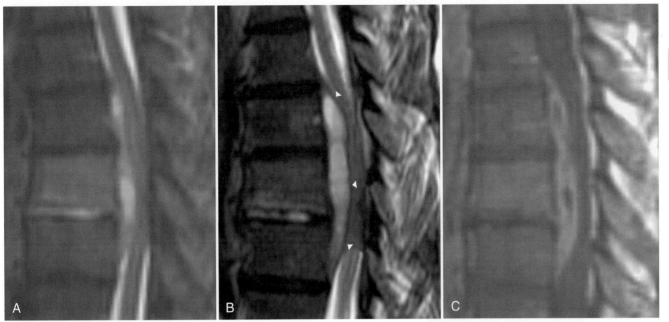

Fig. 39.109 Discitis, osteomyelitis, and epidural abscess. A, Sagittal fat-suppressed image reveals hyperintense signal in the involved disk and hyperintense edema in the vertebral body marrow. Note associated hyperintense epidural collection that displaces the spinal cord. **B,** Sagittal T2-weighted image reveals the discitis and involvement of the inferior endplate of the vertebral body above. The epidural abscess is hyperintense, and the hypointense contour of the dura is well seen *(arrowheads)*. **C,** Sagittal T1-weighted postcontrast image demonstrates intense enhancement of the abscess.

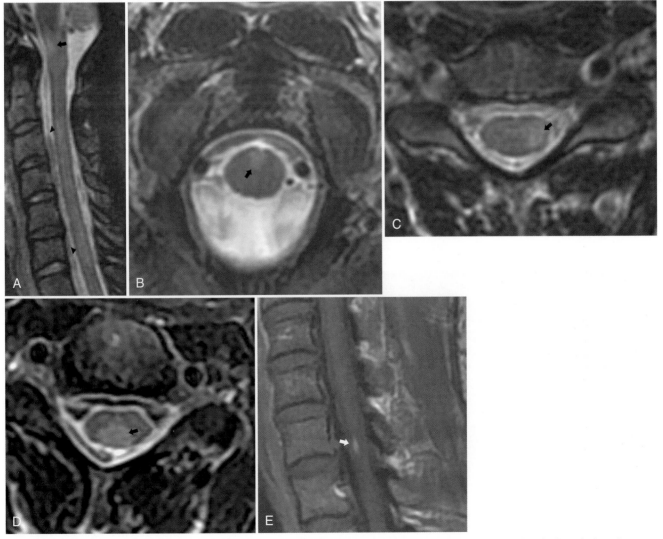

Fig. 39.110 Multiple sclerosis. A, Sagittal fat-suppressed image reveals multiple hyperintense demyelinating lesions in the spinal cord parenchyma *(arrowheads)*, including at the cervicomedullary junction *(arrow)*. On axial T2-weighted images, hyperintense demyelinating lesions are seen in the **(B)** anterior, **(C)** lateral, and **(D)** posterior columns of the cord *(arrows)*. **E,** Sagittal T1-weighted postcontrast image reveals an enhancing lesion in the cord parenchyma *(arrow)*.

infection, syphilis, antiparasitic and antifungal drugs, and even intravenous heroin use (Sahni et al., 2008). The imaging modality of choice is MRI. Acutely, there is T2 hyperintense signal change and cord swelling. In more severe cases, hemorrhage and necrosis may also occur. Following gadolinium administration, diffuse or multifocal patchy enhancement is seen. In the subacute and chronic stages, the swelling and enhancement subside, and the T2 hyperintense signal decreases in extent. In the chronic stage, there may be a variable amount of faint residual T2 hyperintensity. In more severe cases, focal cord atrophy or myelomalacia may be seen.

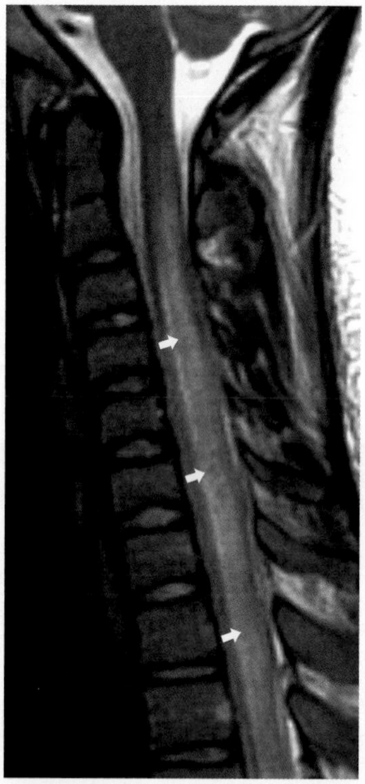

Spinal sarcoidosis and vacuolar myelopathy are described online at http://www.expertconsult.com.

Trauma

Traumatic lesions to the spine are discussed online, available at http://www.expertconsult.com.

Metabolic and Hereditary Myelopathies

Here we group metabolic disorders that potentially cause myelopathy, as well as hereditary and degenerative diseases that result in myelopathy by progressive loss of spinal neurons and/or degeneration of spinal cord pathways. Some of the pathologies result in characteristic signal alterations of the spinal cord, such as that seen in subacute combined degeneration due to vitamin B_{12} deficiency. Others (most degenerative diseases) do not alter the signal characteristics but cause cord atrophy, with or without atrophy of other CNS structures.

The most common entities belonging to this group of myelopathies (subacute combined degeneration, adrenomyeloneuropathy, spinocerebellar ataxias, Friedreich ataxia, amyotrophic lateral sclerosis, and hereditary spastic paraplegia) are discussed online at http://www.expertconsult.com.

Metabolic and Hereditary Myelopathies

Degenerative Spine Disease

Degenerative changes are very commonly seen on neuroimaging studies of the spine. These changes may involve the intervertebral discs, the vertebral bodies, and the posterior elements (facet joints, ligamentum flavum) in various combinations.

Degenerative Disk Disease. In young people, the intervertebral disks have a fluid-rich center (nucleus pulposus) that appears hyperintense on T2-weighted images (Fig. 39.122). With aging, the nucleus pulposus loses water, becoming progressively more hypointense, and the disk flattens. This

Fig. 39.111 Acute disseminated encephalomyelitis (ADEM). Sagittal T2-weighted image shows a diffuse hyperintense lesion spanning the length of the cervical cord *(arrows)*. Note the enlarged caliber of the cord, which is due to swelling.

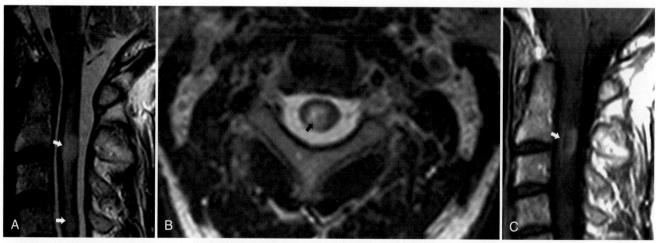

Fig. 39.112 Transverse myelitis. A, Sagittal T2-weighted image demonstrates a longitudinal hyperintense spinal cord lesion spanning three vertebral segments *(arrows)*. **B,** On an axial T2-weighted image, the lesion involves more than two-thirds of the cord's cross-sectional area *(arrow)*. **C,** Sagittal T1-weighted postcontrast image shows an enhancing area within the lesion *(arrow)*.

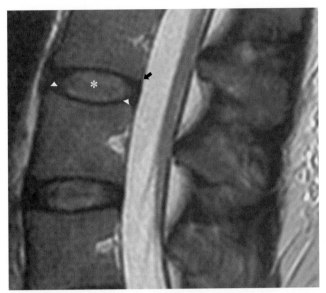

Fig. 39.122 Normal intervertebral disks. Sagittal T2-weighted image demonstrates normal disk height. Note the T2 hyperintense nucleus pulposus (*) and the hypointense annulus fibrosus *(arrowheads)*. The disk does not extend beyond the borders of the vertebral body *(arrow)*.

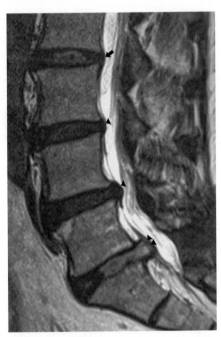

Fig. 39.123 Disk bulge, protrusion, and herniation. Sagittal T2-weighted image demonstrates examples for all stages of disk pathology. Going from rostral to caudal, a disk bulge *(arrow)*, a small and more prominent protrusion *(arrowheads)*, and a herniation *(double arrowhead)* are seen.

phenomenon is no longer considered to be abnormal but an age-related involutional change. However, the often concurrent weakening of the annulus fibrosus raises the chance of annular tear and resultant disk abnormalities.

The nomenclature of disk abnormalities (Fardon and Milette, 2001) is complex (Fig. 39.123). A *disk bulge* is symmetrical presence of disk tissue "circumferentially" (50% to 100%) beyond the edges of the ring apophyses. On sagittal

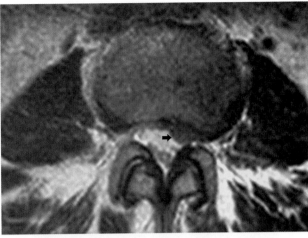

Fig. 39.124 Disk protrusion. Axial T2-weighted image shows a left paracentral disk protrusion *(arrow)* that indents the thecal sac and narrows the left lateral recess.

views, disk bulges have a "flat-tire" appearance. Disk bulges are not categorized as herniations and in the majority of cases do not have any clinical significance.

The term *disk protrusion* refers to extension of a disk past the borders of the vertebral body. A disk protrusion (1) is not classifiable as a bulge, and (2) any one distance between the edges of the disk material beyond the disk space is *less than* the distance between the edges of the base when measured in the same plane. We distinguish between focal and broad-based disk protrusions depending on whether the base of protrusion is less or more than 25% of the entire disk circumference. Disk protrusions may or may not be clinically significant. Whether they affect the neural structures depends on multiple factors. In a congenitally narrow spinal canal, even a small disk protrusion may result in spinal cord or cauda equina compression. In a normal spinal canal, a central disk protrusion may not do anything other than indent the thecal sac. A protrusion of the same size, however, may cause nerve root compression when situated in the lateral recess (Fig. 39.124) or neural foramen (paracentral or lateral disk protrusion).

Disk extrusion refers to a herniation in which any one distance between the edges of the disk material beyond the disk space is *greater than* the distance between the edges of the base measured in the same plane. It occurs when the inner content of the disk, the nucleus pulposus, herniates through a tear of the outer annulus fibrosus. If the extruded disk material loses its continuity with the disk of origin, it is referred to as a *sequestrated* or *free fragment*. Sometimes it is difficult to determine whether continuity exists or not. The term *migration* is used when there is displacement of disk material away from the site of extrusion, regardless of whether it is sequestrated or not, so it may be applied to displaced disk material irrespective of its continuity with the disk of origin (Fig. 39.125). On T2-weighted images, an annular tear may be appreciated as a dotlike or linear hyperintensity against the hypointense background of the annulus fibrosus. This is sometimes also referred to as a *high intensity zone* (HIZ).

Disk herniation frequently reaches considerable size and clinical significance owing to compression of the exiting/descending nerve roots of the spinal cord (Fig. 39.126). Disk protrusions and extrusions/herniations may compromise the spaces to various degrees. As a general guide, spinal canal or neural foraminal stenosis of less than one-third of their original diameter is mild; between one- and two-thirds is

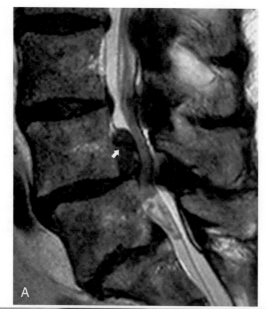

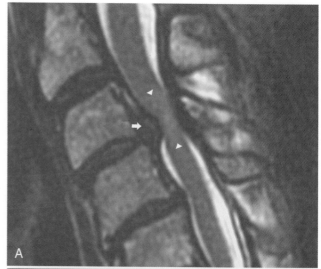

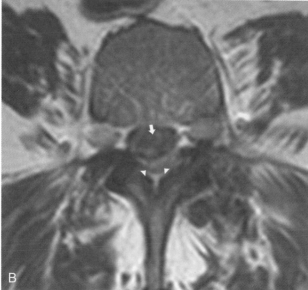

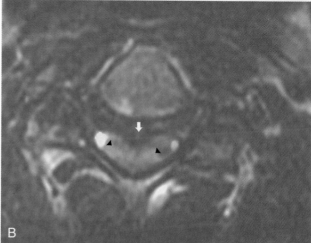

Fig. 39.125 Disk migration. A, Sagittal T2-weighted image shows disk material that did not stay at the level of the disk of origin but migrated cranially *(arrow).* **B,** Axial T2-weighted image demonstrates the migrated disk material *(arrow)* and the compressed thecal sac *(arrowheads).*

Fig. 39.126 Disk herniation, spinal cord compression. A, Sagittal T2-weighted image demonstrates a disk herniation at the C3–C4 level that compresses the cervical spinal cord *(arrow).* Note the hyperintense signal abnormality in the compressed cord parenchyma *(arrowheads).* **B,** Axial T2-weighted image shows the herniation, which has a central component *(arrow).* The hyperintense signal change in the cord is also well seen *(arrowheads).*

moderate; and stenosis involving more than two-thirds of the original caliber is considered severe.

Disk abnormalities are most common in the lumbar spine, particularly at the L4/5 and L5/S1 levels, and second most common at the cervical levels C5/6 and C6/7. These regions represent the more mobile parts of the spinal column.

Degenerative Changes of the Vertebral Bodies. The bone marrow of the vertebral bodies undergoes characteristic changes with age that are well demonstrated by MRI. In younger people, it is largely red marrow composed of hemopoietic tissue. In this age group, the only area of fatty conversion, appearing as a linear T1 hyperintensity, is at the center of the vertebral body around the basivertebral vein. In people older than 40 years, additional foci of fatty marrow changes appear T1 hyperintense in other regions of the vertebral body.

The size and extent of these fatty deposits increases with advancing age.

In degenerative disk disease, characteristic degenerative changes often occur in the adjacent vertebral body endplates as well, seen as linear areas of signal change in these regions (Fig. 39.127). The process of degenerative endplate changes has been thought to occur in stages which have their characteristic MRI signal change patterns. These patterns were traditionally referred to as *Modic type 1, 2,* and *3 endplate changes* (for review see Rahme and Moussa, 2008). This nomenclature has been largely abandoned. The most common change, formerly Modic type 2, is a linear hyperintensity in the endplate region of variable width on T1- as well as T2-weighted images, with corresponding hypointense signal loss on STIR sequences. These changes have been attributed to degenerative fat deposition in these regions.

Besides signal changes, vertebral bodies may also undergo morphological changes. In cases of disk protrusion or extrusion, the bone of the vertebral body may grow along the disk and form osteophytes or spurs. These may contribute to the

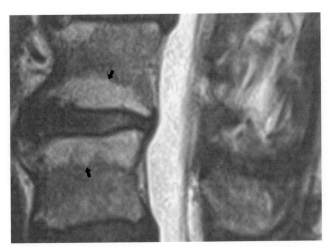

Fig. 39.127 Degenerative endplate change. Sagittal T2-weighted image reveals hyperintense bands of signal change parallel with the disk space in the endplate region of the adjacent vertebral bodies *(arrows)*.

narrowing of spaces and compromise of the neural elements. Large osteophytes may fuse across vertebral bodies, forming spondylotic bars.

Degenerative Changes of the Posterior Elements. Facet joint arthropathy and ligamentum flavum hypertrophy are common findings in degenerative disease of the spine. In facet arthropathy, the synovial surface of the joint becomes poorly defined, and hyperintense synovial fluid may accumulate. The joint becomes hypertrophied. Sometimes the synovial fluid accumulation results in outpouching of the synovium, which emerges from the joint, forming a synovial cyst. When prominent enough, this cyst may compromise the diameter of the spinal canal and (rarely) compress the neural elements (Fig. 39.128). Hypertrophy of the T2 hypointense ligamentum flavum is also frequent and may contribute to compromise of the spaces and neural elements.

Spondylolysis, Spondylolisthesis. Spondylolysis and spondylolisthesis are pathologic changes that often occur together and are most common in the lumbar spine. *Spondylolysis* refers to a defect in the pars interarticularis of the vertebral arch resulting in separation of the articular processes from the vertebral body. A traumatic etiology is common, but it may happen in the setting of advanced degenerative disease as well. A common cause is stress microfractures resulting from episodes of axial loading force on the erect spine, such as when landing after a jump, diving, weight lifting, or due to rotational forces. This abnormality can be visualized with CT or MRI. On sagittal views, the pars defect is well seen; on axial images, the spinal canal may appear slightly elongated at the level of the spondylolysis.

Spondylolisthesis is shifting of one vertebral body relative to its neighbor, either anteriorly (anterolisthesis) or posteriorly (retrolisthesis). It is often associated with spondylolysis (Fig. 39.129). Four grades of spondylolisthesis are distinguished, depending on the degree of shifting. *Grade I spondylolisthesis* refers to shifting over less than one-fourth of a vertebral body's anteroposterior diameter; grade II is shifting over one-fourth to one-half the diameter; grade III is up to three-fourths; and the most severe, grade IV, is shifting over the full vertebral body diameter.

Isolated spondylolysis results in elongation of the spinal canal, whereas spondylolisthesis causes segmental spinal

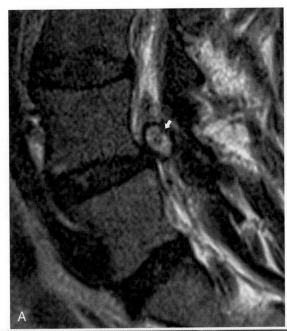

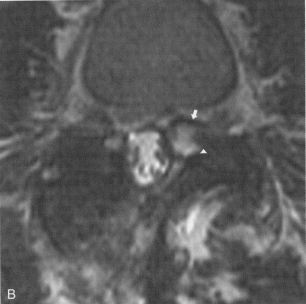

Fig. 39.128 Synovial cyst. A, Sagittal T2-weighted image demonstrates a hyperintense cyst with hypointense rim in the spinal canal *(arrow)*. **B,** Axial T2-weighted image reveals that this cyst *(arrow)* arises from the left facet joint *(arrowhead)*, consistent with a synovial cyst. It narrows the left lateral recess and neural foramen.

canal narrowing, the extent of which depends on the degree of listhesis. In severe cases, there is compression of the spinal cord or cauda equina, and the changes also frequently cause narrowing of the neural foramina and compromise of the exiting nerve roots at the involved level.

INDICATIONS FOR COMPUTED TOMOGRAPHY OR MAGNETIC RESONANCE IMAGING

Structural neuroimaging studies are probably the most commonly ordered diagnostic tests in both inpatient and outpatient neurological practice. Imaging greatly helps with the

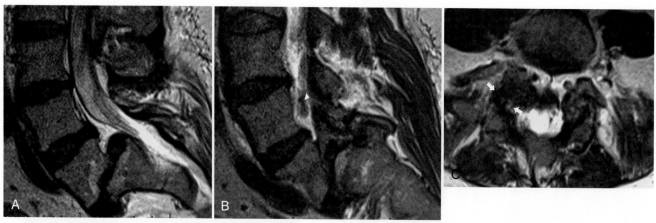

Fig. 39.129 Spondylolysis, grade 2 anterolisthesis. A, Sagittal T2-weighted image demonstrates grade 2 anterolisthesis of the L5 vertebral body on S1. **B,** Sagittal T2-weighted image reveals separation of the L4/L5 facet joint *(arrowhead)* and forward displacement of the L5 articular process *(arrow)*. **C,** Axial T2-weighted image also reveals the spondylolysis *(arrows)*.

diagnosis of various neurological diseases and does so in a relatively quick and noninvasive way. This section (available online at http://www.expertconsult.com) summarizes the most common indications for obtaining a neuroimaging study in clinical neurological practice. Selection of the imaging study should be guided by the patient's history and objective findings on neurological examination, as opposed to shooting in the dark and obtaining "all-inclusive" imaging studies of the entire neuraxis. The availability and cost of the various techniques should also be factored into the decision of what tests to obtain in a given clinical situation.

Neuroimaging in Various Clinical Situations

This section, including a summary (eTable 39.3) on selection of imaging modalities in various clinical situations, based on the current American College of Radiology (ACR) Appropriateness Criteria, is available online at http://www.expertconsult.com.

REFERENCES

The complete reference list is available online at https://expertconsult .inkling.com/.

40 Vascular Imaging: Computed Tomographic Angiography, Magnetic Resonance Angiography, and Ultrasound

Peter Adamczyk, David S. Liebeskind

CHAPTER OUTLINE

COMPUTED TOMOGRAPHIC ANGIOGRAPHY
Methods
Limitations
Applications

MAGNETIC RESONANCE ANGIOGRAPHY
Methods
Limitations
Applications

ULTRASOUND
Methods
Techniques
Applications

COMPUTED TOMOGRAPHIC ANGIOGRAPHY

Computed tomographic angiography (CTA) is a relatively rapid, thin-section, volumetric, spiral (helical) CT technique performed with a time-optimized bolus of contrast medium to enhance visualization of the cerebral circulation. This approach may be tailored to illustrate various segments of the circulation from arterial segments to the venous system. The ongoing development of multidetector CT scanners has advanced CTA, with increasing numbers of detectors used in recent years to further improve image acquisition and visualization.

Methods

Helical CT scanner technology, providing uninterrupted volume data acquisition, can rapidly image the entire cerebral circulation from the neck to vertex of the head within minutes. Typical CT parameters use a slice (collimated) thickness of 1 to 3 mm with a pitch of 1 to 2, which represents the ratio of the table speed per rotation and the total collimation. Data are acquired as a bolus of iodinated contrast medium traverses the vessels of interest. For CTA of the carotid and vertebral arteries in the neck, the helical volume extends from the aortic arch to the skull base. Typical acquisition parameters are 7.5 images per rotation of the X-ray tube, 2.5-mm slice thickness, and a reconstruction interval (distance between the centers of two consecutively reconstructed images) of 1.25 mm. For CTA of the circle of Willis and proximal cerebral arteries, the data acquisition extends from the skull base to the vertex of the head. Typical acquisition parameters for this higher spatial resolution scan are 3.75 images per rotation, 1.25-mm slice thickness, and an interval of 0.5 mm. A volume of contrast ranging from 100 to 150 mL is injected into a peripheral vein

at a rate of 2 to 3 mL/sec and followed by a saline flush of 20 to 50 mL. Adequate enhancement of the arteries in the neck or head is obtained approximately 15 to 20 seconds after injection of the contrast, although this may vary somewhat in each case. Image acquisition uses automated detection of bolus arrival and subsequent triggering of data acquisition. The resulting axial source images are typically post-processed for two-dimensional (2D) and three-dimensional (3D) visualization using one or more of several available techniques including multiplanar reformatting, thin-slab maximum-intensity projection (MIP), and 3D volume rendering. More recent CT with 320 detector rows enables dynamic scanning, providing both high spatial and temporal resolution of the entire cerebrovasculature (4D CTA). The cervical vessels are imaged by acquisition of an additional spiral CT scan analogous to 64-detector row CT. An increasing spectrum of clinical applications utilizing this advanced technique remains under investigation (Diekmann et al., 2010).

Limitations

Contrast-Induced Nephropathy

Careful consideration must be made for performing contrast-enhanced CT studies in patients with renal impairment. Exposure to all contrast agents may result in acute renal failure, called *contrast-induced nephropathy* (CIN), which is typically reversible but may potentially result in adverse outcomes. The incidence of renal injury appears to be associated with increased osmolality of contrast agents, which have been steadily declining with the newer generations of nonionic agents. Patients with a creatinine level above 1.5 gm/dL or estimated glomerular filtration rate below 60 mL/min/1.73 m^2 remain at a higher risk for developing CIN. Treatment for this condition relies on prevention of this disorder, and agents such as *N*-acetylcysteine and intravenous (IV) saline and/or sodium bicarbonate may reduce the incidence of CIN. Avoidance of volume depletion and discontinuation of potential nephrotoxic agents such as nonsteroidal anti-inflammatory drugs or metformin is recommended for patients prior to the procedure. Patients on hemodialysis are recommended to undergo dialysis as soon as possible afterwards to reduce contrast exposure (Asif and Epstein, 2004; Kim et al., 2010).

Metal Artifacts

Metallic implants such as clips, coils, and stents are generally safe for CT imaging, but it should be noted that they may lead to severe streaking artifacts, limiting evaluation. These artifacts occur because the density of the metal is beyond the normal range of the processing software, resulting in incomplete attenuation profiles. Several processing methods for reducing the artifact signal are available, and operator-dependent techniques such as gantry angulation adjustments and use of thin sections to reduce partial volume artifacts may help decrease

459

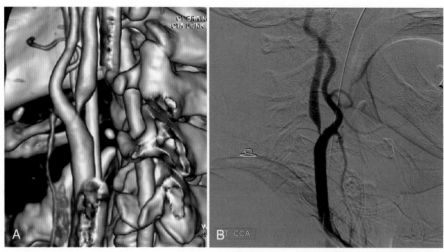

Fig. 40.1 Computed tomographic angiography (CTA) compared to digital subtraction angiography (DSA) in a patient with proximal internal carotid artery (ICA) stenosis. **A,** Three-dimensional reconstructed CTA image of left ICA reveals severe stenosis distal to the ICA bifurcation. **B,** DSA confirms severe stenosis seen on CTA due to an atherosclerotic plaque.

this signal distortion. Generally, knowledge of the composition of metallic implants may help in determining the potential severity of artifacts on CT. Cobalt aneurysm clips produce much more artifact than titanium clips. For patients with stents, careful consideration must be made in evaluating stenosis, as these implants may lead to artificial lumen narrowing on CTA. The degree of artificial lumen narrowing decreases with increasing stent diameter. Lettau et al. evaluated patients with various types of stents and found that CTA may be superior to magnetic resonance angiography (MRA) at 1.5T for stainless steel and cobalt alloy carotid stents, whereas MRA at 3T may be superior for nitinol carotid stents (Lettau et al., 2009; van der Schaaf et al., 2006). Data remain limited for patients undergoing intracranial stent placement but, compared with digital subtraction angiography (DSA), inter-reader agreement for the presence of in-stent stenosis is noted to be inferior (Goshani et al., 2012).

Applications

Extracranial Circulation

Carotid Artery Stenosis. In evaluating occlusive disease of the extracranial carotid artery, CTA complements DSA and serves as an alternative to MRA (Fig. 40.1). In the grading of carotid stenosis using the North American Symptomatic Carotid Endarterectomy Trial (NASCET) criteria, Randoux and colleagues (2001) found that the rate of agreement between 3D CTA and DSA was 95%. In addition, CTA was significantly correlated with DSA in depicting the length of the stenotic segment. In reference to DSA, multiple studies have demonstrated a sensitivity of 77%–100% and a specificity of 95%–100% for CTA in detecting severe (70%–99%) stenosis (Binaghi et al., 2001; Magarelli et al., 1998). Data for moderate (50%–69%) stenoses remain less reliable (Wardlaw et al., 2006). For detection of a complete occlusion, the sensitivity and specificity has been found to be 97% and 99%, respectively (Koelemay et al., 2004). Saba et al. (2007) evaluated the use of multidetector CTA and carotid ultrasound in comparison to surgical observation for evaluating ulceration, which is a severe complication of carotid plaques. CTA was found to be superior, with 93.75% sensitivity and 98.59% specificity compared to carotid ultrasound, which demonstrated 37.5% sensitivity and 91.5% specificity. Furthermore, another study found that plaque ulceration on CTA had a high sensitivity

(80.0%–91.4%) and specificity (92.3%–93.0%) for the prediction of intraplaque hemorrhage, an important marker of atherosclerotic disease progression, as defined on magnetic resonance imaging (MRI) (U-King-Im et al., 2010).

Fibromuscular dysplasia (FMD), which often involves a unique pattern of stenoses in the cervical vessels, may be detected by CTA, although no large studies have evaluated the sensitivity and specificity for detection. This disorder, which characteristically demonstrates a string-of-beads pattern of vascular irregularity on angiography, has been reliably demonstrated on carotid artery evaluations from case reports. This may potentially reduce the need for more invasive angiographic imaging in the future, although further studies in this area are required (de Monye et al., 2007).

Currently, either CTA or MRA is used to evaluate suspected carotid occlusive disease, with the choice of method determined by clinical conditions (e.g., pacemaker), accessibility of CT and MR scanners, and additional imaging capabilities (CT or MR perfusion brain imaging).

Carotid and Vertebral Dissection. Dissections of the cervicocephalic arteries, including the carotid and vertebral arteries, account for up to 20% of ischemic strokes in young adults (Leys et al., 1995). CTA findings include demonstration of a narrowed eccentric arterial lumen in the presence of a thickened vessel wall, with occasional detection of a dissecting aneurysm. In subacute and chronic dissection, CTA has been shown to detect a reduction in the thickness of the arterial wall, recanalization of the arterial lumen, and reduction in size or resolution of dissecting aneurysm. Compared with DSA, CTA of the anterior and posterior circulations has been found to have a sensitivity of 51%–100% and a specificity of 67%–100% (Provenzale et al., 2009; Pugliese et al., 2007). CTA is likely superior to MRI in evaluating aneurysms of the distal cervical internal carotid artery (ICA), a common site of dissection, because MRI findings are often complicated by the presence of flow-related artifacts (Elijovich et al., 2006). Furthermore, it has been suggested that CTA may better delineate the features of cervical vertebral artery dissections (Vertinsky et al., 2008). CTA depiction of dissections at the level of the skull base may be complicated in some cases because of beam hardening and other artifacts that obscure dissection findings, including similarities in the densities of the temporal and sphenoid bones with the dissected vessel.

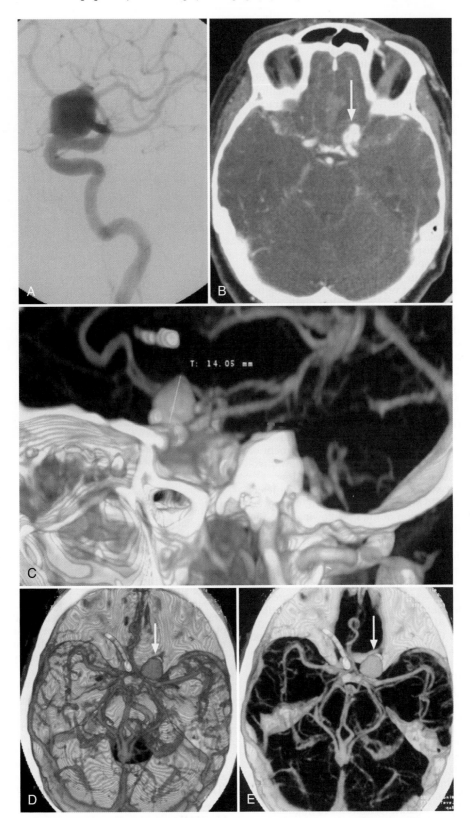

Fig. 40.7 Left internal carotid artery (ICA) aneurysm. Comparison of computed tomographic angiography (CTA) postprocessed images with catheter angiography. **A,** Catheter angiography lateral view, following left ICA injection, shows aneurysm originating from supraclinoid portion of ICA. **B,** CTA axial source image reveals lobulated aneurysm *(arrow)*. **C–E,** CTA three-dimensional (3D) volume-rendered images with transparency feature for user-selected tissue regions (called *4D angiography*). **C,** Lateral view from left side of patient demonstrates relationship of the aneurysm, measuring 14 mm from neck to dome, to the anterior clinoid process. **D,** View of aneurysm *(arrow)*, skull base, and circle of Willis from above. **E,** Same view as **D** but edited to remove most of skull base densities and improve visibility of vessels.

because flowing blood spends more time in the slab than that in a 2D TOF section, a vessel passing through the slab may lose its vascular contrast upon exiting the slab.

In TOF-MRA, stationary material with high signal intensity, such as subacute thrombus, can mimic blood flow. PC-MRA is useful in this situation because the high signal from stationary tissue is eliminated when the two data sets are subtracted to produce the final flow-sensitive images. This technique provides additional information that allows for delineation of flow volumes and direction of flow in various structures from proximal arteries to the dural venous sinuses. In the 2D phase-contrast technique, flow-encoding gradients are applied along two or three axes. A projection image displaying the vessel against a featureless background is produced. Compared with the 2D techniques, 3D PC-MRA provides higher spatial resolution and information on flow directionality along each of three flow-encoding axes. The summed information from all three flow directions is displayed as a speed image, in which the signal intensity is proportional to the magnitude of the flow velocity. The data set in TOF-MRA or PC-MRA may be used to visualize the course of vessels in 3D by mapping the hyperintense signal from the vessel-containing pixels onto a desired viewing plane using a MIP algorithm, producing a projection image. MIP images are generated in several viewing planes and then evaluated together to view the vessel architecture. A presaturation band is applied and represents a zone in which both flowing and stationary nuclei are saturated by a radiofrequency pulse that is added to the gradient recalled echo (GRE) pulse sequence. The downstream signal of a vessel that passes through the presaturation zone is suppressed because of the saturation of the flowing nuclei. Presaturation bands may be fixed or may travel, keeping the same distance from each slab as it is acquired. In general, the placement of presaturation bands can be chosen so as to identify flow directionality and help distinguish arterial from venous flow.

Contrast-enhanced MRA (CE-MRA) uses scan parameters that are typical of 3D TOF-MRA but uses gadolinium to overcome the problem of saturation of the slow-flowing blood in structures that lie within the 3D slab (Fig. 40.8). The scan time per 3D volume is in the order of 5 to 10 minutes, and data are acquired in the first 10 to 15 minutes after the bolus infusion of a gadolinium contrast agent (0.1–0.2 mmol/kg). Presaturation bands usually are ineffective at suppressing the downstream signal from vessels when gadolinium is present. In 3D CE-MRA (called *fast, dynamic,* or *time-resolved CE-MRA*), the total scan time per 3D volume (usually about 30–50 partitions) is reduced to 5 to 50 seconds (Fain et al., 2001; Turski et al., 2001). Data are acquired as the bolus of the gadolinium contrast agent (0.2–0.3 mmol/kg and 2–3 mL/sec infusion rate) passes through the vessels of interest, taking advantage of the marked increase in intravascular signal (first-pass method). Vessel signal is determined primarily by concentration of injected contrast, analogous to conventional angiography. Because 3D CE-MRA entails more rapid data acquisition, and hence higher temporal resolution, than TOF-MRA, spatial resolution may be reduced. The most common approaches to synchronizing the 3D data acquisition with the arrival of the gadolinium bolus in the arteries are measurement of the bolus arrival time for each patient using a small (2 mL) test dose of contrast followed by a separate synchronized manual 3D acquisition by the scanner operator (Fain et al., 2001). Another method rapidly and repeatedly acquires 3D volumes (<10 sec per volume) in the neck, beginning at the time of contrast bolus injection to ensure that at least one 3D volume showing only arteries will be acquired (Turski et al., 2001). Subtraction of preinjection source images from arterial phase images, termed *digital subtraction MRA,* is sometimes used to increase vessel-to-background contrast.

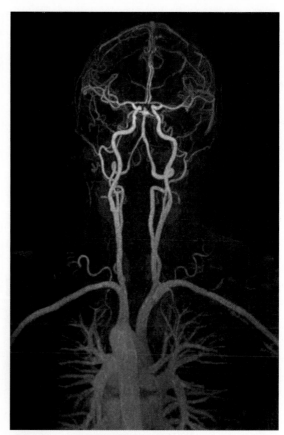

Fig. 40.8 3T contrast-enhanced magnetic resonance angiography (CE-MRA) of the cerebrovascular system.

The advent and increasing availability of MRI scanners with 3.0 tesla (T) or even higher field strengths (up to 7T) in selected centers may also be used to improve MRA by capitalizing on higher signal-to-noise ratios and parallel imaging (Nael et al., 2006). Parallel imaging at 3T or greater can be used to improve spatial resolution, shorten scan time, reduce artifacts, and increase anatomical coverage in first-pass CE-MRA. Recent investigation with 7T TOF-MRA demonstrated that such ultrahigh field strength allows vivid depiction of the large vessels of the circle of Willis with significantly more first- and second-order branches and can even distinguish diseased diminutive vessels in hypertensive patients (Hendrikse et al., 2008a; Kang et al., 2009, 2010). The 4D time-resolved MRA (4D MRA) is a more recent contrast-enhanced vascular imaging method under investigation that uses novel processing techniques to achieve subsecond temporal resolution while maintaining high spatial resolution. Dynamic MRA scans may be obtained up to 60 times faster and with higher spatial resolution at 3T. The resulting images may attain the diagnostic performance of conventional DSA, allowing for better characterization of various vascular lesions (Hope et al., 2010; Parmar et al., 2009; Willinek et al., 2008).

Limitations

Nephrogenic Systemic Fibrosis

Clinicians should be aware that a rare but serious complication of contrast-enhanced MRI studies includes the development of nephrogenic systemic fibrosis (NSF). This condition is characterized by widespread thickening and hardening of the skin, with the potential for rapid systemic progression and immobility over several weeks. Although the precise mechanism remains unclear, NSF was first noted in 1997 and occurs exclusively in patients with renal failure. The majority of reported cases involved exposure to a gadolinium chelate within 2 to 3 months prior to disease onset in dialysis-dependent patients. A large percentage of cases have been specifically associated with gadodiamide (Omniscan), with a possible dose-dependent effect, although it should be noted that cases have been reported with all gadolinium agents. Careful consideration must be made for gadolinium administration in patients with renal impairment (glomerular filtration rate <30 mL/min/1.73 m^2), especially those on dialysis. The risks and benefits should be carefully discussed prior to any contrast-enhanced procedures, and the dose of gadolinium should be minimized. Additionally, for patients on hemodialysis, prophylactic dialysis is generally recommended as soon as possible, ideally within 3 hours after contrast administration (Kuo et al., 2007).

Metal Implant Contraindications

Limitations due to the presence of metallic materials (clips, stents, coils) remain a common concern in patients undergoing vascular imaging. Aneurysm clips made from martensitic stainless steels remain a contraindication for MRI procedures, because excessive magnetic forces may displace these implants and cause serious injury. However, most clips are now made of metals that are nonferromagnetic, and all patients with any metallic implants require screening to determine whether they are safe to undergo an MRI study. For the majority of coils and stents that have been tested, it is unlikely that these implants would become moved or displaced as a result of exposure to MRI systems operating at 1.5T or even 3T. Additionally, it is often unnecessary to wait an extended period of time after a procedure to perform an MRI study in a patient with an implant made of nonferromagnetic material unless there are concerns associated with MRI-related heating. Dental materials including wires and prostheses do not appear to pose a risk, although they may result in artifact on MRI. Artifacts from metal may have varied appearances on MRI related to the type or configuration of the piece of metal. Artifact sizes may increase at 3T compared to 1.5T, depending on the implant type and composition, but these distortions may be substantially reduced by optimizing imaging parameters. Patients who are deemed unsafe for MRI upon screening

may be considered for CT evaluation (Olsrud et al., 2005; Shellock, 2002).

Applications

Extracranial Carotid and Vertebral Circulation

Time-Of-Flight MRA. Internal carotid artery stenosis grading methods used in the landmark NASCET and ECST trials remain the most widely applied and were determined by angiography (European Carotid Surgery Trialists' Collaborative Group, 1998; Ferguson et al., 1999). However, DSA has the drawbacks of being an invasive and costly modality. MRA has become increasingly used as a noninvasive imaging alternative for carotid stenosis as it avoids the radiation and iodinated contrast exposure associated with both DSA and CTA. Furthermore, images are often higher in quality and less operator dependent when compared with ultrasound imaging. Despite these advantages, TOF-MRA remains relatively insensitive to slow flow and may be associated with increased scan times and signal voids, resulting in decreased quality images and overestimation of stenoses. Compared with 2D TOF-MRA, the 3D TOF method is less likely to overestimate the degree of stenosis, particularly if original (Fig. 40.9) or reformatted source images are evaluated rather than the MIP images (Norris and Rothwell, 2001).

In a 2008 meta-analysis of 37 studies, TOF-MRA was noted to have a sensitivity of 91.2% with a specificity of 88.3% for the detection of high-grade (70% to 99%) ICA stenosis. For the detection of ICA occlusions, the sensitivity of TOF-MRA was 94.5% and the specificity was 99.3%. For moderately severe (50% to 69%) stenoses, TOF-MRA had a sensitivity of only 37.9% and a specificity of 92.1% (Debrey et al., 2008). These results were similar to a more recent 2014 study which determined that 3D TOF-MRA had a sensitivity of 91.7% and specificity of 98.5% for high-grade stenoses. For ICA occlusions, 3D TOF-MRA was found to be highly sensitive (100%), with a specificity of 98.7% (Weber et al., 2014). These results suggest that TOF MRA may serve as a useful imaging alternative for the detection of high-grade carotid stenoses.

Atherosclerotic narrowing of the vertebral artery commonly involves the origin or distal intracranial portion. For TOF-MRA evaluation of posterior-circulation cerebrovascular disease, the vertebral origins usually are not evaluated for the same reasons

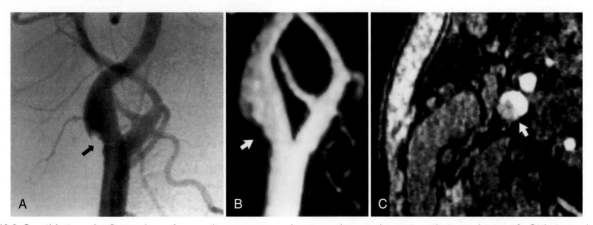

Fig. 40.9 Carotid stenosis. Comparison of magnetic resonance angiogram and source image to catheter angiogram. **A,** Catheter angiogram of the right carotid system shows narrowing *(arrow)* at the origin of the internal carotid artery. Findings suggest intraluminal thrombus. **B,** Three-dimensional (3D) time-of-flight (TOF) angiogram demonstrates similar narrowing *(arrow)*. **C,** Axial 3D TOF source image at the site of stenosis shows clearly that the lumen is narrowed *(arrow)* by approximately 50%. In this case, there is agreement between the narrowing shown on source image and that detected by the maximum-intensity projection image **(B)**.

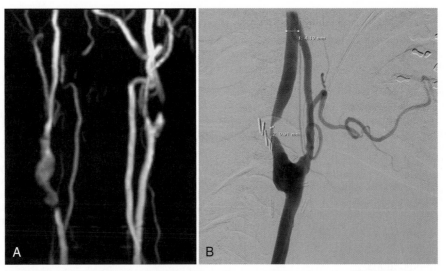

Fig. 40.10 Carotid stenosis. Comparison of contrast-enhanced magnetic resonance angiography (CE-MRA) with conventional catheter angiography. **A,** CE-MRA reveals flow gap in proximal left internal carotid artery (ICA) suggestive of high-grade stenosis. **B,** Digital subtraction angiography (DSA) of the left carotid system confirms greater than 70% stenosis.

the common carotid origins are not evaluated. However, sequential 2D TOF-MRA of the neck is useful in determining whether proximal occlusion is present and in demonstrating flow direction in the vertebral arteries in patients with suspected subclavian steal. A 2D TOF study obtained with no presaturation band shows flow enhancement in both vertebral arteries, whereas a study obtained with a superiorly located walking presaturation band shows flow only in the vertebral artery with normal anterograde flow. While published data remain limited for evaluation of vertebral artery stenosis, a small study investigating 1.5 T TOF-MRA noted a sensitivity of 94% and specificity of 96% for >29% stenosis when compared with DSA. For >49% stenosis, the sensitivity and specificity were similar at 95% and 96%, respectively. In this investigation, 22% of patients had an overestimated degree of stenosis (Sadikin et al., 2007). Although TOF-MRA may be fairly accurate, evaluation for stenosis may be more reliable with CE-MRA.

The evaluation of cervical artery dissection is more commonly performed with MRI in combination with CE-MRA as will be described later. However, TOF-MRA may be a viable alternative for patients who are contraindicated from contrast imaging. Using combined MRI and CE-MRA as a gold standard, a recent paper observed that TOF-MRA had a sensitivity of 93% to 97% and a specificity of 96% to 98% (Coppenrath et al., 2013).

Three-Dimensional Contrast-Enhanced MRA. Compared with 2D and 3D TOF-MRA, 3D CE-MRA delineates carotid arterial stenosis better (Fig. 40.10). Surface morphology (e.g., ulcerated plaque), nearly occluded vessels (e.g., "string sign"), and arterial occlusions are more easily identified (Etesami et al., 2012; Weber et al., 2014). Additional advantages of 3D CE-MRA include greater anatomical coverage (Fig. 40.11) and more accurate identification of intraplaque hemorrhage, a marker for disease progression. When compared with pathology, Qiao et al. (2011) noted that 3T CE-MRA demonstrated a sensitivity of 90% and specificity of 98% for intraplaque hemorrhage evaluation. For high-grade stenosis, which can cause intravascular flow gaps on TOF MIP images, the addition of CE-MRA to the imaging protocol provides sensitivity and specificity equivalent to CTA in determining the severity of stenosis (relative to DSA as the reference standard).

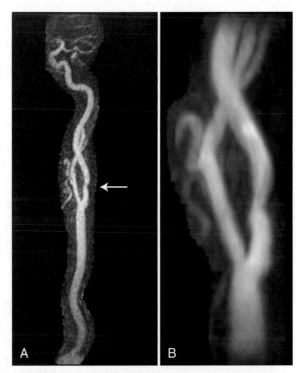

Fig. 40.11 Similar appearance of mild stenosis *(arrow)* of left internal carotid artery on oblique maximum-intensity projection **(MIP) images. A,** Three-dimensional (3D) contrast-enhanced magnetic resonance angiography (CE-MRA). **B,** 3D time-of-flight (TOF) MRA. Note the greater coverage of the carotids afforded by CE-MRA compared with TOF-MRA. *(From Bowen, B.C., 2007. MR angiography versus CT angiography in the evaluation of neurovascular disease. Radiology 245, 357–361.)*

A systematic review of 21 CE-MRA studies found that for the detection of high-grade (≥70%–99%) ICA stenoses, CE-MRA had a sensitivity of 94.6% with a specificity of 91.9%. For the detection of complete ICA occlusions, CE-MRA demonstrated a sensitivity of 99.4% and specificity of 99.6%.

TABLE 41.1 Glossary: PET and SPECT Tracers

Abbreviation	Tracer	Target process/structure
[^{99m}Tc]ECD	[^{99m}Tc]ethylcysteinatedimer	Cerebral blood flow
[^{18}F]FDG	[^{18}F]2-fluoro-2-deoxy-D-glucose	Cerebral glucose metabolism
[^{18}F]FET	[^{18}F]O-(2-fluoroethyl)-L-tyrosine	Amino acid transport
[^{18}F]FLT	[^{18}F]3'-deoxy-3'-fluorothymidine	Proliferation
[^{123}I]FP-CIT	[^{123}I]N-ω-fluoropropyl-2β-carbomethoxy-3β-(4-iodophenyl)nortropane	Dopamine transporter
[^{99m}Tc]HMPAO	[^{99m}Tc]hexamethylpropyleneamine oxime	Cerebral blood flow
[^{123}I]IBZM	[^{123}I]iodobenzamide	Dopamine D2/D3 receptor
[^{123}I]MIBG	[^{123}I]metaiodobenzylguanidine	Cardiac sympathetic innervation
[^{11}C]MET	[^{11}C]methionine	Amino acid transport (protein synthesis)
[^{11}C]PIB	[^{11}C]Pittsburgh compound B	Amyloid-beta plaques

susceptible to partial volume effects if the object or lesion size is below two times the scanner resolution (as a rule of thumb). Today's PET systems are either constructed as hybrid PET/CT or, more recently, PET/MRI systems. Although the clinical utility of the latter still needs to be defined, integrated PET/MRI allows for a comprehensive, synchronous imaging of several morphological, functional, and molecular parameters in a single scanning session. Possible applications are manifold, reaching from cross-validation of imaging techniques and multi-modal neurobiological activation studies, over methodological synergies (e.g., integrated motion and partial volume corrections of PET by MRI) to optimized patient comfort, throughput and diagnostics by one-stop shop multiparametric imaging (e.g., in neurodegeneration, epilepsy, neurooncology, and stroke) (Catana et al., 2012). Time will tell whether integrated PET/MRI can replicate the tremendous success of integrated PET/CT in clinical oncology.

Commonly used radionuclides in neurological PET studies are carbon-11 (^{11}C, half-life = 20.4 minutes), nitrogen-13 (^{13}N, half-life = 10.0 minutes), oxygen-15 (^{15}O, physical half-life = 2.03 minutes), and fluorine-18 (^{18}F, half-life = 109.7 minutes), which are all cyclotron products. Whereas the relatively long half-life of ^{18}F allows shipping ^{18}F-labeled tracers from a cyclotron site to a distant PET site, this is not possible in the case of ^{15}O and ^{11}C. This clearly limits the clinical use of ^{15}O-labeled water, molecular oxygen, and carbon dioxide for quantification of CBF, cerebral metabolic rate of oxygen, and oxygen extraction fraction. This also applies to clinically very interesting ^{11}C-labeled tracers like [^{11}C]raclopride (dopamine D$_2$/D$_3$ receptor), [^{11}C]flumazenil (GABA$_A$ receptor), [^{11}C]methionine (amino acid transport), and [^{11}C]PIB (amyloid-beta). Thus, ^{18}F-labeled substitutes have been proposed and are currently under investigation, including several amyloid-beta ligands recently approved by the FDA.

In this chapter on perfusion and metabolism, we will primarily focus on PET studies using the glucose analog, 2-deoxy-2-(^{18}F)fluoro-d-glucose ([^{18}F]FDG), to assess cerebral glucose metabolism. With the rate of glucose metabolism being closely related to maintenance of ion gradients and transmitter turnover (in particular, glutamate), [^{18}F]FDG represents an ideal tracer for assessment of neuronal function and its changes (Sokoloff, 1977). After uptake in cerebral tissue by specific glucose transporters, [^{18}F]FDG is phosphorylated by hexokinase. Since [^{18}F]FDG-6-P is neither a substrate for transport back out of the cell nor can it be metabolized further, it is virtually irreversible trapped in cells. Therefore, the distribution of [^{18}F]FDG in tissue imaged by PET (started 30–60 minutes after injection to allow for sufficient uptake; 5- to 20-minute scan duration) closely reflects the regional distribution of cerebral glucose metabolism and, thus, neuronal function. By use of appropriate pharmacokinetic models and a plasma input function (i.e., [^{18}F]FDG concentration in arterial or arterialized venous plasma), the absolute cerebral metabolic rate of glucose (CMRglc in μmol/min/100 g tissue) can be estimated. In the case of [^{18}F]FDG, absolute quantification is usually not necessary for routine clinical studies, since the diagnostic information can often be obtained from the cerebral pattern of [^{18}F]FDG uptake or relative estimates of regional glucose metabolism gained by normalizing regional [^{18}F]FDG uptake to the uptake of a suitable reference region unaffected by disease.

Radiolabeled amino acids like [^{11}C]methionine ([^{11}C]MET) and O-(2-[^{18}F]fluoroethyl)-L-tyrosine ([^{18}F]FET) are increasingly used for neurooncological applications (Herholz et al., 2012). Cerebral uptake of these amino acids reflects transport by sodium-independent L-transporters which are driven by concentration gradients and, thus, by intracellular amino acid metabolism and protein synthesis. Although only [^{11}C]MET is actually incorporated into proteins, cerebral uptake of [^{11}C]MET and [^{18}F]FET is commonly used as a surrogate marker of protein synthesis and proliferation. Opposed to [^{18}F]FDG, cerebral uptake of amino acids is very low under normal conditions but greatly increased in neoplastic cells, allowing for an excellent imaging contrast of most brain tumors (Glaudemans et al., 2013; Herholz et al., 2012).

Single-Photon Emission Computed Tomography

The first SPECT measurements were performed in the 1960s (Kuhl and Edwards, 1964). SPECT employs gamma-emitting radionuclides that decay by emitting a single gamma ray. Typical radionuclides employed for neurological SPECT are technetium-99m (^{99m}Tc; half-life = 6.02 hours) and iodine-123 (^{123}I; half-life = 13.2 hours). Gamma cameras are used for SPECT acquisition, whereby usually two or three detector heads rotate around the patient's head to acquire two-dimensional planar images (projections) of the head from multiple angles (e.g., in 3-degree steps). Whereas radiation collimation is achieved by coincidence detection in PET, hardware collimators with lead septa are placed in front of the detector heads in the case of SPECT scanners. Finally, 3D image data reconstruction is done by conventional reconstruction algorithms. With combined SPECT/CT systems, a CT transmission scan can replace less accurate calculated attenuation correction.

The different acquisition principles imply that SPECT possesses a considerably lower sensitivity than PET. Thus, rapid temporal sampling (image frames of seconds to minutes) as a prerequisite for pharmacokinetic analyses is the strength of PET, whereas a single SPECT acquisition usually takes 20 to 30 minutes. Furthermore, the spatial resolution of modern SPECT is only about 7 to 10 mm, deteriorating with increasing distance between object and collimator (i.e., higher resolution for cortical than subcortical structures; distance between patient and collimator should be minimized for optimal resolution). Thus, SPECT is more susceptible to partial volume effects than PET, which can be a particular drawback when it comes to imaging small structures or lesions (e.g., brain tumors). Nevertheless, brain-dedicated SPECT instruments that allow for optimized spatial and temporal sampling and pharmacokinetic data quantification have been proposed (Meyer et al., 2008), and further technical developments are underway (Jansen and Vanderheyden, 2007). The important advantages of SPECT over PET are the lower costs and broad availability of SPECT systems and radionuclides. While [123I]-labeled tracers (e.g., [123I]FP-CIT ([123I]ioflupane, DaTSCAN) for dopamine transporter (DAT) imaging) can easily be shipped over long distances, technetium-99m can be eluted onsite from molybdenum-99 ([99Mo])/[99mTc] generators and used for labeling commercially available radiopharmaceutical kits.

We will focus on the two most widely used CBF tracers, hexamethylpropyleneamine oxime ([99mTc]HMPAO) and ethylcysteinate dimer ([99mTc]ECD). Owing to their lipophilic nature and thus high first-pass extraction, they are radiotracers are rapidly taken up by the brain. They are quasi-irreversibly retained after conversion into hydrophilic compounds (enzymatic de-esterification of [99mTc]ECD; instability, and possibly interaction with glutathione in the case of [99mTc]HMPAO). Differences in uptake mechanisms may explain slight differences in biological behavior (e.g., in stroke), with [99mTc]HMPAO being more closely correlated to perfusion, while [99mTc]ECD uptake is also influenced by metabolic activity. Despite the fact that cerebral radiotracer uptake is virtually complete within just 1 to 2 minutes after injection, SPECT acquisition is usually started after 30 to 60 minutes to allow for sufficient background clearance.

Given the fact that the CBF is closely coupled to cerebral glucose metabolism, and thus to neuronal function (with a few rare exceptions), [99mTc]HMPAO and [99mTc]ECD are used to assess neuronal activity. However, since cerebral autoregulation is also affected by many other factors (e.g., carbon dioxide level) and possibly diseases, cerebral glucose metabolism represents a more direct and probably less variable marker of neuronal activity. Given the technical limitations mentioned earlier, [18F]FDG PET is generally preferred to CBF SPECT. One important exception, however, is the use of ictal CBF SPECT in the assessment of patients with epilepsy. [123I]FP-CIT SPECT scans for assessment of nigrostriatal integrity in suspected parkinsonism or dementia with Lewy bodies are typically acquired 3 hours after tracer injection and evaluated by visual inspection and semi-quantitative region-of-interest analyses as outlined by the respective practice guidelines (Djang et al., 2012) (see also Chapter 42).

CLINICAL APPLICATIONS
Dementia and Mild Cognitive Impairment

Early and accurate diagnosis of dementia is of crucial importance for appropriate treatment (including possible enrollment into treatment trials and avoidance of possible side effects of treatments), for prognosis, and for adequate counseling of patients and caregivers. The diagnostic power of [18F]FDG PET in this situation is well established (Bohnen et al., 2012; Herholz, 2003). In clinical practice, [18F]FDG PET

studies are interpreted by qualitative visual readings. To achieve optimal diagnostic accuracy, these readings should be supported by voxel-based statistical analyses in comparison to aged-matched normal controls (e.g., Frisoni et al., 2013; Herholz et al., 2002a; Minoshima et al., 1995). PET studies should always be interpreted with parallel inspection of a recent CT or MRI scan to detect structural defects (e.g., ischemia, atrophy, subdural hematoma) that cause regional hypometabolism.

Alzheimer Disease

The typical finding in Alzheimer disease (AD), the most frequent neurodegenerative dementia, is bilateral hypometabolism of the temporal and parietal association cortices, with the temporoparietal junction being the center of impairment. As the disease progresses, frontal association cortices also get involved (Figs 41.1 and 41.2). The magnitude and extent of the hypometabolism increases with progressing disease, with relative sparing of the primary motor and visual cortices, the basal ganglia, and the cerebellum (often used as reference regions). The degree of hypometabolism is usually well correlated with the dementia severity (Herholz et al., 2002a; Minoshima et al., 1997; Salmon et al., 2005). Furthermore, cortical hypometabolism is often asymmetrical, corresponding to predominant clinical symptoms (language impairment if dominant or visuospatial impairment if nondominant hemisphere is affected). Voxel-based statistical analyses consistently show that the posterior cingulate gyrus and precuneus are also affected, which is an important diagnostic clue even in the earliest AD stages (Minoshima et al., 1997). The hippocampus is particularly affected by AD pathology and,

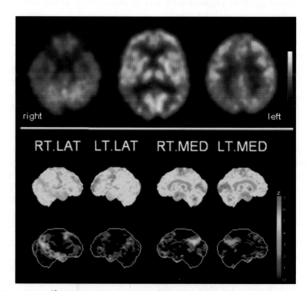

Fig. 41.1 [18F]FDG PET in early Alzheimer disease. Early disease stage is characterized by mild to moderate hypometabolism of temporal and parietal cortices and posterior cingulate gyrus and precuneus. Distinct asymmetry is often noticed, as in this case. As disease progresses, frontal cortices also become involved. *Top*, Transaxial PET images of [18F]FDG uptake (color coded, see color scale on right; orientation in radiological convention as indicated). *Bottom*, Results of voxel-based statistical analysis using Neurostat/3D-SSP. Three-dimensional stereotactic surface projections of [18F]FDG uptake *(upper row)* and statistical deviation of the individual's examination (as z score) from age-matched healthy controls *(lower row)*. Data are color coded in rainbow scale (see lower right for z scale). Given are right and left lateral and mesial views.

consequently, neurodegeneration. This likely also contributes to posterior cingulate/precuneus hypometabolism by diaschisis. However, studies on hippocampal metabolism in AD yielded conflicting results, often showing no significant hypometabolism. This may be due to the relatively low [^{18}F]FDG uptake, small size, and AD-related atrophy of this structure, which render visual and voxel-based statistical analyses insensitive. Region-based analyses (e.g., using automated hippocampal masking) can help overcome these limitations

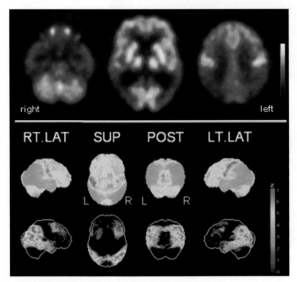

Fig. 41.2 [^{18}F]FDG PET in advanced Alzheimer disease. Advanced disease stage is characterized by severe hypometabolism of temporal and parietal cortices and posterior cingulate gyrus and precuneus. Frontal cortex is also involved, while sensorimotor and occipital cortices, basal ganglia, thalamus, and cerebellum are spared. Mesiotemporal hypometabolism is also apparent. *Top*, Transaxial PET images of [^{18}F]FDG uptake. *Bottom*, Results of voxel-based statistical analysis using Neurostat/3D-SSP. Given are right and left lateral, superior, and posterior views (see **Fig. 41.1** for additional details).

and provide valuable incremental diagnostic information (Mosconi et al., 2005).

The logopenic variant primary progressive aphasia (lvPPA), which is characterized by most prominent deficits in word retrieval and sentence repetition, is commonly assumed to also be caused by AD. LvPPA patients typically show a strongly leftward asymmetric hypometabolism of the temporoparietal cortex (Gorno-Tempini et al., 2011; Lehmann et al., 2013; Madhavan et al., 2013) (Fig. 41.3). Conversely, patients with posterior cortical atrophy (PCA), another nonamnestic presentation of AD with predominant visuospatial and visuoperceptual deficits, typically exhibit a rightward asymmetric temporoparietal hypometabolism with strong involvement of the lateral occipital cortex (Lehmann et al., 2013; Spehl et al., 2014) (Fig. 41.4).

A meta-analysis of recent [^{18}F]FDG-PET cross-sectional case-control studies (n = 562, in total) revealed a very high sensitivity (96%) and specificity (90%) of [^{18}F]FDG PET for the diagnosis of AD (Bohnen et al., 2012). In [^{18}F]FDG PET studies with autopsy confirmation in patients with memory complaints, the pattern of temporoparietal hypometabolism as assessed by visual readings alone showed a high sensitivity of 84% to 94% for detecting pathologically confirmed AD, with a specificity of 73% to 74% (Jagust et al., 2007; Silverman et al., 2001). Visual inspection of [^{18}F]FDG PET was found to be of similar accuracy to a clinical follow-up examination performed 4 years after PET. Moreover, when [^{18}F]FDG PET disagreed with the initial clinical diagnosis, the PET diagnosis was considerably more likely to be congruent with the pathological diagnosis than the clinical diagnosis (Jagust et al., 2007). In a large multicenter trial, voxel-based statistical analyses of cortical [^{18}F]FDG uptake differentiated AD from dementia with Lewy bodies (DLB; see later section Dementia with Lewy Bodies) with 99% sensitivity and 71% specificity (97% accuracy) and from frontotemporal dementia (FTD) with 99% sensitivity and 65% specificity (97% accuracy) (Mosconi et al., 2008). However, the use of an additional hippocampal analysis (being relatively preserved in DLB and FTD) greatly improved specificity (100% and 94% for AD vs DLB and FTD, respectively), yielding an overall classification accuracy of 96% for the aforementioned patient groups and controls

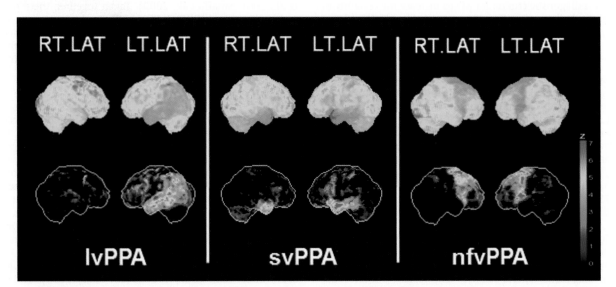

Fig. 41.3 [^{18}F]FDG PET in the different variants of primary progressive aphasia (PPA). [^{18}F]FDG PET scans in logopenic variant PPA (lvPPA) are characterized by a leftward asymmetric temporoparietal hypometabolism, whereas the semantic variant PPA (svPPA) involves the most rostral part of the temporal lobes. Patients with the nonfluent variant PPA (nfvPPA) typically show leftward asymmetric frontal hypometabolism with inferior frontal or posterior fronto-insular emphasis. Results of voxel-based statistical analysis using Neurostat/3D-SSP. Given are right and left lateral views (see **Fig. 41.1** for additional details).

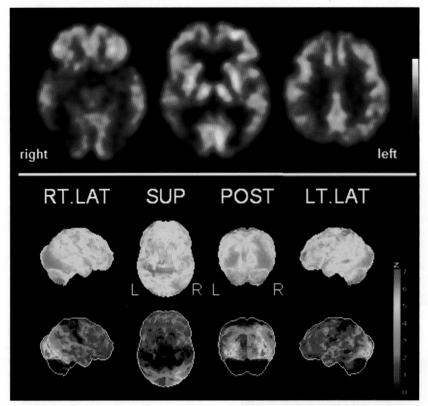

Fig. 41.4 [^{18}F]FDG PET in posterior cortical atrophy (PCA). Patients with PCA usually show a rightward asymmetric temporoparietal hypometabolism with strong involvement of the lateral occipital cortex. Results of voxel-based statistical analysis using Neurostat/3D-SSP. Given are right and left lateral, superior, and posterior views (see **Fig. 41.1** for additional details).

(Mosconi et al., 2008). Patterns of hypoperfusion observed with CBF SPECT in AD are very similar, but according to meta-analyses (Dougall et al., 2004; Frisoni et al., 2013) and direct comparisons (Herholz et al., 2002b), [^{18}F]FDG PET provides a higher diagnostic accuracy. Based on these results, [^{18}F]FDG PET was incorporated as a biomarker of neuronal injury into the latest diagnostic criteria for AD to increase the certainty of the clinical diagnosis of *possible* or *probable AD* (McKhann et al., 2011).

Mild Cognitive Impairment

The syndrome of mild cognitive impairment (MCI) (Petersen et al., 1999) represents a risk state for dementia. More than half of subjects progress to manifest dementia within 5 years, with AD being the most frequent underlying cause, particularly in the group with amnestic MCI (Gauthier et al., 2006). Several studies demonstrated that an AD-like [^{18}F]FDG PET pattern can be observed in high frequency among MCI patients (e.g., Anchisi et al., 2005; Drzezga et al., 2005; Mosconi et al., 2008). Meta-analyses showed that [^{18}F]FDG PET (sensitivity 76–79%, specificity 74%) performs better on prediction of rapid progression to AD than CBF SPECT and MRI (Frisoni et al., 2013; Yuan et al., 2009; Zhang et al., 2012), whereas amyloid-beta imaging offers a superior sensitivity (82–94%). Consequently, [^{18}F]FDG PET (as amyloid-beta PET) was also incorporated as a biomarker of neuronal injury into the most recent diagnostic criteria for MCI due to AD (Albert et al., 2011).

Finally, it has been demonstrated that cognitively normal healthy controls at risk for AD (ApoE ε4 carrier and/or positive maternal family history) exhibited a significantly reduced glucose metabolism in those cortical areas typically affected by AD (Mosconi et al., 2007; Reiman et al., 1996; Small et al., 1995), preceding a possible onset of AD by decades (Reiman et al., 2004). Follow-up studies in subjects at risk for AD also demonstrated that the subsequent decline in cerebral glucose metabolism in AD-typical regions was significantly greater than that in non-at-risk subjects (Mosconi et al., 2009; Reiman et al., 2001; Small et al., 2000). Taken together, these results emphasize that [^{18}F]FDG PET is not only a very powerful method for accurate diagnosis of manifest AD and prediction of progression in MCI but may also be useful for defining preclinical stages of AD (e.g., in prevention and treatment trials) (Sperling et al., 2011).

Dementia with Lewy Bodies

Dementia with Lewy Bodies (DLB) is considered the second most frequent cause of neurodegenerative dementia. The typical [^{18}F]FDG PET pattern observed in DLB resembles the pattern observed in AD with additional hypometabolism of the primary visual cortex and the occipital association cortex (Albin et al., 1996) (Fig. 41.5). The latter has been linked to the occurrence of typical visual hallucinations in DLB patients (particularly in those with relatively preserved posterior temporal and parietal metabolism) (Imamura et al., 1999). Occipital hypometabolism was found to be a valuable diagnostic feature to separate clinically diagnosed patients with AD and DLB (sensitivity 83%–92%, specificity 91%–93%) (Higuchi et al., 2000; Ishii et al., 1998a; Lim et al., 2009). This was substantiated in a study with autopsy confirmation (sensitivity 90%, specificity 80%) (Minoshima et al., 2001). Recent studies have demonstrated that regional metabolism of the hippocampus (Ishii et al., 2007; Mosconi et al., 2008) and mid to posterior cingulate gyrus (so-called cingulate island sign) (Lim

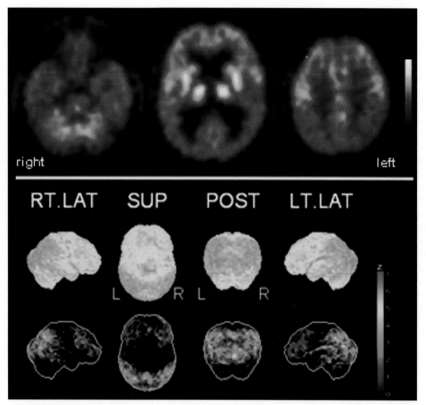

Fig. 41.5 [¹⁸F]FDG PET in dementia with Lewy bodies (DLB). This disorder affects similar areas as those affected by Alzheimer disease (AD). Occipital cortex is also involved, which may distinguish DLB from AD; in turn, the mesiotemporal lobe is relatively spared in DLB. A very similar, if not identical, pattern is observed in Parkinson disease with dementia (PDD). *Top*, Transaxial PET images of [¹⁸F]FDG uptake. *Bottom*, Results of voxel-based statistical analysis using Neurostat/3D-SSP. Given are right and left lateral, superior, and posterior views (see **Fig. 41.1** for additional details).

et al., 2009) is relatively preserved in DLB compared to AD, offering a high specificity for DLB. However, differences between AD and DLB may be hard to appreciate in routine clinical examination of individual patients. In this situation, PET or SPECT examinations of nigrostriatal integrity (most notably [¹²³I]FP-CIT SPECT) can be very helpful in differentiating between AD and DLB (McKeith et al., 2007). A recent meta-analysis indicated a pooled sensitivity and specificity of [¹²³I]FP-CIT SPECT for DLB of 87% and 94%, respectively (Papathanasiou et al., 2012). Furthermore, in a direct comparison of [¹⁸F]FDG PET and dopamine transporter (DAT) SPECT, the latter was found to be superior for the differential diagnosis of DLB versus AD (Lim et al., 2009). In line with this, striatal DAT loss is defined as a *suggestive feature* in the current diagnostic criteria for DLB, while occipital hypometabolism is a *supportive feature* (McKeith et al., 2005). Of note, nigrostriatal projections may also be damaged in FTD (Rinne et al., 2002) and atypical parkinsonian syndromes with dementia (e.g., PSP and CBD; see later section, Parkinsonism). Concerning a possible prodromal stage of DLB, it has been shown that primary visual cortex hypometabolism is associated with clinical core features of DLB in as yet nondemented memory clinic patients (Fujishiro et al., 2012). Those who converted to DLB during follow-up showed a more pronounced lateral occipital and parietal hypometabolism (Fujishiro et al., 2013).

DLB is clinically distinguished from Parkinson disease (PD) with dementia (PDD) by the so-called 1-year rule. In line with the notion that both diseases most likely represent manifestations of the same disease spectrum (Lewy body disease spectrum) (Lippa et al., 2007), [¹⁸F]FDG PET studies in PDD (Peppard et al., 1992; Vander Borght et al., 1997) found results very similar to those in DLB. In fact, in a direct comparison of

both groups, there were only minor differences, if any (Yong et al., 2007). However, according to a recent meta-analysis about two-thirds of DLB patients but only one-third of PDD patients show a positive amyloid-beta PET scan (Donaghy et al., 2015), suggesting a differential contribution of amyloid-beta to the manifestation of cognitive impairment and its timing in PD and DLB (reviewed in Meyer et al., 2014). Recent [¹⁸F]FDG PET studies also support the notion that PD with MCI (PD-MCI) represents a prodromal stage of PDD (Litvan et al., 2012): Similar to the pattern observed in PDD, PD-MCI patients typically exhibit a decreased temporoparietal, occipital, precuneus, and frontal metabolism when compared to healthy controls and, to a lesser extent, to PD patients without MCI (Garcia-Garcia et al., 2012; Hosokai et al., 2009; Pappatà et al., 2011). These changes are more pronounced in multidomain compared to single-domain MCI (Huang et al., 2008; Lyoo et al., 2010) and correlate with overall cognitive performance across patients with PD, PD-MCI, and PDD (Garcia-Garcia et al., 2012; Meyer et al., 2014). Finally, conversion from PD to PDD was predicted by hypometabolism in posterior cingulate, occipital cortex (BA18/19) and caudate nucleus, while hypometabolism of the primary visual cortex (BA17) was also observed in cognitively stable PD patients. Converters showed a widespread metabolic decline in several cortical and subcortical areas on follow-up imaging (Bohnen et al., 2011).

Frontotemporal Dementia

FTD probably represents the third most common overall cause of neurodegenerative dementia. FTD refers to a heterogeneous group of syndromes characterized by predominant deficits in behavior, language, and executive functions that are caused by a progressive degeneration of frontal and/or temporal lobes. FTD can be clinically subdivided into three major syndromes: behavioral variant frontotemporal dementia (bvFTD; prominent behavioral/cognitive symptoms like disinhibition, apathy, or executive deficits), semantic variant primary progressive aphasia (svPPA; prominent confrontation naming and single-word comprehension deficits), and nonfluent variant primary progressive aphasia (nfvPPA; prominent agrammatism and motor speech difficulties). Although associations between clinical syndromes and underlying pathologies have been described (e.g., tauopathies like Pick disease or corticobasal degeneration in nfvPPA; tau-negative, TDP-43- or FUS-positive aggregates in svPPA and bvFTD), clinical syndromes as well as pathologies may considerably overlap, which hinders predicting the underlying pathology by the clinical phenotype (Kertesz et al., 2005; Kertesz and McMonagle, 2011; Pressman and Miller, 2014). In fact, since patients often develop several syndromes during disease course, leading to a convergence of clinical presentations over time, the clinical fractionation of this "Pick complex" has been challenged (Kertesz et al., 2005; Kertesz and McMonagle, 2011). BvFTD is usually associated with a bilateral, often asymmetrical, frontal hypometabolism which is most pronounced in the mesial (polar) frontal cortex (Fig. 41.6) (Garraux et al., 1999; Salmon et al., 2003). The striatum, thalamus, and temporal and parietal cortices are also affected, although to a lesser extent (Garraux et al., 1999; Ishii et al., 1998b). Despite the fact that bvFTD and AD affect overlapping cortical areas, the predominance of frontal and temporoparietal deficits, respectively, is usually very apparent and allows a clear distinction between FTD and AD. In line with this, a voxel-based statistical analysis provided a diagnostic accuracy of 90% (sensitivity 98%, specificity 86%) for separating FTD (bvFTD and svPPA) and AD

in an autopsy-confirmed study, which was clearly superior to clinical diagnosis alone (Foster et al., 2007). Consequently, frontal or anterior temporal hypoperfusion or hypometabolism was incorporated as a criterion for *probable bvFTD* into the revised diagnostic criteria (Rascovsky et al., 2011). A normal [^{18}F]FDG PET may be particularly helpful to assure a high specificity of the clinical diagnosis of bvFTD by identifying "phenocopies" (Kipps et al., 2009). Patients with svPPA typically show a predominant hypometabolism of the rostral temporal lobes, which is usually leftward asymmetrical (see Fig. 41.3) (Diehl et al., 2004; Rabinovici et al., 2008). This pattern distinguishes patients with svPPA from those with lvPPA that present a more posterior, temporoparietal hypometabolism (as a nonamnestic AD manifestation; see earlier). Finally, opposed to the postrolandic hypometabolism found in lvPPA and svPPA, patients with nfvPPA exhibit a left frontal hypometabolism with inferior frontal or posterior fronto-insular emphasis (see Fig. 41.3) (Josephs et al., 2010; Nestor et al., 2003; Rabinovici et al., 2008). The aforementioned PPA-related patterns of hypometabolism on [^{18}F]FDG PET (or hypoperfusion on SPECT) are also necessary findings to make the diagnosis of *imaging-supported* lvPPA, svPPA, or nfvPPA according to the recently proposed classification (Gorno-Tempini et al., 2011).

Vascular Dementia

Finally, pure vascular dementia (VD) seems to be rather rare in North America and Europe and more prevalent in Japan, at least when several large cortical infarcts are seen as the cause of the dementia (so called: multi-infarct dementia). But Binswanger disease or subcortical arteriosclerotic encephalopathy may be underdiagnosed or mistaken as "vascular changes" in

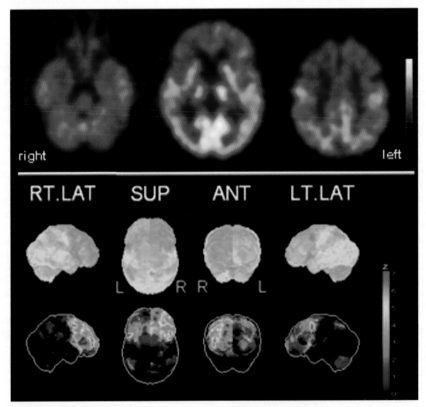

Fig. 41.6 [^{18}F]FDG PET in behavioral variant of frontotemporal dementia (bvFTD). Bifrontal hypometabolism is usually found in FTD, often in a somewhat asymmetrical distribution, as in this case. At early stages, frontomesial and frontopolar involvement is most pronounced, while parietal cortices can be affected later in disease course. *Top*, Transaxial PET images of [^{18}F]FDG uptake. *Bottom*, Results of voxel-based statistical analysis using Neurostat/3D-SSP. Given are right and left lateral, superior, and posterior views (see **Fig. 41.1** for additional details).

AD. [¹⁸F]FDG PET adds little to the diagnosis of VD. In agreement with CT and MRI, PET may show defects of [¹⁸F]FDG uptake corresponding to ischemic infarcts in all cerebral regions, including primary cortices, striatum/thalamus, and cerebellum. Since the latter are usually well preserved in AD, defects in these regions can be an important diagnostic clue. Deficits due to vascular lesions can be considerably larger or cause remote deficits of [¹⁸F]FDG uptake due to diaschisis. Furthermore, cerebral glucose metabolism was reported to be globally reduced (Mielke et al., 1992), but without absolute quantification this finding cannot be reliably assessed.

Parkinsonism

An early and correct differential diagnosis of parkinsonism is of paramount therapeutic and prognostic importance given the possible excellent treatment options and prognosis in patients without nigrostriatal degeneration (e.g., drug-induced parkinsonism, essential tremor) and the limited responsiveness to levodopa and faster progression to disability and death in patients with atypical parkinsonism syndromes (APS) compared to PD (Kempster et al., 2007; O'Sullivan et al., 2008). However, postmortem studies suggest that the clinical diagnosis of PD, as the most frequent cause of parkinsonism, is incorrect in about 25% of patients (Tolosa et al., 2006). Frequent misdiagnoses include secondary parkinsonism and APS like multiple system atrophy (MSA), PSP, and CBD. In turn, cumulative clinicopathological data suggest that about 30% of MSA and PSP and up to 74% of CBD patients are not correctly diagnosed even at late stage (Ling et al., 2010).

Against this background, SPECT and PET are used with two aims: first, to identify patients with progressive nigrostriatal degeneration, which is the common pathological feature in PD, MSA, PSP, and CBD. Second, to differentiate between the latter patient groups. Accurate diagnosis of neurodegenerative parkinsonism can be achieved by imaging nigrostriatal function (most notably [¹²³I]FP-CIT SPECT) (Benamer et al., 2000; Benitez-Rivero et al., 2013; Marshall et al., 2009) (For a more detailed overview on nigrostriatal imaging in parkinsonism please refer to Chapter 42.) However, dopamine transporter imaging does not allow for a reliable differential diagnosis of PD, MSA, PSP, and CBD (Meyer and Hellwig, 2014). Instead, [¹⁸F]FDG PET has gained acceptance as the method of choice here. It surpasses the diagnostic accuracies of other common techniques like imaging cardiac sympathetic innervation (e.g., using [¹²³I]metaiodobenzylguanidine ([¹²³I]MIBG) scintigraphy) or imaging of striatal dopamine D2/D3 receptors (e.g., using [¹²³I]iodobenzamide([¹²³I]IBZM)) (Meyer and Hellwig, 2014). Assessment of regional CBF changes with SPECT may also be used for this purpose (e.g., Eckert et al., 2007). However, since [¹⁸F]FDG PET is technically superior and also widely available, we will focus on [¹⁸F]FDG PET.

[¹⁸F]FDG PET shows disease-specific alterations of cerebral glucose metabolism (e.g., Eckert et al., 2005; Hellwig et al., 2012; Juh et al., 2004; Teune et al., 2010): scans in PD patients often show no major abnormality on first glance. On closer inspection and especially on voxel-based statistical analyses, PD is characterized by a posterior temporoparietal, occipital, and sometimes frontal hypometabolism (especially in PD with mild cognitive impairment and PDD) and a relative hypermetabolism of putamen, globus pallidus, sensorimotor cortex, pons, and cerebellum (Fig. 41.7). Interestingly, temporoparieto-occipital hypometabolism may also be seen in nondemented PD patients (Hellwig et al., 2012; Hu et al., 2000), possibly indicating an increased risk of subsequent development of PDD (see earlier section on Dementia and Mild Cognitive Impairment). Conversely, MSA patients show a marked hypometabolism of striatum (posterior putamen; especially in

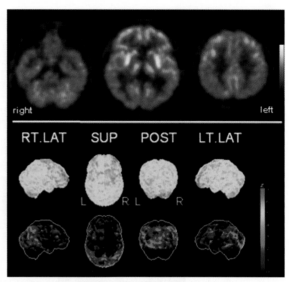

Fig. 41.7 [¹⁸F]FDG PET in Parkinson disease (PD). PD is typically characterized by (relative) striatal hypermetabolism. Temporoparietal, occipital, and sometime frontal hypometabolism can be observed in a significant fraction of PD patients without apparent cognitive impairment. Cortical hypometabolism can be fairly pronounced, possibly representing a risk factor for subsequent development of PDD. *Top,* Transaxial PET images of [¹⁸F]FDG uptake. *Bottom,* Results of voxel-based statistical analysis using Neurostat/3D-SSP. Given are right and left lateral, superior, and posterior views (see **Fig. 41.1** for additional details).

MSA-P), pons and cerebellum (especially in MSA-C) (Fig. 41.8). In the case of PSP, regional hypometabolism is consistently noted in medial, dorso-, and ventrolateral frontal areas (pronounced in anterior cingulate gyrus, supplementary motor, and premotor areas), caudate nucleus, (medial) thalamus, and upper brainstem (Fig. 41.9). Finally, CBD is characterized by a usually highly asymmetric hypometabolism of frontoparietal areas (pronounced parietal), motor cortex, middle cingulate gyrus, striatum, and thalamus contralateral to the most affected body side (Fig. 41.10). The aforementioned results gained from categorical comparisons fit the results gained from spatial covariance analyses. These were employed to detect abnormal, disease-related metabolic patterns in PD, MSA, and PSP (i.e., PDRP, MSARP, and PSPRP, respectively), which were demonstrated to be highly reproducible, to correlate with disease severity and duration, and to allow for prospective discrimination between cohorts (Eckert et al., 2008; Ma et al., 2007; Poston et al., 2012). The expression of two distinctive spatial covariance patterns characterizes PD: one related to motor manifestations (PDRP) and one related to cognitive manifestations (PDCP). The PDRP is already significantly increased in the ipsilateral ("presymptomatic") hemisphere of patients with hemi-parkinsonism (Tang et al., 2010b). Finally, a very recent study (using [¹⁸F]FDG PET and CBF SPECT) demonstrated that PDRP is also increased in REM sleep behavior disorder (RBD), being a significant predictor of phenoconversion to PD or DLB (Holtbernd et al., 2014). Thus, covariance patterns of cerebral glucose metabolism represent very interesting biomarkers for (early) diagnosis and therapy monitoring in parkinsonism (Hirano et al., 2009).

PSP and CBD may be considered to represent different manifestations of a disease spectrum with several common clinical, pathological, genetic, and biochemical features (Kouri et al., 2011). This issue gets even more complex if one considers that FTD is often caused by PSP and CBD pathology (see

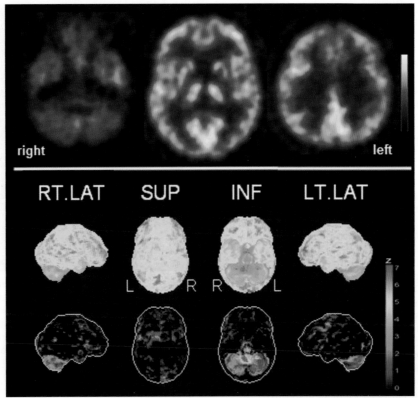

Fig. 41.8 [¹⁸F]FDG PET in multiple system atrophy (MSA). In contrast to Parkinson disease, striatal hypometabolism is commonly found in MSA (see left striatum), particularly in those patients with striatonigral degeneration (SND, or MSA-P). In patients with olivopontocerebellar degeneration (OPCA, or MSA-C), pontine and cerebellar hypometabolism is particularly evident. *Top,* Transaxial PET images of [¹⁸F]FDG uptake. *Bottom,* Results of voxel-based statistical analysis using Neurostat/3D-SSP. Given are right and left lateral, superior, and inferior views (see **Fig. 41.1** for additional details).

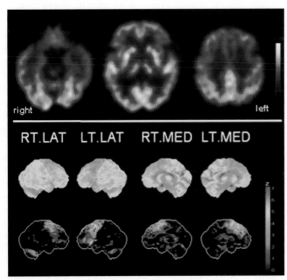

Fig. 41.9 [¹⁸F]FDG PET in progressive supranuclear palsy (PSP). Typical finding in PSP is bilateral hypometabolism of mesial and dorsolateral frontal areas (especially supplementary motor and premotor areas). Thalamic and midbrain hypometabolism is usually also present. In line with overlapping pathologies in FTD and PSP, patients with clinical FTD can show a PSP-like pattern, and vice versa (see **Fig. 41.3**). *Top,* Transaxial PET images of [¹⁸F]FDG uptake. *Bottom,* Results of voxel-based statistical analysis using Neurostat/3D-SSP. Given are right and left lateral and mesial views (see **Fig. 41.1** for additional details).

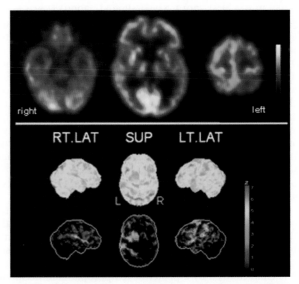

Fig. 41.10 [¹⁸F]FDG PET in corticobasal degeneration (CBD). In line with the clinical presentation, CBD is characterized by a strongly asymmetrical hypometabolism of frontoparietal areas (including sensorimotor cortex; often pronounced parietal), striatum, and thalamus. *Top,* Transaxial PET images of [¹⁸F]FDG uptake. *Bottom,* Results of voxel-based statistical analysis using Neurostat/3D-SSP. Given are right and left lateral and superior views (see **Fig. 41.1** for additional details).

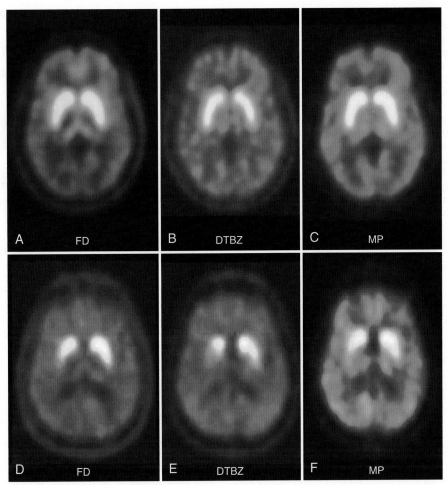

Fig. 42.2 FD uptake, VMAT2 (DTBZ) and DAT (MP) binding in a healthy control *(upper panel)* and an individual with early Parkinson disease (PD) *(lower panel)*. Note the asymmetrical reduction of uptake in the patient with PD, maximally affecting the posterior putamen, with relative sparing of the caudate nucleus.

which the posterior striatum is maximally affected and the caudate nucleus is relatively spared (Fig. 42.2). The degree of abnormality is typically asymmetrical, in keeping with clinical findings, but even patients with clinically unilateral disease have evidence of bilateral striatal dopamine denervation on PET or SPECT (Marek et al., 1996). With disease progression, uptake of all tracers declines according to an exponential function. The rostral-caudal gradient of involvement is maintained throughout the course of the illness, but the asymmetry between sides lessens over time (Nandhagopal et al., 2009). Because the symptoms of PD do not become manifest until loss of approximately 50% of nigral neurons or 80% of striatal dopamine, imaging may be used to detect preclinical abnormalities in individuals at high risk of developing parkinsonism, including persons exposed to the selective nigral toxin, *N*-methyl-4-phenyl-1,2,3,6-tetrahydropridine (MPTP) (Calne et al., 1985); twins of persons with PD (Piccini et al., 1999); family members from pedigrees with dominantly inherited PD (Adams et al., 2005; Nandhagopal et al., 2008); and individuals with REM sleep behavior disorder (Albin et al., 2000). Interestingly, heterozygous mutation carriers from kindreds with recessively inherited PD also demonstrate imaging evidence of dopamine denervation (Hilker et al., 2001; Khan et al., 2002, 2005), of unclear significance. While imaging can be used to assess disease progression, there are numerous examples of discordance between PET or SPECT findings and

clinical observations, particularly in studies designed to assess the effects of potential disease-modifying or cell-based therapies (Fahn et al., 2004; Marek et al., 2002; Olanow et al., 2003; Whone et al., 2003). This has led to caution with respect to the use of imaging as a surrogate marker in such studies (Brooks et al., 2003; Ravina et al., 2005).

By using displacement of [^{11}C]raclopride as a measure of dopamine release, it can be shown that PD patients who go on to develop fluctuations in response to levodopa therapy have a relatively large but poorly sustained increase in synaptic dopamine following levodopa, compared to those who have a stable response to medication, in whom dopamine release is lower in magnitude but more sustained. These differences are evident even at a time when both groups still have a stable response to medication (de la Fuente-Fernandez et al., 2001a). Levodopa-induced dopamine release increases with disease progression and is also increased in patients with medication-induced dyskinesias (de la Fuente-Fernandez et al., 2004). More recently, a contribution from serotonergic terminals to increased dopamine release in the striatum has been demonstrated (Politis et al., 2014). A similar approach has been used to demonstrate increased levodopa-derived dopamine release in the ventral (but not dorsal) striatum of patients with the dopamine dysequilibrium syndrome (Evans et al., 2006). In these subjects, dopamine release correlates with drug-wanting as opposed to drug-liking. Dopamine release is also increased during performance of a gambling task with monetary reward, and this effect is enhanced in PD patients with pathological gambling (Steeves et al., 2009). The same technique has been used to demonstrate dopamine release underlying the placebo effect in PD (de la Fuente-Fernandez et al., 2001b). This finding, initially demonstrated using placebo medication, has been confirmed with sham repetitive transcranial magnetic stimulation, which also induces ventral striatal dopamine release (Strafella et al., 2006).

Postural instability and gait disturbances in PD are less responsive to dopaminergic therapy. PET studies show an association of these features with cholinergic dysfunction. PD patients with falls have lower thalamic cholinergic activity than nonfallers, despite comparable nigrostriatal dopaminergic activity (Bohnen et al., 2009). Reduction in gait speed correlates with a reduction in cortical cholinergic activity (Bohnen et al., 2013). Amyloid deposits have also been associated with postural instability and gait dysfunction (Müller et al., 2013).

PET has been used to investigate depression in PD, with surprising results. Using the selective ligand [¹¹C]DASB, Guttman and colleagues demonstrated widespread reductions in 5HT transporter binding in PD compared to healthy controls, compatible with loss of serotonergic fibers (Guttman et al., 2007). In PD patients with depression, however, 5HT transporter binding was increased, particularly in dorsolateral and prefrontal cortex (Boileau et al., 2008); 5HT transporter binding correlated with clinical ratings of depression. Although not anticipated, this finding is reminiscent of major depression, where 5HT transporter binding is increased in those subjects with negativistic dysfunctional attitude (Meyer et al., 2004).

Dementia in PD (PDD) is associated with marked reductions in cholinergic activity (Bohnen et al., 2003; Hilker et al., 2005), greater than those seen in AD. The pathology of PDD is mixed but often includes cortical Lewy body deposition (with or without evidence of AD pathology), so there has been considerable interest in whether agents that bind to aberrantly folded protein can be used to image dementia with Lewy bodies (DLB) or PDD. Most studies to date have suggested that [¹¹C]PiB binding is increased in DLB but not in PDD. This may seem surprising, as many investigators consider these to represent variations of the same disorder. It is possible that patients with PDD who demonstrate [¹¹C]PiB uptake in fact have concurrent amyloid plaques, as suggested by a relationship to ApoE4 allele and CSF Aβ₄₂ levels (Maetzler et al., 2009), as well as recent postmortem (Burack et al., 2010) and in vitro (Fodero-Tavoletti et al., 2007) studies. However, the pattern of amyloid deposition varies between PD and AD, suggesting that amyloid may play a different role in these illnesses (Campbell et al., 2013). As in other neurodegenerative disorders, there has been great interest in the possibility of an inflammatory component to the pathogenesis and progression of PD. Using the peripheral benzodiazepine ligand, [¹¹C]PK 11195 as a marker of microglial activation, Ouchi et al. (2005) demonstrated increased binding in the substantia nigra of PD patients that correlated with dopaminergic nerve loss and with clinical measures of disease severity. In contrast, Gerhard et al. (2006) found more widespread increases in [¹¹C]PK 11195 binding that did not correlate with either FD uptake or clinical measures of disease progression. However, technical issues make interpretation of these studies difficult. Quantitation with [¹¹C]PK 11195 is difficult, results vary according to the analytical model employed, and binding is apparently not reduced in response to treatment with celecoxib (Bartels et al., 2010). Studies conducted with newer ligands for the TSPO may resolve these issues.

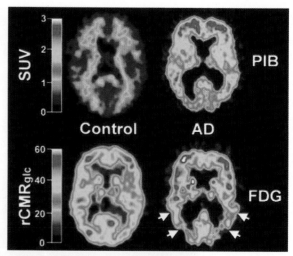

Fig. 42.3 Amyloid binding. *PIB* (Pittsburgh Compound B; *upper panel*) and glucose (2-deoxy-2-(¹⁸F)fluoro-D-glucose [FDG]) metabolism *(lower panel)* in a healthy control subject *(left)* and a patient with Alzheimer disease *(right)*. Note the diffuse increase in amyloid deposition in the patient, combined with reduced glucose metabolism in parietotemporal cortex. *SUV*, Standardized uptake value; *rCMRglc*, regional cerebral metabolic rate for glucose. *(From Klunk, W.E., Engler, H., Nordberg, A., et al., 2004. Imaging brain amyloid in Alzheimer's disease with Pittsburgh Compound-B. Ann Neurol 55, 306–319.)*

Alzheimer Disease

Imaging of amyloid protein has improved our understanding of the aging brain as well as Alzheimer disease (AD). Several radioligands which bind to β-amyloid have been developed, and their uptake is increased in the cortical and subcortical regions in AD (Fig. 42.3). The most commonly employed tracer is [¹¹C]PiB (Klunk et al., 2004). Several fluorine-based amyloid ligands have also been developed, such as [¹⁸F]AV-45 (flobetapir) (Wong et al., 2010) and [¹⁸F]BAY94-9172 (Rowe et al., 2008); these tracers have been shown to bind to multiple sites on β-amyloid (Ni et al., 2013). [¹¹C]-labeled agents require proximity to a cyclotron, whereas the longer half-life of [¹⁸F]-labeled agents allows them to be shipped from regional hubs. [¹⁸F]FDDNP binds to neurofibrillary tangles as well as amyloid plaques (Shoghi-Jadid et al., 2002), resulting in preferential uptake in the hippocampus (Shin et al., 2010). Global [¹¹C]PiB uptake is inversely associated with CSF Aβ₁₋₄₂ levels, while [¹⁸F]FDDNP binding correlates with CSF τ (Tolboom et al., 2009a). Increased [¹⁸F]FDDNP binding seems to correlate better with impairment of episodic memory, while [¹¹C]PiB binding may be associated with more widespread cognitive deficits (Tolboom et al., 2009b). An earlier study showed that binding of [¹¹C]PiB did not correlate with the Mini-Mental State Examination, whereas reduced glucose metabolism does (Jagust et al., 2009). However, a more recent study showed inverse correlations between hemispheric amyloid load, medial temporal glucose metabolism, and verbal memory (Frings et al., 2013). Another study showed that reduced nicotinic acetylcholine receptors were associated with elevated PiB binding and reduced cognitive function (Okada et al., 2013). Both [¹¹C]PiB and [¹⁸F]FDDNP reveal increased uptake in subjects with minimal cognitive impairment (MCI) (Small et al., 2006), although there is some variability reported in the ability of [¹⁸F]FDDNP to differentiate between control, MCI, and AD (Tolboom et al., 2009c). In healthy aging, [¹¹C]PiB binding is increased, particularly in carriers of the ApoE-ε4 allele (Rowe et al., 2010). Binding is also increased in healthy

(Box 43.1), for which comprehensive norms have been published by Heaton and colleagues (Heaton et al., 1991). An advantage to the fixed battery approach is that the information gathered is comprehensive and systematically assesses multiple domains of cognitive functioning. Additionally, if repeated assessments are available, test scores can be directly compared with baseline information, and tests are well validated and normed. Drawbacks of the fixed battery approach include its length (up to 8 hours), because it may be too long for some patients to tolerate and is difficult to afford with the limited reimbursement schedules in managed care. Furthermore, an extended assessment may not be necessary to address the referral question.

In contrast to the fixed battery approach, the flexible battery (or hypothesis-driven) approach allows neuropsychologists to develop a test battery based on the referral question, patient's history, and clinical interview. In the flexible battery approach, a brief set of basic tests is initially administered, and additional tests of more specific abilities are used to conduct in-depth follow-up assessments based on each particular patient's needs. For example, clinicians using the Iowa–Benton method (Tranel, 2008) specifically tailor testing to each patient based on their presenting concern by administering the appropriate portions of a core battery, which are then followed up with tests that assess suspected impairments in more detail (Fig. 43.1). Considerations when selecting tests include age, primary language, level of education, ethnicity/cultural factors, reading level, expected level of global cognitive impairment (to avoid ceiling or floor effects in testing), and physical disabilities (Smith et al., 2008). Although this approach is more tailored to the individual needs of the patient (and is therefore briefer), it can be less comprehensive than the fixed battery approach. Most neuropsychologists' approaches fall somewhere between the use of a set battery and a completely individualized examination.

Test Interpretation

The interpretation of cognitive test results is central to the role of the neuropsychologist and differentiates neuropsychology from all other disciplines. Accurate interpretation of neuropsychological test results depends on a comprehensive understanding of the neuroanatomical correlates of cognition, neurological disease processes, *and* psychometric testing principles. One cannot simply administer a test, look at the score, and declare that the score indicates intact/impaired cognitive

functioning. Test interpretation requires an understanding of test validity and reliability, sensitivity and specificity, likelihood ratios, and score distributions to avoid over- or underdiagnosing cognitive deficits. Substantial intraindividual differences exist in cognitive abilities and a certain number of poor test performances is common among the general population. Cognitive test performances are also impacted by extraneurological factors such as the number of tests administered, where cut scores are placed, the probability of certain test scores occurring, and the demographic characteristics of the patient (Iverson and Brooks, 2011). Proper test interpretation requires that all of these variables are considered and that conclusions are based on recognizable patterns of test results rather than the interpretation of test scores in isolation.

Neuropsychological test interpretation is also dependent on an understanding of the scientific and theoretical concepts that underlie cognitive tests. No cognitive test measures a single isolated aspect of cognitive functioning. Most neuropsychological tests engage multiple cognitive abilities simultaneously. To illustrate, verbal memory tests (e.g., word list memory tasks) assess memory functioning but they are also dependent on the patient's attention, processing speed, and executive functioning. Therefore, an impaired score on a verbal memory task does not necessarily indicate a primary memory impairment. It is the neuropsychologist's task to determine which cognitive deficits are actually causing impaired test performances by analyzing the patient's overall pattern of results across the test battery and by comparing the neuropsychological profile to known patterns of disease. If a score on a verbal memory test does reflect a primary memory deficit, then the neuropsychologist determines whether the impairment is due to a deficit in encoding, storage, or retrieval since the type of memory impairment may be indicative of different disease processes or lesion locations. Neuropsychologists use a similar method of analysis when assessing performances in other cognitive domains.

Test interpretation also requires the integration of neuropsychological test scores with findings from the clinical interview, the patient's history, the neurological examination, neurophysiology and neuroimaging data, and relevant literature. Raw test scores must be compared to an appropriate reference standard. Several reference standards are used in interpreting neuropsychological test scores, including the use of normative data, cut scores, and comparisons with an individual's own prior testing results.

Inferences about individual patients' neuropsychological test scores are often derived by comparing test scores to normative data that are typically collected by test developers as a standardization sample. Normative data are useful for accounting for variables that are likely to influence test performance (e.g., demographic factors) so that accurate and appropriate conclusions are drawn. Confounding variables are accounted for by stratifying test scores according to gender, age, and/or level of education. An individual's raw score is compared with the distribution of scores from his or her peer group to determine where it falls within the range of expected performances. Figure 43.2 and Table 43.2 show a normal distribution and interpretive guidelines for use in neuropsychological interpretation. The usefulness of normative data depends strongly on the size and representativeness of the standardization sample. Clinical interpretation can also be greatly affected by the goodness-of-fit between the individual patient and the standardization sample. Furthermore, it is important to use the most recent norms available, because cohort effects may lead to differences between current patients and those from whom data were collected years ago. When appropriate norms are not available, there is a danger of over- or underdiagnosis of cognitive impairment.

CORE BATTERY   FOLLOW-UP TESTS

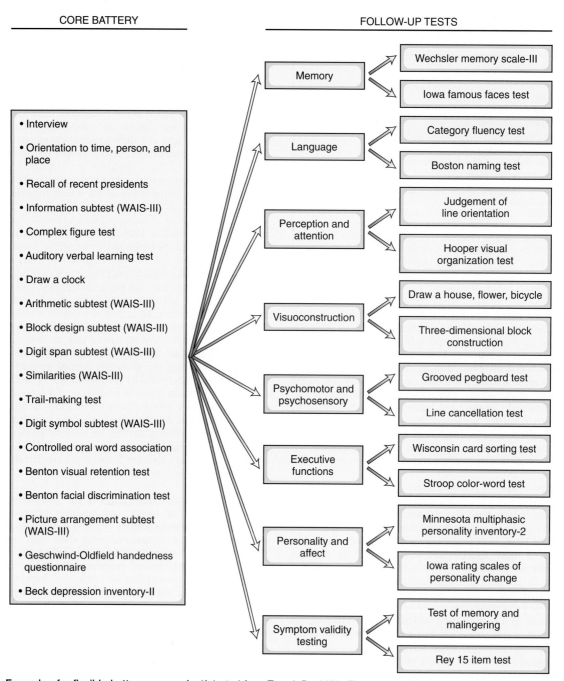

Fig. 43.1 Example of a flexible battery approach. *(Adapted from Tranel, D., 2008. Theories of clinical neuropsychology and brain–behavior relationships, in: Morgan, J.E., Ricker, J.H. (Eds), Textbook of Clinical Neuropsychology. Taylor & Francis, New York, pp. 25–37.)*

Another approach to test interpretation is through the use of cut scores. Tests that rely on cut scores often measure performances with low base rates or deficits very few healthy people demonstrate. Some tests are fairly straightforward in their capability to measure abilities that are largely intact in normal subjects but impaired in disordered patients. For example, most people are able to bisect a line without difficulty, but patients with left-sided visuospatial neglect typically identify the midpoint of the line to be to the right of center. Other tests, however, are more complex and require more sophisticated analyses to develop valid cut scores. Smith et al. (2008) provide an excellent explanation for how cut scores are useful individual statistics that allow inferences about which diagnostic group a patient is likely to belong to

(e.g., AD versus mild cognitive impairment versus healthy). Test validation studies commonly use sensitivity and specificity data with base rate information to calculate likelihood ratios and positive predictive values for individual tests. Likelihood ratios and positive predictive values are differing expressions of the probability that a patient has a particular condition given his or her test score. Smith et al. (2008) put these concepts another way by saying, "the positive predictive value allows for statements such as: 'Based on the patient having earned a score of y on test z, the probability that this patient has the condition of interest is x'" (p. 47). A common example of the application of cut scores can be found in the use of screening instruments to quickly identify potential impairments.

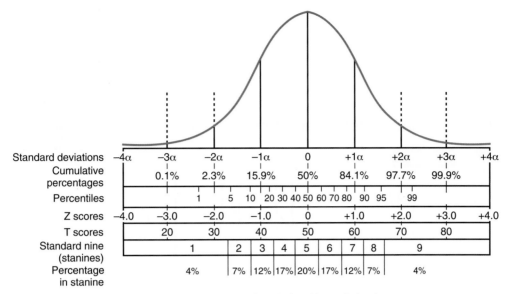

Standard deviations −4α −3α −2α −1α 0 +1α +2α +3α +4α

Cumulative percentages 0.1% 2.3% 15.9% 50% 84.1% 97.7% 99.9%

Percentiles 1 5 10 20 30 40 50 60 70 80 90 95 99

Z scores −4.0 −3.0 −2.0 −1.0 0 +1.0 +2.0 +3.0 +4.0

T scores 20 30 40 50 60 70 80

Standard nine (stanines) 1 2 3 4 5 6 7 8 9

Percentage in stanine 4% 7% 12% 17% 20% 17% 12% 7% 4%

Fig. 43.2 The normal curve and its relationship to derived scores.

TABLE 43.2 Descriptive Terms Associated with Performance within Various Ranges of the Normal Distribution

Qualitative terms	Standard deviation score (i.e. z-score)	T-score	Percentile rank
Severely impaired	<−2.20	<29	<2
Moderately impaired	−2.20 to −1.60	29–34	2–5
Mildly impaired	−1.59 to −1.33	35–37	6–9
Below average	−1.32 to −0.68	38–42	10–24
Average	−0.67 to +0.67	43–57	25–75
Above average	+0.68 to +1.59	58–66	76–94
Superior	+1.60 to +2.20	67–72	95–98
Very superior	>+2.20	>72	>98

Note: The patient's educational history and premorbid level of functioning should be taken into consideration in applying any qualitative label.

The comparison of current performance with past test scores is another important component of test interpretation, especially if cognitive decline is suspected. Rarely, however, do individuals have previous test data available for these comparisons. When no previous test scores are available, evidence of the patient's premorbid intellectual functioning is estimated. Several techniques are available for estimating premorbid intellect, including regression equations that utilize demographic variables as predictors of IQ (e.g., the Barona formula; Barona et al., 1984), irregular-word reading tests that are correlated with IQ (e.g., the North American Adult Reading Test; Blair and Spreen, 1989), and "hold" subtests from intelligence measures that are frequently used as proxies for premorbid functioning (e.g., see Lezak et al., 2012, for review). Most contemporary neuropsychologists use a combination of these strategies, either formally (e.g., Oklahoma Premorbid Intelligence Estimate-3, Schoenberg et al., 2002; Test of Premorbid Functioning, Pearson, 2009) or informally.

Ultimately, feedback about the results of the neuropsychological evaluation, along with diagnostic impressions and treatment recommendations, is communicated to the referring physician and the patient. Some form of written report is typical in neuropsychological evaluations, and these tend to vary in length and level of detail (e.g., <1 to 15 pages). A common structure for neuropsychological report includes sections summarizing the patient interview, collateral interview, medications, medical history, social background, behavioral observations, neuropsychological battery, neuropsychological test results and interpretation, final diagnostic impressions, and treatment recommendations.

BRIEF MENTAL STATUS EXAMINATION

Before referring a patient for a neuropsychological evaluation, the neurologist typically has either clinical or historical evidence of cognitive concerns. This might come from patient self-report or collateral report, an informal mental status examination, or a brief objective screening measure of mental status. Although many mental status examinations are conducted in a nonstandard manner, neurologists are encouraged to use formal cognitive screening measures to develop a standardized method of mental status examination so comparisons across time and patients can be reliably made. The purpose of cognitive screening measures is to determine the need for a more extended evaluation of neuropsychological functioning. Given the limited scope of cognitive screening measures and the psychometric considerations noted earlier, it is not recommended that cognitive screening measures are routinely used as a final summation of a patient's neuropsychological status. Scores from cognitive screeners must be considered in conjunction with clinical observation and judgment to determine whether a referral for neuropsychological evaluation is necessary, since many patients may pass a cognitive screen but still have suspected deficits that warrant more sensitive neuropsychological testing. A few suggested objective screening measures of cognitive functioning that may be useful for neurologists to administer are briefly described in the following.

Montreal Cognitive Assessment

The Montreal Cognitive Assessment (MoCA) was originally developed as a screening tool to correct the shortcomings of the widely used Mini-Mental State Examination (MMSE; see description in self-titled section), which demonstrated an insensitivity to mild cognitive impairment (Nasreddine et al., 2005). The MoCA also improved upon the MMSE by probing more cognitive domains, including executive functioning, immediate and delayed memory, visuospatial abilities, attention, working memory, language, and orientation to time and place (see Figure 43.3 for example). Including more cognitive domains reduces the likelihood that impairments or disorders will be overlooked (e.g., executive dysfunction, a hallmark symptom of vascular dementia). The total score ranges from 0 to 30 points, and a cut score of 26 has demonstrated very good specificity (by correctly identifying 87% of healthy

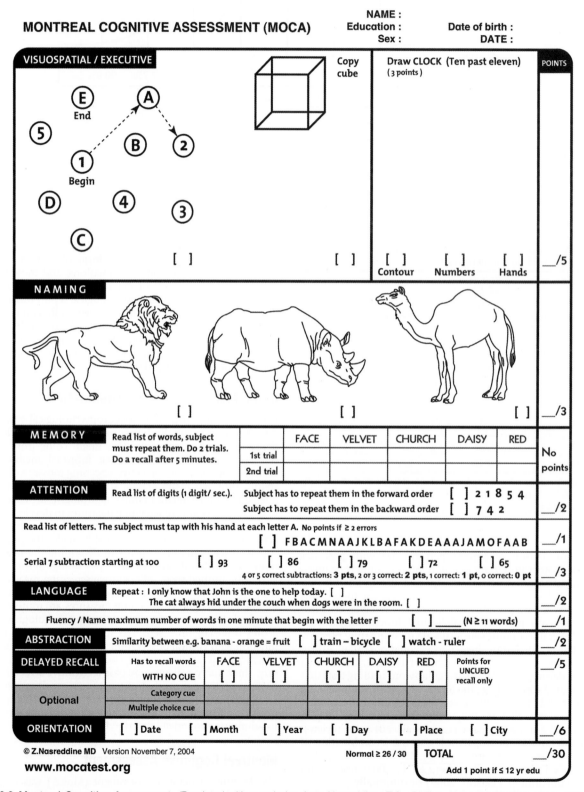

Fig. 43.3 Montreal Cognitive Assessment. *(Reprinted with permission from Nasreddine, Z.S., Phillips, N.A., Bedirian, V., et al., 2005. The Montreal Cognitive Assessment, MoCA: a brief screening tool for mild cognitive impairment. J Am Geriatr Soc 53, 695–699.)*

TABLE 43.3 Montreal Cognitive Assessment (MoCA) score by age and education

Age group (years)	Years of education									Total by age	
	<12			12			>12				
	NO.	MEAD (SD) MEDIAN		NO.	MEAN (SD) MEDIAN		NO.	MEAN (SD) MEDIAN		NO.	MEAN (SD) MEDIAN
<35	20	22.80 (3.38) 23		65	24.46 (3.49) 25		122	25.93 (2.48) 26		207	25.16 (3.08) 26
30–40	37	22.84 (3.18) 23		106	23.99 (2.93) 24		264	25.81 (2.64) 26		408	25.07 (2.95) 25
35–45	55	22.11 (3.33) 23		177	23.02 (3.67) 24		355	25.38 (3.05) 26		588	24.37 (3.51) 25
40–50	77	21.36 (3.73) 22		227	22.26 (3.94) 23		418	25.09 (3.16) 26		723	23.80 (3.80) 24
45–55	77	20.75 (3.80) 21		216	21.87 (3.95) 22		461	24.70 (3.24) 25		755	23.48 (3.84) 24
50–60	62	19.94 (4.34) 20		172	22.25 (3.46) 22		424	24.34 (3.38) 25		659	23.37 (3.78) 24
55–65	60	19.60 (4.14) 20		143	21.58 (3.93) 22		369	24.43 (3.31) 25		573	23.20 (3.96) 23
60–70	57	19.30 (3.79) 19		113	20.89 (4.50) 21		246	24.32 (3.04) 25		418	22.69 (4.12) 23
65–75	38	18.37 (3.87) 19		67	20.57 (4.79) 21		122	24.00 (3.35) 24		228	22.05 (4.48) 23
70–80	14	16.07 (3.17) 17		23	20.35 (4.91) 20		42	23.06 (3.47) 24		79	21.32 (4.78) 22
Total by education	230	20.55 (4.04) 21		608	22.34 (3.97) 23		1,306	24.81 (3.20) 25		2,148	23.65 (3.84) 24

Adapted from Rossetti, H.C., Lacritz, L.H., Cullum, C.M. & Weiner, M.F., 2011. Normative data for the Montreal Cognitive Assessment (MoCA) in a population-based sample. Neurology 77, 1272–5

participants) and excellent sensitivity when differentiating mild cognitive impairment (MCI) (90%) and AD (100%) from healthy comparisons. More importantly, the positive predictive value of the MoCA was 89% for both MCI and AD. Since its inception as a screening measure for MCI, other studies have found the MoCA to outperform the MMSE in screening for general cognitive impairment in Parkinson disease (PD) (Hoops et al., 2009; Nazem et al., 2009), vascular dementia after acute stroke (Dong et al., 2010), and HD (Videnovic et al., 2010) as a measure sensitive to early stages of different types of dementia.

Although the MoCA has demonstrated its utility as a cognitive screener, there are a few caveats worth noting. First, some studies have demonstrated that its reliability is notably low in nonclinical populations (Bernstein et al., 2011), which indicates that it should primarily be used only to detect suspected cognitive impairment in clinical patients. Additionally, the original cut score of 26 used to identify impairment was developed without fully accounting for other variables that affect test performance (e.g., age, education, gender, and race) and the score has also been shown to identify a high number of false positives in certain populations. Rossetti and colleagues (2011) attempted to correct these problems by conducting a normative study of the MoCA in an ethnically diverse sample of healthy participants as presented in Table 43.3. They found that 66% of their sample fell below the cut score of 26, indicating "impairment," and that many of the MoCA items had high failure rates.

The MoCA is free to clinicians (http://www.mocatest.org) and has been translated into 31 different languages and dialects.

Telephone Interview for Cognitive Status—Modified

The Telephone Interview for Cognitive Status—Modified (mTICS) is a relatively brief screening instrument designed to quickly and accurately assess cognition over the telephone, although it can also be used in face-to-face settings. This 13-item measure is heavily weighted toward immediate and delayed free recall, which might make it particularly useful in detecting mild impairments (Duff et al., 2009; Lines et al.,

2003) such as amnestic MCI (Fig. 43.4). Age-, education-, gender-, and race-corrected normative data are available (Hogervorst et al., 2004).

Mini-Mental State Examination

One of the most widely used mental status examinations is the MMSE (Folstein et al., 1975), a 30-point standardized screening tool for assessing orientation, attention, short-term recall, naming, repetition, simple verbal and written commands, writing, and construction (Fig. 43.5). The MMSE has been used in a variety of settings (e.g., community, institutions, general hospital, specialty clinics), with many different neurological and psychiatric conditions (e.g., dementia, stroke, depression), across age ranges, and with different cultural and ethnic subgroups. Demographic variables such as age and education have been shown to systematically influence MMSE scores, so normative data or cut scores should account for these variables. One example of appropriate norms comes from the Epidemiologic Catchment Area study (Crum et al., 1993); these are presented in Table 43.4. Whereas many intact individuals achieve total scores near 30, a cut score of 23 on the MMSE has been shown to have adequate sensitivity and specificity (86% and 91%, respectively) for detecting dementia in community samples (Cullen et al., 2005). However, when working with highly educated patients (i.e., ≥16 years of formal education) a cut score of 27 is recommended (O'Bryant et al., 2008).

Despite its widespread use, the MMSE has some drawbacks. First, it only assesses a limited number of cognitive functions. Second, a potential threat to the test's internal validity is the nonstandardized administration of some of the items. Examples of these frequent adaptations of the MMSE include the use of nonorthogonal (i.e., semantically related) word stimuli for registration and recall, nonstandard scoring of serial 7's, and nonstandard inclusion of spelling *world* backward. Another drawback of the MMSE is that it has "ceiling effects" that can miss cognitive impairments in high-functioning individuals. The MMSE also has difficulty differentiating individuals with MCI from controls and those with dementia (Mitchell, 2009). Finally, because this test relies on a single total score, partial administration of the measure (e.g., due to sensory

Modified Telephone Interview for Cognitive Status (mTICS)

1. What is your name?_____ /2

2. What is your telephone number?_____ /2

3. What is today's date (month, date, year, season, day)? (5 points maximum, 1 point per correct response)

Month:	_____	/1
Date:	_____	/1
Year:	_____	/1
Season:	_____	/1
Day:	_____	/1	/5

4. I'm going to read you a list of 10 words. Please listen carefully and try to remember them. When I am done, tell me as many as you can in any order. Ready? (10 points maximum, 1 point per correctly recalled word)

Cabin	
Pipe	
Elephant	
Chest	
Silk	
Theatre	
Watch	
Whip	
Pillow	
Giant	
TOTAL	

/10

5. Please count backwards from 20 to 1. /2
   20 19 18 17 16 15 14 13 12 11 10 9 8 7 6 5 4 3 2 1

6. Please take 7 away from 100. Now continue to take away 7 from what you have left over until I ask you to stop. (5 points maximum, 1 point per correct response)

93: _____	/1
86: _____	/1
79: _____	/1
72: _____	/1
65: _____	/1	/5

7. What do people usually use to cut paper?_____ /2

8. What is the prickly green plant found in the desert?_____ /2

9. Who is president of the United States now?_____ /2

10. Who is the vice president of the United States now?_____ /2

11. What word is opposite of east?_____ /2

12. Please say this: "Methodist Episcopal" /2
    Correct response (circle one):   YES   NO

13. Please tap your finger 5 times on the part of the phone you speak into. /2
    (2 points if they tap 5 times, 1 point if they tap more or less than 5 times)

14. Please repeat the list of 10 words I read earlier.

Cabin	
Pipe	
Elephant	
Chest	
Silk	
Theatre	
Watch	
Whip	
Pillow	
Giant	
TOTAL	

/10

TOTAL: /50

Fig. 43.4 Modified Telephone Interview for Cognitive Status. *(Data from Welsh, K.A., Breitner, J.C.S., Magruder-Habib, K.M., 1993. Detection of dementia in the elderly using telephone screening of cognitive status. Neuropsychiatry Neuropsychol Behav Neurol 6, 103–110.)*

impairments of the patient) provides no information about cognitive status. This same limitation is true for the MoCA.

Modified Mini-Mental State Examination

Some of the criticisms of the MMSE led to the development of the Modified Mini-Mental State Examination (3MS) (Teng and Chui, 1987), a 15-item extension of the MMSE that assesses orientation (self, time, place), attention (simple and complex), memory (recall and recognition), language (naming, verbal fluency, repetition, following commands, writing), construction, and executive functioning (similarities). It remains relatively brief to administer (10 minutes), and age- and education-corrected normative data are available (Tschanz et al., 2002). Regression-based prediction formulas for the 3MS allow for more accurate assessments of change across time (Tombaugh, 2005). The broader scoring range (0 to 100) has been shown to be more sensitive than that of the MMSE in identifying dementia (McDowell et al., 1997; Tschanz et al., 2002) and other cognitive disorders (Bland and Newman, 2001) in large community samples. A cut score for cognitive impairment is typically 77 (Bland and Newman, 2001; McDowell et al., 1997), and a change of 5 points over the course of 5 to 10 years indicates the presence of clinically meaningful decline (Andrew and Rockwood, 2008).

NEUROPSYCHOLOGICAL CHARACTERISTICS OF NEUROLOGICAL DISEASE

In this section we briefly address the neurocognitive sequelae of some of the major neurological disorders. Although many of these disorders have psychiatric characteristics as well, these will only be briefly discussed. Please see Chapter 9, Behavior and Personality Disturbances, for a more comprehensive discussion on the psychiatric aspects of neurological disorders.

Mild Cognitive Impairment

A major focus of dementia research has been detecting prodromes of cognitive impairment associated with neurodegenerative diseases, with a particular emphasis on characterizing the incipient stages of Alzheimer disease. The diagnostic term mild cognitive impairment was initially defined by Petersen and colleagues (1999) as the presence of subjective memory complaints, a measured deficit in a cognitive domain of approximately 1.5 standard deviations below normative means, otherwise intact cognition, no functional impairments, and the absence of dementia.

This became known as the Petersen criteria and requires the utilization of neuropsychological tests to quantify the deficit using normative data. While MCI originally focused on memory impairment, the concept has evolved to include other cognitive domains. Currently, MCI is typically categorized as either amnestic or nonamnestic with some also specifying whether the cognitive impairment is single- or multi-domain. Both amnestic MCI and nonamnestic MCI are considered to be risk factors for Alzheimer disease with nonamnestic MCI being viewed as a risk factor for other dementias as well. The new DSM-V (APA, 2013) diagnosis of mild neurocognitive disorder is essentially MCI (Petersen et al., 2009). Amnestic MCI is associated with smaller hippocampal and larger inferior lateral ventricle volumes similar to those of Alzheimer neuropathology (England et al., 2014) and approximately half of these cases will convert to Alzheimer dementia (Ferman et al., 2013). However, MCI as a diagnostic concept is extremely heterogeneous, in terms of both cognitive profile and neuropathology (Stephan et al., 2012). Other MCI subtypes are

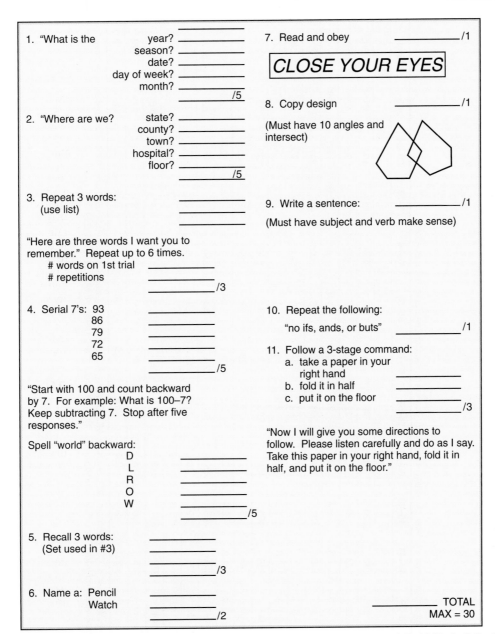

1. "What is the
   year? _____
   season? _____
   date? _____
   day of week? _____
   month? _____
   _____ /5

2. "Where are we?
   state? _____
   county? _____
   town? _____
   hospital? _____
   floor? _____
   _____ /5

3. Repeat 3 words: _____
   (use list) _____
   _____

"Here are three words I want you to
remember." Repeat up to 6 times.
   # words on 1st trial _____
   # repetitions _____
   _____ /3

4. Serial 7's: 93 _____
   86 _____
   79 _____
   72 _____
   65 _____
   _____ /5

"Start with 100 and count backward
by 7. For example: What is 100–7?
Keep subtracting 7. Stop after five
responses."

Spell "world" backward:
   D _____
   L _____
   R _____
   O _____
   W _____
   _____ /5

5. Recall 3 words: _____
   (Set used in #3) _____
   _____ /3

6. Name a: Pencil _____
   Watch _____
   _____ /2

7. Read and obey _____ /1

CLOSE YOUR EYES

8. Copy design _____ /1

(Must have 10 angles and
intersect)

9. Write a sentence: _____ /1

(Must have subject and verb make sense)

10. Repeat the following:
   "no ifs, ands, or buts" _____ /1

11. Follow a 3-stage command:
   a. take a paper in your
      right hand _____
   b. fold it in half _____
   c. put it on the floor _____
   _____ /3

"Now I will give you some directions to
follow. Please listen carefully and do as I say.
Take this paper in your right hand, fold it in
half, and put it on the floor."

_____ TOTAL
MAX = 30

Fig. 43.5 Mini-Mental State Examination. *(Reprinted with permission from Folstein, M.F., Folstein, S.E., McHugh, P.R., 1975. Mini-Mental State: a practical method for grading the cognitive state of patients for the clinician. J Psychiatr Res 12, 189–198.)*

hypothesized to progress to their own dementia outcomes. For example, 20% of nonamnestic MCI cases with impairment in either attention or visuospatial, or both domains have been reported to convert to Lewy body dementia (Ferman et al., 2013). Multi-domain MCI (e.g., deficits in executive functions and processing speed) might be indicative of eventual vascular dementia. Neuropsychological testing is essential for obtaining the necessary information to differentiate MCI subtypes and track their progression into the various forms of dementia.

MCI has attracted so much attention because of its prognostic value, with a 10-fold increase in the rate of dementia for individuals with MCI (Petersen et al., 1999). Patients of memory disorder clinics with MCI progress to dementia at a rate of 10% to 15% per year (Farias et al., 2009), and community dwelling adults at an annual rate of 6% to 10% per year (Petersen et al., 2009), but up to 25% may revert back to normal cognitive baseline at follow-up. It is controversial

whether severity of MCI symptoms does not predict which individuals will convert to dementia (Guo et al., 2013), though impaired olfaction increases the risk of conversion by four times (Conti et al., 2013). Using preclinical staging of AD adds to the predictive validity of who demonstrates conversion (Vos et al., 2013). Having a copy of APOE ε 4 also increases the risk of developing MCI (Brainerd et al., 2013). Individuals with MCI also experience global cognitive decline at over twice the rate of what is observed in nonimpaired individuals (Wilson et al., 2010). For cases that progress to dementia, the average time they would be considered to have MCI is 5.5 years, though they may not be diagnosed early in the process (Wilson et al., 2012). Since not everyone with MCI progresses to dementia, several predictors of the progression from MCI have been identified. Bilingualism has been reported to be a protective factor resulting in later onset of MCI (Bialystok et al., 2014) as are more advanced education and healthy lifestyle behaviors (Lojo-Seoane et al., 2014). Despite

TABLE 43.4 Mini-Mental State Examination Score by Age and Educational Level, Number of Participants, Mean, Standard Deviation, and Selected Percentiles

Age (years)	18-24	25-29	30-34	35-39	40-44	45-49	50-54	55-59	60-64	65-69	70-74	75-79	80-84	≥85	Total
EDUCATIONAL LEVEL															
0–4 yr	17	23	41	33	36	28	34	49	88	126	139	112	105	61	892
Mean	22	25	25	23	23	23	23	22	23	22	22	21	20	19	22
SD	2.9	2.0	2.4	2.5	2.6	3.7	2.6	2.7	1.9	1.9	1.7	2.0	2.2	2.9	2.3
5–8 yr	94	83	74	101	100	121	154	208	310	633	533	437	241	134	3223
Mean	27	27	26	26	27	26	27	26	26	26	26	25	25	23	26
SD	2.7	2.5	1.8	2.8	1.8	2.5	2.4	2.9	2.3	1.7	1.8	2.1	1.9	3.3	22
9–12 yr or H.S. diploma	1326	958	822	668	489	423	462	525	626	814	550	315	163	99	8240
Mean	29	29	29	28	28	28	28	28	28	28	27	27	25	26	28
SD	2.2	1.3	1.3	1.8	1.9	2.4	2.2	2.2	1.7	1.4	1.6	1.5	2.3	2.0	1.9
College experience	783	1012	989	641	354+	259	220	231	270	358	255	181	96	52	5701
Mean	29	29	29	29	29	29	29	29	29	29	28	28	27	27	29
SD	1.3	0.9	1.0	1.0	1.7	1.6	1.9	1.5	1.3	1.0	1.6	1.6	0.9	1.3	1.3
Total	2220	2076	1926	1443	979	831	870	1013	1294	1931	1477	1045	605	346	18,056
Mean	29	29	29	29	28	28	28	28	28	27	27	26	25	24	28
SD	2.0	1.3	1.3	1.8	2.0	2.5	2.4	2.5	2.0	1.6	1.8	2.1	2.2	2.9	2.0

Data from the Epidemiologic Catchment Area household surveys in New Haven, CT; Baltimore, MD; St Louis, MO; Durham, NC; and Los Angeles, CA, between 1980 and 1984. The data are weighted based on the 1980 U.S. population census by age, sex, and race. Adapted from Crum, R.M., Anthony, J.C., Bassett, S.S., et al., 1993. JAMA 269, 2386–2391.

this growing research, no standard for predicting the MCI-to-dementia conversion has yet been established.

Alzheimer Disease

Alzheimer disease-related dementia is the most common type, with prevalence rates of 11% in those of 65 years and older (Hebert et al., 2013) and 68% in memory disorder clinics (Paulino Ramirez Diaz et al., 2005). Definitive diagnosis requires postmortem neuropathological examination of brain tissue for the hallmark signs of plaques and neurofibrillary tangles in the hippocampal and entorhinal regions (Braak and Braak, 1991); however, premortem diagnostic criteria are widely employed in clinical and research settings. Recently, DSM-V (APA, 2013) has changed the terminology for diagnosis of dementia in AD to major neurocognitive disorder due to Alzheimer disease with specified criteria being evidence of significant cognitive decline from a previously higher level of functioning and the cognitive impairments interfering with everyday functioning. The diagnosis is considered probable Alzheimer disease if there is objective evidence of decline in memory and one other cognitive domain, insidious onset and gradual progression of symptoms, and no evidence of other etiology. Evidence of a genetic mutation associated with Alzheimer disease would also result in probable Alzheimer disease diagnosis. However, autosomal dominant cases such as *APP*, *PSEN1*, or *PSEN2* are rare and account for less than 1% of Alzheimer disease patients (Storandt et al., 2014). For research purposes, the National Institute of Neurological and Communicative Disorders and Stroke Alzheimer's Disease and Related Disorders Association (NINCDS-ADRDA) criteria for probable AD are the most commonly used. The National Institutes of Aging–Alzheimer's Association workgroups (McKhann et al., 2011) have recommended diagnosing probable Alzheimer disease dementia when there is a change in cognition that results in functional impairment and there is either an amnestic presentation or a nonamnestic one in the domains of language, visuospatial, or executive function with no evidence of other likely etiologies. The workgroups recommend a diagnosis of possible Alzheimer disease dementia if there is an atypical course such as a lack of evidence of progressive onset or mixed presentation that suggests comorbid etiologies. They also recommend including the incorporation of biomarkers, neuroimaging, and genetic findings into the diagnostic criteria but particularly emphasize the importance of measurable cognitive decline, especially for MCI. The presence of biomarkers without cognitive decline is considered a preclinical AD stage. However, the presence of biomarkers without evidence of early cognitive decline is thought to convey lower risk for dementia than if cognitive deficits are present (Jack et al., 2013). Formal neuropsychological assessment for measuring AD related declines has been demonstrated to have better sensitivity than MRI for tracking disease progression (Schmand et al., 2014). The brief bedside exams mentioned earlier in this chapter also have some degree of utility in detecting cognitive changes, but their comparatively limited scope, low sensitivity, and susceptibility to ceiling effects make them better suited for screening purposes.

Complaints about "memory problems" are what often lead to a clinical evaluation of possible AD and cognitive decline begins 7.5 years prior to diagnosis on average (Wilson et al., 2012). Consistent with patient report and behavioral observations of rapid forgetting of new information, performances across a comprehensive battery of neuropsychological assessment measures are likely to identify stark memory deficits for both verbally (e.g., lists, stories, paired associates) and visually (e.g., concrete or abstract figures) mediated information, including an atypical lack of a primacy effect for information

presented early in lists (Salmon and Bondi, 2009). Recognition memory is also likely to be significantly impaired and intrusion errors are common (e.g., adding extra words to delayed recall trials on word-list memory tasks). Other cognitive deficits are seen in a number of other domains including language functions (e.g., paraphasias, naming), semantic knowledge, visuospatial abilities, and executive functions such as motor planning (Weintraub et al., 2012). Impaired awareness of their own cognitive deficits, known as anosognosia or impaired metacognition, is also common (Rosen et al., 2014). Even though impaired memory is a cardinal feature of AD, it is important to keep in mind that other neurodegenerative dementia syndromes can also result in memory decline and that a nonmemory cognitive deficit may be the primary cognitive presentation of AD, possibly reflecting posterior cortical atrophy. Global cognitive functioning in AD declines at a rate nearly four times faster than what is observed in cognitively intact individuals of the same age (Wilson et al., 2010). Given the pattern of deficits in AD, it is not surprising that measures of semantic fluency, delayed free recall, and global cognitive status demonstrate the highest levels of sensitivity and specificity for detecting patients with early AD (Salmon et al., 2002). Although memory deficits are usually glaring compared to other deficits in AD, general and progressive cognitive decline is common and shows an eightfold increase in rate of decline approximately 3 years prior to death (Yu et al., 2013). As dementia progresses to moderate stages, learning and memory performances are likely to produce floor effects on many standardized neuropsychological measures, and more profound deficits are apparent in other cognitive domains. Deficits in praxis also begin to develop. These pervasive declines in late AD often make formal neuropsychological testing unnecessary or impossible.

Vascular Dementia

Cerebrovascular disease frequently leads to cognitive impairment and vascular factors have garnered significant attention as a modifiable risk factor for dementia. So-called silent brain infarcts, or asymptomatic vascular pathology, are found in up to 35% of individuals with vascular disease (Slark et al., 2012) and are known to double the risk of vascular dementia (VaD) or major neurocognitive disorder due to vascular disease, as described in the DSM-V. Extracerebellar lacunar, large vessel, or strategically placed infarcts and hemorrhage lead to varying degrees of cognitive impairment, and small vessel disease is the most frequently observed vascular pathology that leads to cognitive decline. Recently, the term vascular cognitive impairment (VCI) has been introduced to encompass all cognitive changes attributable to cerebrovascular pathology (i.e., from mild cognitive impairment due to vascular events to VaD; Rincon and Wright, 2013; Sachdev et al., 2014). Cognitive changes can occur abruptly and in a stepwise pattern with coinciding cerebrovascular accidents (CVAs), or they may fluctuate or remain static. Neuroimaging is likely to detect lesions that are a result of a CVA and enhance diagnostic certainty, but imaging is not required to accurately identify dementia with a vascular etiology. Neurological evidence of cerebrovascular pathology (e.g., history of strokes, sensorimotor changes consistent with stroke) in combination with cognitive changes is considered indicative of VaD and the estimated prevalence is 8–12% (Jellinger, 2013).

The clinical presentation of VaD varies depending on the number of infarcts, severity of neural damage following stroke, and location of the CVA. Although many VaD patients may acknowledge "memory problems," which may lead to suspicions of AD, further questioning reveals that these complaints are quite different from those typically seen in AD. If VaD results from a discrete stroke, then the primary cognitive impairment will likely be functionally related to the area of infarct, resulting in focal deficits and a heterogeneous presentation for VaD. Many patients do not experience a notable stroke preceding the onset of VaD, and may not present to memory disorder clinics because their primary symptoms are often dysexecutive in nature (e.g., the patient "just can't figure things out anymore") with accompanying apathy and/or depression being common (Weintraub et al., 2012). Particularly in the frontal regions, increasing lacunae are associated with a higher probability of depression, apathy, atypical behaviors, and other neuropsychiatric symptoms (Kim et al., 2013). Impaired executive functioning is also strongly related to the presence of metabolic syndrome, a significant risk factor for VaD (Falkowski et al., 2014).

Classic dementia symptoms might be reported (e.g., difficulty remembering names, appointments, medications) but changes in instrumental activities of daily living that require complex organizational and problem-solving skills (such as managing finances or following directions) are likely more prominent in a patient with VaD than in one with AD. Depression and apathy are hallmark symptoms and there is evidence that vascular factors are etiologically linked to late life depression (Taylor et al., 2013). Upon first inspection, VaD may initially be cognitively indistinguishable from other dementias in many ways. However, a detailed neuropsychological examination and behavioral observations are likely to reveal a unique pattern of deficits in VaD referred to as the subcortical profile. VaD patients tend to have better long-term verbal memory than their AD counterparts, worse executive functioning, and slowed processing speed, particularly on motor tasks. Impaired complex attention is also prominent (Benedet et al., 2012) and VaD tends to have a rapid initial onset. Free recall might occasionally appear similar in VaD and in AD, but patients with VaD significantly outperform their AD counterparts on tests of recognition memory (Tierney et al., 2001). Better recognition memory suggests encoding processes are relatively intact in VaD patients compared to AD patients, but information retrieval is deficient. This retrieval deficit appears to be quite common in subcortical dementias, with which VaD appears to have several components in common. Patients with VaD also perform more poorly on phonemic fluency tasks relative to semantic fluency tasks, which suggests greater executive dysfunction due to disruption of the frontal subcortical circuitry rather than degeneration in the temporal lobes.

Mixed Dementia

More common than AD and VaD in their pure forms is mixed dementia. While mixed dementia typically refers to a patient having both AD and cerebrovascular pathology, it conceptually can be any case which involves the coexistence of multiple neuropathologies (e.g., amyloid, small vessel ischemic changes, Lewy bodies). For patients diagnosed with VaD, 30% may have insignificant AD neuropathology as well (Lee et al., 2011) and these patients tend to be older than pure VaD cases. Across dementia autopsy studies, 21%–80% of cases had mixed AD and vascular pathology (Jellinger, 2013; Wilson et al., 2012). In older patients (>90 years), having both AD and vascular pathology at autopsy was more likely if they had been diagnosed with mixed dementia rather than AD alone (James et al., 2012). The vast majority of mixed dementia cases are AD and vascular pathology but 5% of cases are AD and Lewy body disease. Persons with multiple pathologies are three times more likely to develop dementia than others with only one identifiable diagnosis (Schneider et al., 2007). There is evidence that mixed dementia cases are more globally

impaired than similarly staged AD patients (Dong et al., 2013). While this may result from interactive effects, there is evidence that vascular and amyloid burden combine independently to impact cognitive impairment (Park et al., 2013).

Frontotemporal Dementia

Frontotemporal dementia (FTD) is another common type of dementia and is in fact the second most common in those younger than age 65 (Arvanitakis, 2010). It is less common in older adults and is frequently misdiagnosed as AD (Beber and Chaves, 2013). The term *frontotemporal lobar degeneration* (FTLD) is also frequently used in connection with FTD but usually refers to the pathological aspects of FTD and not the clinical entity (Hales and Hu, 2013). According to DSM-V (APA, 2013) criteria, FTD has multiple clinical manifestations that include behavioral and language variants. Behavioral observations, neuropsychological testing, and neuroimaging (e.g., frontal or temporal lobe atrophy on computed tomography [CT] or magnetic resonance imaging [MRI], hypoperfusion or hypometabolism on single-photon emission tomography [SPECT] or positron emission tomography [PET]) are used in combination to establish a clinically probable diagnosis of FTD. A definitive diagnosis can be made with histopathological evidence through biopsy or postmortem examination. The latest consensus clinical diagnostic criteria (Rascovsky et al., 2011) define possible FTD as the presence of progressive behavioral and/or cognitive deterioration and three of the following: behavioral disinhibition, apathy or inertia, loss of empathy, perseverative or compulsive behaviors, hyperorality or dietary change, and neuropsychological testing demonstrating executive impairments with intact memory and visuospatial abilities. Probable FTD requires that the patient meet criteria for possible FTD and also has evidence of functional decline and neuroimaging consistent with frontal and anterior temporal atrophy or dysfunction.

Although cognitive deficits are clearly evident on formal testing, the earliest and most common complaints for the behavioral variant of FTD are related to changes in personality and behavior. Increases in impulsivity, poor judgment, stereotypic behaviors, lack of hygiene, and loss of appropriate social behaviors are all prominent. Euphoria and disinhibition are particularly predictive of FTD compared to other dementias (Perri et al., 2014) while apathy is a nonspecific symptom that can occur in all dementias. A formerly mild-mannered and conscientious patient who develops the behavioral variant of FTD may present as overly frank, crass, and uncaring. The patient is usually indifferent to their behavior, but spouses and adult children are usually embarrassed by his or her conduct. Many of these behavioral issues may have underlying cognitive components. Impaired metacognition, or a deficit in monitoring and appreciating behavior, is typical and much more severe than is seen in AD (Rosen et al., 2014). Social impairments likely reflect an inability to cognitively recognize emotions or perspectives in others. Deficits on cognitive testing typically involve impaired executive functions such as mental flexibility, planning deficits, slowed word/design generation, and multiple response errors. Phonemic fluency also tends to be more impaired than semantic fluency. As the disease progresses, even simple go/no go tasks are difficult. Despite the array of cognitive deficits in FTD, memory and visuospatial functioning tend to be well preserved, and some suggest that a lack of deficits in these domains might be one of the best ways to differentiate FTD from other diseases such as AD (Weintraub et al., 2012).

The language variants of FTD are different clinical entities than the behavioral variant (Harciarek and Cosentino, 2013). Confrontation naming, word finding, speech production, comprehension, and/or syntax all gradually worsen over the course of disease. Memory functioning and visuospatial skills are relatively spared. The proposed DSM-V diagnostic criteria suggest that the language variant of FTD be divided into four subtypes: primary progressive aphasia (PPA), semantic variant, nonfluent/agrammatic variant, and logopenic/phonologic variant (APA, 2013). All of these variants except possibly the semantic variant involve some aspect of anomia or impaired object naming that is worse than AD (Reilly et al., 2011) but have otherwise unique neuropsychological profiles. PPA is characterized primarily by the insidious and gradual decomposition of expressive language functions such as word finding, object naming, grammar, and speech production that also affects comprehension later in the disease process (Weintraub et al., 2012). The semantic variant of FTD involves impaired single-word comprehension, object and/or person knowledge, and dyslexia in the presence of spared single-word repetition, motor speech production, and syntax. These patients may appear to have intact expressive and comprehension language functions but are unable to define vocabulary words or concepts. Nonfluent/agrammatic FTD results in impaired motor speech production, grammatical errors, and comprehension of complex sentences, with intact single-word comprehension and object knowledge. Lastly, the logopenic/phonologic variant presents with deficits in spontaneous word retrieval and repetition of sentences and phrases, while single-word comprehension, object knowledge, and motor speech and grammar production are spared. Neuropsychological testing is ideally suited for specifically characterizing deficits and parsing out the complexity of FTD variants and their specific cognitive profiles.

Parkinson Disease with Dementia and Dementia with Lewy Bodies

Parkinson disease with dementia (PDD) and dementia with Lewy bodies (DLB) have been collectively classified as *Lewy body dementias*, given their shared α-synuclein pathology (Lim et al., 2013). While it is believed that all patients with Parkinson disease would eventually develop a Lewy body dementia with sufficient time, the incidence in patients with Parkinson disease is only 12% for DLB and 8.5% for PDD (Savica et al, 2013). The Lewy body dementias are more common in women under 80 years and significantly more common in men over 80 years. DLB accounts for 4.2% of all dementia cases in community settings and 7.5% of dementia diagnoses in specialty clinics (Vann Jones and O'Brien, 2014). DLB is believed to be commonly misdiagnosed, making the actual incidence rate likely higher. Also, there is significant comorbidity with AD as autopsy studies have reported that 27% of cases of likely AD also had Lewy bodies present (Wilson et al., 2012). Incidence peaks at 70–79 years and decreases after that (Savica et al., 2013), making both PDD and DLB two of the young dementias (along with FTD) that do not increase in prevalence with advanced age. The neuropsychological findings in the two disorders are largely similar, so they are often distinguished by differences in the onset of signs and symptoms (Weintraub et al., 2012). The cognitive symptoms of PDD often develop at least 2 years after the onset of motor signs (e.g., bradykinesia, gait instability, tremor, rigidity), while the cognitive symptoms in DLB tend to precede motor features or occur within 1 year of the manifestation of motor signs (Gealogo, 2013). Motor signs develop more quickly in DLB when compared to the insidious onset of PDD signs and symptoms. Although the time course of cognitive symptoms and motor signs in DLB and PDD may serve as a helpful heuristic, caution should be used when differentiating these dementias from one another based on onset alone, since subtle cognitive declines can be detected early in the course of PDD (Tröster, 2008).

The neuropsychological profiles of PDD and DLB are similar. There is considerable heterogeneity in the presentation and progression of cognitive deficits, with some patients displaying only minor cognitive slowing. Rapidly fluctuating attention and level of alertness is a signature symptom (Lee et al., 2012) along with abnormal REM-sleep behaviors and anosmia. Overall, the neuropsychological profile of PDD includes bradyphrenia and significant executive and visuospatial impairments (Ballard et al., 2013). Executive dysfunction—including impairments in decision-making and planning—may be among the earliest signs of cognitive decline in PDD. Language problems such as decreased verbal fluency, poor comprehension, and difficulty producing complex sentences can occur frequently. Regardless of domain, patients with Parkinson disease generally perform better on neuropsychological testing than Alzheimer patients. It has been noted that the visuospatial deficits common in Parkinson disease may account for some impairments observed on neuropsychological testing (Toner et al., 2012). Psychiatric manifestations, including mood disturbances, anxiety, apathy, and psychosis, are also common in PDD (Ballard et al., 2013). Similar psychiatric problems are also observed in patients with DLB, with the most striking symptom in these patients being well-formed visual hallucinations (Weintraub et al., 2012). These hallucinations are typically not frightening to the patient. They can be any visual object but often take human or animal form. Severity of visuospatial deficits predicts likelihood of visual hallucinations (Perri et al., 2014). Importantly, both PDD and DLB patients have strong adverse reactions to antipsychotic medications that make their use contraindicated in this group.

In addition to characterizing the cognitive sequelae of PD and the effects of pharmacological treatment, neuropsychologists are often called upon to evaluate candidates for deep brain stimulation (DBS) of the subthalamic nucleus. DBS in this region is known to result in potential global cognitive decline (Witt et al., 2013) in preoperatively intact patients and may be contraindicated in PDD or DLB patients who are already cognitively impaired. Furthermore, older PD patients with MCI prior to DBS may be at greater risk for postoperative declines (Halpern et al., 2009).

Huntington Disease

The diagnosis of Huntington disease (HD) is dependent upon the manifestation of an unequivocal extrapyramidal movement disorder, although cognitive (Paulsen et al., 2014) and behavioral deficits can be the most debilitating aspect of the disease, place the greatest burden on HD families (Nehl and Paulsen, 2004), and can be present in the absence of motor dysfunction (Paulsen and Long, 2014) (see Fig. 43.6 and Fig 43.7). HD is characterized by insidious and progressive cognitive, emotional-behavioral, and motor symptoms. The symptom presentation for any given individual can include one or all of the HD domains. Cognitive symptoms can include forgetfulness, inattention, executive dysfunction, slowed psychomotor speed, negative emotion recognition, and deficits in time discrimination and production. Emotional-behavioral symptoms may include apathy, depression, aggression, disinhibition, anxiety, and obsessive and perseverative behaviors. In response to findings illustrating the prominence of cognitive outcomes in HD, Brooks and Dunnett (2013) reviewed animal models of basal ganglia cognitive impairments suggesting that translation of cognitive outcomes may provide readouts that better track disease for interventional studies. Additionally, readers are referred to new reviews that provide excellent characterization of the human cognitive

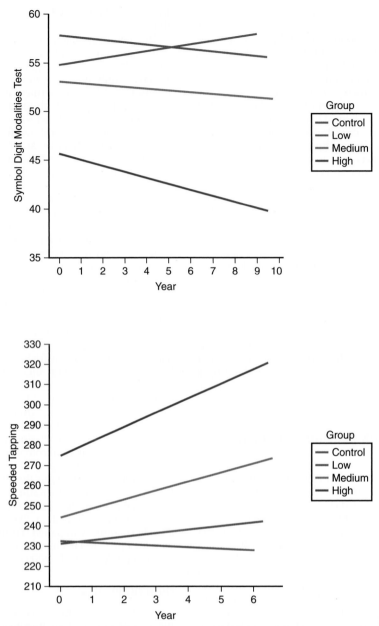

Fig. 43.6 The upper graph shows the fitted curves (based on a linear mixed effects regression fitted model) of the Symbol Digit Modalities Test by year for progression groups (Control, Low probability of near-future diagnosis, Medium probability, High probability). The lower graph shows the fitted curves for speeded tapping. *(From Journal of Neurology, Neurosurgery & Psychiatry, Paulsen, J.S., Smith, M.M., Long, J.D., PREDICT-HD Investigators and Coordinators of the Huntington Study Group, 84, 1233–1239, 2013, with permission from BMJ Publishing Group Ltd.)*

profile of HD (Dumas et al., 2013; O'Callaghan et al., 2014). Efforts to determine the best candidate biomarkers are ongoing.

In a large study of over 1000 research participants with the gene expansion for HD, longitudinal cognitive declines were evident in every test examined (19 tests), with the earliest declines in the Symbol Digit Modality Test, the Smell Identification Test, the Stroop Word Identification Test, and the Trail Making Test evident in a subgroup decades before motor diagnosis (Paulsen et al., 2013, 2014). All cognitive measures examined showed significant changes in the subgroup with the greatest proximity to motor diagnosis, whereas nine of ten cognitive measures showed significant change in the intermediate group (7 to 15 years from motor diagnosis). The

cognitive profile of HD is characterized by bradyphrenia, impairments in executive function, attention, working memory, emotion recognition, smell identification, and the perception and production of time (Paulsen et al., 2013, 2014; Rowe et al., 2010). One author proposed that poor attention in HD may be due to an inability to automatize task performance, which results in the diversion of cognitive resources to tasks that are normally automatic in healthy people (Thompson et al., 2010). This premise is consistent with the well-known deficit HD patients have with procedural learning and memory (Holl et al., 2012) as well as automated behavior such as the Stroop reading task. Memory problems are also frequently reported by patients with HD and their families. Objective deficits in learning and memory have been widely

TABLE 44.1 Actions of Extraocular Muscles

Muscle	Primary	Secondary	Tertiary
Medial rectus	Adduction		
Lateral rectus	Abduction		
Superior rectus	Elevation	Intorsion	Adduction
Inferior rectus	Depression	Extorsion	Adduction
Superior oblique	Intorsion	Depression	Abduction
Inferior oblique	Extorsion	Elevation	Abduction

TABLE 44.2 Yoked Muscle Pairs

Ipsilateral	Contralateral
Medial rectus	Lateral rectus
Superior rectus	Inferior oblique
Inferior rectus	Superior oblique

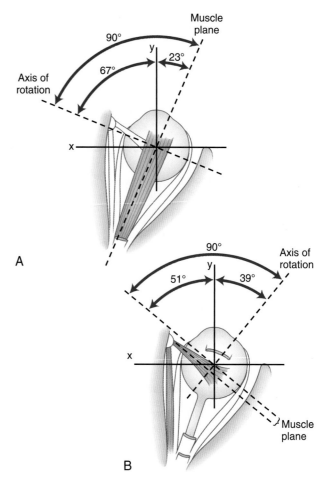

Fig. 44.2 A, Relationship of muscle plane of vertical rectus muscles to x- and y-axes. **B,** Relationship of muscle plane of oblique muscles to x- and y-axes. *(Reprinted with permission from Von Noorden, G.K., 1985. Burian-Von Noorden's Binocular Vision and Ocular Motility, third edn. Mosby, St. Louis.)*

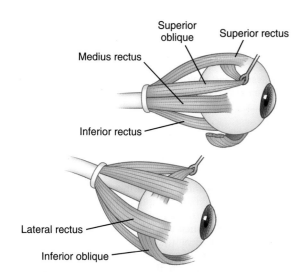

Fig. 44.1 Each eye has six extraocular muscles.

of the globe within the orbit during extraocular muscle contraction.

Images of the same object must fall on corresponding points of each retina to maintain binocular single vision (fusion) and stereopsis (Fig. 44.4). If the visual axes are not aligned, the object is seen by noncorresponding (disparate) points of each retina, and diplopia results (Fig. 44.5). In patients with paralytic strabismus, the image from the nonfixating paretic eye is the false image and is displaced in the direction of action of the weak muscle. Thus, a patient with esotropia has uncrossed diplopia (see Fig. 44.5, *A*), and a patient with exotropia has crossed diplopia (see Fig. 44.5, *B*). After a variable period, the patient learns to ignore or suppress the false image. If suppression occurs before visual maturity (approximately 6 years of age) and persists, central connections in the afferent visual system fail to develop fully, leading to permanent visual impairment in that eye (developmental amblyopia). Amblyopia is more likely to develop with esotropia than with exotropia, because exotropia is commonly intermittent. After visual maturity, suppression and amblyopia do not occur; instead, the patient learns to avoid diplopia by ignoring the false image.

HETEROPHORIAS AND HETEROTROPIAS

When the degree of misalignment, that is, the angle of deviation of the visual axes, is constant, the patient has a comitant strabismus (heterotropia). When it varies with gaze direction, the patient has a noncomitant (paralytic or restrictive) strabismus. In general, comitant strabismus is ophthalmological in origin, whereas noncomitant strabismus is neurological. Some form of ocular misalignment is present in 2% to 3% of preschool children and some form of amblyopia in 3% to 4%.

Most people have a latent tendency for ocular misalignment, *heterophoria*, which may become manifest (*heterotropia*) under conditions of stress such as fatigue, exposure to bright sunlight, or ingestion of alcohol, anticonvulsants, or sedatives. In nonparalytic (comitant) strabismus, the image is projected in the direction opposite the deviation. When such a latent tendency for the visual axes to deviate is unmasked, the diplopia usually is present in most directions of gaze (relatively comitant).

Divergent eyes are designated *exotropic* and convergent eyes are *esotropic*. Vertical misalignment of the visual axes is less common: When the nonfixating eye is higher, the patient is said to have a *hypertropia*, and when it is lower, a *hypotonia* (Donahue, 2007), irrespective of which eye is abnormal; for example, with a right hypertropia, the right eye is higher.

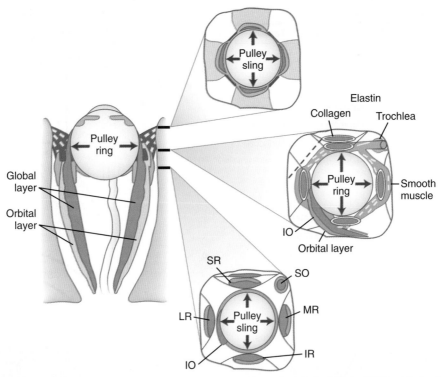

Fig. 44.3 Diagrammatic representation of the structure of orbital connective tissues and their relationship to the fiber layers of the rectus extraocular muscles. Coronal views are represented at levels indicated by the arrows in horizontal section. *IO*, inferior oblique; *IR*, Inferior rectus; *LR*, lateral rectus; *MR*, medial rectus; *SO*, superior oblique; *SR*, superior rectus. *(Redrawn from Demer, J.L., 2002. The orbital pulley system: a revolution in concepts of orbital anatomy. Ann N Y Acad Sci 956, 17–32.)*

Asymptomatic hypertropia on lateral gaze is often a congenital condition or "physiological hyperdeviation."

Comitant Strabismus

New-onset strabismus at school age (after age 6 years) is unusual and warrants evaluation for a neurological disorder. Comitant strabismus occurs early in life; the magnitude of misalignment (deviation) is similar in all directions of gaze, and each eye has a full range of movement (i.e., full ductions). Probably, it occurs because of failure of central mechanisms in the brain that keep the eyes aligned. Infantile (congenital) esotropia may be associated with maldevelopment of the afferent visual system, including the visual cortex, and presents within the first 6 months of life; those with comitant esotropia of more than 40 prism diopters (20 degrees) do not "grow out of it" and require surgical correction (Donahue, 2007). Evidence using cortical motion visual evoked potentials indicates that early correction of strabismus (before 11 months of age) improves visual cortical development (Gerth et al., 2008). Comitant esotropia that manifest between the ages of 6 months and 6 years (average 2½ years) usually is caused by hyperopia (farsightedness) resulting in *accommodative esotropia*: such children with excessive farsightedness must accommodate to have clear vision; the constant accommodation causes excessive convergence and leads to persistent esotropia. Accommodative esotropia responds well to spectacle correction alone. Evidence indicates that high-level stereopsis is restored in these children (unlike those with uncorrected infantile esotropia) if treatment is initiated within 3 months of the onset of constant esotropia (Fawcett et al., 2005).

Occasionally, children with Chiari malformations or posterior fossa tumors present with isolated esotropia before the appearance of other symptoms or signs. Features that suggest a structural cause for the esotropia include presentation after age 6, complaints such as diplopia or headache, incomitance in horizontal gaze, esotropia greater at distance than near, and neurological findings such as abduction deficits, ataxia, optic disc edema, pathological nystagmus, and saccadic pursuit. Adults in whom isolated esotropia develops, particularly when they become presbyopic in their early 40s, should have a cycloplegic refraction to detect *latent hyperopia*. Other causes of adult-onset esotropia include Chiari malformations and acute thalamic hemorrhage (Box 44.1).

Esotropia after the age of 3 months is abnormal and, if constant, usually is associated with development delay, cranial facial syndromes, or structural abnormalities of the eye. It should be corrected early unless contraindicated by one of the above underlying conditions. Intermittent exotropia is common and can be treated with exercises, minus-lens spectacles to stimulate accommodation, or surgery.

Noncomitant (Incomitant) Strabismus

Noncomitant strabismus occurs when the degree of misalignment of the visual axes varies with the direction of gaze as a result of weakness or restriction of one or more extraocular muscles. When a patient with a noncomitant strabismus fixates on an object with the nonparetic eye, the angle of misalignment is referred to as the *primary deviation*. When the patient fixates with the paretic eye, the angle of misalignment is referred to as the *secondary deviation*. Secondary deviation is always greater than primary deviation in noncomitant strabismus because of the Hering law of dual innervation; it may mislead the examiner to believe that the eye with the greater deviation is the weak one (Fig. 44.6).

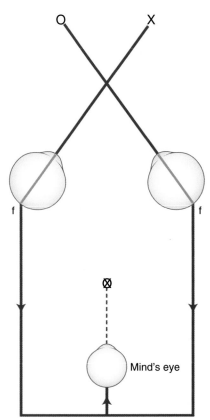

Fig. 44.7 Visual confusion (a rare occurrence). Each fovea (f) views a different object, which is projected to the visual cortex by the cyclopean (mind's) eye and perceived in the same place at the same time.

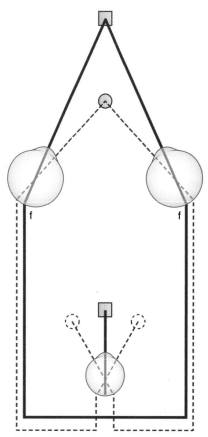

Fig. 44.8 Physiological diplopia. The cyclopean eye views the object *(the square)* as a single object because each fovea (f) fixates it. The images of a nonfixated target *(the circle)* fall on noncorresponding points of each retina, so the object appears double.

diplopia is worse in downgaze, the weak muscle is a depressor. If the diplopia is worse in upgaze, it is an elevator. If one image is tilted, the weak muscle is more likely an oblique rather than a predominantly vertically acting rectus.

Spread of comitance—that is, the tendency for the ocular deviation to "spread" to all fields of gaze—occurs in long-standing cases; then the diplopia no longer obeys the usual rules.

If double vision persists when one eye is covered, the patient has *monocular diplopia*, which may be bilateral. The most common cause of monocular diplopia is an optical aberration (refractive error) and warrants appropriate correction (Box 44.4). Less commonly, monocular diplopia is psychogenic, but occasionally it can be attributed to dysfunction of the retina or cerebral cortex. The *pinhole test* quickly settles the matter. The patient is asked to look through a pinhole; if the cause is refractive, the diplopia abates because optical distortion is eliminated as the light rays entering the eye through the pinhole are aligned along the visual axis and thus not deflected. Oscillopsia (see later discussion) may be misinterpreted as diplopia.

Occasionally, disorders that displace the fovea, such as a subretinal neovascular membrane, can cause binocular diplopia by disrupting the alignment of the photoreceptors *(the dragged-fovea diplopia syndrome or the foveal displacement syndrome)*. The diplopia probably results from rivalry between central and peripheral fusional mechanisms. *Central disruption of fusion* (see later) and *horror fusionis* (in patients with asymmetrical retinal disease) cause intractible diplopia.

Anisoiconia (aniseikonia), defined as a difference of 20% or more between the image size from each eye and usually due to an optical aberration caused by anisometropia or cataract

surgery, can cause diplopia that may resolve with complex optical correction. Small differences in image size, even less than 3%, can cause visual discomfort or asthenopia without frank diplopia.

Clinical Assessment

History

Box 44.5 shows the procedure for assessing patients with diplopia. The following points should be clarified if the patient has not volunteered the information: Is the diplopia relieved by covering either eye? (If not, it is monocular diplopia; see Box 44.4.) Is it worse in the morning or in the evening? Is it affected by fatigue? Are the images separated horizontally, vertically, or obliquely? If obliquely, is the horizontal or vertical component more obvious? Is the distance between images constant despite the direction of gaze, or does it vary? Is the diplopia worse for near vision or for distance? Is one image tilted? Do the eyelids droop? Is the diplopia influenced by head posture? Has this condition remained stable, improved, or deteriorated? Are there any general health problems? Are there associated symptoms such as headache, dizziness, vertigo, or weakness? What medications are taken? Is there a family history of ocular, neurological, autoimmune, or endocrine disease? Has the patient had a "lazy" eye, worn a patch, had strabismus surgery, or had botulinum toxin (Parikh and Lavin, 2011)?

For example, lateral rectus muscle weakness causes diplopia that is worse at distance and worse on looking to the side of the weak muscle. Acutely, superior oblique weakness causes

---

BOX 44.3 Causes of Vertical Diplopia

COMMON CAUSES

- Superior oblique palsy
- Dysthyroid orbitopathy (muscle infiltration)
- Myasthenia
- Skew deviation (brainstem, cerebellar, hydrocephalus)

LESS COMMON CAUSES

- Orbital inflammation (myositis, idiopathic orbital inflammatory syndrome [previously designated "orbital pseudotumor"])
- Orbital infiltration (lymphoma, metastases, amyloid, IgG 4 related disease)
- Primary orbital tumor
- Entrapment of the inferior rectus (blowout fracture)
- Third nerve palsy
- Superior division third nerve palsy
- Atypical third nerve (partial nuclear lesion)
- Aberrant third nerve reinnervation
- Brown syndrome (congenital, acquired)
- Congenital extraocular muscle fibrosis or muscle absence
- Double elevator palsy (monocular elevator deficiency); controversial in origin
- Sagging Eye Syndrome (see its section later in the chapter)

OTHER CAUSES

- Chronic progressive external ophthalmoplegia
- Fisher syndrome
- Botulism
- Monocular supranuclear gaze palsy
- Vertical nystagmus (oscillopsia)
- Stiff person syndrome (associated with hypometric saccades, abduction deficits) (Economides and Horton, 2005)
- Superior oblique myokymia
- Dissociated vertical deviation (divergence)
- Wernicke encephalopathy
- Vertical one-and-a-half syndrome
- Monocular vertical diplopia (see **Box 44.4**)

BOX 44.4 Causes of Monocular Diplopia

- After surgery for long-standing tropia (eccentric fixation)
- Corneal disease (e.g., astigmatism, dry eye, keratoconus)
- Corrected long-standing tropia (eccentric fixation)
- Equipment failure (defective contact lens, ill-fitting bifocals in patients with dementia)
- Foreign body in aqueous or vitreous media
- Iris abnormalities (polycoria, trauma)
- Lens: multirefractile (combined cortical and nuclear cataracts, subluxation)
- Monocular oscillopsia (nystagmus, superior oblique myokymia, eyelid twitching)
- Occipital cortex: migraine, epilepsy, stroke, tumor, trauma (palinopsia, polyopia)
- Psychogenic
- Retinal disease (rarely)

BOX 44.5 Assessment of the Patient with Diplopia

HISTORY

- Define symptoms
- Effect of covering either eye?
- Horizontal or vertical separation of the images?
- Monocular?
- Effect of distance of target (worse at near or far)?
- Effect of gaze direction?
- Tilting of one image?

OBSERVATION

- Head tilt or turn? ("FAT scan")
- Ptosis (fatigue)?
- Pupil size?
- Proptosis?
- Spontaneous eye movements?

EYE EXAMINATION

- Visual acuity (each eye separately, and binocularly if primary position nystagmus present)
- Versions (pursuit, saccades, and muscle overaction)
- Convergence (does miosis occur?)
- Ductions
- Ocular alignment (muscle balance) in the "forced primary position"
- Pupils
- Lids (examine palpebral fissures, levator function, fatigue)
- Vestibulo-ocular reflexes (doll's eye reflex)
- Bell phenomenon
- Prism measurements
- Stereopsis (Titmus stereo test)
- Optokinetic nystagmus

GENERAL NEUROLOGICAL EXAMINATION

OTHER TESTS WHERE INDICATED

- Listen for bruits
- Forced ductions
- Edrophonium (Tensilon) test
- Lights on-off test for *the dragged-fovea diplopia syndrome*
- Ice-pack test for ptosis

"FAT", Family album tomography—review of old photographs for head tilt, pupil size, lids, ocular alignment, etc. For magnification, use ophthalmoscope, magnifying glass, or slit lamp.

General Inspection

Ptosis that fatigues suggests myasthenia gravis (MG). Ptosis associated with a dilated pupil suggests an oculomotor nerve palsy. Lid lag suggests thyroid eye disease or myotonia. Lid retraction suggests thyroid eye disease, aberrant reinnervation after a third nerve palsy, a cyclical third nerve palsy, a dorsal midbrain lesion, hypokalemic periodic paralysis, or chronic corticosteroid use. The association of partial ptosis or elevated upper lid creases, baggy eyelids, superial sulcal enlargement or deformity, and previous blepharoplasty, suggests the sagging eye syndrome (see below). Proptosis suggests an orbital lesion or, if associated with conjunctival injection and periorbital swelling, an inflammatory disorder such as idiopathic orbital inflammatory syndrome (orbital pseudotumor), orbital lymphoma, dural shunt fistula, IgG 4 related disease, or infection. Facial asymmetry suggests a superior oblique palsy that is congenital contralateral to the hemiatrophic side.

Head Posture

Because the weak extraocular muscle cannot move the eye fully, patients compensate by tilting or turning the head in the

---

diplopia that is worse on looking downward to the side opposite the weak muscle and causes difficulty with tasks such as reading, watching television in bed, descending steps, and walking on uneven ground. Medial rectus muscle weakness causes diplopia that is worse for near than for distance vision and is worse to the contralateral side (e.g., with an internuclear ophthalmoplegia- see later).

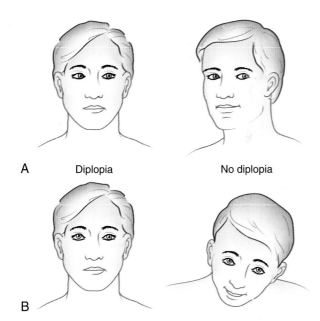

Fig. 44.9 A, Right lateral rectus palsy. A right esotropia is present in primary gaze; however, by turning the head to the right (in the direction of action of the weak right lateral rectus muscle), the patient can maintain both eyes on target (orthotropia), thereby achieving binocular single vision. **B,** Acute right superior oblique muscle palsy. Right eye extorts (excycloduction) because of the unopposed action of the right inferior oblique muscle. When the patient tilts the head to the left and forward (in the direction of action of the weak muscle), the right eye is passively intorted, while the left eye actively intorts to compensate and maintain binocular single vision. The head also tilts forward to compensate for the depressor action of the weak right superior oblique.

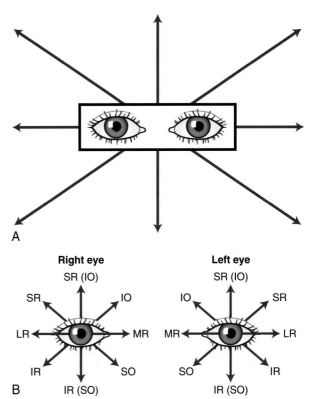

Fig. 44.10 A, The nine diagnostic positions of gaze, used for testing versions (saccades and pursuit). **B,** Ductions are used to test the isolated action of each of the six muscles of each eye (the other five muscles are assumed to be functioning normally). Pure elevation (supraduction) and depression (infraduction) of the eyes are predominantly functions of the superior (SR) and inferior (IR) rectus muscles, respectively, with some help from the oblique muscles. That is, the eyes are rotated directly upward primarily by the SR, with some help from the inferior oblique (IO). The eyes are rotated directly downward primarily by the IR, with some help from the superior oblique (SO). *LR,* Lateral rectus; *MR,* medial rectus.

direction of action of the weak muscle (Fig. 44.9). For example, with right lateral rectus palsy, the head is turned slightly to the right; then on attempted right gaze, the patient turns the head farther to the right (see Fig. 44.9, *A*). With a right superior oblique palsy, the head tilts forward and to the left (see Fig. 44.9, *B*). The rule is as follows: The head turns or tilts in the direction of action of the weak muscle.

Sensory Visual Function

Visual acuity, stereopsis, color vision, and confrontation visual fields should be checked carefully and separately in each eye. Patients with nystagmus should have visual acuity checked binocularly as well, because often it is better than with both eyes viewing than either eye alone.

Stability of Fixation

Fixation and stability of gaze-holding should be checked. This is done by having the patient look at a target and then observing for spontaneous eye movements such as drift, microtremor, nystagmus, opsoclonus, ocular myokymia, ocular myoclonus, or saccadic intrusions.

Versions (Pursuit, Saccades, and Ocular Muscle Overaction)

Pursuit movements are tested by asking the patient to fixate and follow (track) a moving target in all directions (Fig. 44.10, *A*). This test determines the range of eye movement and provides an opportunity to observe for gaze-evoked nystagmus. If spontaneous primary-position nystagmus is present, the effects of the direction of gaze and convergence on the

nystagmus may be determined. Pursuit movements should be smooth and full. Cogwheel (saccadic) pursuit is a nonspecific finding and is normal in infants. When present in only one direction, however, it suggests a defect of the ipsilateral pursuit system.

Saccades (fast eye movements) are tested by asking the patient to look rapidly from one target to another (e.g., from the examiner's nose to a finger or pen) while observing for a delay in initiating the movement (latency) as well as the movement's speed, accuracy, and conjugacy. An internuclear ophthalmoplegia is best detected by this method (Video 44.1). A slow saccade (as in Video 44.1) indicates neurogenic or neuromuscular dysfunction, whereas an incomplete saccade, with normal velocity, indicates limitation of the eye movement by a restrictive disorder (see Box 44.6). If a specific muscle (particularly an oblique) underacts or overacts, this can be observed in eccentric gaze before testing ductions in each eye separately, as shown in Fig. 44.10, *B*. Assessment of disorders of conjugate gaze, which are supranuclear, is discussed later.

Convergence

Convergence is tested by asking patients to fixate on a target moving toward the patient's nasion while observing the alignment of the eyes and constriction of the pupils. Miosis confirms an appropriate effort, whereas its absence suggests less than optimal effort, except in the presence of disorders affecting pupil constriction, such as Adie's pupil, pharmacological mydriasis, etc. (see Chapter 18).

Ductions

Ductions are tested monocularly by having the patient cover one eye and checking the range of movements of the other eye (see Fig. 44.10, *B*). If ductions are not full, the physician should check for restrictive limitation by moving the eye forcibly (see Forced Ductions, later).

Ocular Alignment and Muscle Balance

Before determining ocular alignment, first the examiner must neutralize a head tilt or turn by placing the patient in the "controlled (or forced) primary position"; otherwise, the misalignment may go undetected because of the compensating head posture. Subjective tests of ocular alignment include the red glass, Maddox rod, Lancaster red-green, and Hess screen tests.

With the *red glass test*, the patient views a penlight while a red filter or glass is placed, by convention, over the right eye. This allows easier identification of each image; the right eye views a red light and the left a white light. The addition of a green filter over the left eye, using red-green glasses, further simplifies the test for younger or less reliable patients. The target light is shown to the patient in the nine diagnostic positions of gaze (see Fig. 44.10, *A*). As the light moves into the field of action of a paretic muscle, the images separate. The patient is asked to signify where the images are most widely separated and to describe their relative positions. Interpretation of the results is summarized in Fig. 44.11.

The *Maddox rod test* uses the same principle as the red glass test, but the images are completely dissociated. A point of light seen through the rod, which is a series of half cylinders, is changed to a straight line perpendicular to the cylinders (Fig. 44.12). This dissociation of images (a point of light and a line) breaks fusion, allowing detection of heterophorias as well as heterotropias. Cyclotorsion may be detected by asking if the image of the line is tilted (see Fig. 44.15, *B*). The Maddox rod can be positioned to produce a horizontal, vertical, or oblique line.

A further extension of these tests includes the *Lancaster red-green test* and the *Hess screen test*, which use similar principles. Each eye views a different target (a red light through the red filter and a green light through the green filter). The relative positions of the targets are plotted on a grid screen and analyzed to identify the paretic muscle. These haploscopic tests are used mainly by ophthalmologists to quantitatively follow patients with motility disorders.

The *Hirschberg test*, an objective method of determining ocular deviation in young or uncooperative patients, is performed by observing the point of reflection of a penlight held approximately 30 cm from the patient's eyes (Fig. 44.13); 1 mm of decentration is equal to 7 degrees of ocular deviation. One degree is equal to approximately 2 prism diopters. One prism diopter is the power required to deviate (diffract) a ray of light by 1 cm at a distance of 1 m (Fig. 44.14).

The *cover-uncover test* is determined for both distance (tested at 6 m) and near (tested at 33 cm) vision. The patient is asked to fixate an object held at the appropriate distance. The left eye is covered while the patient maintains fixation on the object. If the right eye is fixating, it remains on target, but if the left eye alone is fixating, the right eye moves onto the object. If the uncovered right eye moves in (adducts), the patient has a right exotropia; if it moves out (abducts), the patient has an esotropia; if it moves down, a right hypertropia; if it moves up, a right hypotropia. The physician should *always*

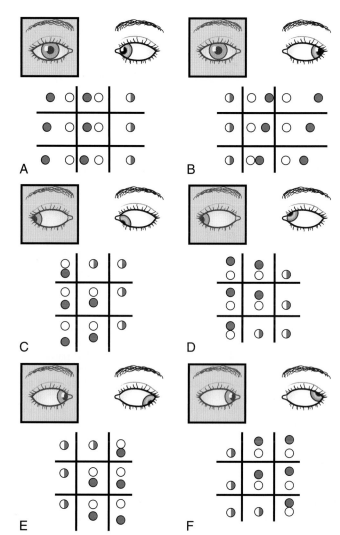

Fig. 44.11 The red glass test. Diplopia fields for each muscle paralysis are shown. By convention, the red glass is placed over the right eye. The charts below each case are displayed as the subject, facing the examiner, indicates the position of the red *(red circle)* and the white *(white circle)* images in the nine diagnostic positions of gaze. **A,** Right lateral rectus palsy. **B,** Right medial rectus palsy. **C,** Right inferior rectus palsy. **D,** Right superior rectus palsy. **E,** Right superior oblique palsy. **F,** Right inferior oblique palsy. *(Reprinted with permission from Cogan, D.G., 1956. Neurology of the Ocular Muscles, second edn. Charles C Thomas, Springfield, IL. Courtesy Charles C Thomas, Publisher, 1956.)*

observe the uncovered eye. The test should be repeated by covering the other eye. If the patient has a tropia, the physician must determine whether it is comitant or noncomitant by checking the degree of deviation in the nine diagnostic cardinal positions of gaze (see Fig. 44.10, *A*). With a lateral rectus palsy, the esotropia increases on looking to the side of the weak muscle and disappears on looking to the opposite side (see Fig. 44.11, *A*). Similarly, with a medial rectus weakness, the patient has an exotropia that increases on looking in the direction of action of that muscle (see Fig. 44.11, *B*). Prisms are used, mainly by ophthalmologists, orthoptists, and optometrists, to measure the degree of ocular deviation (see Fig. 44.14). If the diplopia is due to breakdown of a long-standing (congenital) deviation, prism measurement can detect supranormal fusional amplitudes (large fusional reserves). If

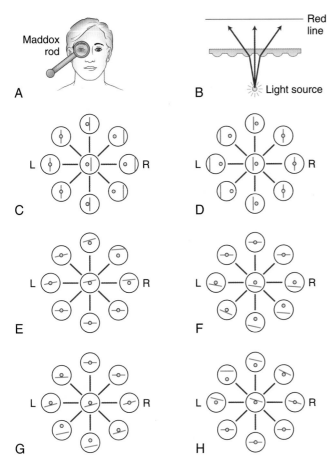

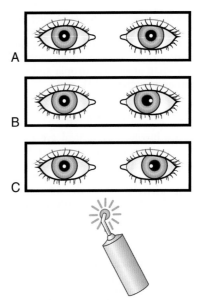

Fig. 44.13 The Hirschberg method for estimating amount of ocular deviation. Displacement of the corneal light reflex of the deviating eye varies with the amount of ocular misalignment. One millimeter is equivalent to approximately 7 degrees of ocular deviation, and 1 degree equals approximately 2 prism diopters. **A,** No deviation (orthotropic). **B,** Left esotropia. **C,** Left exotropia.

Fig. 44.12 The Maddox rod test. (Unlike in Fig. 44.11, the images are displayed as the patient perceives them.) **A,** By convention, the right eye is covered by the Maddox rod, which may be adjusted so the patient sees a red line, at right angles to the cylinders, in the horizontal or vertical plane, as desired (red image seen by the right eye; light source seen by the left eye). **B,** The Maddox rod is composed of a series of cylinders that diffract a point of light to form a line. **C,** Right lateral rectus palsy. **D,** Right medial rectus palsy. **E,** Right superior rectus palsy. **F,** Right inferior rectus palsy. **G,** Right superior oblique palsy. **H,** Right inferior oblique palsy.

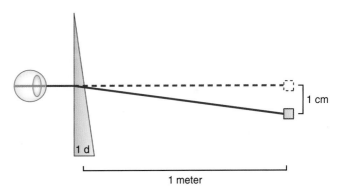

Fig. 44.14 A prism with the power of 1 prism diopter (d) can diffract a ray of light 1 cm at 1 meter.

no manifest deviation of the visual axes is found using the cover-uncover test, the patient is orthotropic. Then the physician may perform the cross-cover test.

During the *cross-cover test* (alternate-cover test), the patient is asked to fixate an object, and then one eye is covered for at least 4 seconds. The examiner should observe the uncovered eye. If the patient is orthotropic, the uncovered eye does not move, but the covered eye loses fixation and assumes its position of rest—latent deviation (heterophoria or phoria). In that case, when the covered eye is uncovered, it refixates by moving back; the uncovered eye is immediately covered and loses fixation. The cross-cover test prevents binocular viewing, and thus foveal fusion, by always keeping one eye covered. Unlike the cover-uncover test, the cross-cover test detects heterophoria. Most normal persons are exophoric because of the natural alignment of the orbits.

Fixation switch diplopia occurs in patients with long-standing strabismus who partially lose visual acuity in the fixating eye, usually as a result of a cataract or refractive error. Such patients normally avoid double vision by ignoring the false image from the nonfixating eye, but a significant decrease in acuity in the

"good" eye forces them to fixate with the weak eye. This causes misalignment of the previously good eye and results in diplopia. Fixation switch diplopia usually can be treated successfully with appropriate optical management.

Dissociated vertical deviation (divergence) is an asymptomatic congenital anomaly that usually is discovered during the cover test. While the patient fixates an object, one eye is covered. The covered eye loses fixation and rises; the uncovered eye maintains fixation but may turn inward. This congenital ocular motility phenomenon usually is bilateral but frequently is asymmetrical and often associated with amblyopia, esotropia, and latent nystagmus (LN). Whether the number of axons decussating in the chiasm is excessive, as suggested by evoked potential studies, remains controversial. Dissociated vertical deviation has no other clinical significance.

The sagging eye syndrome

Age-related involution (atrophy) of orbital connective tissue can cause "sagging" of the orbital pulleys (see earlier) and extraocular muscles, resulting in *the sagging eye syndrome*. It occurs about the age of seventy years: When the orbits are affected symetrically it causes divergence insufficiency and impaired elevation of both eyes; when it occurs asymmetrically it causes a small angle hypertropia and verticular diplopia (Chaudhuri and Demer, 2013).

Three-Step Test for Vertical Diplopia

Eight muscles are involved in vertical eye movements: four elevators and four depressors. The three-step test endeavors to determine whether one particular paretic muscle is responsible for vertical diplopia (Fig. 44.15). Using the cover-uncover test, which is objective, or one of the subjective tests such as the red glass test, the physician can perform the three-step test for vertical diplopia. When using one of the subjective tests, it is important to remember that the hypertropic eye views the lower image.

- *Step 1* determines which eye is higher (hypertropic) in primary position. The patient's head may have to be repositioned (controlled primary position) to neutralize any compensatory tilt. If the right eye is higher, the weak muscle is either one of the two depressors of the right eye (inferior rectus or superior oblique) or one of the two elevators of the left eye (superior rectus or inferior oblique).
- *Step 2* determines whether the hypertropia increases on left or right gaze. If a right hypertropia increases on left gaze, the weak muscle is either the depressor in the right eye, which acts best in adduction (i.e., the superior oblique), or the elevator in the left eye, which acts best in abduction (i.e., the superior rectus), and vice versa.
- *Step 3* determines whether the hypertropia changes when the head tilts to the left or the right. If a right hypertropia increases on head tilt right, the weak muscle must be an intortor of the right eye (superior oblique); if it increases on head tilt left, the weak muscle must be an intortor of the left eye (superior rectus).

Two more optional steps:

- *Step 4* uses one of a number of techniques (e.g., double Maddox rod, visual field blind spots, indirect ophthalmoscopy, fundus photography) to determine whether ocular torsion is present. Establishing the degree and direction of ocular torsion, if any, can differentiate a skew deviation from a superior oblique palsy. Because the primary action of the superior oblique muscle is incyclotorsion (see Table 44.1), an acute palsy typically results in approximately 5 degrees of excyclotorsion of the affected eye due to unopposed action of the ipsilateral inferior oblique muscle. If either eye is intorted, a superior oblique palsy is not responsible, and the patient may have a skew deviation (Donahue et al., 1999).
- *Step 5* is helpful in the acute phase. If the deviation is greater on downgaze, the weak muscle is a depressor; if it is worse on upgaze, the weak muscle is likely to be an elevator. This fifth step is helpful only in the acute stage, because with time the deviation becomes more comitant.

The examiner should be aware of the pitfalls of the three-step test—namely, the conditions in which the rules break down. These include restrictive ocular myopathies (Box 44.6), long-standing strabismus, skew deviation, and disorders involving more than one muscle.

The four fundamental features of the fourth cranial nerve are: (1) it has the longest intracranial course and is the thinnest of all the cranial nerves and thus very susceptible to injury; (2) it is the only cranial nerve that exits the neuraxis dorsally; (3) its nucleus of origin is on the contralateral side

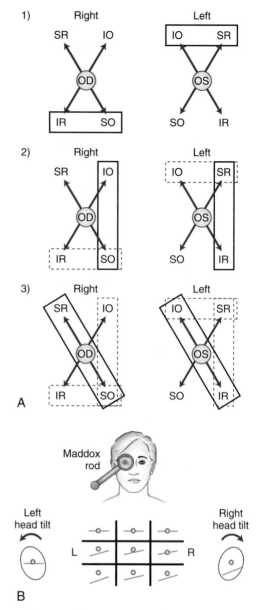

Fig. 44.15 Example of the three-step test in a patient with an acute right superior oblique palsy. A, If a patient has a hypertropia, one of eight muscles may be responsible for the vertical ocular deviation. Identifying the higher eye eliminates four muscles. Step 1: With a right hypertropia, the weak muscle is either one of the two depressors of the right eye (IR or SO) or one of the two elevators of the left eye (IO or SR) *(enclosed by solid line)*. Step 2: If the deviation (or displacement of images) is greater on left gaze, one of the muscles acting in left gaze *(enclosed by solid line)* must be responsible, in this case either the depressor in the right eye (SO) or the elevator in the left eye (SR). Step 3: If the deviation is greater on right head tilt, the incyclotors of the right eye (SR and SO) or the excyclotortors of the left eye (IR and IO) *(enclosed)* must be responsible, in this case, the right SO—that is, the muscle enclosed three times. If the deviation was greater on left head tilt, the left SR would be responsible. *IO,* Inferior oblique; *IR,* inferior rectus; *SO,* superior oblique; *SR,* superior rectus. **B,** The Maddox rod test (displayed as in Fig. 44.12, as the subject perceives the images) in a patient with a right SO palsy shows vertical separation of the images that is worse in the direction of action of the weak muscle and demonstrates subjective tilting of the image from the right eye. When the head is tilted toward the left shoulder, the separation disappears, but when the head is tilted to the right shoulder, to the side of the weak muscle, the separation is exacerbated (Bielschowsky's third step).

---

nystagmus may be dysconjugate because the amplitude is greater in the abducting eye. A torsional component is seen sometimes. Physiological nystagmus is distinguished from pathological nystagmus by its symmetry on right and left gaze and by the absence of other neurological features. It is not present when the angle of gaze is less than 30 degrees from primary position. Oculographic recordings demonstrate a linear slow phase (see Fig. 44.17, B) and may detect transient small-amplitude rebound nystagmus.

Dysconjugate Nystagmus

Dysconjugate (dissociated) nystagmus occurs when the ocular oscillations are out of phase (in different directions). It is seen with internuclear ophthalmoplegia, other brainstem lesions (see earlier discussion of pendular vergence nystagmus under Pendular Nystagmus), and spasmus nutans. Monocular nystagmus also is dysconjugate and may be associated with amblyopia and other forms of vision loss (Box 44.11).

Monocular Nystagmus

Monocular nystagmus may be pendular or jerk and also may be horizontal, vertical, or oblique. Oculographic recordings may reveal small-amplitude oscillations in the fellow eye. Monocular nystagmus may occur in patients with *alternating hemiplegia of childhood* (Egan, 2002), amblyopia, strabismus, monocular blindness, spasmus nutans, internuclear ophthalmoplegia, MS, or (rarely) seizures, and of course when the other eye is completely ophthalmoplegic or absent.

The *Heimann-Bielschowsky phenomenon* is a rare form of monocular vertical pendular oscillation, with a frequency of 1 to 5 Hz, that occurs in an amblyopic eye or after acquired monocular vision loss, such as with cataract. In the latter situation, it may be reversible after successful treatment of the underlying condition or with gabapentin (Rahman et al., 2006).

Superior oblique myokymia may be mistaken for a monocular torsional or vertical nystagmus (see Box 44.11).

Upbeat Nystagmus

Upbeat nystagmus is a spontaneous jerk nystagmus with the fast phase upward while the eyes are in primary position (Video 44.4). It is attributed to interruption of the anterior semicircular canal projections, which are responsible for the upward vestibulo-ocular reflex, causing downward drift of the eyes with corrective upward saccades. The amplitude and intensity of the nystagmus usually increase on upgaze. This finding strongly suggests bilateral paramedian lesions of the brainstem, usually at the pontomedullary or pontomesencephalic junction, the paramedian tract neurons in the lower medulla, or midline cerebellum (vermis). Upbeat nystagmus may result from Wernicke encephalopathy or intoxication with anticonvulsants, organophosphates, lithium, nicotine, or thallium (author's personal observation). Rarely, upbeat nystagmus may be congenital. In infants, upbeat nystagmus may be a sign of anterior visual pathway disease, such as Leber congenital amaurosis (see Chapter 45), optic nerve hypoplasia, aniridia, or cataracts. Small-amplitude upbeat nystagmus may be seen in persons who are carriers of blue-cone monochromatism, whereas affected patients may have intermittent pendular oblique nystagmus. If the intensity of upbeat nystagmus diminishes in downgaze, base-up prisms over both eyes may improve the oscillopsia; Medications such as memantine also may be helpful (Table 44.4). For an extensive list of causes of upbeat nystagmus, see Leigh and Zee's textbook (2006).

A variant of upbeat nystagmus called "bow-tie nystagmus" is reported with posterior fossa medial medullary stroke (Choi et al., 2004) and is characterized by obliquely upward fast phases alternating to the left or right because of the changing direction of each horizontal component (Leigh and Zee, 2006).

Downbeat Nystagmus

Downbeat nystagmus is the most common form of acquired primary position nystagmus; it is a spontaneous downward-beating jerk nystagmus present in primary position and is attributed to either (1) interruption of the posterior semicircular canal projections, which are responsible for the downward vestibulo-ocular reflex (VOR), causing upward drift of the eyes with corrective downward saccades, or (2) impaired cerebellar inhibition of the vestibular circuits for upward eye movements, resulting in uninhibited upward drifting of the eyes, with corrective downward saccades (Video 44.5). The amplitude of the oscillations increases significantly when the eyes are deviated laterally and slightly downward (Daroff sign), particularly when the oscillations are subtle in primary gaze.

Downbeat nystagmus may be apparent only with changes in posture (positional downbeat nystagmus), particularly the head-hanging position. Downbeat nystagmus results from either damage to the commissural fibers between the vestibular nuclei in the floor of the fourth ventricle or bilateral damage to the flocculus that disinhibits the VOR in pitch; frequently it occurs with structural lesions at the craniocervical junction (Box 44.12). MRI of the foramen magnum region (in the sagittal plane) is the imaging investigation of choice. In some cases of unexplained downbeat nystagmus, the cause is a radiographically occult infarction; however, lesions that cause downbeat nystagmus are bilateral. Causes of downbeat nystagmus are listed in Box 44.12. The treatment of downbeat nystagmus involves correction of the underlying cause when possible. When downbeat nystagmus damps on convergence, it may be treated successfully with base-out prisms, reducing the oscillopsia and improving the visual acuity. Medications including clonazepam, and the aminopyridines may help as well (see Table 44.4); 4-aminopyridine is more effective in downbeat nystagmus associated with cerebellar atrophy rather than structural lesions (Huppert et al., 2011), and the sustained release form (dalfampyridine) may be more effective (Claassen et al., 2013).

Both upbeat and downbeat nystagmus may be altered in amplitude and direction by a variety of maneuvers (e.g., convergence, head tilting, changes in posture) and by 3,4-diaminopyridine (Leigh and Zee, 2006).

Periodic Alternating Nystagmus

Periodic alternating nystagmus (PAN) is a horizontal jerk nystagmus in which the fast phase beats in one direction and then

TABLE 44.4 Treatment of Nystagmus and Non-Nystagmus Oscillations*

Nystagmus syndrome	Treatment
Infantile nystagmus syndrome	Prisms Contact lenses Extraocular muscle surgery Kestenbaum-Anderson procedure Tenotomy and reattachment procedure (experimental) Acetazolamide 250–1000 mg bid (Thurtell et al., 2012) Brinzolamide 1% eye drops, 1 drop OU bid (Thurtell et al., 2012) Gabapentin 300–600 mg qid (Shery et al., 2006; Thurtell et al., 2012) Gene therapy (experimental) when the nystagmus is associated with retinal disorders (Leigh and Zee, 2006)
Acquired Pendular Nystagmus	Trihexyphenidyl 5–20 mg tid, benztropine, clonazepam .5–1 mg bid, gabapentin 300 mg qid, isoniazid, memantine 10 mg qid[†] (Leigh and Zee, 2006), valproate, diethylpropion hydrochloride, tenotomy followed by memantine (Tomsak et al., 2006), hand held muscle massager (vibrator) held to the head (Beh et al., 2014)
Convergence-evoked horizontal	Base-in prisms nystagmus
Downbeat nystagmus	Base-out prisms (if nystagmus damps with convergence) Base-down prisms over both eyes if intensity of nystagmus diminishes in upgaze Contact lenses (personal observation) Extraocular muscle surgery realignment (Dohahue, personal communication, and observation) Baclofen 5 mg tid, chlorzoxazone 500 mg tid (Feil et al. 2013), betahistine, clonazepam .5–1mg bid, gabapentin, scopolamine, 4-AMP 5–10 mg tid (dalfampridine, the sustained-release form of 4-AMP @ 10 mg bid may be more effective than 4-AMP [Claassen et al., 2013]) , 3,4-diaminopyridine 10–20 mg bid Brinzolamide 1% eye drops, 1 drop OU bid (personal observation)

Periodic Alternating Nystagmus:
  Congenital
  Acquired
	
	Dextroamphetamine, baclofen 5–10 mg tid (occasionally), 5-HT
	Baclofen 5–10 mg tid, phenytoin, memantine 5–10 mg qid

Upbeat nystagmus	Base-up prisms over both eyes if intensity of nystagmus diminishes in downgaze Baclofen 5–10 mg tid, gabapentin, 4-aminopyridine 5–10 mg tid-qid, memantine 10 mg qid (Thurtell et al., 2010), thiamine
Oculopalatal myoclonus	Chronically patch one eye Baclofen, carbamazepine, cerulein, clonazepam, gabapentin 300 mg qid, memantine 10 mg qid, scopolamine, trihexyphenidyl 5–20 mg tid, valproate
Seesaw Nystagmus	Baclofen, clonazepam .5–1 mg bid, gabapentin, memantine 10 mg qid (Huppert et al., 2011), base-out prisms
Hemi-Seesaw Nystagmus	Memantine (Thurtell et al., 2010)
Ictal nystagmus	AEDs

Episodic nystagmus:
  Episodic ataxia-1
  Episodic ataxia-2
	
	Acetazolamide 125–1000 mg bid
	Acetazolamide 125–1000 mg bid, 4-aminopyridine 5–10 mg tid, (Strupp et al., 2011), dalfampridine 10 mg bid

Oculomasticatory myorhythmia	Antibiotics for Whipple disease; consider gabapentin or memantine
Torsional nystagmus	Gabapentin 300 mg qid, memantine (Thurtell et al., 2010)
Non-nystagmus ocular oscillations	**Treatment**
Opsoclonus	Treat underlying condition when possible, ACTH, vitamin B1, clonazepam, gabapentin, ondansetron, steroids; if paraneoplastic, protein A immunoabsorption
Superior oblique myokymia	Carbamazepine, gabapentin, oxcarbazepine, other AEDs, topical beta-blockers, memantine, base-down prism over the affected eye, muscle/tendon surgery, microvascular decompression
Ocular neuromyotonia	Carbamazepine, oxcarbazepine (Whitted and Lavin, personal observation)
Microflutter	Propranolol, verapamil
Saccadic intrusions	Memantine (Serra et al., 2008)
Square-wave jerks	Valproate, amphetamines, barbiturates, diazepam, clonazepam, memantine (Leigh and Zee, 2006)
Square-wave oscillations	Valproate

ACTH, Adrenocorticotropic hormone; *AEDs*, antiepileptic drugs; *5-HT*, 5-hydroxytryptamine; *APN*, acquired pendular nystagmus; *PAN*, periodic alternating nystagmus; *SSN*, seesaw nystagmus; *4-AMP*, 4-aminopyridine.
*Treat underlying cause when possible.
[†]Memantine is reported to exacerbate MS (Villoslada el al., 2009).

TABLE 44.6 Ocular Bobbing

Type	Movement	Cause
Ocular bobbing (atypical bobbing, horizontal eye movements preserved)	Fast down, slow upward return to primary position	Severe central pontine destruction, central pontine myelinolysis, encephalitis, extra-axial pontine compression (usually a cerebellar hematoma), organophosphate poisoning
Reverse bobbing	Fast up, slow downward return to primary position	Usually nonlocalizing encephalopathy: anoxia, metabolic encephalopathy, head injury, post status epilepticus
Dipping (inverse bobbing)	Slow down, fast upward return to primary position	Anoxic, metabolic, and toxic position encephalopathies, post status epilepticus
Reverse dipping	Slow up, fast downward return to primary position	Cryptococcal meningitis or obtundation (in a patient with acquired immunodeficiency syndrome), pontine stroke
V-pattern pretectal pseudobobbing	Fast downward convergent movements at higher frequency, and slower return to primary position than with typical bobbing	Acute obstructive hydrocephalus

with a seizure disorder and chronic meningitis. Bobbing may be dysconjugate (see Table 44.6).

V-pattern pretectal pseudobobbing, a higher-frequency, more rapid downward convergent movement with a slower than normal return toward primary position, occurs with acute obstructive hydrocephalus and is an indication for urgent decompression. Some patients may exhibit more than one type of bobbing.

Ocular Myoclonus (Oculopalatal Tremor)

Ocular myoclonus is a vertical pendular oscillation with a frequency of approximately 160 Hz, usually associated with similar oscillations of the soft palate (palatal tremor) and sometimes other muscles of branchial origin (Leigh and Zee, 2006). The palatal tremor, referred to as the *oculopalatal syndrome*, occurs after brainstem infarction, particularly of the pons, involving the central tegmental tract. Following a latency of months, hypertrophic degeneration of the inferior olives ensues and the myoclonus begins. The association of a facial nerve palsy and the one-and-a-half syndrome may predict the development of oculopalatal myoclonus, probably because of the proximity of the central tegmental tract to the facial nerve. Also, oculopalatal myoclonus can occur spontaneously in association with progressive ataxia, a fourth ventricular tumor, or hydrocephalus following subarachnoid hemorrhage. Dys-

function of the cerebellar nuclei or their connections (Guillain-Mollaret triangle) and disruption of retinal error signals relayed to the inferior olive may be responsible for oculopalatal myoclonus, which is confined to the muscles of branchial origin. Patients may get some relief from anticonvulsants such as carbamazepine, clonazepam, gabapentin, memantine (Thurtell et al., 2010), valproic acid, and agents such as trihexyphenidyl hydrochloride and cerulein, or by chronically patching one eye. Palatal tremor may respond to botulinum injections. Palatal tremor should be distinguished from pulsations of the uvula that are synchronous with the systolic pulse (Muller sign) in patients with aortic regurgitation (Williams and Steinberg, 2006).

Superior Oblique Myokymia

Superior oblique myokymia is a paroxysmal, rapid, small-amplitude, monocular torsional-vertical oscillation caused by contraction of the superior oblique muscle, predominantly on the right side. Patients may complain of monocular blurring, torsional or vertical oscillopsia, torsional or vertical diplopia, or twitching of the eye. Oculography using magnetic search coils demonstrates both phasic and tonic contractions of intorsion, depression, and to a much lesser extent, abduction of the superior oblique muscle (Leigh and Zee, 2006). MRI demonstrated that the affected superior oblique muscle was smaller in some patients, suggesting antecedent injury to the fourth nerve; this hypothesis is supported by an MRI finding of neurovascular compression of the fourth nerve at its root exit zone.

Superior oblique myokymia may be difficult to detect with the unaided eye and is more easily detected with a direct ophthalmoscope. It may be precipitated by activating the superior oblique muscle when the patient looks down in the direction of action of that muscle or tilts the head toward the affected eye. Superior oblique myokymia has a relapsing-remitting course in otherwise normal, healthy adults. It is reported with adrenoleukodystrophy, lead poisoning, cerebellar astrocytoma, dural arteriovenous fistula, and microvascular compression.

Superior oblique myokymia may respond dramatically to medication such as carbamazepine or gabapentin, propranolol in low dosage, amitriptyline, baclofen, phenytoin, benzodiazepines, or topical beta-blockers used for glaucoma (see Table 44.4). A base-down prism in front of the affected eye may alleviate the patient's symptoms, avoid potential side effects of long-term medication, and obviate superior oblique muscle or tendon surgery occasionally used in resistant cases. Disabling superior oblique myokymia may respond to microvascular decompression of the trochlear nerve at its root exit.

Saccadic Intrusions and Oscillations

Saccadic intrusions such as square wave jerks are brief, unwanted, nonrepetitive saccadic interruptions of fixation (Box 44.14) (Video 44.8). Other intrusions are saccadic pulses (stepless saccades) that interrupt fixation and are followed by a slow drift back on target (glissade), double saccadic pulses (fragment of flutter), and dynamic overshoots (see Fig. 44.29). Macrosaccadic oscillations—macro square wave jerks—are discussed later.

GENERATION AND CONTROL OF EYE MOVEMENTS

A reasonable understanding and interpretation of gaze disorders require an appreciation of the anatomy and physiology

---

BOX 44.14 Saccadic Oscillations

- Flutter (voluntary, involuntary)
- Flutter dysmetria
- Microsaccadic flutter (variant of voluntary flutter?)
- Opsoclonus
- Macro–square wave jerks (now designated *square-wave pulses*)
- Ocular bobbing, reverse and inverse bobbing, dipping, and reverse dipping
- Superior oblique myokymia
- Convergence-retraction nystagmus
- Abduction nystagmus with internuclear ophthalmoplegia
- Tic-like ocular myoclonic jerks (eye tics)

---

of eye movement control. In the words of J. Hughlings Jackson, "The study of the cause of things must be preceded by study of things caused."

Normal visual behavior is accomplished by a continuous cycle of visual fixation and visual analysis interrupted by saccades. Individuals with intact sensory visual systems (optical and afferent) are capable of discerning small details comparable to Snellen acuity of 20/13, provided the image of the target is maintained within 0.5 degree of the center of the fovea. However, 10 degrees from fixation, the resolving power of the retina drops to 20/200. Although the peripheral retina has poor spatial resolution capabilities, it is exquisitely sensitive to movement (temporal resolution). The image of an object entering the peripheral visual field stimulates the retina to signal the ocular motor system to make a rapid eye movement (saccade) and fixate it on the fovea. In the words of American psychologist William James, "The peripheral retina is like a sentinel and when an object of regard falls upon it, it shouts 'hark, who goes there' and calls the fovea to the spot." Visual information concerning spatial resolution (fine detail) and color travels via retinal ganglion (P) cells to the parvocellular layers of the lateral geniculate nucleus (LGN), whereas information concerning temporal resolution (movement) travels via retinal ganglion (M) cells to the magnocellular layer of the LGN. In turn, neurons in the LGN project via the optic radiations to the primary visual area (V1), the striate cortex (area 17).

Visual processing in the cortex begins in the primary visual area from which issues two processing streams (Fig. 44.19, A). The ventral stream, responsible for form and object recognition and emphasizing foveal representation, projects to the temporal lobe via occipital areas V2 and V4. The dorsal stream, responsible for movement recognition, guiding actions in space, and emphasizing peripheral visual field representation, projects to the prestriate cortex; then it relays to the superior temporal sulcus region, which contains cortical areas MT (middle temporal) and MST (middle superior temporal) in monkeys, roughly equivalent to the parietotemporo-occipital junction (PTO) in humans, and detects location, direction, and velocity of objects. Both streams converge on the FEF (frontal eye field) and are involved in controlling saccades (see later discussion). The premotor substrates for conjugate gaze and vergence eye movements are in the brainstem. The substrates specific for vertical gaze, vergence, and ocular counter-rolling are in the mesodiencephalic region, whereas those for horizontal eye movements are mainly in the pons. Our understanding of the mechanisms for eye movements is based on clinicopathological and radiological correlation as well as animal and bioengineering experiments. With the exception of reflexive movements such as the VOR and fast phases of nystagmus, cerebral structures determine *when* and *where* the eyes move, whereas brainstem mechanisms determine *how* they move. In other words, voluntary eye movements are generated in the brainstem but are triggered by the cerebral cortex.

Ocular Motor Subsystems

Eye movements are of two main types: those that redirect gaze to different objects of interest and those that stabilize the image of the target on each retina and maintain binocular foveation during head or target movement, or both. The saccadic system moves the eyes rapidly (up to 800 degrees per second) to fixate new targets (Fig. 44.20, A). Saccades may be generated voluntarily or in response to verbal commands in the absence of a visible target. Reflex saccades may occur in response to peripheral retinal stimuli such as visual threat or retinal error signals, or to sound. Saccades also are the fast components of nystagmus.

The pursuit system enables the eyes to track slowly moving targets (up to 70 degrees per second) to maintain the image stable on the fovea. Specially trained subjects are capable of smooth-pursuit eye movements as fast as 100 degrees per second. Pursuit eye movements are limited more by the target's acceleration than by its velocity. If the target moves too quickly or changes direction abruptly, or if the pursuit system is impaired, the eyes are unable to maintain pace with the target and fall behind. Consequently, the image moves off the fovea, producing a retinal error signal that provokes a corrective (catch-up) saccade and refixates the target. The cycle then repeats itself, resulting in saccadic ("cogwheel") pursuit (see Fig. 44.20, B).

Bidirectionally defective pursuit eye movements, a normal finding in infants, are nonspecific and occur under conditions of stress or fatigue or with sedative medication. However, impaired tracking in one direction suggests a structural lesion of the ipsilateral pursuit system (see Fig. 44.20, B).

Fixation allows the eyes to maintain an image of a stationary target on each fovea at rest. The fixation subsystem shares neural circuitry with the optokinetic and pursuit systems (Leigh and Zee, 2006).

The vestibular eye movement subsystem maintains a stable image on the retina during head movements. The semicircular canals respond to rotational acceleration of the head by driving the VOR to maintain the eyes in the same direction in space during head movements. The otoliths (utricle and saccule) are gravity receptors that respond to linear acceleration and static head tilt (gravity)—that is, with ocular counter-rolling. The vestibular system is discussed further in Chapter 46.

The optokinetic system uses visual reference points in the environment to maintain orientation. It complements the vestibulo-ocular system, which becomes less responsive during slow or sustained head movements, to stabilize images on the retina in situations such as large turns or spinning. When the eyes reach their limit of movement in the orbits, a reflex saccade allows refixation to a point further forward in the direction of head rotation. The sequence repeats itself, resulting in OKN.

In humans, the optokinetic system responds predominantly to fixation and pursuit of a moving target (immediate component) and to a lesser extent velocity storage (delayed component), which involves neural circuitry in the vestibular system. (*Velocity storage* is a mechanism by which the CNS, predominantly the vestibular system including the vestibulocerebellum, prolongs or causes perseveration of short signals generated by the vestibular end-organ to enhance orientation in space. Velocity storage is largely involuntary.) The optokinetic system probably evolved to supplement the vestibular system during sustained rotations.

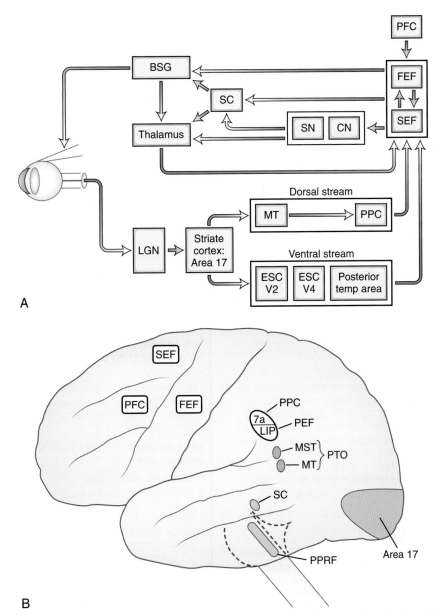

Fig. 44.19 A, Overview of the combined afferent and efferent visual system. **B,** Areas in the human brain that are believed to be important in generating saccades and pursuit. *BSG,* Brainstem saccadic generator; *CN,* caudate nucleus; *ESC,* extrastriate cortex; *FEF,* frontal eye field; *LGN,* lateral geniculate nucleus; *LIP,* lateral intraparietal area; *MST,* medial superior temporovisual area; *MT,* middle temporovisual area; *PEF,* parietal eye field; *PFC,* prefrontal cortex; *PPC,* posterior parietal cortex area; *PPRF,* paramedian pontine reticular formation; *PTO,* parietotemporo-occipital junction; *SC,* superior colliculus; *SEF,* supplementary eye fields in the supplementary motor area; *7a,* area 7a; *SN,* substantia nigra. *(A Redrawn from Stuphorn, V., Schall, J.D., 2002. Neuronal control and monitoring of the initiation of movements. Muscle Nerve 26, 326–339.)*

The vergence system enables the eyes to move disconjugately (converge and diverge), in the horizontal plane, to maintain binocular fixation on a target moving toward or away from the subject. Vergence movements are essential for binocular single vision and stereoscopic depth perception.

The different types of eye movements are listed in Box 44.15.

Horizontal Eye Movements

When gaze is redirected from one point to another, a saccade moves the eyes conjugately. To enable the small, straplike extraocular muscles to move the relatively large globes and overcome inertia and the elastic recoil of the viscous orbital contents, the yoked agonist muscles require a surge or *burst* of innervation (pulse) at the same time as their yoked antagonists are reciprocally inhibited (Fig. 44.21, A). For a leftward saccade, the left lateral rectus and the right medial rectus muscles each receive a pulse of innervation while their antagonists, the left medial and right lateral rectus muscles, are reciprocally inhibited. Excitatory burst neurons (EBNs) contained in the ipsilateral paramedian pontine reticular formation (PPRF) just rostral to the abducens nucleus generate the pulse to initiate the saccade. The EBNs are medium-lead burst cells that discharge about 10 msec before and during all horizontal saccadic eye movements; they discharge preferentially for ipsilateral saccades and create the immediate premotor command, generating pulse activity for saccades.

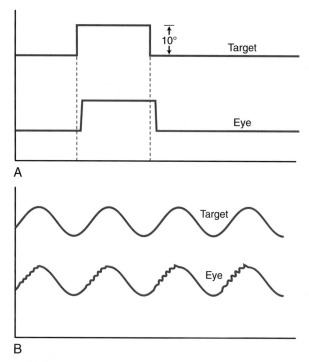

A

B

Fig. 44.20 Simulated eye movement recordings. By convention for horizontal movements, upward deflections represent rightward eye movements, and downward deflections represent leftward eye movements. **A,** Saccades. A target moves rapidly 10 degrees to the right. After a latency of about 200 msec, the eye follows. When the target returns to the center, the sequence is repeated in the opposite direction. **B,** Pursuit. The target moves in a sinusoidal pattern in front of the patient. The eye follows the target after a latency of about 120 msec, but pursuit movements to the right are defective, resulting in the rightward "cogwheel" (saccadic) pursuit. Pursuit to the left is normal.

About half the neurons in the abducens nucleus are interneurons (with different morphological and pharmacological features than the neurons of the abducens nerve) that relay, via the medial longitudinal fasciculus (MLF), to the contralateral medial rectus neurons in the oculomotor nuclear complex (Fig. 44.22). Except just before and during a saccade, the EBNs are tonically suppressed by omnipause neurons located in the nucleus raphe interpositus rostral to the abducens nucleus. The trigger that initiates a saccade also inhibits the omnipause neurons. Subsequently, hypothetical latch neurons in the reticular formation, which receive input from the EBNs, inhibit omnipause neurons until the saccade is complete (Leigh and Zee, 2006). Latch neurons are active during pursuit also. Disorders of latch neurons may result in prematurely terminated saccades and very hypometric saccades in disorders such as Parkinson disease (PD). Thus the omnipause neurons, which receive input from the cerebrum, cerebellum, and superior colliculus (SC), mediate the command for a saccade when they cease discharging and allow the burst cells to fire (Fig. 44.23). While the EBNs discharge, a group of inhibitory cell-burst neurons that lie caudal to the abducens nucleus in the medial rostral medulla and project across the midline to the contralateral abducens nucleus discharge during the saccade to reciprocally inhibit the yoked antagonist muscles (Leigh and Zee, 2006).

To maintain the eyes on target in an eccentric position at the end of a saccade, the agonist muscles for a leftward movement (left lateral and right medial recti) now require a new level of tonic innervation—a position command—achieved by a group

BOX 44.15　Types of Eye Movements

SACCADES (MOVE EYES FROM ONE TARGET TO ANOTHER)

- Intentional saccades (internally triggered, with a goal):
  - Visually guided saccades
  - Memory-guided saccades (with visual/vestibular input)
  - Predictive saccades
  - Target-searching saccades
  - Antisaccades*
- Reflexive saccades (externally triggered):
  - Visually guided saccades
  - Auditory saccades
- Spontaneous saccades (internally triggered, without a goal):
  - During another motor activity
  - At rest
  - When sleeping
- Quick phases of nystagmus:
  - Physiological nystagmus:
    - Vestibular nystagmus
    - Optokinetic nystagmus
  - End-point nystagmus
  - Pathologic nystagmus

EYE MOVEMENTS STABILIZING THE IMAGE OF THE TARGET ON THE FOVEA

- Smooth pursuit:
  - Foveal pursuit
  - Full-field pursuit (slow phase of optokinetic nystagmus)
- Vestibulo-ocular reflex (horizontal, vertical, torsional)
- Convergence

OCULAR OSCILLATIONS THAT MAY INTERFERE WITH VISION

- Double saccadic pulses
- Macrosaccadic oscillations
- Nystagmus (pathological)
- Ocular bobbing
- Ocular dysmetria:
  - Ocular hypometria
  - Ocular hypermetria
  - Ocular lateropulsion
  - Ocular torsipulsion
  - Ocular flutter-dysmetria
- Ocular flutter
- Ocular neuromyotonia
- Ocular tics (myoclonic jerks)
- Oculogyric crisis
- Opsoclonus
- Saccadic pulses
- Square-wave pulses (previously designated *macro–square wave jerks*)
- Square-wave jerks
- Superior oblique myokymia
- Torsional saccades (blips)

*Antisaccades are fast eye movements deliberately made away from a new target. It is a laboratory procedure used to investigate frontal lobe or cognitive function.

of neurons referred to as the *neural integrator*. (An integrator mathematically converts phasic input to tonic output by using reverberating collateral circuits to reexcite neurons. The efficiency of an integrator depends on its time constant [i.e., the duration it can prolong the activity of the input]. The effective time constant is the period necessary for the output to decay to 37% of its initial value after the input signal stops.)

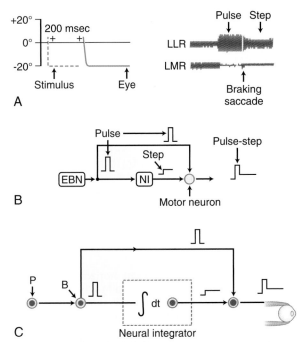

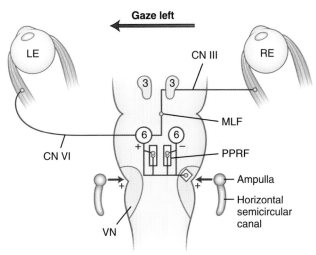

Fig. 44.21 Ocular motor events on gaze left. A, After the appearance of a stimulus 20 degrees to the left of fixation (–20 degrees), the eyes move to the target with a saccade after a latency of 200 msec. Idealized electromyography of the left extraocular muscles shows the activity of the agonist (the left lateral rectus [LLR]) and the antagonist (the left medial rectus [LMR]) muscles. **B,** The pulse originates in the excitatory burst neurons (EBNs) and is mathematically integrated by the neural integrator (NI); both signals are added to produce the pulse-step of the innervation to the ocular motor neurons. **C,** The pause cells (P) discharge continuously, suppressing the burst cells (B), except during a saccade, when they "pause," allowing the burst cells to discharge and generate a pulse. *(Reprinted with permission from Lavin, P.J.M., 1985. Conjugate and disconjugate eye movements, in: Walsh, T.J. [Ed.], Neuro-ophthalmology: clinical signs and symptoms. Lea & Febiger, Philadelphia.)*

Fig. 44.22 A lateral head turn (yaw, or side-to-side) induces movement of the endolymph in the ipsilateral horizontal semicircular canal toward the ampulla (as would warm water caloric stimulation of the external auditory meatus/tympanic membrane), and thus excites the contralateral abducens nucleus and inhibits the ipsilateral abducens nucleus via the vestibular nuclei (VN). Each abducens nucleus innervates the ipsilateral lateral rectus muscle via the abducens nerve and the contralateral medial rectus muscle via the abducens nucleus interneurons, the medial longitudinal fasciculus (MLF), and the neurons for the medial rectus (part of cranial nerve [CN] III nucleus). Neurons in each paramedian pontine reticular formation (PPRF) also have an excitatory input to the ipsilateral abducens nucleus and an inhibitory input to the contralateral abducens nucleus, for saccades and quick phases of nystagmus. *LE,* Left eye; *RE,* right eye. *(Adapted from Lavin, P.J.M., 1985. Conjugate and disconjugate eye movements, in: Walsh, T.J. (Ed.), Neuro-ophthalmology: Clinical Signs and Symptoms. Lea & Febiger, Philadelphia.)*

The NI for horizontal gaze, thought to be partly in the rostral perihypoglossal nuclear complex and the adjacent rostral medial vestibular nucleus (Leigh and Zee, 2006), receives the velocity command signal (pulse) from the EBNs. The NI then mathematically integrates the pulse to a "tonic" position command (step) before relaying it to the ipsilateral abducens nucleus (see Figs. 44.21, *B,* and 44.22).

The cerebellum and the PPRF maintain the output of this NI by controlling the gain, via a positive feedback loop, to keep the eyes on target (Fig. 44.24). The *gain* of a system is the ratio of its output to its input. In this case, the output is the innervation required to maintain eccentric fixation, and the input is the pulse signal (see Fig. 44.21, *C*). If the NI is unable to maintain the gain at unity (output/input = 1), the output falls, causing the eyes to drift off target toward primary position. A corrective saccade then refixates the target, resulting in gaze-evoked (gaze-paretic) nystagmus. Current evidence suggests that all conjugate eye movement commands, including saccades, pursuit, the slow phases of OKN, and the VOR, are initiated as velocity commands and mediated by a final common integrator (Fig. 44.25).

Although its anatomical borders are unclear, the PPRF is defined functionally with the medial aspects of the nuclei gigantocellularis, or pontis centralis oralis and caudalis, and is located just ventral and lateral to the MLF, extending from

the level of the abducens nucleus almost to the trochlear nucleus. The PPRF innervates the ipsilateral abducens nucleus, the rostral medulla (part of the NI), and the midbrain reticular formation (MRF) to coordinate horizontal and vertical eye movements. The PPRF receives direct input from each medial vestibular nucleus, the contralateral FEFs, the ipsilateral posterior parietal region, the SC, and the cerebellum.

A lesion of the abducens nucleus produces paralysis of all ipsilateral versional eye movements. Pontine lesions outside the abducens nucleus may selectively involve certain classes of eye movements while sparing others, demonstrating that the neural signals encoding subclasses of eye movements (e.g., saccades, pursuit, VOR, tonic position) project independently to the abducens nucleus. The PPRF also plays a role in generating vertical eye movements; acute bilateral injury may cause transient vertical and horizontal gaze palsies. Bilateral injury may cause persistent horizontal and vertical selective saccadic palsies. A unilateral lesion, in addition to impairing ipsilateral horizontal saccades, may also cause slowing and oblique misdirection of vertical saccades away from the side of injury. With rare exceptions, lesions of the abducens nucleus that cause an acquired ipsilateral gaze palsy almost always involve the facial nerve fasciculus as it loops around the abducens nucleus and result in an associated facial nerve palsy.

The vestibular system stabilizes the direction of gaze during head movements by virtue of changes in its tonic input to the ocular motor nuclei. This is most clearly illustrated by the horizontal VOR (see Fig. 44.22). Each horizontal semicircular canal innervates the ipsilateral medial vestibular nucleus to inhibit the ipsilateral, and excite the contralateral, abducens

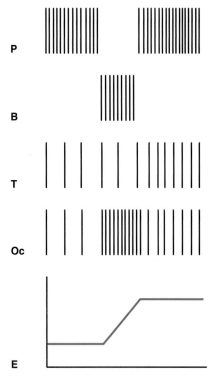

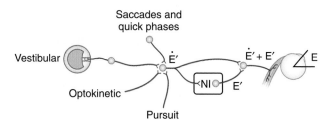

Fig. 44.25 The final common integrator hypothesis. All conjugate eye movements (E) are initiated as eye velocity commands (Ė′) that are converted to eye position commands (E′) by the neural integrator (NI). Both eye velocity and eye position commands are relayed to the motor neurons. *(Adapted from Cannon, S.C., Zee, D.S., 1988. The neural integrator of the oculomotor system, in: Lessell, S., Van Dalen, J.T.W. (Eds), Current Neuro-ophthalmology. Year Book, Chicago.)*

Fig. 44.23 Electrophysiological events during an eye movement. P represents an intraneuronal recording from a pause cell and demonstrates a constant discharge, which ceases just before and during a saccade, allowing an excitatory burst neuron (B) to discharge during pulse. T represents the discharge in a tonic neuron, which increases after the pulse as a result of integration of the pulse to a step. Both the pulse (P) and the tonic output (T) of burst-tonic neurons innervate the oculomotor neurons (Oc). The result is a rapid contraction of the extraocular muscle, which moves the eye from primary position and holds it in an eccentric position (E).

nucleus. The ampulla of the right horizontal semicircular canal is stimulated by turning the head to the right (or warm caloric stimulation). This mechanical information is transduced by the vestibular end-organ to electrical signals and transmitted to the ipsilateral vestibular nucleus. Excitatory information is then relayed to the contralateral abducens nucleus, and inhibitory information to the ipsilateral abducens nucleus, causing the eyes to deviate in the direction opposite to head rotation, thus maintaining the direction of gaze.

Saccades (see Box 44.15), or fast eye movements: In general voluntary saccades are generated in the contralateral frontal region, and reflexive in the contralateral parietal region. Saccades may be classified into four broad groups:

1. Internally triggered saccades, which are voluntary (intentional) and include target-searching, memory-guided, predictive (where the appearance of the target is anticipated), intentional visually guided saccades to an existing target in the peripheral visual field, and antisaccades.
2. Externally triggered saccades are reflexively activated by the appearance of a new target or a sound.
3. Spontaneous saccades, which occur in the absence of a target and are triggered internally by both the FEF and the SC to scan the environment repetitively; they occur at rest, during other motor activities, and during rapid-eye-movement sleep.
4. The quick phases of nystagmus.

A number of specialized areas in the cerebral cortex, identified by both experimental and pathological lesions, by neurophysiological studies (particularly in monkeys), and by transcranial magnetic stimulation, play a major role in controlling saccades (see Fig. 44.19, *B*):

1. The FEF in the precentral gyrus and sulcus (Brodmann area 6 in humans and area 8 in monkeys).
2. The supplementary eye field (SEF) on the dorsomedial aspect of the superior frontal gyrus anterior to the supplementary motor area.
3. The parietal eye field (PEF) in the lateral intraparietal (LIP) area in monkeys is equivalent to an area in the intraparietal sulcus near the angular gyrus region (Brodmann areas 39 and 40) in humans.

Other cortical areas that have a role in controlling saccades include the posterior parietal cortex (PPC), located in Brodmann area 39 in the upper angular gyrus in humans (equivalent to 7a in monkeys); the dorsolateral prefrontal cortex (PFC), area 46; the vestibular cortex in the posterior aspect of the superior temporal gyrus; and the hippocampus in the

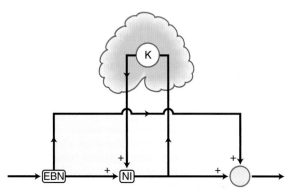

Fig. 44.24 The time constant of the brainstem neural integrator (NI), and therefore the fidelity of its output (innervation for gaze holding) is controlled predominantly by the cerebellum. Dysfunction of the gain control (K) may cause the integrator output to fall (a shortened time constant causes the signal to decay), allowing the eyes to drift back toward primary position. Conversely, an increase in K may result in an unstable integrator and cause the eye to drift eccentrically with an increasing velocity waveform. *EBN,* Excitatory burst neuron; *N,* Ocular motor neuron. *(Adapted from Lavin, P.J.M., 1985. Conjugate and disconjugate eye movements, in: Walsh, T.J. (Ed.), Neuro-ophthalmology: Clinical Signs and Symptoms. Lea & Febiger, Philadelphia. Reprinted by permission of the author and the publisher.)*

medial temporal lobe. These cortical areas and the superior colliculus are parts of a network that collectively produce saccades and determine when different types of saccades occur and where they go; that is, they calculate their direction and amplitude (accuracy). In summary, this network determines where potential targets for orienting are located; where, whether, and when gaze will shift; and coordinates saccades with visually guided reaching and head movements.

Topographically, the FEF is heavily interconnected with areas in both the dorsal and ventral streams of the extrastriate visual cortex (see Fig. 44.19, *A*) and participates in the transformation of visual signals into saccadic motor commands. Many neurons in the FEF that are connected extensively with extrastriate visual cortical areas respond to visual stimuli. The FEF and SC are both activated in the same way at the same time in response to visual stimuli before and during saccades.

Also, the FEF plays a direct role in producing saccades. Subpopulations of neurons in the FEF that discharge specifically before and during saccades innervate the deeper layers of the SC and neural circuits in the brainstem that generate saccades.

The FEF projects to the SC mainly by three pathways: a direct pathway through the posterior aspect of the anterior limb of the internal capsule near the genu, an indirect pathway via the thalamus, and another indirect pathway via the caudate nucleus to neurons in the substantia nigra pars reticulata (SNr). These neurons in the SNr project, in turn, to the SC and tonically suppress saccades by a GABA-ergic mechanism (see Fig. 44.19). Controlled disinhibition of this basal ganglia system is important for normal visually and auditory-guided saccades and is probably essential for saccades to remembered targets. Saccades of different amplitudes and directions are encoded in neurons in the FEF and SC in a retinotopic fashion (i.e., the size and direction of a saccade is determined by which neurons are stimulated). The SC also has some role in reflexive and orienting saccades. The basal ganglia are involved in sequencing complex memory-guided saccades and perhaps predictive saccades.

Neurons in the dorsolateral PFC project to the superior colliculus via the anterior limb, genu, and anterior half of the posterior limb of the internal capsule to suppress unwanted saccades to distracting stimuli when attention is directed at an existing target. Clinically, this system may be evaluated with the antisaccade test (Zee and Lasker, 2004).

The SEF parallels the FEF in several respects and also innervates ocular motor centers in the SC and brainstem. However, the SEF seems to play a less essential or less potent role in saccade production, as ablation of SEF causes only minimal and short-lasting gaze impairment.

The role of the PEF (area LIP in monkeys) is uncertain. Although neural activity in the PEF precedes saccades, the PEF does not directly control the initiation of saccades, but signals areas such as the FEF and SC with the location of potential targets for orienting.

The SC has seven alternating fibrous and cellular layers that are divided broadly into a superficial sensory (dorsal) and a deep, predominantly motor (ventral) division. The superficial sensory division receives a direct orderly input from the retina via the accessory optic tract, bypassing the lateral geniculate body, such that the visual field may be mapped on the surface of the SC (retinotopic). Only about 10% of the retinal ganglion cells project to the SC; the majority of the remainder project to the lateral geniculate body to subserve conscious vision. The deep motor division receives visual input from the striate cortex (area 17) and projects to motor areas in the subthalamic region and brainstem. The deeper division also receives input directly from the FEF and PPC and indirectly

via the basal ganglia, as well as somatosensory and auditory input. Stimulation of the SC drives the eyes contralaterally to a point in the visual field corresponding to the retinal projection to that site. Thus the SC is essentially a sensory map overlying a corresponding motor map and represents the visual fields (Leigh and Zee, 2006). The SC may also play a role in relaying excitatory information from part of the inferior parietal lobule (IPL), which has some influence in initiating saccades. Isolated lesions of the SC produce minimal but specific defects of saccades. However, when combined with experimental lesions of the FEFs, significant contralateral saccadic defects result. Purely vertical saccades require bilateral simultaneous stimulation of corresponding points of the SC or of the FEFs.

Control of smooth-pursuit eye movements is also complex (see Fig. 44.19) but essentially consists of three components: sensory, motor, and attentional-spatial. The stimulus for pursuit is movement of an image across the fovea at velocities greater than 3 to 5 degrees per second. The sensory component includes the striate cortex (area 17), which receives information from the retinal ganglion (M) cells via the magnocellular layer of the lateral geniculate body (nucleus) and the optic radiations. The striate cortex projects to the prestriate cortex (parieto-occipital areas 18 and 19) and then to the superior temporal sulcus region, which contains cortical areas MT and MST in monkeys, equivalent to the PTO (parieto-tempero-occipital) junction in humans. This sensory subsystem encodes for location, direction, and velocity of objects moving in the contralateral visual field and is the major afferent input driving smooth pursuit. It projects bilaterally to the pursuit motor subsystem, which is also located in the PTO region, as well as to the FEF and SEF. This pursuit pathway is indirect and focuses attention on small moving targets. A direct pathway bypassing the attentional-spatial subsystem enables large moving objects, such as full-field OKN stimuli, to generate smooth pursuit contralaterally even when the subject is inattentive. The SC contributes to pursuit drive also. The PTO projects via the internal sagittal stratum and the posterior limb of the internal capsule to the ipsilateral dorsolateral and lateral pontine nuclei. The pursuit pathways control ipsilateral tracking and so must either remain on the same side or undergo a double decussation at least once. In 1992, Johnston and co-workers suggested the pursuit pathways project from the pontine nuclei to the contralateral flocculus and medial vestibular nucleus and then back to the ipsilateral abducens nucleus (Fig. 44.26).

Pursuit defects fall into four categories:

1. Retinotopic defects: Lesions of the geniculostriate pathway cause impaired pursuit in both directions in the contralateral visual field defect. Defects also occur with lesions of areas MST or MT; these patients have apparently normal visual fields but selective "blindness" for movement.
2. Impaired pursuit, worse in the ipsilateral direction in both hemifields, occurs with lesions in the lateral aspect of area MST and the foveal representation of area MT in monkeys, similar to a focal PTO lesion in humans. Lesions in the FEFs, posterior thalamus, midbrain, ipsilateral pons, contralateral cerebellum, contralateral pontomedullary junction, and the ipsilateral abducens nucleus also can impair pursuit in both hemifields, but worse in the ipsilateral direction.
3. Symmetrically impaired pursuit in both horizontal directions occurs with focal lesions in the parieto-occipital region (area 39), medication (e.g., anticonvulsants, sedatives, and psychotropic agents), alcohol, fatigue, inattention, schizophrenia, encephalopathy, a variety of neurodegenerative disorders, and age (infants and the elderly).

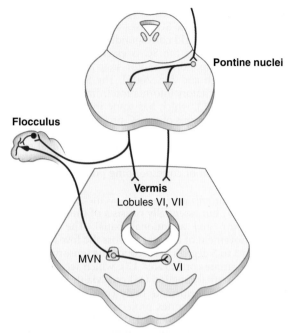

Fig. 44.26 Postulated double decussation of pursuit pathways in the brainstem and cerebellum. The first decussation consists of excitatory mossy fiber projections from the pontine nuclei to granule cells, which excite basket cells and stellate cells in the contralateral cerebellar flocculus. The basket and stellate cells inhibit Purkinje cells, which in turn inhibit neurons in the medial vestibular nucleus (MVN). The second decussation consists of excitatory projections from the MVN to the opposite abducens nucleus (VI). *(Reprinted with permission from Johnston, J.L., Sharpe, J.A., Morrow, M.J., 1992. Paresis of contralateral smooth pursuit and normal vestibular smooth eye movements after unilateral brainstem lesions. Ann Neurol 31, 495–502.)*

4. An acute nondominant (e.g., parietal, frontal) hemisphere lesion associated with a hemispatial neglect syndrome causes transient loss of pursuit beyond the midline into contralateral hemispace.

The cerebellum coordinates the ocular motor system to drive the eyes smoothly and accurately and is richly supplied by afferent fibers conveying ocular information (e.g., velocity, position, neural integration) from the vestibular system, the afferent visual system, the PPRF, and the MRF. The dorsal vermis and fastigial nuclei determine the accuracy of saccades by modulating saccadic amplitude; also, they adjust the innervation to each eye selectively to ensure precise conjugate movements. Lesions of the dorsal vermis and fastigial nuclei result in saccadic dysmetria (often, overshoot dysmetria that is greater centripetally), macrosaccadic oscillations, and disorders of vergence (see following section).

Selective cerebellar lesions have differential effects on eye movements. Bilateral lesions of the fastigial and globose (interpositus) nuclei cause hypermetria of externally triggered saccades but do not affect internally triggered saccades. Bilateral lesions of the posterior vermis (lobules VI and VII) cause hypometric horizontal and vertical saccades and impaired pursuit. Unilateral lesions of the posterior vermis cause hypometric ipsilateral and hypermetric contralateral saccades, whereas unilateral lesions of the caudal fastigial nucleus cause hypermetric ipsilateral and hypometric contralateral saccades.

The flocculus, part of the vestibulocerebellum, is responsible for matching the saccadic pulse and step appropriately and for stabilizing images on the fovea. It adjusts the output of the NI and participates in long-term adaptive processing to ensure that eye movements remain appropriate to the stimulus. For example, the amplitude (gain) and even the direction of the slow phases of the VOR are adjusted by the flocculus. Lesions of the flocculus result in gaze-holding deficits such as gaze-evoked, rebound, and downbeat nystagmus. Floccular lesions also impair smooth pursuit, cancellation (suppression) of the VOR by the pursuit system during combined head and eye tracking, and the ability to suppress nystagmus (and vertigo) by fixation. The nodulus, also part of the vestibulocerebellum, influences vestibular eye movements and vestibular optokinetic interaction. Lesions of the nodulus in monkeys and humans produce PAN.

Vergence Eye Movements

In humans and other animals capable of binocular fusional vision, dysconjugate (vergence) eye movements are necessary to maintain ocular alignment on an approaching or retreating object (convergence and divergence, respectively). Electromyography demonstrates that divergence is an active movement, although not as dynamic or as much under voluntary control as convergence. The principal driving stimuli for vergence movements, relayed from the occipital cortex, are accommodative retinal blur (unfocused) and fusional disparity (diplopia). Each of these stimuli can operate independently. Also, during convergence, each eye extorts (more so in downgaze) to facilitate stereoscopic perception (Brodsky, 2002). In addition, the pupils change size synkinetically as part of the near reflex to increase the depth of field and sharpen the focus of the optical system.

Although the precise locations of the convergence and divergence centers are unknown, important areas include the paramedian thalamus, the midbrain pretectum, the nucleus reticularis tegmenti pontis (NRTP), and the dorsal vermis. A group of neurons just lateral to the third cranial nerve nuclear complex fire in relation to the angle of convergence. Lesions to the pretectal region cause accommodative and vergence abnormalities. Lesions to the dorsal cerebellar vermis cause small-angle esodeviations in primates. The NRTP is contiguous with the PPRF and forms part of a feedback loop by relaying visual information to the cerebellum via a cerebropontocerebellar pathway; the NRTP may also function as a vergence integrator. Experimental lesions of the NRTP in monkeys can cause sustained convergence or pendular convergence-divergence oscillations.

Unilateral stimulation of areas 19 and 22 of the preoccipital cortex caused bilateral convergence, accommodation, and miosis in macaque monkeys. The occipitomesencephalic pathway, involved in vergence, travels more ventrally in the diencephalon and midbrain than does the light reflex pathway and is less susceptible to compression by extrinsic lesions (dorsal midbrain syndrome) (see Chapter 21).

Vertical Eye Movements

The pathways involved in controlling vertical gaze are not fully known, and some of the neural connections discussed here are speculative. The third and fourth cranial nerves innervate the extraocular muscles responsible for both vertical and torsional eye movements. The premotor substrate for vertical and torsional eye movements lies in the midbrain reticular formation (MRF), but some vertical saccades are programmed in the PPRF and relayed to the MRF via a juxta-MLF pathway, presumably to coordinate horizontal, vertical, and oblique trajectories as well as head movement. Lesions of the PPRF can impair both horizontal and vertical saccades and cause a pseudo-PSP syndrome (see Supranuclear Gaze Disturbances).

The rostral interstitial nucleus of the medial longitudinal fasciculus (riMLF) on each side contains EBNs for both upward and downward saccades but only for ipsilateral torsional saccades. The EBNs for upward saccades are probably caudal, ventral, and medial in the riMLF and project to the elevator muscles (superior rectus and inferior oblique) bilaterally, with axons crossing within the oculomotor nucleus (Fig. 44.27, *A*) and not in the posterior commissure (PC) as previously thought (Bhidayasiri et al., 2000). The EBNs for downward saccades are more rostral, dorsal, and lateral in the riMLF and

project only to the ipsilateral depressor muscles (inferior rectus and superior oblique) (see Fig. 44.27, *B*). The EBNs for vertical saccades project also to the interstitial nucleus of Cajal (INC), which plays a major role in neural integration for vertical and torsional gaze (Bhidayasiri et al., 2000). From the INC, the pathways project dorsally and laterally to cross in the PC before turning ventrally to the oculomotor and trochlear nerve nuclei (see Fig. 44.27). The axons to the elevator muscles travel more dorsally and thus are more susceptible to extrinsic compression, such as from a pinealoma.

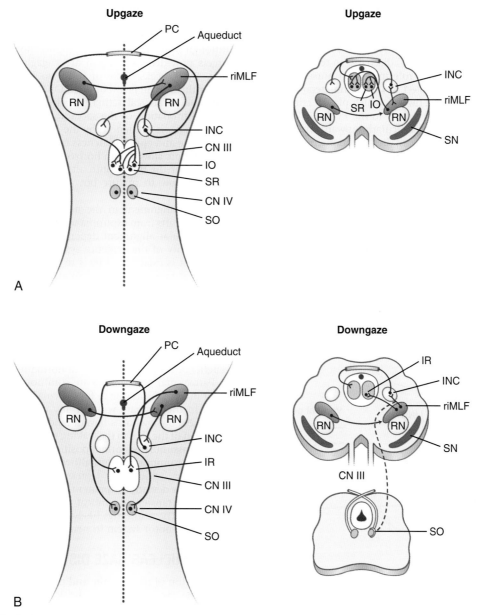

Fig. 44.27 Hypothetical pathways involved in controlling vertical eye movements. A, Upward eye movements. Burst neurons for upward saccades are shown projecting from the medial rostral interstitial nucleus of the medial longitudinal fasciculus (riMLF) to the elevator muscles, superior recti and inferior obliques bilaterally, with axons crossing within the oculomotor nucleus. **B,** Burst neurons for downward saccades are shown projecting only to the ipsilateral depressor muscles, the inferior rectus and superior oblique. The axons of the burst neurons for upward saccades also project to the interstitial nucleus of Cajal (INC), which plays a role in neural integration for vertical and torsional gaze. From the INC, the axons project dorsally and laterally to cross in the posterior commissure before turning ventrally to the oculomotor and trochlear nerve nuclei. *CN III,* Third nerve nuclear complex; *CN IV,* fourth nerve nucleus; *IO,* inferior oblique subnucleus; *IR,* inferior rectus subnucleus; *PC,* posterior commissure; *RN,* red nucleus; *SN,* substantia nigra; *SO,* superior oblique nucleus; *SR,* superior rectus subnucleus. *(Redrawn from Bhidayasiri, R., Plant, G.T., Leigh, R.J., 2000. A hypothetical scheme for the brainstem control of vertical gaze. Neurology 54, 1985–1993.)*

Although the riMLF is key for vertical saccades, the MRF also has a role because of its reciprocal connections with the SC. Each riMLF also receives input from the nucleus of the posterior commissure, the FEF, the SC, the fastigial nucleus of the cerebellum, and the contralateral riMLF; the latter fibers cross in a commissure ventral to the aqueduct (see Fig. 44.27). Each riMLF is supplied by a branch of the proximal posterior cerebral artery (the posterior thalamosubthalamic paramedian artery). Sometimes a single anomalous posterior thalamosubthalamic paramedian artery, (the *artery of Percheron*) supplies both riMLFs; thus, occlusion from a single embolus (seen most frequently with *Top of the Basilar Syndrome*) causes bilateral midbrain/thalamic infarction. Vertical saccades require bilateral supranuclear innervation from the FEF or SC, or both.

The NI for vertical and torsional eye movements (Leigh and Zee, 2006) is located in the INC. Burst-tonic and tonic neurons in the region of the INC discharge in relation to vertical eye position and play a role in vertical pursuit and eye position. These neurons project to the contralateral INC and the ocular motor nuclei via the PC, which plays a critical role in vertical gaze (Fig. 44.28). Injury to the PC limits all types of vertical eye movements, particularly upward movements, although the vertical VORs and Bell phenomenon (ocular deviation, usually upward, on forced eyelid closure) may be relatively spared.

Retinal slip, the sensory stimulus for vertical pursuit, is encoded by the dorsolateral pontine nuclei and relayed to the flocculus and posterior vermis before converging, via the INC, on the midbrain (see Figs. 44.26 and 44.27). The commands for vertical pursuit pass through the pons and cerebellum before turning rostrally to reach the relevant ocular motor neurons in the midbrain.

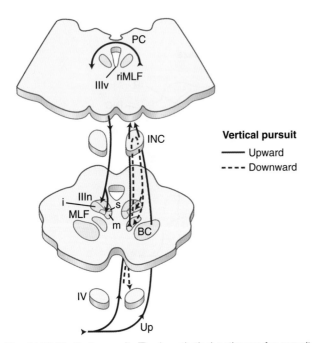

Fig. 44.28 Vertical pursuit. The hypothetical pathways for pursuit reach the midbrain via the dorsal lateral pontine nuclei and travel upward in the brachium conjunctivum (BC) and the medial longitudinal fasciculus (MLF). The interstitial nucleus of Cajal (INC) is involved in pursuit and may also be the neural integrator for vertical position commands. *(Reprinted with permission from Ranalli, P.J., Sharpe, J.A., Fletcher, W.A., 1988. Palsy of upward and downward saccadic, pursuit, and vestibular movements with a unilateral midbrain lesion: pathophysiological correlations. Neurology 38, 114–122.)*

DEVELOPMENT OF THE OCULAR MOTOR SYSTEM

At birth, the vestibular system is the most developed of the ocular motor subsystems and is easily tested by rotating the infant, held at arm's length, with the head tilted 30 degrees forward. In normal neonates, the eyes tonically in the same direction as head movement; reflex saccades develop by 2 to 3 weeks after birth. Smooth-pursuit movements may be detected in neonates but only with large targets (such as a human face) at low velocities. These findings, although not well quantified, are consistent with histological maturation of the fovea after at least 8 weeks of age. Also, neonates can generate the smooth-pursuit component of OKN with full-field stimulation.

Fixation is not well developed until about 2 months, although some infants younger than 1 month of age can fixate targets provided the stimuli are engaging and the infant is alert. By 9 weeks, 90% of full-term infants can fixate and follow the human face. Full-field OKN and larger targets stimulate the parafoveal retina, which matures earlier than the fovea. Stimulation of the saccadic system, also immature in the neonate, is influenced by the infant's attention as well as by the size and appropriateness of the target. Vertical saccades mature more slowly than horizontal saccades and may not be detected for the first month after birth. Vergence movements are also slow to mature but are seen after about the first month.

Ocular alignment in the newborn is usually poor, with transient shifts from esotropia to exotropia during the first few weeks. Ocular alignment depends on both visual input and the maturity of the vergence system. In most infants, ocular alignment is established by 3 to 4 weeks of age but may be delayed as late as 5 months. Small-angle esotropia and intermittent esotropia may spontaneously resolve in infants younger than 20 weeks of age; constant esotropia greater than 40 prism diopters is unlikely to resolve spontaneously. Esotropia after 3 months and exotropia after 5 months are considered abnormal and require appropriate evaluation. Large-angle exotropia may be associated with craniofacial, genetic, or other neurological abnormalities.

Paroxysmal phenomena are common in infancy and may occur in as many as one in four. Ocular motor anomalies may occur in the neonate without any pathological significance. About 2% of newborns have a tendency for tonic downward deviation of the eyes in the waking state; during sleep, however, the eyes assume the normal position, and the VORs are intact. Other uncommon abnormalities seen in newborns include opsoclonus, which may regress through a phase of ocular flutter, skew deviation, apparent bilateral internuclear ophthalmoplegia, transient downbeat nystagmus, and tonic upward deviation. These findings likely represent delayed maturity of the ocular motor system in neonates.

SUPRANUCLEAR GAZE DISTURBANCES

Interruption of the saccadic and pursuit pathways before they reach the eye-movement generators in the MRF and PPRF results in a loss of voluntary eye movements but relatively spares reflex movements such as the VOR, optokinetic response, and the Bell phenomenon (see earlier). This constellation of findings is referred to as a *supranuclear gaze palsy* and classically occurs in progressive supranuclear palsy (PSP) as well as a variety of disorders listed in Table 44.7.

A *pseudo-PSP syndrome*, characterized by a selective saccadic palsy (sometimes associated with ataxia, dysarthria, and dysphagia) that progresses over several months can follow aortic or cardiac surgery under hypothermic circulatory arrest. It has

psychiatric evaluation. Strategies such as the use of cycloplegia (homatropine eye drops) to prevent accommodative spasm, thus inhibiting the near triad, may be helpful.

Disorders of Divergence

Divergence insufficiency (DI) is characterized by sudden-onset esotropia and uncrossed horizontal diplopia at distance, in the absence of other neurological symptoms or signs. The esotropia may be intermittent or constant, but the patients can fuse at near. The esodeviation is greater at distance than near but is comitant in all directions. Versions and ductions are full, and saccadic velocities, if measured quantitatively, appear normal. Fusional divergence is reduced. The origin of DI is unclear, but it may result from a break in fusion in a patient with a congenital esophoria, usually coming on later in life; also, it occurs in patients with midline cerebellar disease particularly hereditary spinocerebellar ataxia (Morrison et al., 2008). The condition is easily treated with base-out prisms for the distance correction and rarely requires extraocular muscle surgery. DI in the elderly occurs with the sagging eye syndrome (see above); it is recognized by the associated signs of involutional changes such as ptosis and/or elevated upper lid creases, superior sulcus enlargement or deformity or baggy eyelids; it is differentiated from DI of neurogenic origin by the absence of nystagmus, saccadic dysmetria and ataxia.

Divergence paralysis, a controversial entity that may be difficult to distinguish from divergence insufficiency, occurs usually in the context of a severe head injury or other cause of raised ICP. Such patients have horizontal diplopia at distance too, but quantitatively; abducting saccades are slow. Patients with bilateral palsies of the sixth cranial nerve who recover gradually may go through a phase in which the esotropia becomes comitant with full ductions, mimicking divergence paralysis. Divergence paralysis can also occur with Fisher syndrome, Chiari malformations, pontine tumors, and excessive sedation from drugs.

Central disruption of fusion, or post-traumatic fusion deficiency, can occur after moderate head injury and causes intractable diplopia despite the patient's ability to fuse intermittently and, even briefly, achieve stereopsis. The diplopia fluctuates and varies among crossed, uncrossed, and vertical. Versions and ductions may be full, but vergence amplitudes are reduced greatly. Prism therapy or surgery is ineffective, but an eye patch or centrally frosted lens may provide symptomatic relief. The location of injury is presumed to be in the midbrain. Also, central disruption of fusion is reported with brainstem tumors, stroke, following removal of long-standing cataracts, uncorrected aphakia, and neurosurgical procedures. This condition must be distinguished from bilateral fourth cranial nerve palsies, when diplopia is constant and associated with cyclodiplopia and excyclotropia (>12 degrees), and also from psychogenic disorders of vergence (see Disorders of Convergence).

A congenital inability to fuse is associated with amblyopia or congenital esotropia.

The hemislide (hemifield slip) phenomenon causes diplopia in patients with large visual field defects, particularly dense bitemporal hemianopias or, occasionally, heteronymous altitudinal defects. Because of loss of overlapping areas of visual field, patients have difficulty maintaining fusion and can no longer suppress any latent ocular deviation.

Cyclical esotropia, also called *circadian, alternate-day,* or *clock-mechanism esotropia,* usually begins in childhood, although it can occur at any age and can also follow surgery for intermittent esotropia. The cycles of orthotropia and esotropia may run 24 to 96 hours, similar to many other cyclical or periodic biological phenomena of obscure mechanisms.

Patients with cyclical esotropia can decompensate into a constant esotropia that can be corrected surgically.

Ocular neuromyotonia is a brief episodic myotonic contraction of one or more muscles supplied by the ocular motor nerves, most commonly the oculomotor nerve. It may occur spontaneously or be provoked by prolonged gaze in a particular direction. Usually it results in esotropia of the affected eye accompanied by failure of elevation and depression of the globe. When the oculomotor nerve is affected, there may be associated signs of aberrant reinnervation (see Chapter 104). The pupil may be fixed to both light and near stimuli or become myotonic. Ocular neuromyotonia occurs most often after radiation therapy for sellar region tumors. Less often it is associated with compressive lesions such as pituitary adenomas, cavernous sinus meningiomas or aneurysms, thyroid orbitopathy, radiation of a frontal lobe lesion (Whitted et al., 2013), following myelography with thorium dioxide, with Paget disease of the skull base, or with neurovascular compression by a dolichoectatic basilar artery. Demyelinating lesions in the region of the third cranial nerve fascicle also can cause "paroxysmal spasm" of the muscles innervated by the oculomotor nerve but usually are accompanied by other findings such as eyelid retraction or paroxysmal limb dystonia. Occasionally, no cause can be found. Ocular neuromyotonia may respond to carbamazepine or other antiepileptic drugs. It should be distinguished from superior oblique myokymia and the spasms of cyclical oculomotor palsy.

Cyclical oculomotor palsy is characterized by paresis alternating with "cyclic" spasms of both the extra- and intraocular muscles supplied by the oculomotor nerve. It is a rare condition usually noted in the first 2 years of life, although the majority of cases are believed to be congenital and are often associated with other features of birth trauma. During the spasms, which last 10 to 30 seconds, the upper eyelid elevates, the globe adducts, and the pupil and ciliary muscle constrict, causing miosis and increased accommodation (Loewenfeld, 1999); the paretic phase usually lasts longer. Signs of aberrant oculomotor reinnervation (see Chapter 104) usually are present. Spasms, often heralded by twitching of the upper lid, may be precipitated by intentional accommodation or adduction. Cycles occur irregularly, vary from 1.5 to 3 minutes in duration, persist during sleep, may be suppressed by topical cholinergic agents (eserine, pilocarpine), and are abolished by topical anticholinergic agents (atropine, homatropine) or general anesthesia. The cycles usually persist throughout life, but the spasms of the extraocular muscles may abate, leaving only intermittent miosis.

Symptomatic cyclical oculomotor palsy may occur in later life in patients with underlying lesions involving the third cranial nerve, but the features and cycles are atypical. The mechanism of cyclical spasms is unclear but is discussed elsewhere (Loewenfeld, 1999).

Gaze-evoked phenomena such as end-point nystagmus, the oculoauricular phenomenon, and orbicularis oculi myokymia are physiological or benign. Others, such as gaze-evoked nystagmus or tinnitus, are pathological (Box 44.21) and may be the result of damage to the horizontal neural integrator.

EYE MOVEMENT RECORDING TECHNIQUES

Oculographic techniques provide clinicians and researchers with objective and quantitative means of analysis that have led to a better understanding of eye movement neurophysiology and ocular motility disorders. Quantitative oculography can measure saccadic latency, velocity, accuracy, pursuit and VOR gain, and nystagmus slow-phase velocity; it can detect unsuspected oscillations and intrusions and identify different nystagmus waveforms. Oculography is used to record both

---

BOX 44.21 Gaze-Evoked Phenomena

PHYSIOLOGICAL PHENOMENA

- Blinks
- End-point nystagmus
- Flaring of the nostrils during vertical saccades
- Mentalis contraction during horizontal saccades (personal observation)
- Oculoauricular phenomenon: retraction of ear during lateral gaze (or convergence)
- Orbicularis oculi myokymia
- Phosphenes (more intense in patients with optic neuritis, retinal/vitreous detachment: Moore lightning streaks)

PATHOLOGICAL SENSORY PHENOMENA

- Gaze-evoked amaurosis in the eye ipsilateral to an orbital apex tumor
- Gaze-evoked tinnitus with cerebellopontine angle tumors or following posterior fossa surgery
- Reverse-Tullio phenomenon (gaze-evoked swooshing sound) caused by end-organ damage in a patient with Tullio

phenomenon (sound-evoked nystagmus and vertigo) (personal observation)

- SUNCT (sudden unilateral conjunctival injection and tearing) syndrome with saccades
- Tinnitus with periodic saccadic oscillations
- Vertigo

PATHOLOGICAL MOTOR PHENOMENA

- Convergence retraction nystagmus on attempted upgaze (dorsal midbrain syndrome)
- Facial twitching, clonic limb movements, blepharoclonus, lid nystagmus, involuntary laughter and seizures
- Gaze-evoked nystagmus
- Neuromyotonia
- Retraction of the globe in Duane syndrome
- Superior oblique myokymia
- Synkinetic movements with cyclical oculomotor palsy and with aberrant reinnervation of the oculomotor nerve (see Chapter 104)

---

spontaneous and induced eye movements to a target, such as a projected light in front of the subject, or to vestibular and optokinetic stimuli.

Electro-oculography, also known as *electronystagmography* (Chapter 46), is a popular method of quantitative oculography but has a limited range and is unreliable for vertical eye movements because of eyelid artifact. Infrared oculography is more accurate but not ideal for vertical eye movements. The most quantitatively accurate technique involves the scleral search coil.

REFERENCES

The complete reference list is available online at https://expertconsult .inkling.com.

45 Neuro-Ophthalmology: Afferent Visual System

Matthew J. Thurtell, Robert L. Tomsak

CHAPTER OUTLINE

NEURO-OPHTHALMOLOGICAL EXAMINATION OF THE AFFERENT VISUAL SYSTEM
Examination of Visual Acuity
Contrast Vision Testing
Light-Stress Test
Color Vision Testing
Examination of the Pupils
Light Brightness Comparison
Visual Field Testing
Interpretation of Visual Field Defects
ANCILLARY DIAGNOSTIC TECHNIQUES
Perimetry
Ophthalmic Imaging
Electrophysiology
NONORGANIC (FUNCTIONAL) VISUAL DISTURBANCES
Diagnostic Techniques
Prognosis

From a conceptual standpoint, it is useful to consider vision as having two components: *central* or *macular* vision (high acuity, color perception, light-adapted) and *peripheral* or *ambulatory* vision (low acuity, poor color perception, dark-adapted). Light, refracted by the cornea and lens, is focused on the retina. For the best possible vision, the image of the object of regard must fall onto the *fovea*, which is the most sensitive part of the macula. The cone photoreceptors, which mediate central and color vision, are greatest in density at the fovea. The cone system functions optimally in conditions of light adaptation. Visual acuity and cone density fall off rapidly as eccentricity from the fovea increases. For example, the retina 20 degrees eccentric to the fovea can only resolve objects equivalent to Snellen 20/200 (6/60 metric) optotypes or larger. Rod photoreceptors are present in highest numbers approximately 20 degrees from the fovea and are more abundant than cones in the more peripheral retina; rods function best in dim illumination. The total extent of the normal peripheral visual field in each eye is approximately 60 degrees superior, 60 degrees nasal, 70 to 75 degrees inferior, and 100 degrees temporal to fixation (Fig. 45.1) (see Chapter 16).

Each eye sends visual information, transduced by the retina, to both hemispheres of the brain by the optic nerves, each of which contains over 1 million axons. Axons that arise from the ganglion cells of the nasal retina of each eye decussate in the optic chiasm to the contralateral optic tract. Axons from the temporal retina do not decussate. The percentages of crossed and uncrossed axons in the human optic chiasm are approximately 53% and 47%, respectively. Because of the optical properties of the eye, the nasal retina receives visual information from the temporal visual field, while the temporal retina receives visual information from the nasal visual field (see Fig. 45.1). Similarly, the superior retina receives

information from the inferior visual field, and vice versa. These points are clinically important in evaluating visual loss (see Chapter 16).

Visual information stratifies further in the lateral geniculate nucleus (LGN), which is the only way station between the retinal ganglion cells and the primary visual cortex. The LGN, a portion of the thalamus, has six layers. Axons from ipsilateral retinal ganglion cells synapse in layers 2, 3, and 5; contralateral axons synapse in layers 1, 4, and 6. Layers 1 and 2 of the LGN are the *magnocellular layers* and these receive input from M retinal ganglion cells. The magnocellular pathway is concerned mainly with movement detection, detection of low contrast, and dynamic form perception. After projecting to the primary visual cortex (visual area 1, V1, or Brodmann area 17), information from the M pathway is distributed to V2 (part of area 18) and V5 (junction of areas 19 and 37). Layers 3 to 6 of the LGN are the *parvocellular layers* and receive input from P retinal ganglion cells, which are color selective and responsive to high contrast. Information from the P pathway is distributed to V2 and V4 (fusiform gyrus) (Trobe, 2001). Superior fibers that leave the LGN go straight back to the primary visual cortex; inferior fibers loop anteriorly around the temporal horn of the lateral ventricle (*Meyer loop*). Since these fibers pass close to the tip of the temporal lobe, temporal lobectomy sometimes damages these fibers causing a "pie in the sky" homonymous visual field defect.

The primary visual cortex (striate cortex, V1, or Brodmann area 17) is in the occipital lobe. Fibers from the macula project to the portion of the visual cortex closest to the occipital poles, while fibers from the peripheral retina project to the visual cortex lying more anteriorly. The nonoverlapping part of the most peripheral temporal visual field (*monocular temporal crescent*) arises from unpaired crossed axons from the nasal retina that project to the most anteromedial portion of the visual cortex. The primary visual cortex has interconnections with visual association areas concerned with color, motion, and object recognition (Trobe, 2001).

NEURO-OPHTHALMOLOGICAL EXAMINATION OF THE AFFERENT VISUAL SYSTEM

The neuro-ophthalmological examination makes use of ophthalmic tools and techniques, but aims at neurological diagnosis. Since many neurologists are not familiar with ophthalmic examination techniques, and ophthalmologists are often not experienced with neurological localization, the neuro-ophthalmological subspecialty provides a bridge between the two disciplines.

Examination of Visual Acuity

Visual acuity is the spatial resolution of vision. Visual acuity should always be measured in each eye individually and with the best possible optical correction (i.e., with the patient's glasses); other optical means such as a pinhole device or refraction may be needed if optical correction is not available (Wall and Johnson, 2005). The resulting measure, called *best-corrected visual acuity*, is the only universally interpretable measurement of central visual function. Ideally, visual acuity

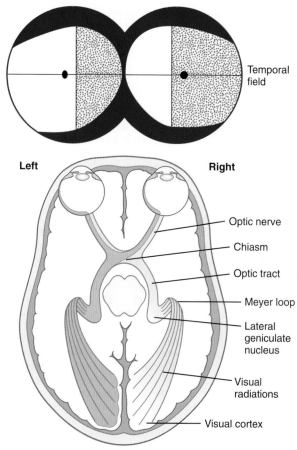

Fig. 45.1 Visual pathways.

should be measured both at distance (usually 20 feet or 6 m) and near (usually 14 inches or 0.33 m). The notation *20/20* (6/6 metric) indicates that the patient (numerator) is able to see the optotypes seen by a normal person at 20 feet (denominator). A visual acuity of 20/60 (6/18 metric) indicates that the patient sees an optotype at 20 feet that a normal person would see at 60 feet.

A disparity between the distance and near visual acuities is often indicative of a specific problem. For example, the most common cause of better distance than near acuity is uncorrected presbyopia. Common causes of better near than distance acuity include myopia and congenital nystagmus. In the latter disorder, convergence needed for near vision dampens the nystagmus.

When measuring near vision, the reading card should be held at the specified distance of 14 inches (or 0.33 m) to control for variation in image size on the retina. The medical record should clearly specify if a nonstandard distance is used. Two types of near cards are readily available; one has numbers and the other has written text (Fig. 45.2). Both are useful, but in neurological practice, a near card with text measures visual acuity as well as reading ability to some degree. A disparity between the measurements from the two types of near card might suggest a disturbance of some other cortical function, such as language function (see Chapter 12).

Contrast Vision Testing

Contrast vision, the ability to distinguish adjacent areas of differing luminance, can be evaluated by assessing the perception of lines or optotypes of different sizes (spatial frequencies)

with varying degrees of contrast. Contrast vision can be impaired in numerous diseases of the eye (e.g., cataract) and retrobulbar visual pathways (e.g., optic neuropathies). Special charts—the Pelli–Robson chart (sensitivity) and Sloan chart (acuity)—are required to assess contrast vision.

Light-Stress Test

In some disorders of the macula, abnormalities are not apparent with the direct ophthalmoscope. The light-stress (or photo-stress) test is a useful method for determining whether reduced central vision is a consequence of macular dysfunction (Wall and Johnson, 2005). Prior to the test, the best-corrected visual acuity is measured in each eye. Then, with the eye with decreased vision occluded, the other eye is exposed to a bright light for 10 seconds. Immediately thereafter, the patient is instructed to read the next largest line on the eye chart, and the recovery period is timed. The same procedure is followed for the eye with decreased vision, and the results are compared. Fifty seconds is the upper limit of normal for visual recovery, although most normal subjects recover within several seconds. In patients with macular disease, the recovery period often takes several minutes.

Color Vision Testing

Dyschromatopsia, especially if asymmetrical between the eyes, is an indication of optic nerve dysfunction, but can also occur with retinal disease (Almog and Nemet, 2010). Symmetrical acquired dyschromatopsia might indicate a retinal degeneration, such as a cone–rod dystrophy. Congenital dyschromatopsia occurs in about 8% of men and 0.5% of women.

Techniques for assessing color vision range from the simple to the sophisticated. A gross color vision defect is identifiable at the bedside by assessing for red desaturation. The clinician holds a bright red object in front of each of the patient's eyes individually, and asks for a comparison of both brightness and color intensity. Asking for a comparison of red saturation on each side of fixation sometimes detects a subtle hemianopia. Formal measurements of color vision can be obtained with pseudoisochromatic color plates (e.g., Ishihara or Hardy–Rand–Rittler plates) or with sorting tests (e.g., Farnsworth–Munsell test).

Examination of the Pupils

Examination of the pupils involves assessing pupil size and shape, the direct and consensual reactions to light, and the near response. The examination should also include an assessment for a relative afferent pupillary defect (RAPD). If a difference in pupil size (*anisocoria*) is noted, look for ptosis and ocular motility deficits, keeping in mind the possibility of Horner syndrome or third cranial nerve palsy. Record findings in an easily understood format (Table 45.1).

Measurements of pupil size and light reaction are made in dim illumination with the patient fixating on an immobile distant target. If there is anisocoria, it is useful to measure pupil size in both darkness and bright light. Anisocoria due to oculosympathetic paresis (Horner syndrome) is often greater in the dark, because the affected pupil does not dilate well. Conversely, anisocoria due to parasympathetic denervation (e.g., Adie tonic pupil) is often more evident in bright light, because the affected pupil does not constrict well (see Chapter 18).

When measuring light reactions or assessing for an RAPD, the brightest light available should be used. The near reaction can be elicited by having the patient look at their thumb,

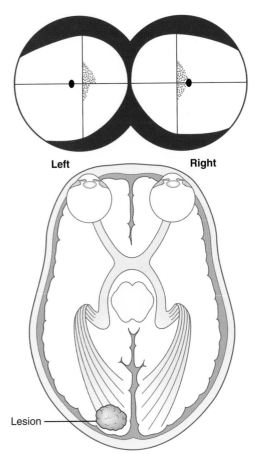

Left   Right

Lesion

Fig. 45.10 Congruent paracentral right homonymous hemianopia from a left occipital pole lesion.

Perimetry

Numerous techniques for examining the visual fields are available (Wall and Johnson, 2005), but a detailed discussion of these is beyond the scope of this chapter. Examination of the entire visual field requires a perimeter; the tangent screen measures only the central 30 degrees of the visual field at a distance of 1 m. Perimeters can be divided into those that use a moving (kinetic) stimulus and those that use a static stimulus. Most static perimeters are automated and driven by computer. Static perimeters can determine the visual threshold at defined points in the visual field (threshold static perimetry) or may evaluate these points using stimuli of set luminance (suprathreshold static perimetry). The Goldmann perimeter is the most commonly used kinetic perimeter (see Fig. 45.11, *A* for a normal Goldmann visual field), although kinetic perimetry can also be performed with both the Humphrey and Octopus perimeters. The Humphrey and Octopus perimeters are the most commonly used static perimeters (see Fig. 45.11, *B* for a normal Humphrey visual field). Threshold static perimeters are the most sensitive and quantitative, allowing for a comparison of the patient's responses with those of age-matched normal controls, but testing can be time consuming and tiring for the patient. To gain useful information from static perimetry, the patient must be alert, cooperative, and able to maintain steady central fixation. Many patients with neurological disorders are unable to concentrate for an examination that can take as long as 15 minutes per eye and, thus, static perimetry findings may be unreliable in such patients. Recent refinements in testing strategy have made it possible to reduce testing time and thereby increase reliability, but many neuro-ophthalmologists continue to use Goldmann perimetry to assess the visual fields in selected patients.

Ophthalmic Imaging

Photographs of the ocular fundus may be obtained to identify and document ophthalmoscopic findings. Retinal vascular abnormalities, such as occlusions (e.g., central retinal artery occlusion) and microvascular disease (e.g., diabetic retinopathy), may be evaluated when red-free fundus photographs are taken following intravenous injection of fluorescein (*fluorescein angiography*). Fundus autofluorescence photography allows for topographical mapping of lipofuscin in the retinal pigment epithelium layer. Lipofuscin is a fluorescent pigment that accumulates in retinal pigment epithelial cells following photoreceptor degradation and, thus, autofluorescence may be used to detect subtle abnormalities in patients with retinal degenerations (Schmitz-Valckenberg et al., 2008). Since optic nerve head drusen exhibit autofluorescence, they may be detected on fundus autofluorescence even when they are not visible on ophthalmoscopy (Kurz-Levin and Landau, 1999).

Optical coherence tomography (OCT) uses light waves to generate high-resolution cross-sectional images of the optic nerve and retina. Since the retinal layers have differing optical reflectivity, they can be distinguished using OCT. The thickness of the layers can be determined from OCT and compared with age-matched normal controls. Measurement of the peripapillary retinal nerve fiber layer and macular ganglion cell layer thicknesses with OCT may help with the detection of mild optic neuropathy (Fig. 45.12). Measurement of the thickness of retinal layers or identification of architectural changes on OCT can aid the diagnosis and management of retinal disease.

Electrophysiology

Electrophysiology may help in the investigation of unexplained visual loss or in identification of subclinical optic

hemianopias usually result from occipital lobe infarcts (Fig. 45.10), but can sometimes occur with more anterior retrochiasmal lesions (Kedar et al., 2007).

Rule 8

Even a complete unilateral homonymous hemianopia does not decrease visual acuity, because the macular cortex in the opposite hemisphere is still functioning. If the input to both macular cortices is impaired, central acuity is often diminished (*cortical blindness*), but the visual acuities should be equally diminished. If the visual acuities are not similar, the clinician should search for another (or additional) explanation for the asymmetry.

ANCILLARY DIAGNOSTIC TECHNIQUES

Ancillary diagnostic tests may be obtained to further characterize and determine the cause of visual loss. Formal visual field testing (perimetry) allows for characterization and quantification of visual field defects. Ophthalmic imaging techniques may not only be used to image the ocular fundus and blood vessels, but now allow for measurement of the thickness of individual retinal layers and detection of subtle architectural abnormalities. Electrophysiological techniques may be used to objectively evaluate the function of the retina and optic nerves. Imaging techniques for evaluating the afferent visual pathways and cortical areas involved in visual processing are discussed in Chapter 39.

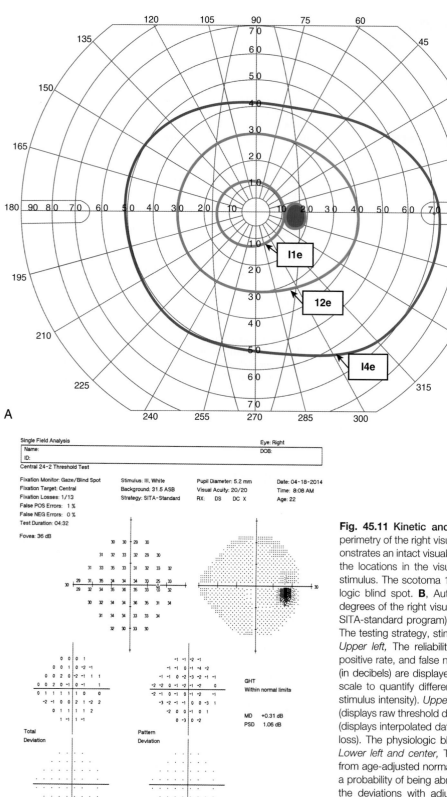

Fig. 45.11 Kinetic and automated static perimetry. A, Kinetic perimetry of the right visual field using the Goldmann perimeter demonstrates an intact visual field. The isopters (I1e, I2e, and I4e) indicate the locations in the visual field where the subject perceived each stimulus. The scotoma 10–20 degrees right of center is the physiologic blind spot. **B,** Automated static perimetry of the central 24 degrees of the right visual field using the Humphrey perimeter (24-2 SITA-standard program) demonstrates an intact visual field. *Upper,* The testing strategy, stimulus size, and stimulus color are indicated. *Upper left,* The reliability indices (number of fixation losses, false positive rate, and false negative rate) and the foveal visual threshold (in decibels) are displayed. The decibel (dB) is a logarithmic relative scale to quantify differential light sensitivity (1 dB = 0.1 log-unit of stimulus intensity). *Upper center and right,* Threshold sensitivity plot (displays raw threshold data for each test location) and grayscale plot (displays interpolated data; darker areas indicate areas of visual field loss). The physiologic blind spot is 10–20 degrees right of center. *Lower left and center,* The total deviation plots indicate deviations from age-adjusted normal values at each test location (in dB and as a probability of being abnormal). The pattern deviation plots indicate the deviations with adjustment for generalized depression of the visual field (e.g., due to refractive error, media opacity, or pupillary miosis). *Lower right,* The mean deviation (MD; mean of all total deviation values) is a global indicator of the severity of visual field loss. Negative values indicate greater visual field loss. The pattern standard deviation (PSD) provides a measure of the uniformity of the visual field loss, such that diseases causing highly focal defects (e.g., glaucoma) will have a high PSD, whereas those causing diffuse visual field loss will have a low PSD.

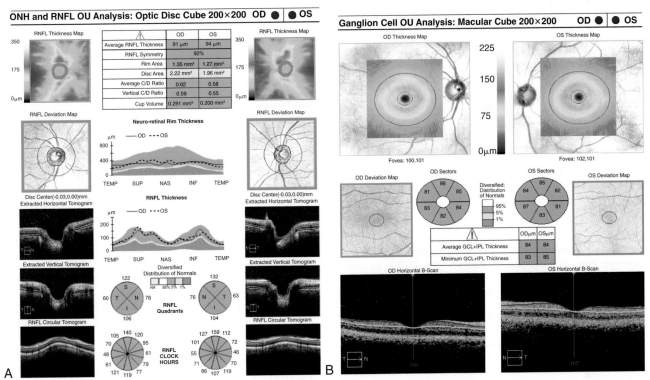

Fig. 45.12 Optical coherence tomography of the optic nerves and macula. A, Optical coherence tomography of the optic nerve head (OHN) and retinal nerve fiber layer (RNFL) from the right eye (OD) and left eye (OS), obtained using the Cirrus optic disc cube protocol. The top panel shows the RNFL thickness map, with the average RNFL thickness (in micrometers), optic disc area, and the cup-to-disc (C/D) ratio for each eye. Neuro-retinal rim and RNFL thicknesses are plotted below for quadrants of the optic nerves (S, superior; N, nasal; I, inferior; T, temporal) compared with the distribution from age-matched normal controls. The RNFL thicknesses fall within the normal range in both eyes. **B,** Optical coherence tomography showing the macular ganglion cell analysis from the right eye and left eye, obtained using the Cirrus macular cube protocol. The top panel shows the ganglion cell thickness map for each eye. The ganglion cell layer thicknesses are plotted below for the six sectors of the macula compared with the distribution from age-matched controls. The ganglion cell layer thicknesses fall within the normal range for both eyes.

nerve dysfunction. Measurement of *visual-evoked potentials* (VEP) has long been used for the evaluation of demyelinating optic neuropathies, which produce a delayed P-100. However, VEP findings can be misleading; a low-amplitude VEP could be misinterpreted as indicating optic neuropathy in a patient with retinal disease. *Electroretinography* (ERG) is useful for evaluation of suspected retinal dysfunction, especially when ophthalmoscopic findings are subtle or absent. *Full-field ERG* evaluates the response of the entire retina to flashes of light. A variety of stimuli are presented in differing states of light adaptation, allowing for evaluation of different retinal elements, including the rod and cone photoreceptors. Since full-field ERG evaluates the response of the entire retina, it may not be abnormal in patients with focal retinal dysfunction (e.g., macular dysfunction). *Multi-focal ERG* allows for the topographic evaluation of macula ERG responses and is more sensitive for detecting macular dysfunction (Sutter and Tran, 1992); multi-focal ERG findings can be grossly abnormal even when ophthalmoscopic changes are absent or subtle.

NONORGANIC (FUNCTIONAL) VISUAL DISTURBANCES

Nonorganic (functional) visual disturbances can have a variety of manifestations (Box 45.3). Like other nonorganic conditions, they can be a challenge to diagnose and manage (Friedman et al., 2010).

BOX 45.3 Some Forms of Nonorganic Visual Disturbance

Visual acuity loss (one or both eyes)
Visual field loss (unilateral or bilateral)
Color perception abnormalities
Convergence/accommodative insufficiency
Spasm of the near triad
Loss of depth perception
Diplopia
Night blindness
Photophobia
Pharmacological pupils
Voluntary nystagmus

Diagnostic Techniques

A careful social and family history must be obtained when evaluating a patient with suspected nonorganic visual disturbance, especially regarding abuse, peer pressure, and visually impaired friends and family members. Different examination approaches are needed, depending on the type of nonorganic visual disturbance. For example, if a patient reports total blindness, the clinician should examine the pupils, check for the optokinetic response using an optokinetic drum, and oscillate a large mirror in front of the patient to try inducing

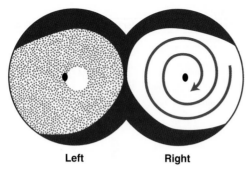

Left   Right

Fig. 45.13 Two common visual field abnormalities with nonorganic visual loss. *Left*, Concentric (tubular) constriction. *Right*, Spiraling of an isopter (seen only with kinetic visual field testing).

pursuit eye movements. If the patient claims visual loss in one eye, the clinician should examine the pupils to assess for an RAPD, attempt the mentioned tests with the good eye occluded, and test stereopsis. Specialized ophthalmic techniques such as a "fogging" refraction can also be helpful in this setting, but these require the assistance of an ophthalmologist.

Testing of visual fields in patients with suspected nonorganic visual loss may reveal one of several patterns, including tubular constriction, cloverleaf constriction, spiraling of an isopter, crossing isopters, or inverted isopters (Fig. 45.13). Confrontation or tangent screen testing done at different distances can be useful in evaluating a patient with visual field constriction, since the visual field area should increase as the distance between the patient and clinician increases. Lack of expansion of visual field area with increasing distance from the clinician suggests nonorganic visual field constriction (see Fig. 45.4). Cloverleaf constriction is best detected on automated static perimetry and cannot be produced by organic disease. Spiraling, crossing, and inversion of isopters can be detected using kinetic perimetry and cannot be produced by organic disease. Kinetic perimetry with both eyes opened in a patient with suspected nonorganic monocular visual loss may demonstrate nonphysiologic visual field constriction on the side of the reported visual loss.

The use of VEPs to diagnose nonorganic visual loss can be unreliable. If the VEP is normal, useful information is gained, but factitious abnormalities in the VEP can be induced if the patient defocuses their vision during the test. Therefore, an abnormal VEP is not always diagnostic of organic visual disturbance.

A variety of nonorganic ocular motor disturbances can be encountered. Spasm of the near triad is a common nonorganic ocular motor disturbance that is characterized by inappropriate appearance of the near triad (convergence, pupillary miosis, and lens accommodation). The patient will often report intermittent binocular horizontal diplopia and blurring of vision. The diagnosis can be verified by identifying pupillary miosis on attempted lateral gaze. Voluntary nystagmus is another common nonorganic ocular motility finding, which is characterized by high-frequency back-to-back horizontal saccades without an intersaccadic interval. It can be confused with ocular flutter (see Chapter 44). Unlike ocular flutter, it is usually initiated by a convergence effort, associated with eyelid flutter, and difficult to sustain for more than several seconds.

Prognosis

About half of patients with nonorganic visual disturbance improve with time and reassurance. Factors that indicate a good prognosis include youth and the presence of anxiety, whereas older age and depression are usually associated with a poor prognosis.

REFERENCES

The complete reference list is available online at https://expertconsult .inkling.com/.

46 Neuro-otology: Diagnosis and Management of Neuro-otological Disorders

Kevin A. Kerber, Robert W. Baloh

CHAPTER OUTLINE

HISTORICAL BACKGROUND

EPIDEMIOLOGY OF VERTIGO, DIZZINESS, AND HEARING LOSS

NORMAL ANATOMY AND PHYSIOLOGY

HISTORY OF PRESENT ILLNESS

PHYSICAL EXAMINATION
General Medical Examination
General Neurological Examination
Neuro-otological Examination

SPECIFIC DISORDERS CAUSING VERTIGO
Peripheral Vestibular Disorders
Central Nervous System Disorders
Vertigo in Inherited Disorders
Familial Hearing Loss and Vertigo

COMMON CAUSES OF NONSPECIFIC DIZZINESS

COMMON PRESENTATIONS OF VERTIGO
Acute Severe Vertigo
Recurrent Attacks of Vertigo
Recurrent Positional Vertigo

HEARING LOSS
Conductive Hearing Loss
Sensorineural Hearing Loss
Central Hearing Loss

SPECIFIC DISORDERS CAUSING HEARING LOSS
Meniere Disease
Cerebellopontine Angle Tumors
Superior Canal Dehiscence
Otosclerosis
Noise-Induced Hearing Loss
Genetic Disorders
Ototoxicity

COMMON PRESENTATIONS OF HEARING LOSS
Asymmetrical Sensorineural Hearing Loss
Sudden Sensorineural Hearing Loss
Hearing Loss with Age

TINNITUS

LABORATORY INVESTIGATIONS IN DIAGNOSIS AND MANAGEMENT
Dizziness and Vertigo
Hearing Loss and Tinnitus

MANAGEMENT OF PATIENTS WITH VERTIGO
Treatments of Specific Disorders
Symptomatic Treatment of Vertigo

MANAGEMENT OF PATIENTS WITH HEARING LOSS AND TINNITUS

Dizziness is a term patients use to describe a variety of symptoms including spinning or movement of the environment (vertigo), lightheadedness, presyncope, or imbalance. Patients may also use the term for other sensations such as visual distortion, internal spinning, nonspecific disorientation, and anxiety.

Patients may experience dizziness in isolation or with other symptoms. Neurological causes should be considered when other neurological signs and symptoms are present and also whenever specific peripheral vestibular or general medical disorders have not been identified. It is critical to ask the patient about associated symptoms, since they may be the key to diagnosis. *Vertigo*, a sensation of spinning of the environment, indicates a lesion within the vestibular pathways, either peripheral or central. Associated ear symptoms such as hearing loss and tinnitus can suggest a peripheral localization (i.e., inner ear, eighth nerve). Many different types of hearing loss occur with or without dizziness, and an understanding of common auditory disorders is important to the practicing neurologist. With an understanding of the neuro-otological bedside examination, specific findings can often be identified.

In this chapter, we provide background information regarding dizziness, vertigo, and hearing loss and the clinical information necessary for making specific diagnoses. We also include details on testing and management of these patients.

HISTORICAL BACKGROUND

In 1861, Prosper Meniere was the first to recognize the association of vertigo with hearing loss and thus to localize the symptom to the inner ear (Baloh, 2001). Caloric testing, the most widely used test of the vestibulo-ocular reflex (VOR), was introduced by Robert Barany in 1906. He was later awarded the Nobel Prize for proposing the mechanism of caloric stimulation. Barany also provided the first clinical description of benign paroxysmal positional vertigo (BPPV) in 1921. Endolymphatic hydrops was identified in postmortem specimens of patients with Meniere disease in 1938. A method for measuring eye movements in response to caloric and rotational stimuli (electronystagmography) was introduced in the 1930s, and in the 1970s digital computers began to be used to quantify eye movement responses.

Neuroimaging in the late 1970s and 1980s greatly expanded our understanding of causes of dizziness and vertigo. Prior to this time, stroke was considered an exceedingly rare cause of vertigo (Fisher, 1967). Though it remains a controversial topic even today, infarctions within the cerebellum and brainstem have been identified on imaging studies in patients with isolated vertigo. Imaging studies continue to lead to new discoveries of causes of vertigo, as demonstrated by the recently described disorder of superior canal dehiscence (SCD). But the most common causes of vertigo—Meniere disease, BPPV, and vestibular neuritis—still have no identifiable imaging characteristics.

Over the past 25 years, our understanding of the mechanisms for the common neuro-otological disorders has been greatly enhanced. BPPV can now be readily identified and cured at the bedside with a simple positional maneuver, and variants have also been described (Aw et al., 2005; Fife et al., 2008). The head-thrust test can be used at the bedside to identify a vestibular nerve lesion, and because of this it has particular utility in helping distinguish vestibular neuritis from a posterior fossa stroke (Halmagyi and Curthoys, 1988; Kattah et al., 2009; Newman-Toker et al., 2008; Nuti et al., 2005). Controversies regarding Meniere disease have been clarified, and medical and surgical treatments have improved (Minor et al., 2004). It is now clear that patients with recurrent episodes of vertigo without hearing loss, a condition once called *vestibular Meniere disease*, do not actually have Meniere disease.

Migraine is now recognized as an important cause of dizziness, even in patients without simultaneous headaches. In fact, benign recurrent vertigo (patients with recurrent episodes of vertigo without accompanying auditory symptoms or other neurological features) is usually a migraine equivalent (Oh et al., 2001b). A more detailed description of the rotational vertebral artery syndrome has led to appreciation of the high metabolic demands of the inner ear and its susceptibility to ischemia (Choi et al., 2005). Genetic research has identified ion channel dysfunction in disorders such as episodic ataxia and familial hemiplegic migraine, and patients with these disorders also commonly report vertigo (Jen et al., 2004a). It is hoped that identifying specific genes causing vertigo syndromes will lead to a better understanding of the mechanisms and also create the opportunity to develop specific treatments in the future.

EPIDEMIOLOGY OF VERTIGO, DIZZINESS, AND HEARING LOSS

Approximately 30% of people will experience moderate to severe dizziness at some point in their life (Neuhauser et al., 2005). Though most people report nonspecific forms of dizziness, nearly 25% of these people report true vertigo. Dizziness is more common among females and older people and has important healthcare utilization implications because up to 80% of patients with dizziness seek medical care at some point. In the United States, the National Centers for Health Statistics report 7.5 million annual ambulatory visits to physician offices, hospital outpatient departments, and emergency departments (EDs) for dizziness, making it one of the most common principal complaints (Burt and Schappert, 2004).

Hearing loss affects approximately 16% of adults (age >18 years) in the United States (Lethbridge-Cejku et al., 2006). Men are more commonly affected than women, and the prevalence of hearing loss increases dramatically with age, so that by age 75, nearly 50% of the population reports hearing loss, which is a common cause of disability. The most common type of hearing loss is sensorineural, and both idiopathic presbycusis and noise-induced forms are common etiologies. Bothersome tinnitus is less frequent in the U.S. population, with about 3% reporting it, although this increases to about 9% for subjects older than 65 (Adams et al., 1999). The most common type of tinnitus is a high-pitched ringing in both ears.

NORMAL ANATOMY AND PHYSIOLOGY

The inner ear is composed of a fluid-filled sac enclosed by a bony capsule with an anterior cochlear part, central chamber (vestibule), and a posterior vestibular part (Fig. 46.1). Endolymph fills up the fluid-filled sac and is separated by a membrane from the perilymph. These fluids primarily differ in their composition of potassium and sodium, with the endolymph resembling intracellular fluid with a high potassium and low sodium content, and perilymph resembling extracellular fluids with a low potassium and high sodium content.

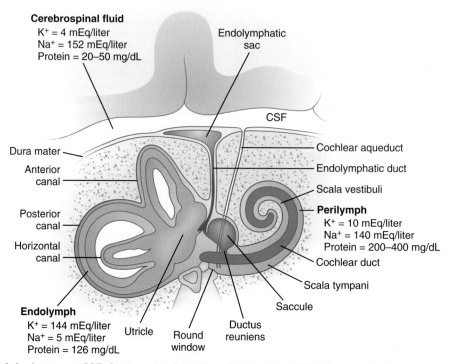

Fig. 46.1 Anatomy of the inner ear. *CSF*, Cerebrospinal fluid. *(From Baloh, R.W., 1998. Dizziness, Hearing Loss, and Tinnitus. F.A. Davis Company, Philadelphia, Figure 6, p. 16.)*

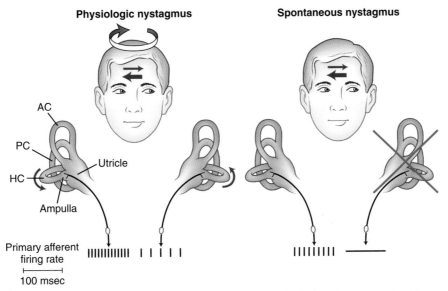

Fig. 46.2 **Primary afferent nerve activity associated with rotation-induced physiological nystagmus and spontaneous nystagmus resulting from a lesion of one labyrinth.** Thin straight arrows indicate the direction of slow components; thick straight arrows indicate the direction of fast components; curved arrows show the direction of endolymph flow in the horizontal semicircular canals. *AC,* Anterior canal; *HC,* horizontal canal; *PC,* posterior canal. *(From Baloh, R.W., 1998. Dizziness, Hearing Loss, and Tinnitus. F.A. Davis Company, Philadelphia, Figure 16, p. 36.)*

Perilymph communicates with the cerebrospinal fluid (CSF) through the cochlear aqueduct.

The cochlea senses sound waves after they travel through the external auditory canal and are amplified by the tympanic membrane and ossicles of the middle ear (Baloh and Kerber, 2011). The stapes, the last of three ossicles in the middle ear, contacts the oval window, which directs the forces associated with sound waves along the basilar membrane of the cochlea. These forces stimulate the hair cells, which in turn generate neural signals in the auditory nerve. The auditory nerve enters the lateral brainstem at the pontomedullary junction and synapses in the cochlear nucleus. The trapezoid body is the major decussation of the auditory pathway, but many fibers do not cross to the contralateral side. Signals then travel to the superior olivary complex. Some projections travel from the superior olivary complex to the inferior colliculus through the lateral lemnisci, and others terminate in one of the nuclei of the lateral lemniscus. Next, fibers travel to the ipsilateral medial geniculate body, and then auditory radiations pass through the posterior limb of the internal capsule to reach the auditory cortex of the temporal lobe.

The peripheral vestibular system is composed of three semicircular canals, the utricle and saccule, and the vestibular component of the eighth cranial nerve (Baloh and Kerber, 2011). Each semicircular canal has a sensory epithelium called the *crista;* the sensory epithelium of the utricle and saccule is called the *macule.* The semicircular canals sense angular movements, and the utricle and saccule sense linear movements. Two of the semicircular canals (anterior and posterior) are oriented in the vertical plane nearly orthogonal to each other; the third canal is oriented in the horizontal plane (horizontal canal). The crista of each canal is activated by movement occurring in the plane of that canal. When the hair cells of these organs are stimulated, the signal is transferred to the vestibular nuclei via the vestibular portion of cranial nerve VIII. Signals originating from the horizontal semicircular canal then pass via the medial longitudinal fasciculus along the floor of the fourth ventricle to the abducens nuclei in the middle brainstem and the ocular motor complex in the rostral brainstem. The anterior (also referred to as the *superior*) and posterior canal impulses pass from the vestibular nuclei to the ocular motor nucleus and trochlear nucleus, triggering eye movements roughly in the plane of each canal. A key feature is that once vestibular signals leave the vestibular nuclei they divide into vertical, horizontal, and torsional components. As a result, a lesion of central vestibular pathways can cause a pure vertical, pure torsional, or pure horizontal nystagmus.

The primary vestibular afferent nerve fibers maintain a constant baseline firing rate of action potentials. When the baseline rate from each ear is symmetrical (or an asymmetry has been centrally compensated), the eyes remain stationary. With an uncompensated asymmetry in the firing rate, resulting from either increased or decreased activity on one side, slow ocular deviation results. By turning the head to the right, the baseline firing rate of the horizontal canal is physiologically altered, causing an increased firing rate on the right side and a decreased firing rate on the left side (Fig. 46.2). The result is a slow deviation of the eyes to the left. In an alert subject, this slow deviation is regularly interrupted by quick movements in the opposite direction (nystagmus), so the eyes do not become pinned to one side. In a comatose patient, only the slow component is seen because the brain cannot generate the corrective fast components ("doll's eyes").

The plane in which the eyes deviate as a result of vestibular stimulation depends on the combination of canals that are stimulated (Table 46.1). If only the posterior semicircular canal on one side is stimulated (as occurs with BPPV), a vertical-torsional deviation of the eyes can be observed, which is followed by a fast corrective response generated by the conscious brain in the opposite direction. However, if the horizontal canal is the source of stimulation (as occurs with the horizontal canal variant of BPPV), a horizontal deviation with a slight torsional component (because this canal is slightly off the horizontal plane) results. If the vestibular nerve is lesioned (vestibular neuritis) or stimulated (vestibular paroxysmia), a horizontal greater than torsional nystagmus is seen that is the vector sum of all three canals—the two vertical canals on one side cancel each other out.

TABLE 46.1 Physiological Properties and Clinical Features of the Components of the Peripheral Vestibular System

Localization	Component(s)	Triggered eye movements	Common clinical conditions	Localizing features
SEMICIRCULAR CANALS				
Posterior canal	PC	Vertical, torsional	BPPV-PC	Nystagmus
Anterior canal	AC	Vertical, torsional	BPPV-AC, SCD	Nystagmus, fistula test
Horizontal canal	HC	Horizontal ≫ torsional	BPPV-HC, fistula	Nystagmus
VESTIBULAR NERVE				
Superior division	AC, HC, utricle	Horizontal > torsional	VN, ischemia	Nystagmus, head-thrust test
Inferior division	PC, saccule	Vertical, torsional	VN, ischemia	Nystagmus
Common trunk (cranial nerve 8)	AC, HC, PC, utricle, saccule	Horizontal > torsional	VN, VP, ischemia	Nystagmus, head-thrust test, auditory findings
Labyrinth	AC, HC, PC, utricle, saccule	Horizontal > torsional	EH, labyrinthitis	Nystagmus, auditory findings

AC, Anterior canal; *BPPV*, benign paroxysmal positional vertigo; *EH*, endolymphatic hydrops; *HC*, horizontal canal; *PC*, posterior canal; *SCD*, superior canal dehiscence; *VN*, vestibular neuritis; *VP*, vestibular paroxysmia.

Over time, either an asymmetry in the baseline firing rates resolves (the stimulation has been removed) or the central nervous system (CNS) compensates for it. This explains why an entire unilateral peripheral vestibular system can be surgically destroyed and patients only experience vertigo for several days to weeks. It also explains why patients with slow-growing tumors affecting the vestibular nerve, such as an acoustic neuroma, generally do not experience vertigo or nystagmus.

HISTORY OF PRESENT ILLNESS

The history and physical examination provide the most important information when evaluating patients complaining of dizziness (Colledge et al., 1996; Lawson et al., 1999). Often, patients have difficulty describing the exact symptom experienced, so the onus is on the clinician to elicit pertinent information. The first step is to define the symptom. No clinician should ever be satisfied to record the complaint simply as "dizziness." For patients unable to provide a more detailed description of the symptom, the physician can ask the patient to place their symptom into one of the following categories: movement of the environment (vertigo), lightheadedness, or strictly imbalance without an abnormal head sensation. Because patient descriptions about dizziness can be unreliable and inconsistent (Newman-Toker et al., 2007), other details about the symptom become equally important. The physician should also ask the following questions: Is the symptom constant or episodic, are there accompanying symptoms, how did it begin (gradual, sudden, etc.), and were there aggravating or alleviating factors? If episodic, what was the duration and frequency of attacks, and were there triggers? Table 46.2 displays the key distinguishing features of common causes of dizziness. One key point is that any type of dizziness may worsen with position changes, but some disorders such as BPPV only occur after position change.

PHYSICAL EXAMINATION
General Medical Examination

A brief general medical examination is important. Identifying orthostatic drops in blood pressure can be diagnostic in the correct clinical setting. Orthostatic hypotension is probably the most common general medical cause of dizziness among patients referred to neurologists. Identifying an irregular heart rhythm may also be pertinent. Other general examination measures to consider in individual patients include a visual assessment (adequate vision is important for balance) and a musculoskeletal inspection (significant arthritis can impair gait).

General Neurological Examination

The general neurological examination is very important in patients complaining of dizziness, because dizziness can be the earliest symptom of a neurodegenerative disorder (de Lau et al., 2006) and can also be an important symptom of stroke, tumor, demyelination, or other pathologies of the nervous system.

The cranial nerves should be thoroughly assessed in patients complaining of dizziness. The most important part of the examination is the ocular motor examination (described in more detail in the Neuro-otological Examination section). One should ensure that the patient has full ocular ductions. A posterior fossa mass can impair facial sensation and the corneal reflex on one side. Assessing facial strength and symmetry is important because of the close anatomical relationship between the seventh and eighth cranial nerves. The lower cranial nerves should also be closely inspected by observing palatal elevation, tongue protrusion, and trapezius and sternocleidomastoid strength.

The general motor examination determines strength in each muscle group and also assesses bulk and tone. Increased tone or cogwheel rigidity could be the main finding in a patient with an early neurodegenerative disorder. The peripheral sensory examination is important because a peripheral neuropathy can cause a nonspecific dizziness or imbalance. Temperature, pain, vibration, and proprioception should be assessed. Reflexes should be tested for their presence and symmetry. One must take into consideration the normal decrease in vibratory sensation and absence of ankle jerks that can occur in elderly patients. Coordination is an important part of the neurological examination in patients with dizziness because disorders characterized by ataxia can present with the principal symptom of dizziness. Observing the patient's ability to perform the finger-nose-finger test, the heel-knee-shin test, and rapid alternating movements adequately assesses extremity coordination (Schmitz-Hubsch et al., 2006).

TABLE 46.2 Distinguishing Among Common Peripheral and Central Vertigo Syndromes

Cause	History of vertigo	Duration of vertigo	Associated symptoms	Physical examination
PERIPHERAL				
Vestibular neuritis	Single prolonged episode	Days to weeks	Nausea, imbalance	"Peripheral" nystagmus, positive head-thrust test, imbalance
BPPV	Positionally triggered episodes	<1 minute	Nausea	Characteristic positionally triggered burst of nystagmus
Meniere disease	May be triggered by salty foods	Hours	Unilateral ear fullness, tinnitus, hearing loss, nausea	Unilateral low-frequency hearing loss
Vestibular paroxysmia	Abrupt onset; spontaneous or positionally triggered	Seconds	Tinnitus, hearing loss	Usually normal
Perilymph fistula	Triggered by sound or pressure changes	Seconds	Hearing loss, hyperacusis	Nystagmus triggered by loud sounds or pressure changes
CENTRAL				
Stroke/TIA	Abrupt onset; spontaneous	Stroke, >24 hours; TIA, < 24 hours	Brainstem, cerebellar	Spontaneous "central" nystagmus; gaze-evoked nystagmus; focal neurologic signs; negative head-thrust test; skew deviation
MS	Subacute onset	Minutes to weeks	Unilateral visual loss, diplopia, incoordination, ataxia	"Central" types or rarely "peripheral" types of spontaneous or positional nystagmus; usually other focal neurologic signs
Neurodegenerative disorders	May be spontaneous or positionally triggered	Minutes to hours	Ataxia	"Central" types of spontaneous or positional nystagmus; gaze-evoked nystagmus; impaired smooth pursuit; cerebellar, extrapyramidal and frontal signs
Migraine	Onset usually associated with typical migraine triggers	Seconds to days	Headache, visual aura, photo-/phonophobia	Normal interictal exam; ictal examination may show "peripheral" or "central" types of spontaneous or positional nystagmus
Familial ataxia syndromes	Acute-subacute onset; usually triggered by stress, exercise, or excitement	Hours	Ataxia	"Central" types of spontaneous or positional nystagmus Ictal, or even interictal, gaze-evoked nystagmus; ataxia; gait disorders

BPPV, Benign paroxysmal positional vertigo; *MS*, multiple sclerosis; *TIA*, transient ischemic attack.

Neuro-otological Examination

The neuro-otological examination is a specialty examination expanding upon certain aspects of the general neurological examination and also includes an audio-vestibular assessment.

Ocular Motor (see Chapter 44)

The first step in assessing ocular motor function is to search for spontaneous involuntary movements of the eyes. The examiner asks the patient to look straight ahead while observing for nystagmus or saccadic intrusions. Nystagmus is characterized by a slow- and fast-phase component and is classified as spontaneous, gaze-evoked, or positional. The direction of nystagmus is conventionally described by the direction of the fast phase, which is the direction it appears to be "beating" toward. Recording whether the nystagmus is vertical, horizontal, torsional, or a mixture of these provides important localizing information. Spontaneous nystagmus can have either a

peripheral or central pattern. Although central lesions can mimic a "peripheral" pattern of nystagmus (Lee and Cho, 2004; Newman-Toker et al., 2008), unusual circumstances are required for peripheral lesions to cause "central" patterns of nystagmus. The peripheral pattern of spontaneous nystagmus is unidirectional; that is, the eyes beat only to one side (Video 46.1). Peripheral spontaneous nystagmus never changes direction. It is usually a horizontal greater than torsional pattern because of the physiology of the asymmetry in firing rates within the peripheral vestibular system whereby the vertical canals cancel each other out. The prominent horizontal component results from the unopposed horizontal canal. Other characteristics of peripheral spontaneous nystagmus are suppression with visual fixation, increase in velocity with gaze in the direction of the fast phase, and decrease with gaze in the direction opposite of the fast phase. Some patients are able to suppress this nystagmus so well at the bedside, or have partially recovered from the initiating event, that spontaneous nystagmus may only appear by removing visual fixation.

Several simple bedside techniques can be used to remove the patient's ability to fixate. Frenzel glasses are designed to remove visual fixation by using +30 diopter lenses. An ophthalmoscope can be used to block fixation. While the fundus of one eye is being viewed, the patient is asked to cover the other eye. Probably the simplest technique involves holding a blank sheet of paper close to the patient's face (so as to block visual fixation) and observing for spontaneous nystagmus from the side. (See Video 46.1.)

Saccadic intrusions are spontaneous, involuntary saccadic movements of the eyes, without the rhythmic fast and slow phases characteristic of nystagmus. *Saccades* are fast movements of the eyes normally under voluntary control and used to shift gaze from one object to another. Square-wave jerks and saccadic oscillations are the most common types of saccadic intrusions. *Square-wave jerks* refer to small-amplitude, involuntary saccades that take the eyes off a target, followed after a normal intersaccadic delay (around 200 ms) by a corrective saccade to bring the eyes back to the target. Square-wave jerks can be seen in neurological disorders such as cerebellar ataxia, Huntington disease (HD), or progressive supranuclear palsy (PSP), but they also occur in normal individuals. If the square-wave jerks are persistent or of large amplitude (macro-square wave jerks), pathology is more likely.

Saccadic oscillations refer to back-to-back saccadic movements without the intersaccadic interval characteristic of square-wave jerks, so their appearance is that of an oscillation. When a burst occurs only in the horizontal plane, the term *ocular flutter* is used (Video 46.2). When vertical and/or torsional components are present, the term *opsoclonus* (or so-called dancing eyes) is used. The eyes make constant random conjugate saccades of unequal amplitude in all directions. Ocular flutter and opsoclonus are pathological findings typically seen in several different types of CNS diseases involving brainstem–cerebellar pathways. Paraneoplastic disorders should be considered in patients presenting with ocular flutter or opsoclonus. (See Video 46.2.)

Gaze Testing

The patient should be asked to look to the left, right, up, and down; the examiner looks for gaze-evoked nystagmus in each position (Video 46.3). A few beats of unsustained nystagmus with gaze greater than 30 degrees is called *end-gaze nystagmus* and variably occurs in normal subjects. Gaze-evoked downbeating nystagmus (Video 46.4), vertical nystagmus that increases on lateral gaze, localizes to the craniocervical junction and midline cerebellum. Gaze testing may also trigger saccadic oscillations. (See Videos 46.3 and 46.4.)

Smooth Pursuit

Smooth pursuit refers to the voluntary movement of the eyes used to track a target moving at a low velocity. It functions to keep the moving object on the fovea to maximize vision. Though characteristically a very smooth movement at low frequency and velocity testing, smooth pursuit inevitably breaks down when tested at high frequencies and velocities. Though smooth pursuit often becomes impaired with advanced age, a longitudinal study of healthy elderly individuals found no significant decline in smooth pursuit over 9 years of evaluation (Kerber et al., 2006). Patients with impaired smooth pursuit require frequent small saccades to keep up with the target; thus, the term *saccadic pursuit* is used to describe this finding (see Video 46.3). Abnormalities of smooth pursuit occur as the result of disorders throughout the CNS and with tranquilizing medicines, alcohol, inadequate concentration or vision, and fatigue. However, in a cognitively intact individual presenting with dizziness or imbalance symptoms, bilaterally impaired smooth pursuit is highly localizing to the cerebellum. Patients with early or mild cerebellar degenerative disorders may have markedly impaired smooth pursuit with mild or minimal truncal ataxia as the only findings.

Saccades

Saccades are fast eye movements (velocity of this eye movement can be as high as 600 degrees per second) used to quickly bring an object onto the fovea. Saccades are generated by the burst neurons of the pons (horizontal movements) and midbrain (vertical movements). Lesions or degeneration of these regions leads to slowing of saccades, which can also occur with lesions of the ocular motor neurons or extraocular muscles. Severe slowing can be readily appreciated at the bedside by instructing the patient to look back and forth from one object to another. The examiner observes both the velocity of the saccade and the accuracy. Overshooting saccades (missing the target and then needing to correct) indicates a lesion of the cerebellum (Video 46.5). Undershooting saccades are less specific and often occur in normal subjects. (See Video 46.5.)

Optokinetic Nystagmus and Fixation Suppression of the Vestibulo-ocular Reflex

Optokinetic nystagmus (OKN) and fixation suppression of the vestibulo-ocular reflex (VOR suppression) can also be tested at the bedside. OKN is a combination of fast (saccadic) and slow (smooth pursuit) movements of eyes and can be observed in normal individuals when, for example, watching a moving train. OKN is maximally stimulated with both foveal and parafoveal stimulation, so the proper laboratory technique for measuring OKN uses a full-field stimulus by having the patient sit stationary while a large rotating pattern moves around them. This test can be approximated at the bedside by moving a striped cloth in front of the patient, though this technique only stimulates the fovea. Patients with disorders causing severe slowing of saccades will not be able to generate OKN, so their eyes will become pinned to one side. VOR suppression can be tested at the bedside using a swivel chair. The patient sits in the chair and extends his or her arm in the "thumbs-up" position out in front. The patient is instructed to focus on the thumb and to allow the extended arm to move with the body so the visual target of the thumb remains directly in front of the patient. The chair is then rotated from side to side. The patient's eyes should remain locked on the thumb, demonstrating the ability to suppress the VOR stimulated by rotation of the chair. Nystagmus will be observed during the rotation movements in patients with impairment of VOR suppression, which is analogous to impairment of smooth pursuit. Both OKN and VOR suppression can also be helpful when examining patients having difficulty following the instructions for smooth pursuit or saccade testing.

Vestibular Nerve Examination

Often omitted as part of the cranial nerve examination in general neurology texts, important localizing information can be obtained about the functioning of the vestibular nerve at the bedside. A unilateral or bilateral vestibulopathy can be identified using the *head-thrust test* (Halmagyi et al., 2008) (Fig. 46.3 and Video 46.6). To perform the head-thrust test, the physician stands directly in front of the patient, who is seated on the exam table. The patient's head is held in the examiner's hands, and the patient is instructed to focus on the examiner's nose. The head is then quickly moved about 5 to 10 degrees to one side. In patients with normal vestibular function, the VOR results in movement of the eyes in the

COMMON CAUSES OF NONSPECIFIC DIZZINESS

Patients with nonspecific dizziness are probably referred to neurologists more frequently than patients with true vertigo. These patients are usually bothered by lightheadedness (wooziness), presyncope, imbalance, motion sensitivity, or anxiety. Side effects or toxicity from medications are common causes of nonspecific dizziness. Bothersome lightheadedness can be a direct effect of the medication itself or the result of lowering of the patient's blood pressure. Ataxia can be caused by antiepileptic medications and is usually reversible once the medication is decreased or stopped. Patients with peripheral neuropathy causing dizziness report significant worsening of their balance in poor lighting and also the sensation that they are walking on cushions. Drops in blood pressure can be caused by dehydration, vasovagal attacks, or as part of an autonomic neuropathy. Patients with panic attacks can present with nonspecific dizziness, but their spells are invariably accompanied by other symptoms such as sense of fear or doom, palpitations, sweating, shortness of breath, or paresthesias. Other medical conditions such as cardiac arrhythmias or metabolic disturbances can also cause nonspecific dizziness. In the elderly, confluent white matter hyperintensities have a strong association with dizziness and balance problems. Presumably the result of small vessel arteriosclerosis, decreased cerebral perfusion (Marstrand et al., 2002) has been identified in these patients even when blood pressure taken at the arm is normal. Patients with dizziness related to white matter hyperintensities on MRI usually feel better sitting or lying down and typically have impairment of tandem gait. Since many elderly patients are taking blood pressure medications, at least a trial of lowering or discontinuing these medications is warranted.

COMMON PRESENTATIONS OF VERTIGO

Patients present with symptoms rather than specific diagnoses. The most common presentations of vertigo are the following.

Acute Severe Vertigo

The patient presenting with new-onset severe vertigo probably has vestibular neuritis but stroke should also be a concern. An abrupt onset and accompanying focal neurological symptoms suggest an ischemic stroke. If no significant abnormalities are noted on the general neurological examination, attention should focus on the neuro-otological evaluation. If no spontaneous nystagmus is observed, a technique to block visual fixation should be applied. The direction of the nystagmus should be noted and the effect of gaze assessed. If a peripheral vestibular pattern of nystagmus is identified, a positive head-thrust test in the direction opposite the fast phase of nystagmus is highly localizing to the vestibular nerve. By far the most common cause of this presentation is vestibular neuritis. A central vestibular lesion (e.g., ischemic stroke) becomes a serious concern if there are "red flags" such as other central signs or symptoms, direction-changing nystagmus, vertical nystagmus, a negative head-thrust test (i.e., no corrective saccade after the head-thrust test to the direction opposite the fast phase of spontaneous nystagmus), a skew deviation, or substantial stroke risk factors (Kattah et al., 2009; Lee et al., 2006b). Vertebral artery dissection can lead to an acute vertigo presentation, but the most common symptom is severe, sudden-onset occipital or neck pain, with additional neurological signs and symptoms (Arnold et al., 2006). If hearing loss accompanies the episode, labyrinthitis is the most likely diagnosis, but auditory involvement does not exclude the possibility of a vascular cause, because the anterior inferior cerebellar artery supplies both the inner ear and brain. When hearing loss and facial weakness accompany the acute onset of vertigo, one should closely inspect the outer ear for vesicles characteristic of herpes zoster (Ramsay Hunt syndrome). An acoustic neuroma is a slow-growing tumor, so only rarely is it associated with acute-onset vertigo. Migraine can mimic vestibular neuritis, though the diagnosis of migraine-associated vertigo hinges on recurrent episodes and lack of progressive auditory symptoms.

Recurrent Attacks of Vertigo

In patients with recurrent attacks of vertigo, the key diagnostic information lies in the details of the attacks. Meniere disease is the likely cause in patients with recurrent vertigo lasting longer than 20 minutes and associated with unilateral auditory symptoms. If the Meniere-like attacks present in a fulminate fashion, the diagnosis of autoimmune inner-ear disease should be considered. Transient ischemic attacks (TIA) should be suspected in patients having brief episodes of vertigo, particularly when vascular risk factors are present and other neurological symptoms are reported (Josephson et al., 2008). Case series of patients with rotational vertebral artery syndrome demonstrate that the inner ear and possibly central vestibular pathways have high energy requirements and are therefore susceptible to levels of ischemia tolerated by other parts of the brain (Choi et al., 2005). Crescendo TIAs can be the harbinger of impending stroke or basilar artery occlusion. As with acute severe vertigo, accompanying auditory symptoms do not exclude the possibility of an ischemic disorder. Migraine and the migraine equivalent, BRV, are characterized by a history of similar symptoms, a normal examination, family or personal history of migraine headaches and/or BRV, other migraine characteristics, and typical triggers. Attacks are otherwise highly variable, lasting anywhere from seconds to days. If the attacks are consistently seconds in duration, the diagnosis of vestibular paroxysmia should be considered. Multiple sclerosis may be the cause when patients have recurrent episodes of vertigo and a history of other attacks of neurological symptoms, particularly when fixed deficits such as an afferent pupillary defect or internuclear ophthalmoplegia are identified on the examination.

Recurrent Positional Vertigo

Positional vertigo is defined by the symptom being *triggered*, not simply worsened, by certain positional changes. Physicians often confuse vestibular neuritis with BPPV because vestibular neuritis patients can often settle into a relatively comfortable position and then experience dramatic worsening with movement. The patient complaining of recurrent episodes of vertigo triggered by certain head movements likely has BPPV, but this is not the only possibility. BPPV can be identified and treated at the bedside, so positional testing should be performed in any patient with this complaint. Positional testing can also uncover the other causes of positionally triggered dizziness (Bertholon et al., 2002). The history strongly suggests the diagnosis of BPPV when the positional vertigo is brief (<1 minute), has typical triggers, and is unaccompanied by other neurological symptoms. A burst of vertical torsional nystagmus is specific for BPPV of the posterior canal (Aw et al., 2005). If the Dix–Hallpike test is negative, the examiner should search for the horizontal canal variant of BPPV with supine positional testing. Central positional nystagmus occurs as the result of disorders affecting the posterior fossa, including tumors, cerebellar degeneration, Chiari malformation, or MS. The nystagmus of these disorders is typically downbeating and persistent, though a pure torsional nystagmus may occur as well. Patients with loss of one vertebral artery may develop vertigo or significant dizziness after head turns to the direction opposite the intact artery because the bony structures of the spinal column can pinch off the remaining vertebral artery (Choi et al., 2005). Central types of nystagmus develop as a result, and vertigo can be the most prominent symptom. Finally, migraine can also closely mimic BPPV and central positional nystagmus (von Brevern et al., 2005). Patients with migraine as the cause typically report a longer duration of symptoms once the positional vertigo is triggered, and the nystagmus may be of a central or peripheral type. The mechanisms are not clear, but the disorder is benign because it is usually self-limited and not progressive. Associations between migraine and typical BPPV have also been made, but the link between these disorders is unclear.

HEARING LOSS

Neurologists generally do not encounter patients principally bothered by auditory symptoms such as hearing loss or tinnitus, as opposed to patients with dizziness, who are frequently referred for evaluation. Nevertheless, an understanding of the auditory system, certain disorders causing auditory symptoms, and audiograms can enhance the diagnostic abilities of the neurologist.

Conductive Hearing Loss

Conductive hearing loss results from lesions involving the external or the middle ear. The tympanic membrane and ossicles act as a transformer, amplifying the airborne sound and effectively transferring it to the inner-ear fluid. If this normal pathway is obstructed, transmission can occur across the skin and through the bones of the skull (bone conduction) but at the cost of significant energy loss. Patients with a conductive hearing loss can hear speech in a noisy background better than a quiet background, since they can understand loud speech as well as anyone. The most common cause of conductive hearing loss is impacted cerumen in the external canal. The most common serious cause of conductive hearing loss is otitis media, which can result from either infected fluid (suppurative otitis) or noninfected fluid (serous otitis) accumulating in the middle ear and impairing conduction of airborne sound. With chronic otitis media, a cholesteatoma may erode the ossicles. Otosclerosis produces progressive conductive hearing loss by immobilizing the stapes with new bone growth in front of and below the oval window. Other common causes of conductive hearing loss are trauma, congenital malformations of the external and middle ear, and glomus body tumors.

Sensorineural Hearing Loss

Sensorineural hearing loss results from lesions of the cochlea, the auditory division of the acoustic nerve, or both and results in inability to normally perceive both bone- and air-conducted sound. The spiral cochlea mechanically analyzes the frequency content of sound. For high-frequency tones, only sensory cells in the basilar turn are activated, but for low-frequency tones, all sensory cells are activated. Therefore, with lesions of the cochlea and its afferent nerve, the hearing levels for different frequencies are usually unequal, and the phase relationship between different frequencies may be altered. Patients with sensorineural hearing loss often have difficulty hearing speech that is mixed with background noise, and they may be annoyed by loud speech. Distortion of sounds is common with sensorineural hearing loss. A pure tone may be heard as noisy, rough, or buzzing, or it may be distorted so that it sounds like a complex mixture of tones.

Central Hearing Loss

Central hearing loss results from lesions of the central auditory pathways. These lesions involve the cochlear and dorsal olivary nuclear complexes, inferior colliculi, medial geniculate bodies, auditory cortex in the temporal lobes, and interconnecting afferent and efferent fiber tracks. As a rule, patients with central lesions do not have impaired hearing levels for pure tones, and they understand speech so long as it is clearly spoken in a quiet environment. If the listener's task is made more difficult with the introduction of background or competing messages, performance deteriorates more markedly in patients with central lesions than it does in normal subjects. Lesions involving the eighth nerve root entry zone or cochlear nucleus (demyelination or infarction in the lateral pontomedullary region), however, can cause unilateral hearing loss for pure tones. Because about half of afferent nerve fibers cross central to the cochlear nucleus, this is the most central structure in which a lesion can result in a unilateral hearing loss.

SPECIFIC DISORDERS CAUSING HEARING LOSS
Meniere Disease

Auditory symptoms in Meniere disease consist of a fluctuating sense of fullness and pressure along with tinnitus and decreased hearing in one ear. In the early stages, the hearing loss is completely reversible, but in later stages a residual hearing loss remains. Tinnitus may persist between episodes but usually increases in intensity immediately before or during the acute episode. It is typically described as a roaring sound like the sound of the ocean or a hollow seashell. The hearing loss on the audiogram appears in the early stages as a low-frequency loss. However, as the disorder progresses, a more complete hearing loss occurs. In about one-third of patients, the disorder becomes bilateral. Eventually, severe permanent hearing loss develops, and the episodic nature spontaneously disappears. When the progression of hearing loss (particularly when bilateral) is fulminant and rapidly progressive, the diagnosis of autoimmune inner-ear disease should be considered. Also see the section on Meniere disease under Specific Disorders Causing Vertigo.

Cerebellopontine Angle Tumors

Acoustic neuromas (vestibular schwannoma) account for about 5% of intracranial tumors and more than 90% of cerebellopontine angle tumors. These tumors usually begin in the internal auditory canal, producing symptoms by compressing the nerve in its narrow confines. As the tumor grows, it protrudes through the internal auditory meatus, stretches adjacent nerves over the surface of the mass, and deforms the cerebellum and brainstem. By far the most common symptoms associated with acoustic neuromas are slowly progressive unilateral hearing loss and tinnitus from compression of the cochlear nerve. Rarely, acute hearing loss occurs, possibly from compression of the labyrinthine vasculature. Vertigo occurs infrequently, but approximately half of patients with an acoustic neuroma complain of mild imbalance or disequilibrium. An epidermoid tumor, meningioma, facial nerve schwannoma, or metastatic disease can also cause mass lesions within the cerebellopontine angle. The audiometric pattern is variable; however, patients with cerebellopontine angle tumors causing hearing loss usually have poor speech discrimination, acoustic reflex decay, and pure tone decay rather than a marked asymmetry of pure tones.

Superior Canal Dehiscence

Patients with SCD may experience conductive hyperacusis (hearing their eye move or the impact of their feet during walking or running) and autophony (hearing their own breath and voice sounds) in the affected ear. An air/bone gap, with preserved acoustic reflexes, may be identified on standard audiograms. The Weber tuning fork test typically lateralizes to the affected ear, and the Rinne turning fork test may show bone conduction greater than air conduction (see Specific Disorders Causing Vertigo).

Otosclerosis

Otosclerosis is a metabolic disease of the bony labyrinth that usually manifests by immobilizing the stapes, thereby producing a conductive hearing loss. A positive family history for otosclerosis is reported in 50% to 70% of cases. Bilateral involvement is usual, but about one-fourth of cases are unilateral. Although conductive hearing loss is the hallmark of otosclerosis, a combined conductive-sensorineural hearing loss pattern is frequent. Although otosclerosis is primarily a disorder of the auditory system, vestibular symptoms and signs are more common than generally appreciated.

Noise-Induced Hearing Loss

Noise-induced hearing loss is extremely common. About one-third of individuals with hearing loss can attribute at least part of the loss to noise exposure. The loss almost always begins at 4000 Hz, creating the typical notched appearance on the audiogram, and does not affect speech discrimination until late in the disease process. Typically, levels of noise exposure greater than 85 dB are required to cause the changes in the ear induced by loud noise. Examples of noise greater than 85 dB that are common sources of exposure include motorcycles, firecrackers, factory machinery, and music concerts.

Genetic Disorders

Many genetic causes of hearing loss have been identified, including syndromic and nonsyndromic phenotypes and inheritance types that are autosomal dominant, autosomal recessive, and mitochondrial. Typically these disorders start early in life and cause profound hearing loss. Vestibular symptoms are not common but may not be thoroughly assessed in affected individuals.

Ototoxicity

The most common medications causing hearing loss are aminoglycoside antibiotics, loop diuretics, and cisplatin. Impaired elimination of these drugs, such as occurs in patients with renal insufficiency, predisposes to ototoxicity. Patients receiving high-dose salicylate therapy frequently complain of hearing loss, tinnitus, and dizziness. These symptoms and signs are rapidly reversible after cessation of the salicylate ingestion.

COMMON PRESENTATIONS OF HEARING LOSS
Asymmetrical Sensorineural Hearing Loss

Evaluation of patients identified as having an asymmetrical sensorineural hearing loss is primarily the search for a tumor in the area of the internal auditory canal or cerebellopontine angle, or more rarely other lesions of the temporal bone or brain. With an asymmetry of hearing defined as 15 dB or greater in two or more frequencies or a 15% or more asymmetry in speech discrimination scores, approximately 10% of patients will have lesions identified on MRI (Cueva, 2004). A simple management guide that has been proposed is to order an MRI if there is a ≥15 dB asymmetry at 3,000 Hz, or instead a follow-up audiogram if the asymmetry is <15 dB at 3,000 Hz (Saliba et al., 2011). Acoustic neuromas are by far the most common abnormality found. Other causative lesions may include glomus jugulare tumors, ectatic basilar artery with brainstem compression, or petrous apex cholesterol granuloma. Auditory brainstem response testing shows a sensitivity and specificity around 70%, with a false-positive rate of 77%, but a false-negative rate of 29% (Cueva, 2004).

Sudden Sensorineural Hearing Loss

The etiology of sudden sensorineural hearing loss is similar to both Bell palsy and vestibular neuritis in that a viral cause is presumed in the majority of cases, but proof of a viral pathophysiology in a given case is difficult to obtain. The hearing loss can abruptly develop or evolve over several hours. Acoustic neuromas may be found in around 5% of patients with this presentation (Aarnisalo et al., 2004), but one should also be aware of false-positive MRIs, particularly for lesions smaller than 6 mm (Arriaga et al., 1995). Focal ischemia to the cochlea, cochlear nerve, or the root entry zone can also cause an abrupt loss of hearing over several minutes. In the setting of a patient at risk for stroke, this cause should be considered early, because it can be the harbinger of basilar artery occlusion (Toyoda et al., 2002). Sudden-onset bilateral hearing loss can rarely result from bilateral lesions of the primary auditory cortex in the transverse temporal gyri of Heschl. Deficits can range from auditory agnosia for speech or nonspeech sounds, with relatively normal hearing thresholds, to rare cases of cortical deafness characterized by markedly elevated pure-tone thresholds.

Hearing Loss with Age

The bilateral hearing loss commonly associated with advancing age is called *presbycusis*. It is not a distinct entity but rather represents multiple effects of aging on the auditory system. It may include conductive and central dysfunction, but the most consistent effect of aging is on the sensory cells and the neurons of the cochlea. The typical audiogram appearance in patients with presbycusis is that of symmetrical hearing loss, with the tracing gradually sloping downward with increasing frequency. The most consistent pathology associated with presbycusis is a degeneration of sensory cells and nerve fibers at the base of the cochlea.

TINNITUS

Tinnitus is a noise in the ear that is usually audible only to the patient, although occasionally the sound can be heard by the examining physician. It is a symptom that can be associated with a variety of disorders that may affect the ear or the brain. The most important piece of information is whether the patient localizes it to one or both ears or if it is nonlocalizable. Tinnitus localized to one ear is probably more likely to have an identifiable cause than when localized to both ears or nonlocalizable. The characteristics of the tinnitus should be described by the patient, as this can provide helpful information. For an example, the typical tinnitus associated with Meniere disease is described as a roaring sound like listening to a seashell. The tinnitus associated with an acoustic neuroma is typically a high-pitched ringing or like the sound of steam blowing from a teakettle. If the tinnitus is rhythmic, the patient should be asked whether it is synchronous with the pulse or with respiration. Recurrent rhythmic or even nonrhythmic clicking sounds in one ear can indicate stapedial palatal myoclonus. However, the most common form of tinnitus is a bilateral high-pitched sound that is usually worse at night when it is quiet and there is less background noise to mask it. Tinnitus can be worse when the patient is under stress or with the use of caffeine.

LABORATORY INVESTIGATIONS IN DIAGNOSIS AND MANAGEMENT
Dizziness and Vertigo

The history and physical examination should determine what diagnostic tests if any are necessary in patients presenting with dizziness or vertigo. Studies have repeatedly shown that MRI, audiogram, and vestibular tests are not more likely to be abnormal in unselected patients complaining of dizziness when compared to age-matched controls (Colledge et al., 1996, 2002; Hajioff et al., 2002; Lawson et al., 1999; Yardley et al., 1998). Many disorders causing dizziness can be diagnosed and even treated at the bedside, with no further diagnostic tests indicated.

General Tests

General tests such as blood work, chest X-ray, or electrocardiograms are only indicated when searching for a specific abnormality. If a patient has otherwise unexplained nonspecific dizziness, ruling out metabolic causes is indicated.

Imaging

Brain imaging is commonly ordered in patients complaining of dizziness. Though a CT scan can rule out a large mass, smaller lesions cannot be excluded because of artifact and poor resolution in the posterior fossa (Chalela et al., 2007). MRI is the imaging modality of choice but is expensive and generally a much less practical test than CT. Determining which patients should have an MRI can be difficult, which is why an understanding of the common peripheral vestibular disorders is important. Patients identified as having BPPV, vestibular neuritis, or Meniere disease do not require an imaging study. Additionally, patients with normal neurological and neuro-otological examinations reporting episodes of dizziness dating back more than several months are highly unlikely to have a relevant abnormality on MRI. Though studies suggest improved hearing preservation after surgery in patients with acoustic neuromas when diagnosed early, this does not mean that every patient complaining of dizziness requires an MRI to exclude this cause. Acoustic neuromas are rare, whereas dizziness and vertigo are extremely common. On the other hand, for any patient experiencing focal neurological symptoms or having unexplained neurological deficits or an otherwise rapid, unexplained progression of symptoms, an MRI should be strongly considered to rule out a mass lesion, stroke, structural abnormality, or MS. In dizzy patients with gradually progressive hearing loss, MRI may also be helpful.

Vestibular Testing

Eye Movement Recording
Methods of Recording Eye Movements. Eye movement recordings can be made with *electronystagmography* (ENG) or video-nystagmography (VNG). ENG equipment is less expensive to purchase, and the test provides reliable clinical infor-

mation (Furman et al., 1996). Artifacts from lid movements or muscle action potentials are common; thus the "noise" is greater in ENG than in VNG. Probably the main clinical advantage of video-oculography (VOG) is the ability to go back and observe the actual video recording of the eye movements. Measuring torsional eye movements is also possible with VNG, although systems for doing so are still being developed. Disadvantages of VNG are the inability to measure eye movements with the eyes closed and difficulties stabilizing the head gear.

Eye Movement Subtests.
A standard test battery includes a search for pathological nystagmus or saccadic intrusions with fixation and with eyes open in the darkness, tests of visual ocular control (saccades, smooth pursuit, OKN), and the bithermal caloric test (Baloh and Kerber, 2011).

Recording Pathological Spontaneous Eye Movements.
Once the equipment has been set up and calibrated, the patient is asked to look straight ahead, both when fixating on a target and in darkness with eyes open (removing fixation). In this manner, spontaneous nystagmus or saccadic intrusions can be recorded. Patients are then instructed to look about 30 degrees from the midline in each direction, maintaining gaze for about 10 to 20 seconds in each direction. Gaze-evoked nystagmus is demonstrated when nystagmus not seen in the primary position appears with gaze. The most common type of gaze-evoked nystagmus has approximately equal amplitude in all directions and results from either medication toxicity or cerebellar dysfunction. In patients with a partially compensated peripheral vestibular lesion, nystagmus in one direction may be present. Small-amplitude nystagmus with gaze more than 30 degrees is typically a physiological nystagmus appearing in normal individuals and is referred to as *end-gaze nystagmus*. Positional testing using both the head-hanging positions and supine positions is used to search for positional nystagmus. A characteristic burst of nystagmus is seen in patients with BPPV. Persistent positional nystagmus (i.e., no burst) is a common finding when recordings are made with eyes open in darkness. When the average slow-phase velocity exceeds 4 deg/sec, it is abnormal but nonlocalizing. When patients are able to suppress this nystagmus when presented with a visual target, a peripheral cause is suggested.

Visual Ocular Motor Control
Saccades. By presenting the patient with visual targets that move 10 to 30 degrees in the horizontal and vertical planes, measurements of saccade onset, velocity, and accuracy can be made. Patients are instructed to "jump" from target to target. Normal subjects, elderly and young alike, achieve a highly reproducible pattern of saccadic velocity that has a nonlinear relationship between peak velocity and amplitude of the eye movement. Velocities initially increase from about 5-degree to 30-degree movements, and then a maximum velocity is achieved. Saccade velocity remains intact through late age in individuals without focal neurological disease. Slowing of saccades can occur with lesions anywhere in the diffuse central pathways involved in generating saccades, but the most pronounced slowing occurs with lesions affecting the brainstem (pretectal and paramedian pontine gaze centers or ocular motor neurons) and the extraocular muscles. Typical disorders with slowing of saccades are PSP and HD. Slowing can also result if the patient has taken tranquilizing drugs. A lesion of medial longitudinal fasciculus results in slowing of the adducting eye, often more easily appreciated with quantitative measures than bedside testing. Normal subjects consistently undershoot target jumps larger than 20 degrees and will require a small corrective saccade to achieve the final position. Overshooting saccades, however, are rare and do not

consistently occur in normal patients. Overshooting saccades typically are seen in patients with cerebellar dysfunction.

Smooth Pursuit. Recordings of smooth pursuit are made by having the patient follow a target back and forth. The slope of this eye/target velocity relationship represents the gain of the smooth pursuit system, which depends on the velocity and frequency of the target movements. Higher velocity and frequency testing results in lower gains. Though each laboratory must establish normal values, typically normal subjects have very high mean gains (0.92 ± 0.05 at 0.2 Hz, 22.6 deg/sec). Though a patient's age is typically considered when interpreting results, a recent study shows smooth-pursuit gains can be well maintained in subjects well into their ninth decade (Kerber et al., 2006).

Optokinetic Nystagmus. Laboratory testing of OKN uses a full-field visual stimulus (typically a patterned drum) that moves at a constant velocity and frequency around the subject, who is either instructed to follow the target (resulting in large-amplitude nystagmus) or stare through it (resulting in small-amplitude nystagmus). This stimulus also causes a sensation of self-rotation called *circular vection* even though the peripheral vestibular system is not being stimulated. The OKN gain is measured by comparing the slow-component velocity of the eye movement to the target velocity. As with smooth-pursuit testing, gain drops off with increasing frequency and velocity of the target in normal subjects. The normal and abnormal ENG appearance of saccades, smooth pursuit, and OKN are demonstrated in (Fig. 46.5).

Bithermal Caloric Testing. With the bithermal caloric test, each ear is irrigated alternately for a fixed duration (30 to 40 seconds) with a constant flow of water that is either 7°C above or below body temperature. The external auditory canal should first be inspected to make sure that cerumen does not occlude it and that the tympanic membrane is intact. The different temperatures of the water induce a movement of the endolymph mainly within the horizontal semicircular canal, because this canal is anatomically closest to the tympanic membrane. The resulting temperature gradient from one side of the canal to the other causes flow of the endolymph that triggers a very low-frequency stimulus of the horizontal canal.

The advantages of this test method are that the endolymph can be triggered to flow in both directions (ampullopetal and ampullofugal), each ear can be stimulated separately, and the test is tolerated by most patients. Limitations include the need for constant temperature baths and plumbing to maintain continuous circulation of the water through the infusion hose, the interindividual variability of caloric vestibular responses, and only being able to apply a single frequency stimulus.

The conventional method for measuring caloric stimulation is to compare the maximum slow-phase velocities achieved on one side to that of the other side, using the vestibular paresis formula

$$\frac{(R30° + R44°) - (L30° + L44°)}{(R30° + R44° + L30° + L44°)} \times 100.$$

Directional preponderance is also calculated using the formula

$$\frac{(L30° + R44°) - (L44° + R30°)}{(L30° + R44° + L44° + R30°)} \times 100.$$

Dividing by the total response normalizes the measurements to remove the large variability in absolute magnitude of normal caloric responses. Typically, the finding of significant vestibular paresis of 25% to 30% with bithermal caloric stimulation suggests a lesion in the vestibular system that is located anywhere from the end-organ to the vestibular nerve root entry zone in the brainstem. This finding is a strong indicator of a unilateral peripheral lesion, but it must be placed in the context of the patient's clinical history and bedside examination; a caloric paresis can also occur in central vestibular disorders. A recent study found a high rate of significant vestibular paresis (as measured by the caloric test) in patients with acute vertigo presentations caused by stroke (Newman-Toker et al., 2008). It is also common to find a caloric asymmetry in control subjects without dizziness (particularly those with migraine or diabetes) who undergo this test. A significant directional preponderance on caloric testing (>30%) indicates an imbalance in the vestibular system but is nonlocalizing, occurring with both peripheral and central lesions.

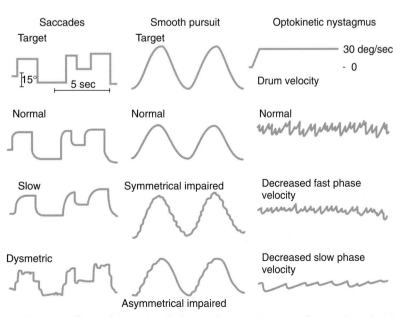

Fig. 46.5 Electronystagmographic recordings of normal and abnormal saccades, smooth pursuit, and optokinetic nystagmus. *(From Baloh, R.W., 1998. Dizziness, Hearing Loss, and Tinnitus. F.A. Davis Company, Philadelphia, Figure 37, p. 84.)*

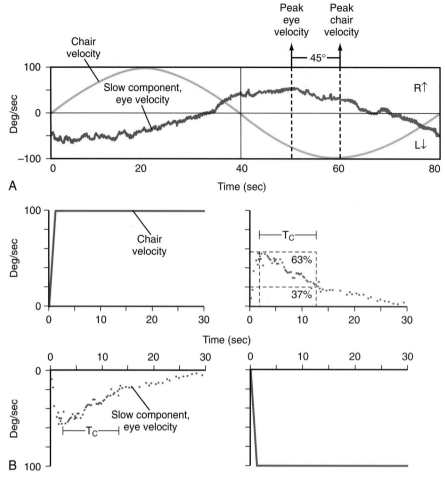

Fig. 46.6 Plots of slow-component eye velocity versus time for nystagmus induced by sinusoidal angular rotation in the horizontal plane at 0.0125 Hz and a peak velocity of 100 deg/sec **(A)** and by step changes in angular velocity of 100 deg/sec occurring with an acceleration of approximately 140 deg/sec² **(B)**. Subject is seated on a motorized rotating chair with eyes open in darkness. Eye movements are recorded with electronystagmography. Fast components are identified and removed, and slow component eye velocity is measured every 20 msec. The gain of the response (peak slow-component eye velocity/peak chair velocity) is about 0.6 for both types of stimulation. The phase lead with sinusoidal stimulation is the difference in timing between the peak eye velocity and peak chair velocity (in this case 45 deg). The time constant (T_C) is the time required for the response to decay to 37% of its initial value (about 10 seconds in **B**). *(From Baloh, R.W., 1998. Dizziness, Hearing Loss, and Tinnitus. F.A. Davis Company, Philadelphia, Figure 36, p. 81.)*

Rotational Testing. For rotational testing, the patient sits in a motorized chair that rotates under the control of a computer, and the patient's head and body move in unison with the chair. The chair is in a dark room, so visual fixation is removed. Eye movements induced by the vestibular system stimulating movements of the patient's head and body within the chair are recorded using ENG or VNG. The computer precisely controls the velocity and frequency of rotations so that the VOR can be measured at multiple frequencies in a single session. Sinusoidal and step (impulse) changes in angular velocity are routinely used (Fig. 46.6). In clinical testing, generally only rotations about the vertical axis are used, which maximally stimulates the horizontal canals. Off-vertical rotation can be used to measure the function of the vertical semicircular canals and otoliths, but typically this is only done in research studies. For sinusoidal rotations, results are reported as gain (peak slow-component eye velocity divided by peak chair velocity) and phase (timing between the peak velocity of eye and head) at different frequencies.

Because both inner ears are stimulated at the typically low velocities and frequencies used, rotational testing is most effective at determining a bilateral peripheral vestibular

hypofunction that leads to a decreased gain and increased phase. Unilateral vestibular hypofunction can be suggested by a normal gain with increased phase on standard testing or a decreased unilateral gain with shortened time constant on impulse (rapid movement) testing. Normal rotational testing results in gains around 0.5 at low-frequency rotation (0.05 Hz), with gains approaching 1.0 at higher-frequency rotations (>1 Hz). Even patients with partial loss of bilateral vestibular function may have gains in the normal range at the higher-frequency rotations, probably owing to the contribution of additional sensory systems (Jen et al., 2005; Wiest et al., 2001). The main disadvantage of rotational chair testing is the expense associated with setting it up. As a result, this vestibular test is typically only available at large academic centers. Because of this, portable devices using either passive (examiner-generated) head rotations or active (patient-generated) head turns have been developed, but the quality of evidence to support the use of these tests is low (Fife et al., 2000).

Rotational chair testing can also be used to measure the patient's ability to suppress the VOR and a combined measure of both OKN and rotational testing (visual VOR).

Quantivative Head-Thrust Testing. New devices that enable quantitative measurement of the vestibular-ocular reflex as elicited by the head-thrust test have been developed (MacDougall et al., 2009; Newman-Toker et al., 2013b). The devices consist of goggles that contain a video camera to measure eye movement velocity and an accelerometer to measure head movement velocity. Because of its ability to determine eye and head velocity, the device-based head-thrust test is mainly focused on measuring the VOR gain to each side rather than on the presence or absence of corrective saccades, which are the focus of the non-device-based head-thrust test. The quantitative measure of the head-thrust test is an advantage of the device because corrective saccades can be imperceptible, so-called "covert" saccades (Weber et al., 2008). The head-thrust test uses much higher acceleration than caloric testing to elicit eye movements via the vestibular system so that a direct comparison of the results of these tests is not entirely appropriate. However, one comparison found that a clinically significant abnormal device-based head-thrust test result is unlikely to occur in subjects with only a mild caloric asymmetry (Mahringer and Rambold, 2014).

Posturography. Posturography is a method for quantifying balance. This testing consists of measuring sway while standing on a stable platform and also with tilt or linear displacement of the platform, both with eyes open and eyes closed, and also with movement of the visual surround. Posturography is not a diagnostic test and is of little use for localizing a lesion. It can be helpful for following the course of a patient and may serve as a quantitative measure of the response to therapy or in research studies. Posturography may be useful for identifying people at risk for falling, though whether it is better at this than a careful clinical assessment is unclear (Piirtola and Era, 2006). Posturography may be helpful in identifying patients with factitious balance disorders (Gianoli et al., 2000).

Vestibular Evoked Myogenic Potentials. It has long been known that the sacculus, which during the course of its evolution functioned as an organ of hearing and still does in primitive vertebrates, can be stimulated by loud sounds. As a result of this stimulation, a signal travels via the inferior trunk of the vestibular nerve to cranial nerve VIII and into the brainstem. From there, inhibitory postsynaptic potentials travel to the ipsilateral sternocleidomastoid muscle (SCM), essentially allowing the individual to reflexively turn towards the sound. To generate this vestibular evoked myogenic potential (VEMP) response, intense clicks of about 95 to 100 dB above normal hearing level (NHL) are required (Welgampola and Colebatch, 2005). The response is measured from an activated ipsilateral SCM. Tonic contraction of the muscle is required to demonstrate the inhibitory response. The amplitude of the response and also the threshold needed to generate it are measured. Because the absolute amplitudes vary greatly from patient to patient, the more reliable abnormality is detecting a side-to-side difference in an individual. Additionally, responses are unreliable in subjects older than 60 years and in patients with middle ear abnormalities. Abnormal VEMP responses can be detected in most disorders affecting the peripheral vestibular system, but this test may help identify disorders that selectively affect the inferior vestibular nerve (Halmagyi et al., 2002) or SCD (Minor, 2005). Because caloric and rotational testing mainly stimulate the horizontal semicircular canal (which sends afferent responses via the superior vestibular nerve), the rare disorder affecting only the inferior vestibular nerve will not be identified with these tests. In patients with SCD, VEMP testing leads to increased amplitudes and lowered thresholds due to the low-impedance pathway created by the third window.

Hearing Loss and Tinnitus
Auditory Testing

Audiological assessment is the basis for quantifying auditory impairment. Most neurologists rely on bedside assessments of hearing. In defining an auditory abnormality, tuning forks are no substitute for a complete audiological battery. Audiological testing is most reliable in defining peripheral or cochlear auditory disturbances and often may provide useful information, based on subtests, to diagnose retrocochlear disorders such as an acoustic neuroma. Tests for central auditory dysfunction are more difficult and poorly understood. Detailed descriptions of audiological tests, both peripheral and central, are provided in standard texts (Katz et al., 2009).

The basic audiological evaluation establishes the degree and configuration of hearing loss, assesses ability to discriminate a speech signal, and provides some insight into the type of loss and possible cause. The test battery consists of pure-tone air- and bone-conduction thresholds, speech thresholds, speech discrimination testing, and immittance measures.

Pure-Tone Testing. Pure-tone air-conduction thresholds provide a measure of hearing sensitivity as a function of frequency and intensity. When a hearing loss is present, the pure-tone air conduction test indicates reduced hearing sensitivity. Pure tones are defined by their frequency (pitch) and intensity (loudness). Normal hearing levels for pure tones are defined by international standards. Brief-duration pure tones at selected frequencies are presented through earphones (air conduction) or a bone-conduction oscillator on the mastoid bone (bone conduction). The audiogram indicates the lowest intensity at which a person can hear at a given frequency and displays the degree (in decibels) and configuration (sensitivity loss as a function of frequency) of a hearing loss. Thresholds in audiology are usually defined as the lowest-intensity signal a person can detect approximately 50% of the time during a given number of presentations. Bone-conduction tests are intended to be a direct measure of inner-ear sensitivity. Pure-tone bone-conduction thresholds are obtained when a stimulus is presented by bone conduction.

Comparison of air- and bone-conduction thresholds establishes the type of hearing loss. Conductive loss results from disorders in the outer or middle ear. The audiogram of patients with SCD may also have an air/bone gap, even though there is no abnormality of the outer or middle ear. This exception results from the third window created by the dehiscence which increases bone conduction. Sensorineural loss is associated with disorders of the cochlear and eighth cranial nerves. Mixed loss is a conductive and sensorineural loss coexisting in the same ear. Typical audiogram pure-tone patterns seen in patients with four common causes of sensorineural hearing loss are shown in Fig. 46.7.

Speech Testing. The speech reception threshold (SRT) is the lowest-intensity level at which the listener can identify or understand two-syllable spoken words 50% of the time. This test provides a check on the validity of the pure-tone test, as it should agree (±5 dB) with an average of the two best pure-tone thresholds in the speech range (500–2000 Hz). Once the SRT is determined, the audiologist measures speech discrimination ability by presenting a standardized list of 50 phonetically balanced monosyllabic words at volume levels approximately 35 to 40 dB above SRT. The speech discrimination score is reported as the percentage of words the subject can correctly repeat back to the audiologist.

Pure tone, SRT, and speech discrimination testing comprise the major routine measures of hearing. Considering these tests together can also provide localizing information. In patients

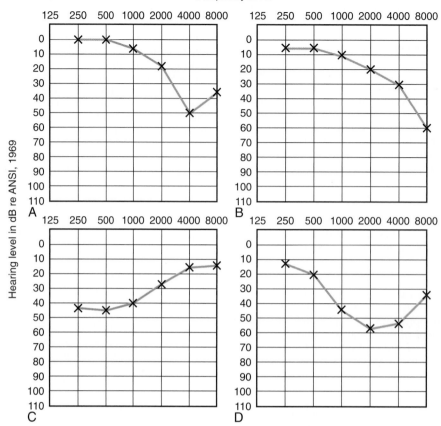

Fig. 46.7 Audiograms illustrating four characteristic patterns of sensorineural hearing loss. **A,** Notched pattern of noise-induced hearing loss. **B,** Downward-sloping pattern of presbycusis. **C,** Low-frequency trough of the Meniere syndrome. **D,** Pattern of congenital hearing loss. *(From Baloh, R.W., 1998. Dizziness, Hearing Loss, and Tinnitus. F.A. Davis Company, Philadelphia, Figure 39, p. 95.)*

with retrocochlear lesions, speech discrimination can be severely reduced even when pure-tone levels are normal or near normal, whereas in patients with cochlear lesions, discrimination tends to be proportional to the magnitude of hearing loss.

Middle Ear Testing. Immittance measures assess the status of the middle ear and confirm information obtained in other tests of the battery. The basic immittance battery consists of tympanometry, static immittance, and acoustic reflex thresholds. Data from the tympanogram permit determination of the static compliance of the middle ear system. A result of "type A tympanogram" means that mobility of the tympanic membrane and middle ear structures is within normal limits.

Acoustic Reflex Testing. Acoustic reflex measures the contraction of the stapedius muscle (innervated by the seventh cranial nerve) in response to a loud sound. The afferent limb of the reflex arch is through the auditory portion of the eighth cranial nerve, and the efferent portion of the reflex arch is through the seventh cranial nerve. The stapedius muscle normally contracts on both sides when an adequate sound is presented in one ear. As a result of contraction of the stapedius muscle, the tympanic membrane tightens or stiffens, thereby increasing the impedance or resistance of the eardrum to acoustic energy and resulting in a slight attenuation of sound transmitted through the middle ear system. In a normal subject, the acoustic reflex occurs in response to a pure tone between 70 and 100 dB above hearing level or when a white

noise stimulus is presented at 65 dB above hearing level. Patients with conductive hearing loss due to middle ear pathology do not have reflexes because the lesion prevents a change in compliance with stapedius muscle contraction. With cochlear lesions, the acoustic reflex may be present at sensation levels less than 60 dB above the auditory pure-tone threshold, which is a form of abnormal loudness growth or recruitment. Cochlear hearing losses must be moderate or severe before the acoustic reflex is lost. In contrast, patients with retrocochlear or eighth cranial nerve lesions often have abnormal acoustic reflexes with normal hearing. The reflex may be absent or exhibit an elevated threshold or abnormal decay. Reflex decay is present if the amplitude of the reflex decreases to half its original size within 10 seconds of stimulation at 1000 Hz, 10 dB above reflex threshold. Observation of the pattern of acoustic reflex testing, along with hearing evaluation, permits inferences to support the presence of a cochlear, conductive, or retrocochlear lesion of the seventh or eighth cranial nerves.

Evoked Potentials (see Chapter 34). Brainstem auditory evoked potentials are also known as *brainstem auditory evoked responses* or *auditory brainstem responses* (ABRs). These physiological measures can be used to evaluate the auditory pathways from the ear to the upper brainstem. In addition, ABR threshold testing, although not a test of hearing sensitivity, may be used to determine behavioral threshold sensitivity in infants or uncooperative patients. The most consistent and reproducible potentials are a series of five submicrovolt waves that occur within 10 milliseconds of an auditory stimulus. These potentials are recorded by averaging 1000 to 2000 responses from click stimuli by use of a computer system and amplifying the response. The anatomical correlates of the five reliable potentials have been only roughly approximated. Wave I of the brainstem auditory evoked potential is a manifestation of the action potentials of the eighth cranial nerve and is generated in the distal portion of the nerve adjacent to the cochlea. Wave II may be generated by the eighth cranial nerve or cochlear nuclei. Wave III is thought to be generated at the level of the superior olive, and waves IV and V are generated in the rostral pons or in the midbrain near the inferior colliculus. The complex anatomy of the central auditory pathway, with multiple crossing of fibers from the level of the cochlear nuclei to the inferior colliculus, makes interpretation of central disturbances in the evoked responses difficult.

Abnormal interwave latencies (I–III or I–V) are seen with retrocochlear lesions (cerebellopontine angle tumors) and can even be seen when only mild or no hearing loss is detected on pure tone audiometry. However, compared to brain MRI with gadolinium, the sensitivity of the ABR test is low, particularly with small tumors (Cueva, 2004). The least specific finding is the absence of all waves. This occurs in some patients with acoustic neuroma and in some with cerebellopontine angle meningiomas. Such patients often have marked hearing deficits with poor discrimination, suggesting retrocochlear disease. The absence of all waves should not occur unless a severe hearing loss exists.

Other Tests. Electrocochleography is a method of recording the stimulus-related electrical potentials associated with the inner ear and auditory nerve, including the cochlear microphonic, summating potential (SP), and compound action potential (AP) of the auditory nerve. The amplitude of the SP and compound AP is measured; an increased SP/AP ratio suggests increased endolymphatic pressure. This test is sometimes used in an attempt to distinguish Meniere disease from other causes of dizziness and hearing loss but lacks a rigorous analysis of its usefulness when there is clinical uncertainty.

MANAGEMENT OF PATIENTS WITH VERTIGO
Treatments of Specific Disorders

BPPV can be diagnosed and treated at the bedside, requiring no further treatment. Once repositioning is confirmed to be successful (see Fig. 46.4), patients are instructed to avoid head-hanging positions such as those used by dentists and hairdressers. These positions can cause the particles to reaccumulate in the posterior semicircular canals. For patients with horizontal canal BPPV, the "barbeque" rotation, Gufoni maneuver, or forced prolonged position can be used (Fife et al., 2008; Kim et al., 2012a; Tirelli and Russolo, 2004; Vannucchi et al., 1997). The management of patients with vestibular neuritis is primarily symptomatic. Prolonged use of sedating medications to treat symptoms is not recommended, because it can slow down the vestibular compensation process. Randomized controlled trials have found that vestibular physical therapy improves outcomes in patients with unilateral vestibulopathy, though very few of these studies were specifically performed in a vestibular neuritis population (Hillier and McDonnell, 2011). A course of corticosteroids has been shown to improve recovery of the caloric response but has not been shown to improve functional or symptom outcome (Fishman et al., 2011). The early treatment of Meniere disease continues to be a low-salt diet and diuretics, though the evidence to support these interventions is weak (Minor et al., 2004). Minimally invasive intratympanic gentamicin injections can be used for patients with debilitating symptoms. Surgical ablation of the

labyrinth and sectioning of the vestibular nerve are other options. Patients with vestibular paroxysmia may benefit from carbamazepine or a similar antiepileptic medication (Hufner et al., 2008). The third window in patients with SCD can be surgically repaired, but this is usually only recommended in patients debilitated by the symptoms (Minor, 2005).

Patients identified as having a small infarction in the posterior fossa should be closely monitored, as herniation or recurrent stroke can occur. Patients identified within 3 hours of an infarction are candidates for intravenous tissue plasminogen activator (tPA). Stenting of a symptomatic (i.e., TIA or nonsevere stroke) stenosis of the basilar artery or an intracranial vertebral artery has been shown to be substantially inferior to medical management (Chimowitz et al., 2011). Patients identified with demyelinating lesions may be candidates for disease-modifying treatments even after presenting with a clinically isolated syndrome. Patients with episodic ataxia are typically highly responsive to treatment with acetazolamide, and there is anecdotal evidence of benefit of the use of acetazolamide in patients with BRV, a migraine equivalent. Patients with migraine-associated dizziness should first attempt to identify and eliminate triggers of their symptoms and also obtain adequate sleep and cardiovascular exercise. If these general measures are not adequate in controlling symptoms, a migraine prophylactic medication could be tried. Small trials of triptan medications in patients with migrainous vertigo suggest safety of these medicines but no significant benefit (Neuhauser et al., 2003).

Symptomatic Treatment of Vertigo

The commonly used antivertiginous drugs and their dosages are listed in Table 46.3 (Huppert et al., 2011). It is often difficult to predict which drugs or combinations of drugs will be most effective in individual patients, and large trials are lacking. Additionally, the mechanisms of these medications

TABLE 46.3 Medical Therapy for Symptomatic Vertigo*

Class	Dosage[†]
ANTIHISTAMINES	
Meclizine	25 mg PO q 4–6 h
Dimenhydrinate	50 mg PO or IM q 4–6 h, or 100 mg suppository q 8 h
Promethazine	25–50 mg PO or IM or as a suppository q 4–6 h
ANTICHOLINERGIC AGENT	
Scopolamine	0.2 mg PO q 4–6 h, or 0.5 mg transdermally q 3 days
BENZODIAZEPINES	
Diazepam	5 or 10 mg PO, IM, IV q 4–6 h
Lorazepam	0.5–2 mg PO, IM, IV q 6–8 h
PHENOTHIAZINE	
Prochlorperazine	5 or 10 mg PO or IM q 6 h, or 25 mg suppository q 12 h
BENZAMIDE	
Metoclopramide	5 or 10 mg PO, IM, or IV q 4–6 h

IM, intramuscular; *IV*, intravenous; *PO*, oral.
*Huppert et al. (2011).
[†]Usual adult starting dosage; maintenance dosage can be increased by a factor of 2-3. The most common side effect is drowsiness.

are not specific to the vestibular system, so side effects are common. Anticholinergic or antihistamine drugs are usually effective in treating patients with mild to moderate vertigo, and sedation is minimal. If the patient is particularly bothered by nausea, the antiemetics prochlorperazine and metoclopramide can be effective and combined with other antivertiginous medications. For severe vertigo, sedation is often desirable, and drugs such as promethazine and diazepam are particularly useful, though prolonged use is not recommended.

MANAGEMENT OF PATIENTS WITH HEARING LOSS AND TINNITUS

Hearing aids continue to become more effective and better designed for patient comfort and acceptance, although cost remains the major limiting factor in their more widespread use. Cochlear implants have revolutionized the approach to treatment of profound sensorineural loss. The management of tinnitus remains difficult, and specific treatments are often ineffective. Patients with a specific cause for the problem usually have the most potential for improvement. Idiopathic high-pitched tinnitus may diminish with avoidance of caffeine, other stimulants, and alcohol. A masking device used in quiet environments may also provide some relief. For patients with intolerable idiopathic tinnitus, a trial of a tricyclic amine antidepressant may be of benefit.

REFERENCES

The complete reference list is available online at https://expertconsult .inkling.com/.

pathological process is likely to have extended into the neocortex and explains why the clinical context in which bladder dysfunction is seen in PD is common in patients with cerebral symptoms, as well as with adverse effects of longstanding treatment with dopaminergic agents.

Thirty-eight to 71% of PD patients report lower urinary tract symptoms (LUTS) (Andersen, 1985; Berger et al., 1987). Storage symptoms are the most common problem seen in more than 60% of patients of PD and they have a considerable impact on quality of life in PD (Araki et al., 2000a; Campos-Sousa et al., 2003; Sakakibara et al., 2001b). Nocturia (56.7%) is the most common symptom, followed by urinary urgency and these together are the commonest nonmotor symptoms in PD. The most common abnormality in urodynamic studies is detrusor overactivity (Araki et al., 2000b). It is thought that neuronal loss in the substantia nigra would disinhibit the normal effect of basal ganglia on the micturition reflex, resulting in detrusor overactivity. Dopaminergic receptor stimulation through D1 provides the main inhibitory influence on the micturition reflex (Yoshimura et al., 2003) in health. However, this is poorly reflected with dopaminergic stimulation in patients with PD.

Overactive bladder (OAB) is currently believed to be the main reason for urological symptoms in PD. Many patients with PD have nocturnal polyuria (NP) which may be a significant cause of nocturia and may be associated with excessive production of urine at night, perhaps related to loss of circadian rhythm in PD (Batla and Panicker, 2012; Suchowersky et al., 1995). NP would not be expected to improve with antimuscarinics directed to help OAB symptoms. In addition to neurogenic bladder dysfunction, prostatic enlargement may occur concomitantly in some men with PD and contribute to bladder dysfunction. Pelvic floor weakness, stress incontinence, and bradykinesia of pelvic floor muscles causing "pseudo-dyssynergia" may be other key factors to consider. A study evaluating the management of benign prostatic obstruction in men with PD highlights the importance of proper patient selection involving neurological and urological input before proceeding with transurethral resection of the prostate (Roth et al., 2009).

Other factors that may contribute to LUTS in PD include associated vascular disease, cervical spondylosis and myelopathy, diabetes mellitus, congestive cardiac failure or pedal edema, and use of diuretic drugs. These may be commonly associated and difficult to dissect out from inherent bladder dysfunction in PD. Sleep disturbances and disturbed circadian rhythm may be closely associated with nocturia (Cochen De Cock et al., 2010; Gomez-Esteban et al., 2006; Menza et al., 2010). Sleep apnea has been proven to be contributory to nocturia (Saunders and Schuckit, 2006). The management must hence be individualized and also aim to address the associated features.

Multiple System Atrophy

MSA must be suspected if bladder symptoms dominate the clinical picture at onset of a parkinsonism condition. As many as 41% of MSA patients present with LUTS and 97% have LUTS during the disease course (Sakakibara et al., 2001d, 2010, 2011; Sammour et al., 2009). These include daytime frequency (45% of women, 43% of men), night-time frequency (65%, 69%), urinary urgency (64% of men), urgency incontinence (66% of women, 75% of men,) (Saunders, 2006).

The bladder affection in MSA is much earlier and more disabling as compared to PD. Although OAB symptoms of urgency and frequency occur in both conditions, patients with MSA are more likely to have a high (>100 mL) PVR (Hahn and Ebersbach, 2005; Regier, 2008), detrusor–sphincter dyssynergia, an open bladder neck at the start of bladder filling on videocystometrogram (Sakakibara et al., 2001a), and a neurogenic EMG of the anal sphincter (Kirby et al., 1986; Palace et al., 1997; Roth et al., 2009; Tison et al., 2000).

Pure Autonomic Failure

Although not affecting basal ganglia predominantly, pure autonomic failure (PAF) is a synucleinopathy similar to MSA. Neurodegeneration is mainly in the postganglionic autonomic neurons with Lewy bodies confined primarily to the autonomic ganglia neurons. Nocturia and voiding dysfunction are common and bladder emptying is often affected. Bladder dysfunction in PAF appears to be as common as but less severe than in MSA and this could possibly reflect slower progression of the disease (Sakakibara et al., 2000). Orthostatic hypotension, erectile dysfunction, and constipation are common in addition.

Bowel Dysfunction

Additional text available at http://expertconsult.inkling.com.

Sexual Dysfunction

Experimental evidence from animals and humans shows that dopaminergic mechanisms are involved in determining libido and inducing penile erection. In animal studies, the medial preoptic area of the hypothalamus has been shown to regulate sexual drive, and selective stimulation of dopamine D2 receptors in this region increases sexual activity in rats (Andersson, 2001). The cause of ED in PD is unclear, but it is a significant problem and in one study was shown to affect 60% of a group of men, compared with 37.5% of age-matched healthy men. ED usually affects men later in the course of PD, with onset years after the diagnosis of neurological disease has been established. A survey of relatively young patients with PD (mean age, 49.6 years) and their partners revealed a high level of sexual dysfunction, with the most severely affected couples being those in which the patient was male.

ED may be the first symptom in men with MSA, predating the onset of any other neurological symptoms by several years. The disorder appears chronologically to be distinct from the development of postural hypotension. The reason for the apparently early selective involvement of neural mechanisms for erection is not known. Preserved erectile function in a man with parkinsonism strongly contradicts the diagnosis of MSA. The available literature on female sexual problems in movement disorders is limited (Jacobs et al., 2000; Oertel et al., 2003).

Hypersexuality due to sexual compulsive behavior in some patients with PD treated with dopamine agonists and L-dopa as part of an impulse control disorder (Giovannoni et al., 2000) is a well-recognized phenomenon, and the DOMINION study, which systematically assessed 3,090 individuals with PD for impulse control disorders, found that impulse control disorder was identified in 13.6% of the patients; specifically, pathological gambling in 5.0%, compulsive sexual behavior in 3.5%, compulsive buying in 5.7%, and binge-eating disorder in 4.3% (Weintraub et al., 2010).

Brainstem Lesions

Voiding difficulty is a rare but recognized symptom of a posterior fossa tumor and has been reported in series of patients with brainstem disorders (Fowler, 1999). In an analysis of urinary symptoms of 39 patients who had had brainstem strokes, lesions that resulted in micturition disturbance usually were dorsally situated (Sakakibara et al., 1996)—a finding consistent with the known location of the brainstem centers involved with control of the bladder. The proximity in the dorsal pons between the pontine micturition center and the medial longitudinal fasciculus means that a disorder of eye movements, such as an internuclear ophthalmoplegia, is highly likely in patients with a pontine disorder causing a voiding difficulty.

Spinal Cord Lesions

Bladder Dysfunction

Spinal cord disorders are the most common cause of neurogenic bladder dysfunction. Trans-spinal pathways connect the pontine micturition centers to the sacral cord. Intact connections are necessary to affect the reciprocal activity of the detrusor and sphincter needed to switch between storage and voiding. After disconnection from the pons, this synergistic activity is lost, resulting in detrusor–sphincter dyssynergia.

Initially after acute spinal cord injury, there usually is a phase of neuronal shock of variable duration characterized clinically by complete urinary retention, with urodynamics demonstrating an acontractile detrusor. Gradually over the course of weeks, new reflexes emerge to reinitiate bladder emptying and cause detrusor contractions in response to low filling volumes. The neurophysiology of this recovery has been studied in cats and it has been proposed that after spinal injury, C fibers emerge as the major afferents, forming a spinal segmental reflex that results in automatic voiding. It is assumed that the same pathophysiology occurs in humans. In support of this assumption is the observed response to intravesical capsaicin (a C-fiber neurotoxin) in patients with acute traumatic spinal cord injury (SCI) or chronically progressive spinal cord disease from multiple sclerosis (MS). The abnormally overactive, small-capacity bladder that characterizes spinal cord disease causes patients to experience urgency and frequency. However, patients with complete transection of the cord may not complain of urinary urgency. If detrusor overactivity is severe, incontinence is highly likely. Poor neural drive on the detrusor muscle during attempts to void, together with an element of detrusor–sphincter dyssynergia, contributes to incomplete bladder emptying. This difficulty may exacerbate the symptoms of the overactive bladder. Although the neurological process of voiding may have been as severely disrupted as the process of storage, the symptoms of difficulty emptying can be minor compared with those of urge incontinence. Only on direct questioning may the patient admit to having difficulty initiating micturition, an interrupted stream, or possibly a sensation of incomplete emptying.

Because bladder innervation arises more caudally than innervation of the lower limbs, any form of spinal cord disease that causes bladder dysfunction is likely to produce clinical signs in the lower limbs as well, unless the lesion is limited to the conus. This rule is sufficiently reliable to be of great value in determining whether a patient has a neurogenic bladder caused by spinal cord disease.

Spinal Cord Injury (SCI)

After SCI, bladder dysfunction can be of such severity as to cause ureteric reflux, hydronephrosis, and eventual upper urinary tract damage. Before the introduction of modern treatments, renal failure was a common cause of death after SCI. The bladder problems of persons with SCI, therefore, must be managed aggressively to lessen the possibility of upper tract disease and to provide the patient with adequate bladder control for a fully rehabilitated life. People with SCI often are

young and otherwise fit and it may be best for them to undergo surgery on the lower urinary tract with a view to fulfilling these two aims rather than to be treated medically.

Multiple Sclerosis

The pathophysiological consequences of progressive MS affecting the spinal cord for the bladder are similar to those of SCI, but the medical context of increasing disability is such that management must be quite different. Estimates of the proportion of patients with MS who have LUTS vary according to the severity of the neurological disability in the group under study, but a figure of about 75% is frequently cited (Marrie et al., 2007). Several studies have shown that urinary incontinence is considered to be one of the worst aspects of the disease, with 70% of a self-selected group of patients with MS responding to a questionnaire classifying the impact bladder symptoms had on their life as "high" or "moderate" (Hemmett et al., 2004). A strong association has been recognized between bladder symptoms and the presence of clinical spinal cord involvement, including paraparesis and upper motor neuron signs on examination of the lower limb in patients with MS. A similar observation has been made in patients with a similar condition, acute disseminated encephalomyelitis (ADEM) (Panicker et al., 2009).

Considering the multitude of symptoms in MS, not surprisingly, LUT symptoms may be overlooked in the clinical management of MS. The North American Research Committee On Multiple Sclerosis questionnaire survey found that of more than 5,000 patients with MS in North America with troublesome urinary symptoms only 43% had been referred to urological services and 51% had been treated with antimuscarinic medications (Mahajan et al., 2010). Recently, a screening tool for patients with bladder problems related to MS has been developed and validated called the "Actionable Bladder Symptom Screening Tool" (Burks et al., 2013). It must be remembered as well that there may be several factors contributing to LUT symptoms in pwMS (see Table 47.1).

Often incomplete bladder emptying and an overactive bladder coexist, the residual urine exacerbating symptoms. Whereas the symptoms of an overactive bladder are a reliable indicator of underlying LUT dysfunction (DO), patient reports of incomplete bladder emptying are often not. In a cohort of patients studied by Betts et al. (1993), patients who thought they did not empty their bladders were found to most often be correct; however, only half those who thought they did were wrong. It is for this reason measurement of the post void residual volume is such a critical investigation in the management of LUT symptoms in patients with MS (see Fig. 47.1) (Fowler et al., 2009).

A particular problem in MS is that neurological symptoms may deteriorate acutely when the patient has an infection and pyrexia, including urinary tract infection. As MS progresses it is not uncommon for recurrent infections to result in deficits which accumulate and lead to progressive neurological deterioration (Buljevac et al., 2002).

Bowel Dysfunction

Additional text available at http://expertconsult.inkling.com.

Sexual Dysfunction

Male Sexual Dysfunction
The level and completeness of a spinal cord lesion determine erectile and ejaculatory capability after SCI. With a complete cervical lesion, psychogenic erections are lost, but the capacity for spontaneous or reflex erections may be intact. With low

47

spinal cord lesions, particularly if the cauda equina is involved, little or no erectile capacity may be retained. Theoretically, a lesion below spinal level L2 leaves psychogenic erections intact, but in practice it is uncommon for men with such a lesion to have erections adequate for intercourse. Psychogenic erections are more likely to be preserved in incomplete lesions. Preservation of ejaculation function after a spinal cord lesion is unusual. Although earlier studies indicated a much lower figure, it is now known that 60% to 65% of men with MS have ED, often coexisting with urinary symptoms, with urodynamically demonstrable overactivity in a majority of those affected. Typically, in the early stages of MS, the chief complaint is of difficulty sustaining an erection for intercourse. With advancing neurological disability, erectile function may cease, and difficulty with ejaculation may develop or become manifest. A study of pudendal evoked potentials in men with MS found that those with severely delayed latencies (i.e., with more severe spinal cord disease) were more likely to be unable to ejaculate. Though it has been said that a diagnosis of MS should be considered in a young man presenting with impotence, this possibility seems unlikely in the absence of clinical spinal cord disease. In one series, only a single patient had erectile difficulties at the time of the first symptoms of MS, and neurological disease did not develop subsequently in any of the men who presented with ED.

Female Sexual Dysfunction. Studies of women with SCI at different levels, both complete and incomplete, have advanced current understanding of the neural pathways involved in female sexual response. It has been hypothesized that the sensory experience of orgasm may have an autonomic basis, because orgasmic capacity is preserved in a proportion of affected women, particularly with higher cord lesions (Sipski et al., 2001); fMRI studies in SCI patients suggest preservation of vagal pathways. Sexual dysfunction in women with MS is common (affecting 50% to 60%), although probably underdiagnosed, with the incidence increasing with worsening disability. Neurogenic problems during intercourse include decreased lubrication and reduced orgasmic capacity. A double-blind, randomized placebo-controlled crossover study of sildenafil citrate in treating females with sexual dysfunction due to MS did not show any overall benefit with this drug, which has been shown to be far more effective in men with MS (Dasgupta et al., 2004). In women with advanced disease, additional problems may include lower limb spasticity, loss of pelvic sensation, genital dysesthesia, and fear of incontinence (Hulter and Lundberg, 1995).

Impaired Sympathetic Thoracolumbar Outflow

The fibers that travel from the thoracolumbar sympathetic chain emerge from the T10–L2 spinal levels and course through the retroperitoneal space to the bifurcation of the aorta, from which they enter the pelvic plexus. Loss of sympathetic innervation of the genitalia causes disorders of ejaculation, with either failure of emission or retrograde ejaculation; the ability to experience the sensation of orgasm may be retained. As the sympathetic thoracolumbar fibers are particularly likely to be injured by the procedure of retroperitoneal lymph node dissection or by surgeries involving an anterior approach to the lumbar spine, complaints of loss of ejaculation are common after these surgeries.

Conus and Cauda Equina Lesions

The cauda equina contains the sacral parasympathetic outflow together with the somatic efferent and afferent fibers. Damage

to the cauda equina leaves the detrusor decentralized, rather than denervated, because the postganglionic parasympathetic innervation is unaffected. This distinction may explain why the bladder dysfunction after a cauda equina lesion is unpredictable and why even detrusor overactivity has been described (Podnar, 2014).

Inability to evacuate the bowel may be a severe problem, and manual evacuation may be necessary for the long term. Additional denervation of the anal sphincter can result in incontinence of flatus and feces. Damage to the cauda equina results in sensory loss and both men and women complain of perineal sensory loss and loss of erotic genital sensation for which no effective treatment is available. In men, ED is also a complaint (Podnar et al., 2006).

Disturbances of Peripheral Innervation
Diabetic Neuropathy

Bladder involvement once was considered an uncommon complication of diabetes, but the increase in use of techniques for studying bladder function has shown that such involvement is common, although often asymptomatic. Bladder dysfunction does not occur in isolation, and other symptoms and signs of generalized neuropathy are necessarily present in affected patients. The onset of the bladder dysfunction is insidious, with progressive loss of bladder sensation and impairment of bladder emptying over years, eventually culminating in chronic low pressure urinary retention (Hill et al., 2008). Urodynamic studies demonstrate impaired detrusor contractility, reduced urine flow, increased postmicturition residual volume, and reduced bladder sensation. It seems likely that vesical afferent and efferent fibers are involved, causing reduced awareness of bladder filling and decreased bladder contractility.

Diabetes is the most common cause of ED. Surveys of andrology clinics have found that 20% to 31% of men attending are diabetic. The prevalence of ED increases with age and duration of diabetes, and the problem is known to be associated with severe retinopathy, a history of peripheral neuropathy, amputation, cardiovascular disease, raised glycosylated hemoglobin, and the use of antihypertensives such as betablockers. A large population study of men with early-onset diabetes found that 20% had ED. Whether its pathogenesis in diabetic patients results mainly from neuropathy or involves a significant microvascular contribution, or whether the two processes are co-dependent, is not yet resolved. Age-matched studies of women with and without diabetes suggest that diabetic women also may be affected by specific disorders of sexual function, including decreased vaginal lubrication and capacity for orgasm.

Amyloid Neuropathy

Autonomic manifestations are common and these include erectile dysfunction, orthostatic hypotension, bladder dysfunction, distal anhydrosis and abnormal pupils. LUTS generally appear early on and are present in 50% of patients within the first 3 years of the disease. Patients most often complain of difficulty in bladder emptying and incontinence (Andrade, 2009). Often, however, bladder dysfunction may be asymptomatic and uncovered only during investigations. Urodynamic studies have demonstrated reduced bladder sensations, underactive detrusor, poor urinary flow and opening of the bladder neck. Bladder wall thickening may be seen in ultrasound scan. As many as 10% of patients with FAP type I may proceed to end-stage renal disease (Lobato, 2003) and may complain of polyuria. Urinary incontinence has been shown to be associated with higher post-liver transplant mortality (Adams et al., 2000).

Reduced libido and erectile dysfunction are common and phosphodiesterase inhibitors may have the adverse effect of accentuating orthostatic hypotension and should therefore be used with caution.

Additional text available at http://expertconsult.inkling.com.

Immune-Mediated Neuropathies

Approximately a quarter of all patients with Guillain–Barré syndrome have bladder symptoms. These symptoms usually occur in the patients with more severe neuropathy and appear after limb weakness is established. Both detrusor areflexia and bladder overactivity have been described.

Autoimmune Autonomic Ganglionopathy

Patients with autoimmune autonomic ganglionopathy present with rapid onset of severe autonomic failure, with orthostatic hypotension, gastrointestinal dysmotility, anhidrosis, bladder dysfunction, erectile dysfunction and sicca symptoms and may have ganglionic acetylcholine receptor (AChR) antibodies. Bladder dysfunction generally manifests with voiding difficulty and incomplete emptying. Severity and distribution of autonomic dysfunction appear to depend upon the level of antibody titers (Gibbons and Freeman, 2009).

Myotonic Dystrophy

Although myotonic activity has not been found in the sphincter or pelvic floor of patients with myotonic dystrophy, bladder symptoms may be prominent and difficult to treat, presumably because bladder smooth muscle is involved. With advancing disease, megacolon and fecal incontinence also may become intractable problems.

Urinary Retention in Young Women

Urinary retention or symptoms of obstructed voiding in young women in the absence of overt neurological disease have long puzzled urologists and neurologists alike, and in the absence of any convincing organic cause, the condition was once said to be hysterical. The typical clinical picture is that of a young woman in the age range of 20 to 30 years who presents with retention and a bladder capacity greater than 1 liter. Although patients retaining such quantities may be uncomfortable, they do not have the sensation of extreme urgency that might be expected. Many affected women have previously experienced an interruption of the urinary stream but are unaware that this is abnormal; therefore, a voiding history can be misleading unless taken carefully. Other clinical neurological features or findings on laboratory investigations that would support a diagnosis of MS are lacking, and MR images of the brain, spinal cord, and cauda equina are normal. The lack of sacral anesthesia makes a cauda equina lesion improbable. An association between this syndrome and polycystic ovaries was described in the original description of the syndrome.

In some young women with urinary retention, concentric needle electrode examination of the striated muscle of the urethral sphincter reveals complex repetitive discharges and myotonia-like activity, decelerating bursts. Sometimes known as Fowler syndrome, it had been managed symptomatically only for a long time. However, it is now known that these patients respond particularly favorably to sacral neuromodulation (DasGupta and Fowler, 2004; Wiseman et al., 2003).

Day 1		Time / Volume (mL)						Total Fluid intake	Episodes of leakage
26,4,2009	Time	6 AM	10 AM	12:30 PM	3:30 PM	5 PM		1700	4
Time out of bed (am)- 6 AM	Volume	160	120	130	190	140			
	Time	7 PM	8:45 PM	2:30 AM	4 AM				
Time to bed (pm)- 9 PM	Volume	150	170	200	180				
	Time								
	Volume								

Fig. 47.2 Bladder diary recorded over 24 hours, demonstrating increased daytime and night-time urinary frequency, low voided volumes, and incontinence. These findings are seen in patients with detrusor overactivity. (From Panicker, J.N., Kalsi, V., de Seze M., 2010. Approach and evaluation of neurogenic bladder dysfunction, in: Fowler, C.J., Panicker, J.N., Emmanuel, A, (Eds), Pelvic Organ Dysfunction in Neurological Disease: Clinical Management and Rehabilitation. Cambridge University Press, New York.)

DIAGNOSTIC EVALUATION

History

History forms the cornerstone for evaluation and should address both storage and voiding dysfunction. Patients with storage dysfunction complain of frequency for micturition, nocturia, urgency and urgency incontinence. Urgency, frequency and nocturia, with or without incontinence, is called the overactive bladder syndrome, urge syndrome or urgency-frequency syndrome (Abrams et al., 2002). Patients experiencing voiding dysfunction report hesitancy for micturition, a slow and interrupted urinary stream, the need to strain to pass urine, and double voiding. Patients may be in complete urinary retention. The history of voiding dysfunction is often unreliable and patients may be unaware of incomplete bladder emptying. Therefore, the history should be supplemented by a bladder scan (see the section Bladder Scan).

Bladder Diary

The bladder diary supplements the history taking and records the frequency for micturition, volumes voided, episodes of incontinence, and fluid intake over the course of a few days (Fig. 47.2).

Physical Examination

Findings on clinical examination are critical in deciding whether a patient's urogenital complaints are neurological in origin. As the spinal segments that innervate the bladder and genitalia are distal to those that innervate the lower limbs, bladder disturbances generally have been shown to correlate with lower limb deficits. The possible exceptions are lesions of the conus medullaris and cauda equina, where findings may be confined to saddle anesthesia and absence of sacral cord mediated reflexes such as the anal reflex or bulbocavernosus reflex. Akinetic rigidity, cerebellar ataxia, and postural hypotension should raise the suspicion of MSA, in conditions characterized by early and severe urinary incontinence and erectile dysfunction.

Examination for evidence of peripheral neuropathy is important. Peripheral neuropathy, notably diabetic, is the common cause of male erectile dysfunction and as the neuropathy progresses, abnormalities and innervation of the detrusor muscle develop also. Clear evidence for peripheral neuropathy is likely before the innervation of the bladder is involved.

The neurological examination is complete only after an inspection of the lumbosacral spine. Congenital malformations of the spine can sometimes present with pelvic organ

TABLE 47.3 Urological Procedures That May Be Performed to Treat Various Causes for Incontinence

Stress incontinence: pelvic floor weakness	Bladder neck suspension TVT TOT
Stress incontinence: sphincter incompetence	Artificial sphincter
Urgency incontinence (detrusor overactivity)	Botulinum toxin Sacral neuromodulation Augmentation cystoplasty ?Myomectomy
Intractable incontinence	Urinary diversion with stoma

TOT, Transobturator tape; *TVT,* tension-free vaginal tape.

Nerve Root Stimulators

In patients who have suffered a complete spinal cord transection, but in whom the caudal section of the cord and its roots are intact, the implantation of a nerve root stimulator may be considered. This device was pioneered by Professor Giles Brindley and his collaborators, and several thousand have now been implanted worldwide. The principle on which they work is that the stimulating electrodes are placed around the lower sacral roots (S2 to S4) and activated by an external switching device. The stimulating electrodes are usually applied intrathecally to the anterior roots, and the posterior roots are cut at the same time. After the implant, adjustments are made to the stimulation parameters so that the patient obtains maximum benefit in terms of making the bladder contract for voiding, assisting defecation, or even producing a penile erection. Although such devices are highly effective in selective cases, the additional neurological deficit caused by the need for sectioning of the dorsal roots and consequent loss of reflex erections has reduced its acceptance.

Permanent Indwelling Catheters

There comes a point when the patient is no longer able to perform self-catheterization, or when incontinence is refractory to management. It is at this stage that an indwelling catheter becomes necessary. The most immediate solution is an indwelling Foley catheter, held in place by an inflatable balloon in the bladder proximal to the catheter opening. The long-term ill effects of these devices are well known. One of the major problems may be catheter bypassing, which occurs when strong detrusor contractions produce a rapid urine flow that cannot drain sufficiently quickly. A common response to this would be to use a wider caliber catheter, with the effect that the bladder closure mechanism becomes progressively stretched and destroyed. The detrusor contraction may be of sufficient intensity to extrude the 10- or 20-mL balloon from the bladder, causing further damage to the bladder neck and resulting in a totally incompetent outlet. Bladder stones and recurrent infections are also more likely in patients with an indwelling catheter.

A preferred alternative to an indwelling urethral catheter is a suprapubic catheter. This can be inserted by a urologist; however, extreme care is required as these patients often have small, contracted bladders and this contributes to the risk of bowel perforation during catheter placement. Although by no means a perfect system, a suprapubic catheter is a better long-term alternative to a urethral catheter as it preserves urethral integrity, and helps to promote perineal hygiene and sexual functions.

The option of intermittent bladder drainage using a catheter valve, as opposed to continuous drainage into a leg bag, depends upon whether the bladder has a reasonable capacity to store urine.

External Devices

If incontinence is the major problem and the bladder empties completely, some men are able to wear an external device such as a penile sheath.

Other Options

Beta-3-Receptor Agonists. The recent licensing of an oral beta-3-receptor agonist, mirabegron, offers a new approach to the management of the overactive bladder (Chapple et al., 2014). It remains to be seen whether mirabegron will be effective in neurological patients reporting overactive bladder symptoms; it is a potentially attractive option, being devoid of the central side effects that may be reported with anti-muscarinics.

Cannabinoids. Positive anecdotal reports on the effect of cannabis in controlling bladder symptoms in patients with MS and identification of the cannabinoid receptor in animals and human studies led to studies of cannabis-based medicinal extracts in this group. An open label study in patients with advanced MS produced promising results, with diminished frequency, nocturia, and incontinence (Freeman et al., 2006). A license was recently granted in the United Kingdom for the use of a cannabis-based medicine to treat spasticity in MS, but this does not cover bladder dysfunction.

Vanilloids. Despite the initial enthusiasm for its use, intravesical vanilloid therapy, capsaicin and resiniferatoxin, generally has been superseded by botulinum toxin therapy. Only a few centers worldwide offer resiniferatoxin treatment and, therefore, this treatment is not discussed further here.

Stepwise Approach to Neurogenic Bladder Dysfunction

The treatment options offered to a patient should reflect the severity of bladder dysfunction, which generally parallels the extent of neurological disease (Fig. 47.8). However, beyond a certain point, incontinence may become refractory to all treatment options and it is at this stage that a long-term indwelling catheter should be offered. Although most patients can be managed along these lines, there are specific situations where specialist urology services should be involved earlier on in the journey of the patient (Box 47.1).

Urinary Tract Infections

The presence of asymptomatic bacteria alone in a patient performing intermittent self-catheterization should not be an indication for antibiotics (Fowler et al., 2009). The usual indication would be presence of associated symptoms (local or systemic) and certainly if there was involvement of the upper urinary tract (pyelonephritis). In an individual with recurrent urinary tract infections (more than two in 6 months, or more than three in a year), the catheterization technique should be reviewed and, if optimal, it is worthwhile to exclude a urological cause such as a bladder stone. In individuals with proven recurrent urinary tract infections and when no urological structural abnormality has been identified, it is reasonable to start prophylactic low-dose antibiotics for a finite duration. Rotation of antibiotics is one approach for minimizing antibiotic resistance developing. It is also important to distinguish *relapsing* from *remitting* infections, and ensure that it is not the undertreatment of a causative organism that is the underlying

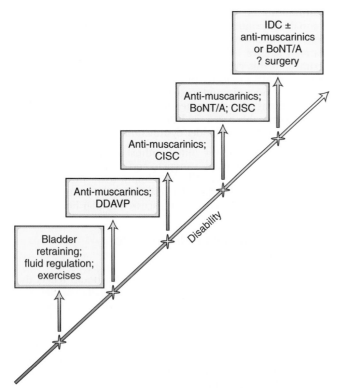

Fig. 47.8 Stepwise approach to neurogenic bladder dysfunction and its relation to progression of disabilities (see text for details). *BoNT/A,* Botulinum toxin A; *CISC,* clean intermittent self-catheterization; *DDAVP,* desmopressin; *IDC,* indwelling catheter.

cause of the symptoms. There is debate about the pros/cons of introducing CISC as a preventative measure against UTIs, as well as the threshold above which CISC should be recommended (e.g., a residual volume of 150 mL). The input of a specialist nurse in lower urinary tract dysfunction who teaches CISC is particularly helpful here.

The value of cranberry juice in preventing urinary tract infections in neurogenic patients is debatable.

MANAGEMENT OF NEUROGENIC SEXUAL DYSFUNCTION

The first step in approaching sexual dysfunction of neurogenic origin is providing an opportunity for patients and their partners to openly discuss their sexual dysfunction. The topic can often be broached during the consultation while discussing concomitant bladder or bowel troubles. An explanation of the neurological basis for sexual dysfunction often relieves anxiety about the problem and removes assumptions that the problem is essentially psychological in origin.

Sexual dysfunction in neurological disease can occur due to several different causes (Box 47.2) (Foley and Werner, 2000). Primary sexual dysfunction results from the actual neurological lesions directly affecting the neural pathways for sexual functions. For example, lesions in the spinal cord may cause loss of tactile sensations from the genitalia. Physical disabilities, such as spasticity or pain, resulting from the neurological disease can interfere with sexual functions as well. This is known as secondary sexual dysfunction. Sexual dysfunction arising from the psychological, emotional, or cultural impact of living with a neurological disease is known as tertiary sexual dysfunction. A holistic approach to managing sexual dysfunction involves identifying all these contributory factors.

Management of Erectile Dysfunction

Sexual dysfunction in men most commonly manifests with erectile dysfunction. The evidence generally points to spinal cord involvement as the major cause of erectile dysfunction in neurological conditions such as MS. Cord involvement may initially result in a partial deficit so that erectile dysfunction is variable, with preserved nocturnal penile erections and erections on morning waking. It is only in the past 10 to 20 years that neurological teaching has recognized the error of the view that "if a man can get an erection at any time, erectile dysfunction is likely to be psychogenic." With increasing neurological disability, there may be a total failure of erectile function and also difficulty with ejaculation. Few men with complete spinal cord injury can ejaculate and difficulty with ejaculation may become apparent when erectile dysfunction is successfully treated. The treatment of erectile dysfunction was transformed

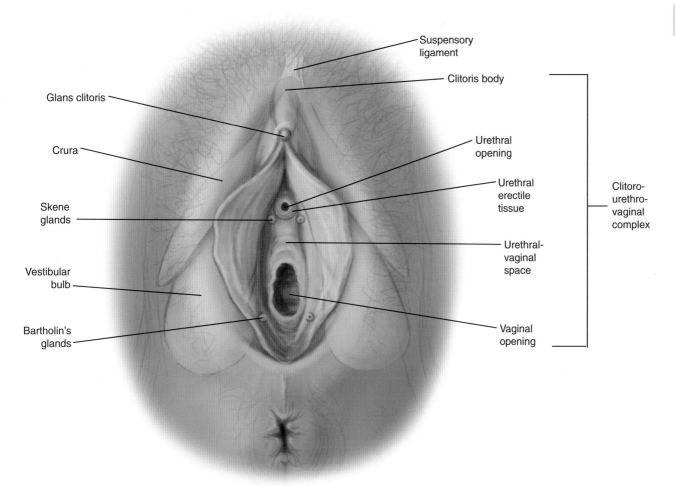

Fig. 48.3 Anatomy of the clitoris.

facilitating vaginal orgasm (Courtois and Charvier, 2013; Courtois et al., 2013b; Masters and Johnson, 1966).

Sexual arousal can also be activated by psychogenic stimuli feeding into the sacral pathway or synapsing with the TL pathway traveling through the paravertebral sympathetic chain feeding into the utero-vaginal plexus.

Orgasm and Resolution

Orgasm is characterized by rhythmic contractions of perineal muscles perceived as clitoral, vulvar, vaginal, and anal pulsations, and by various signs of autonomic discharge, including hypertension, tachycardia, hyperventilation, flushing, shivering, red skin spots, and the like (Courtois et al., 2011b; Masters and Johnson, 1966). Given the resemblance between these responses in men and women (see Fig. 48.4), the neural pathway governing climax in women is suggested to be identical to emission and ejaculation, that is, involving the concurrent activation of the hypogastric nerves and sympathetic chain (Courtois and Charvier, 2013; Courtois et al., 2013b).

Following orgasm, the resolution phase clears out vasocongestion and restores cardiovascular and autonomic responses back to normal (Masters and Johnson, 1966).

Brain Regulation of Sexual Responses

Brain structures control sexual reflexes through excitatory or inhibitory influences (Hubscher et al., 2004, 2010; Johnson et al., 2011) and participate in the perceptual, cognitive-emotional, and rewarding effect of orgasm (Cacioppo et al., 2012; Georgiadis and Kringelbach, 2012).

The medial preoptic area (MPOA) (Marson, 2004; Marson and McKenna, 1994), the paraventricular nucleus (PVN), and the arcuate nucleus of the hypothalamus exert excitatory influences on sexual reflexes, while the nucleus paragigantocellularis (nPGI) exerts tonic inhibition (see Figs 48.1 and 48.4). Excitatory inputs from the MPOA can be conveyed through connection with the PVN and the periaqueductal gray (PGA), both inhibiting the inhibitory nPGI (Meston et al., 2004).

The perception of sexually stimulated body areas and visual imagery during climax are associated with activity in the parietal lobe and visual cortex (Hostege et al., 2003). Independent but overlapping cortical representation of the clitoris, vagina, cervix, and breast is found on the homunculus parietal lobe (Komisaruk et al., 2011). Generalized arousal characterizing climax is associated with activity in the thalamus, and visceral perception with activity in the ventroposterior thalamus (Hostege et al., 2003). Cardiovascular activity and respiratory events (Georgiadis et al., 2009) are recorded in the brainstem, and muscular spasms in the cerebellum. Cerebellar projections participate in the cardiovascular (Georgiadis et al., 2009) and motor aspects of orgasm (Georgiadis et al., 2007; Hostege et al., 2003). Ventrolateral pontine activity is partly responsible for climactic pelvic floor contractions (Huynh et al., 2013).

The emotional and phenomenological experience of orgasm is associated with deactivation of the prefrontal,

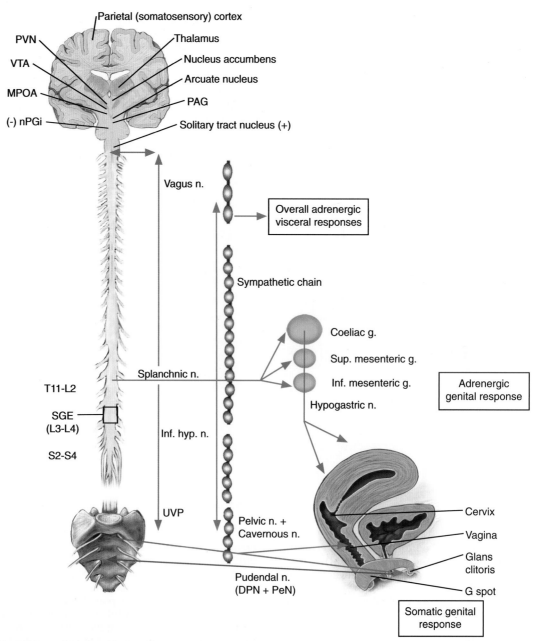

Fig. 48.4 Innervation of the female genital and reproductive system. Genital stimulation of the glans clitoris, G spot, and vagina is conveyed through the dorsal clitoral nerve (afferent pudendal nerve) to the sacral segments S2–S4 of the spinal cord, where they synapse with the preganglionic pelvic nerve, running through the uterovaginal plexus and synapsing with the post-ganglionic cavernous nerve to initiate clitoral erection and vaginal lubrication. Deeper vaginal and cervix stimulation is conveyed through the thoracolumbar segments T11–L2 running through the splanchnic nerves and descending the inferior sympathetic chain (inferior hypogastric nerve) feeding into the uterovaginal plexus to trigger clitoral erection and vaginal lubrication. Psychogenic inputs can further travel from the brain (1) to the sacral segments or (2) the thoracolumbar segments T11–L2 descending the inferior sympathetic chain (inferior hypogastric nerve) feeding into the uterovaginal plexus, or (3) the vagus nerve innervating the genitals. At the threshold of orgasm, intraspinal connections are believed to be established, as in men, between the sacral and TL segments to activate (1) the hypogastric nerve innervating the uterus and responsible for uterine contractions and (2) the entire sympathetic chain responsible for the overall adrenergic visceral responses (e.g., hypertension, tachycardia, hyperventilation, red skin spots) in addition to the adrenergic and somatic genital responses of climax. The SGE, which is also identified in women, may presumably participate in the coordination of events in women. *DCN,* Dorsal clitoral nerve; *g,* ganglia; *MPOA,* medial preoptic area of the hypothalamus; *n,* nerve; *nPGi,* nucleus paragigantocellularis; *PAG,* periaqueductal gray; *PeN,* perineal nerve; *PVN,* paraventricular nucleus; *UVP,* uterovaginal plexus; *VTA,* ventrotegmental area.

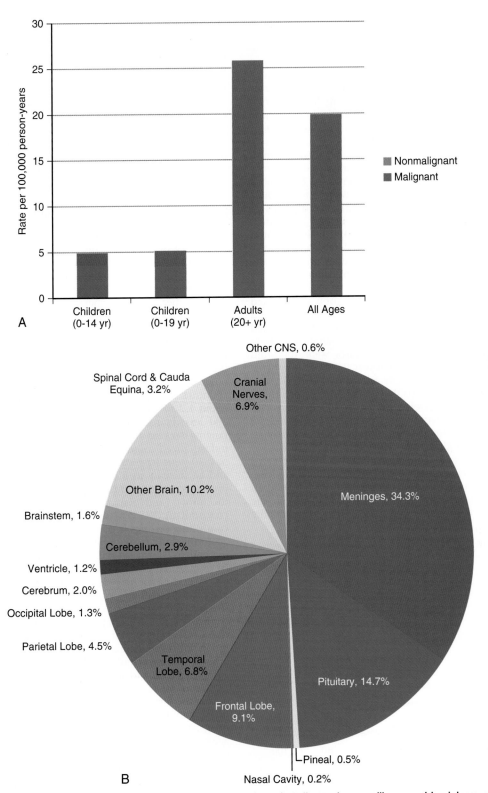

Fig. 49.2 Central nervous system malignancy incidence rates by age (years) at diagnosis: surveillance, epidemiology, and end results; Central Brain Tumor Registry of the United States (CBTRUS). A, Incidence rates are age standardized to the United States 2000 standard population. **B,** Histological classification of central nervous system brain tumors (CBTRUS, 2012). *(Data from Central Brain Tumor Registry of the United States, Hinsdale, IL. Available at:* http://www.cbtrus.org. *Accessed May 2014.)*

of any cause in persons with the disorder; specific etiological disorders or factors include status epilepticus, accidents due to seizures, treatment-related factors, suicide, aspiration pneumonia, and SUDEP. A large population-based epilepsy cohort in Sweden found an 11-fold increased risk of pre-mature mortality compared with general population and sibling controls (Fazel et al., 2013). Of these deaths, 16% were due to external causes such as motor vehicle accidents and suicide. Psychiatric comorbidity was strongly associated with external causes of death.

SUDEP generally is considered to be the most common cause of epilepsy-related death, with a relative frequency of 1 per 1000 epilepsy cases (Opeskin and Berkovic, 2003). Risk factors that have been consistent across studies include male sex, generalized tonic-clonic seizures, early age of onset of seizures, refractory treatment, and being in bed at the time of death. Proposed mechanisms for SUDEP include central apnea, acute neurogenic pulmonary edema, and cardiac arrhythmia precipitated by seizure discharges acting via the autonomic nervous system. Other causes of death in epilepsy can be classified as those in which epilepsy is secondary to an underlying disease (cerebrovascular disease) or is an unrelated disorder (ischemic heart disease). Age-specific mortality rates for Rochester, Minnesota, are shown in Fig. 49.3. Graphed curves for mortality data were similar in configuration to those for age-specific prevalence data, but rates were 1000-fold lower. This finding suggests that each year, 0.1% of the patients with epilepsy die of causes directly related to their epilepsy.

Status epilepticus affects 105,000 to 152,000 persons annually in the United States (DeLorenzo et al., 1996). Status epilepticus represents a neurological emergency, and despite improvements in treatment, the mortality rate is still high. Population-based studies have reported 30-day case-fatality ratios between 8% and 22%. Short-term fatality after status epilepticus is associated with the presence of an underlying acute etiological disorder. Fatality ratios are lowest in children (short-term mortality rate 3% to 9%) and highest in the elderly (short-term mortality rate 22% to 38%). Case-fatality ratios for those surviving the initial 30 days after status epilepticus are 40% within the next 10 years.

Morbidity Rates

Figure 49.3 also shows morbidity measures for epilepsy in Rochester, Minnesota, by age group. Age-specific incidence of epilepsy was high during the first year of life, declined during childhood and adolescence, and then increased again after age 55. The cumulative incidence of epilepsy was 1.2% through age 24 and steadily increased to 4.4% through age 85 years. Age-specific prevalence increased with advancing age; nearly 1.5% of the population older than 75 years had active epilepsy.

Point prevalence and average age-adjusted annual incidence rates for epilepsy are available from a number of community surveys (Banerjee et al., 2009). In general, the prevalence of convulsive disorders is about 3 to 9 per 1000 population in industrialized countries. Some of the variation can be attributed to methodological differences in studies. Developing countries have reported higher prevalence rates of up to 41 per 1000. In general, males have higher rates than females, and recent studies have found no significant racial predilection. The overall lifetime prevalence of a nonfebrile seizure, as opposed to active epilepsy, is 5% in both industrialized and developing countries. Average annual age-adjusted incidence rates for epilepsy are about 50 per 100,000, with a range of 16 to 70 per 100,000 population in industrialized countries. A slight male excess is reported, which averages about 1.2 to 1. Surveys from developing countries are fewer and less rigorous and report much higher incidence rates, ranging between 43 and 190 cases per 100,000 per year. Within industrialized countries, temporal trends in epilepsy over the past 30 years have shown a decrease in incidence in children and an increase in incidence rates for the elderly. Improved prenatal care and immunization may explain the changes for the former, and perhaps longer life expectancy with more concomitant CNS disease for the latter. Overall prognosis for controlling seizures is good, with more than 70% of patients achieving long-term remission. Age-specific incidence rates for epilepsy from several surveys showed a sharp decrease from maximal rates in infancy to adolescence and thereafter a slow decline for new cases throughout life. In other studies, rates were essentially constant after infancy or showed an irregular rise with age. In Rochester, Minnesota, however, the configuration was U-shaped, with a marked increase in incidence rates at the age of 75 and older (Fig. 49.4). This configuration reflects generalized tonic-clonic disorders, together with absence and myoclonic seizures for the left arm of the U and complex partial and generalized tonic-clonic epilepsies for the right arm. Myoclonic seizures were the major type diagnosed during the first year of life; they also were the most common in the 1 to 4 years age group but rarely occurred after 4 years of age. Absence (petit mal) seizures peaked in the 1 to 4 years age group and did not begin in patients older than 20. Both complex partial and generalized tonic-clonic seizures had fairly consistent incidence rates of 5 to 15 per 100,000 in persons 5 to 69 years of age, after low maxima at ages 1 to 4 years; for age 70 and older, the rates of each were sharply higher. Generalized tonic-clonic seizure rates had a similar configuration for both primary and secondary seizures. Simple partial seizures increased only slightly with age.

Febrile Seizures

In the United States and Europe, the risk of a child's developing febrile seizures has been about 2%, ranging between 1% and 4%. Surveys from Japan and the Mariana Islands showed

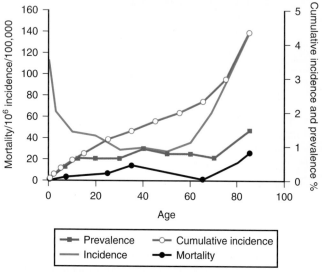

Fig. 49.3 Measures of epilepsy (Rochester, Minnesota, 1935–1984): age-specific incidence per 100,000 person-years; cumulative incidence (percent); age-specific prevalence (percent); and age-specific mortality per 100,000 person-years. *(From Hauser, W.A., Annegers, J.F., Rocca, W.A., 1996. Descriptive epidemiology of epilepsy: contribution of population-based studies from Rochester, Minnesota. Mayo Clin Proc. 71, 576–586.)*

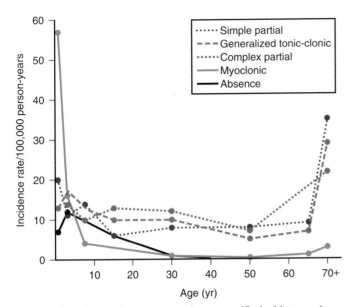

Fig. 49.4 Epilepsy. Average annual age-specific incidence rates per 100,000 population by clinical type of seizure—absence, myoclonic, generalized, simple, complex partial. *(From Kurtzke, J.F., Kurland, L.T., 2004. The epidemiology of nervous system disease, in: Baker and Joynt's Clinical Neurology on CD-ROM. Lippincott Williams & Wilkins, London.)*

rates of 7% and 11%, respectively. As with epilepsy in general, a male preponderance of 1.2 to 1 for febrile convulsions was observed. In most studies, recurrent febrile seizures occur in approximately one-third of the cases, and overall the risk of subsequent epilepsy is approximately 2% to 4% for simple and 11% for complex febrile seizures.

MULTIPLE SCLEROSIS
Mortality Rates and Survival

Over the past four decades, mortality for multiple sclerosis (MS; see Chapter 80) has declined steadily in North America and Western Europe and remained stable or increased in Eastern Europe. There is some variability in mortality data within population-based cohort studies but overall average time to death from MS onset ranges between 24 and 45 years (Scalfari et al., 2013). SMRs range from 1.3 to 2.9 for MS compared with the general population.

As to cause of death, approximately 50% of patients with MS die of complications related to their disease. Koch-Henriksen and colleagues (1998) in Denmark, as well as Smestad and colleagues (2009) in Norway, attributed more than half of all deaths in a large population cohort to MS or its complications. An overall SMR of 2.5 for all causes was calculated for the Norwegian cohort (Smestad et al., 2009). Infections were the most common cause of death; survival was age dependent and not related to disease course. As more patients with MS survive to older ages, however, a greater proportion of them can be expected to die of causes unrelated to MS and thus will not be coded as dying from MS (underlying cause). This last point is supported by analysis of contributory causes of death for patients with MS in Denmark and in the United States. The estimated 25-year survival of the population with MS in Rochester, Minnesota, was 76.2%, compared with 87.7% for the general U.S. white population of similar age and gender. Survival for men was less than that for women. This survival figure was slightly greater than earlier estimates

for Rochester. The Danish National MS Registry data provided a median survival of 30 years from onset of the disease. Median survival times for U.S. World War II veterans from MS disease onset were 43 years (white females), 30 years (black males), and 34 years (white males) (Wallin et al., 2000). The male rates did not differ significantly, and when relative survival ratios were calculated, none of the three groups were significantly different; indicating the excess for the white females was more attributable to gender than to disease.

Morbidity Rates

The prevalence surveys for Europe and the Mediterranean basin from the later twentieth century appear to separate into clusters within two zones: one to the north, with rates of 30 per 100,000 and higher, considered to represent high frequency, and the other to the south, with rates less than 30 per 100,000 but greater than 4 per 100,000 population, classified as medium frequency.

The northernmost parts of Scandinavia and the Mediterranean basin were medium-prevalence regions in 1980. More recent surveys of Italy and its islands, however, have documented prevalence rates of 60 per 100,000 and higher; therefore, this country is now clearly within the high-frequency band (Kurtzke, 2005). This increase in prevalence appears to be recent, because some of the earlier Italian surveys with lower rates were well done. This change is not limited to Italy—indeed, all of Europe from northernmost Norway to the Mediterranean regions now falls in the high-frequency zone, as documented by Pugliatti et al. (2006) in Fig. 49.5.

Although clearly intra- and international diffusion of this disease has occurred in recent years, the general worldwide distribution of MS may still be described within three zones of frequency or risk. As of 2004, the high-risk zone, with prevalence rates of 30 per 100,000 population and above, included essentially all of Europe, the United States, Canada, Israel, and New Zealand, plus southeastern Australia and easternmost Russia. These regions are bounded by areas of medium frequency, with prevalence rates between 5 and 29 per 100,000, consisting now of Russia from the Ural mountains into Siberia, as well as the Ukraine. Also in the medium zone still fall most of Australia and perhaps Hawaii, all of Latin America, the North African littoral, and white people in South Africa; even northern Japan seems now to be of medium prevalence. Low-frequency areas, with prevalence rates below 5 per 100,000, still comprise all other known areas of Asia, Africa, Alaska, and Greenland (Kurtzke, 2005). MS clearly is a place-related disorder. All of the high- and medium-risk areas are found in Europe or the European colonies: Canada, the United States, Australia, New Zealand, Israel, South Africa, and probably Latin America. MS probably originated in northwestern Europe and was brought to the other lands by European settlers. In Europe itself, although the disease clearly has shown geographical clustering in some countries, there is evidence even within these clusters of diffusion over time, as well as the notable spread throughout the continent. The annual incidence rate for MS in high-risk areas at present is approximately 3 to 6 per 100,000 population, whereas in low-risk areas it is approximately 1 per 1,000,000. Medium-risk areas have an incidence near 1 per 100,000. In Denmark during the years 1939 to 1945, age-specific incidence rates rose rapidly, from essentially zero in childhood to a peak at about age 27 of more than 9 per 100,000 for females and almost 7 per 100,000 for males. Beyond age 40, little difference between the sexes was seen; in both, rates declined equally to 0 by age 65. The most recent evidence indicates that women of all races in the United States now have incidence rates 3 times higher than men, and black people have the highest incidence rates

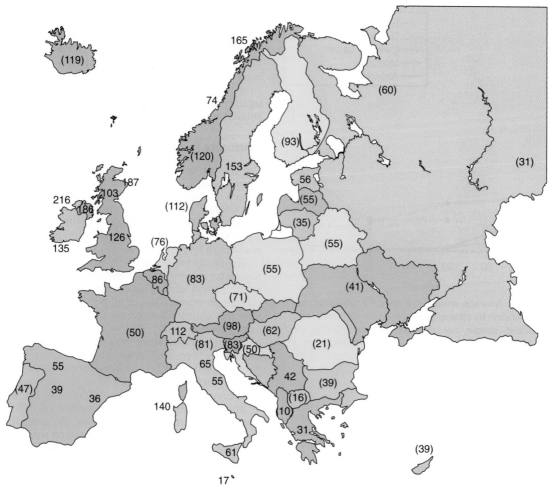

Fig. 49.5 Multiple sclerosis (MS) prevalence rates in Europe (adjusted to the 1966 European population; in brackets, crude rates when adjustment not possible). *(From Pugliatti, M., Rosati, G., Carton H., et al., 2006. The epidemiology of multiple sclerosis in Europe. Eur J Neurol 13, 709.)*

compared to all other groups. The incidence rates for Hispanic people (8.2 per 100,000), Asian people (3.3 per 100,000), and Native American people (3.1 per 100,000) are in the moderate to high range (Wallin et al., 2012).

The U.S. World War II veteran series showed a markedly elevated risk for residents who lived in the northern region of the country (Fig. 49.6). This was seen for both sexes among white people and for black men, with a north-to-south difference of almost 3 to 1. Veterans of the Vietnam War and later conflicts still showed a gradient, but it was much less (Wallin et al., 2004). All southern states then were calculated to lie within the high-frequency zone, with prevalence rates that were estimated at well over 30 per 100,000 population. For all races and both sexes, the north-to-south difference was only 2 to 1. This is not a "regression to the mean" with a decreased prevalence in the north, but rather reflects an even greater increase in the south. This diffusion is in accord with the intra- and international changes for Europe as noted. MS is geographically a slowly spreading disease, the reason(s) for which must be environmental.

Genetic Studies

Family studies in MS have provided a means of assessing environmental factors against a set genetic background. Such

studies have shown that the risk for multiple family members with MS is 3% to 4% for primary relatives and 20% to 30% for monozygotic twins. This finding is in contrast with the general population prevalence of approximately 0.1%. The increased family frequency may be related to shared environment, as opposed to shared genetic factors, because close relatives would be expected to share similar environmental influences. However, further evidence that MS is under some genetic control includes the following:

1. An excess of MS-concordant monozygous twins in most twin studies. The difference in concordance rates between monozygotic and dizygotic twins is attributable primarily to genetic factors. Moreover, a recent study found no evidence for genetic, epigenetic, or transcriptome differences in identical twins discordant for MS (Baranzini et al., 2010). The maximum concordance rate for MS in monozygotic twins in high-risk areas is approximately 30%. This indicates that although genes play a role in MS, the maximal effect of genes is at most 30%.

2. The association of HLA alleles (specifically the HLA DR2 haplotype) and MS, and the higher frequency of HLA sharing in affected sibling pairs. There is a dose effect of the DRB1*1501 on MS susceptibility. The interplay between MHC alleles via epistasis within racial groups could be a factor but has not been extensively studied.

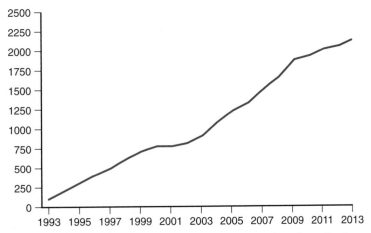

Fig. 50.1 Rapid growth of clinical testing for genetic disease. This graph plots the number of genetic diseases for which clinical testing was available over the period of 1993–2013, illustrating an approximate 20-fold increase in the number of testable disorders. *(Data from GeneTests. Available at http://www.genetests.org/.)*

diagnostic information available today. This is becoming more true as the use of clinical exome and genome sequencing becomes increasingly widespread. In this chapter we will discuss these essential basics and present examples of how genetic information has informed our understanding of disease definition and etiology, show how it is utilized in the practice of neurology today, and how it will be used even more extensively in the future. Given the massive acceleration in technology, from microarrays to the methods enabling complete and efficient human genome sequencing, this future is closer than most realize and the era of genomic medicine is fast approaching.

GENE EXPRESSION, DIVERSITY, AND REGULATION

The basic principles of molecular genetics are outlined in Fig. 50.2 and Table 50.1, and more detailed descriptions can be found elsewhere (Alberts et al., 2008; Griffiths et al., 2002; Lodish et al., 2008; Strachan and Read, 2003). To briefly summarize, deoxyribonucleic acid (DNA), found in the nucleus of all cells, comprises the raw material from which heritable information is transferred among individuals, with the simplest heritable unit being the gene. DNA is composed of a series of individual nucleotides, all of which contain an identical pentose (2′-deoxyribose)-phosphate backbone but differ at an attached base that can be adenine (A), guanine (G), thymine (T), or cytosine (C). A and G are purine bases and pair with the pyrimidine bases T and C, respectively, to form a double-stranded helical structure which allows for semiconservative bidirectional replication, the means by which DNA is copied in a precise and efficient manner. In total, there are approximately 3.2 billion base pairs in human DNA. By convention, a DNA sequence is described by listing the bases as they are expressed from the 5′ to 3′ direction along the pentose backbone (e.g., 5′-ATGCAT-3′), as this is the order in which it is typically used by the cellular machinery, also called the *sense strand* (compare to RNA, later). The opposite paired, or *antisense*, strand is arranged antiparallel (3′ to 5′) and can also be referred to when discussing sequence; however, by convention this is generally not done unless that strand is also transcribed into RNA.

The expression of a gene is tightly and coordinately regulated (Fig. 50.2), an important consideration for understanding the molecular mechanisms of disease. The typical gene

contains one or more *promoters*, DNA sequences that allow for the binding of a cellular protein complex that includes RNA polymerase and other factors that faithfully copy the DNA in the 5′ to 3′ direction in a process known as *transcription*. The resulting single-stranded molecule contains a ribose sugar unit in its backbone and thus the resulting molecule is termed *ribonucleic acid*, or RNA. RNA also differs from the template DNA by the incorporation of uracil (U) in place of thymine (T), as it also pairs efficiently with adenine, and thymine serves a secondary role in DNA repair that is not necessary in RNA. The sequence of the RNA matches the sense DNA strand and is therefore complementary to (and hence derived from) the antisense strand.

Transcribed coding RNA must be processed to become protein-encoding *messenger RNA* (mRNA), a term used to differentiate these RNAs from all other types of RNA in the cell. To become mature, RNA is stabilized by modification at the ends with a 7-methylguanosine 5′ cap and a long poly-A 3′ tail. A further critical stage in the maturation of the RNA molecule involves a rearrangement process termed *RNA splicing* (Fig. 50.3). This is necessary because the expressed coding sequences in DNA, called *exons*, of virtually every gene are discontinuous and interspersed with long stretches of generally nonconserved intervening sequences referred to as *introns*. This, along with other mechanisms, likely plays an evolutionary role in the development of new genes by allowing for the shuffling of functional sequences (Babushok et al., 2007). Nascent RNA molecules are recognized by the *spliceosome*, a protein complex that removes the introns and rejoins the exons. Not every exon is utilized at all times in every RNA derived from a single gene. Exons may be skipped or included in a regulated manner through alternative splicing, which occurs in nearly 95% of all genes to create different isoforms of that mRNA. The dynamic nature of this observation is critical to a complete understanding of cellular gene expression. DNA is essentially a storage molecule, and with few exceptions in the absence of mutagens, its sequence remains static and, aside from epigenetic events, is therefore limited to a genetic regulatory role as a transcriptional rheostat. Current estimates place the number of individual human genes at just over 22,000 (Pertea and Salzberg, 2010), so it is difficult to reconcile biological and clinical diversity with simple variations in expression. Alternative splicing provides a means of dramatically elevating this diversity by enabling a single gene to encode multiple proteins with a wide array of functions.

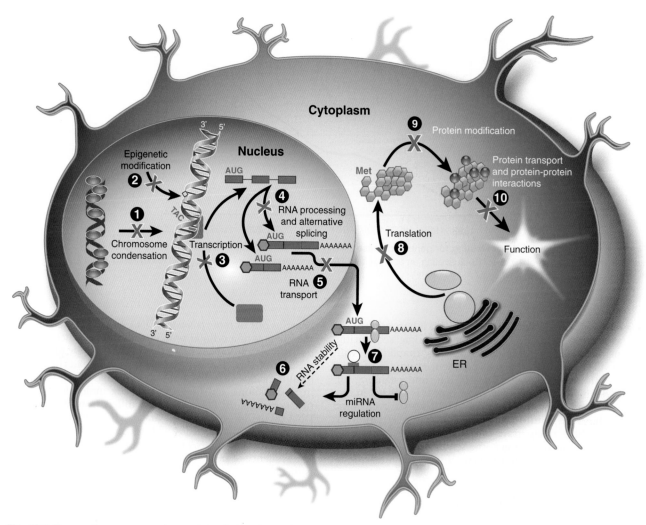

Fig. 50.2 Neuronal gene expression and regulation. A generic human neuron is depicted. **(1)** DNA bound to histones forms transcriptionally inactive chromatin, which can be relieved through the action of various proteins and enzymes. **(2)** Epigenetic modifications *(yellow)* are heritable changes to the DNA or its associated histones that alter gene expression without changing the DNA sequence and can result from various environmental stimuli or perturbations. **(3)** Active DNA is bound by RNA polymerase in a process regulated by protein factors, and the genetic information contained within the DNA is converted to RNA via the process of transcription. An example of a three-nucleotide codon *(red)* is shown on the antisense DNA strand being converted to its complement on the sense strand of the RNA. **(4)** Nascent RNA undergoes processing to become messenger RNA (mRNA) with the addition of a 5′ cap structure *(green)* and a poly-A tail, as well as undergoing RNA splicing which removes noncoding sequences and can generate transcript diversity through the use of alternative exons (see text). **(5)** Mature mRNA is exported from the nucleus to the cytoplasm and/or to a specific subcellular location. **(6)** Over time, mRNA is subject to degradation within the cell, and its inherent stability can be dynamic, changing in relation to the state of the cell. **(7)** Short noncoding RNAs, called *micro-RNAs* (miRNAs) *(pink)*, can target cellular protein complexes *(white)* to specific mRNAs and regulate their activity by promoting degradation or blocking translation (see text). **(8)** The mRNA is bound by ribosomes (either free or associated with the endoplasmic reticulum) and undergoes translation into protein. The three-nucleotide codon *(red)* directs the incorporation of a single amino acid into the newly synthesized protein (in this example methionine, met). **(9)** The protein undergoes post-translational chemical modifications *(pink)* to generate a functional protein for use by the cell. **(10)** Mature protein interacts with other proteins and/or is transported to its site of activity within the cell. All direct steps in this pathway are potential sites for disease-modifying therapies *(red X's)*, depending on the gene in question.

Supporting this, recent analysis of RNA complexity in human tissues suggests that there are at least seven alternative splicing events per multi-exon gene, generating over 100,000 alternative splicing events (Pan et al., 2008). Because alternative splicing and other forms of RNA processing can be subject to complex layers of temporal and spatial regulation, particularly in the human brain (Licatalosi and Darnell, 2010; Ward and Cooper, 2010), it is a robust source for both biological diversity and disease-causing mutations (see Polymorphisms and Point Mutations).

DNA to RNA to Protein

The central dogma of genetics has been that DNA is transcribed into RNA that is then translated into protein—the "business" end of the process. So, following its transcription from DNA in the nucleus, mRNA is transported out of the nucleus to the cytoplasm, and possibly to a specific subcellular location depending on the mRNA, where it can be deciphered by the cell. This takes place via interaction with a complex known as the *ribosome*, which binds the mRNA and converts

TABLE 50.1 Glossary of Genetic Terminology

Allele	Alternate forms of a locus (gene)	Lyonization	The process of random inactivation of one of the pair of X chromosomes in females
Anticipation	Earlier onset and/or worsening severity of disease in successive generations	Marker	Sequence of DNA used to identify a gene or a locus
Antisense	Nucleic acid sequence complementary to mRNA	Megabase	1,000,000 bases or base-pairs
Chromosome	Organizational unit of the genome consisting of a linear arrangement of genes	Meiosis	Process of cellular division that produces gametes containing a haploid amount of DNA
Cis-acting	A regulatory nucleotide sequence present on the molecule being regulated	Mendelian	Obeying standard single-gene patterns of inheritance (e.g., recessive or dominant)
Codon	A three-nucleotide sequence representing a single amino acid	Microarray	A glass or plastic support (e.g., slide or chip) to which large numbers of DNA molecules can be attached for use in high-throughput genetic analysis
Complex disease	Disease exhibiting non-Mendelian inheritance involving the interaction of multiple genes and the environment		
De novo	A mutation newly arising in an individual and not present in either parent	Missense	DNA mutation that changes a given codon to represent a different amino acid
Diploid	A genome having paired genetic information; half-normal number is haploid	Mitosis	Process of cellular division during which DNA is replicated
DNA	Deoxyribonucleic acid; used for storage, replication, and inheritance of genetic information	Nonsense	DNA mutation that changes a given codon into a translation termination signal
		Penetrance	The likelihood of a disease-associated genotype to express a specific disease phenotype
Dominant	Allele that determines phenotype when a single copy is present in an individual	Phenotype	The clinical manifestations of a given genotype
Endophenotype	Subset of phenotypic characteristics used to group patients manifesting a given trait	Polymorphism	Sequence variation among individuals, typically not considered to be pathogenic
Epigenetic	Relating to heritable changes in gene expression resulting from DNA, histone, or other modifications that do not involve changes in DNA sequence	Probe	DNA sequence used for identifying a specific gene or allele
		Promoter	DNA sequences that regulate transcription of a given gene
Exome	Portion of the genome representing only the coding regions of genes	Protein	Functional cellular macromolecules encoded by a gene
Exon	Segment of DNA that is expressed in at least one mature mRNA	Recessive	Allele that determines phenotype only when two copies are present in an individual
Expressivity	The range of phenotypes observed with a specific disease-associated genotype	Relative risk	The ratio of the chance of disease in individuals with a specific genetic susceptibility factor over the chance of disease in those without it
Frameshift	DNA mutation that adds or removes nucleotides, affecting which are grouped as codons		
Gene	Contiguous DNA sequence that codes for a given messenger RNA and its splice variants	Resequencing	A method of identifying clinically relevant genetic variation in a candidate gene of interest by comparing the sequence in individuals with disease to a reference sequence
Genome	A complete set of DNA from a given individual		
Genotype	The DNA sequence of a gene	RNA	Ribonucleic acid; expressed form of a gene, called *messenger* or *mRNA* if protein coding
Haplotype	A group of alleles on the same chromosome close enough to be inherited together		
		Sense	Nucleic acid sequence corresponding to mRNA
Hemizygous	Genes having only a single allele in an individual, such as the X chromosome in males	Silent	DNA mutation that changes a given codon but does not alter the corresponding amino acid
Heteroplasmy	A mixture of multiple mitochondrial genomes in a given individual	SNP	Single nucleotide polymorphism
Heterozygous	Genes having two distinct alleles in an individual at a given locus	Splicing	RNA processing mechanism where introns are removed and exons joined to create mRNA; in alternative splicing, exons are utilized in a regulated manner within a cell or tissue
Homozygous	Genes having two identical alleles in an individual at a given locus		
Intron	Segment of DNA between exons that is transcribed into RNA but removed by splicing	Trans-acting	A regulatory protein that acts on a molecule other than that which expressed it
Kilobase	1000 bases or base-pairs	Transcription	Cellular process where DNA sequence is used as template for RNA synthesis
Linkage disequilibrium	The co-occurrence of two alleles more frequently than expected by random chance, suggesting they are in close proximity to one another		
		Transcriptome	The complete set of RNA transcripts produced by a cell, tissue, or individual
Locus	Location of a DNA sequence (or a gene) on a chromosome or within the genome	Translation	Cellular process where mRNA sequence is converted to protein

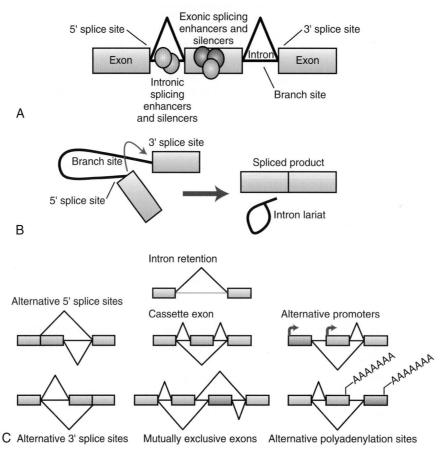

CONSTITUTIVE AND ALTERNATIVE SPLICING

Fig. 50.3 RNA splicing. A, A generic precursor RNA is shown, consisting of three exons *(blue)* with intervening introns *(dark lines)*. Representative sequences recognized by the protein complexes that mediate splicing are shown (5′ and 3′ splice sites and the branch site). Binding of these complexes may be influenced either positively or negatively by regulatory sequences and their associated proteins *(circles)* located in either the introns or exons. Splicing pattern is shown by angled lines spanning introns. **B,** Splicing occurs via the complex-mediated association of the 5′ splice site and the branch site, with subsequent attack of the 3′ splice site by the upstream exon *(arrow)*, which joins it to the downstream exon and releases the intron. **C,** Possible alternative splicing patterns for various mRNAs are shown. Constitutive exons are in blue. Alternatively utilized exons are shown in orange or purple. A retained intron is shown by an orange line.

its genetic information into protein via the process of *translation*. The ribosome initiates translation at a pre-encoded start site and converts the mRNA sequence into protein until a designated termination site is reached. Sequence information is read in three-nucleotide groups called *codons*, each of which specifies an individual amino acid. With the four distinct bases, there are mathematically 64 possible codons, but these have an element of redundancy and code for only 20 different amino acids and 3 termination signals (UAG, UGA, and UAA), also called *stop codons*. The *start codon* is ATG and codes for methionine. These amino acids are joined by the ribosome to synthesize a protein. This protein, which may undergo further modification, will ultimately carry out a programmed biological function in the cell. Regulation of this process is highly coordinated and important in learning, for example, where activity-dependent translation at the synapse underlies some aspects of synaptic plasticity, which may go awry in certain disorders such as fragile X syndrome and autism (Morrow et al., 2008).

Over the past decade, the discovery of several classes of functional non-protein coding RNAs has added additional complexity to our understanding of how the genetic code is manifest at the level of cellular function. Of these, microRNAs (miRNAs) are increasingly being recognized as vital players in gene regulation and neurological disease (Weinberg and Wood, 2009). Nascent miRNA molecules are processed to form short (approximately 22-nucleotide) RNA duplexes that target endogenous cellular machinery to specific coding RNAs and induce post-transcriptional gene silencing through a diverse repertoire including RNA cleavage, translational blocking, transport to inactive cell sites, or promotion of RNA decay (Filipowicz et al., 2008; Weinberg and Wood, 2009). Depending on the cell and the context, miRNA activity can result in specific gene inactivation, functional repression, or more subtle regulatory effects and may involve multiple RNAs in a given biological pathway (Flynt and Lai, 2008). Estimates suggest that miRNAs may regulate 30% of protein-coding genes, implicating these molecules as important targets for future research into the biology of neurological disease (Filipowicz et al., 2008; Weinberg and Wood, 2009).

For a specific disease-related gene, the DNA sequence present within an individual is referred to as their *genotype*, and the expression of that code often results in a feature (or features) that can be observed or measured, known as the *phenotype*. Genes are further organized into higher-order structures termed *chromosomes*, which together compose the entire set of DNA, or *genome*, of the individual. The human genome is diploid, meaning we possess 23 pairs of chromosomes, 22

TABLE 50.3 Selected Online Clinical Neurogenetics Resources

Disease-specific and gene-specific resources	GeneCards: The Human Gene Compendium Crown Human Genome Center, Department of Molecular Genetics, The Weizmann Institute of Science, Rehovot, Israel http://www.genecards.org	Genomic variation and other genome resources	Catalog of Published Genome-Wide Association Studies US National Human Genome Research Institute http://www.genome.gov/gwastudies/
	GeneReviews University of Washington, Seattle, WA, USA US National Center for Biotechnology Information http://www.ncbi.nlm.nih.gov/books/NBK1116/		ClinVar Database US National Center for Biotechnology Information https://www.ncbi.nlm.nih.gov/clinvar/
	GeneTests Bio-Reference Laboratories, Inc., Elmwood Park, NJ, USA http://www.genetests.org/		Database of Genomic Variants The Centre for Applied Genomics, Canada http://dgv.tcag.ca/dgv/app/home
	The Genetic Testing Registry US National Center for Biotechnology Information http://www.ncbi.nlm.nih.gov/gtr/		Ensembl Databases European Molecular Biology Laboratory— European Bioinformatics Institute Wellcome Trust Sanger Institute, UK http://www.ensembl.org/
	Locus Specific Mutation Databases Human Genome Variation Society, Australia http://www.hgvs.org/dblist/glsdb.html		Exome Variant Server National Heart Lung and Blood Institute Grand Opportunity Exome Sequencing Project http://evs.gs.washington.edu/EVS/
	Neuromuscular Disease Center Washington University, St. Louis, MO, USA http://neuromuscular.wustl.edu/		International HapMap Project http://hapmap.ncbi.nlm.nih.gov/index.html
	Online Mendelian Inheritance in Man Johns Hopkins University, Baltimore, MD, USA http://omim.org/		National Center for Biotechnology Information Databases US National Center for Biotechnology Information http://www.ncbi.nlm.nih.gov/
Clinical genetic testing and clinical trials	ClinicalTrials.gov US National Institutes of Health http://clinicaltrials.gov/		Single Nucleotide Polymorphism Database US National Center for Biotechnology Information http://www.ncbi.nlm.nih.gov/projects/SNP/
	GeneTests Bio-Reference Laboratories, Inc., Elmwood Park, NJ, USA http://www.genetests.org/		1000 Genomes Project http://www.1000genomes.org/
	The Genetic Testing Registry US National Center for Biotechnology Information http://www.ncbi.nlm.nih.gov/gtr/		University of California, Santa Cruz (UCSC) Genome Bioinformatics University of California, Santa Cruz, Santa Cruz, CA, USA http://genome.ucsc.edu/

clinically relevant insofar as disproportionate activation of an abnormal X chromosome could potentially lead to clinical phenotypes in female carriers of recessive X-linked disorders. Usually though, skewing occurs, so that the pathogenic allele is less expressed than the other normal allele.

Recessive X-linked transmission is characterized by the presence of disease in males only (Fig. 50.8). Affected males cannot pass the disease on to their sons, but all their daughters must inherent the abnormal X chromosome and are, therefore, *obligate carriers*. A carrier female has a 50% chance of passing the disease allele to a child, but all males receiving it will be affected. Dominant X-linked transmission (see Fig. 50.8) is similar, except carrier females are affected and transmit the disease to 50% of their children irrespective of their sex. Affected males usually show a more severe phenotype, or may even exhibit lethality, and transmit the disease to all of their daughters and none of their sons.

Over 100 X-linked disorders with neurological phenotypes are known (OMIM, 2014). The majority of these X-linked disorders are recessive, and as seen for the autosomal diseases, mutation type varies widely among the different disorders. Some examples include X-linked adrenoleukodystrophy (ATP-binding cassette subfamily D member 1, commonly caused by missense and frameshift mutations), Duchenne muscular dystrophy (dystrophin, commonly caused by deletions), Emery–Dreifuss muscular dystrophy-1 (emerin, often caused by nonsense mutations), Menkes disease (ATPase, Cu^{++}-transporting, alpha-polypeptide, commonly caused by frameshifts, nonsense mutations, and splicing mutations), Fabry disease (alpha-galactosidase A, commonly caused by point mutations, gene rearrangements, and splicing mutations), and Pelizaeus-Merzbacher disease (proteolipid protein-1, often caused by duplications and missense mutations). X-linked dominant disorders include Rett syndrome (methyl-CpG-binding protein-2, often due to missense and nonsense mutations), incontinentia pigmenti (inhibitor of kappa light polypeptide gene enhancer in B cells, kinase gamma [IKBKG], often due to deletions), and Aicardi syndrome (gene unknown). More detailed lists can be found using the recommended online resources (see Table 50.3).

MENDELIAN DISEASE GENE IDENTIFICATION BY LINKAGE ANALYSIS AND CHROMOSOME MAPPING

As mentioned previously, patterns of inheritance can be utilized to locate genes responsible for disease. Traditionally, genes showing Mendelian patterns of inheritance can be physically mapped and identified through linkage analysis (Altshuler et al., 2008; Pulst, 2003) (Fig. 50.9). In this technique, one attempts to find a known region of DNA, termed a *marker*, which is co-inherited (segregates) with the disease being studied and subsequently uses the location of that marker to find the disease gene. Although, in principle, two points on the same chromosome theoretically segregate independently from one another, the recombination process that mediates this (termed *crossing-over* because maternal and paternal chromosomes swap segments during gamete formation) is statistically more likely to separate points that are far apart from one another than those that are close. Segments of DNA that segregate together are described as being linked. If the degree of linkage exceeds that expected by chance, the regions are said to be in *disequilibrium* and are therefore in close proximity. By using naturally occurring DNA polymorphisms as locational markers, the physical mapping of an unknown disease gene is possible, although the mapped region will likely contain other genes as well. Depending on the size of the family, the generational distance of affected individuals sampled, and the density of the markers being used, the region containing the disease gene is narrowed down to a size more amenable to further detailed analysis. Subsequent analysis, usually DNA sequencing of likely candidate genes, is then performed to locate a mutation that segregates with the affected members of the original family. Many genes important to neurological disease have been identified in this way, including the genes for HD, Duchenne muscular dystrophy, Wilson disease, neurofibromatosis type 1, Von Hippel–Lindau syndrome, torsion dystonia 1, Friedreich ataxia, myotonic dystrophy type 1, hyperkalemic periodic paralysis, familial advanced sleep-phase syndrome, and many others. Although still useful clinically for large families, utilization of this technique is not possible for many diseases because of small family sizes and/or lack of power due to insufficient generational separation between affected individuals in the pedigree. Recent advances in next-generation sequencing technology have allowed for the utilization of entire exomic or genomic sequence for the purposes of mapping, allowing for disease gene identification in families of smaller size (see Genome/Exome Sequencing in Clinical Practice and Disease Gene Discovery).

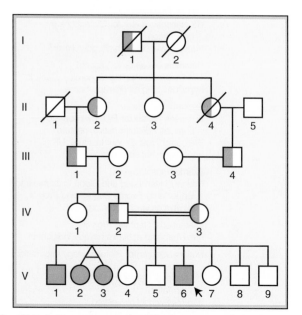

Fig. 50.7 Autosomal recessive inheritance. A pedigree diagram is shown, using standard nomenclature as described in Fig. 50.6. Carriers of disease are indicated by half-filled icons. Individuals V-2 and V-3 illustrate the diagramming of monozygotic twins. Consanguineous mating is indicated by a doubled line. An autosomal recessive pedigree demonstrates indirect transmission of disease without a sex preference, often in a single generation (occasionally described as horizontal). On average, 25% of offspring of two carriers are affected.

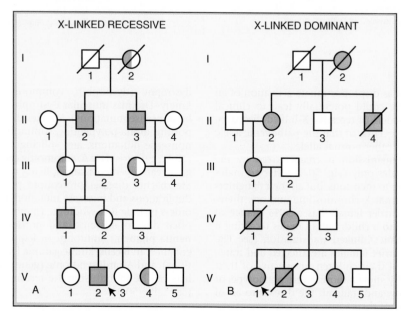

Fig. 50.8 X-linked inheritance. A, X-linked recessive disease. A pedigree diagram is shown using standard nomenclature as described in Fig. 50.6. Carriers of disease are indicated by half-filled icons. Disease manifests only in hemizygous males. Fathers cannot pass the disease to their sons, but all daughters of an affected male are obligate carriers of disease. Carrier females have a 50% chance to pass on the disease gene and can have affected sons. In some cases, a female carrier can be mildly symptomatic, usually due to nonrandom lyonization. **B,** X-linked dominant disease. A pedigree diagram is shown using standard nomenclature as described in Fig. 50.6. Disease manifests in heterozygous females (although severity may be affected by lyonization). The mutant gene is either lethal in males (as shown here) or has a much more severe phenotype. Affected females pass on the disease 50% of the time.

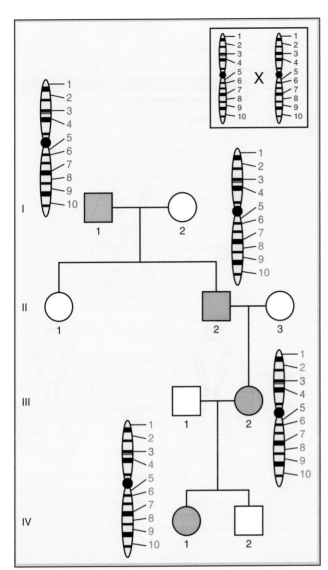

Fig. 50.9 Linkage analysis. A pedigree is depicted as in Fig. 50.6, showing autosomal dominant inheritance of disease *(filled icons).* Transmission of the chromosome containing the mutant gene *(purple line)* is illustrated for all affected individuals. Numbers represent the location of specific chromosomal markers (e.g., single nucleotide polymorphisms or other sequences). Purple numbers represent markers originally from the mutant chromosome in individual I-1. With each mating, there is potential crossing over between regions of homologous chromosomes *(inset),* likely resulting in the separation of markers spaced far apart along the chromosome. In this example, examination of all affected individuals shows the disease segregates with marker 3, and the two are therefore in linkage disequilibrium, suggesting they are near one another. Once identified, the marker location can be used to select candidate genes for sequencing to identify the causative gene and mutation in the family.

NON-MENDELIAN PATTERNS OF INHERITANCE

In rare instances, pedigree analysis of affected families has revealed patterns of inheritance that do not conform to the classic Mendelian patterns thus far described and, therefore, must result from other mechanisms. In this section, we will discuss the more common and clinically relevant ways in which single-gene disorders can be transmitted in a non-Mendelian fashion: mitochondrial inheritance, imprinting, and uniparental disomy. It is important to recognize that this

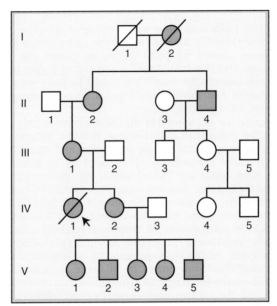

Fig. 50.10 Mitochondrial (maternal) inheritance. A pedigree diagram is shown using standard nomenclature as described in Fig. 50.6. As the mutant gene is carried in the mitochondrial genome, disease is passed on to all the offspring of affected females (see text). Males can be affected but cannot pass on disease. Severity and onset of the disease may be affected by heteroplasmy, the proportion of abnormal mitochondria per cell, as illustrated by a severe phenotype seen in patient IV-1.

is not all inclusive. Other examples exist, such as developmental events that can potentially lead to disease or syndromic conditions through formation of a *mosaic,* an individual with cells of different genotypes derived from a common cell, or a *chimera,* an individual who contains cells of different distinct genotypes (e.g., from separate fertilizations). Such rare events will not be discussed further. Additionally, the non-Mendelian heritability of diseases that are *polygenic,* or involve multiple genes, and other forms of complex disorders will be discussed in later sections.

Mitochondrial Disorders

Mitochondria are double-membraned organelles responsible for energy production within the cell via the process of oxidative phosphorylation, which relies on the transfer of electrons through a chain of protein complexes within the inner mitochondrial membrane. Disruption of mitochondrial function can lead to a variety of diseases with multisystem involvement, including prominent neurological symptoms (DiMauro and Hirano, 2009; Zeviani and Carelli, 2007). Mitochondria possess their own genome with 37 genes. Because mitochondria are cytoplasmic and the majority of cytoplasm within the zygote is derived from the egg and not the sperm, disorders involving mitochondrial DNA are inherited through the maternal line (Fig. 50.10). A single cell contains many mitochondria which all replicate independently of the nuclear DNA, so it is possible that a mutation in the mitochondrial genome may be present in some of the mitochondria but not others, a condition termed *heteroplasmy.* This proportion can affect whether a disease is expressed and, if so, what tissues are affected if a minimum threshold of abnormal mitochondria is reached. Heteroplasmy may also change over time as cells divide and the mitochondria are redistributed. Some examples of such disorders include MELAS (mitochondrial encephalomyopathy, lactic acidosis, and stroke-like episodes, caused by point mutations within the gene encoding mitochondrial tRNA^{LEU}), MERRF (myoclonic epilepsy with ragged red fibers, caused by point mutations within the gene-encoding mitochondrial tRNA^{LYS}), and LHON (Leber hereditary optic neuropathy, most often caused by point mutations in either of two mitochondrial genes encoding complex I subunits, ND4 or ND6).

Because the mitochondria themselves contain only a few genes, the majority of mitochondrial proteins, including the machinery responsible for the replication and repair of the mitochondrial genome, are all encoded by nuclear genes. Since these genes are located within the nuclear genome, despite the fact that their mutation gives rise to dysfunctional mitochondria, the disease will show a Mendelian pattern of inheritance. Some examples include infantile-onset SCA (twinkle on chromosome 10, autosomal recessive, caused by missense mutations), progressive external ophthalmoplegia A2 (adenine nucleotide translocator 1 on chromosome 4, autosomal dominant, caused by missense mutations), and Charcot–Marie–Tooth type 2A2 (mitofusin-2 on chromosome 1, autosomal dominant, often caused by missense mutations). Interestingly, various mutations, commonly missense, of the nuclear gene DNA polymerase gamma (POLG) on chromosome 15, which encodes the polymerase responsible for both replication and repair of the mitochondrial genome, cause a wide variety of diverse phenotypes with different modes of inheritance (Hudson and Chinnery, 2006). These include the autosomal recessive Alpers syndrome of encephalopathy, seizures, and liver failure, an autosomal dominant form of chronic progressive external ophthalmoplegia, and autosomal recessive phenotypes of cerebellar ataxia and peripheral neuropathy, among others.

Imprinting

For most genes, expression is controlled by distinct cellular processes that operate irrespective of the gene's parental origin. However, for some genes, expression in the offspring differs, depending on whether the allele was maternally or paternally inherited, and such genes are described as being imprinted (Spencer, 2009). *Imprinting* arises from epigenetic modifications such as DNA or histone methylation, which are parent-specific alterations that do not change the actual DNA sequence (Fig. 50.11). One example of this is sex-specific DNA methylation that occurs for some genes during the formation of gametes. In the offspring, the methylated gene is bound by histone proteins forming transcriptionally inactive heterochromatin. This allows all gene expression to be driven by the allele derived from the other parent. This can be dynamic depending on the gene, and the magnitude of differential expression between the alleles can vary based on stage of development, tissue type, and possibly other factors. Deletion of an imprinted region or defective imprinting in gametogenesis can lead to disease as illustrated by observations involving chromosome 15q (Lalande and Calciano, 2007). In this example, differential methylation affects the expression of multiple genes, and loss of maternal patterning can lead to Angelman syndrome, characterized by intellectual impairment, epilepsy, ataxia, and inappropriate laughter, while loss of the paternal pattern causes Prader–Willi syndrome, associated with intellectual impairment, obesity, and behavioral problems. The most common mechanism involves de novo deletion of the imprinted region from one parent, although in some cases, defective imprinting can also occur during gametogenesis. In the majority of cases, defective imprinting occurs spontaneously and is therefore unlikely to recur in families; however, imprinting defects can rarely be due to

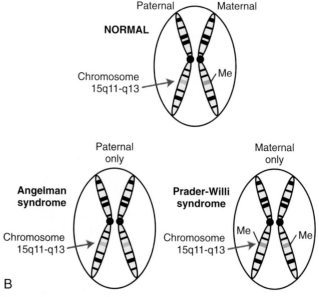

Fig. 50.11 Epigenetics in human disease. A, Imprinting. Gene expression on human chromosome 15q11-q13 is subject to epigenetic regulation via imprinting. The region contains the loci for two neurological diseases, Prader–Willi syndrome and Angelman syndrome (see text). When inherited from the father, gene expression occurs from the Prader–Willi locus *(blue arrow)*, and this also inactivates genes at the Angelman locus via a presumed antisense-RNA mechanism *(dashed arrow)*. In contrast, when inherited from the mother, a specific site on the chromosome called the *imprinting center (circle)* becomes methylated (Me). This methylation causes transcriptional inactivation of the genes within the Prader–Willi locus *(X)*, which correspondingly allows transcription from genes at the Angelman locus *(purple arrow)*. If imprinting does not properly occur, either Angelman or Prader–Willi syndrome will arise depending on whether the maternal or paternal expression pattern is absent. **B,** Uniparental disomy. During gamete/zygote formation, errors in chromosomal segregation or chromosomal rearrangement can result in retention of all or part of a chromosome inherited from the same parent. Although there is no loss of genetic information, the epigenetic imprinting pattern is lost, and therefore correct gene expression patterns are not retained. For chromosome 15q11-q13, for example, this can give rise to Angelman or Prader–Willi syndrome depending on whether the duplicated chromosome is that of the father or the mother, respectively.

small deletions involving sequences important for regulating parent-specific methylation.

Uniparental Disomy

Uniparental disomy arises when pairs of chromosomes are inherited from the same parent, either in their entirety or in large segments due to segregation errors or chromosomal rearrangement (Kotzot, 2008) (see Fig. 50.11). The uniparentally

tests are vastly more comprehensive and cost-effective (Coppola and Geschwind, 2012; Fogel et al., 2014), on the order of approximately $5,000 for over 21,000 genes. In the short term, the use of broader gene panels that take advantage of the less expensive next-generation sequencing technology (approximately $2,000 for ~200 genes) will likely form a transition step between current methodologies and sequencing of the complete exome or genome (Nemeth et al., 2013). Regardless, the clinical examination should be used to precisely define the patient's phenotype, which will in turn suggest the most high-yield conditions for genetic testing. This systematic approach is of immense benefit in resource management and the education of current and future physicians should include discussion on the implementation and utilization of such strategies in clinical practice (Fogel et al., 2013).

The types of single-gene testing available vary per laboratory and gene (Table 50.9). The most comprehensive (and expensive) testing type commonly available is full individual gene sequencing, where all coding regions, as well as approximately 50 bases in each intron/exon junction, are sequenced for the presence of mutation. This will detect all coding point mutations and splice-site mutations as well as small insertions and deletions but will miss more detailed structural variation. Importantly, novel coding mutations can be detected in this way. Targeted sequence analysis (also called *select exon testing*) consists of specific sequencing reactions designed to only detect one or a few previously identified mutations. This will not detect any sequence variations outside of the limited region of the gene being searched. For repeat disorders, there are specific tests to identify the relevant expansions using either polymerase chain reaction (PCR) or Southern blotting, a hybridization-based DNA sizing technique. Larger deletions or duplications (e.g., copy number variations) can be detected by quantitative PCR methods or by comparative genomic hybridization. It is important to be aware of the type of testing being ordered; in some cases, such as select exon testing, a negative result does not exclude mutations elsewhere in the gene being tested. Interpretation of these genetic results may be straightforward, for example, if no variants are present or if known pathogenic changes are found. In contrast, interpretation may be complicated if novel sequence variants of unknown pathological significance are identified. Inconclusive results may require interpretation by a specialist and/or further testing to determine the likelihood of pathogenicity.

Common diseases must be approached in a different manner, because detailed phenotype alone cannot always predict the mutation to test for, particularly when assessing genomic variation. Still, the goal remains to develop strategies incorporating known genetic information into a systematic protocol designed to maximize diagnostic capability while minimizing cost and unnecessary testing (Lintas and Persico, 2009). Tests such as chromosomal microarray analysis are clinically available to search genome-wide for disease-causing CNVs and are recommended for sporadic causes in disorders such as intellectual disability or autism where CNVs have been found responsible for a reasonable percentage of disease (Geschwind and Spence, 2008; Miller D.T., et al., 2010). Use of such testing in sporadic adult-onset disease is less clear, so the physician is advised to refer to current published guidelines for the disease in question before ordering. For more specific phenotypes, other available tests include those assessing for CNVs (often called simply *deletions/duplications*) involving individual genes or specific chromosomal regions. Overall, interpretation of CNV results can be challenging, particularly if the CNV was previously unreported. Here, the parents will often need to be evaluated to determine whether the CNV in question is inherited or de novo. As already discussed for DNA sequence changes, such findings may require interpretation by

TABLE 50.9 Types of Genetic Testing

Type of test	Sequence variant(s) identified	Sequence variant(s) missed or not accurately determined
Gene sequencing	Point mutations* Frameshifts Splicing mutations[†] Polymorphisms	Noncoding variants[‡] Copy number variations[§] Repeat expansions
Select exon sequencing (Targeted mutation analysis)	Known predefined variants *Target region only*[#,**] Point mutations* Frameshifts Splicing mutations[†] Polymorphisms	*Variants outside target region*[**] Point mutations* Frameshifts Splicing mutations[†] Polymorphisms Noncoding variants[‡] Copy number variations[§] Repeat expansions
Repeat expansion testing[¶] (Targeted mutation analysis)	Repeat expansion in the specific gene tested	Point mutations* Frameshifts Splicing mutations[†] Polymorphisms Noncoding variants[‡] Copy number variations[§]
Gene copy number variation (Deletion/duplication testing)	Copy number variation[§] of gene tested	Point mutations* Frameshifts Splicing mutations[†] Polymorphisms Noncoding variants[‡] Repeat expansions
Chromosomal microarray analysis[††] (Comparative genomic hybridization)	Genome-wide copy number variations[‡‡]	Point mutations* Frameshifts Splicing mutations[†] Polymorphisms Noncoding variants[‡] Repeat expansions
Clinical exome sequencing[††]	Point mutations* Frameshifts Splicing mutations[†] Polymorphisms	Noncoding variants[‡] Copy number variations[§] Repeat expansions[#]
Clinical genome sequencing[††]	Point mutations* Frameshifts Splicing mutations[†] Polymorphisms Noncoding variants[‡] Copy number variations[§]	Repeat expansions[#]

*Includes missense, nonsense, and silent mutations.
[†]Includes only those involving splice sites and exonic splicing regulatory sequences.
[‡]Includes promoter mutations and noncoding splicing regulatory elements.
[§]Arbitrarily defined here as any deletion/duplication/insertion larger than detectable by Sanger sequencing.
[¶]Targeted mutation analysis using either polymerase chain reaction (PCR) and/or Southern blot is preferred, as sequencing may be inaccurate due to the large size of many repeat regions.
[#]Potentially detectable by genomic sequencing methods with appropriate read lengths.
[**]Size and number of region(s) targeted varies per individual test.
[††]Genome-wide testing method.
[‡‡]Minimum size of CNVs detected and density of genomic coverage varies per test.

a specialist and/or further testing to determine the likelihood of pathogenicity.

Clinical genome and/or exome sequencing are becoming more routinely available in the clinic but have not yet achieved widespread use (Coppola and Geschwind, 2012). Like CNV analysis, clinical exome sequencing appears to be appropriate in the principal evaluation of sporadic neurodevelopmental cases, such as severe intellectual disability (de Ligt et al., 2012), and in the evaluation of patients with early-onset and/or familial disorders (Coppola and Geschwind, 2012); however, use in sporadic adult-onset disease will likely be disease-specific (Fogel et al., 2014) and should await the publication of specific guidelines. Genome sequencing is the more comprehensive of the two methods and capable of detecting more types of mutation, as well as structural variation, but its use will hinge on the development of accurate and efficient bioinformatic techniques for translating the expected massive genomic variation per patient (millions of SNPs and hundreds of CNVs across the whole genome) into clinically meaningful results. How such a pipeline would operate has not yet been established, but we expect that the cost should be equivalent to that of an MRI study within 5 years. Incorporation of such testing into a clinical evaluation will also depend on other elements such as cost of testing and time of analysis, but these factors are not expected to vary much from clinical exome sequencing or other methods of genetic testing currently in use.

Genetic Counseling

Establishing a precise genetic diagnosis will definitively establish the means of inheritance of a disorder and is extremely useful in genetic counseling and family planning, particularly for disorders that show incomplete penetrance. However, unlike other tests typically ordered by physicians, a positive diagnosis carries implications not only for individual patients but for the entire family. Genetic counseling, therefore, should be provided in all cases where genetic testing is recommended, by an experienced neurologist, a geneticist, or a licensed genetic counselor. Follow-up counseling should also be provided to all patients with a positive test result and, in many cases, offered to other family members who may be at risk for disease or as carriers. Physicians must be aware of the various ethical implications involved in such testing (Ensenauer et al., 2005). One area of particular importance in this regard involves considerations of genetic testing in asymptomatic individuals, especially minors. This stems in part from concerns that have been raised regarding risks of depression and suicide in asymptomatic individuals diagnosed with fatal genetic disease, although this is not well established, and further study will be important for determining best practices. For minors, standard practice dictates that unless there is disease-modifying therapy available for them, they should not be tested if asymptomatic until they reach an age to consent to such testing and are properly counseled as to the implications. Counseling regarding prenatal testing and assisted reproduction are other topics of relevance to patients of reproductive age. Current reproductive medicine techniques such as in vitro fertilization and preimplantation genetic testing, by assuring that offspring will not harbor the mutation in question, can aid couples concerned about the risk for passing on inherited conditions. Other ethical considerations may also apply, depending on the disease and specific family/patient circumstances.

Prognosis and Treatment

A confirmed genetic diagnosis can contribute clinically useful data concerning patient prognosis, as it allows information

from published case studies to be utilized in the care of an individual patient. This can aid in the identification of specific clinical features to focus on for surveillance in the development of a particular genetic disorder, such as cognitive decline in a patient with isolated chorea found to have HD or cardiac testing in an autistic patient with chromosome 15q duplication. A genetic diagnosis may also alert the clinician to potential life-threatening comorbidities such as adrenal insufficiency in X-linked adrenoleukodystrophy or cardiomyopathy in Friedreich ataxia. Review of case studies in a particular disorder may help answer questions regarding life expectancy or future disability, such as years of disease prior to loss of ambulation in the various SCAs. Lastly, there are important positive psychological aspects to establishing a definitive diagnosis, particularly for patients who have undergone many fruitless clinical evaluations.

Although the majority of genetic diseases are not curable, therapies do exist for many of them. Defining the genetic etiology of a patient's disease allows for utilization of the published literature on symptomatic treatments and pharmacotherapy that may benefit a specific condition. Phenylketonuria is an excellent example of this, since dietary restriction of phenylalanine initiated soon after birth will prevent cognitive impairment and enable virtually normal development (Burgard et al., 1999). More importantly, new clinical trials are being developed frequently and can be offered to patients with an established diagnosis. Many disease-based patient registries exist to facilitate this.

The ultimate goal of translational neuroscience is to utilize advances in our understanding of disease at the molecular level to aid in the treatment of patients in the clinic. Recent new treatments, which take advantage of the molecular aspects of these disorders, show promise in the clinic and the laboratory. Such treatments include enzyme replacement therapy for metabolic disorders such as the severe fatal glycogen storage disorder Pompe disease, where use of recombinant acid α-glucosidase in 18 infants prior to 6 months of age enabled all to live to the age of 18 months, a 99% reduction in death, as well as reduced their risk of death or invasive ventilation by 92% compared to historical controls (Kishnani et al., 2007). Work in animal models has suggested potential new pharmacological treatments, such as a recent research study which demonstrated that the use of histone-deacetylase inhibitors can unsilence expanded frataxin alleles in a Friedreich ataxia mouse model, restoring wild-type gene expression levels and reversing cellular transcription changes associated with frataxin deficiency (Rai et al., 2008), leading to the use of such compounds in clinical trials (Gottesfeld et al., 2013). Targeted molecules have been designed to correct specific disease-causing biological defects, as shown by recent work where antisense oligonucleotides were used to block mutations that promote splicing defects in the ataxia-telangiectasia mutated (ATM) gene in cell lines from patients with ataxia-telangiectasia, leading to restoration of functional protein (Du et al., 2007), and such molecules are poised for clinical study (Du et al., 2011). Such newer techniques may markedly exceed the therapeutic benefit of current options, such as in Duchenne muscular dystrophy where patients can expect only moderate short-term benefit (up to 2 years) from the gold standard, glucocorticosteroid treatment (Manzur et al., 2008; Wood et al., 2010). Newer molecular strategies such as dystrophin splice-modulation, which promotes exon skipping via antisense oligonucleotides to bypass point mutations or frameshifts, may potentially resolve the primary defect and has shown promising results in early clinical trials (Kinali et al., 2009; Wood et al., 2010). Novel treatments aimed at genetic modification of disease are also in development, as was seen in a recent study where investigators used

Classes of Igs differ in their ability to fix complement. In humans, IgM, IgG1, and IgG3 antibodies are capable of activating the complement cascade. Different Ig classes also differ in their transport properties and ability to bind to phagocytes. Fc binding to Fc receptors (FcR) present on macrophages, dendritic cells, neutrophils, NK cells, and B cells initiates signaling within the cell only when the receptors are cross-linked by immune complexes containing more than one IgG molecule. Different Fc receptors (FcR) mediate different cellular responses, some being predominantly stimulatory, while others are inhibitory.

Genetics of the Immune System

Antigen Receptor Gene Rearrangements

During B- and T-cell development, multiple gene rearrangements occur to form their respective antigen receptors, the Ig and the TCR. Diversity of the antigen receptors is due to diversity in their principal components, the variable (V) gene segment and the joining (J) gene segments. One of the many V gene segments is juxtaposed by chromosomal rearrangements with one of the J segments (and when present, with the diversity [D] segment) to form the complete variable region gene. Recombinational inaccuracies at the joining sites of the V, D, and J regions further increase the diversity of the antigen receptors.

Constant (C) gene segments are present in all receptors. The V, D, J, and C gene segments along with the intervening noncoding gene segments between the J and C regions are initially transcribed into mature RNA. Through a process of RNA splicing, the noncoding gene segments are excised, and the V(D)JC messenger RNA (mRNA) is translated into protein. After binding antigen, B cells undergo somatic mutations that further increase the diversity and the affinity of antigen binding (affinity maturation). This phenomenon does not occur in T cells. During isotype switching in B cells, further rearrangements lead to recombination of the same variable region gene with new constant region genes (see Fig. 51.1).

Major Histocompatibility and Human Leukocyte Antigens

Major histocompatibility complex gene products or the human leukocyte antigens (HLAs) serve to distinguish self from nonself. In addition, they serve the important function of presenting antigen to the appropriate cells. The MHC class I gene product contains an MHC-encoded α chain, and a smaller non-MHC-encoded β_2-microglobulin chain. The MHC class II gene product consists of two polypeptide chains, α and β, which are noncovalently linked. Both class I and class II proteins are stabilized by intrachain disulfide bonds. Class I antigens are expressed on all nucleated cells, whereas class II antigens are constitutively expressed only on dendritic cells, macrophages, and B cells and are also expressed on a variety of activated cells including T cells, endothelial cells, and astrocytes.

In humans, class I molecules are HLA-A, B, and C, whereas the class II molecules are HLA-DP, DQ, and DR. Several alleles are recognized for each locus; thus, the HLA-A locus has at least 20 alleles, and HLA-B has at least 40. The number of alleles for the D region appears to be as extensive as that for HLA-A, HLA-B, and HLA-C. In view of the extensive polymorphisms present, the chances of two unrelated individuals sharing identical HLA antigens are extremely low. The reasons for the extensive diversity and evolutionary pressure that lead to this are not fully understood.

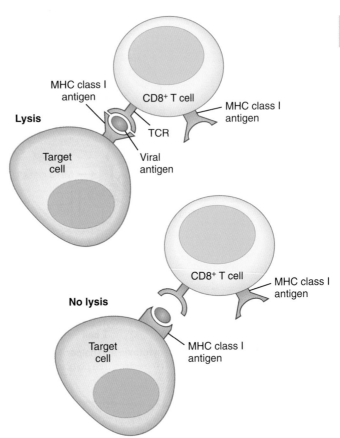

Fig. 51.2 The phenomenon of major histocompatibility complex (MHC) restriction. For antigen-specific cytolysis of virus-infected targets to occur, T cells should be sensitized to the virus and share the same class I human leukocyte antigen (HLA) with the target cell. In the lower part of the figure, the MHC class I antigen expressed on the CD8+ T cell is different from the MHC class 1 antigen expressed on the target cell; therefore, lysis does not occur. *TCR,* T-cell receptor.

Class I antigens regulate the specificity of cytotoxic CD8+ T cells, which are responsible for killing cells bearing viral antigens or foreign transplantation antigens (Fig. 51.2). The target cells share class I MHC genes with the cytotoxic cell. Thus, the cytotoxic cell that is specific for a particular virus is capable of recognizing the antigenic determinants of the virus only in association with a particular MHC class I gene product. The function of class II MHC gene products appears to be to regulate the specificity of T-helper cells, which in turn regulate DTH and antibody response to foreign antigens. Similarly, an immunized T-cell population will recognize a foreign antigen only if it is presented on the surface of an APC that shares the same class II MHC antigen specificity as the immunized T-cell population. Thus, the functional specificity of the T-cell population is restricted by the MHC molecules they recognize. CD8+ T cells (cytotoxic) and CD4+ T cells (helper) are referred to as *MHC class I* and *MHC class II restricted T cells*, respectively (Fig. 51.3).

The analysis of the three-dimensional structure of the class I and class II molecules has confirmed the notion that these molecules are carriers of immunogenic peptides that are processed by APCs and presented on the cell surface (Fig. 51.4). Both MHC class I and class II molecules share similarities in crystal structure that allow them to accept and retain immunogenic peptides in grooves, or pockets, and present them to T cells.

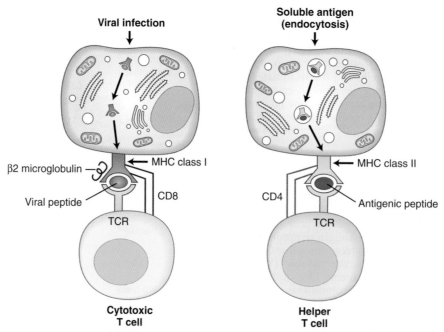

Fig. 51.3 Antigenic recognition of cytotoxic and helper T cells. The cytotoxic T cell recognizes viral peptides associated with human leukocyte antigen-A (HLA-A), HLA-B, or HLA-C molecules. The coreceptor for the helper T cell is the CD4 molecule. *MHC*, Major histocompatibility complex; *TCR*, T-cell receptor.

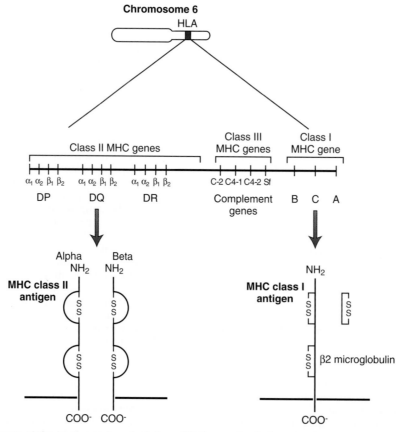

Fig. 51.4 Schematic diagram of the human leukocyte antigen (HLA) complex in humans, located on chromosome 6. The HLA class I gene (HLA-A, -B, and -C) codes for a single heavy-chain molecule. The β_2-microglobulin is coded by genes on a different chromosome. The HLA class II genes (DR, DP, and DQ) form the $\alpha\beta$ heterodimer. The HLA class III genes include those encoding for members of the complement family of proteins. *MHC*, Major histocompatibility complex.

ORGANIZATION OF THE IMMUNE RESPONSE
Initiation of the Immune Response

Antigen Presentation

One of the crucial initial steps in the immune response is the presentation of encountered antigens to the immune system. Antigens are carried from their site of arrival in the periphery by way of lymphatics or blood vessels to the lymph nodes and spleen. There, antigens are then taken up by cells of the monocyte–macrophage lineage and by B cells, processed intracellularly, and presented not as whole molecules but as highly immunogenic peptides.

Accessory Molecules for T-Cell Activation

The interaction of MHC–peptide complex with T cells, although necessary, is insufficient for T-cell activation. Other classes of molecules are involved in T-cell antigen recognition, activation, intracellular signaling, adhesion, and trafficking of T cells to their target organs. The distinction between the functions of these classes of molecules is not absolute, and many may be involved in interactions between other cells of the immune system.

CD3. Molecules whose primary role is signaling include the CD3 molecule. The CD3 molecule is part of the TCR complex. Although the TCR interacts with the MHC–peptide complex on APCs, the signals for the subsequent enactment of T-cell activation and proliferation are delivered by the CD3 antigen. The cytoplasmic tail of the CD3 proteins contains one copy of a sequence motif important for signaling functions, called the *immunoreceptor tyrosine-based activation motif* (ITAM). Phosphorylation of the ITAM initiates intracellular signaling events. In experimental situations, anti-CD3 antibodies can nonspecifically activate these intracellular signals, producing activated T cells in the absence of antigen.

CD4 and CD8. CD4 or CD8 antigens are expressed on mature T cells and serve an accessory role in signaling and antigen recognition. CD4 binds to a nonpolymorphic site on the MHC class II β chain, and CD8 binds to the α3 domain of the MHC class I molecule. Signals for cell division that are delivered to the nucleus are mediated by second messengers. When the receptor binds its ligand, it causes the activation of protein kinases. These kinases add phosphate groups to other proteins that ultimately signal the cell to divide. CD4, CD8, and CD3 on T cells and CD19 on B cells are examples of receptors that are linked to kinases. CD4 is the cell surface receptor for human immunodeficiency virus (HIV-1), and the fact that certain non-T cells such as microglia and macrophages can express low levels of CD4 may explain the propensity of the virus for the central nervous system (CNS).

Costimulatory Molecules. Costimulatory molecules serve as a "second signal" to facilitate T-cell activation. Costimulatory pathways that are critical for T-cell activation include the B7–CD28 and CD40–CD154 pathways. Members of the integrin families including vascular cell adhesion molecule 1 (VCAM-1), intercellular adhesion molecule (ICAM-1), and leukocyte function antigen 3 (LFA-3) can provide costimulatory signals, but they also play critical roles in T-cell adhesion, facilitate interaction with the APCs, mediate adhesion to nonhematopoietic cells such as endothelial cells, and guide cell traffic (Fig. 51.5).

The B7–CD28 interaction is one of the most extensively studied costimulatory systems. The B7 molecules are expressed on antigen-presenting cells, and their expression is induced in activated cells. There are two forms of B7, B7-1 (CD80) and

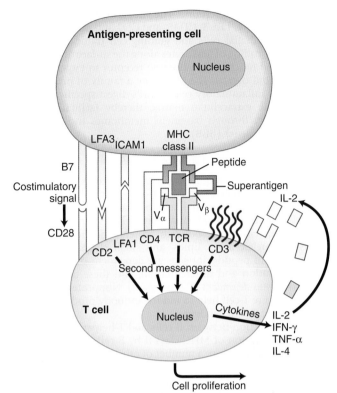

Fig. 51.5 Antigen-driven activation of helper T cells. Proliferation of T cells requires the delivery of a number of concordant signals. Along with stimulation through the T-cell receptor–CD3 complex, the presence of appropriate costimulatory signals via CD28 antigen, adhesion molecules, leukocyte function antigen 1 (LFA1) and CD2, and the coreceptor molecule CD4 are essential for T-cell activation and proliferation. The membrane events of antigen recognition lead to activation of second messengers. The second messengers signal the nucleus and cell to divide and secrete cytokines. Interleukin 2 (IL-2) acts as an autocrine growth stimulator, thereby amplifying the response. *ICAM,* Intercellular adhesion molecule; *IFN-γ,* interferon γ; *MHC,* major histocompatibility complex; *TCR,* T-cell receptor; *TNF,* tumor necrosis factor.

B7-2 (CD86), that share some homology but have different expression kinetics. The B7 molecules interact with their ligand, CD28, which is constitutively expressed on most T cells. Binding of the CD28 molecule mediates intracytoplasmic signals that increase expression of the growth factor, IL-2, and enhance expression of the anti-apoptotic molecule, Bcl-xL. An alternate ligand for B7 is CTLA-4, which is homologous to CD28 in structure, but in contrast to CD28, CTLA-4 functions to inhibit T-cell activation. Costimulatory molecules may deliver either a stimulatory (positive) or inhibitory (negative) signal for T-cell activation (Brunet et al., 1987). Examples of molecules delivering a positive costimulatory signal for T-cell activation include the B7-CD28, CD40-CD154 pathways. Examples of molecular pathways delivering a negative signal for T-cell activation include B7–CTLA4 and PD1–PD ligand (Khoury and Sayegh, 2004). The delicate balance between positive and negative regulatory signals can determine the outcome of a specific immune response.

Cell Migration. Molecules primarily involved in cell migration into tissues include chemokines, integrins, selectins, and matrix metalloproteinases (MMPs). Chemokines constitute a large family of chemoattractant peptides that regulate the vast spectrum of leukocyte migration events through interactions with chemokine receptors. The integrin family includes VCAM-1, ICAM-1, LFA-3, CD45, and CD2 and mediates adhesion to endothelial cells and guiding cell traffic. L-Selectins facilitate the rolling of leukocytes along the surface of endothelial cells and function as a homing receptor to target peripheral lymphoid organs. The MMPs are a family of proteinases secreted by inflammatory cells; MMPs digest specific components of the extracellular matrix, thereby facilitating lymphocyte entry through basement membranes including the blood–brain barrier (BBB).

Accessory Molecules for B-Cell Activation

Like T cells, B cells require accessory molecules that supplement signals mediated through cell-surface Igs. Signaling molecules whose functions are likely to be analogous to CD3 are linked to Ig. Unlike T cells that may only respond to peptide antigens, B cells can respond to proteins, peptides, polysaccharides, nucleic acids, lipids, and small chemicals. B cells responding to peptide antigens are dependent on T-cell help for proliferation and differentiation, and these antigens are termed *thymus-dependent* (T-dependent). Nonprotein antigens do not require T-cell help to induce antibody production and are therefore T-independent.

The interaction between B cells and T-helper (CD4+) cells requires expression of MHC class II by B cells and is antigen dependent. In addition, a number of other molecules mediate adhesion between T and B cells and induce signaling for B-cell activation. These include B7 expressed on B cells interacting with CD28 on T cells and CD40 on B cells interacting with CD154. Interaction of T-helper and B cells occurs in the peripheral lymphoid organs, initially in the primary follicles and later in the germinal centers of the follicle. Activation of B cells induces activation of transcription factors (c-Fos, JunB, NFκB, and c-Myc), which in turn promote proliferation and Ig secretion. Cytokines elicited from the T-helper cell induce isotype switching in B cells, producing stronger and long-lived memory responses, in contrast to weak IgM responses to T-independent antigens.

Further generation of high-affinity antibody-producing B cells and memory B cells occurs in the germinal center of lymphoid follicles through a process called *affinity maturation*. As the amount of available antigen lessens, B cells that do not express high-affinity receptors for antigen are eliminated by apoptosis. Some B cells lose the ability to produce Ig but survive for long periods and become memory B cells.

Regulation of the Immune Response

Cytokines

Cytokines play a major role in regulating the immune response. Cytokines are broadly divided into the following categories, which are not mutually exclusive: (1) growth factors such as IL-1, IL-2, IL-3, and IL-4 and colony-stimulating factors; (2) activation factors, such as interferons (α, β, and γ, which are also antiviral); (3) regulatory or cytotoxic factors, including IL-10, IL-12, transforming growth factor beta (TGF-β), lymphotoxins, and tumor necrosis factor alpha (TNF-α); and (4) chemokines that are chemotactic inflammatory factors, such as IL-8, MIP-1α, and MIP-1β.

Cytokines are necessary for T-cell activation and for the amplification and modulation of the immune response. A limited representation of the cytokines that participate in the immune response is shown in Table 51.1. Secretion of IL-1 by macrophages results in stimulation of T cells. This leads to synthesis of IL-2 and IL-2 receptors and finally to the clonal expansion of T cells. Only activated T cells express the IL-2 receptor (CD25); therefore, the cytokine-induced expansion

favors antigen-activated cells only. T-cell activation causes secretion of interferon gamma (IFN-γ), which induces expression of MHC class I and class II molecules on many cell types including APCs. This, in turn, increases the T-cell response to the antigen. Secretion of IL-2 also results in activation of NK cells that mediate lysis of tumor cell targets. In addition, IL-3 is released, resulting in stimulation of hematopoietic stem cells. The signal for differentiation of B cells to form antibody-secreting cells involves clonal expansion and differentiation of virgin memory B cells. IL-4 and B-cell differentiation factors secreted by T cells induce differentiation and expansion of committed B cells to become plasma cells.

IFN-α and IFN-β are both type I interferons. IFN-α is produced by macrophages, whereas IFN-β is produced by fibroblasts. Both inhibit viral replication by causing cells to synthesize enzymes that interfere with viral replication. They also can inhibit the proliferation of lymphocytes by unknown mechanisms.

Although the emphasis has been on factors that cause expansion and differentiation of lymphocytes, there are cytokines that can downregulate immune responses. Thus, IFN-α and IFN-β, in addition to possessing antiviral properties, can modulate antibody response by virtue of their antiproliferative properties. Similarly, TGF-β (a cytokine produced by T cells and macrophages) can also decrease cell proliferation. IL-10, a growth factor for B cells, inhibits the production of IFN-γ and thus may have anti-inflammatory effects.

CD4+ T-helper cells differentiate into T_H1 or T_H2 phenotypes, as well as a recently described T_H17 subset, which secrete characteristic cytokines and stimulate specific functions. T_H1 cells secrete IFN-γ, IL-2, and TNF-α. These cytokines exert proinflammatory functions and, in T_H1-mediated diseases such as MS, promote tissue injury. IL-2, TNF-α, and IFN-γ mediate activation of macrophages and induce DTH. T_H1 cell differentiation is driven by IL-12, a cytokine produced by monocytes and macrophages. In contrast, the T_H2 cytokines IL-4, IL-5, IL-6, IL-10, and IL-13 promote antibody production by B cells, enhance eosinophil functions, and generally suppress cell-mediated immunity (CMI). T_H3 cells secrete TGF-β, which inhibits proliferation of T cells and inhibits activation of macrophages. Cytokines of the T_H1 type may inhibit production of T_H2 cytokines and vice versa. More recently, a subset of T cells that predominantly produce IL-17 has been described (Yao et al., 1995). These cells are believed to represent a distinct subset from IFN-γ-producing T_H1 cells, evidenced by the dependence of T_HIL-17 cells on IL-6 and TGF-β for differentiation (Bettelli et al., 2006; Mangan et al., 2006; Veldhoen et al., 2006) and IL-23 for expansion (Aggarwal et al., 2003; Langrish et al., 2005), as opposed to T_H1 cells, which are dependent on IL-12 and IL-2, respectively, for differentiation and expansion. Both T_H1 and T_H2 cytokines have been shown to suppress the development of T_H17 cells (Harrington et al., 2005; Park et al., 2005). T_H17 cells facilitate the recruitment of neutrophils and participate in the response to Gram-negative organisms. These cells may also play a role in the initiation of autoimmune disease. Th17 cells produce a range of cytokines and may produce IL-10, IL-21, and IL-9 (classic Th17), or IL-23, IFN-g, and GM-CSF (alternative Th17) that are more pathogenic (Peters et al., 2011). Interestingly, recent data showed that modest increase in sodium chloride concentration induces SGK1 expression in T cells with increased IL-23R expression and TH17 cell generation in vitro (Wu et al., 2013), suggesting that increased dietary salt intake might represent an environmental risk factor for the development of autoimmune diseases through the induction of pathogenic TH17 cells (Kleinewietfeld et al., 2013).

Another effector T-cell subset, T_H9 cells, has recently been described (Dardalhon et al., 2008; Veldhoen et al., 2008).

TABLE 51.1 An Abridged List of Cytokines Involved in Interactions Between the Immune and Nervous Systems

Cytokine	Cell source	Cells principally affected	Major functions
IL-1	Most cells; macrophages, microglia	Most cells; T cells, microglia, astrocytes, macrophages	Costimulates T- and B-cell activation Induces IL-6, promotes IL-2 and IL-2R transcription Endogenous pyrogen, induces sleep
IL-2	T cells	T cells, NK cells, B cells	Growth stimulation
IL-3	T cells	Bone marrow precursors for all cell lineages	Growth stimulation
IL-4	T cells	B cells, T cells, macrophages	MHC II upregulation Isotype switching (IgG1, IgE)
IL-6	Macrophages, endothelial cells, fibroblasts, T cells	Hepatocytes, B cells, T cells	Inflammation, costimulates T-cell activation MHC I upregulation, increases vascular permeability Acute phase response (Schwartzman reaction)
IL-10	Macrophages, T cells	Macrophages, T cells	Inhibition of IFN-γ, TNF-α, IL-6 production Downregulation of MHC expression (macrophages)
IL-12	Macrophages, dendritic cells	T cells, NK cells	Costimulates B-cell growth, CD4$^+$ T$_H$1 cell differentiation, IFN-γ synthesis, cytolytic function
IL-17	T cells	Neutrophils, T cells, epithelial cells, fibroblasts	Host defense against gram-negative bacteria, induction of neutrophilic responses Induction of proinflammatory cytokines
IFN-γ	T cells, NK cells	Astrocytes, macrophages, endothelial cells, NK cells	MHC I and II expression Induces TNF-α production, isotype switching (IgG$_2$) Synergizes with TNF-α for many functions
TNF-α	Macrophages, microglia (T cells)	Most cells, including oligodendrocytes	Cytotoxic (e.g., for oligodendrocytes), lethal at high doses Upregulates MHC, promotes leukocyte extravasation Induces IL-1, IL-6, cachexia; endogenous pyrogen
Lymphotoxin (TNF-β)	T cells	Most cells (shares receptor with TNF-α)	Cytotoxic (at short range or through contact) Promotes extravasation
TGF-β	Most cells; macrophages, T cells, neurons	Most cells	Pleiotropic, antiproliferative, anticytokine Promotes vascularization, healing

IFN, Interferon; *Ig,* immunoglobulin; *IL,* interleukin; *MHC,* major histocompatibility complex; *NK,* natural killer; *TGF,* tumor growth factor; *TNF,* tumor necrosis factor.

Driven by the combined effects of TGF-β and IL-4, T$_H$9 cells produce large amounts of IL-9 and IL-10. It has been shown that IL-9 combined with TGF-β can contribute to T$_H$17 cell differentiation, and T$_H$17 cells themselves can produce IL-9 (Elyaman et al., 2009).

Traditionally, T$_H$ cell subsets have been distinguished by their patterns of cytokine production, but identification of distinguishing surface molecule markers has been a major advance in the field. Tim (T cell, immunoglobulin, and mucin-domain containing molecules) represents an important family of molecules that encode cell-surface receptors involved in the regulation of T$_H$1 and T$_H$2 cell–mediated immunity. Tim-3 is specifically expressed on T$_H$1 cells and negatively regulates T$_H$1 responses through interaction with the Tim-3 ligand galactin-9, also expressed on CD4$^+$ T cells (Monney et al., 2002; Sabatos et al., 2003; Zhu et al., 2005). Tim-2 is expressed on T$_H$2 cells (Chakravarti et al., 2005), and appears to negatively regulate T$_H$2 cell proliferation, although this has not been fully established. Tim-1 is expressed on T$_H$2 cells > T$_H$1 cells, and interacts with Tim-4 on APCs to induce T-cell proliferation (Meyers et al., 2005).

Chemokines

Chemokines are a recently discovered and extensively studied group of molecules that aid in leukocyte mobility and directed movement. Chemokines may be grouped into two subfamilies based on the configuration and binding of the two terminal cysteine residues. If the two residues participating in disulfide bonding are adjacent, they are termed the *C-C family* (e.g., MCP, MIP-1α, RANTES). Those separated by one amino acid, are C-X-C family members (e.g., IL-8), where X indicates a nonconserved amino acid. An important recent discovery is that two chemokine receptors, CCR-5 and CXCR-4, can act as coreceptors for strains of HIV. Chemokines are produced by a variety of immune and nonimmune cells. Monocytes, T cells, basophils, and eosinophils express chemokine receptors, and these receptor–ligand interactions are critical to the recruitment of leukocytes into specific tissues.

Termination of an Immune Response

The primary goal of the immune response is to protect the organism from infectious agents and generate memory T- and B-cell responses that provide accelerated and high-avidity secondary responses on re-encountering antigens. It is desirable to terminate these responses once an antigen has been cleared. In parallel, the immune system must constantly function to prevent autoimmune activation and maintain self-tolerance. A number of systems operate to prevent uncontrolled responses. Here we discuss termination of individual components of the immune response. Following is a discussion of the mechanisms that maintain self-tolerance, many of which are also involved in immune-response termination.

B-Cell Inhibition

In most instances, an antigen is cleared either by cells of the reticuloendothelial system or through the formation of antigen–antibody complexes. These complexes can themselves result in the inhibition of B-cell differentiation and proliferation through binding of the Fc receptor to the CD32 (FcγRIIB) receptor on the surface of the B cell.

Immunoglobulin

The variable regions of the Ig and the TCR molecule represent novel proteins that can act as antigens. Antigenic variable regions are called *idiotopes*, and responses against such antigens are called *anti-idiotypic*. Niels Jerne's network hypothesis postulates that anti-idiotypic responses serve to regulate the immune response; however, the extent to which this operates is unclear.

T Cells

Termination of the T-cell immune response is mediated by several mechanisms including anergy, deletion, and suppressor cell activity. Anergy or functional unresponsiveness occurs when there is insufficient T-cell activation. Repeated stimulation of T cells may lead to activation-induced cell death through apoptosis. Cytokine-mediated regulation can also serve to terminate the immune response, notably by secretion of T_H2 and T_H3 cytokines. Regulatory cells (discussed in the following section) generally inhibit the immune response through secretion of cytokines, through cytotoxic mechanisms, or by modulation of the function of APCs.

A combination of the above described mechanisms cooperate to maintain self-tolerance, particularly peripheral tolerance, and are discussed later.

SELF-TOLERANCE

An organism's ability to maintain a state of unresponsiveness to its own antigens is termed *self-tolerance*. Self-tolerance is maintained through three principal mechanisms: deletion, anergy, and suppression. Self-tolerance may be broadly categorized as either central or peripheral tolerance. Similar mechanisms may also be used to induce tolerance to a foreign antigen or terminate an immune response.

Central Tolerance

Bone marrow stem cells migrate to the thymus, thereby becoming thymocytes, or T cells. In this location, T-cell VDJ germline genetic elements recombine to create α and β chains, which in turn form the TCR. Thymocytes then undergo a process of education that involves positive and negative selection. Positive selection of thymocytes occurs in the thymus cortex when the cells are in the double-negative stage, CD4$^-$ CD8$^-$. The cortex contains dendritic and epithelial cells that present MHC antigens to the developing thymocytes. T cells with receptor having no affinity to MHC will fail to receive signals needed for maturation and will die in situ. Those with low affinity toward MHC survive and become single-positive thymocytes depending on their affinity toward MHC I (CD8$^+$) or MHC II (CD4$^+$). In the thymus medulla, thymocytes that display a high affinity toward self-antigen are deleted by apoptosis, a process called *negative selection*. Most T-cell education occurs in the thymus; however, extrathymic sites may exist.

Peripheral Tolerance

Self-reactive lymphocytes may escape central tolerance; therefore, peripheral mechanisms exist to maintain self-tolerance.

This is termed *peripheral tolerance*. Peripheral tolerance is maintained through clonal anergy or clonal deletion. It is not clear to what extent each of these mechanisms functions in maintaining human self-tolerance; however, extensive research has been done to elucidate the mechanisms through which anergy and deletion work. In addition, self-tolerance may be maintained despite the presence of antigen-responsive lymphocytes. It is postulated that this is due to the presence of suppressor T cells or other factors that may interfere with a successful lymphocyte response.

Anergy Due to Failure of T-Cell Activation

In normal circumstances, an APC presents antigen as a peptide + MHC complex (signal one). In the absence of signal one, the T cell dies because of neglect. If signal one is presented in the absence of costimulatory signals (signal two), the T cell becomes anergic. An example of this situation occurs when an antigen is presented by nonprofessional APCs that lack the appropriate costimulatory molecules (Fig. 51.6). However, when a T cell is activated, it upregulates the expression of an alternate costimulatory molecule, CTLA-4. CTLA-4 engagement by CD80 and CD86 on the surface of APCs sends a negative signal to the T cell, inhibiting cell growth and proliferation. Animals deficient for CTLA-4 expression on their T lymphocytes have an uncontrolled lymphoproliferative phenotype with autoreactivity (Waterhouse et al., 1995).

Apoptosis

Apoptosis is the process in which a cell undergoes programmed cell death. As opposed to necrosis, when interruption of the supply of nutrients triggers cell death, apoptosis may be triggered by various signals including withdrawal of growth factors, cytokines, exposure to corticosteroids, and repeated exposure to antigens. Mediators of apoptosis include the Bcl family of genes, which are mostly antiapoptotic, and the Fas family of genes, which are proapoptotic. Activated T cells also express Fas ligand (CD95L or FasL) and Fas (CD95); ligation of Fas and FasL induces apoptosis of the T cells.

Repeated stimulation with an antigen may also induce apoptosis via the Fas/FasL pathway, a process termed *activation-induced cell death* (AICD). Therefore, an autoreactive T lymphocyte may encounter large doses of self-antigen in the periphery and consequently may be deleted by AICD. Mice lacking Fas or FasL develop a lupus-like syndrome (Zhou et al., 1996), and mutations in the Fas gene were associated with an autoimmune disease with lymphoproliferation in humans (Drappa et al., 1996).

IL-2 is the prototypical growth factor, inducing clonal expansion of antigen-stimulated lymphocytes; paradoxically, disruption of the IL-2 gene leads to accumulation of activated lymphocytes and autoimmune syndromes (Sadlack et al., 1993). This is because IL-2 induces the transcription and surface expression of Fas ligand (FasL). Interactions of Fas with FasL lead to cell death (Fig. 51.7). Therefore, IL-2 plays a dual role in T-cell regulation, reflecting a possible role for cytokine concentration and timing of exposure. Other cytokines that mediate apoptosis and cell death are TNF-α and IFN-γ. Complete absence of either of these cytokines results in deficient T-cell apoptosis, inability to terminate the immune response, and uncontrolled autoimmune disease.

Regulatory T Cells

Regulatory T cells (T_{reg}) function to downregulate CD4 and CD8 T-cell responses. Regulatory T cells can be of the CD4$^+$ or CD8$^+$ subtypes. Regulatory T cells can be generated under similar conditions used to generate anergic cells, and it has

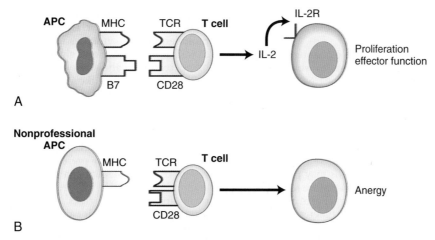

Fig. 51.6 A two-signal model of T-cell activation. Activation of the T-cell receptor (TCR) by an antigen major histocompatibility complex (MHC) provides signal 1, which is sufficient to induce the T cell to enter the cell cycle and begin blast transformation, which is characterized by an increase in cell size. Signal 2, the costimulatory signal, can be provided to the T cell through interaction of CD28 with molecules of the B7 family found on the surface of bone marrow-derived antigen-presenting cells (APCs). **A,** In this instance, TCR signals are complemented, enabling the T cell to proliferate, produce cytokines, and develop mature effector functions. **B,** In the absence of a second signal, T-cell activation is abortive, and the cell becomes anergic. Signal 2 might not be delivered if the APC does not express a costimulatory ligand on its surface, perhaps because a nonprofessional APC, such as an epithelial cell, is presenting antigen. *IL,* Interleukin.

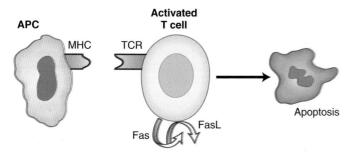

Fig. 51.7 Activation of the T cell leads to coexpression of the death receptor Fas (CD95) and its ligand (FasL), resulting in death of the cell and neighboring cells. *APC,* Antigen-presenting cell; *MHC,* major histocompatibility complex; *TCR,* T-cell receptor.

been postulated that they are the same entity (Lombardi et al., 1994). Several populations of regulatory or suppressor T cells have been described in humans. CD4$^+$ regulatory T cells, also called Tregs, were initially identified by expression of CD4 and high levels of CD25 (Baecher-Allan et al., 2001; Dieckmann et al., 2001; Levings et al., 2001; Stephens et al., 2001; Yagi et al., 2004). Most Tregs also express GITR, CD103, CTLA-4, lymphocyte activation gene 3 (LAG-3), and low levels of CD45RB, although no single marker is specific for Tregs. The expression of the transcription factor Foxp3 correlates with regulatory function of CD4$^+$ T cells in mice (Littman and Rudensky, 2010) and deletion of Foxp3 results in loss of suppressive phenotype. In humans, immune dysfunction/ polyendocrinopathy/enteropathy/X-linked (IPEX) syndrome is an autoimmune syndrome consisting of lymphoproliferation, thyroiditis, insulin-dependent diabetes mellitus, enteropathy, and other immune disorders. Most cases of IPEX syndrome are caused by mutations in *FOXP3*.

Other types of regulatory T cells include CD8$^+$CD28$^-$ T cells (Koide and Engleman, 1990), IL-10-producing T$_H$2 cells (Bacchetta et al., 1994), and TGF-β producing T$_H$3 cells (Kitani et al., 2000, Levings et al., 2001, Roncarolo and Levings, 2000). In humans, there is little evidence for antigen-specific

suppressor cell responses. Regulatory T cells suppress T-cell proliferation through a variety of mechanisms, including the production of immunosuppressive cytokines (T$_H$2 or TGF-β) or through T–T cell interactions, including the expression of inhibitory molecules such as CTLA-4. Regulatory cells play an important role in the control of the immune response in autoimmune disorders, and the function of regulatory T cells may be enhanced by immunomodulatory therapies.

IMMUNE SYSTEM AND CENTRAL NERVOUS SYSTEM

Immune Privilege in the Central Nervous System

Immunological reactions in the CNS differ from those in the rest of the body because of its unique architecture, cellular composition, and molecular expression. The CNS has been termed an *immunologically privileged site* because of the relative improved survival of allografts within this region. Indeed, the same factors that play a role in immunological tolerance in the CNS play a role in immune-mediated diseases involving the CNS, infections of the CNS, tumor survival, and therapies.

Important factors relevant to immunological responses in the CNS are: (1) absence of lymphatic drainage, limiting the immunological circulation; (2) the blood–brain barrier, which limits the passage of immune cells and factors; (3) the low level of expression of MHC factors, particularly MHC II in the resident cells of the CNS; (4) low levels of potent APCs, such as dendritic or Langerhans cells; and (5) the presence of immunosuppressive factors such as TGF-β (Wilbanks and Streilein, 1992) and CD200 (Webb and Barclay, 1984).

Because of the lack of a lymphatic system, antigens drain along perivascular spaces. Monocyte-derived CNS resident cells, termed *microglia*, play an important role in immune surveillance in these areas. The BBB is composed of tight junctions between endothelial cells and a layer of astrocytic foot processes that prevent entry of inflammatory cells and other factors into the CNS. Entry of inflammatory cells across the BBB is facilitated by upregulation of adhesion molecules ICAM-1 and VCAM-1 on endothelial cells. T cells must be activated before crossing the BBB. Entry is facilitated by expression of receptors for adhesion molecules, including α4-integrin.

The CNS houses cells that are capable of antigen presentation under certain conditions in vitro, but to what extent this occurs in vivo remains under debate. In the CNS, endogenous expression of MHC class I and class II on APCs such as microglia is low, and in oligodendrocytes and astrocytes, it is almost undetectable. Neurons express MHC class I only when damaged and in the presence of IFN-γ (Neumann et al., 1995). Expression of MHC antigens on both microglia and astrocytes is enhanced by the presence of cytokines, TNF-α, and IFN-γ. Under certain conditions, microglial cells may play a role as APCs in the nervous system (Perry, 1994). More recently, populations of perivascular dendritic cells capable of antigen presentation have been identified in rodents (Greter et al., 2005), with analogous populations demonstrated in humans; however, their role in human disease is unclear.

Immune privilege in the CNS is also influenced by the constitutive expression of a number of immunoregulatory factors, some of which are common to immune privilege in the anterior chamber of the eye. Anterior chamber immune privilege is due in part to expression of TGF-β in the aqueous of the eye. In the CNS, TGF-β is produced by astrocytes and microglia and may play a role in downregulating immune responses locally. Neurons are also capable of producing TGF-β, which in animal models has been shown to facilitate the differentiation of regulatory T cells (Liu et al., 2006). Increased expression of Fas ligand in the CNS compared with the peripheral nervous system (PNS) may increase apoptosis of T cells, thereby downregulating the immune response (Moalem et al., 1999). Some CNS tumors express large amounts of TGF-β, which may play a role in protecting them from immune surveillance. CNS tumors may also express Fas or Fas ligand, facilitating protection from immune surveillance. Some populations of neurons express a cell surface marker named *CD200*. CD200 is a nonsignaling molecule but serves to inhibit activation of cells including microglia and macrophages that express the CD200 receptor (CD200R) (Hoek et al., 2000; Wright et al., 2000). CD200 has been shown to downregulate inflammatory responses in models of MS (Liu et al., 2010) and uveitis (Banerjee and Dick, 2004; Broderick et al., 2002). Fractalkine (CXCL1) is a chemokine that is constitutively expressed on some populations of neurons. Interaction with its receptor, CX3CR1, present on microglia and NK cells, serves to downregulate microglial-mediated neurotoxicity both in vitro and in animal models of Parkinson disease and ALS (Cardona et al., 2006). In the animal model of MS, absence of fractalkine or its receptor resulted in a reduction of NK cells in the CNS and exacerbation of disease, supporting the view that NK cells play an inhibitory role in CNS inflammation (Huang et al., 2006).

Neuroglial Cells and the Immune Response

Neuroglial cells including microglia and astrocytes participate in immune responses within the CNS, and there is increasing evidence that these cells play a central role in initiating and propagating immune-mediated diseases of the CNS.

Microglia are derived from bone marrow cells during ontogeny (Hickey and Kimura, 1988) and reside within the CNS as three principal types of cells: perivascular microglia, parenchymal microglia, and Kolmer cells, which reside in the choroid plexus. Microglia have mitotic potential and can differentiate from bone marrow-derived cells to perivascular microglia and parenchymal microglia. Compared to macrophages, microglia are relatively radioresistant. Microglia may exist in either a resting (ramified) form or activated or phagocytic forms within the CNS. Activated microglia express higher levels of MHC class II and produce higher levels of proinflammatory cytokines including TNF-α, IL-6, and IL-1, as well as nitric oxide and glutamate. Microglia express chemokine receptors and various pattern recognition receptors (PRRs) including Toll-like receptors. PRRs recognize pathogen-associated molecular patterns (PAMPs) expressed by a variety of microbes, and interaction results in microglial activation. The primary functions of microglia are immune surveillance for foreign antigens and phagocytic scavengers of cellular debris. Microglia, particularly perivascular microglia, may also participate in antigen presentation within the CNS under certain conditions. Microglia play a role in regulating the programmed elimination of neural cells during brain development and, in some cases, enhance neuronal survival by producing neurotrophic and anti-inflammatory cytokines. Microglia may also play a role in neuroregeneration and repair. However, there is overwhelming evidence that microglia play a deleterious role in several neurodegenerative diseases: MS, ALS, Parkinson disease, and HIV-associated dementia. Their role in Alzheimer disease (AD) is less clear. Overactivation of microglia, possibly by microbes or other environmental factors through PRRs, may result in a chronic proinflammatory milieu in the CNS, leading to progressive neurodegeneration. Strategies to downregulate such responses are under investigation (Block et al., 2007).

Astrocytes play multiple roles in the CNS, including their role in the glia limitans at the BBB and physical support of neuronal and axonal structures, as well as provision of growth factors. Astrocytes secrete cytokines including TGF-β and are also influenced by IL-1 and interferons to divide and express proteins such as costimulatory molecules and Toll-like receptors on their surfaces. There is increasing evidence against the role of astrocytes in antigen presentation within the CNS. Astrocytes play a critical role in converting glutamate to glutamine, a less toxic substance, so impairment of astrocyte function may result in increased glutamate-mediated neurotoxicity. Astrocytes also produce chemokines including stromal-derived factor-1 (SDF-1), which plays a significant role in HIV-associated dementia.

Cells of the CNS not only respond to inflammatory stimuli but also are also capable of producing cytokines and other inflammatory factors, often directly under the influence of lymphocytes. These observations led to the conclusion that the brain is not an immunologically sequestered organ but that it interacts, produces immunologically active factors, and is closely involved with the systemic immune response.

PUTATIVE MECHANISMS OF HUMAN AUTOIMMUNE DISEASE

Why does autoimmune disease occur? It largely results as a culmination of interactions between genetic predisposition, environmental factors, and failure of self-tolerance maintenance mechanisms. Some diseases such as MS are termed *immune-mediated* because no definitive autoantigen has been demonstrated. Other diseases are clear cases of molecular mimicry such as Gd1b-mediated axonal neuropathy, in which the self-antigen attacked by the immune system is similar to that of an environmental antigen (in this case the Penner O:19 serotype of *Campylobacter jejuni*). Thus autoimmune diseases may be mediated by heterogeneous mechanisms, and in some cases more than one mechanism may be operating.

Autoimmune diseases may be classified as T- or B-cell-mediated. Some, such as myasthenia gravis (MG), are mediated through a combination of both. In many B-cell-mediated diseases, an autoantigen has been identified, to which the B cell produces autoantibodies. Examples are MG, in which sera

influenza virus hemagglutinin (Markovic-Plese et al., 2005), and EBV (Lang et al., 2002). PLP shares common sequences with *Haemophilus influenzae* (Olson et al., 2001). Semliki Forest virus (SFV) peptides mimic MOG (Mokhtarian et al., 1999).

The lesions in ADEM resemble those of MS. The CNS white matter contains perivascular inflammatory infiltrates as well as demyelination. The most likely mechanism by which this disease occurs is molecular mimicry. Experimental evidence has shown that T cells isolated from patients with ADEM are 10 times more likely to react with MBP than controls, likening this disease to EAE in animal models (Pohl-Koppe et al., 1998). We have recently found that 30% of patients with ADEM demonstrate serum antibodies to MOG, which were absent in MS patients (O'Connor et al., 2007). Because of the monophasic nature of ADEM, it appears that the immunological response occurs acutely, but in contrast to MS, further amplification of inflammation within the CNS is suppressed.

MRI demonstrates multifocal white matter lesions involving the cerebrum, brainstem, cerebellum, and spinal cord, which may or may not enhance with gadolinium. Lesions generally resolve over time. CSF is characterized by normal pressure, moderately elevated cell count ($5-100/\mu L$), moderately elevated protein ($40-100$ mg/dL), and normal glucose. The presence of red blood cells may indicate a diagnosis of hemorrhagic leukoencephalitis. Oligoclonal bands may very rarely be present, and these cases should be followed for the development of MS.

Acute episodes of ADEM should be treated with intravenous corticosteroids. The usual dose is 1 g/day of methylprednisolone for 5 days in adults. Refractory cases have been treated with plasmapheresis or cyclophosphamide. Cases that are suspicious for MS should be followed with MRI.

Neuromyelitis Optica

Neuromyelitis optica (NMO), or Devic disease, is a rare subtype of demyelinating disease characterized by clinical episodes of optic neuritis and transverse myelitis and demonstration of contiguous lesions in the spinal cord (Wingerchuk et al., 2006). It was originally considered to be a form of multiple sclerosis; however, increasing evidence demonstrates a distinct pathogenesis and response to treatment. The presence of serum antibodies targeting the aquaporin-4 water channel present on the surface of the glia limitans at the BBB has been shown to be a sensitive and specific marker of NMO (Lennon et al., 2004). Injection of aquaporin-4 antibodies into animal models of disease has demonstrated enhanced complement deposition around blood vessels, loss of aquaporin-4, and astrocyte and myelin damage (Kutzelnigg et al., 2005). This study, as well as others, indicates increasing recognition of the role of glial pathology in MS. There is no FDA-approved treatment for NMO. Intravenous steroids are typically used for acute relapses, and are administered at a dose of 20–30mg/kg (up to 1g/day) for a 3- to 5-day period. Plasmapheresis may be used as first- or second-line treatment for acute attacks, and five exchanges are administered every other day or as tolerated. NMO titers may be reduced following plasmapheresis, suggesting that the antibody is linked to relapses. IVIG (up to 2g/kg divided into 2–5 doses) has been used as third-line therapy by some investigators. Prophylactic therapies used for NMO include Rituximab (anti-CD20 antibody), azathioprine, mycophenolate mofetil, and mitoxantrone. Some MS therapies including beta-interferon, fingolimod and natalizumab may worsen disease in NMO patients, reinforcing that immune mechanisms may be distinct in these two diseases.

Immune-Mediated Neuropathies

The immune-mediated neuropathies are a large and heterogeneous group of diseases. We shall focus on acute inflammatory demyelinating polyneuropathy (AIDP) and chronic inflammatory demyelinating polyneuropathy (CIDP), which may be defined by the time to peak disability; in the former, 4 weeks, and in the latter, 2 months. Although AIDP and CIDP share many characteristics, the question of whether one is a continuum of the other is still under debate. AIDP or Guillain–Barré syndrome (GBS) usually presents with symmetrical ascending weakness and may be associated with autonomic dysfunction and respiratory depression. Sensory systems may be involved and may present with paresthesias or numbness. Demyelination and axonal damage may be involved to varying degrees. If the patient's symptoms continue to progress beyond 4 weeks, the illness is termed *CIDP*.

AIDP is the most common acute paralytic disease in the Western world, with a mean annual incidence of 1.8 per 100,000 persons. There is an increasing incidence with age. Mortality was generally due to respiratory failure and has now been significantly reduced with the introduction of positive-pressure ventilation. Epidemics have been found, most notably in northern China, where a high incidence has been associated with *C. jejuni* infections (McKhann et al., 1993).

AIDP or GBS is characterized pathologically by an endoneurial lymphocytic, monocytic, and macrophage infiltrate. Several autoantibodies to myelin glycolipids, including GM1, GD1a, and GD1b, have been identified. Antibody-mediated demyelination due to complement fixation has been identified in pathology specimens. In some cases, axonal damage is present and is believed to be a result of bystander damage. Activation of calcium-dependent processes within the nerve, including calpain activation, has been shown in animal models to augment axonal degeneration (O'Hanlon et al., 2003). GBS is primarily an antibody-mediated disease, as evidenced by the fact that many patients improve after treatment with plasmapheresis, and that serum from GBS patients causes demyelination after transfer into experimental animals and peripheral nerve cultures. The Miller–Fisher variant of GBS is characterized by ophthalmoplegia, ataxia, and areflexia and is associated with the presence of GQ1b antibodies in the serum.

The occurrence of AIDP has been linked to many infectious diseases, including *C. jejuni*, herpesvirus, *Mycoplasma pneumonia*, and many other bacterial and viral infections, as well as vaccinations. The incidence of infection has been reported to be 90% in the 30 days before occurrence of GBS. *Campylobacter jejuni* is one of the most commonly identifiable agents, and molecular mimicry and host susceptibility play a role in disease pathogenesis. Autoantibodies not present in controls have been identified in the sera of GBS patients associated with *C. jejuni*, including autoantibodies to the gangliosides GM1, GD1a, GD1b, and GQ1b (Sheikh et al., 1998).

In contrast to AIDP, in CIDP no specific autoantibodies have yet been discovered. The histopathological picture is similar to AIDP; however, most studies identify fewer inflammatory infiltrates. Nerve biopsy reveals mixed demyelination and axonal changes. Onion bulbs may be present, indicating attempts at remyelination. There is little laboratory evidence that this disease is antibody mediated, but paradoxically, patients do improve with plasmapheresis. There is indirect evidence that CIDP is T-cell mediated; however, this area is still under investigation.

Treatment of AIDP involves supportive care and cardiac and respiratory monitoring. Plasmapheresis or intravenous immunoglobulin (IVIG) have been used for acute treatment of AIDP and have been shown to be equally effective in shortening recovery time. Plasmapheresis is a short-term immunotherapy that nonspecifically removes antibodies from the circulation. IVIG is an immunomodulating agent commonly used in the treatment of allergic and autoimmune diseases. It works in part through the presence of Fc fragments that interact with the inhibitory Fc receptor, FcγRIIB, which is also induced on macrophages following IVIG administration (Samuelsson et al., 2001). Additionally, IVIG may displace low-affinity autoantibodies from the nerve. High-dose steroids have not been found to be effective in AIDP.

In contrast to AIDP, CIDP responds well to high-dose oral corticosteroids. Both plasmapheresis and IVIG are also used with success. Immunosuppressants such as cyclosporine A, cyclophosphamide, azathioprine, and rituximab have had positive outcomes in refractory cases but require further testing in controlled studies. Future therapies for AIDP or CIDP may target complement activation or inhibition of axonal calpain activation.

Autoimmune Myasthenia Gravis

Myasthenia gravis is a disorder of the neuromuscular junction. It is an autoimmune disorder, and 80% to 90% of cases have detectable autoantibodies to the α subunit of the acetylcholine receptor (AChR). MG is characterized by fluctuating weakness and fatigability, primarily in muscles innervated by the cranial nerves, but may occur in skeletal and respiratory muscles. MG has a biphasic age distribution. Most cases occur in women between the ages of 20 and 40 years, the remainder in older patients, with an equal sex distribution. Thymomas occur in 10% to 15% of cases; most are in the older age group. Some 75% of patients will have a thymic abnormality, 85% being thymic hyperplasia. MG is often associated with other autoimmune diseases, thyroid disorders, rheumatoid arthritis (RA), pernicious anemia, and SLE. A similar syndrome, Lambert–Eaton, is associated with antibodies against the presynaptic voltage-gated calcium channel, generally in the setting of small cell cancer of the lung.

Autoimmune MG is caused by the presence of α_1 nicotinic acetylcholine receptor (nAChR) antibodies and is a B-cell-mediated disease. Eighty percent to 90% of patients have detectable autoantibodies. These are polyclonal and may be of any IgG subtype. Transfer of serum from myasthenic patients to experimental animals results in neuromuscular blockade. The mechanism by which antibody mediates neurological symptoms is controversial. Possible mechanisms include neuromuscular blockade or damage to the AChR from complement-mediated damage after attachment of the IgG antibody. There is, however, poor correlation between serum antibody titers and disease course and severity.

Although the B cell is the effector cell producing antibodies, experimental evidence has shown that autoreactive T cells are necessary for the disease to occur (Yi and Lefvert, 1994). Removal of the thymus results in improvement of disease in 80% to 90% of myasthenic patients. The role of thymic abnormalities remains unclear, and patients with thymomas have antibodies to additional skeletal muscle proteins such as the ryanodine receptor and titin, as well as the neuromuscular junctional protein, MuSK. Patients may also display symptoms of neuromyotonia. Antibodies directed towards α_3-nAChR are associated with autoimmune autonomic neuropathy.

A large body of research is targeted at understanding the reasons for the failure of T-cell and subsequent failure of B-cell tolerance in MG. Both normal and myasthenic thymus glands contain myoid cells and epithelial cells that express the AChR. T cells expressing the $V_\beta 5.1^+$ TCRs are overrepresented, both in the core of germinal centers and in perifollicular areas of hyperplastic thymuses, suggesting a role in the

autoimmune response (Truffault et al., 1997). Failure of central or thymic tolerance may play an important role in disease pathogenesis.

Genetic factors play a role in the pathogenesis of autoimmune MG, but monozygotic twins demonstrate less than 50% concordance rate. There is a moderate association of MG with the HLA antigens B8 and DRw3 in young women. The stronger association with HLA-DQw2 remains controversial. There is an unusually high incidence of other autoimmune diseases such as SLE, RA, and thyroid diseases in first-degree relatives of myasthenic patients, suggesting the presence of shared autoimmune genes.

Therapies in MG are targeted toward alleviating symptoms with acetylcholinesterase inhibitors and using strategies to reduce the damage being done by the immune system. Thymectomy is recommended for patients 15 to 65 years old, with 80% to 90% remission rate (Durelli et al., 1991). The thymus plays an important role in T-cell education in the developing human; therefore, prepubertal thymectomy is discouraged. A variety of anticholinesterase inhibitors provide temporary symptomatic relief in most patients. Pyridostigmine bromide (Mestinon) and neostigmine bromide (Prostigmin) are the most commonly used agents and must be taken daily.

MG is an antibody-mediated disease and therefore responds to therapies that nonspecifically target antibodies. Both plasmapheresis and treatment with IVIG are used for acute MG exacerbations or in preparation for surgery (Gajdos et al., 1997). Because the autoantigen is known in MG, investigational therapies may target specific molecules such as the B-cell surface Ig or the TCR and deliver immunotoxins.

Corticosteroids are used at various stages of treatment and have multiple effects on the immune system, including reducing AChR antibody levels. Immunosuppressives such as cyclosporine, azathioprine, and mycophenolate are used to augment treatment when symptoms are not adequately controlled by the previously mentioned methods, but the decision to use such agents must balance the need and the side effects. Rituximab has also been used for severe generalized MG. Emerging therapy options may include belimumab, eculizumab and granulocyte–macrophage colony-stimulating factor. However, one pilot study of etanercept indicated lack of benefit with this agent.

Inflammatory Muscle Diseases

Polymyositis (PM), dermatomyositis (DM), and inclusion body myositis (IBM) are all inflammatory and presumably immune-mediated diseases of the muscle and the surrounding connective tissue. Each has its own unique clinical and immunohistological features. Both PM and DM are more common in females, whereas IBM is more common in males. DM in adults is associated with an increased risk of cancer, and therefore a full cancer screening should be part of patient management.

PM is thought to result from a multitude of causes, including systemic autoimmune connective-tissue disorders and viral and bacterial infections. PM is characterized histopathologically by an endomysial inflammatory infiltrate containing predominantly CD8+ T cells. There is relative sparing of blood vessels. In one subtype of PM, T cells with γδ receptors have been identified surrounding non-necrotic muscle fibers (Hohlfeld et al., 1991).

In contrast, DM is characterized by perifascicular atrophy. There is hypoperfusion and subsequent degeneration of the muscle fibers in the periphery of the fascicle, secondary to microvascular damage. Damage to capillaries, resulting in muscle fiber ischemia, is mediated by complement.

Immunofluorescence studies have revealed immune-complex deposition within the endothelium, indicating that this is an antibody-mediated disease; therefore, the disease differs from PM (Kissel et al., 1986).

As with PM, IBM is mediated by CD8$^+$ T cells. However, in contrast to PM, the muscle biopsy in IBM may also demonstrate the presence of characteristic autophagic "rimmed" vacuoles. Amyloid deposits may be demonstrated in the muscle, similar to those seen in AD, suggesting similarities in the pathogenesis of these two disease (Askanas et al., 1992).

Various autoantibodies directed against nuclear and cytoplasmic cell components are found in up to 30% of inflammatory myopathies. Most are nonspecific for connective-tissue disease. Viruses including coxsackie B are implicated in the pathogenesis of disease, and both PM and DM patients may have anti-Jo-1 antibodies to the viral enzyme, histidyl-tRNA synthetase (Mathews and Bernstein, 1983). More recently, the presence of B cells, and in particular antibody-secreting plasma cells with V-D-J rearrangements, has been demonstrated in muscle biopsies from both IBM and PM and to a lesser extent in DM (Greenberg et al., 2005).

The mainstay of treatment of PM and DM is corticosteroids. Dosages may vary from 60 to 100 mg/day of prednisone, and duration is determined by clinical outcome. Alternative treatment options for the inflammatory myositis diseases include IVIG, methotrexate, azathioprine, cyclophosphamide, cyclosporine, and in extreme cases, total lymphoid or whole-body irradiation (Mastaglia et al., 1998). A recent study of rituximab in polymyositis in over 200 adults and children with PM/DM, suggested a benefit (Oddis et al., 2013). Mortality rates vary between 15% and 35% and are generally due to cardiac or respiratory failure. Because there is a higher incidence of malignancy with PM and DM, screening for breast, lung, hematological, ovary, stomach, and colon carcinoma should be performed on patients with these diagnoses. IBM may be more resistant to corticosteroid therapy and is often diagnosed after an assumed PM fails to respond to treatment.

Alzheimer Disease and Amyotrophic Lateral Sclerosis

It may seem strange to include AD and ALS in a chapter on neuroimmunology. These diseases have traditionally been considered neurodegenerative, but recent studies and therapies have suggested a role for the immune system in disease pathogenesis and protection.

β-Amyloid plaques and neurofibrillary tangles consisting of hyperphosphorylated tau protein are the hallmarks of AD. Clearance of amyloid plaques consisting of amyloid-β-fibrils is considered a primary goal of therapy. Amyloid plaques are often surrounded by activated microglia and reactive astrocytes, and are associated with complement activation, leading to the hypothesis that the immune response participates in the clearance of amyloid deposits. Further studies in animal models of AD demonstrated that immunization with amyloid-β peptide resulted in the induction of amyloid-β-specific antibodies, which enhanced the clearance of amyloid plaques (Janus et al., 2000; Morgan et al., 2000). Passive transfer of amyloid-β-specific antibodies yielded similar results. Amyloid plaque clearance is believed to occur through either microglial- and complement-mediated clearance or through direct antibody–amyloid interactions. These studies led to a clinical trial investigating an amyloid-β vaccine administered in conjunction with an adjuvant, which enhanced T$_H$1 responses. Although cognitive testing results were favorable, 6% of patients developed meningoencephalitis, which is generally believed to be a result of T-cell responses to amyloid-β

(Gilman et al., 2005; Orgogozo et al., 2003). Thus, induction of an antibody and microglial-mediated clearance of amyloid in the absence of a prominent T$_H$1 response is the current goal of therapy. An intriguing study has recently demonstrated that nasal administration of glatiramer acetate (Copaxone), which induces a predominantly T$_H$2 cellular response, to a murine model of AD resulted in the clearance of amyloid-β plaques in association with activated microglia, but in the absence of antibody formation (Frenkel et al., 2005). Recently, phase III trials of two monoclonal antibodies against Aβ, bapineuzumab and solanezumab, failed to significantly improve clinical outcomes in patients with mild to moderate AD (Doody et al., 2014; Salloway et al., 2014). Future immunotherapeutic strategies for AD include modified vaccines and strategies to induce activation of microglial cells in the absence of deleterious side effects.

In ALS, a new avenue of investigation has emerged: exploring the role of microglia in disease pathogenesis and, in particular, on disease progression. Pathological analysis and neuroimaging using positron electron tomography (PET) studies have demonstrated activated microglia in areas of severe motor neuron loss. Studies in the animal model of ALS have demonstrated that the presence of the SOD1 mutation in microglia enhanced disease progression (Boillee et al., 2006). Use of minocycline, which acts in part by inhibiting microglial activation, has shown some initial promise in the treatment of ALS. Cyclooxygenase-2 (COX-2) inhibitors have reduced disease severity in animal models of ALS but have been ineffective in humans. Lymphocytes, including T cells, do not appear to play a significant role in this disease, and this is reinforced by the failure of studies using T-cell-targeted therapies including total lymphoid irradiation (TLI) or cyclophosphamide. Thus, possible future therapies for ALS include strategies to downregulate microglial activation.

IMMUNE RESPONSE TO INFECTIOUS DISEASES

The immune response within the CNS must carefully balance the need to eliminate the pathogen and the risk of inducing bystander damage to the delicate and vital nervous tissues. This is believed to be the reason the CNS immune response deviates from that in the rest of the body, and it remains an immune-privileged site. The result is that many pathogens are not completely eliminated and may persist to cause further symptoms. Examples of this are CNS syphilis, Lyme neuroborreliosis, herpes zoster, HIV, and *Mycobacterium tuberculosis*. Lyme *Borrelia* incites IFN-γ production, with correspondingly low levels of IL-4 in the CSF, thus predisposing the CNS tissue to bystander damage.

The portal of entry and site of replication of the pathogen plays a critical role in elimination of the infection. In the case of viral meningitis, the portal of entry is the mucosal membrane, usually the nasopharynx. This incites a strong local immune response to the proliferating organism, and by the time the virus disseminates to the leptomeninges, a sufficient immune response has been mounted in the periphery to eliminate the pathogen. However, in the case of viral encephalitis, the CNS invasion is so sudden that the peripheral immune system has insufficient time to react, and the weak CNS immune response is often inadequate, resulting in a poor outcome.

HIV-associated dementia (HAD) is a clinical disorder characterized by cognitive, behavioral, and motor dysfunction in AIDS patients. HIV infection of the brain is characterized by multinucleated giant cells, astrogliosis, microglial nodules, and neuronal loss in the cortex and basal ganglia. The HIV protein gp120 can bind directly to CXCR4 on neurons, resulting in neuronal signaling and apoptosis. Neurodegeneration is also thought to occur through production of neurotoxic factors by HIV-infected microglia and astrocytes. HIV infection results in production of proinflammatory cytokines (IL-6, IL-1, and TNF-α), nitric oxide, and MMPs by microglia, as well as increased glutamate by dysfunctional astrocytes. Astrocyte production of SDF-1 (CXCR4 ligand), which is subsequently cleaved by MMP-2 to produce a truncated protein, c-SDF, is neurotoxic in vitro. In summary, glial-mediated neurotoxicity plays a significant role in the pathogenesis of HAD and is an active area of investigation.

TUMOR IMMUNOLOGY

The immunological response to tumors has elicited much interest in the past 10 years. This field provides opportunities for understanding the cause and immunological features of tumors and venues for treatment.

The body uses a mechanism called *tumor immunosurveillance* to prevent the formation of tumors or inhibit further growth. The main effector cells are CTLs, NK cells, and TNF-α-producing macrophages. Tumor-reactive antibodies have also been identified in patients but are thought to play a lesser role. It has been recognized that tumors express tumor-specific antigens that may be recognized by the previously mentioned cells. However, tumor cells may escape the body's natural surveillance mechanisms, resulting in cancer. Tumor cells escape surveillance mechanisms by masking or modulating antigens on their surface, downregulating class I and II molecules (thereby inhibiting antigen presentation), and expressing immunosuppressant factors.

Tumors in the CNS have similar abilities to evade the immune system, and it has been shown that some gliomas produce high levels of TGF-β, an immunosuppressant. Downregulation of class II MHC may also occur, but this remains controversial. It has recently been established that gliomas may express high levels of FasL, allowing for local apoptosis of Fas-bearing cells including lymphocytes. Increased expression of the inhibitory costimulatory molecule, B7H1, on gliomas has been shown to play a role in downregulating T-cell (Wintterle et al., 2003). Glioma patients have been shown to express increased frequencies of CD4+CD25+Foxp3+ regulatory T cells. Treatment with daclizumab (anti-CD25 antibody) in a murine model of glioma reduced regulatory T-cell function and enhanced host tumor immunity, so daclizumab therapy in CNS tumors merits additional investigation.

Additional therapies are being designed to exploit the body's natural tumor immunosurveillance mechanisms. One avenue of research is vaccination with killed tumor cells or tumor antigens. Another technique employs genetic engineering to transfect tumors with plasmids bearing genes for costimulatory molecules to enhance the tumor APC ability. Injection of cytokines such as IL-2 and TNF-α, which enhance lymphocyte and NK function, has been attempted, with variable results. Dendritic cells pulsed with tumor antigens to induce NK cell-mediated tumor killing is a promising new therapy for CNS gliomas and is under investigation.

Overall, strategies to enhance host tumor immunosurveillance and reduce inhibitory responses mediated by CNS tumors are promising new avenues of treatment.

Paraneoplastic Syndromes

Neurological paraneoplastic disorders are defined as neurological syndromes arising in association with a distant cancer. These are mediated by antibodies produced by the immune system in reaction to a tumor antigen, which cross-react with neural tissue. It is likely that aberrant, primitive, or hamartomatous

antigens are expressed by the tumor cells. Enhanced cellular infiltrates are found in tumors associated with paraneoplastic syndrome compared to those not associated with a paraneoplastic syndrome. Therefore, one can postulate that the immune system is more active in these situations. Cancers associated with paraneoplastic syndromes are generally associated with a better outcome. Several autoantibodies associated with paraneoplastic syndromes have been identified. The anti-Hu antibody arises in association with small-cell cancer of the lung and cross-reacts with neurons; it is linked to a syndrome of encephalomyelitis and/or sensory neuropathy. Similarly, anti-Yo antibody produces cerebellar degeneration due to cross-reactivity with Purkinje cell cytoplasm and is associated with breast and ovarian cancer. Opsoclonus-myoclonus syndrome is associated with anti-Ri antibody and is found in cases of cancer of the ovary and breast. Cases of paraneoplastic and immune-mediated brainstem and limbic encephalitis have recently been reported to be caused by antibodies targeting LGI1, a neuronal-secreted protein that interacts with presynaptic ADAM23 and postsynaptic ADAM22 (Lai et al., 2010). NMDA receptor encephalitis typically presents with seizures and psychiatric symptoms, but a recent case report describes a patient presenting with optic neuritis and transverse myelitis mimicking neuromyelitis optica (Kruer et al., 2010). Antibodies directed against voltage-gated potassium channels (VGKC) are also associated with acquired neuromyotonia, or Isaac syndrome, and Morvan syndrome, characterized by neuromyotonia and insomnia. Lambert–Eaton myasthenic syndrome is caused by antibodies directed against the P/Q type of voltage-gated calcium channels and is generally found in the setting of small-cell cancer of the lung. The same antibodies have also been associated with cases of lung cancer-associated cerebellar ataxia. Stiff person syndrome is associated with antibodies to glutamic acid decarboxylase (GAD), and both autoimmune and paraneoplastic forms, principally associated with breast cancer, have been described.

ANTIBODY-ASSOCIATED NEUROLOGICAL SYNDROMES

In the past 10 years, more sophisticated techniques have led to greater insights into the study of antibodies in CNS diseases. Antiphospholipid (APL) syndrome, or Hughes syndrome, results in CNS symptoms that include chorea, strokes, bleeding, migraine headaches, and epilepsy (Asherson, 2006). These result in part from the underlying systemic problems of coagulopathy and thrombocytopenia, but more direct effects of autoantibodies directed against neuronal antigens have been implicated both in APL syndrome and in CNS lupus. One study found that antibodies directed against the NR2A and NR2B subunits of the NMDA receptor were found in a subset of patients with CNS lupus and could facilitate apoptotic death of neurons (DeGiorgio et al., 2001).

Recently, antibodies against the *N*-methyl-D-aspartate subtype of ionotropic glutamate receptors [*N*-methyl-D-aspartate receptor (NMDAR) antibodies] have been reported, predominantly in young women who developed a subacute-onset encephalopathy, commonly associated with a prominent movement disorder and frequently an underlying ovarian teratoma (Dalmau et al., 2007), although two recent reports suggest a much higher incidence of nonparaneoplastic cases in children (Dale et al., 2009; Florance et al., 2009). Additional reports have confirmed these findings, and the mainstay of treatment in patients with NMDAR antibody-associated syndromes includes removal of underlying tumors, and immunotherapy with either steroids, IVIG, or plasmapheresis acutely. In patients with refractory disease, chronic immunosuppression with rituximab or mycophenolate mofetil is used. Other neuronal antibodies including those to AMPA receptor, GABAB receptor, LGII, and Caspr2 have been recently associated with neuropsychiatric syndromes, increasing the potential role for immunotherapy in these antibody-associated disorders.

Sydenham chorea is associated with *Streptococcus pyogenes* (β-hemolytic streptococcal) infections, and there is considerable evidence for a causative role of antibodies that cross-react with streptococcal antigens and neurons in the basal ganglia. This association has led to the postulation that molecular mimicry mechanisms related to streptococcal infections may result in other movement disorders, including Tourette syndrome and the clinical entity of pediatric autoimmune neuropsychiatric disorders associated with streptococcal infection (PANDAS), which encompasses tics and obsessive-compulsive disorder in children. Evidence for an immune-mediated mechanism is inconclusive (Harris and Singer, 2006).

Antibodies directed against glutamate receptor 3 (GluR3) are associated with Rasmussen encephalitis, a form of severe intractable epilepsy localized to one hemisphere and partially responsive to immunotherapy. The presence of antibodies directed against voltage-gated potassium channels in a small group of patients with intractable epilepsy has been demonstrated (Majoie et al., 2006), and more recently, other antibodies including GAD65 and CRMP-5 as well as VGKC have been described in patients with chronic epilepsy, with some response to immunotherapy (Quek et al., 2012).

IMMUNOLOGY OF CENTRAL NERVOUS SYSTEM TRANSPLANT

Recently, there has been much research in the field of CNS transplantation, with the use of fetal dopaminergic striatal cells, various types of genetically engineered cells, and the potential of stem cell transplantation. A major factor in the survival of these grafts is their lack of immunogenicity in the relatively immune-privileged site of the CNS. Therefore, transplant grafts in the CNS tend to have longer survival times than peripheral grafts; however, this is not absolute, and rejection can undoubtedly occur.

Factors that influence CNS graft survival include type of graft (xenogenic, allogeneic, genetically modified tissue, or stem cell populations); location of the graft, with the periventricular areas being the most susceptible to rejection; presence of antigen-presenting cells within the graft, which can be eliminated in purified grafts; and host immunosuppression.

Immunosuppressive strategies currently under investigation include the immunophilins, daclizumab, and cyclosporine. Successful immunosuppression must be balanced against the risk of graft toxicity.

Neural stem cells (NSCs) are increasingly being investigated in neurodegenerative diseases (Gincberg et al., 2012). In addition to their effects on repair, studies in the animal model of MS found that these cells suppress disease (Einstein et al., 2003, 2007; Pluchino et al., 2003, 2005; Yang et al., 2009) through immunomodulatory mechanisms. Some studies suggested that NSCs can directly inhibit T-cell proliferation in response to concanavalin A (ConA) or to MOG peptide (Einstein et al., 2003; Pluchino et al., 2005) by inducing T-cell apoptosis (Pluchino et al., 2005; Yang et al., 2009) or through nitric oxide- and PGE2-mediated T-cell suppression (Wang et al., 2009). Neural stem cells can express costimulatory molecules, CD80 and CD86, particularly after exposure to the proinflammatory cytokines IFN-γ and TNF-α (Imitola et al., 2004). Thus, NSCs are not conventional immune cells, but under certain conditions, they can interact with immune cells.

Mesenchymal stem cells (MSCs) are also being investigated for treatment of neurologic diseases including MS and ALS. Their therapeutic benefit is thought to be by induction of immune tolerance and the release of molecules fostering tissue repair. There are phase II trials of MSCs in MS ongoing.

SUMMARY

The field of immunology has progressed significantly in the past 30 years. This knowledge is currently being applied to immune-mediated diseases in neurology. In this rich environment, we can expect many advances in the field of neuroimmunology, including new therapies and better strategies for the treatment of neurological diseases.

REFERENCES

The complete reference list is available online at https://expertconsult .inkling.com/.

52 Neuroendocrinology

Paul E. Cooper, Stan H.M. Van Uum

CHAPTER OUTLINE

NEUROPEPTIDES, NEUROTRANSMITTERS, AND NEUROHORMONES

NEUROPEPTIDES AND THE IMMUNE SYSTEM

NONENDOCRINE HYPOTHALAMUS
Temperature Regulation
Appetite
Emotion and Libido
Biological Rhythms

ENDOCRINE HYPOTHALAMUS: THE HYPOTHALAMIC–PITUITARY UNIT
Functional Anatomy
Blood Supply

ANTERIOR PITUITARY
Hypothalamic Control of Anterior Pituitary Secretion
Abnormalities of Anterior Pituitary Function
Pituitary Tumors and Pituitary Hyperplasia
Other Tumors
Hypophysitis

POSTERIOR PITUITARY
Physiology
Diabetes Insipidus
Syndrome of Inappropriate Antidiuretic Hormone Secretion
Cerebral Salt Wasting

APPROACH TO THE PATIENT WITH HYPOTHALAMIC-PITUITARY DYSFUNCTION
History and Physical Examination
Assessment by Imaging Studies
Endocrinological Investigation
Treatment of Pituitary Tumors
Treatment of Hypopituitarism

NEUROENDOCRINE TUMORS
Pheochromocytomas
Carcinoid Tumors

Neuroendocrinology is the study of the coordinated interaction of the nervous, endocrine, and immune systems to maintain the constancy of the internal milieu (homeostasis). In practical clinical terms, it concentrates mainly on the functions of the hypothalamus and its interaction with the pituitary gland.

NEUROPEPTIDES, NEUROTRANSMITTERS, AND NEUROHORMONES

One of the features of the neuroendocrine system is that it uses neuropeptides as both neurotransmitters and neurohormones. The term *neurotransmitter* is applied traditionally to a substance that is released by one neuron and acts on an adjacent neuron in a stimulatory or inhibitory fashion. The effect usually is rapid, brief, and confined to a small area of the neuron surface. In contrast, a *hormone* is a substance that is released into the bloodstream and usually travels to a distant site to act over seconds, minutes, or hours to produce its effect over a large area of the cell or over many cells. *Neuropeptides* can act in either fashion. For example, the neuropeptide vasopressin, produced by the neurons of the supraoptic and paraventricular nuclei, is released into the bloodstream and has a hormonal action on the collecting ducts in the kidney. Vasopressin is also released within the central nervous system (CNS), where it acts as a neurotransmitter (Landgraf and Neumann, 2004). Similarly, the neuropeptide substance P acts as a neurotransmitter in primary sensory neurons that convey pain signals, and more as a neurohormone in the hypothalamus.

The influence of neurohormones and neuropeptides on the brain can be divided into two broad categories: organizational and activational. *Organizational effects* occur during neuronal differentiation, growth, and development and bring about permanent structural changes in the organization of the brain and therefore brain function. An example of this is the structural and organizational changes brought about in the brain by prenatal exposure to testosterone. *Activational effects* are those that change pre-established patterns of neuronal activity, such as an increased rate of neuronal firing caused by exposure of a neuron to substance P or vasopressin.

Numerous neuropeptides are found in the brain, where they have a wide variety of effects on neuronal function (Table 52.1). Current understanding of all the actions of neuropeptides in the nervous system is far from complete.

NEUROPEPTIDES AND THE IMMUNE SYSTEM

It has been known for many years that stress, through activation of the hypothalamic–pituitary–adrenal axis, modulates the function of the immune system (Tsigos and Chrousos, 2002; Wrona, 2006). Infections in the periphery convey information to the central nervous system through humoral (cytokines and bacterial toxins) and neuronal routes to bring about behaviors that enhance survival (McCusker and Kelley, 2013. Certain peptides and their receptors, once thought to be unique to either the immune or the neuroendocrine system, actually are found in both.

Cytokines—interleukins (IL)-1, -2, -4, and -6 and tumor necrosis factor (TNF)—are synthesized by glial cells in the CNS in response to cell injury. IL-1 and the other cytokines, through their ability to stimulate the synthesis of nerve growth factor, may be important promoters of neuronal damage repair. Circulating cytokines have been thought to play a role in the hypothalamus to activate the hypothalamic–pituitary-adrenal axis in response to inflammation elsewhere in the body (see the section Fever, later in this chapter) and inhibit the pituitary–thyroid and pituitary–gonadal axes in response to systemic disease.

Several other hormones and neuropeptides have modulatory effects on immune function. Similarly, immunocompetent cells contain hormones and neuropeptides that may

TABLE 52.1 Neuropeptides Found in the Brain and Their Effects on Brain Function*

Neuropeptide	Central nervous system function and selected function outside the central nervous system	Neuropeptide	Central nervous system function and selected function outside the central nervous system
HYPOTHALAMIC PEPTIDES MODULATING PITUITARY FUNCTION		β-Lipotropic hormone	Skin tanning
Corticotropin (ACTH)-releasing hormone (CRH)	Regulation of ACTH secretion Integration of behavioral and biochemical responses to stress Modulatory effects on learning and memory	Melanocyte-stimulating hormone (α- and γ-)	Weight loss Skin tanning Increased sexual desire Anti-inflammatory effect Important mediator of leptin control on energy homeostasis
Growth hormone-releasing hormone (GHRH)	Regulation of growth hormone secretion	Oxytocin	Anxiety and mood Active/passive stress coping Maternal behavior, aggression Pair bonding
Growth hormone release-inhibiting hormone (somatostatin)	Regulation of growth hormone secretion	Vasopressin	Active/passive stress coping Anxiety Spatial memory Social discrimination, social interaction Pair bonding Activation of the hypothalamic–pituitary–adrenal (HPA) axis
Ghrelin	Regulation of growth hormone secretion Regulation of feeding		
Thyrotropin-releasing hormone (TRH)	Regulation of thyroid-stimulating hormone secretion May be involved in depression Enhances neuromuscular function (in the periphery)	Neurophysins	
		BRAIN–GASTROINTESTINAL TRACT PEPTIDES	
Gonadotropin-releasing hormone (luteinizing hormone-releasing hormone) (GnRH)	Regulates gonadotropin secretion Influences sexual receptivity	Vasoactive intestinal polypeptide	Cerebral blood flow Potent anti-inflammatory factor
Prolactin-releasing peptide	Stimulates prolactin secretion	Somatostatin	
Neurotensin	Endogenous neuroleptic Regulates mesolimbic, mesocortical, and nigrostriatal dopamine neurons Thermoregulation Analgesia	Insulin	Feeding behavior Modulatory effect on learning and memory Hunger
		Glucagon	Inhibition of feeding
Neuropeptide Y	Stimulates hunger, food intake, and drinking Sexual behavior Locomotion Memory	Pancreatic polypeptide	
		Gastrin	
		Cholecystokinin	Feeding behavior Satiety Modulates dopamine neuron activity Facilitation of memory processing (especially under stress)
Orexins (hypocretins)	Stimulate CRH and antidiuretic hormone (ADH) Inhibit GHRH Stimulate GnRH May stimulate preovulatory prolactin release Inhibit TRH release Inhibit hunger and food intake	Tachykinins (e.g., substance P)	Substance P co-localizes with serotonin and is involved in nociception
		Secretin	Modulates motor and other functions in brain, facilitating GABA
PITUITARY PEPTIDES		Thyrotropin-releasing hormone	
Prolactin	Maternal behavior Mood Anxiety	Bombesin	Thermoregulation Inhibition of feeding Modulatory effect on learning and memory
Growth hormone			
Thyroid-stimulating hormone		Orexins (hypocretin)	Gastric and gastrointestinal motility and secretion Pancreatic hormone release Regulation of energy homeostasis Feeding behavior Locomotion and muscle tone Wakefulness/sleep
Follicle-stimulating hormone			
Luteinizing hormone	Elevated levels may promote neurodegeneration		
Pro-opiomelanocortin		Galanin	Modulates release of gonadotropin-releasing hormone, prolactin, insulin, glucagons, growth hormone, and somatostatin Affects feeding, sexual behavior, and anxiety Potent anticonvulsant effects
ACTH			
ACTH-like intermediate lobe peptides			
β-Endorphin	Analgesic mechanisms Feeding Thermoregulation Learning and memory	Leptin	Satiety factor

Continued on following page

TABLE 52.1 Neuropeptides Found in the Brain and Their Effects on Brain Function *(Continued)*

Neuropeptide	Central nervous system function and selected function outside the central nervous system	Neuropeptide	Central nervous system function and selected function outside the central nervous system
GROWTH FACTORS		Calcitonin gene-related peptide	Migraine and other vascular headaches
Insulin-like growth factors (IGF) 1 and 2		**OTHER NEUROPEPTIDES**	
Nerve growth factors	Axonal plasticity	Angiotensin	Hypertension Thirst
OPIOID FAMILY		Synapsins	
Endorphins	Analgesia	Calcitonin gene–related peptide	Migraine and other vascular headaches
Enkephalins (met-, leu-)	Analgesic mechanisms Feeding Temperature control Learning and memory Cardiovascular control	Calcitonin	
		Sleep peptides	Regulation of sleep cycles
Dynorphins		Orexins (hypocretin)	Sleep–wake regulation Narcolepsy Energy homeostasis
Kytorphin			
NEUROPEPTIDES MODULATING IMMUNE FUNCTION		Carnosine	
ACTH		**PRECURSOR PEPTIDES**	
Endorphins		Pro-opiomelanocortin	
Interferons		Proenkephalins (A and B)	
Neuroleukins		Calcitonin gene product	
Thymosin		Vasoactive intestinal polypeptide gene product	
Thymopeptin			
OTHER NEUROPEPTIDES		Proglucagon	
Atrial natriuretic factors	?Role in cerebral salt wasting	Proinsulin	
Bradykinins	Cerebral blood flow		

ACTH, Adrenocorticotropic hormone; *GABA,* γ-aminobutyric acid.
*This is only a partial list of all of the neuropeptides that have been found in the brain, and not all of the putative functions have been listed.

affect neuroendocrine and brain cells (Table 52.2). Despite speculation about the ability of the psyche to influence immunological function and therefore disease outcome, conclusive evidence suggesting a clinically significant effect remains lacking (Padgett and Glaser, 2003).

NONENDOCRINE HYPOTHALAMUS
Temperature Regulation

The hypothalamus plays a key role in ensuring that body temperature is maintained within narrow limits by balancing the heat gained from metabolic activity and the environment with the heat lost to the environment (Nakamura, 2011; Romanovsky, 2007). A theoretical schema of the mechanisms of hypothalamic temperature regulation is depicted in Fig. 52.1. Although numerous neurotransmitters and peptides alter body temperature, their physiological roles remain unclear.

Hypothalamic injury can cause disordered temperature regulation. One potentially serious consequence is the hyperthermia that may occur when the preoptic anterior hypothalamic area is damaged or irritated by ischemia, subarachnoid hemorrhage, trauma, or surgery. In some patients, the marked impairment of heat-loss mechanisms and the resulting hyperthermia may be fatal. In those individuals who survive, temperature control usually returns to normal over a period of days to weeks. Chronic hyperthermia of hypothalamic origin

is extremely uncommon; it may occur with continued impairment of ability to dissipate heat adequately or with difficulty sensing temperature elevations. Chronic hypothalamic hyperthermia does not respond to salicylates and other antipyretics because it is not prostaglandin mediated. Hypothermia, both acute and chronic, can be due to hypothalamic injury, the most common causes being head trauma, infarction, and demyelination. Other entities to be considered in the differential diagnosis are severe hypothyroidism, Wernicke disease, and drug effect. Some patients with no apparent hypothalamic structural abnormalities may have episodes of recurrent hypothermia. The cause of this syndrome is unclear, although the response of some patients to anticonvulsant agents and of others to clonidine or cyproheptadine suggests a possible neurotransmitter abnormality. Agenesis of the corpus callosum in association with episodic hyperhidrosis and hypothermia (Shapiro syndrome) is caused in some individuals by an abnormally low hypothalamic "set point." These symptoms may respond to clonidine (a centrally acting α₂-adrenergic agonist). A similar condition associated with hyperthermia (so-called reverse Shapiro syndrome) has been found to respond with normalization of temperature to low-dose L-dopa, higher doses causing hypothermia. Large lesions in the posterior hypothalamus may impair both heat production (by altering the set point) and heat loss (by damaging the outflow from the preoptic anterior hypothalamic area). This results in poikilothermia, a condition in which body temperature varies with the environmental temperature.

Drugs:
  Dopamine receptor blockers
  Phenothiazines such as chlorpromazine
  Butyrophenones such as haloperidol
  Metoclopramide
  Reserpine
  α-Methyldopa
  Monoamine oxidase inhibitors
  Tricyclic antidepressants (unusual, probably idiosyncratic)
  Benzodiazepines (unusual, probably idiosyncratic)
  Verapamil
  Cocaine
  Fluoxetine
  Amoxapine
Hormones:
  Estrogens
  Thyrotropin-releasing hormone (as can occur in primary
    hypothyroidism)
  Pituitary tumor
  Prolactin-secreting adenoma
  Interference of flow of dopamine down the pituitary stalk by
    large pituitary or parapituitary tumor
Chest wall stimulation
Chronic skin disease (e.g., severe acne)
Tumors of chest wall
Chronic renal failure
Cirrhosis
Ectopic production
Hypothalamic disease
Pseudocyesis
Idiopathic

Headache—nonspecific, tension-type like, felt at the vertex and
  behind the eyes
Impaired glucose tolerance or diabetes mellitus
Enlargement of hands and feet
Enlargement of the jaw, with increased spacing between the
  teeth and malocclusion
Hypertension
Menstrual irregularities
Soft-tissue growth:
  Thick skin
  Dough-like feel to palm (e.g., during handshake)
  Carpal tunnel syndrome
Arthralgia and osteoarthritis
Proximal muscle weakness
Hyperhidrosis

diameter) stage. In men, the insidious onset of erectile dysfunction and reduced libido usually means that these tumors are found late, often only after they have produced signs and symptoms of optic nerve compression. Galactorrhea is a rare accompaniment of elevated prolactin in men.

Serum prolactin levels increase after generalized tonic-clonic seizures and complex partial seizures due to temporary lack of hypothalamic dopaminergic inhibition of prolactin release but show no change after virtually all cases of psychogenic, absence, or simple or complex partial seizures of frontal lobe origin. After a seizure, prolactin levels peak at 15 to 20 minutes and then decrease to baseline levels within 60 minutes. The increase should be at least two times baseline. Caution should be exercised in interpreting early-morning prolactin levels, because a 50% to 100% increase in prolactin is normal just before waking. Furthermore, prolactin elevations are far from specific for epilepsy, and some tendency for the elevation to attenuate in patients with frequent seizures has been observed.

Because prolactin secretion is under strong inhibitory control by the hypothalamus, anything that interferes with the free flow of blood down the pituitary portal veins can reduce the exposure of the pituitary to the dopamine released by the hypothalamus. This results in raised peripheral blood prolactin levels. In patients with this condition, prolactin levels commonly range from 50 to 150 ng/mL (usually <100 ng/mL; normal, <25 ng/mL); such elevations can be seen, for example, in patients with granulomatous disease involving the pituitary stalk. However, probably the most common situation in which this occurs is in patients in whom the pituitary stalk is "kinked" by a pituitary adenoma. In such circumstances, this may lead to the erroneous assumption that the pituitary

adenoma is secreting prolactin, and long-term therapy with bromocriptine might be undertaken. We have seen such patients whose tumors continued to grow despite normalization of prolactin levels. The mistake with these patients is to assume that a prolactin-secreting macroadenoma would result in a moderately elevated prolactin level. Microprolactinomas usually produce prolactin levels in excess of 200 ng/mL, and patients with macroadenomas that secrete prolactin often have much higher levels, not infrequently in excess of 1000 ng/mL.

Patients taking neuroleptic medications also may have elevated prolactin levels, and occasionally the elevation is enough to cause galactorrhea or amenorrhea. In such patients, it may be uncertain whether symptoms are secondary to drug-induced hyperprolactinemia or to a microadenoma. Unless there is a documented normal prolactin level before start of the drug, our practice is to perform an MRI study of the pituitary to look for a tumor. Occasionally we will perform dynamic pituitary testing with thyrotropin-releasing hormone and metoclopramide. In most patients, drug-induced hyperprolactinemia responds normally to stimulation with these agents. The treatment of drug-induced hyperprolactinemia is difficult if the causative drug cannot be stopped. Some patients may benefit from the use of atypical antipsychotics with reduced or no action at dopamine receptors (at normal therapeutic doses).

Gigantism and Acromegaly. Presence of excessive amounts of circulating GH before closure of the epiphyses leads to gigantism. If the epiphyses have closed, only tissue still capable of responding to GH will grow, leading to the clinical syndrome of acromegaly; its clinical features are summarized in Box 52.3. Of particular note for the neurologist and the neurosurgeon is the frequent complaint of headache and symptoms related to carpal tunnel syndrome. It is not uncommon to find patients with acromegaly in whom surgery for carpal tunnel release was performed 3 to 5 years before diagnosis of their disease.

Most cases of gigantism and acromegaly are due to excess GH production by a pituitary adenoma. Rare cases of ectopic GH production have been described; for example, excessive GHRH production by pancreatic tumors can cause acromegaly. Excess production of GHRH by the hypothalamus could theoretically cause an identical clinical syndrome.

Cushing Disease and Nelson Syndrome. The term *Cushing syndrome* refers to the clinical picture resulting from exposure

BOX 52.4 Common Clinical Features of Cushing Disease

Truncal obesity—arms and legs tend to be thin; excess fat
 deposition in preauricular and supraclavicular fat pads
Hypertension
Impaired glucose tolerance and diabetes mellitus
Menstrual irregularities or amenorrhea
Excessive hair growth
Acne
Proximal myopathy
Abdominal striae (purplish)
Osteoporosis
Thin skin with excessive bruising

to excessive corticosteroids, either endogenous or exogenous. If the clinical manifestations are caused by excessive production of ACTH from the pituitary, the condition is referred to as *Cushing disease.* Common clinical features of Cushing disease are listed in Box 52.4. The syndrome of hyperpigmentation and local compression of parapituitary structures that occurs in approximately 10% of patients with Cushing disease who have been treated with bilateral adrenalectomy is called *Nelson syndrome.* Given the generally good results from surgery on the pituitary gland in Cushing disease, Nelson syndrome is now quite uncommon.

The diagnosis of Cushing syndrome, although simple in theory, often is quite difficult in practice (Findling and Raff, 2005). It is also often difficult for tests to distinguish between true Cushing syndrome and so-called pseudo-Cushing syndrome due to alcoholism, depression, and eating disorders.

As a screening test, the most sensitive and specific screening tool is an 11pm salivary cortisol determination. Unfortunately, this test may not be readily available in all clinical centers, and 24-hour urine collections for urinary free cortisol are still used. The sensitivity and specificity of the 24-hour collection can be increased by doing two collections on consecutive days. A third screening test is the 1-mg overnight dexamethasone suppression test. For years now, the 2-day low dose dexamethasone suppression test has been pivotal in the diagnosis of Cushing disease. For this test, 0.5 mg of dexamethasone is given every 6 hours for 8 doses; during the second 24 hours of administration, the normal response is suppression of cortisol production, as reflected by reduced urinary levels of 17-ketogenic steroids or urinary free cortisol, and of serum ACTH and cortisol. Patients with Cushing disease usually show a similar suppression only when the dose of dexamethasone is increased to 2 mg every 6 hours for 8 doses. The formal dexamethasone suppression test is cumbersome, requiring 6 consecutive days of collection of urine for urinary-free cortisol levels. Various modifications of this test may be useful and less cumbersome. More detailed discussion can be found in the literature, both for screening (Findling and Raff, 2005) and for diagnosis (Lindsay and Nieman, 2005) of Cushing syndrome.

In Cushing disease, ACTH levels usually are in the normal range or moderately elevated. Failure to suppress on high-dose dexamethasone and unmeasurable ACTH levels are seen with primary adrenal problems such as adenoma or carcinoma. Ectopic ACTH production usually is insuppressible, and the ACTH levels tend to be much higher than those seen in typical pituitary Cushing disease, although many exceptions to these rules have been found. In well-documented cases of ectopic ACTH production and primary adrenal problems, dexamethasone suppression test results have been compatible with a diagnosis of pituitary ACTH production. Intermittent excess

ACTH production also can give rise to false-negative results in patients who actually have Cushing disease.

Even when all test results point to a pituitary source for the excessive ACTH production, care must still be taken in diagnosing the patient as having Cushing disease. An abnormality of the sella may or may not be present on CT or MRI. Intermediate-lobe cysts or clefts may mimic the appearance of adenoma on CT or MRI. In such cases, simultaneous sampling from the petrosal sinuses bilaterally and from the inferior vena cava can help localize the excessive ACTH production.

The pituitary glands of some patients with biochemical Cushing disease do not show adenoma formation but demonstrate evidence of hyperplasia of the cells that secrete ACTH. Although this picture can be due to ectopic production of CRH, the hypothalamic peptide that stimulates release of ACTH, or to excessive release of CRH from the hypothalamus, such etiologies affect less than 0.3% of patients with Cushing disease who have pituitary surgery.

Excessive Secretion of Thyroid-Stimulating Hormone. Elevated levels of thyroid-stimulating hormone (TSH) are seen most commonly with primary hypothyroidism. The resulting pituitary hypertrophy infrequently can be of sufficient magnitude to cause visual field defects. Hyperthyroidism due to excessive TSH secretion is a rare (accounting for less than 1% of all pituitary tumors) but well-recognized entity, and these tumors are usually large and readily visible on CT scans.

Pituitary resistance to thyroid hormone also may produce a clinical picture of hyperthyroidism with high-normal or mildly elevated TSH levels. Unlike in the case of TSH-secreting tumors, which are relatively autonomous, the TSH levels in patients with pituitary resistance usually respond well to stimulation with thyrotropin-releasing hormone or to suppression with dexamethasone or dopamine.

Gonadotropin-Secreting Tumors. Many pituitary tumors formerly classified as nonfunctioning are actually gonadotropin- or gonadotropin subunit-producing tumors. The usual presentation is a macroadenoma in an elderly man; however, they occur in persons of all ages and both sexes, with a male preponderance.

Many of these tumors secrete only FSH, and only rarely do they secrete LH alone. Some may secrete both LH and FSH, and others secrete biologically inactive gonadotropin subunits: the α subunit, LH-αβ subunit, or FSH-β subunit. Most clinical radioimmunoassays used to measure LH and FSH require the α and β subunits to be associated before they register in the assay. As a result, subunit secretion is not detected in such assays. FSH levels usually are elevated in patients with FSH-secreting tumors, and testosterone or estradiol levels almost always are low. In patients with LH-secreting tumors, LH levels usually are elevated, and estradiol or testosterone levels may be high. Despite high sex steroid levels, these patients often have no clinical gonadal-related symptoms. Patients with tumors that secrete both LH and FSH usually have normal or high sex steroid levels, but again, they are often clinically asymptomatic. Because subunits are biologically inactive, they do not interfere directly with hormonal function, although by means of pressure effects on the pituitary, subunit-secreting tumors can cause hypopituitarism.

Long-standing primary hypogonadism that is not replaced adequately may cause pituitary enlargement secondary to gonadotroph hyperplasia. Rarely, this may lead to gonadotroph tumor development. Most of the time, the pituitary enlargement is asymptomatic and regresses in response to sex steroid replacement.

An overall review of pituitary dysfunction can be found in the article by Levy (2004).

TABLE 52.5 Classification of Pituitary Adenomas

Tumor	Frequency (%)
Growth hormone cell adenoma	14.0
Prolactin cell adenoma	27.2
Growth hormone–prolactin cell adenoma	8.4
Corticotroph cell adenoma	8.1
Thyrotroph cell adenoma	1.0
Gonadotroph cell adenoma	6.4
Clinically nonfunctioning adenoma	31.2
Plurihormonal adenoma	3.7

Modified from Thapar, K., Kovacs, K., Muller, P.J., 1995. Clinical-pathological correlations of pituitary tumours. Clin Endocrinol Metab 9, 243–270.

Pituitary Tumors and Pituitary Hyperplasia

Pituitary tumors account for approximately 15% of all intracranial tumors. Although most are benign, they can be locally invasive. Only rarely is true malignancy evidenced by metastases. The old classification of pituitary adenomas into chromophobe, acidophil, and basophil has been supplanted by a more functional classification based on findings of immunological and electron microscopic examinations (Table 52.5). Hyperplasia of various cellular elements of the pituitary is relatively rare and usually only seen in cases of ectopic hypothalamic-releasing hormone production (Ironside, 2003).

Most pituitary tumors that have been removed surgically and examined have been found to be monoclonal in origin. This finding suggests that a majority of pituitary tumors arise from a single cell in which a mutation either activated a proto-oncogene or inactivated a tumor suppressor gene. Around 2% of pituitary adenomas occur in a familial setting, in the absence of any other tumor, and are referred to as familial isolated pituitary adenomas (FIPA). Some 15%–30% of such families harbor inactivating germ-line mutations in the aryl hydrocarbon receptor-interacting protein (AIP) gene, which is associated with early onset, aggressive macroadenomas, most of which secrete somatotropin (growth hormone) (Williams et al., 2014). Almost half of pituitary tumors show aneuploidy (usually more or [rarely] fewer than the normal number of chromosomes). The significance of this to tumor formation is uncertain. The cell cycle inhibitory proteins p14ARF and p16^{INK4a} are coded for by the CDKN2A (cyclin-dependent kinase inhibitor) gene. This gene has been found to have reduced expression in a majority of human pituitary tumors. PTTG (pituitary tumor-transforming gene) expression is increased in certain human pituitary tumors, but whether these changes in gene expression play a role in tumor induction or whether they are the result of tumor formation is unclear.

The G proteins are a family of proteins comprising α, β, and γ subunits that bind to guanine nucleotides. A variety of mutations involving single amino acid substitutions in the portion of the Gs gene that encodes the Gs α subunit have been identified in nearly 40% of GH-secreting tumors. These mutations inhibit the breakdown of the α subunit, thereby mimicking the effect of specific growth factors and leading to increased adenylate cyclase activity and elevated intracellular cyclic adenosine monophosphate levels. Nevertheless, no single mutation or alteration of function seems to explain tumor formation in more than the occasional case. Somatostatin inhibits both GH and cyclic adenosine monophosphate

production, and this may be the mechanism by which it shrinks GH-secreting pituitary tumors.

Levy and Lightman (2003) suggest that although some pituitary tumors may be due to genetic abnormalities, it is possible that a majority of pituitary tumors are not "tumors" in the usual sense but rather represent an over-response to normal trophic factors that has failed to normalize once the growth stimulus has returned to normal.

Other Tumors

Gliomas, meningiomas, chordomas, teratomas, and dermoid and epidermoid tumors all can occur in the region of the sella turcica, and local compressive effects may produce a clinical picture resembling that of primary pituitary tumors. The pituitary gland is the site of metastatic deposits in 4% of cancer patients. Usually these metastases are asymptomatic; when symptoms do occur, however, they most often are related to disturbance of posterior pituitary function.

Craniopharyngiomas are only one-third as common as pituitary tumors. They are thought to arise from residual rests of Rathke pouch tissue. Most commonly found in a suprasellar location, they also occur anywhere along the pituitary–hypothalamic axis, including within the sella. Craniopharyngiomas can appear at any age; however, approximately a third of cases arise before the age of 15 years. Because these tumors produce no hormones, patients usually present with signs of local compression, especially of the visual system, or with hypothalamic dysfunction such as growth failure or diabetes insipidus (DI). Almost half of affected children show evidence of growth failure. Three-fourths of patients, both adults and children, have visual symptoms, and these are more common in patients requiring complex treatment (Yeun et al., 2014).

Hypophysitis

Hypophysitis from infection or granulomatous disease such as sarcoidosis can result in hypopituitarism. Lymphocytic hypophysitis, a sterile inflammation of the pituitary of probable autoimmune origin, is seen almost exclusively in women, particularly during pregnancy. Usually it causes hypopituitarism, although it can cause hyperprolactinemia and may be a cause of the empty sella syndrome.

POSTERIOR PITUITARY
Physiology
Vasopressin

Vasopressin, or antidiuretic hormone (ADH), an essential hormone in fluid and electrolyte homeostasis, is synthesized in the magnocellular neurons of the supraoptic and paraventricular nuclei as a large precursor molecule, which is cleaved enzymatically to yield vasopressin and neurophysin. The function of this latter peptide is unknown.

Four vasopressin-containing pathways have been recognized in the brain: (1) hypothalamo-neurohypophysial, (2) paraventricular nucleus to the zona incerta of the median eminence, (3) paraventricular nucleus to the limbic system (amygdala), and (4) paraventricular nucleus to the brainstem and spinal cord. The best-characterized of these is the hypothalamo-neuro-hypophysial (hypophysial-portal) pathway. Virtually all of the neurons from the supraoptic nuclei contribute to this pathway, whereas only a portion of paraventricular nuclei terminate in the posterior pituitary. Some of the vasopressin-containing fibers from the paraventricular nuclei appear to be more involved in ACTH regulation than in fluid balance. Vasopressin-containing fibers also project widely outside the hypothalamus, where (as some evidence suggests) they may participate in memory.

Oxytocin

Oxytocin, like vasopressin, is synthesized in magnocellular neurons of the supraoptic and paraventricular nuclei as a large precursor molecule that is cleaved into oxytocin and a specific neurophysin. Many of the physiological stimuli of vasopressin also result in oxytocin release, and although in supraphysiological doses, oxytocin does have ADH-like properties, its physiological role in these circumstances remains obscure. The only specific stimulus that causes the release of oxytocin but not vasopressin is suckling. Oxytocin's role in normal lactation and parturition in the human remains to be defined clearly. Oxytocin receptors are found in the limbic system, particularly in the amygdala, and for this reason oxytocin has been implicated in emotion. Lim and Young (2006) have shown that in mammals it plays a role in a variety of complex social behaviors as well as helping regulate the response to stress.

Thirst and Drinking

Certain cells of the anterior hypothalamus are sensitive to changes in the osmolality of the blood bathing them and respond by signaling the cells of the supraoptic and paraventricular nuclei to alter their secretion of vasopressin. These cells are most sensitive to osmotic substances that do not diffuse freely into cells, such as sodium, sucrose, and mannitol. Substances such as urea produce less osmotic stimulation because they diffuse freely. Glucose, in addition to diffusing freely, actually inhibits ADH release. These cells respond with marked increases in ADH secretion not only to increased osmolality, and hence dehydration, but also to hypotension.

Water homeostasis cannot be maintained by antidiuresis alone but also requires thirst and the drinking behavior induced by it. A drinking center is thought to be located near the feeding center in the lateral hypothalamus. Angiotensin may play an important role in stimulating drinking in humans and animals.

Sodium Homeostasis and Atrial Natriuretic Peptide

Sodium homeostasis is extremely important for normal functioning of the organism. Most of the regulation of body sodium takes place in the kidney. Sodium reabsorption is under control of the renin–angiotensin–aldosterone system. In normal physiological circumstances, aldosterone, the principal mineralocorticoid produced by the adrenal gland, is affected in only a minor way by ACTH.

The human heart has been shown to synthesize and secrete atrial natriuretic peptide, which has diuretic, natriuretic (serving to increase urinary sodium excretion), and vasorelaxant properties. In addition to atrial natriuretic peptide, the brain contains brain natriuretic peptide and C-type natriuretic peptide. Judging from the pattern of their distribution in the brain, these substances may have important roles in the central control of the cardiovascular system. The natriuretic peptides seem to act as natural antagonists to the central actions of angiotensin II.

Diabetes Insipidus

Diabetes insipidus (DI) is a clinical syndrome characterized by severe thirst, polydipsia, and polyuria. Central DI must be distinguished from nephrogenic DI (an inability of the kidney to respond to ADH) and from compulsive water drinking (Baylis, 1995). Distinguishing among these entities normally

is done using a water deprivation test. A urine osmolality of greater than 750 mmol/L after water deprivation excludes the diagnosis of DI. Central DI is characterized by an increase in osmolality to greater than 750 mmol/L after administration of desamino-D-arginine-vasopressin (DDAVP). In nephrogenic DI, little change in osmolality occurs after DDAVP administration. The polyuria induced by chronic compulsive water drinking may produce a renal tubular concentrating defect because of medullary washout—that is, the loss of sodium and other solutes from around the loops of Henle. This can make it difficult to differentiate partial DI of central or renal cause from polydipsia. Treatment by gradual fluid restriction, with or without DDAVP, can be used to reverse the medullary washout, thereby increasing the sensitivity of the test.

The water deprivation test must be strictly supervised by a physician familiar with the technique. Severe and potentially fatal dehydration can occur rapidly in patients with complete DI, especially children. Similarly, patients with compulsive water drinking given DDAVP and allowed access to water can drink themselves into hyponatremic coma.

Etiology

Approximately a third of patients with central DI have no demonstrable disease of the hypothalamic–posterior pituitary unit. The remaining patients have damage to the supraoptic-hypophysial–portal pathway from trauma, surgery, tumors, inflammatory lesions (which may be granulomatous or infectious), or vascular lesions. In patients with polyuria, the urine should be examined to ensure that a solute diuresis, as with hyperglycemia, has not occurred, or that a type of nephrogenic DI has not been induced by hypokalemia, hypercalcemia, or lithium carbonate therapy. In the acute care setting on a neurosurgical ward, administration of mannitol may be one of the more common causes of polyuria. The investigation of DI has been well summarized by Diederich and colleagues (2001).

Management

Patients with DI excrete mainly water, and therefore water replacement alone is the mainstay of their management. Patients who are alert and have intact thirst mechanisms should be given free access to water. Only if urine output exceeds 7 L/day is treatment necessary. In most circumstances, DDAVP given as a nasal solution or as an oral or sublingual tablet is the treatment of choice. To avoid water intoxication, under-replacement is preferable in these patients, who should be allowed to modulate their water balance by drinking.

The unconscious patient can present a problem in management. When calculating such a patient's fluid needs, the clinician should be aware that the urine in DI is electrolyte poor. Thus, the electrolyte requirements of such a patient are little different from those of other patients. The bulk of the urinary replacement should be given as 5% dextrose in water. The administration of 5% dextrose in 0.2 NaCl or solutions with even higher salt concentrations presents a high solute load to the kidney and tends to exacerbate the polyuria.

Syndrome of Inappropriate Antidiuretic Hormone Secretion

Etiology and Pathophysiology

The syndrome of inappropriate ADH secretion (SIADH) is characterized by low serum sodium, high urine sodium, and relative or absolute hyperosmolarity of urine to serum. Before

Index

Page numbers followed by "*f*" indicate figures, "*t*" indicate tables, and "*b*" indicate boxes.

A

A vigilance test, for delirium, 28
A wave, 385, 385*f*
A2BP1. *see* Ataxin 2 binding protein 1 (A2BP1)
AAASPS (African American Antiplatelet Stroke Prevention Study), 953
ABA (applied behavior analysis), for autism spectrum disorder, 1306
Abacavir (Ziagen), for HIV infection, 1108*t*–1109*t*
Abasia, 1999
ABCA1 gene, in Tangier disease, 1338
ABCD1 gene, in adrenomyeloneuropathy, 1493–1494
Abciximab
    for acute ischemic stroke, 958
    for preventing stroke recurrence, 954
Abdominal examination, for coma, 39
Abdominal migraine, 1719
Abducens fascicle
    anatomy of, 1727
    clinical lesions of, 1727
Abducens nerve, 1727–1728
    anatomy of, 1721*f*, 1727
    clinical lesions of, 1727–1728
        of abducens nucleus, 1727
        abducens palsy as
            appearance of, 1727, 1727*f*
            isolated, 1728
        of brainstem fascicle, 1728
        of cavernous sinus, 1728
        of orbital apex, 1728
        of petrous apex, 1728
        of subarachnoid space and Dorello canal, 1728
Abducens nucleus
    anatomy of, 1727
    clinical lesions of, 1727
    in horizontal eye movements, 554, 555*f*
Abducens palsy
    appearance of, 1727, 1727*f*
    isolated, 1728
Abductor pollicis brevis muscle, in carpal tunnel syndrome, 1802, 1803*f*
Abetalipoproteinemia, 1229, 1338, 1818.*e*9
    ataxia due to, 1468
ABILHAND-Kids, for cerebral palsy, 1311
ABLV (Australian bat lyssavirus), 1141.*e*1
Abnormal test result, 344
Abrupt drug withdrawal, for medication overuse headache, 1708
Abscess
    brain
        bacterial, 1150–1151
            clinical presentation of, 1150
            diagnosis of, 1150, 1151*f*
            management of, 1149*t*, 1150–1151
            risk factors for, 1150
        with congenital heart disease, 836

Abscess *(Continued)*
        fungal, 1154–1155
            clinical presentation of, 1154–1155
            diagnosis of, 1155
            etiology of, 1154
            management of, 1154*t*, 1155
        due to neonatal meningitis, 1965
    epidural
        spinal, 1151–1152, 1759–1760
            clinical presentation of, 1151
            diagnosis of, 1151–1152, 1152*f*
            etiology of, 1151
            management of, 1149*t*, 1152
            risk factors for, 1151
            structural imaging of, 452
    HIV-associated, 1117, 1119*f*
    lumbosacral plexopathy and, 1788–1789
    root, 1695
    spinal cord, epidural, 1151–1152
        clinical presentation of, 1151
        diagnosis of, 1151–1152, 1152*f*
        etiology of, 1151
        management of, 1149*t*, 1152
        risk factors for, 1151
        structural imaging of, 436.*e*1, 436.*e*2*f*
Absence epilepsy
    childhood, 1520*t*–1521*t*, 1535, 1576–1577
    juvenile, 1577
Absence seizures, 14, 14*t*
    EEG of, 1569
    generalized, 1569, 1570*f*
    simple *versus* complex, 1569
Abulia, 34–35, 35*t*
Acanthamoeba spp., granulomatous amebic encephalitis due to, 1155, 1156*t*
Acanthocytes, 1448
    for Huntington disease, 1448
Acanthocytic syndromes, neurological complications of, 824
ACAS (Asymptomatic Carotid Atherosclerosis Study), 961–962
Acceleration concussion, 851
Accessory deep peroneal nerve, nerve conduction studies with, 371
Accommodative retinal blur, and vergence, 558
ACE (Aspirin in Carotid Endarterectomy) trial, 953
Acephalgic migraine, 1696
Aceruloplasminemia, 1455
Acetaminophen (Tylenol)
    for chronic pain, 723, 725*t*
    for tension-type headache, 1713
Acetazolamide
    for cerebral edema, 1272
    for hypokalemic periodic paralysis, 1524, 1524*t*
Acetazolamide-sensitive myotonia, 1526
Acetylcholine (ACh)
    in basal ganglia, 1425–1426
    in myasthenia gravis, 1898

Acetylcholine receptor (AChR)
    in basal ganglia, 1426
    in myasthenia gravis, 1898
Acetylcholine receptor antibodies (AChR-abs), in myasthenia gravis, 1901–1902
Acetylcholine receptor (AChR) deficiency, congenital myasthenic syndromes due to, 1911
Acetylcholinesterase, in chemical imaging, 505*t*, 506
Acetylcholinesterase (AChE) deficiency, congenital myasthenic syndrome due to, 1911
Acetylcholinesterase Inhibitor Drugs, 1401–1403
Acetylcholinesterase inhibitors, 1397–1398
    for myasthenia gravis, 692
Acetylsalicylic acid (Aspirin), for chronic pain, 725*t*
aCGH (array comparative genomic hybridization), molecular diagnostics and, 1030
ACh. *see* Acetylcholine (ACh)
Achalasia, in autonomic disorders, 1870–1871
AChE. *see* Acetylcholinesterase (AChE) deficiency
Achondroplasia, 1738, 1738*b*
    pseudo, 1738
AChR. *see* Acetylcholine receptor (AChR)
Achromatopsia, 123
Acid maltase deficiency
    hypotonic infant due to, 310
    myopathy due to, 1941–1942
Acidosis, lactic, 1354
Acid-sensing ion channels (ASICs), in nociception, 296
aCL (anticardiolipin) antibodies, 947
    and retinal vein occlusion, 947.*e*1*f*
Acoustic neuroma
    acoustic noise and, 1022
    hearing loss due to, 595–597
    in neurofibromatosis, 1546, 1546*f*
Acoustic reflex testing, for hearing loss, 602
Acquired Creutzfeldt-Jakob disease, 1374–1378
Acquired demyelinating polyradiculoneuropathy, 1778, 1778*f*
Acquired horizontal gaze palsy, 564–565
Acquired immunodeficiency syndrome
    cerebral toxoplasmosis in, 1116*f*
    sleep disorders in, 1671
Acquired immunodeficiency syndrome-associated neuropathies, sensory, 320
Acquired neuromyotonia
    channelopathy in, 1536
    muscle hypertrophy due to, 282–283
Acquired ocular motor apraxia, 564
Acquired pendular nystagmus (APN), 544, 546*t*
Acquired supranuclear monocular elevator palsy, 568

Acromegaly, 705, 705b, 1856–1857
  medical management of, 711
  radiotherapy for, 711
Acrylamide, occupational exposure to, 1238
ACST (Asymptomatic Carotid Surgery Trial), 961–962
ACTH. see Adrenocorticotropic hormone (ACTH)
Actigraphy, sleep disorders, 1675–1676, 1677f
Actinomyces spp., meningitis due to, 1147–1148
Action myoclonus, after anoxic-ischemic encephalopathy, 1203t
Action semantics, disturbance in, 117
Action tremor, 218, 230
Actionable Bladder Symptom Screening Tool, 610
Activated protein C (APC) resistance, ischemic stroke due to, 946
Activated rigidity, 227–228
"Activating procedures," for EEG, 350, 351f
Activation, painful stimuli and, 722
Activation factors, in immune response, 682
Activational effects, of neurohormones and neuropeptides, 696
Activation-induced cell death (AICD), 684
Active motor threshold (AMT), in transcranial magnetic stimulation, 392
Activity-dependent plasticity, 722
Actometer, 1675–1676
Acupuncture, in rehabilitation, 802
Acute angle-closure glaucoma, 1694
Acute chorioretinitis, 1157
Acute coronary syndrome, in neurointensive care, 752–753, 753f
Acute disseminated encephalomyelitis (ADEM), 1183
  clinical features of, 1184
  hemiplegia due to, 264
  laboratory and clinical features of, 1184–1185, 1184f
  MRI of, 691
  para-infectious, 1184
  postvaccination, 1184
  seizures due to, 1582–1583
  structural imaging of
    of brain, 440
    of spinal cord, 452, 454f
  versus viral nervous system disease, 1124t
Acute hemorrhagic leukoencephalitis, 1185
Acute illness myopathy, 1955
Acute inflammatory demyelinating polyradiculoneuropathy, sensory abnormalities due to, 319t, 320–321
Acute intermittent porphyria (AIP), psychiatric manifestations of, 103–104
Acute ischemic stroke
  CT angiography of, 461–462, 461f–462f, 462b
  MR angiography of, 472
  power motion-mode Doppler of, 480
  transcranial Doppler of, 480
  ultrasonography of, 480
Acute lymphocytic leukemia, intracerebral hemorrhage due to, 969–971
Acute meningitis, parasitic, 1155
  diagnosis of, 1155, 1156t
  etiology and clinical presentation of, 1155
  management of, 1155
Acute motor axonal neuropathy (AMAN), 1819
Acute motor neuron disease, 1136
Acute motor-sensory axonal neuropathy (AMSAN), 1819

Acute necrotizing myopathy, 1194
Acute pandysautonomia, 1886
Acute promyelocytic leukemia, intracerebral hemorrhage due to, 969–971
Acute quadriplegic myopathy (AQM), 1955
Acute radiation encephalopathy, 1245
Acute-phase proteins, in innate immune system, 676
Acyclovir
  for herpes simplex, 1967
  for viral infections, 1127t
Acylcarnitine profile, in inborn errors of metabolism, 1326t
ADAGIO (Attenuation of Disease Progression with Azilect Given Once-Daily) trial, 1432
Adaptation theory, of sleep, 1628
Adaptive aids, in rehabilitation, 787–788, 788b, 788f
Adaptive immunity, 676–677
ADAS (Alzheimer Disease Assessment Scale), 76, 77t
ADCME (autosomal dominant cortical myoclonus and epilepsy), 1535
Addiction, deep brain stimulation for, 405–406
Addison disease
  due to autonomic disorders, 1890–1891
  neurological complications of, in adults, 833
  neurological complications of, in children, 847
ADEM. see Acute disseminated encephalomyelitis (ADEM)
Adenoma
  pituitary, 707, 707t
    management of, 1061f, 1064
      radiotherapy for, 711
      surgical, 711
    neurological complications of, in adults, 831, 831f
    structural imaging of, 418t–419t, 426–427, 427f, 427.e1f
  sebaceum, in tuberous sclerosis, 1539
Adenosine A$_{2A}$ receptors, in basal ganglia, 1426
Adenosine triphosphate (ATP), in nociception, 296
Adenovirus, 1133–1135
Adenylosuccinate lyase deficiency, 1339
  intellectual disability associated with, 1310t
Adhesive arachnoiditis, chronic, 1763, 1763.e1b
ADI-R (Autism Diagnostic Interview-Revised), 1304
ADNFLE (autosomal dominant nocturnal frontal lobe epilepsy), 1520t–1521t, 1532–1533
Adolescence
  with inborn errors of metabolism, 1333
  stroke in, oral contraceptives and, 1006
Adolescents
  headache in, 1718–1719
    tension-type, 1719
  migraine in, 1718–1719
ADOS-2 (Autism Diagnostic Observation Schedule- 2), 1304
ADPEAF (autosomal dominant partial epilepsy with auditory features), 1520t–1521t
Adrenal glands, neurological complications of, in adults, 833

β-adrenergic blockers
  for exertional headache, 1714
  for migraine prophylaxis, 1702
    chronic, 1707
    menstrual, 1704
Adrenocorticotropic hormone (ACTH), 697t–698t
  in Cushing disease, 706
  hypothalamic peptides controlling release of, 702t
  immunoregulatory effects of, 699t
Adrenocorticotropic hormone (ACTH)-like intermediate lobe peptides, 697t–698t
Adrenocorticotropic hormone (ACTH) deficiency, treatment of, 711
Adrenoleukodystrophy (ALD), 1332, 440.e1, 1326.e1t–1326.e2t, 440.e1f
  genetics and paradox of disease definition in X-linked, 671–672
Adrenomyeloneuropathy (AMN), 1493–1494, 1818.e8–1818.e9
  key characteristics of, 1487t
Adson test, 324–325
Adult hexosaminidase-A deficiency, 1517
Adult polyglucosan body disease, 1517–1518
Adult-onset hydrocephalus, 1275–1276, 1276f
Advance sleep phase state (ASPS), 1654
Adventitious movements, in comatose patient, 46
AEDs. see Antiepileptic drugs (AEDs)
Affective agnosia, 139–140
Affective disorders
  in multiple sclerosis, 1167
  during rehabilitation, 810
    incidence of, 810
    treatment of, 810
Afferent inhibition, short-latency and long latency, in transcranial magnetic stimulation, 393, 394t
Afferent visual system
  ancillary diagnostic techniques, 579–581
    electrophysiology, 579–581
    ophthalmic imaging, 579, 581f
    perimetry, 579, 580f
  neuro-ophthalmological examination of, 573–579, 574f
    color vision testing in, 574
    contrast vision testing in, 574
    light brightness comparison in, 576
    light-stress test in, 574
    pupil examination in, 574–576, 575t, 576b, 576f
    visual acuity examination in, 573–574, 575f
    visual field testing in, 576–577, 577f
  nonorganic (functional) disturbances of, 581–582, 581b
    diagnostic techniques, 581–582
    prognosis, 582
    visual field testing in, 582, 582f
  visual field defects in, 577–579, 577b
    binasal hemianopia as, 578, 578f
    bitemporal hemianopia as, 578
    from chiasmal disease, 578, 578f
    from compressive optic neuropathy, 577, 578f
    homonymous hemianopia as
      congruous, 578–579, 579f
      cortical blindness, 579
      incongruous, 578f
      visual acuity with, 579
    inferior altitudinal, 577, 578f
    monocular temporal crescent syndrome, 578

Afferent visual system (*Continued*)
    from nonarteritic anterior ischemic
        optic neuropathy, 577, 578*f*
    from optic neuritis, 577, 578*f*
    pseudobitemporal hemianopia, 578,
        578*f*
    scotoma
        cecocentral, 577–578, 578*f*
        junctional, 578
Affinity maturation, 679, 682
African American Antiplatelet Stroke
    Prevention Study (AAASPS), 953
African sleeping sickness (trypanosomiasis),
    1155, 1634
    sleep disorders in, 1671
AGAT (arginine:glycine amidinotransferase)
    deficiency, 1341
Age
    and nerve conduction studies, 370
    and sleep patterns, 1621–1622, 1622*f*
    and stroke, 920–921
Age-adjusted rate, 635–636
Age-related involutional changes, structural
    imaging of, 445–446, 446*f*
Age-specific rates, 635–636
Ages and Stages Questionnaire (ASQ), 66
Aggression
    after stroke, 90
    after traumatic brain injury, 91
    in Alzheimer disease, 78
    in autism spectrum disorder, 1307*t*
    in epilepsy, 89
    in Huntington disease, 82*t*, 83
Aging
    EEG with, 359
    falls due to, 20–22
    hearing loss with, 597
    with neurological disabilities, functional
        outcomes with, 813
Agitated delirium, 30
Agitation, in Alzheimer disease, 1398
Agnosia, 122–127
    affective, 139–140
    auditory, 125–127
        amusia as, 126–127
        cortical deafness as, 125
        nonverbal as, 126
        phonagnosia as, 126
        pure word deafness as, 126, 126*f*
    color, 123
    defined, 122
    tactile, 127
        tactile aphasia as, 127
    verbal auditory, in autism spectrum
        disorder, 1302–1303
    visual, 122–125
        Balint syndrome and simultanagnosia
            as, 123
        cortical visual distortions as, 123
        cortical visual disturbances as, 122–123
        Klüver-Bucy syndrome as, 125
        optic aphasia as, 124–125
        prosopagnosia as, 125
        visual object, 123–124
            apperceptive, 123–124, 124*f*
            associative, 124
Agouti-related protein, in appetite, 700
Agrammatic variant, of frontotemporal
    dementia, 522–523
Agrammatism, 131
Agraphesthesia, 127
Agraphia, 139, 140*f*
    alexia with, 138, 139*t*
Agricultural workers, brain tumors in, 1022

Agyria, 1299–1300
AICA (anterior inferior cerebellar artery)
    syndrome, 929
Aicardi syndrome, 1294*t*
AICD. *see* Activation-induced cell death
    (AICD)
AIDS dementia complex (ADC), 1110–1111
Air embolism, ischemic stroke due to, 945
Air-conduction thresholds, 601
Airway assistance, in neurointensive care,
    750–752
Airway management, for acute ischemic
    stroke, 963
Akathisia, 244
Akinesia, 121, 224
Akinetic mutism, 59, 1370
Akinetic-rigid syndrome, 224–225
Akinetopsia, 123
Alberta Stroke Program Early CT Score
    (ASPECTS), 461–462, 462*b*, 462*f*
    posterior circulation (pc)-ASPECTS,
        461–462, 462*f*
Albuminocytological dissociation,
    1818–1819
Alcohol
    and brain tumors, 1023
    and headache, 199
    hypoglycemia and, 1219–1220
Alcohol abuse, seizures due to, 1583
Alcohol block, for trigeminal neuralgia, 1717
Alcohol consumption, as risk factor for
    stroke, 923
Alcohol-related hypersomnolence,
    1634–1635
Alcohol-withdrawal syndromes, 1233–1234
Alcoholic cerebellar degeneration, 1235
Alcoholic neuropathy, 1234, 1852
    clinical features of, 1234
    laboratory studies and pathology of, 1234
    treatment of, 1234
Alcoholism
    ataxia due to, 1461
    neurological complications of, 1233*b*
    other diseases associated with, 1233–
        1235, 1233*b*
Aldosterone, during sleep, 1631, 1631*f*
Alemtuzumab (Campath/Lemtrada), for
    multiple sclerosis, 1178–1179
Alert, 34
Alertness, 23
Alexia
    with agraphia, 138, 139*t*, 927–928
    aphasic, 138–139, 139*f*
    defined, 137–138
    without agraphia, 137–138, 138*f*, 138*t*
Alfentanil, half-life of, 1203*t*
Alice in Wonderland syndrome, 123, 540
Alien hand syndrome, 59–60
Alien limb phenomenon, 121
Alkylating agents
    for brain tumors, 1051, 1052*t*–1053*t*
    reducing resistance to, 1051
Allele, 651*t*
Allen and Ferguson classification system, 888
Allergy(ies)
    and brain tumors, 1023–1024
    functional symptoms in, 1993*t*
Allesthesia, visual, 123
Allgrove syndrome (Four-A Syndrome), 1517
Allodynia, 296, 1777
    cutaneous, in migraine, 1697
    in peripheral nerve disorders, 1795
Allyl chloride, occupational exposure to,
    1238

Almotriptan, for migraine, 1701*t*, 1700.*e*1*t*
    in children and adolescents, 1719
Alopecia, in viral CNS disease, 1124*t*
Alpha activity, sleep staging, 1619*f*
Alpha coma, in hypoxia, 357, 358*f*
Alpha motoneurons, 1494
Alpha rhythm, on EEG, 349–350, 349*f*
Alphaviruses, equine encephalitis viruses as,
    1139
Alprostadil injection, for erectile dysfunction,
    621
ALS. *see* Amyotrophic lateral sclerosis (ALS)
[¹⁸F]Altanserin , in chemical imaging, 506
Alteplase, for acute ischemic stroke, 956–957
Altered peptide ligands (APL), for multiple
    sclerosis, 690
Altered states of consciousness, EEG of,
    356–357
Alternate response tasks, for delirium, 28
Alternate-cover test, for diplopia, 537
Alternating hemiplegia of childhood, 265
    genetic basis for, 1520*t*–1521*t*
    headache due to, 1719
    stroke *versus*, 1002
Alternating leg muscle activation, 1668
Alternating sequence, Luria's test of, 59*f*, 64
"Alternating windmill nystagmus", 542*t*, 547
Aluminum, occupational exposure to, 1242
Aluminum chloride hexahydrate in
    anhydrous ethyl alcohol (Drysol), for
    hyperhidrosis, 1873*t*
Alveolar ventilation, during sleep, 1630*t*
Alzheimer, Alois, 1385–1386
Alzheimer dementia
    genetics of, 663, 663*t*
        copy number variation in, 668*t*
        genome-wide association studies of, 664,
            663.*e*1*t*–663.*e*2*t*
Alzheimer disease (AD), 1385–1399, 1390*f*
    agitation as, 1398
    β-amyloid plaques in, 693
    atypical, 1387–1388
    behavior and personality disturbances in,
        77–79
        aggression as, 78
        apathy as, 78
        atypical antipsychotics for, 77
        depression as, 78, 78*t*
        environmental interventions for, 77–78
        psychosis as, 78–79, 79*f*, 79*t*
        redirection for, 77–78, 78*t*
        versus schizophrenia, 79*t*
    behavioral observations in, 521
    biomarkers in, 1391–1394
        hypothetical model for, 1393*f*
        longitudinal tracking of, 1393–1394
    clinical features, 1387
    clinical presentation of
        cognitive deficits in, 521
        memory deficits in, 521
    diagnosis of
        biomarkers, 1411*f*, 1418–1419
        biopsy studies, 1419
        diagnostic criteria and, 1419
        functional, 488–490, 488*f*–489*f*
        imaging
            chemical, 508–509, 508*f*
            structural, 1391, 1391*f*
        neurological examination, 1384–1385
    diagnostic approach in, 1383–1385
    diagnostic criteria for, 521, 1389
    differential diagnosis of, *versus* dementia
        with Lewy bodies, 490–491
    EEG of, 359

Alzheimer disease (AD) *(Continued)*
  epidemiology of, 1386–1387
  frontal variant, 1388
  genetics, 1394
  hippocampal sparing, 1397
  historical background of, 1384*t*,
      1385–1386
  immune mediation in, 693
  language in, 140
  and mild cognitive impairment, 490
  mitochondrial disorders, 1363
  National Institute on Aging Criteria for
      Preclinical, 1381*t*
  neurofibrillary tangles in, 693
  neuropsychiatric features of, 1388–1389
  neuropsychological characteristics of, 521
  neuropsychology, dementia, 1389–1391
  pathology of, 1395–1397, 1396*f*
  patient safety, 1398–1399
  psychiatric manifestations of, 106
  seizures due to, 1583
  sleep dysfunction in, 1634
      treatment of, 1685*b*
  smell loss and, 194
  structural imaging of, 446, 446.e1*f*
  subjective cognitive impairment, 1382–
      1383, 1385*t*
  transcranial magnetic stimulation for, 396
  treatment, 1397–1399
Alzheimer Disease Assessment Scale (ADAS),
    76, 77*t*
Alzheimer type II astrocyte, in hepatic
    encephalopathy, 1215
Amantadine (Symmetrel)
  for chronic disorder of consciousness, 55
  for fatigue, in multiple sclerosis, 1182
  for neuropathic pain, 918*t*–919*t*
  for Parkinson disease, 1433*t*–1434*t*
Amaurosis fugax, 927
  due to giant-cell arteritis, 1692
Amblyopia
  developmental, 529
  tobacco-alcohol or nutritional, 1234
Ambulation, after stroke, 811
Amerge, for migraine, 1701*t*
American Spinal Injury Association/
    International Medical Society of
    Paraplegia (ASIA/IMSOP) Impairment
    Scale, 883, 883*b*
American trypanosomiasis, associated with
    peripheral neuropathy, 1864.e6–1864.e7
Amine precursor uptake and decarboxylation
    (APUD) cells, 712
Amino acid analysis, in inborn errors of
    metabolism, 1326*t*
Amino acids
  in chemical imaging, 505*t*, 506
  for hepatic encephalopathy, 1212,
      1215–1216
Aminoacidopathies, 1335
γ-Aminobutyric acid
  in basal ganglia, 1422–1423
  in REM sleep, 1624.e1*f*
γ-Aminobutyric acid (GABA)-
    benzodiazepine, in hepatic
    encephalopathy, 1212
γ-Aminobutyric acid (GABA)$_A$ receptors, in
    chemical imaging, 505*t*, 506
  of epilepsy, 509
Amiodarone
  myopathy due to, 1954
  neuropathy due to, 1858–1860
Amitriptyline (Elavil)
  for chronic pain, 725*t*
  for depression, in multiple sclerosis,
      1183

Amitriptyline (Elavil) *(Continued)*
  for migraine prophylaxis, 1702–1703
    chronic, 1707
  for neuropathic pain, 918*t*–919*t*
  for tension-type headache, 1713
AML (angiomyolipoma), renal, in tuberous
    sclerosis, 1542–1543
Ammonia
  alternative pathways to reduce
      accumulation of, 1331*f*
  in hepatic encephalopathy, 1212, 1214*f*
  in inborn errors of metabolism, 1326*t*
Amnesia
  anterograde, 62
  retrograde, 62
    functional, 2002
    transient, 63
      global, 926
      versus epilepsy, 1590
Amnestic shellfish poisoning (ASP), 1253
Amnestic syndromes, 61–63, 62*b*, 1408
Amniotic fluid embolism, ischemic stroke
    due to, 945
Amphetamines, and stroke in children,
    1000–1001
Amphiphilic drug myopathy, 1954
  due to amiodarone, 1954
  due to chloroquine, 1954
Amphiphysin antibody, blood tests for, 344
Ampicillin, for neonatal meningitis, 1965
Amsler grid, in visual field testing, 577,
    577*f*
AMT (α-[^{11}C] Methyl-L-tryptophan), in
    chemical imaging, 506
  of epilepsy, 509
AMT (active motor threshold), in
    transcranial magnetic stimulation, 392
Amusia, 126–127
Amusia, 126–127
Amygdala
  in behavior and personality disturbances,
      73–75
  in memory, 61, 62*f*
Amyloid, CNS vasculitis due to, 1017
Amyloid angiopathy, cerebral
  intracerebral hemorrhage due to, 971–972
  ischemic stroke due to, 945
  microbleeds in, 974*f*
Amyloid deposition
  in chemical imaging, 505*t*, 506
  of Alzheimer disease, 508–509, 508*f*
  in inclusion body myositis, 1952–1953,
      1953*f*
Amyloid hypothesis, 1395
Amyloid imaging, 1392
Amyloid neuropathy
  bowel dysfunction due to, 612.e1
  neurogenic bladder dysfunction due to,
      611–612
  sensory abnormalities due to, 320
Amyloid plaques, in Alzheimer disease,
    1396
β-Amyloid plaques, in Alzheimer disease,
    693
Amyloid polyneuropathy, familial,
    1818.e4–1818.e5, 1818.e4*t*
  apolipoprotein A1 amyloidosis, 1818.e5
  diagnosis of, 1818.e5
  gelsolin amyloidosis, 1818.e5
  transthyretin, 1818.e4–1818.e5
  treatment of, 1818.e5
Amyloid precursor protein (APP)
  chromosome 21, 1394, 1395*f*
Amyloidogenic pathway, 1395
Amyloidopathy, in sleep disorder, 1656*f*
Amyloidosis, neurological complications of,
    825

Amyotrophic lateral sclerosis (ALS), 5,
    1506–1515
  adult hexosaminidase-A deficiency, 1517
  adult polyglucosan body disease,
      1517–1518
  Allgrove syndrome (Four-A Syndrome),
      1517
  atypical features of, 1509–1510
  behavior and personality disturbances in,
      83–84
    depression as, 85, 85*f*
    personality change as, 85–86
    pseudobulbar affect as, 85
  classification of, 1507*b*
  clinical features of, 1508–1509
    atypical, 1509–1510
    cognitive impairment as, 1509
    dysphagia as, 155, 1509
    facial and bulbar weakness as, 280
    flail arm or flail person in the barrel
        variant in, 1508
    foot drop as, 1508
    frontotemporal dementia as, 1509
    head drop as, 1508, 1509*f*
    hemiplegia as, 267
    joint contractures, 1509
    monomelic presentation as, 1508
    muscle cramps as, 1508
    muscle weakness as, 1508
    pseudobulbar palsy as, 1508
    pseudoneuritic presentation (flail leg)
        as, 1510
    respiratory failure as, 1514
    sialorrhea as, 1508
    spasticity as, 1508
    tongue atrophy as, 1509*f*
  copy number variation in, 668*t*
  diagnosis of, 1511
    diagnostic classification of, 383
    needle electromyography of, 383
  differential diagnosis of, 1511–1512, 1511*t*
    versus benign focal amyotrophy, 1499
    versus Kennedy disease, 1503*b*,
        1504–1505
    versus progressive muscular atrophy,
        1505–1506
  etiology of, 1507–1508
    aberrant RNA processing in, 1508
    glutamate excitotoxicity and free radical
        injury in, 1507–1508
    immunological and inflammatory
        abnormalities in, 1508
    mitochondrial dysfunction in, 1508
    neurofilament and microtubule
        dysfunction in, 1508
    protein aggregation in, 1507
  familial, 1515–1516
  genome-wide association studies of,
      663.e1*t*–663.e2*t*
  heritability of, 663, 663*t*
  human immunodeficiency virus type
      1-associated motor neuron disorder,
      1518
  immune mediation in, 693
  laboratory studies of, 1510–1511
  microglia in, 693
  natural history of disease, 1510
  neurodegenerative disorders, 1342
  paraneoplastic motor neuron disease,
      1518
  Parkinsonism-Dementia complex,
      1516–1517
  pathology of, 1507
  prognosis of, 1510
  rTMS for, 399–400
  sleep dysfunction in, 1659

Amyotrophic lateral sclerosis (ALS)
(Continued)
spinocerebellar ataxia type 3 (Machado-Joseph disease), 1517
sporadic or acquired, 1507b
symptomatic, 714
treatment of, 1512–1515, 1512b, 1513t
aggressive symptomatic in, 1513–1514
home care and hospice care in, 1514–1515
multidisciplinary team approach in, 1514
nutritional care in, 1514
physical rehabilitation in, 1514
presentation of the diagnosis in, 1512
respiratory care in, 1514
specific pharmacotherapy in, 1512–1513
speech and communication management in, 1514
treatment of, ethical considerations in, 716
Western Pacific, 1516–1517
Amyotrophy
diabetic, monoplegia due to, 272
monomelic, monoplegia due to, 272
neuralgic, hereditary, 1818
Anabolic-androgen steroid abuse, ischemic stroke due to, 939
Analgesia, in neurointensive care, 749–750, 751t
Analgesics
and medication overuse headache, 1707
opioid, for chronic pain, 727–729, 727t
for traumatic brain injury, 875t–876t
Anaplasia, 1028
Anaplasma phagocytophilum, meningitis due to, 1147–1148
Anaplastic astrocytoma, 418t–419t, 420–421
Anarthria, 145
Anatomical localizations, 1, 5–6
Ancrod, for acute ischemic stroke, 960
Andersen-Tawil syndrome (ATS), 1520t–1521t, 1527
skeletal muscle disorders in, 1939
Androgen-insensitivity syndrome, 1504
Anemia
in autonomic disorders, 1872
megaloblastic, neurological complications of, 824
neurological complications of, 824
pernicious, 1226
causes of, 1226–1227
laboratory studies for, 1227
Anencephaly, 1282, 1293
Anergy, due to failure of T-cell activation, in self-tolerance, 684, 685f
Anesthesia, and intraoperative monitoring, 410
Anesthesia dolorosa, 1716
Anesthetic management, with myasthenia gravis, 1909
Anesthetics, for traumatic brain injury, 875t–876t
Aneuploidy, 656
Aneurysmal subarachnoid hemorrhage, ultrasound of, 482–483, 483f
Aneurysms
aortic, 818
coiled intracranial, 472–473
lumbosacral plexopathy and, 1789
mycotic, cerebral, due to infective endocarditis, 817–818, 817f
posterior communicating artery, 1721–1723

Aneurysms (Continued)
postoperative, 464
pseudo-, traumatic, 867
recurrence of, MRA imaging of, 472–473, 473f
traumatic, 867
"Angel dust", 1258
Angelman syndrome, 662, 662f
copy number variation in, 668t
Angiitis
in adults, 821
CNS, ischemic stroke due to, 941–942
granulomatous, intracerebral hemorrhage due to, 972–974
primary
of CNS
in children, 841
postpartum, 1989
and stroke in children, 1000
Angioendotheliomatosis, neoplastic, ischemic stroke due to, 944
Angiofibromas, facial, in tuberous sclerosis, 1539
Angiogenesis inhibitors, for brain tumors, 1053–1054, 1054b
Angiography
cerebral, 202
digital subtraction, for carotid artery stenosis, 460f, 463
Angiokeratoma corporis diffusum, 943, 1818.e7
Angiomas
facial cutaneous, in Sturge-Weber syndrome, 1546
retinal, in von Hippel-Lindau disease, 178, 178f
Angiomyolipoma (AML), renal, in tuberous sclerosis, 1542–1543, 1543f
Angiopathy, cerebral, 1016
amyloid
intracerebral hemorrhage due to, 971–972
ischemic stroke due to, 945
microbleeds in, 974f
Angioplasty and stenting
for carotid artery disease, 763–765
for ischemic stroke, 762–763
Angiostrongylus cantonensis, acute meningitis due to, 1155
Angiotensin, 697t–698t
Angiotropic lymphoma, ischemic stroke due to, 944
Anglo-Scandinavian Cardiac Outcomes Trial-Lipid Lowering Arm (ASCOT-LLA) studies, 922
Angular velocity, in rotational testing, 600, 600f
Angulated fibers, with denervation, 1916, 1916f
Anhedonia, 1994
ANI (asymptomatic neurocognitive impairment), HIV-associated, 1110–1111
Animal models, in inborn errors of metabolism, 1333
Animal neurotoxins, 1247–1249
from snakes, 1248
Animal toxins, 1914
from snake, 1914
Anion gap, in inborn errors of metabolism, 1326t
Aniridia, copy number variation in, 668t
Aniseikonia, 533

Anisocoria, 574
due to efferent pathological conditions, 180
episodic, 186
evaluation of, 182f
greater in dark, 184–186
due to Horner syndrome, 184–185, 184f–185f
due to iritis, 185–186
due to pupillary light-near dissociation, 186
episodic, 186
greater in light, 180–184
due to iris sphincter injury and ischemia, 183
due to pharmacological mydriasis, 183–184
due to postganglionic parasympathetic dysfunction, 180–182, 183f
due to preganglionic parasympathetic dysfunction, 182–183
physiological (central, simple, benign), 179
Anisoiconia, 533
Anisotropic diffusion, 417.e4
Ankle-foot orthoses, 789, 790f
Ankylosing hyperostosis, 1751
Ankylosing spondylitis
clinical presentation of, 1762
pathogenesis of, 1762
spinal neurological complications of, 1762, 1762t, 1762.e1f–1762.e2f
ANNAs (antineuronal antibodies), in paraneoplastic neurological syndromes, 1187
ANO5 gene, 1926
Anodal conduction block, 366
Anomia, 130
color, 123
optic, 124–125
Anomic aphasia, 134–135, 136t
Anorectal angle, in control of defecation, 606
Anorexia nervosa, 701
Anosmia, 193
Anosognosia, 927–928
after traumatic brain injury, 90
in frontotemporal dementia, 79–80
Anoxic-ischemic encephalopathy, 1201–1208
approach to prediction of prognosis for, 1203–1205, 1205b, 1205f
clinical examination for, 1202–1203, 1203t
clinical syndromes after, 1203t
laboratory and electrophysiological testing for, 1205–1206
management of, 1203, 1204b, 1204f, 1204t
pathophysiological concepts of, 1201–1202, 1202f
sedative and analgesic medications and, 1203t
Anoxic vegetative state, 54
Antalgic gaits, 261
Anterior cerebral artery (ACA), infarction of, hemiplegia due to, 264
Anterior cerebral artery ischemia, drop attacks due to, 18
Anterior cerebral artery syndromes, 928, 928f
Anterior choroidal artery syndrome, 928
Anterior cingulate circuit, 96
Anterior cingulate cortex, in delirium, 26
Anterior column, 889

Anterior communicating artery
  CT angiography of, 988*f*
  with vasospasm, 994*f*
Anterior communicating artery aneurysm
  syndrome, amnestic syndrome and,
  62–63
Anterior cord syndrome, 884, 884*f*
Anterior ethmoidal nerve, 1721*f*
Anterior horn cell disorders, needle
  electromyography of, 382*f*, 383
Anterior horn syndrome, 274
Anterior inferior cerebellar artery syndrome,
  214*b*, 215*f*, 929
Anterior interosseous nerve syndrome, 270,
  1804
Anterior ischemic optic neuropathy
  arteritic, optic disc in, 167
  nonarteritic, 163–165
    fundus photograph of, 168*f*
    optic disc edema due to, 163–165
    visual field defects in, 165*f*, 577, 578*f*
    visual loss due to, 159–161
Anterior limb of internal capsule (ALIC),
  lesioning of, 405
Anterior median spinal vein,
  1007.*e1*–1007.*e2*
Anterior medulloradicular arteries, 1007.*e1f*
Anterior operculum syndrome, dysphagia in,
  152–153
Anterior pituitary, 703–707
  hyperfunction of, 704–706
    Cushing disease and Nelson syndrome
      due to, 705–706, 706*b*, 711
    due to gonadotropin-secreting tumors,
      706, 711
    excessive secretion of thyroid-
      stimulating hormone due to, 706,
      711
    gigantism and acromegaly due to, 705,
      705*b*, 711
    hyperprolactinemia due to, 704–705,
      705*b*, 710–711
    precocious puberty due to, 704–706
  hypofunction of, 703–706, 704*b*, 704*t*
  hypophysitis of, 707
  hypothalamic control of, 702*t*, 703
  other tumors of, 707
  tumors and hyperplasia of, 707, 707*t*
    medical management of, 710–711
    radiotherapy for, 711
    surgery for, 711
Anterior radiculomedullary veins,
  1007.*e1*–1007.*e2*
Anterior spinal artery (ASA), anatomy of,
  1007.*e1*, 1007.*e1f*
Anterior spinal artery (ASA) syndrome, 274,
  1007
"Anterior subcortical aphasia syndrome",
  136
Anterior sulcal artery, 1007.*e1*, 1007.*e1f*
Anterior thalamic nucleus, in memory, 62*f*
Anterior tibial compartment syndrome, 1809
Anthracenones, in plants, 1250*t*
Anti-AMPA receptor encephalitis, 1198–1199
  brain MRI of, 1198–1199
  immunotherapy for, 1199
Antiapoptotic agents, for traumatic brain
  injury, 857, 858*f*
Antibiotics, for hepatic encephalopathy, 1216
Antibodies
  in adaptive immune response, 677
  blood tests for, 344
  paraneoplastic antineuronal, 1187
Antibody-associated neurological syndromes,
  694–695
Antibody-mediated diseases, 686–687

Antibody screening, for toxoplasmosis, 1967
Anticardiolipin (aCL) antibodies, 947
  and retinal vein occlusion, 947.*e1f*
Anti-CASPR2 associated encephalitis, 1199
Anticholinergic agent, for vertigo, 603–604,
  603*t*
Anticholinergic intoxication, delirium due
  to, 30
Anticholinesterase drugs, for myasthenia
  gravis, 1904*t*
Anticipation
  defined, 651*t*
  in Kennedy disease, 1504
  in myotonic dystrophy, 289–290, 1934,
    1977
Anticoagulants
  intracerebral hemorrhage due to, 969–971
    management of, 980
  for preventing stroke recurrence, 954–955
Anticoagulation
  with atrial fibrillation, 815
  during pregnancy, 1988
Anticonvulsants, for chronic pain, 725–726
Anti-CV2 antibody, blood tests for, 344
Antidepressants
  for chronic pain, 723–726, 725*t*
  for functional symptoms, 2007–2008
  for migraine prophylaxis, 1702–1703
    in children and adolescents, 1719
    menstrual, 1704
  for neuropathic pain, 918*t*–919*t*
  tricyclic, 111–112
    for chronic pain, 723–725, 725*t*
Anti-DPPX encephalitis, 1199–1200
Antiemetics, for migraine in children and
  adolescents, 1719
Antiepileptic drugs (AEDs), 1984
  and anxiety, 88
  for brain metastases, 1086
  and depression, 88
  for epilepsy
    absorption, elimination half-life,
      formulations of, 1600*t*
    adverse effects of, 1605
    based on age and gender, 1602
    discontinuation of, 1606
    efficacy by seizure type of, 1601*t*
    hepatic metabolism, enzyme induction/
      inhibition, pharmacokinetic
      interactions, and protein binding
      in, 1603*t*
    initiation of, 1599–1602
    mechanism of action of, 1604*t*
    pharmacoresistance, tolerance, and
      seizure aggravation with,
      1602–1605
    therapeutic drug monitoring in,
      1605–1606
  for migraine prophylaxis, 1703
  for neuropathic pain, 918*t*–919*t*
  and neuropsychological functioning, 526
  psychotropic effects of, 88, 89*t*
  teratogenic effect of, 1985
  transcranial magnetic stimulation for, 396
  for traumatic brain injury, 91
Antifolates, for brain tumors, 1051,
  1052*t*–1053*t*
Anti-GABA_A receptor encephalitis, 1199
Anti-GABA_B receptor encephalitis, 1198
Antigen presentation, 681
  in CNS, 686
Antigen-presenting cells (APCs)
  in CNS, 685
  innate immune system, 676
Antigen receptor, gene rearrangements of,
  679

Antigen recognition, of cytotoxic and helper
  T cells, 680*f*
Antigliadin antibodies, blood tests for, 344
Anti-glutamic acid decarboxylase antibodies,
  ataxia and, 1464
Antihistamines, for vertigo, 603–604, 603*t*
Anti-Hu antibody, blood tests for, 344
Antihypertensive therapy, for intracerebral
  hemorrhage, 981
Anti-idiotypic responses, 684
Anti-inflammatory medications, for
  Alzheimer disease, 1398
Anti-intrinsic factor antibodies, in cobalamin
  deficiency, 1227
Anti-LGI1 limbic encephalitis, 1199
Anti-Ma1 antibody, blood tests for, 344
Anti-Ma2 antibody, blood tests for, 344
Antimicrotubular myopathies, 1954
Antimicrotubule agents, for brain tumors,
  1052*t*–1053*t*
Anti-muscarinic medications, for neurogenic
  bladder, 617, 617*t*
Antineuronal antibodies, blood tests for,
  344
Anti-NMDAR encephalitis, 1196–1198, 1198*f*
  diagnosis of, 1198
  symptoms of, 1196–1197
  treatment for, 1200
Anti-parietal cell antibodies, in cobalamin
  deficiency, 1227
Antiphospholipid (aPL) antibodies
  diseases associated with, 947, 947.*e1f*
  as risk factor for stroke, 924
Antiphospholipid antibody, oral
  contraceptives and, 1974
Antiphospholipid antibody syndrome
  during pregnancy, 1988
  and stroke in children, 1005–1006
Antiphospholipid (aPL) antibody syndrome
  (APAS), 694
  diagnosis of, 947
  ischemic stroke due to, 947
  migraines due to, 942
  neurological complications of, 827, 827*f*
  treatment of, 947
Antipsychotic side effects, 112.*e1t*
Antipsychotics, 1403
  atypical, for Alzheimer disease, 77
Antiquitin, 1231
Antiretroviral therapy, for HIV disease,
  1106–1107, 1108*t*–1109*t*
Anti-Ri antibody, blood tests for, 344
Antiseizure prophylaxis, for traumatic brain
  injury, 875*t*–876*t*
Antisense strand, 649, 650*f*, 651*t*
Anti-striational muscle antibodies (StrAbs),
  in myasthenia gravis, 1902
Antithrombin deficiency, ischemic stroke due
  to, 945–946
Antithrombotic therapy, for cerebral
  ischemia, 957*t*
Antithyroglobulin antibodies, 102–103
Antithyroid microsomal antibodies, 102–103
Antithyroid peroxidase antibodies, 102–103
α_1-Antitrypsin deficiency, and stroke in
  children, 1001
Anti-Yo antibodies, 1189
Anton syndrome, 122, 161
  inverse, 122
Antoni A areas, 1041
Antoni B areas, 1041
Anxiety
  after traumatic brain injury, 91, 91*t*
  in Alzheimer disease, 1403
  in autism spectrum disorder, 1307*t*
  in epilepsy, 88

Autosomal dominant ataxias, 1471–1479
  episodic, 1471
  gene mutations and phenotype-genotype
    correlations in, 1473–1477, 1473*f*,
    1474*t*
  imaging and other laboratory studies in,
    1472, 1472*f*–1473*f*
  neuropathology of, 1472–1473
  pathogenesis of, 1478–1479, 1478*f*
  spinocerebellar, clinical features of,
    1471–1472, 1471*t*
Autosomal dominant cortical myoclonus
  and epilepsy (ADCME), 1535
Autosomal dominant disorders, 657–658,
  658*f*
Autosomal dominant epilepsy with auditory
  features (ADEAF), 1578
Autosomal dominant lateral temporal
  epilepsy, in anti-LGI1 limbic
  encephalitis, 1199
Autosomal dominant leukodystrophy, copy
  number variation in, 668*t*
Autosomal dominant nocturnal frontal lobe
  epilepsy (ADNFLE), 1520*t*–1521*t*,
  1532–1533
Autosomal dominant partial epilepsy with
  auditory features (ADPEAF),
  1520*t*–1521*t*
Autosomal dominant polycystic kidney
  disease, intracranial aneurysm in,
  983–984
Autosomal recessive ataxia, with ocular
  motor apraxia, 564
Autosomal recessive cerebellar ataxias
  (ARCA), 1465–1470, 1465*t*
  with abetalipoproteinemia, 1468
  ataxia-telangiectasia as, 1468–1469,
    1468*f*
  ataxia-telangiectasia-like disorder as, 1469
  Cayman, 1468
  of Charlevoix-Saguenay, 1469
  in childhood and young adult-onset
    metabolic disorders, 1470, 1470*t*
  Friedreich, 1465–1467, 1465*t*, 1466*f*
  in infantile-onset spinocerebellar ataxia,
    1467
  with isolated vitamin E deficiency,
    1467–1468
  with Marinesco-Sjögren syndrome, 1469
  in mitochondrial, 1467
  with oculomotor apraxia
    type 1, 1469
    type 2, 1469
  other DNA repair defects causing, 1469
  type 1, 1469–1470
  type 2, 1470
Autosomal recessive cerebellar ataxias type 1
  (ARCA1), 1469–1470
Autosomal recessive cerebellar ataxias type 2
  (ARCA2), 1470
Autosomal recessive disorders, 658, 660*f*
Autosomal recessive hereditary inclusion
  body myopathy, 1933–1934
Autosomal recessive spastic ataxia of
  Charlevoix-Saguenay (ARSACS), 1469
AV (atrioventricular block), syncope due to,
  10
[¹⁸F]AV-45, in Alzheimer disease, 508–509
Avanafil, for erectile dysfunction, 632
AVDO₂. *see* Arteriovenous oxygen difference
  (AVDO₂)
AVED (ataxia with isolated vitamin E
  deficiency), 1467–1468
Avellis syndrome, 1722*t*, 1732

AVM. *see* Arteriovenous malformation (AVM)
Awareness, 23
A-waves of Lundberg, in intracranial pressure
  monitoring, 745, 745*f*
Axert, for migraine, 1701*t*
Axial dystonia, 235
Axial muscle weakness, 280
Axillary freckling, in neurofibromatosis type
  1, 1544, 1545*f*
Axon discontinuity conduction block, 910
Axonal degeneration, 1792, 1793*f*
Axonal dysfunction, sports and performance
  concussion and, 861
Axonal injury, traumatic, 853–854, 854*f*
Axonal polyneuropathies
  needle electromyography of, 383
  nerve conduction studies of, 375, 375*f*
Axonal shearing, 855
Axonal transport, abnormalities, 1347
Axon-loss mononeuropathy
  needle electromyography of, 383
  nerve conduction studies of, 374, 374*f*
Axonopathy, 1792, 1793*f*
Axonotmesis, 371–373, 905, 1801
Axons
  growth of, 1288–1289
  myelinated, 371
    versus demyelinated, 1159–1160, 1160*f*
  of peripheral nerve, 903–904, 904*f*
  tangential migration along, 1284–1286
AZA. *see* Azathioprine (AZA)
Azathioprine (AZA)
  for dermatomyositis, polymyositis, and
    immune-mediated necrotizing
    myopathy, 1951–1952
  for myasthenia gravis, 1903*t*, 1906

B
B cells
  in immune system, 677–678
  in multiple sclerosis, 1162
  and T-helper cells, 682
B value, in diffusion-weighted imaging,
  415
B7-CD28 pathways, in T-cell activation, 681,
  681*f*
B19 parvovirus, 1135
Babinski-Nageotte syndrome, 1722*t*,
  1734
Baclofen
  for chronic pain, 726, 734
  for dystonia, 1452*t*
  for neuropathic pain, 918*t*–919*t*
  for spasticity, 799*t*
    in multiple sclerosis, 1182
Bacterial infections, 1147–1152
  brain abscess as, 1150–1151
    clinical presentation of, 1150
    diagnosis of, 1150, 1151*f*
    management of, 1149*t*, 1150–1151
    risk factors for, 1150
  meningitis as, 1147–1150
    clinical presentation of, 1148
    diagnosis of, 1148–1149
    etiology of, 1147–1148
    management of, 1149–1150,
      1149*t*–1150*t*
    pathogens of, 1148*t*
    versus viral, 1149
  and neuropathy, 1864.*e*4–1864.*e*6
  spinal epidural abscess as, 1151–1152
    clinical presentation of, 1151
    diagnosis of, 1151–1152, 1152*f*

Bacterial infections (*Continued*)
    etiology of, 1151
    management of, 1149*t*, 1152
    risk factors for, 1151
  versus viral nervous system disease, 1124*t*
Bacterial meningitis, 1147–1150
  acute, 1147
  in children, 1147
  clinical presentation of, 1148
  diagnosis of, 1148–1149
  etiology of, 1147–1148
  management of, 1149–1150, 1149*t*–1150*t*
  neoplastic, 1149
  pathogens of, 1148*t*
  recurrent, 1763
  and stroke in children, 1000
  subacute or chronic, 1147–1148
  versus viral, 1149
Bacteroides spp., brain abscess from, 1150
Bailey, Percival, 1026–1027
Balamuthia mandrillaris, 1156*t*
  granulomatous amebic encephalitis due
    to, 1155
Balance
  neural substrate of, 20–22
  in screening neurological examination, 5*t*
Balanced forearm orthosis, 787–788
Balint syndrome, 123, 1387–1388
Ballism, 240, 240*b*, 1449–1450
Ballistic movements, for functional tremor,
  1998
Balloon angioplasty, for cerebral vasospasm,
  774, 774*f*, 994–995
Balloon cells, in tuberous sclerosis, 1540
Balloon remodeling, for cerebral aneurysms,
  770, 770*f*–771*f*
Ball-valve tumor, and headache, 1688
Balo concentric sclerosis, 1175, 1175*f*
Baltic myoclonus, 1579
Band heterotopia, 1300.*e*2
Banna virus, 1139
Barany, Robert, 583
Barbiturates, 1256*b*
  drug dependence with, 1256
  psychotropic effects of, 89*t*
Bariatric surgery
  complications after, 1235–1236
  neuropathy and, 1854–1855
Barium swallow test, modified, for
  dysphagia, 157
Baroreceptors, 1868
Baroreflex failure, 1883–1885,
  1883*f*–1884*f*
  acute, 1883
  chronic, 1883–1884
Baroreflex function, tests of, 1872–1874,
  1874*t*
Bartholin glands, 624
Bartter syndrome, 1520*t*–1521*t*
Basal bodies, in ependymoma, 1036
Basal energy expenditure (BEE), in
  neurointensive care, 755
Basal ganglia
  anatomy, 1423
  biochemistry of, 1425–1426, 1426*t*
  functional organization of,
    1423–1425
  in memory, 61
  motor system anatomy of, 262
  movement disorders and, 1422–1426,
    1425*f*
Basal ganglia aphasia, 136
Basal ganglia calcification, mitochondrial
  disorders, 1355–1356

Basal ganglia disorders, 223
  dysphagia in, 154–155
  falls due to, 20
Basal ganglia lesions, 608–609
  bowel dysfunction due to, 609.e1
  multiple system atrophy due to, 609
  Parkinson disease due to, 608–609
  pure autonomic failure due to, 609
  sexual dysfunction due to, 609
Base rate information, in neuropsychological
    evaluation, 514
Basilar artery aneurysms
  imaging of, 986f, 992f
  stent-assisted coil embolization for, 992f
  symptoms of, 990
Basilar artery migraine, syncope due to, 12
Basilar artery occlusion, 481
  pc-ASPECTS for, 462, 462f
Basilar artery stenosis
  three-dimensional contrast magnetic
    resonance angiography of, 469, 469f
  vertigo due to, 603
Basilar impression, 1740, 1740.e1f
Basilar invagination, 1740
Basilar membrane, 585
Basilar migraine, 1697, 1878
Basilar syndrome, 930
Bassen-Kornzweig syndrome, 1229, 1338,
    1818.e9
Batson plexus, 1007.e2
Battle's sign, with coma, 39
[18F]BAY94-9172, in Alzheimer disease,
    508–509
B-cell activation, accessory molecules for,
    682
B-cell inhibition, 684
B-cell lymphoma, peripheral neuropathy
    associated with, 1192–1193
B-cell-mediated autoimmune disease,
    686–687
BCL-6, in CNS lymphoma, 1042
BCNU, for brain tumors, 1052t–1053t
BDI (Beck Depression Inventory), 76, 76t
Beals syndrome, 1739
Beck Depression Inventory (BDI), 76, 76t
Becker muscular dystrophy (BMD),
    1923–1924
  clinical characteristics of, 1923
  copy number variation in, 668t
  diagnosis of, 1923–1924
  leg weakness in, 291
  molecular defects of, 1919–1924,
    1920t–1921t
  treatment of, 1924
Becker myotonia, 1526
Becker nevus associated with extracutaneous
    involvement, 1553
BEE. see Basal energy expenditure (BEE)
BEHAVE-AD (Behavioral Pathology in
    Alzheimer Disease Rating Scale), 76, 77t
Behavior, changes in, due to brain tumor,
    1047
Behavior and personality disturbances,
    73–91
  after stroke, 89–90
    aggression as, 90
    depression as, 89–90
    pseudobulbar affect as, 90
    psychosis as, 90
  after traumatic brain injury, 90–91,
    90t–91t
    anosognosia as, 90
    anxiety as, 91
    apathy as, 91
    depression as, 90–91
    personality change as, 91

Behavior and personality disturbances
    (Continued)
  in Alzheimer disease, 77–91
    aggression as, 78
    apathy as, 78
    atypical antipsychotics for, 77
    depression as, 78, 78t
    environmental interventions for,
    77–78
    psychosis as, 78–79, 79f, 79t
    redirection for, 77–78, 78t
    versus schizophrenia, 79t
  amygdala in, 73–75
  in amyotrophic lateral sclerosis, 83–84
    depression as, 85, 85f
    personality change as, 85–86
    pseudobulbar affect as, 85
  assessment of, 75–76, 77t
  associated with cerebral dysfunction,
    77–91
  with cerebral dysfunction, 75–76
  in dementia with Lewy bodies, 82
    psychosis as, 82
  in epilepsy, 86–89, 88t, 526
    aggression as, 89
    anxiety as, 88
    depression as, 88, 89t
    psychosis as, 88–89
  frontosubcortical circuitry and, 73–75,
    74b, 74f, 74t–75t
  in frontotemporal dementia, 79–80,
    522
    anosognosia as, 79–80
    behavioral disruption as, 79
    relationship to anatomy, 80
  in Huntington disease, 82–83, 82t
    aggression as, 83
    apathy as, 83
    depression as, 82–83
    obsessive-compulsive traits as, 83
    psychosis as, 83
    suicide as, 83
  with motor circuit dysfunction, 74b
  in multiple sclerosis, 83–84
    anxiety as, 84, 84b
    depression as, 83–84
    euphoria as, 84
    pseudobulbar affect as, 84, 85t
  in Parkinson disease, 80–82, 80t
    apathy as, 81
    depression as, 81
    impulse control disorders as, 81
    neuropsychiatric effects of deep brain
    stimulation in, 81–82, 82.e1t–
    82.e3t, 82.e4b
    psychosis as, 81, 81t
  prevalence of, 73, 74t
  in Tourette syndrome, 83
  in vascular dementia, 80
    additional disorders in, 80
    depression as, 80
Behavioral abnormalities, in delirium, 26
Behavioral disabilities, during rehabilitation,
    804–810
Behavioral disorders, during rehabilitation,
    809–810
    treatments in, 809–810, 809b–810b
Behavioral disruption, in frontotemporal
    dementia, 79
Behavioral impairment, structural imaging
    for, 458.e5
Behavioral Pathology in Alzheimer
    Disease Rating Scale (BEHAVE-AD),
    76, 77t
Behavioral variant frontotemporal dementia
    (bvFTD), 79

Behçet disease, neurological complications
    of
  in adults, 822
  in children, 841
Behçet syndrome, ischemic stroke due to,
    940
Beighton score, 1737–1738, 1738t
Bell palsy, in pregnancy, 1978
Bell phenomenon, 563, 1729–1730
  with combined vertical gaze
    ophthalmoplegia, 205
  variant of, 565
Bell's Palsy, 1722t, 1730
Benediction posture, 1805
Benedikt syndrome, 929–930, 1721, 1722t
Benign calf amyotrophy, 1498
Benign congenital hypotonia, 309
Benign epilepsy
  with centrotemporal spikes, 1574, 1575f
  familial neonatal, 1572
Benign familial infantile seizures (BFIS),
    1520t–1521t
Benign familial neonatal-infantile seizures
    (BFNIS), 1520t–1521t
Benign familial neonatal seizures (BFNS),
    1520t–1521t, 1533–1534, 1533f
Benign fasciculations, 285
Benign focal amyotrophy, 1498–1499
  differential diagnosis of, 1499
  treatment of, 1499
Benign focal epilepsy of childhood with
    rolandic spikes, effect of sleep on,
    1655
Benign lymphocytic meningitis, recurrent,
    1763–1764
Benign paroxysmal positional vertigo
    (BPPV), 583, 589–591
  treatment of, 589–590, 590f, 603
Benign paroxysmal torticollis, 1719
Benign paroxysmal vertigo, 1719
Benign recurrent vertigo, 584
Benign rolandic epilepsy, 352, 354f, 1574
Benign sleep myoclonus of infancy, 1661
Benson, D. Frank, 130
Bent spine syndrome, 280
Benton, Arthur, 511
Benzamide, for vertigo, 603–604, 603t
Benzodiazepine receptor, in chemical
    imaging, 505t, 506
  of epilepsy, 509
Benzodiazepines
  for alcohol withdrawal, 1234
  commonly used, 1257b
  drug dependence with, 1256
  for dystonia, 1452t
  hepatic encephalopathy and, 1212
  psychotropic effects of, 89t
  for spasticity, in multiple sclerosis, 1182
  for vertigo, 603–604, 603t
Benztropine
  for dystonia, 1452t
  for Parkinson disease, 1433t–1434t
O6-benzylguanine, to reduce resistance to
    alkylating agents, 1051
Beriberi, 1231
  infantile, 1231
  wet and dry, 1231
Beta activity, on EEG, 349–350, 349f
Beta motoneurons, 1494
Beta-2-transferrin, 1689–1690
Bethanechol, for bladder dysfunction, 796t
Betz cells, 1487
Bevacizumab, for brain tumors, 1053–1054
  complications of, 1048
BFIS (benign familial infantile seizures),
    1520t–1521t

BFNIS (benign familial neonatal-infantile seizures), 1520t–1521t
BFNS (benign familial neonatal seizures), 1520t–1521t, 1533–1534, 1533f
BG-12, for multiple sclerosis, 1179–1180
BH4 (tetrahydrobiopterin), in inborn errors of metabolism, 1331–1332
Biballism, 240
Bickerstaff encephalitis, ataxia due to, 1462
Bilateral independent periodic discharges, 362, 362f
Bimanual Fine Motor Function Classification, for cerebral palsy, 1311
Bimanual upper extremity therapy, in rehabilitation, 801
Binocular diplopia, 2000
Binswanger disease, 492–493, 1413
    structural imaging of, 432–434, 434f
Biochemical tests, for global developmental delay, 69
Biofeedback, instrumented, in rehabilitation, 802
Biologic therapy, for brain tumor, complications of, 1048
Biological rhythms, hypothalamus in, 702
Biomarkers
    for anoxic-ischemic encephalopathy, 1206
    in neurogenetic evaluation, 672t
Biot breathing, 41, 1645–1648
Biotin, for inborn errors of metabolism, 1339
Biphasic illness, in viral CNS disease, 1124t
Bipolar stimulation, for nerve conduction studies, 366
Bismuth toxicity, ataxia due to, 1461–1462
Bitemporal hemianopia, 547–548
Bithermal caloric testing, 599
Blackouts, 1995–1996, 1995t, 1996f
Bladder
    atonic, 896t, 896.e1f
    in autonomic disorders, 1895
    neurogenic, 896–897, 896.e1f
    neurological control of, 605, 606f
        storage phase of, 605
        voiding phase of, 605
Bladder diary, 612, 612f
Bladder dysfunction
    due to cortical lesions, 607–608
    due to spinal cord lesions, 610
    due to spinal lesions, 278
    and multiple system atrophy, 609
    neuromedical problems during rehabilitation for, 796–797, 796t
    and Parkinson disease (PD), 608–609
Bladder impairment, in multiple sclerosis, 1166
    treatment of, 1182–1183
Bladder incontinence, due to spinal cord lesions, 630
Bladder scan, 613, 613f
Blaschko lines, in hypomelanosis of Ito, 1551–1552
Blast injury
    models of, 851
    traumatic brain injury due to, 867
Blastomyces dermatitidis, meningitis due to, 1153
Blastomycosis, 1154t
Bleeding disorders
    intracerebral hemorrhage due to, 969–971
    and stroke in children, 996, 999
        treatment of, 1005
Blepharoclonus, 227
Blepharoplasts, in ependymoma, 1036

Blepharospasm, 188, 235, 1453
    orbital myectomy, 1453
Blindness
    cortical, 122, 161
        transient, 159
    day, 159
    visual hallucinations in, 122–123
Blindness, cortical, 579
Blindsight, 58, 122
Blink reflex, 386
Blocking tics, 240
Blood, in autonomic disorders, 1872
"Blood doping," ischemic stroke due to, 939
Blood gas, in inborn errors of metabolism, 1326t
Blood oxygen level-dependent (BOLD) effect
    in functional magnetic resonance imaging, 486
    for presurgical brain mapping, 499
Blood pressure
    acute ischemic stroke and, 963
    on brain edema, 1269–1270, 1270f
    high, management of, 922t
    during sleep, 1630, 1630t
    for traumatic brain injury, 875t–876t
Blood pressure evaluation, for coma, 38
Blood pressure management, in neurointensive care, 753–754, 753t
    for acute ischemic stroke, 753t, 754
    for intracerebral hemorrhage, 753t, 754
    for subarachnoid hemorrhage, 753t, 754
    for traumatic brain injury, 753t, 754
Blood pressure monitoring, in neurointensive care, 743
Blood studies, for acute ischemic stroke, 963–964
Blood-brain barrier (BBB)
    antiretroviral therapy and, 1107
    and chemotherapy delivery, 1051
    function, chemical imaging of, 505t
    and immune privilege of CNS, 685–686
    in multiple sclerosis, 1160–1161
    new delivery strategies for, 1055
    in spinal cord injury, 882
Blood-brain interfaces, 1262–1267
    anatomical sites of central nervous system infection in, 1265–1266, 1265t
    arachnoid granulations and absorption of cerebrospinal fluid in, 1266, 1266f
    cerebral blood vessels and neurovascular unit in, 1262–1264, 1262t, 1263f, 1264b
    cerebrospinal fluid pressure in, 1266
    composition of cerebrospinal fluid in, 1266–1267
    gap junctions on ependymal and pial surfaces in, 1266
    production of cerebrospinal fluid and interstitial fluid in, 1264–1265
    water molecules, as basis for magnetic resonance imaging in, 1265
Blood-oxygen-level dependent (BOLD) signal, 1392–1393
Blue native polyacrylamide gel electrophoresis (BN-PAGE), for mitochondrial disorders, 1357
Blue toe syndrome, ischemic stroke due to, 945
Blunt injury, traumatic brain injury due to, 867
BMD. see Becker muscular dystrophy (BMD)

B-mode imaging, 477
    high-resolution, 478
        of atherosclerotic plaques, 478–479, 478f
        of intima-media thickening, 481–482
        of transient ischemic attack, 480–481
BN-PAGE (blue native polyacrylamide gel electrophoresis), for mitochondrial disorders, 1357
Bobath hands-on approach, 786–787
Bobath slings, 787–788
Bombesin, 697t–698t
Bon-bon sign, 239
Bone conduction, 596, 601
Bone marrow suppression, due to pediatric chemotherapy, 1083.e2
Bone marrow transplantation, neuropathies related to, 1848–1849
Bones, disorders of, 1736–1765
Bonnet syndrome, 122–123
Bortezomib
    for brain tumors, 1053
    neuropathy due to, 1860
Botulinum toxin type A (Botox)
    for diplopia, 539–540
    dysphagia due to, 154
    for hyperhidrosis, 1873t
    for migraine prophylaxis, 1703
    for myasthenia gravis, 1908–1909
    for neurogenic bladder, 618
    for spasticity, in multiple sclerosis, 1182
Botulism, 1913–1914
    clinical features of, 1913–1914
    electromyographic findings in, 1914
    forms of, 1913
    infantile, 1914
        hypotonic infant due to, 312
    repetitive nerve stimulation for, 388
    treatment of, 1914
Bouche de tapir, 1931
Bovine spongiform encephalopathy (BSE), 1376f–1377f
"Bow-tie nystagmus", 542t, 545
Bowel
    in autonomic disorders, 1895
    neurological control of, 606
Bowel dysfunction, 608, 608.e1
    due to basal ganglia lesions, 609.e1
    due to conus and cauda equina lesions, 611
    due to spinal cord injury, 610.e1
    due to spinal lesions, 278
    multiple sclerosis and, 610
    neuromedical problems during rehabilitation for, 796–797
Bowel impairment, in multiple sclerosis, 1166
Bowel incontinence, due to spinal cord lesions, 630
Bowlus maneuver, 2000
BPPV (benign paroxysmal positional vertigo), 583, 589–590
    treatment of, 589–590, 590f
Braak staging system, for Parkinson disease, 1430
Brachial monomelic amyotrophy, 1498
Brachial neuritis, 328
Brachial plexitis, monoplegia due to, 271
Brachial plexopathy, 328
    brachial neuritis (neuralgic amyotrophy, Parsonage-Turner syndrome) as, 328
    in cancer patients, 328
    metastatic, 1100–1101

Brachial plexus
  differential diagnosis of, 272.e2
  disorders of, 1779–1786
    anatomical features of, 1779–1780,
      1780f
    clinical features and diagnosis of,
      1780–1781
    electrodiagnostic studies of, 1781
    idiopathic brachial plexopathy as,
      1784–1786
      diagnosis of, 1785
      pathophysiology and etiology of,
        1785
      treatment and prognosis of,
        1785–1786
    metastatic and radiation-induced,
      1783–1784
      metastatic plexopathy, 1783
      radiation-induced plexopathy, 1784
    neurogenic thoracic outlet syndrome as,
      1782–1783, 1783f
    neurological examination of, 1781
    radiological studies of, 1781
    traumatic plexopathy as, 1782
      early management of, 1782
      long-term management of, 1782
    pre- and post-fixed, nerve conduction
      studies with, 371
Brachial plexus entrapment, of lower trunk,
  1801t
Brachial plexus injury, in newborn,
  1969–1970, 1969f
  management of, 1970
Brachial plexus neuropathy, in pregnancy,
  1979
Brachialgia, due to nerve root pain, 324
Brachycephaly, 1739t
Brachytherapy, for brain tumors, 1050
Bracing
  for Duchenne muscular dystrophy, 1923
  in rehabilitation, 789–790
  for spinal muscular atrophy, 1503
Bradycardia, in neurointensive care, 753
Bradykinesia, 224
  treatment of, 716
Bradykinins, 697t–698t
Bradyphrenia, 226
Bragg peak, 1068–1069
Brain
  degeneration of, with atrophy, 444.e1
  imaging of, prior to lumbar puncture, for
    meningitis, 1148
  neuropeptides in, 697t–698t
  normal, 1345f–1346f
Brain abscess
  bacterial, 1150–1151
    clinical presentation of, 1150
    diagnosis of, 1150, 1151f
    management of, 1149t, 1150–1151
    risk factors for, 1150
  with congenital heart disease, 836
  fungal, 1154–1155
    clinical presentation of, 1154–1155
    diagnosis of, 1155
    etiology of, 1154
    management of, 1154t, 1155
  HIV-associated, 1117, 1119f
  structural imaging of, 436.e1, 436.e2f
Brain arteriovenous malformations
  MR angiography of, 464
  Spetzler-Martin Grading system for,
    474–475, 475t
Brain atrophy, imaging of, in multiple
  sclerosis diagnosis, 1169–1170, 1171f
Brain biopsy, risk-to-benefit analysis of,
  345–346, 346f

Brain death, 51–54
  clinical determination of, 53f
  clinical findings not compatible with, 52b
  CT angiography of, 464
  EEG of, 359
  electroencephalogram of, 54
  lack of confounding factors for, 51, 52t
  ultrasound of, 483–484, 484f
Brain edema, 1261–1278
  cytotoxic, 1262t, 1268–1269,
    1268f–1269f
    defined, 1261
    molecular cascade in, 1267
  defined, 1261
  due to acute ischemic stroke, 964, 965f
  due to idiopathic intracranial
    hypertension, 1274
  effect of blood pressure and osmolality
    changes on, 1269–1270, 1270f
  interstitial, 1262t
    molecular cascade in, 1267
  molecular cascade in, 1267–1268, 1267f
  neuroinflammation and, 1268
  treatment of, 1272
  vasogenic, 1262t, 1268
    molecular cascade in, 1267
  in venous occlusion and intracerebral
    hemorrhage, 1270, 1271f–1272f
Brain herniation, coma and, 46–47
Brain metastases, 1084–1091
  clinical presentations of, 1085
  differential diagnosis of, 1085
  epidemiology of, 1084, 1085f
  management of, 1086–1091
    chemotherapy in, 1091
    multiple, 1088
    radiation therapy in, 1086–1088
      prophylactic, 1087
      with stereotactic radiosurgery,
        1089–1090
      toxicity of, 1087
      whole-brain, 1089
    recurrent, 1091
    re-irradiation in, 1091
    stereotactic radiosurgery in, 1089–1090
    supportive care in, 1086, 1086t
    surgery in, 1087–1088
    treatment paradigms in, 1090–1091
    whole-brain radiotherapy in, 1089
  multiple, 1085–1086, 1088
  neuroepidemiology of, incidence
    proportions in, 638
  neuroimaging of, 1085–1086
  pathophysiology and pathology of,
    1084–1085
  recurrent, 1085f
    treatment options for, 1091
Brain microcirculation, 924
Brain monitoring, in neurointensive care,
  744–745, 744t
  cerebral blood flow monitoring for, 744t,
    747–748
    laser Doppler flowmetry for, 744t, 748
    thermal diffusion flowmetry for, 744t,
      748
    xenon-133, 744t, 747
  electroencephalogram for, 744t, 747
  global techniques for, 745–747
  intracranial pressure monitoring in, 744t,
    745–746, 745f
  jugular oximetry for, 744t, 746–747
  local cerebral oxygenation monitoring for,
    748
    brain tissue PO₂ for, 744t, 748
    near-infrared spectroscopy for, 744t, 748
  microdialysis for, 744t, 748–749

Brain monitoring, in neurointensive care
    (Continued)
  multimodality monitoring for, 744, 748,
    749f
  regional/focal techniques for, 747–749
  somatosensory evoked potentials for, 744t,
    748
  transcranial Doppler for, 744t, 748
Brain neoplasms, during pregnancy,
  1982–1983
Brain pathways, in sensory system, 314
Brain stimulation, in rehabilitation,
  803–804
Brain tissue PO₂, in neurointensive care,
  744t, 748
Brain tumors
  alcohol and, 1023
  allergies and, 1023–1024
  challenges in studies of, 1018, 1019b
  classification of, 1018
  clinical features and complications of,
    headache as, 1687
  clinical features of, 1045–1047, 1046f
    age in, 1045
    aphasia as, 1046
    ataxia as, 1045–1046
    focal motor symptoms in, 1045
    headaches as, 1046–1047
    limb weakness as, 1045–1046
    mental status and behavioral changes
      as, 1047
    nausea and vomiting as, 1047
    seizures as, 1046
    visual problems as, 1046
  coffee and, 1023
  epidemiology of, 1018–1025
    analytical, 1020–1025
      from allergies, 1023–1024
      genetic susceptibility in, 1025
      genetic syndromes in, 1024–1025,
        1025t
      from head trauma, 1022
      from infections, 1023–1024
      methodological challenges in, 1021
      from N-nitroso compounds,
        1022–1023
      occupational studies in, 1022
      radiation in, 1021–1022
      study designs in, 1020–1021
      from tea and coffee, 1023
      from tobacco and alcohol, 1023
      from vitamins, 1023
    descriptive, 1018–1020
      gender and race in, 1019–1020, 1019f
      geographical trends and migrant
        studies in, 1020, 1020f
      incidence in, 1018–1019
      mortality and prognostic factors in,
        1019, 1019f
      for primary central nervous system
        lymphoma, 1020
      temporal trends in, 1020
  established treatment strategies for,
    1049–1051
    chemotherapy as, 1051, 1052t–1053t
    radiation therapy as, 1050–1051
    surgery as, 1049–1050
  excessive sleepiness due to, 1633
  familial clustering of, 1024–1025
  focal, symptoms of, 1045
  functional neuroimaging of, 495–497,
    495f–496f
    magnetic resonance spectroscopy for,
      497
    recurrent, 496–497, 496f
  genetic polymorphisms and, 1025

Brain tumors (*Continued*)
genetic susceptibility and, 1025
genetic syndromes and, 1024–1025, 1025*t*
head trauma and, 1022
immunity and, 1023–1024
infections and, 1023–1024
management of, 1055–1064
of cranial and peripheral nerves, 1060–1061
malignant peripheral nerve sheath tumor, 1061
schwannoma and neurofibroma, 1060–1061
for embryonal tumors, 1059–1060
medulloblastoma as, 1059–1060
supratentorial primitive neuroectodermal tumors, 1060
for germ cell tumors, 1063
for meningeal tumors, 1061–1062
hemangiopericytoma, 1062
meningioma, 1061–1062, 1061*f*
for neuraxis tumors derived from hematopoietic system, 1062–1063
for neuroepithelial tumors, 1055–1060, 1056*f*
astrocytic tumors, 1055–1058
choroid plexus tumors, 1058–1059
ependymal tumors, 1058
oligodendroglial tumors, 1058
for neuronal and mixed neuronal-glial tumors, 1059
for peripheral neuroblastic tumors, 1059
for pineal parenchymal tumors, 1059
for sellar region tumors, 1063–1064
craniopharyngioma as, 1063–1064
pituitary adenoma as, 1064
metastatic, 1045
intracerebral hemorrhage due to, 969, 970*f*
structural imaging of, 428, 428*f*–429*f*
morbidity rates in, 638, 639*f*
mortality rates and survival in, 637
N-nitroso compounds and, 1022–1023
neuroepidemiology of, 637
new treatment strategies for, 1051–1055, 1054*b*
occupation and, 1022
pediatric, 1065, 1066*t*
astrocytic, 1070–1076, 1070*b*
anaplastic astrocytoma and glioblastoma as, 1075–1076, 1076*f*
diffuse astrocytoma as, 1073, 1074*f*, 1074*t*
diffuse intrinsic pontine glioma as, 1073–1075
optic pathway glioma as, 1071–1072, 1072*f*
pilocytic astrocytoma as, 1070–1071, 1071*f*
pleomorphic xanthoastrocytoma as, 1075
subependymal giant cell astrocytoma as, 1072–1073
of choroid plexus, 1082–1083, 1083*f*
craniopharyngioma as, 1081–1082, 1082*f*
embryonal, 1065–1070
atypical teratoid/rhabdoid tumor as, 1069–1070
medulloblastoma as, 1065–1069
primitive neuroectodermal tumor as, 1065–1069
ependymoma as, 1078–1079, 1079*f*

Brain tumors (*Continued*)
germ cell tumor as, 1079–1080, 1080*f*
neuronal and mixed neuronal-glial, 1076–1077
central neurocytoma as, 1077.*e*1–1077.*e*2, 1077.*e*2*f*
desmoplastic infantile astrocytoma or ganglioglioma as, 1077.*e*1
dysembryoplastic neuroepithelial tumor as, 1077.*e*1, 1077.*e*1*f*
ganglioglioma as, 1077, 1077*f*
oligodendroglioma as, 1077–1078
treatment-related complications in, 1083.*e*1–1083.*e*2
due to chemotherapy, 1083.*e*2
due to radiation therapy, 1083.*e*1–1083.*e*2
due to surgery, 1083.*e*1
primary, 1045
radiation and, 1021–1022
seizures due to, 1582
structural imaging of, 417, 418*t*–419*t*
tea and, 1023
tobacco and, 1023
treatment for, complications of, 1047–1048
vitamins and, 1023
Brain volume, in autism spectrum disorder, 1306
Brain warts, 1287
Brain-computer interfaces, in rehabilitation, 804
Brainstem, in sensory system, 314
Brainstem arousal centers, 1624*f*
Brainstem auditory evoked potential (BAEP), 365.*e*3–365.*e*4
for intraoperative monitoring, 407, 408*f*
monitoring interpretation of, 409
in neurological disease, 365.*e*3–365.*e*4, 365.*e*4*f*–365.*e*5*f*
normal, 365.*e*3, 365.*e*4*f*
Brainstem control
of eye movements, 552
of upper motor neurons, 1485
Brainstem encephalitis, paraneoplastic, 1190
Brainstem ischemia/infarction, 587*t*, 592–593
Brainstem lesions
bladder dysfunction due to, 609–610
hemiplegia due to, 265–266
monoplegia due to, 268
differential diagnosis of, 272.*e*1
sensory, 318–319
Brainstem locomotor centers, 250–251
Brainstem nuclei, in control of upper motor neurons, 1485
Brainstem processes, dysphagia due to, 155
Brainstem reflexes, and brain death, 52
Brainstem reticular formation, in control of upper motor neurons, 1485
Brainstem syndromes, 205–216
involving ocular motor nuclei, 208
sixth cranial nerve nucleus, 208
third cranial nerve nucleus, 208
ischemic stroke syndromes as, 210–216, 210*f*
medullary, 212–216, 216*b*
midbrain, 211–212, 212*b*
pontine, 212, 214*b*
thalamic, 210–211, 211*b*
ocular motor syndromes as, 205–208
combined vertical gaze ophthalmoplegia as, 205–206, 206*b*
downgaze paresis as, 206

Brainstem syndromes (*Continued*)
global paralysis of gaze as, 207–208, 208*b*
horizontal gaze paresis as, 207
internuclear ophthalmoplegia as, 207
one-and-a-half syndrome as, 208
upgaze paresis (dorsal midbrain or Parinaud syndrome) as, 206, 206*b*
other and associated syndromes, 208–210
diencephalic syndrome (Russell syndrome) as, 208–209
foramen magnum syndrome as, 209
syringobulbia as, 209–210
tectal deafness as, 209
thalamic syndrome as, 209
Brainstem tumor, 1027*t*
pediatric, 1074*t*
Branch retinal artery occlusion, 177
Branchio-oto-renal syndrome, 594
BRB-N (Brief Repeatable Battery of Neuropsychological Tests), for multiple sclerosis, 1167
Breastfeeding
antiepileptic drugs and, 1987
and migraine, 1976
with multiple sclerosis, 1982
with myasthenia gravis, 1977
Breath-holding spells, 15
Breathing
apneustic, 41
ataxic, 41–42
Biot, 41
cluster, 41
Kussmaul, 41
paradoxical, 742–743
short-cycle periodic, 41
sleep disorders, classification of, 1635
Brief mental status examination, 515–518
Mini-Mental State Examination as, 517–518, 519*f*, 520*t*
Modified, 518
Montreal Cognitive Assessment as, 515–517, 516*f*, 517*t*
Telephone Interview for Cognitive Status-Modified as, 517, 518*f*
Brief Repeatable Battery of Neuropsychological Tests (BRB-N), for multiple sclerosis, 1167
Bright light, visual loss in, 159
Brightness-mode (B-mode) imaging, 477
high-resolution, 478
of atherosclerotic plaques, 478–479, 478*f*
of intima-media thickening, 481–482
of transient ischemic attack, 480–481
Brindley, Giles, 619
Broca, Paul, 131
Broca aphasia, 59, 131–132, 131*t*
Broca area, 129*f*, 131
Bromism, 1904
Bromocriptine
for acromegaly, 711
for menstrual migraine prophylaxis, 1705
for neuroleptic malignant syndrome, 700
for Parkinson disease, 1432–1435
for prolactinoma, 710–711
for TSH-secreting and gonadotropin-secreting tumors, 711
Bronchial asthma, sleep disturbances in, 1670
Bronchogenic cyst, 1043–1044
Bronchopulmonary dysplasia (BPD), neurological complications of, 841–842

Brown-Séquard plus, 885
Brown-Séquard syndrome, 266, 884–885,
    884f–885f
    paraplegia due to, 273–274
Brucella spp., meningitis due to, 1147–1148,
    1148t
Brugada syndrome, 1669–1670
    syncope due to, 10–11
Bruininks-Oseretsky Test of Motor
    Proficiency, for developmental
    coordination disorders, 1316
Bruns nystagmus, 542t, 548
Bruxism, 1661
BSE (bovine spongiform encephalopathy),
    1376f–1377f
Buccal nerve, 1726f
Buccolingual apraxia, 147
Buerger disease, ischemic stroke due to,
    941–942
Bulbar function, in ataxia, 219
Bulbar muscles
    clinical presentation of, 280
    differential diagnosis of, 289–290
Bulbar symptoms, ataxia and, 217
Bulbocavernosus reflex, 616, 886
    stimulation of, for rehabilitation,
    632
Bulimia nervosa, 701
Bunina bodies, 1507
Bunyaviruses, California serogroup of viruses
    as, 1139
Bupropion, 111–112
    for neuropathic pain, 918t–919t
Burning feet syndrome, 848
Burning hand syndrome, 886
Burning pain, treatment of, 715
Burns, effects of, 1247
Bursitis, arm and neck pain due to, 331
Burst fractures, 889
    structural imaging for, 454.e1, 454.e1f
Burst suppression pattern, in hypoxia, 357,
    358f
Burst-tonic neurons, in vertical eye
    movement, 560, 560f
Butalbital-containing products, and
    medication overuse headache, 1707
Butt-first maneuver, 285
bvFTD (Behavioral variant frontotemporal
    dementia), 79

C

C. *see* Constant (C) gene segments
C5 radiculopathy, 1771
C6 radiculopathy, 1771–1772
C7 radiculopathy, 1771–1772
C8/T1 roots entrapment, 1801t
Cabergoline
    for Parkinson disease, 1432–1435
    for prolactinoma, 710–711
Cachectic atrophy, 1918, 1918f
CACL1A3 gene, in hypokalemic periodic
    paralysis, 1937
CACNA1A gene
    in familial episodic ataxia, 1530
    in familial hemiplegic migraine,
    1528–1529
CACNA1H gene, in childhood absence
    epilepsy, 1535
CACNA1S gene, in hypokalemic periodic
    paralysis, 1523
CACNB4 gene
    in familial episodic ataxia, 1530
    in juvenile myoclonic epilepsy,
    1534–1535
Cacosmia, 193

CADASIL (cerebral autosomal dominant
    arteriopathy with subcortical infarcts
    and leukoencephalopathy), 942–943,
    943f, 1416, 434.e1, 434.e1f
CADASILM (cerebral autosomal dominant
    arteriopathy with subcortical infarcts,
    leukoencephalopathy and migraine),
    942–943
Café-au-lait spots, in neurofibromatosis type
    1, 1544, 1545f
Caffeine, for hypnic headache, 1714
Caffeine-contracture test, for malignant
    hyperthermia, 1527–1528
CAG expansion disorders, pathogenesis of,
    1478
CAG repeat expansion, in Huntington
    disease, 1446
Caisson disease
    ischemic stroke due to, 945
    spinal cord infarction due to, 1009
Cajal-Retzius neurons, of fetal brain, 1291,
    1291f
Calcitonin, 697t–698t
Calcitonin gene product, 697t–698t
Calcitonin gene-related peptide (CGRP),
    697t–698t
    in complex regional pain syndrome, 738
Calcitonin gene related peptide (CGRP)
    antagonists, for migraine, 1701–1702
Calcium, in uremic encephalopathy, 1217
Calcium channel abnormalities,
    hypokalemic periodic paralysis as
    familial type 1, 1937
    secondary, 1937–1938
Calcium channel blockers
    for cluster headache maintenance
    prophylaxis, 1710
    for migraine prophylaxis, 1702
Calcium channels, 1936–1937
    voltage-gated, 1521
Calcium disturbances, neurological
    complications of, 830–831
Calcium metabolism, disorders of,
    1224
Calcium-activated neutral protease
    (CANP-3), 1925
Calf amyotrophy, benign, 1498
California serogroup of viruses, 1137t,
    1139
Call-Fleming syndrome, 1016
    ischemic stroke due to, 944–945
Callosal agenesis, 1298–1299, 1299f
    clinical features of, 1294t
    EEG of, 1299
    pathogenesis of, 1298
Callosal apraxia, 118
    testing for, 120
Caloric requirement, in neurointensive care,
    755
Caloric testing, 583
    brain death and, 52
    for coma, 45, 46t
    for vestibular disorders, 599
Caloric-induced nystagmus, 544
Calpain-3 deficiency, 1925
Calpains, 960.e1
Calvarial metastases, 1095
CAM (confusion assessment method),
    28–29, 28b
Campath (alemtuzumab), for multiple
    sclerosis, 1178–1179
Campath-1H, for multiple sclerosis, 690
Camptocormia, 228, 229f, 253–254
Canalithiasis, 591
Canavan disease, 1328.e1t–1328.e2t,
    1326.e1t–1326.e2t

Cancer
    ischemic stroke due to, 947
    metastatic and radiation-induced brachial
    plexopathy with, 1783–1784
    metastatic plexopathy, 1783
    radiation-induced plexopathy, 1784
    and stroke in children, 997–998, 998f
Cancer-associated retinopathy (CAR),
    177–178, 1195
Candidate gene association study, 663–664
Candidate gene resequencing, 665–666
Candidiasis, 1154t
Canes, in rehabilitation, 787
Cannabinoids, for neurogenic bladder, 619
CANP-3. *see* Calcium-activated neutral
    protease (CANP-3)
CAP (cyclic alternating pattern), in sleep,
    1617–1620
Capecitabine, for leptomeningeal metastases,
    1099
Capgras syndrome
    after stroke, 100–101
    in delirium, 26
Capillary telangiectasia, structural imaging
    for, 447.e1
CAPRIE (Clopidogrel *versus* Aspirin in
    Patients at Risk of Ischemic Events),
    953–954
Capsaicin, for chronic pain, 726
Capsaicin cream, for neuropathic pain,
    918t–919t
Capsular warning syndrome, 927
Caput medusa, 447.e1
Caput succedaneum, in newborn, 1968,
    1969t
CAR (cancer-associated retinopathy),
    177–178
Carbamazepine (Tegretol)
    for chronic pain, 725
    for epilepsy
        absorption, elimination half-life,
            formulations of, 1600t
        efficacy by seizure type of, 1601t
        hepatic metabolism, enzyme induction/
            inhibition, pharmacokinetic
            interactions, and protein binding
            of, 1603t
        mechanism of action of, 1604t
    during pregnancy, 1985
    for glossopharyngeal neuralgia, 1717
    levonorgestrel and, 1974
    for neuropathic pain, 918t–919t
    during pregnancy, 1985
    and vitamin K deficiency, 1986
    psychotropic effects of, 89t
    for tremor, in multiple sclerosis, 1182
    for trigeminal neuralgia, 736, 1716
Carbidopa
    for dystonia, 1452t
    for Parkinson disease, 1433t–1434t
Carbidopa levodopa, and entacapone
    (Stalevo), for Parkinson disease, 1435
Carbohydrate metabolism, disorders of,
    1336, 1940–1942
    β-enolase deficiency as, 1941
    α-glucosidase deficiency (acid maltase
        deficiency), 1941–1942
    lactate dehydrogenase deficiency as, 1941
    myophosphorylase deficiency as,
        1940–1941
    phosphofructokinase deficiency as, 1941
    phosphoglycerate kinase deficiency as,
        1941
    phosphoglycerate mutase deficiency as,
        1941
    treatment of, 1942

Carbon-11 (^{11}C), for positron emission tomography, 504

Carbon disulfide, occupational exposure to, 1238–1239

Carbon monoxide, occupational exposure to, 1239

Carbon monoxide poisoning
parkinsonism due to, 1442
structural imaging for, 444.*e1*

Carboplatin, for brain tumors, 1052*t*–1053*t*

Carcinoid syndrome, 712

Carcinoid tumors, 712

Carcinomatous meningitis, 1149
headache due to, 1687–1688

Cardiac arrest
induced hypothermia after, 1203
complications of, 1203, 1204*f*
out-of-hospital protocol for, 1203, 1204*b*
studies on, 1203, 1204*t*
neurological complications of, 816

Cardiac arrhythmias
with acute ischemic stroke, 963
in neurointensive care, 753
sleep and, 1669
syncope due to, 10

Cardiac catheterization
cardiogenic embolism due to, 935
neurological complications of, in adults, 816–817, 817*f*

Cardiac cephalalgia, headache due to, 1694, 1714

Cardiac disease, during pregnancy, 1987

Cardiac disorders, neurological complications of, in adults, 815–818

Cardiac evaluation
for stroke in children, 1004–1005
of stroke patient, 951–952

Cardiac examination, for coma, 39

Cardiac monitoring, for acute ischemic stroke, 963

Cardiac output
decreased, syncope due to, 11
during sleep, 1630*t*

Cardiac rhabdomyoma, in tuberous sclerosis, 1542, 1543*f*

Cardiac surgery
cardiogenic embolism due to, 935
neurological complications of, in adults, 816–817, 817*f*

Cardiac transplantation, neurological complications of, 837

Cardiogenic embolism
in adults, 815
ischemic stroke due to, 933–935, 934*b*, 935*f*

Cardioinhibitory sinus syndrome, drop attacks due to, 17–18

Cardiology, functional symptoms in, 1993*t*

Cardiomyopathy
familial, with subsarcolemmal vermiform deposits, 1927
with inborn errors of metabolism, 1326

Cardiovascular care, in neurointensive care, 752–754
for acute coronary syndrome, 752–753, 753*f*
for cardiac arrhythmias, 753
for congestive heart failure, 753

Cardiovascular changes, during sleep, 1630–1631

Cardiovascular disease, sleep disorders in, 1669–1670

Cardiovascular features, of autonomic disorders, 1870

[^{11}C]Carfentanil, in chemical imaging, 506
of epilepsy, 509

Carmustine, for brain tumor, complications of, 1048

Carnitine cycle, disorders of, 1337

Carnitine deficiency, 1362

Carnitine deficiency myopathy, 1942–1943, 1943*f*

Carnitine palmitoyl transferase (CPT) deficiency, myopathy due to, 1942

Carnitine palmitoyltransferase I (CPT-I) deficiency, 1325–1326

Carnitine profile, for inborn errors of metabolism, 1326*t*

L-Carnitine replacement, 1354

Carnosine, 697*t*–698*t*

Carotid arteries, CTA of, 459

Carotid artery, ischemic stroke due to, coils and kinks of, 945

Carotid artery angioplasty and stenting, 763–765
clinical trials for, 763–765, 764*b*
procedure for, 763, 763*f*–764*f*

Carotid artery disease (CAD), 763–765
asymptomatic, as risk factor for stroke, 923

Carotid artery dissection
CT angiography of, 460
magnetic resonance angiography of, 469, 470*f*–471*f*

Carotid artery stenosis
asymptomatic, as risk factor for stroke, 923
CT angiography of, 460, 460*f*
MR angiography of
three-dimensional contrast enhanced, 468*f*
time-of-flight, 467, 467*f*
surgical therapy for
asymptomatic, 961–962
symptomatic, 960–961

Carotid artery stenting (CAS)
for acute ischemic stroke, 962–963, 962*f*
ultrasound monitoring of, 484

Carotid Artery Surgery Asymptomatic Narrowing Operations *versus* Aspirin (CASANOVA) trial, 961–962

Carotid artery syndromes, 927

Carotid endarterectomy (CEA)
for carotid artery stenosis
asymptomatic, 961–962
symptomatic, 960–961
dysphagia after, 153
ultrasound monitoring of, 484, 484*f*

Carotid hypersensitivity syndrome, 1732

Carotid Occlusion Surgery Study, 961

Carotid Revascularization Endarterectomy *versus* Stenting Trial (CREST), 765, 963

Carotid sinus, 1731

Carotid sinus hypersensitivity, 1878
syncope due to, 10

Carotid sinus massage, syncope due to, 10

Carotid ultrasonography, 477–479, 478*f*–479*f*

Carotid-cavernous fistulas (CCFs)
grading scale for, 779*b*
neurointerventional therapy for, 778–779, 778*f*–779*f*

Carpal tunnel syndrome (CTS), 328–329, 1802–1803
due to hypothyroidism, 832
monoplegia due to, 269
nerve conduction studies of, 1803, 1803*t*
predisposing factors for, 1803
in pregnancy, 1978
sensory abnormalities due to, 319*t*, 321
symptoms of, 1802, 1803*f*
treatment of, 1803
work-related, 1802–1803

Carrier, of allele, 658

CARS-2 (Childhood Autism Rating Scale-Second Edition), 1304

Cartilage oligomeric matrix protein (COMP), in pseudoachondroplasia, 1738

CASANOVA (Carotid Artery Surgery Asymptomatic Narrowing Operations *versus* Aspirin) trial, 961–962

Case-control ratios, for multiple sclerosis, 643*f*

Case-control study design, for brain tumors, 1020–1021

Castleman disease, 1193

Catalepsy, 121

Catamenial epilepsy, 1584

Cataplexy, 1640–1641
differential diagnosis of, 1643*b*
versus seizures, 1592
excessive sleepiness due to, 1633
falls due to, 19
orexin A in, 194
treatment of, 1679

Cataracts, with global developmental delay, 69*t*

Catathrenia (expiratory groaning), 1667

Catatonia, 34–35, 35*t*

Catecholaminergic myocardial stunning, 1881–1882

Category fluency test, for Alzheimer disease, 1387

Catheter angiography, of intracranial aneurysm, 989*f*

Cauda equina lesions, 276–277, 277*f*
differential diagnosis of, 272.*e2*
neurogenic bladder dysfunction due to, 611
sphincter EMG for, 615

Cauda equina syndrome, 886, 886*f*, 886*t*
acute, 1758
due to inflammatory spondyloarthropathies, 1762
due to L4 radiculopathy, 1771
lower back pain and leg pain due to, 337

Caudate hemorrhage, 977, 978*t*, 979*f*

Caudate nucleus, in basal ganglia, 1423

Causalgia, dystonia with, 1455

Cautious gaits, 260

Caveolin-3 deficiency, 1925

Cavernomas, structural imaging of, 447.*e1*

Cavernous angiomas, intracerebral hemorrhage due to, 968–969, 969*f*

Cavernous hemangiomas, structural imaging of, 447.*e1*

Cavernous malformations
seizures due to, 1582, 1582*f*
spinal, 1013
and stroke in children, 996

Cavernous sinus
abducens nerve in
anatomy of, 1727
clinical lesions of, 1728
oculomotor nerve in, 1720
lesions in, 1723, 1723.*e1f*

Cavernous sinus *(Continued)*
and pituitary fossa, 703*f*
trochlear nerve in
anatomy of, 1724
clinical lesions of, 1725
Cavernous sinus metastases, 1095*t*
Cavernous sinus thrombosis, 964–966
Cayman ataxia, 1468
Caytaxin, in Cayman ataxia, 1468
CBF. *see* Cerebral blood flow (CBF)
CBI (cerebellar inhibition), in transcranial magnetic stimulation, 394, 394*t*
CBS (Clot Burden Score), on CT angiography, 461, 461*f*
CBTRUS (Central Brain Tumor Registry of the United States), 1018
C-C family, of chemokines, 683
CCA. *see* Congenital contractural arachnodactyly (CCA)
CCA (common carotid artery), volume flow rate in, 479, 479*f*
CCNU, for brain tumors, 1052*t*–1053*t*
CCR5
in HIV disease, 1103, 1106
in immune response, 683
CCT (central conduction time), in AMT (active motor threshold), in transcranial magnetic stimulation, 391–392
in cervical myelopathy and other spinal cord lesions, 397
in multiple sclerosis, 397
CD (celiac disease), ataxia due to, 1464
CD3, in T-cell activation, 681
CD4, in T-cell activation, 681
CD4 molecules, in HIV disease, 1103, 1103*t*
CD4 T cells, in immune response, 677
CD4+ T-cells, in myasthenia gravis, 1899
CD8, in T-cell activation, 681
CD8+ cytotoxic cells, in inclusion body myositis, 1953
CD8 T cells, in immune response, 677
CD40-CD154 pathways, in T-cell activation, 681
CD45, in immune response, 678
CD200, in CNS, 686
CDCV. *see* Common disease-common variant (CDCV) model
CDI (Child Development Inventory), 66
Cefotaxime, for neonatal meningitis, 1965
Celecoxib (Celebrex), for chronic pain, 725*t*
Celiac disease (CD)
ataxia due to, 1464
neurological complications of, 828
Celiac plexus block, 729*t*
Cell death, after spinal cord injury, 882
Cell growth, interference with pathways regulating, 1051–1053
Cell invasion inhibitors, for brain tumor, 1053–1054, 1054*b*
Cell membrane, electrical polarity of, 1289
disorders of, 1289
Cell migration, in T-cell activation, 681–682
Cell proliferation, methods of assessing, 1030
Cell-mediated immunity (CMI), 677, 682
Cellular lineage, disorders of, 1293
Cellular prion protein (PrP^C), 1366–1367, 1366*f*
Cellular swelling, brain edema due to, 1267
Cellular telephone, and brain tumors, 1021–1022
CE-MRA (contrast-enhanced MRA), 466, 466*f*, 468–469, 468*f*–471*f*
3D, 466, 470–471
4D, for arteriovenous malformations, 475
for arteriovenous malformations, 474–475

CE-MRA (contrast-enhanced MRA) *(Continued)*
of carotid and vertebral circulation, 466
after stent placement, 469, 471*f*
with basilar artery stenosis, 469, 469*f*
with carotid artery dissection, 469, 470*f*–471*f*
with carotid stenosis, 468*f*
with fibromuscular dysplasia, 469
with vertebral artery dissection, 469, 470*f*
for cerebral aneurysms, 472, 473*f*
of coiled intracranial aneurysms, 467
fast, dynamic, or time-resolved, 466
sensitivity and specificity of, 468–469
Center for Epidemiologic Studies Depression Scale (CES-D), 76*t*
Centimetering technique, in nerve conduction studies, 369, 369*f*–370*f*
Centractin, 1282
Central Brain Tumor Registry of the United States (CBTRUS), 1018
Central conduction time (CCT), in transcranial magnetic stimulation, 391–392
in cervical myelopathy and other spinal cord lesions, 397
in multiple sclerosis, 397
Central cord syndrome, 274, 276*f*, 883–884, 883*f*
Central core disease, 1520*t*–1521*t*, 1946, 1947*f*
hypotonic infant due to, 313
Central disruption of fusion, 533, 571
Central European encephalitis hyperimmunoglobulin, 1131*t*
Central motor conduction measurements, with transcranial magnetic stimulation, 391–392, 394*t*
cerebellar inhibition in, 394, 394*t*
interhemispheric inhibition (IHI), 393–394, 394*t*
intracortical facilitation in, 393, 394*t*
short-interval, 393, 394*t*
intracortical inhibition in
long-interval, 392, 394*t*
short-interval, 393, 394*t*
MEP recruitment curve in, 392, 394*t*
motor excitability measurements in, 392–394, 394*t*
motor thresholds in, 392, 394*t*
other inhibitory phenomena of the motor cortex, 393–394, 394*t*
short-latency and long latency afferent inhibition in, 393, 394*t*
silent period in, 392, 392*f*, 394*t*
stimulation parameters for diagnostic use of, 391–394, 394*t*
surround inhibition in, 393, 394*t*
Central nervous system
fungal infections of, 1152–1155
granulomatous angiitis of, intracerebral hemorrhage due to, 972–974
immune privilege in, 685–686
malformations of
clinical expression of, 1293–1300, 1294*t*
etiology of, 1291–1292
molecular genetic classification of, 1292–1293
neurodegenerative disorders of, 1342, 1343*t*
primary angiitis of, and stroke in children, 1000

Central nervous system *(Continued)*
vasculitis, 1015–1017
due to amyloid, 1017
due to cutaneous herpes zoster infection, 1017
due to drug abuse, 1017
due to lymphoma, 1017
isolated, 1015–1017
approach to diagnosis of, 1016
clinical findings in, 1015
laboratory findings in, 1016
pathology of, 1015–1016
therapy for, 1016–1017
types of, 1015
Central nervous system infections, in newborn, 1965–1968
meningitis as, 1965
management of, 1965
prognosis of, 1965, 1966*f*
viral and parasitic infections of, 1966–1968
congenital rubella as, 1966, 1966*f*
cytomegalovirus as, 1967
herpes simplex as, 1967
human immunodeficiency virus as, 1967–1968
toxoplasmosis as, 1967
Central nervous system lymphoma, pathology and molecular genetics of, 1041–1042, 1042*f*
Central nervous system transplant, immunology of, 695
Central neuroblastomas, 1028
Central neurocytoma
management of, 1059
pathology and molecular genetics of, 1036
pediatric, 1077.*e*1–1077.*e*2, 1077.*e*2*f*
structural imaging of, 418*t*–419*t*, 426.*e*1
Central neurogenic hyperventilation, 41, 42*f*
Central pain
arm and neck pain due to, 324
neuromedical problems during rehabilitation for, 797
Central pontine myelinolysis, structural imaging of, 440.*e*2
Central positional nystagmus, 590–591
Central post-stroke pain, 322
Central retinal artery occlusion, 176*f*–177*f*
Central sleep apnea syndrome, 1649, 1649.*e*2
treatment of, 1647*f*
Central tolerance, 684
Centralspindlin, 1282
Centrifugal conduction, along nociceptive axons, 296
Centripetal conduction, along nociceptive axons, 297
Centripetal nystagmus, 547
Centro-median-parafascicular complex (CM-Pfc) deep brain stimulation
for neuropsychiatric disorders, 403*t*
for Tourette syndrome, 405
Centronuclear myopathy, 1947–1948
hypotonic infant due to, 313
ocular weakness due to, 288–289
Cephalalgias, 1691
cardiac, headache due to, 1694, 1714
trigeminal-autonomic, 1709, 1711–1713
Cephalhematoma, in newborn, 1968, 1969*t*
Cephalic sensation, with seizures, 1565
Cephaloceles, 1282, 1293–1295, 1295*f*
Cephalosporin, with metronidazole, for brain abscess, 1151
CERAD Behavior Rating Scale for Dementia (C-BRSD), 76, 77*t*
Cercopithecine herpesvirus 1, 1132.*e*1

Cerebellar ataxia, 221*b*, 1461, 1465–1480
  acquired, 1461–1464, 1462*t*
    autoimmune causes of, 1463–1464
      and anti-glutamic acid decarboxylase
        antibodies, 1464
      with gluten sensitivity, 1464
      paraneoplastic cerebellar degeneration
        as, 1463–1464
      superficial siderosis as, 1464, 1464*f*
    clinical approach to, 1480–1483
    due to hypothyroidism, 1461
    due to infectious and transmissible
      diseases, 1462–1463, 1463*f*
    toxic causes of, 1461–1462
      alcohol as, 1461
      anticonvulsants as, 1462
      chemotherapeutic agents as, 1461
      heavy metals as, 1461–1462
      solvents as, 1462
  associated with Hodgkin lymphoma, 1200
  clinical approach to, 1480–1483
  Friedreich, 1465–1467, 1466*f*
    with abetalipoproteinemia, 1468
    ataxia-telangiectasia as, 1468–1469,
      1468*f*
    ataxia-telangiectasia-like disorder as,
      1469
    Cayman, 1468
    of Charlevoix-Saguenay, 1469
    in childhood and young adult-onset
      metabolic disorders, 1470, 1470*t*
    in infantile-onset spinocerebellar ataxia,
      1467
    with isolated vitamin E deficiency,
      1467–1468
    in Marinesco-Sjögren syndrome, 1469
    in mitochondrial, 1467
    with oculomotor apraxia type 1, 1469
    with oculomotor apraxia type 2, 1469
    other DNA repair defects causing, 1469
    type 1, 1469–1470
    type 2, 1470
  gait disorders due to, 256
  gene mutations and phenotype-genotype
      correlations in
    imaging and other laboratory studies in,
      1472, 1472*f*–1473*f*
    neuropathology of, 1472–1473
  inherited
    autosomal dominant, 1471–1479
      episodic, 1471
      gene mutations and phenotype-
        genotype correlations in,
        1473–1477, 1473*f*, 1474*t*
      imaging and other laboratory studies
        in, 1472, 1472*f*–1473*f*
      neuropathology of, 1472–1473
      pathogenesis of, 1478–1479, 1478*f*
      spinocerebellar, 1471–1472, 1471*t*
    autosomal recessive, 1465–1470, 1465*t*
    of childhood, 1463*f*
    gene mutations and phenotype-
      genotype correlations in, 1473–
      1477, 1473*f*, 1474*t*
    mitochondrial disease and, 1470–1471
    sporadic (idiopathic), 1480–1483
    of unknown origin, 1479–1480
  molecular testing of, 1480–1482
  neurological signs of, 217–219
    abnormalities of muscle tone and
      strength as, 218
    cognitive-affective changes as, 219
    disorders of speech and bulbar function
      as, 219

Cerebellar ataxia *(Continued)*
    limb incoordination as, 218
      action tremor as, 218
      cerebellar outflow (rubral, wing-
        beating) tremor as, 218
      dysdiadochokinesia as, 218
      dysmetria as, 218
      kinetic (intention) tremor as, 218
    oculomotor disturbances as, 218–219
      disorders of pursuit as, 219
      disorders of saccades as, 219
      nystagmus as, 219
      other saccadic intrusions as, 219
      vestibulo-ocular reflex as, 219
    stance and gait as, 218
  prevalence rates of, 1482*f*
  sporadic (idiopathic), 1480–1483
    defined, 1461
    non-cerebellar deficits, 1480
    in sporadic cortical cerebellar atrophy,
      1480
  transcranial magnetic stimulation for, 396
  x-linked, 1479
"Cerebellar cognitive affective syndrome",
  1485
Cerebellar degeneration
  alcoholic, 1235
  paraneoplastic, 1188–1189, 1463–1464
    ataxia due to, 1463–1464
    channelopathy in, 1536
    clinical findings in, 1188–1189
    immune responses in, 1189, 1189*f*
    treatment of, 1189
    tumor association of, 1189
Cerebellar development, disorders of,
    1300.*e*2–1300.*e*3
  Chiari malformation as, 1300.*e*3
  Dandy-Walker malformation as,
    1300.*e*2–1300.*e*3
  focal cerebellar dysplasia, 1300.*e*3,
    1300.*e*3*f*
  global cerebellar hypoplasia as, 1300.*e*3,
    1300.*e*3*f*
  selective cerebellar hemispheric aplasia as,
    1300.*e*2
  selective vermal aplasia as, 1300.*e*2
Cerebellar disorders, 217–222
  falls due to, 19
  structural imaging of, 444
  transcranial magnetic stimulation for, 396
Cerebellar dysplasia, focal, 1300.*e*3, 1300.*e*3*f*
Cerebellar fits, in coma, 46
Cerebellar hemispheric aplasia, selective,
  1300.*e*2
Cerebellar hemorrhage, 978*t*, 979, 979.*e*1*f*
  headache due to, 1692
  surgical therapy for, 981–982, 982.*e*1*f*
Cerebellar hypoplasias, global, 1300.*e*3
  clinical features of, 1294*t*
Cerebellar inhibition (CBI), in transcranial
  magnetic stimulation, 394, 394*t*
Cerebellar ischemia/infarction, vertigo due
  to, 587*t*, 592–593
Cerebellar liponeurocytoma, pathology and
  molecular genetics of, 1035
Cerebellar mutism, 1083.*e*1
Cerebellar neuroblastomas, 1028
Cerebellar outflow tremor, 1444–1445
Cerebellar pathways, impairment of, in
  multiple sclerosis, 1166
Cerebellar tonsillar herniation, in Chiari I
  malformation, 1741, 1743*t*
  upper limits of normal, 1743*t*
Cerebellar tonsils, low-lying, 448–449

Cerebellar tumor, 1027*t*
Cerebellar-sensory ataxias, 221*b*
Cerebellopontine angle tumors, 603, 1027*t*
  hearing loss due to, 596–597
Cerebellum
  disorders, including degenerative ataxias,
    1461–1483
  in horizontal eye movements, 555, 556*f*,
    558
  magnetic stimulation of, 394
  in memory, 61
  motor system anatomy of, 262
Cerebral abscess
  due to neonatal meningitis, 1965
  structural imaging of, 436.*e*1, 436.*e*2*f*
Cerebral amebiasis, 1157
Cerebral amyloid angiopathy, 1391–1392,
    1416
  intracerebral hemorrhage due to, 971–972
  ischemic stroke due to, 945
  microbleeds in, 974*f*
  structural imaging of, 436.*e*1, 436.*e*1*f*
Cerebral aneurysms
  CT angiography of, 463–464, 464*f*–465*f*
  MR angiography of, 472–473, 472*f*–473*f*
  mycotic, due to infective endocarditis,
    817–818, 817*f*
  neurointerventional therapy for, 768–774
    alternative treatments for, 773–774,
      773*f*
    endovascular treatment modalities for,
      769–771
      balloon remodeling as, 770,
        770*f*–771*f*
      coil embolization as, 769–770,
        770*f*–772*f*
    ruptured, 768–769
    unruptured, 769
Cerebral angiography, 202
  for threatened stroke, 952–953, 952*f*
Cerebral angiopathy, 1016
Cerebral arteriography, risk-to-benefit
  analysis of, 345
Cerebral arteriovenous fistulas, 777–779
  carotid-cavernous, 778–779, 778*f*–779*f*,
    779*b*
  cranial dural, 777–778, 777*b*
Cerebral arteriovenous malformations,
  775–777
  embolization procedure for, 775–777,
    776*f*
    with ethylene vinyl alcohol copolymer,
      776–777
    with N-butyl cyanoacrylate, 776
    with polyvinyl alcohol, 775–776
  stereotactic radiosurgery for, 777
Cerebral autosomal dominant arteriopathy
  with subcortical infarcts,
  leukoencephalopathy and migraine
  (CADASILM), 942–943
Cerebral autosomal dominant arteriopathy
  with subcortical infarcts and
  leukoencephalopathy (CADASIL),
  942–943, 1416
  during pregnancy, 1988
Cerebral blood flow (CBF)
  and brain death, 54
  in hepatic encephalopathy, 1212
  monitoring, in neurointensive care, 744*t*,
    747–748
    laser Doppler flowmetry for, 744*t*, 748
    thermal diffusion flowmetry for, 744*t*,
      748
    xenon-133, 744*t*, 747

Cerebral blood flow (CBF) (Continued)
  during sleep, 1630, 1630t
  in SPECT, 488
    for epilepsy, 497
    tracers for, 497
  sports and performance concussion and, 861
Cerebral blood vessels, and neurovascular unit, 1262–1264, 1262t, 1263f, 1264b
Cerebral contusion, intracerebral hemorrhage due to, 975
Cerebral cortex
  association, 57
  in cognition, 57–58
  differential diagnosis of, 272.e1
  functional subtypes, 94, 96f
  in horizontal eye movements, 556
  lesions in, consciousness and, 59
  in pain pathway, 721
  primary sensory, 57
  in sensory system, 314
Cerebral disorders
  falls due to, 19
  hypotonic infant due to, 309
Cerebral dysgenesis, with congenital heart disease, 835
Cerebral edema, 1961
  during treatment of diabetic ketoacidosis, 1221, 1221f
Cerebral glucose metabolism, 1218
  as marker of neuronal activity, 488
Cerebral hypoplasia, 1283, 1283f
Cerebral infarction, 483
  headache due to, 1692
  hyperhidrosis after, 1872t
Cerebral ischemia
  clinical syndromes of, 925–931
    anterior cerebral artery syndromes as, 928, 928f
    anterior choroidal artery syndrome as, 928
    carotid artery syndromes as, 927
    lacunar syndromes as, 928
    middle cerebral artery syndromes as, 927–928
    posterior cerebral artery syndromes as, 930–931, 931f
    thalamic infarction syndromes as, 931, 931.e1f
    transient ischemic attacks as, 925–927, 926b, 926t
    vertebrobasilar system syndromes as, 929–931, 929f, 930.e1f
    watershed ischemic syndromes as, 931
  crescendo episodes of, 927
  headache due to, 1692
  pathophysiology of, 924–925
Cerebral lesions
  hemiplegia due to, 263–265, 263t
  monoplegia due to, 268
  sensory deficit due to, 319
    cortical, 319
    thalamic, 319
Cerebral lymphoma, functional neuroimaging of, 495–496, 496f
Cerebral malaria, 1155
Cerebral malformations, with congenital heart disease, 835
Cerebral microbleeds, 971, 973f–974f
Cerebral oxygen extraction rate (O₂ER), in neurointensive care, 746
Cerebral oxygenation, in traumatic brain injury, 875t–876t

Cerebral palsy, 1311–1313
  clinical features of, 1311
  defined, 1311
  diagnosis and etiology of, 1311–1312
  disorders that mimic, 1312b
  due to hypoxic ischemic encephalopathy, 1311–1312
  evaluation of, 1313f
  metabolic or genetic causes of, 1312
  neuroimaging for, 1312
  prevention and management of, 1312–1313
  risk factors for, 1311–1312
Cerebral parenchymal hematoma, structural imaging of, 444
Cerebral perfusion pressure (CPP), 745
  after traumatic brain injury, 872, 875t–876t
Cerebral salt wasting, 709–710
Cerebral salt-wasting syndrome (CSWS), in neurointensive care, 755, 755t
Cerebral sensory lesions, 319
  cortical, 319
  thalamic, 319
Cerebral small vessel disease, 1416
Cerebral toxoplasmosis
  HIV-associated, 1115, 1116f
  structural imaging of, 436.e5
Cerebral tumor, 1027t
Cerebral vascular malformations, CT angiography of, 464
Cerebral vasculitides
  classification of, 936b
  ischemic stroke due to, 938–939
Cerebral vasospasm, 774–775
  balloon angioplasty for, 774, 774f
  intra-arterial vasodilators for, 774–775
  subarachnoid hemorrhage with, 994–995, 994f
  syncope due to, 12
  transcranial Doppler ultrasonography of, 748
Cerebral venous sinus thrombosis, 434–435, 435f
Cerebral venous thrombosis (CVT), 964–967
  aseptic, 966, 966f
  CT angiography of, 463
    multidetector-row, 463
  MR angiography of, 473–474, 474f
  during pregnancy, 1989–1990
  septic, 964–966, 966.e1f
  therapeutic measures for, 966–967
Cerebritis, 1265–1266, 1265t
  structural imaging of, 436.e1, 436.e2f
Cerebrocerebellar networks, 97
Cerebrohepatorenal disease, 1294t
Cerebrospinal fluid (CSF), 584–585
  absorption of, 1266, 1266f
  composition of, 1266–1267
  for Creutzfeldt-Jakob disease, 1371
  culture of, 1148–1149
  for inborn errors of metabolism, 1325, 1327t
  movement ventricles and around the spinal cord, 1264
  pressure, 1266
  production of, 1264–1265
Cerebrospinal fluid (CSF) analysis
  for HIV-associated neurocognitive disorders, 1111
  in multiple sclerosis diagnosis, 1170, 1172t
Cerebrospinal fluid (CSF) circulation
  abnormalities, headache due to, 1687
  disorders, structural imaging of, 447–449

Cerebrospinal fluid (CSF) examination, for leptomeningeal metastases, 1096–1097, 1097t
Cerebrospinal fluid (CSF) leak, headaches due to, imaging studies of, 1689, 1689f, 1689.e1f
Cerebrospinal fluid (CSF) lymphocytosis, transient syndrome of headache with neurological deficits and, 1690
Cerebrospinal fluid (CSF) pathway obstruction, headache due to, 1687
Cerebrospinal fluid (CSF) pleocytosis, migrainous syndrome with, 1690
Cerebrospinal fluid (CSF) rhinorrhea, headache due to, 1689–1690
Cerebrospinal fluid (CSF) tests, for headache, 202
Cerebrospinal fluid (CSF) volume, headache due to low, 1688–1690
Cerebrotendinous xanthomatosis (CTX), 1338, 1557–1558
  clinical features of, 1557b
  neurological features of, 1557
  treatment of, 1557–1558
  xanthomas in, 1557
Cerebrovascular accidents (CVAs), 521
Cerebrovascular disease
  headache due to, 1692
  ischemic. see Ischemic cerebrovascular disease
  neuroepidemiology of, 636–637
    morbidity rates in, 636–637
    mortality rates in, 636, 636f
    transient ischemic attacks in, 637
  during pregnancy, 1987–1990
    antiphospholipid antibody syndrome as, 1988
    arteriovenous malformations as, 1987
    cerebral venous thrombosis as, 1989–1990
    intracranial hemorrhage as, 1987
    ischemic stroke as, 1987–1988
    postpartum stroke as, 1988–1989
Cerebrovascular dysregulation, after traumatic brain injury, 872
Cerebrovascular ischemia, syncope due to, 12
Cerebrovascular occlusive diseases, structural imaging of, 432–435
Cerebrovascular reactivity, ultrasound for, 483
Cerovive, 960.e1
Ceruloplasmin, in copper deficiency, 1236
Cervical artery dissection, MR angiography of, 468
Cervical cord neuropraxia, 886
Cervical dystonia, 1452–1453
  botulinum toxin injections for, 155
Cervical myelopathy, transcranial magnetic stimulation for, 397
Cervical osteoarthritis, 1752
  vertebral artery stroke caused by, 1754–1755
Cervical radiculopathy, 1752–1753
  clinical presentation of, 1752–1753
  imaging of, 1752–1753, 1753f
  treatment of, 1753
Cervical segmental arteries, 1007.e1f
Cervical spinal cord injury, dysphagia due to, 155–156
Cervical spine
  and headaches, 1695
  imaging of, headache and, 202
Cervical spine fractures, 887–889
  subaxial, 888–889
Cervical spine injury, headache after, 1690

Dementia (*Continued*)
neuroleptic sensitivity, 1401
neuropsychiatric symptoms, 1401
neuropsychology, 1401
parkinsonism, 1400
pathology, 1401, 1402*f*
prodromal, 1399
REM sleep behavior disorder,
1400–1401
treatment, 1401–1403
and mild cognitive impairment, 488–493
mild cognitive impairment and, 1380–
1383, 1382*f*
mixed, neuropsychological characteristics
of, 522
multi-infarct, 1414
neurodegenerative associated with
Parkinsonism, 1399–1405
non-degenerative, 1420, 1420*b*
with Parkinson disease, *versus* dementia
with Lewy bodies, 491
Parkinson disease with, 107
chemical imaging of, 508
cognitive symptoms of, 523
motor signs of, 523
neuropsychological characteristics of,
523
parkinsonian, 1399*t*, 1400
preclinical stage of, 1381
pugilistica, 1419
redirection for, 77–78, 78*t*
seizures due to, 1583
semantic, behavior and personality
disturbances in, 80
and sleep dysfunction, 1656–1658
synucleinopathies as, 1399–1404
tauopathies as, 1404–1405
transcranial magnetic stimulation for, 396
treatment of, 717
urinary incontinence in, 608
vascular, 492–493
neuropsychological characteristics of,
521–522
young onset, 1420–1421, 1421*t*
"Dementia pugilistica", 865
Demyelinated axons, myelinated axons
versus, 1159–1160, 1160*f*
Demyelinating diseases
hemiplegia due to, 264–265
inflammatory, 1159–1186
site-restricted forms of, 1186
Demyelinating polyneuropathies
needle electromyography of, 383
nerve conduction studies of, 375–376,
375*f*
Demyelination, segmental, 1792–1794,
1794*f*
Demyelinative mononeuropathy, nerve
conduction studies of, 373–374,
373*f*
Dendrites, growth of, 1288–1289
Dendritic branching, 1288
Dendritic injury, traumatic, 853–854
Dendritic ramification, 1288
Denervation, of muscle, 1916
angulated fibers in, 1916, 1916*f*
checkerboard or mosaic pattern due to,
1916, 1917*f*
group atrophy due to, 1916, 1917*f*
reinnervation after, 1916, 1917*f*
target fiber in, 1916, 1917*f*
Dengue fever, 1145
Denis, Leigh, 1349
Dense MCA sign, 950, 950*f*

Dent disease, 1520*t*–1521*t*
Dental causes, of craniofacial pain, 1695
Dental imaging studies, headache and, 202
Dentatorubral-pallidoluysian atrophy
(DRPLA), 1448, 1471, 1477
2-deoxy-2-[^{18}F] FDG, 487
Deoxycytidine analogue, for brain tumors,
1051
Deoxyguanosine kinase deficiency,
1326.*e1t*–1326.*e2t*
Deoxyribonucleic acid (DNA), 649, 650*f*,
651*t*
Deoxyribonucleic acid viruses, encephalitis
and meningitis due to, 1121–1135
Depersonalization, 1994
DepoCyt (cytarabine), for leptomeningeal
metastases, 1099
Deprenyl, for Parkinson disease, 1432
Deprenyl and Tocopherol Antioxidative
Therapy of Parkinsonism (DATATOP)
trial, 1432
Depression, 92–114, 226, 92.*e1b*
after traumatic brain injury, 90–91, 91*t*
in Alzheimer disease, 78, 78*t*, 1398
in amyotrophic lateral sclerosis, 85, 85*f*,
1513*t*
assessment of, 76, 76*t*
biology of, 98–99
cerebral vascular disease, stroke and,
99–101, 100*b*
clinical symptoms and signs suggesting
neurological disease, 99
deep brain stimulation for, 405
versus delirium, 32, 32*t*
dementia with Lewy bodies in, 107
due to degenerative disorders, 105–109
Alzheimer disease as, 106
epilepsy, 107–109
frontotemporal dementia as, 106–107
Huntington disease as, 107
idiopathic Parkinson disease, 107
Lewy body dementia as, 107
due to epilepsy, 88, 89*t*, 526
due to vascular disease, stroke and
cerebral, 99–101, 100*b*
functional imaging studies of, 99
functional symptoms of, 1994
in Huntington disease, 82–83, 82*t*,
107
infectious
with Creutzfeldt-Jakob disease,
101–102
with Human Immunodeficiency Virus,
101
with neurosyphilis, 102
interferon-alpha and, 1145–1146
medication treatment for, 112*t*
metabolic and toxic, 102–105, 102.*e1t*
drug abuse as, 104
multiple sclerosis as, 104–105
porphyrias as, 103–104
systemic lupus erythematosus as, 104
thyroid disease as, 102–103
vitamin B$_{12}$ and folic acid deficiency as,
103
Wilson disease as, 103
in multiple sclerosis, 83–84, 525, 1167
treatment of, 1183
neuroanatomy corresponding, 93*t*
cortical networks, 94–97
neurological and systematic causes of,
99.*e2t*
in Parkinson disease, 80*t*, 81, 107
chemical imaging of, 508

Depression (*Continued*)
principles
of differential diagnosis, 92–93, 93*t*
of neuropsychiatric evaluation, 93–94,
95*f*
during rehabilitation
incidence of, 810
treatment of, 810
rTMS for, 398
seizures due to, 1583
in stroke, 89–90
treatment modalities and, 111–114
electroconvulsive therapy as, 113
psychiatric neurosurgery (psychosurgery)
as, 113–114
repetitive transcranial magnetic
stimulation as, 113
vagus nerve stimulation as, 113
treatment principles of, 114
in vascular dementia, 80
Depression-related cognitive impairment
(DRCI), 110
Depsipeptide, for brain tumor, 1053
Derealization, 1994
Dermatome, 1766
Dermatomyositis, 1949–1950
antibodies in, 1950
associated with neoplasia, 1951
associated with other collagen vascular
diseases, 1951
creatine kinase in, 1949
dysphagia in, 150
EMG of, 1949
histological feature of
perifascicular atrophy as, 1949,
1949*f*–1950*f*
plasmacytoid dendritic cells as, 1950
immune mediation in, 692
interferon-stimulated gene 15 in, 1950
needle electromyography of, 384
paraneoplastic, 1194
prognosis for, 1951–1952
of skin, 1949
treatment for, 693, 1951–1952
weakness and pain as, 1949
Dermoid cysts
pathology and molecular genetics of,
1043
structural imaging of, 446.*e8*
Desamino-D-arginine-vasopressin (DDAVP),
for diabetes insipidus, 708
Desipramine (Norpramin)
for chronic pain, 725*t*
for neuropathic pain, 918*t*–919*t*
Desmin deficiency, 1925, 1927
Desmin myopathy, 1927
Desmin storage myopathy, 1927
Desminopathy, familial, 1927
Desmoplasia, 1028
Desmoplastic infantile astrocytoma (DIA),
1077.*e1*
Desmoplastic infantile ganglioglioma (DIG),
1077.*e1*
Desmopressin
for bladder dysfunction, in multiple
sclerosis, 1183
for diabetes insipidus, in neurointensive
care, 755
for neurogenic bladder, 617–618
Desmoteplase, for acute ischemic stroke, 958
Desmoteplase in Acute Ischemic Stroke
(DIAS) study, 958
Desomorphine, 1254
Determinant spreading, 687–688

Detrusor leak-point pressure (DLPP), 896
Detrusor muscles, neurological control of, 605, 606f
Detrusor overactivity, 607–608, 614f, 616
  in Parkinson disease, 609
Detrusor-external sphincter dyssynergia (DESD), 896, 896t
Detrusor-sphincter dyssynergia, 607, 610
Development
  of axons and dendrites, 1288–1289
  biosynthesis of neurotransmitters in, 1290
    disorders of, 1290
  Cajal-Retzius neurons and subplate neurons of fetal brain in, 1291, 1291f
  concepts of, 66
  electrical polarity of cell membrane in, 1289
    disorders of, 1289
  embryological and fetal, 1279–1281
  of fissures and sulci, 1287–1288, 1288b, 1288f
    disorders of, 1288
  mitotic proliferation of neuroblasts (neuronogenesis) in, 1282–1283
    disorders of, 1283, 1283f
  molecular, 1279
  myelination in, 1290–1291
    disorders of, 1290–1291
  neuroblast migration in, 1284–1287, 1284f–1285f
    disorders of, 1286–1287, 1286f
      early, 1299–1300
      late, 1300.e2
    major mechanisms of, 1284–1286, 1285f
  neurulation in, 1281–1282
    disorders of, 1282
  programmed cell death (apoptosis) in, 1283–1284
    disorders of, 1283–1284
  synaptogenesis in, 1289–1290
    disorders of, 1289–1290
  typical and atypical, 66, 67t
Developmental coordination disorders (DCD), 1315–1317
  comorbid conditions with, 1316
  diagnosis of, 1315–1316, 1316b
  evaluation and etiology of, 1316–1317, 1316b
  handedness in, 1316
  motoric difficulties in, 1315, 1316b
  natural history of, 1316t–1317t
  treatment for, 1317
  visuospatial learning disabilities in, 1317b
Developmental delay
  global. see Global developmental delay (GDD)
  red flags for, 66
Developmental disabilities, 1301–1323
  autism spectrum disorders as, 1301–1306
    clinical features of, 1302–1304
      abnormalities of play as, 1303
      age and, 1303
      communication and, 1303
      IQ and, 1302–1303
      restricted range of behaviors, interests, and activities as, 1303–1304
      social communication dysfunction as, 1303
    diagnosis of, 1304–1306
    diagnostic criteria of, 1301, 1302b
    epidemiology of, 1301–1302
    etiology of, 1305–1306
      genetic, 1305–1306
      neuropathology, 1306

Developmental disabilities (Continued)
    evaluation of, 1304
    management of, 1306, 1307t
    medical comorbidities in, 1304–1305
    medical disorders associated with, 1304b
    prognosis of, 1306
    severity levels for, 1303t
  cerebral palsy as, 1311–1313
    clinical features of, 1311
    diagnosis and etiology of, 1311–1312
    prevention and management of, 1312–1313
  intellectual disability as, 1307–1311
    autism spectrum disorder and, 1302–1303
    clinical features of, 1307
    cognitive and behavioral problems in, 1309t
    comorbidities in, 1307–1308
    defined, 1307
    diagnosis and etiology of, 1307–1308
    environmental factors in, 1308
    epidemiological studies on, 1307–1308
    genetic defects in, 1308
    management of, 1308–1311
    metabolic disorders associated with, 1310t
    mild, 1307
    moderate, 1307
    neuroimaging for, 1308
    prevalence of, 1307
    profound, 1307
    severe, 1307
  learning disabilities as. see Learning disabilities
  prognosis for, 71
Developmental disorders, of nervous system, 1279–1300
  cerebellar, 1300.e2–1300.e3
    Chiari malformation as, 1300.e3
    Dandy-Walker malformation as, 1300.e2–1300.e3
    focal cerebellar dysplasia, 1300.e3, 1300.e3f
    global cerebellar hypoplasia as, 1300.e3, 1300.e3f
    selective cerebellar hemispheric aplasia as, 1300.e2
    selective vermal aplasia as, 1300.e2
  clinical expression of, 1293–1300, 1294t
  due to ischemic encephalopathy in fetus, 1292
  due to midline malformations of forebrain, 1295–1299
    agenesis of corpus callosum as, 1294t, 1298–1299, 1299f
    colpocephaly as, 1294t, 1299
    holoprosencephaly as, 1294t, 1296–1298, 1296t, 1297f
    isolated arhinencephaly and Kallmann syndrome as, 1298
    rhombomeric deletions and ectopic genetic expression as, 1298
    septo-optic-pituitary dysplasia as, 1294t, 1298
  etiology of, 1291–1292
  of fissures and sulci, 1288
  genetic loci and mutations in, 1279, 1280t–1281t
  of membrane polarity, 1289
  molecular genetic classification of, 1292–1293
  of myelination, 1290–1291
  of neurite growth, 1288–1289

Developmental disorders, of nervous system (Continued)
    of neuroblast migration, 1286–1287, 1286f
      early, 1299–1300
      late, 1300.e2
      lissencephaly as, 1286, 1299–1300
        in Miller-Dieker syndrome, 1286, 1294t, 1300.e1, 1300.e1f
        in Walker-Warburg syndrome, 1294t, 1300.e1–1300.e2
        X-linked recessive, with abnormal genitalia, 1300.e2
      pachygyria as, 1286–1287, 1294t
      periventricular nodular heterotopia as, 1286, 1300.e2
      polymicrogyria as, 1286–1287
      schizencephaly as, 1300.e2
      subcortical laminar heterotopia as, 1286, 1300.e2
    of neuronogenesis, 1283, 1283f
    of neurotransmitter synthesis, 1290
    of neurulation, 1282
      anencephaly (aprosencephaly with open cranium) as, 1282, 1293
      cephalocele as, 1282, 1293–1295, 1295f
      congenital aqueductal stenosis as, 1294t, 1295, 1295b
      meningomyelocele (spinal dysraphism, rachischisis, spina bifida cystica) as, 1282, 1295
    of programmed cell death, 1283–1284
    of symmetry and cellular lineage, 1293
      hemimegalencephaly as, 1293, 1294t
    of synaptogenesis, 1289–1290
    uniqueness of, 1281
Developmental dyscalculia, 1317–1318
  clinical features of, 1317
  evaluation and etiology of, 1317–1318
  management of, 1318
Developmental history, 3, 66
Developmental milestone, 66, 67t
Developmental quotient, 66
Deviation
  contraversive ocular, 565
  dissociated vertical, 537
  eye
    downward, 44
    inward, 44
    lateral, 44
    skew, 44
  periodic alternating gaze, 565
  physiological hyper-, 529–530
  primary and secondary, 530, 532f
  psychogenic ocular, 565
  skew, 563, 569
    with combined vertical gaze ophthalmoplegia, 205
    contraversive, 569
    ipsiversive, 569
    paroxysmal, 569
    periodic alternating, 569
  transient gaze, 564
Devic disease, 166, 691
Devic syndrome, 1982
Dexamethasone
  for brain metastases, 1086
  for cerebral edema, 1272
  for meningitis, 1149–1150
  for migraine, 1702
  for spinal cord compression, 1093
Dexamethasone suppression test, for Cushing disease, 706
Dexterity, loss of, 1485
  due to upper motor neuron impairment, 1485

Dextrose, for neonatal seizures, 1958
DFNA9 (deafness, familial, non-syndromic, type A), vertigo due to, 594
DFNB4 (deafness, familial, non-syndromic, type B), vertigo due to, 594
D-2-hydroxyglutaric aciduria, 1328.e1t
DIA (desmoplastic infantile astrocytoma), 1077.e1
Diabetes
　erectile dysfunction in, 611
　gastrointestinal dysfunction in, 1871
　hypoglycemia with, 1219
　as risk factors of Alzheimer disease, 1386
Diabetes insipidus (DI), 708
　central and nephrogenic, 708
　etiology of, 708
　management of, 708
　in neurointensive care, 755
　neurological complications of, in adults, 832
Diabetes mellitus (DM)
　and holoprosencephaly, 1296
　neurological complications of
　　in adults, 833–834
　　　in central nervous system, 833–834
　　　due to hypoglycemia, 834
　　　in peripheral nervous system, 833
　　in children, 847–848
　as risk factor, for stroke, 921–922, 948
Diabetic amyotrophy, 1842
　leg pain due to, 340
　monoplegia due to, 272
Diabetic autonomic neuropathy, 1841–1842
Diabetic ketoacidosis (DKA)
　hyperglycemia due to, 1220
　　complications of treatment of, 1221, 1221f
　neurological complications of
　　in adults, 834
　　in children, 847
Diabetic mononeuropathy multiplex, in adults, 833
Diabetic neuropathies, 1839–1845, 1840b
　clinical features of, 1840–1843
　laboratory findings of, 1843
　neurogenic bladder dysfunction due to, 611
　pathogenesis of, 1844
　pathology of, 1843–1844
　sensory abnormalities due to, 320
　treatment of, 1844–1845
Diabetic papillopathy, 172, 172f
Diabetic polyradiculoneuropathy, 1773–1774
　in adults, 833
Diagnosis
　assessment of cause of symptoms in, 5–6
　　anatomical localization in, 5–6
　　differential diagnosis in, 6
　　laboratory investigations in, 6
　chief complaint in, 2
　differential, 6
　examination in, 4–5
　　general physical, 5
　　neurological, 4–5, 5t
　experienced neurologist's approach to, 7
　history in
　　family, 4
　　of present illness, 2–3
　　of previous illness, 3
　　social, 4
　key to accurate, 1
　and management, 7
　neurological interview in, 1–2

Diagnosis (Continued)
　phenomenology in, 1
　review of patient-specific information in, 3–4
　review of systems in, 3
　spot, 1
　steps in, 1, 2f
Diagnostic and Statistical Manual of Mental Disorders (DSM), 92
Diagnostic and Statistical Manual of Mental Disorders-V (DSM-V), 76
Dialysis
　neurological complications of, in adults, 829–830
　for uremic encephalopathy, 1217
Dialysis dementia, progressive, in children, 848
Dialysis dementia syndrome, in adults, 829–830
Dialysis disequilibrium syndrome, 1218
　in adults, 829
　in children, 848
Dialysis encephalopathy, 1218
3,4-Diaminopyridine (3,4-DAP), for Lambert-Eaton syndrome, 1913
Diaphragmatic weakness, clinical presentation of, 280
Diarrhea, in autonomic disorders, 1870–1871
Diary, for Parkinson disease, 1436f
DIAS (Desmoteplase in Acute Ischemic Stroke) study, 958
Diaschisis, 500
　with neglect, 501
　reversal of, 500–501, 501f
Diastematomyelia, 1746, 1746.e1f
Diazepam
　for dystonia, 1452t
　for spasticity, 799t
Dichlorphenamide, for hypokalemic periodic paralysis, 1524
Diclofenac sodium (Voltaren), for chronic pain, 725t
Dicrotic wave, in intracranial pressure monitoring, 745
Didanosine (ddl, Videx), for HIV infection, 1108t–1109t
Dideoxynucleosides, neuropathy due to, 1860–1861
Diencephalic epilepsy, 1881
Diencephalic pupils, 42
Diencephalic seizures, 1881
Diencephalic syndrome, 208–209
Diet
　for inborn errors of metabolism, 1330
　and migraine, 1700
　as protective factors of Alzheimer disease, 1387
Dietary measures, for autonomic disorders, 1891–1892
Differential diagnosis, 6
Diffuse astrocytoma
　pathology and molecular genetics of, 1029f
　pediatric, 1073, 1074f, 1074t
Diffuse axonal injury (DAI), 871–872, 872f
　structural imaging of, 444, 445f
Diffuse glioma, 1030–1031
　molecular characteristics of, 1032–1033
Diffuse idiopathic skeletal hyperostosis (DISH), 1751, 1751.e1f
Diffuse intrinsic pontine glioma (DIPG), 1073–1075

Diffusion tensor imaging (DTI), 502, 502f, 670f, 417.e4, 417.e4f
　in disorders of consciousness, 55
　sports and performance concussion in, 862
Diffusion-weighted imaging (DWI)
　for Creutzfeldt-Jakob disease, 1371–1372, 1372f
　for stroke in children, 1004
Diffusion-weighted magnetic resonance imaging, 417.e3
　of ischemic stroke, 429
Diflunisal (Dolobid), for chronic pain, 725t
DIG (desmoplastic infantile ganglioglioma), 1077.e1
DiGeorge syndrome, copy number variation in, 668t
Digital span test, for delirium, 28
Digital subtraction angiography (DSA), 459–460, 463, 447.e1
　for carotid artery stenosis, 460f, 463
　for transient ischemic attack, 480–481
Dihydroergotamine (DHE)
　for cluster headaches, 1710
　for migraine, 1701, 1701t
　　in children and adolescents, 1719
　　menstrual, 1704
Dihydropyrimidine dehydrogenase deficiency, 1339
[11C]Dihydrotetrabenazine (DTBZ), in chemical imaging, 505
Dilated cardiomyopathy, cardiogenic embolism due to, 933–934
Dilator pupillae, neural control of, 179
Dimethyl fumarate, for multiple sclerosis, 1179–1180
DIP (drug-induced parkinsonism), 1442
Diphasic dyskinesias, in Parkinson disease, 1435
Diphenhydramine, for migraine, 1702
Diphtheritic neuropathy, 1864.e5–1864.e6
Diplopia, 529, 531f, 532–533
　in anisoiconia, 533
　assessment of patient with, 534b
　binocular, 533
　clinical assessment for, 533–539
　　convergence in, 535–536
　　cover-uncover test in, 536–537, 537f
　　cross-cover test in, 537
　　of ductions, 535f, 536
　　　forced, 539, 539b
　　edrophonium (Tensilon) test, 539
　　fatigability in, 539
　　general inspection in, 534
　　of head posture, 534–535, 535f
　　Hess screen test in, 536
　　Hirschberg test in, 536, 537f
　　history in, 533–534
　　Lancaster red-green test in, 536
　　Maddox rod test in, 536, 537f
　　of ocular alignment and muscle balance, 536–537
　　pinhole test in, 533
　　red glass test in, 536, 536f
　　sagging eye syndrome in, 537–538
　　of sensory visual function, 535
　　of stability of fixation, 535
　　three-step test for vertical diplopia in, 538–539, 538f, 539b
　　versions (pursuit, saccades, and ocular muscle overaction), 535, 535f
　crossed, 529, 531f
　fixation switch, 537
　in foveal displacement syndrome, 533

Diplopia (*Continued*)
  monocular, 533, 534*b*
  in myasthenia gravis, 1899
  ophthalmoplegia due to
    acute bilateral, 540*b*
    chronic bilateral, 540*b*
  physiological, 532, 533*f*
  related disorders to, 540–541
    asthenopia as, 540
    "interstate illusions" (highway
        hallucinosis) as, 540
    mal de débarquement as, 540
    micropsia as, 540
    monocular elevator deficiency (double
        elevator palsy) as, 540, 568
      acquired, 568
    oscillopsia as, 540
    palinopsia as, 540–541, 541*f*
    polyopia as, 540
    superior oblique myokymia as, 541, 551
      detection of, 551
      versus monocular nystagmus, 545
      treatment of, 546*t*, 551
    tortopia as, 541
    triplopia as, 540
  rules for evaluation of, 532*b*
  signs associated with, 539, 539*b*
  spread of comitance in, 533
  treatment of, 539–540
  uncrossed, 529, 531*f*
  and vergence, 558
  vertical, 532–533, 534*b*
    three-step test for, 538–539, 538*f*, 539*b*
  visual confusion with, 532, 533*f*
Dipole source localization methods, in EEG,
    350–351
[¹¹C]Diprenorphine, in chemical imaging,
    506
  of epilepsy, 509
"Dipstick" test, 613
Dipyridamole, for preventing stroke
    recurrence, 954
Direct cortical electrostimulation (DCES),
    499–500
Direct cortical stimulation, for intraoperative
    monitoring, 407
Direct nerve stimulation, for intraoperative
    monitoring, 407
Direct wave, in transcranial magnetic
    stimulation, 391
Directional preponderance, 599
Disability, defined, 714
Disc bulge, 455, 455*f*
Disc DeKompressor, 733
Disc extrusion, 455, 456*f*
Disc herniation, structural imaging of,
    455*f*–456*f*
Disc migration, 455, 456*f*
Disc protrusion, 455, 455*f*
Discitis
  lumbar, lower back pain due to, 341
  structural imaging of, 452, 452*f*
Discourse, 128
Disease gene discovery, genome/exome
    sequencing in, 666–669, 669*t*
Disease modifiers, 664
Disease modifying therapy, for multiple
    sclerosis, 1177–1180, 1181*f*
Disease progression, slowing of, as goal of
    treatment, 714
Disequilibrium, in linkage analysis,
    659–660, 661*f*
Disfacilitation hypothesis, of NREM sleep,
    1625.*e1*
DISH. *see* Diffuse idiopathic skeletal
    hyperostosis (DISH)

Disinhibition, in frontotemporal dementia,
    79
Disk herniation, 1769–1772
  clinical features of, 1770–1771, 1770*f*
  diagnosis of, 1771–1772, 1772*f*
  lumbar, 1757, 1757*f*
  soft, 1769
  spondylosis and, 1769–1770
  thoracic, 1755, 1755*f*
  treatment of, 1772
  type of, 1769*f*
Diskogram, for lower back and leg pain,
    336*t*
Diskography, 729*t*
Disopyramide, neuropathy due to, 1861
Disorders of consciousness
  chronic, 54–55
  decision-making and bioethics in, 56
  imaging in, 55–56
  prolonged, 54–55
Disorganized thinking, in delirium, 25
Disorientation, in delirium, 26
Dissecting aneurysm, 985, 986*f*–988*f*
Disseminated encephalomyelitis, acute, 1183
  clinical features of, 1184
  laboratory and clinical features of,
    1184–1185, 1184*f*
  para-infectious, 1184
  postvaccination, 1184
Disseminated intravascular coagulation
    (DIC), neurological complications of,
    826
Dissociated sensory loss, 318
Dissociated vertical deviation, 537
Dissociation apraxia, 117
  testing for, 119–120
Dissociative (nonepileptic) attacks, 1995–
    1996, 1995*t*, 1996*f*
  specific advice for, 2007
Dissociative seizure/motor disorder, 1992
Distal latency, of compound muscle action
    potential, 367–368, 367*f*
Distal muscular dystrophies, 1920*t*–1921*t*,
    1933–1934
Distal myopathies, 1933–1934
  Laing, 1934
  Markesbery-Griggs, 1920*t*–1921*t*, 1927,
    1933
  Miyoshi, 1933
  Nonaka, 1933–1934
  Udd, 1933
  Welander, 1933
  Williams, 1934
Distal renal tubular acidosis with deafness,
    594
Distal segment changes, in wallerian
    degeneration, 906
Distal sensory polyneuropathy (DSPN),
    HIV-associated, 1119
Distal symmetrical polyneuropathy,
    1840–1841, 1864.*e2*
Disturbed night sleep, 1641
Disturbed recent memory, in delirium, 28
Disulfiram, neuropathy due to, 1861
Ditropan (oxybutynin), for bladder
    dysfunction, in multiple sclerosis,
    1182–1183
Diuretics, for cerebral edema, 1272
Diurnal variation, of ischemic events, 924
Divalproex sodium, for chronic migraine
    prophylaxis, 1707
Divergence
  disorders of, 571
  dissociated vertical, 537

Divergence insufficiency, 571
Divergence paralysis, 571
Divergent eyes, 529–530
Diversity (D) segment, 679
Dix-Hallpike test, 595–596
Dizziness
  definition, 583
  epidemiology of, 584
  historical background of, 583–584
  history of present illness with, 586, 587*t*
  laboratory investigations in diagnosis and
      management, 598–603
    general tests, 598
    imaging in, 598
    vestibular testing, 598–601
      bithermal caloric testing, 599
      eye movement recording for, 598
      eye movement subtests for, 598
      posturography for, 601
      quantitative head-thrust testing for,
        601
      recording pathological spontaneous
        eye movements for, 598
      rotational testing, 600, 600*f*
      vestibular evoked myogenic potentials
        for, 601
      visual ocular motor control for,
        598–599, 599*f*
  nonspecific, common causes of, 587*t*,
    595
  physical examination of, 586–591
    general medical examination, 586
    general motor examination, 586
    general neurological examination, 586
    neuro-otological examination, 587–591
      auditory examination, 591
      fistula testing, 591
      of gait, 591
      gaze testing, 588
      ocular motor, 587–588
      optokinetic nystagmus and fixation
        suppression of the vestibulo-
        ocular reflex, 588
      positional testing, 589–591, 590*f*
      saccades, 588
      smooth pursuit, 588
      vestibular nerve examination,
        588–589, 589*f*
DKA. *see* Diabetic ketoacidosis (DKA)
DMD. *see* Duchenne muscular dystrophy
    (DMD)
DMPK. *see* Myotonic dystrophy protein
    kinase (DMPK)
DNA repair defects, ataxia due to, 1469
DNA sequencing
  in disease gene discovery, 666–667,
    669*t*
  exome, 669
  next-generation, 666–667
  Sanger, 666–667
DNA testing, for inborn errors of
    metabolism, 1328
DNA-based diagnosis, of mitochondrial
    disorders, 1357–1358
DNAJB6 deficiency, 1925
Docetaxel, for brain tumors, 1051
DOK-7 mutations, congenital myasthenic
    syndrome due to, 1911–1912
Dolichoectasia, 985, 986*f*
  ischemic stroke due to, 945
Doll's eye maneuver
  with coma, 44–45
  with combined vertical gaze
      ophthalmoplegia, 205
Doll's eye phenomenon, with coma,
    44–45

Doll's eye test, 588–589

"Doll's eyes", 585

Doll's head maneuver, with combined vertical gaze ophthalmoplegia, 205

Dolutegravir (Tivicay), for HIV infection, 1108t–1109t

Dominant allele, 651t, 657

Dominant intermediate CMT (DI-CMT), 1817

Dominant optic atrophy, 161–162

Dominant X-linked transmission, 659, 660f

Donepezil (Aricept), 1397
  for dystonia, 1452t

Doose syndrome, 1574

Dopa decarboxylase, in chemical imaging, 505t

Dopa-responsive dystonia, 244–245

Dopamine
  in ADHD, 1320
  in basal ganglia, 1426
  in chemical imaging, 505, 505f, 505t
  deficiency of, 632

Dopamine agonists (DAs), for Parkinson disease, 1427

Dopamine β-hydroxylase (DBH) deficiency, 1887

Dopamine depleters, for dystonia, 1452t

Dopamine dysequilibrium syndrome, chemical imaging of, 507–508

"Dopamine hypothesis," in psychosis, 97

Dopamine (D₂) receptor agonist, for menstrual migraine prophylaxis, 1705

Dopamine receptors
  in basal ganglia, 1426
  in chemical imaging, 505–506, 505t
  of epilepsy, 509

Dopamine release
  in Parkinson disease, 507–508
  in placebo effect, 507–508

Dopamine transmission, in chemical imaging of epilepsy, 509

Dopamine Transport (DAT) Scan, 1401

Dopamine transporter deficiency, 1326.e1t–1326.e2t

Dopamine transporter (DAT) imaging, 505, 505f, 505t
  of Parkinson disease, 506–507, 507f

Dopaminergic function, in chemical imaging, 505, 505f

Dopaminergic nerve terminal, in chemical imaging, 505, 505f

Dopaminergic neurons (DA), in wakefulness, 1623–1624, 1624f

Dopaminergic therapy, 1403

Dopa-responsive dystonia (DRD), 1454

Doppler ultrasound
  continuous-wave, 476–477
  microembolic signals in, 476–477
    of transient ischemic attacks, 481
  power, 477
    for high-grade stenosis, 479
    of transient ischemic attack, 480–481
  power motion-mode, 480
  pulsed-wave, 476–477
  transcranial
    of acute ischemic stroke, 480
    and brain death, 484
    of cervical carotid stenosis, 481
    and increased ICP, 483–484, 484f
    of intracranial atherosclerotic plaque, 482, 482f
    microembolic signals detected by, 481
    in neurointensive care, 744t, 748

Doppler ultrasound (Continued)
    for periprocedural monitoring, 484
    and thrombolytic agents, monitoring the effect of, 480
    of vasospasms, 483

Dorello canal, abducens nerve in
  anatomy of, 1727
  clinical lesions of, 1728

Dorsal cerebellar syndrome, 929, 929f

Dorsal column stimulators, 917

Dorsal midbrain syndrome, 206, 206b, 570

Dorsal polyganglionopathy, 1792, 1793f

Dorsal ramus, 1766, 1767f

Dorsal root ganglion (DRG)
  acquired disorders of, 1778–1779
  anatomy of, 1767
  in pain pathway, 721

Dorsal roots, 1767, 1767f

Dorsal scapular nerve entrapment, 1801t

Dorsal stream, 552
  in visual system, 58

Dorsal vermis
  in horizontal eye movements, 558
  and vergence, 558

Dorsolateral prefrontal cortex (DLPFC)-subcortical circuit, 96

Dorsomedial pattern generator, in swallowing, 149

Dose Escalation Study of Desmoteplase in Acute Ischemic Stroke (DEDAS), 958

Dose failure, in Parkinson disease, 1435

Double cortex, 1286

Double crush syndrome, 1807–1808

Double elevator palsy, 540, 568
  acquired, 568

Double hockey stick sign, in Creutzfeldt-Jakob disease, 1372f

Double vision, 2000
  due to brain tumor, 1046

Double-blind placebo-controlled studies, 713–714

Doublecortin (DCX) gene, 1286, 1300.e2

Down syndrome, 656
  cognitive and behavioral problems in, 1309t
  and stroke in children, 998

Downbeat nystagmus, 542t, 545
  causes of, 545, 547b
  treatment of, 546t

Downgaze, forced, 569

Downgaze paralysis, 568

Downgaze paresis, 206

Downward deviation, of eyes, 44

Doxepin (Sinequan), for chronic pain, 725t

Dragging gait, 1996, 1998f, 1999

Draw a Person test, 1315.e1b

DRCI (depression-related cognitive impairment), 110

DRD (dopa-responsive dystonia), 1454

DRD2 gene, in delirium, 28

DRD3 gene, in delirium, 28

Dream anxiety attacks, 1666–1667

Dreams, 1623

DRG. see Dorsal root ganglion (DRG)

Drinking, in posterior pituitary in, 708

Dronabinol, 1257
  for spasticity, 799t

Dronedarone, for preventing stroke recurrence, 955

Drop attacks, 17–22, 926–927
  causes and types of, 18b
  defined, 17, 1571
  due to Chiari malformation, 18

Drop attacks (Continued)
  due to otolith crisis, 19
  due to posterior fossa abnormalities, 18
  due to seizures, 18
  due to syncope, 17–18
  due to third ventricular abnormalities, 18
  due to transient ischemic attacks, 18
    from anterior cerebral artery ischemia, 18
    from vertebrobasilar insufficiency, 18
  with loss of consciousness, 17–18, 18b
  medical history with, 17
  neurological examination for, 17
  without loss of consciousness, 18–19, 18b

Dropped head syndrome, 280, 281f

Droxidopa, for autonomic disorders, 1894

DRPLA (dentatorubral-pallidoluysian atrophy), 1448

DRS-R-98 (Delirium Rating Scale-Revised-98), 28–29

Drug abuse
  CNS vasculitis due to, 1017
  drug dependence and, 1254–1258
    with anticholinergics, 1258
    with hallucinogens, 1257
    with inhalants, 1258
    with marijuana, 1257
    with opioids, 1254–1255
    with phencyclidine, 1258
    with psychostimulants, 1255–1256
    with sedatives, 1256–1257
  effects on nervous system, 1254–1260
    cognitive, 1259–1260
    fetal, 1260
    miscellaneous, 1260
    neurological complications, 1258–1260
      infection as, 1258
      seizures as, 1258
      stroke as, 1259
      trauma as, 1258
  and stroke, 939, 940f

Drug addiction, deep brain stimulation for, 405–406

Drug dependence, 1254–1258
  with anticholinergics, 1258
  with hallucinogens, 1257
  with inhalants, 1258
  with marijuana, 1257
  with opioids, 1254–1255
  with phencyclidine, 1258
  with psychostimulants, 1255–1256
  with sedatives, 1256–1257

Drug effects, in newborns, 1970–1972, 1970t
  passive addiction and withdrawal syndrome as, 1971–1972
  risk for intracranial hemorrhage as, 1971
  teratogenic effects and intrauterine growth retardation as, 1971, 1971f

Drug intoxication, delirium due to, 30, 30t

Drug withdrawal, delirium due to, 30, 30t

Drug-induced autophagic lysosomal myopathy, 1954

Drug-induced dysautonomia, 1887

Drug-induced hyperthermia, hypothalamus in, 700

Drug-induced neuropathies, 1858–1864, 1859t

Drug-induced parkinsonism (DIP), 1442

Drug-resistant epilepsy, 1594–1595

Drug-resistant seizures, 1594–1595

Drugs
    associated with idiopathic intracranial
        hypertension, 1273, 1273b
    for autonomic disorders, 1893–1894,
        1893b
    hypoglycemia and, 1219–1220
    and stroke in children, 1000–1001
    and viral nervous system disease,
        1124t
Drusen
    optic disc, 173–174, 174f
    of optic nerve head, 162
Drysol (aluminum chloride hexahydrate in
        anhydrous ethyl alcohol), for
        hyperhidrosis, 1873t
DSA (digital subtraction angiography),
        459–460, 463
    for carotid artery stenosis, 460f, 463
    for transient ischemic attack, 480–481
DSM (Diagnostic and Statistical Manual of
        Mental Disorders), 92
DSPN (distal sensory polyneuropathy),
        HIV-associated, 1119
DSPS (delayed sleep phase state), 1654
d₄T, for HIV infection, 1108t–1109t
DTBZ ([¹¹C]dihydrotetrabenazine), in
        chemical imaging, 505
DTH. see Delayed-type hypersensitivity
        (DTH)
Dual innervation, Hering law of, 528–530
Duchenne muscular dystrophy (DMD),
        1921–1923
    cardiac involvement in, 1922
    contractures in, 1922
    copy number variation in, 668t
    creatine kinase in, 1922, 1922f
    falls in, 1921–1922
    genetic counseling for, 1924
    Gower maneuver in, 1921
    leg weakness in, 291
    molecular defects of, 1919–1924,
        1920t–1921t
    muscle biopsy for, 1922, 1922f–1923f
    pseudohypertrophy in, 1921, 1922f
    treatment of, 1922–1923
        bracing for, 1923
        pharmacological, 1923
        physical therapy for, 1922–1923
        surgery for, 1923
Ductions, assessment of, for diplopia, 535f,
        536
    forced, 539, 539b
Duloxetine, for neuropathic pain,
        918t–919t
Duplex ultrasonography, 477–478, 477f
    color flow, 477, 478f
    sensitivity of, 479
    transcranial color-coded, 480
    of transient ischemic attack, 480–481
Duplications, 673–674, 673t
Dural arteriovenous fistula (DAVF), 464
    carotid-cavernous, neurointerventional
        therapy for, 778–779, 778f–779f,
        779b
    cranial, neurointerventional therapy for,
        777–778, 777b
    MR angiography of, 475–476, 475f
    spinal, 477f, 1010
        classification of, 1010b
        neurointerventional therapy for, 780
        structural imaging for, 451.e1
Dural ectasia, in Marfan syndrome, 1739
Dural metastases, 1094–1095
Dural sinus occlusion, MR angiography of,
        473–474, 474f
Dural tail sign, with meningioma, 424

Dural tumor, 1027t
Dural venous sinus thrombosis, 966
D-wave, in transcranial magnetic
        stimulation, 391
Dying-back polyneuropathy, 1792
Dynorphins, 697t–698t
Dysarthria, 128
    ataxia and, 217
    ataxic, 145
    classification of, 146t
    defined, 145
    examination for, 145
    flaccid, 145, 146t
    functional, 2000–2001
    hyperkinetic, 146, 146t
    hypokinetic, 145, 146t
    management of, 146
    mixed, 146
    spastic, 145, 146t
    spastic-flaccid, 146
    treatment of, 716
    unilateral upper motor neuron, 145
Dysautonomia, 1870–1871, 1881
    neuromedical problems during
        rehabilitation for, 795–796
    therapy for, 1891–1895
Dyscalculia, 1317–1318
    clinical features of, 1317
    evaluation and etiology of, 1317–1318
    management of, 1318
Dyschromatopsia, 574
Dyscognitive phenomena, with seizures,
        1565
Dysconjugate nystagmus, 545, 545b
Dysdiadochokinesia, 4–5, 218
Dysembryoplastic neuroepithelial tumor
        (DNET), 1077.e1, 1077.e1f
    pathology and molecular genetics of,
        1035
Dysesthesia, 315
Dysferlin deficiency, 1925
Dysfibrinogenemia, ischemic stroke due to,
        946
Dysgraphia, 1316–1317
Dyskinesia
    in Parkinson disease, 1435
    paroxysmal, 1532
    paroxysmal nonkinesigenic, 1456
Dyslexia, 1313–1315
    atypical features in, 1314b
    clinical features of, 1313–1314,
        1314t
    connectivity abnormalities in, 1315
    deep, 138–139
    developmental, double-deficit hypothesis
        of, 1314
    diagnosis and etiology of, 1314–1315
    functional imaging of, 1315
    genetic component of, 1314
    letter-by-letter, 138–139
    management of, 1315
    pathological studies of, 1314
    phonological, 139
    reading process, 139f
    structural imaging of, 1314
    surface, 139
Dyslipidemias, 1338
    as risk factor, for stroke, 922
Dysmetria, 218
    flutter, 542t, 549f, 550
    ocular, 549f, 550
    overshoot, 549f
    saccadic, 558
    undershoot, 549f
Dysmyelinating diseases, 1159
Dysosmia, 193

Dysphagia
    assessment, 157f
    defined, 148
    evaluation of, 156–157
        cervical auscultation, 156
        clinical examination in, 156, 156t
        diagnostic tests, 156, 156b
            EMG recording as, 157
            modified barium swallow test, 157
            3-ounce water swallow test, 157
            pharyngeal manometry as, 157
            timed swallowing tests as, 156–157
            videoendoscopy as, 157
            videomanofluorometry as, 157
    mechanical, 149, 149b
    in muscular dystrophy
        myotonic, 150
        oculopharyngeal, 1932
    neurogenic, 151–156, 152b
        in amyotrophic lateral sclerosis, 155
        due to brainstem processes, 155
        due to cervical spinal cord injury,
            155–156
        due to cranial neuropathies, 155
        due to other processes, 156
        due to stroke, 152–153
        in multiple sclerosis, 153–154
        in other basal ganglia disorders,
            154–155
        in Parkinson disease, 154
    neurologic, 148–157
    neuromuscular, 149–151, 150b
        in inflammatory myopathies, 150–151
        in mitochondrial disorders, 151
        muscular dystrophy
            oculopharyngeal, 150
            other, 150
        in myasthenia gravis, 151
    rehabilitation for, 794–795
    swallowing and
        neurophysiology of, 148–149
        normal, 148
        testing, 156b
Dysphagia limit, 157
Dysphasias, 128
Dysphonia, functional, 2001
Dysplasia, septo-optic, structural imaging for,
        446.e5
Dysplasminogenemias, ischemic stroke due
        to, 946
Dyspraxia, 115, 1316–1317
Dysregulation, after traumatic brain injury,
        91t
Dysrhythmic breathing, 1645–1648
Dysthyroid orbitopathy, 832
Dystonia, 235–237, 1451–1456
    adult-onset primary focal and segmental,
        1452–1453
        epidemiology and clinical features,
            1452–1453
        medical treatment of, 1453
        pathogenesis, 1453
        treatment, 1453
    cervical, 1452–1453
        botulinum toxin injections for, 155
    childhood-onset generalized, 1451–1452
        epidemiology and clinical features of,
            1451
        pathogenesis of, 1451–1452
        pathology of, 1451
        treatment of, 1452, 1452t
    classification of, genetic, 1451t
    common symptoms of, 235–237
    deep brain stimulation for, 404
    dopa-responsive, 1454
    embouchure, 1452–1453

Dystonia *(Continued)*
etiological classification of, 236*b*
examination of, 237
functional, 1999, 1999*f*
gravidarum, 1980
isolated foot, 1452–1453
limb, 1455
muscle pain due to, 303
myoclonus, 1454
neurodegeneration with brain iron
accumulation, 1455
oromandibular, 1452–1453
posttraumatic, 1455
in pregnancy, 1980
rTMS for, 399
tardive, 1450–1451
task-specific, 1452–1453
transcranial magnetic stimulation for,
395–396
truncal, pure, 1452–1453
in Wilson disease (hepatolenticular
degeneration), 1454–1455
clinical features of, 1454–1455
pathogenesis, 1455
pathology, 1455
treatment, 1455
Dystonia-parkinsonism
rapid-onset (DYT12), 1454
x-linked (DYT3; Lubag), 1453–1454
Dystonic gait, 257
Dystonic paraparesis, 256
Dystonic posturing, 1564, 1564.*e2f*
Dystonic tics, 240
Dystonic tremor, 231
Dystonic writer's cramp, 231
α-Dystroglycan, 1919
β-Dystroglycan, 1919
α-Dystroglycanopathies, 1926
Dystroglycans, 1919
Dystrophin, 1919
Dystrophin deficiency, 1919–1924
Becker muscular dystrophy due to. *see*
Becker muscular dystrophy (BMD)
Duchenne muscular dystrophy due to. *see*
Duchenne muscular dystrophy
(DMD)
other phenotypes associated with, 1924
Dystrophinopathy. *see* Dystrophin deficiency

E

EAAT (excitatory amino acid transporter)
proteins, in amyotrophic lateral
sclerosis, 1507–1508
EAE. *see* Experimental autoimmune
encephalomyelitis (EAE)
Eagle syndrome, 1722*t*, 1731
Eales disease, ischemic stroke due to, 944
EAOH (Early-onset ataxia with ocular motor
apraxia and hypoalbuminemia), 564
Ear
normal anatomy and physiology of,
584–586, 584*f*–585*f*, 586*t*
nose, and throat, functional symptoms in,
1993*t*
Earlier *versus* Later L-Dopa (ELLDOPA) trial,
1435
Early delayed radiation encephalopathy,
1245
Early life cognitive abilities, as protective
factors of Alzheimer disease, 1386
Early myoclonic encephalopathy, 1572
Early Start Denver Model (ESDM), for
autism spectrum disorder, 1306

EARLY STIM trial, 404
Early-onset ataxia with ocular motor apraxia
and hypoalbuminemia (EAOH), 564
Early-onset myasthenia gravis (EOMG),
1899, 1900*t*
EAS (external anal sphincter), in control of
defecation, 606
Eastern equine encephalitis (EEE), 1137*t*,
1139
Eating disorders, sleep-related, 1662–1663
EBNs (excitatory burst neurons), in eye
movements
horizontal, 553, 555*f*
vertical, 558–559, 559*f*
Ebola virus, 1145.*e1*
EBV. *see* Epstein-Barr virus (EBV)
Eccentric muscle contraction, muscle pain
due to, 303–304
[99mTc]ECD (ethylcysteinate dimer) , for
SPECT, 488
Echinococcus genus, CNS lesions due to, 1157
Echo train length, in fast spin echo imaging,
417.*e1*
Echoplanar imaging, in MRI, 417.*e2*–417.*e3*
Echopraxia, 121
Eclampsia
defined, 1990
and ischemic stroke, 1988
Eclamptic encephalopathy, 1990–1991
ECMO (extracorporeal membrane
oxygenation), and stroke in children,
997
ECoG (electrocorticography), for
intraoperative monitoring, 407
ECST (European Carotid Surgery Trial), 961
"Ecstasy", 1256
ECT (electroconvulsive therapy), for major
depressive disorder, 113
Ectopic genetic expression, 1298
Eczema, and brain tumors, 1024
Edema, in complex regional pain syndrome,
738
Edinger-Westphal nuclei, 179
EDMD. *see* Emery-Dreifuss muscular
dystrophy (EDMD)
Edrophonium chloride test, for myasthenia
gravis, 1901, 1901*f*
Edrophonium (Tensilon) test, for diplopia,
539
EDS. *see* Ehlers-Danlos syndrome (EDS)
EDSS (Expanded Disability Status Scale), for
multiple sclerosis, 1166
Education, as protective factors of Alzheimer
disease, 1386
Edurant (rilpivirine), for HIV infection,
1108*t*–1109*t*
EEE (Eastern equine encephalitis), 1137*t*,
1139
EEG. *see* Electroencephalography (EEG)
Efavirenz (Sustiva), for HIV infection,
1108*t*–1109*t*
Effendi system, modified, 888
EFHC1 gene, in juvenile myoclonic epilepsy,
1534
EGFR (epidermal growth factor receptor), in
diffuse gliomas, 1033
EGFR (epidermal growth factor receptor)
inhibitors, for brain tumor, 1053
Ehlers-Danlos syndrome (EDS), 1555–1557,
1556*f*, 1737–1738
classic, 1737
diagnosis of, 1737–1738
incidence of, 1737
intracranial aneurysm in, 983–984

Ehlers-Danlos syndrome (EDS) *(Continued)*
ischemic stroke due to, 943
neuromuscular symptoms of, 1737
neurovascular features of, 1556–1557
and stroke in children, 998
type IX, 1559
vascular (autosomal dominant), 1737
Ehrlichia chaffeensis, meningitis due to,
1147–1148
Eigenvectors, in diffusion tensor imaging,
417.*e4*
Ejaculation, 607, 622, 624*f*
disorders, treatment of, 633
SSRI, 633
vibrostimulation as, 633
impact of spinal cord lesions on, 628
premature, 633
Ejaculation dysfunction, management of,
621
Elavil, for dystonia, 1452*t*
Elbow
epicondylitis of, 331
"golfer's", 331
olecranon bursitis of, 331
pain in, 331
"tennis", 331
Elderly
delirium in, 33
falls in, 21, 21*t*
gait patterns in, 260
sleep pattern and, 1621–1622
Electrical current, effects of, 1246
Electrical injuries, of peripheral nerves, 909
Electrical polarity, of cell membrane, 1289
disorders of, 1289
Electrical stimulation, for chronic disorder of
consciousness, 55
Electrocardiogram (ECG), for stroke in
children, 1004–1005
Electrocardiography, for coma, 48
Electrocerebral inactivity, in brain death, 359
Electrocerebral silence, in brain death, 54,
359
Electrocochleography, 603
Electroconvulsive therapy (ECT)
for depression, 398
for major depressive disorder, 113
Electrocorticography (ECoG), for
intraoperative monitoring, 407
Electrodes
for nerve conduction studies, 367
positioning of, for EEG, 350
Electrodiagnostic examination (EDX), 366
for amyotrophic lateral sclerosis, 1510
for lower motor neuron impairment, 1495
needle electromyelography in, 381–384
of anterior horn cell disorders, 382*f*,
383
of lower motor disorders, 381–383,
382*f*
of mononeuropathies, 382–383, 382*f*
of myopathic disorders, 382*f*, 384, 384*t*
of peripheral polyneuropathies, 382*f*,
383
of plexopathies, 382, 382*f*
of radiculopathies, 382, 382*f*
of upper motor neuron lesions, 382*f*,
384
nerve conduction studies in
of axon-loss mononeuropathy, 374,
374*f*
of axonal polyneuropathies, 375, 375*f*
of demyelinating polyneuropathies,
375–376

Electrodiagnostic examination (EDX) (Continued)
  of demyelinative mononeuropathy, 373–374, 373f
  of focal nerve lesions, 371–375
  of generalized polyneuropathies, 375–376
  of preganglionic (intraspinal canal) lesions, 374–375
Electrodiagnostic studies, for peripheral nerve disorders, 1798, 1799f
Electrodiagnostic technologist, 407
Electrodiagnostic testing, for myasthenia gravis, 1902
Electroencephalography (EEG), 348–365
  alpha rhythm on, 349–350, 349f
  for anoxic-ischemic encephalopathy, 1202, 1206
  beta activity on, 349–350, 349f
  for brain death, 54
  clinical uses of, 351–359
    for aging and dementia, 359
    for altered states of consciousness, 356–357
    for brain death, 359
    for epilepsy, 352–355
      benign rolandic, 352, 354f
      epileptiform activity in, 352
      excessive focal or generalized slow-wave activity in, 352
      focal-onset (partial), 352, 353f
      generalized seizures, 352, 352f
      in Lennox-Gastaut syndrome, 352, 354f
      myoclonic, juvenile, 352, 352f
      petit mal, 352, 353f
      West syndrome as, 352, 353f
    for focal cerebral lesions, 355–356, 355f
    for hypoxia, 357
      alpha coma in, 357, 358f
      burst suppression pattern in, 357, 358f
      periodic pattern in, 357, 358f
    for infectious diseases, 357–359
    for metabolic encephalopathies, 357, 357f
  for coma, 48–49
  common types of abnormalities on, 350
    epileptiform discharges as, 350
    focal polymorphic slow activity as, 350
    generalized polymorphic slow activity as, 350
    intermittent monomorphic slow activity as, 350
    voltage attenuation as, 350
  continuous monitoring in intensive care unit, 359–365, 360b
    "ictal-interictal continuum", 361–362, 362f
    for nonconvulsive seizures, 360–361, 360f
      electrographic identification of, 361, 361b, 361f
    periodic discharges, 362, 362f–363f
    quantitative, 362–365, 364f, 364t
    stimulus-induced rhythmic, periodic/ictal discharges, 362, 363f
  for delirium, 29
  delta activity on, 349–350
  of dissociative (nonepileptic) attack, 1995
  for epilepsy, 1593–1594, 1593f
    epileptiform activity in, 1593
    prolonged recordings, 1594–1595

Electroencephalography (EEG) (Continued)
  epileptiform activity in, 348
  for global developmental delay, 69
  for hepatic encephalopathy, 1211
  for hypotonic infant, 307
  for intraoperative monitoring, 407
    monitoring interpretation of, 409
  invasive, recordings in, 1598
  magnetoencephalography as, 365.e1
  for neonatal hypoxic-ischemic brain injury, 1960, 1962
  for neonatal seizures, 1957
    amplitude-integrated, 1957
    interictal, 1957
  in neurointensive care, 744t, 747
  normal activities on, 349–350, 349f
  for patients with syncope, 13
  physiological principles of, 348–349
  prior to epilepsy surgery, 1596
  recording techniques for, 350–351
    "activating procedures" in, 350, 351f
    dipole source localization methods in, 350–351
    electrode positioning in, 350
    long-term, 351
    mathematical techniques in, 350–351
    montages in, 350
    during sleep, 350
    technological advances in, 350
    time-locked digital video image in, 351
    topographic maps in, 350, 351f
  rhythmic delta waves on, 356, 356f
  slow activity on
    focal polymorphic, 350
    generalized polymorphic, 350
    intermittent monomorphic, 350
    newborns and young children, 349–350
  in sporadic Creutzfeldt-Jakob disease, 1371f
  theta activity on, 349–350
  video-, 1596
Electrolyte disturbances, neurological complications of, 830–831
Electrolyte metabolism, encephalopathy due to disorders of, 1221–1225
Electrolytes, in neurointensive care, 754–755, 755t, 756f
Electromagnetic field (EMF) radiation, and brain tumors, 1021
Electromyographic findings, in botulism, 1914
Electromyography (EMG), 366, 615–616
  for hypotonic infant, 308
  for intraoperative monitoring, 407
    interpretation of, 409
    neurotonic discharge in, 409
  for lower back and leg pain, 335–337, 336t
  for muscle weakness, 286
  pelvic floor, 615
    of penilo-cavernosus reflex, 616
    of pudendal nerve terminal motor latency (PNMTL), 616
    of pudendal somatosensory evoked potentials, 616
  specialized electrodiagnostic studies in, 385–390
    A wave as, 385, 385f
    blink reflex as, 386
    F wave as, 385, 385f
    H reflex as, 385–386, 386f
    repetitive nerve stimulation as, 386–390
      principles of, 386–387
      rapid, 388, 388t, 389f
      slow, 387–388, 387f, 388t

Electromyography (EMG) (Continued)
    single-fiber electromyography as, 388–390
      fiber density in, 389
      jitter in, 389–390, 390f
      stimulation, 388–389
      voluntary, 388–389
  sphincter
    for cauda equina lesions, 615
    for multiple system atrophy, 615, 615f
    for urinary retention in young women, 615–616
Electron microscopy, 1029
Electron-transferring flavoprotein (ETF), 1337
Electroneuromyography, 366
Electronystagmography (ENG), 572, 598, 599f
Electro-oculography, 572
Electrophysiological testing, for headache, 202
Electroretinography (ERG), 579–581
  full-field, 579–581
  multi-focal, 579–581
Elementary motor, of seizures, 1564
Eletriptan, for migraine, 1701t, 1700.e1t
Elevated glucose, as risk factors of Alzheimer disease, 1386
ELLDOPA (earlier versus Later L-Dopa)) trial, 1435
Elliptical pendular nystagmus, 544
Elvitegravir (EVG), for HIV infection, 1108t–1109t
EMA (epithelial membrane antigen), 1030
Embolic protection device (EPD), for carotid artery, angioplasty and stenting, 763, 763f–764f
Embolism, cardiogenic
  in adults, 815
  ischemic stroke due to, 933–935, 934b, 935f
Embolization
  for cerebral arteriovenous malformations, 775–777, 776f
    with ethylene vinyl alcohol copolymer, 776–777
    with n-butyl cyanoacrylate, 776
    with polyvinyl alcohol, 775–776
  coil, for cerebral aneurysms, 769–770, 770f
  tumor, 780–782
    clinical evidence on, 782
    materials for, 781–782
    procedure for, 781–782, 781f–782f
    vessel selection for, 782
Embouchure dystonia, 1452–1453
Embryological development, of nervous system, 1279–1281
  mitotic proliferation of neuroblasts (neurogenesis) in, 1282–1283
    disorders of, 1283, 1283f
  neurulation in, 1281–1282
    disorders of, 1282, 1293–1295
Embryonal spinal tumor, structural imaging for, 450.e1
Embryonal tumors
  management of, 1059–1060
  pathology and molecular genetics of, 1038–1039
  pediatric, 1065–1070
    atypical teratoid/rhabdoid tumor as, 1069–1070
    medulloblastoma as, 1065–1069
    primitive neuroectodermal tumor as, 1065–1069

External stenotic lesions, ultrasound of, 481–482
External-pressure headache, 1715
Extraaxial primary brain tumors, 418t–419t, 423–426
Extra-axial tumor, 1027t, 1039–1041
  hemangiopericytoma and solitary fibrous tumor as, 1040–1041
  meningioma as, 1039, 1040f
Extracorporeal membrane oxygenation (ECMO), and stroke in children, 997
Extracranial circulation
  CT angiography of, 460
  MR angiography of, 467–469, 467f
Extracranial hemorrhage, in newborn, 1968, 1969t
Extracranial/intracranial (EC/IC) bypass surgery, for coronary artery occlusions, 961
Extradural tumors, structural imaging of, 449, 450f
Extramedullary intradural spinal tumors, 450
Extramedullary lesions, arm and neck pain due to, 327
Extraocular muscle weakness
  clinical presentation of, 280
  differential diagnosis of, 288–289
Extraocular muscles, 553
  actions of, 528–529, 529f, 529t
  anatomy of, 528–529, 529f–530f
  yoked pairs of, 528–529, 529t
Extraparenchymal tumors, headache due to, 1687–1688
Extrapyramidal diseases, 223
Eye examination, for coma
  abnormalities in resting position in, 44
  eye deviation in, 44
  general, 39
  ocular motility in, 43–45, 47
  pupil reactivity in, 42–43, 43f–44f, 47
  pupil size in, 42–43, 43f–44f, 47
  reflex ocular movements in, 44–45, 45t–46t, 47
  spontaneous eye movements in, 44, 47
Eye movements
  with coma
    reflex, 44–45, 45t, 47
    roving, 44
    spontaneous, 44, 47
  horizontal, 553–558, 555f–556f
    cerebellum in, 555, 556f, 558
    flocculus in, 558
    palsy of
      acquired, 564–565
      familial, 564
  ocular motor subsystems in, 552–553, 554f
  recording of, 598
    pathological spontaneous, 598
  recording techniques for, 571–572
  saccades as, 552, 556–557
    abducens nucleus in, 554, 555f
    cerebral cortex in, 556
    cerebrum in, 554
    classification of, 556–557
    electrophysiological events during, 556f
    excitatory burst neurons in, 553, 555f
    final common integrator hypothesis for, 555, 556f
    frontal eye field in, 552, 557
    gain of, 555
    hippocampus in, 556
    inhibitory cell-burst neurons in, 554
    interneurons in, 554, 555f

Eye movements (*Continued*)
    latch neurons in, 554
    lateral intraparietal area in, 556
    medial longitudinal fasciculus in, 554, 555f
    midbrain reticular formation in, 555
    neural integrator in, 554, 555f–556f
    ocular motor events in, 555f
    oculomotor neurons in, 556f
    omnipause neurons in, 554
    paramedian pontine reticular formation in, 553, 555, 555f
    parietal eye field in, 556–557
    pause cells in, 555f
    posterior parietal cortex in, 556
    prefrontal cortex, 556
    rostral medulla in, 554
    spontaneous, 556
    superior colliculus in, 554
    supplementary eye field in, 556–557
    vestibular cortex, 556
    vestibular nuclei in, 555f
    vestibular system in, 555–556
  simulated eye movement recordings of, 554f
  smooth-pursuit
    control of, 557, 558f
    defects, 557–558
  subtests for, 598
  types of, 554b
  vergence, 553f, 558
  vertical, 558–560, 559f–560f
    disorders of, 567–570, 569f
    paralysis of, 567–568
Eye protrusion, 186–187
Eyelid
  anatomy and neural control, 186
  normal position of, 186f
Eyelid abnormalities, 186–189
  with cerebral hemisphere lesions, 187t
  clinical presentation and examination, 186–187, 186b
  dynamic, 188–189
    apraxia of lid opening as, 188, 188f
    blepharospasm as, 188, 188f
    hemifacial spasm, 188–189
  pathologically narrowed palpebral fissures as, 188
  pathologically widened palpebral fissures as, 187–188
Eyelid myoclonia, with absence seizure, 1569
Eyelid retraction
  on downgaze, 187
  lower, 188
Eyestrain, 532
Ezetimibe, necrotizing myopathy due to, 1954
Ezogabine/retigabine, for epilepsy
  absorption, elimination half-life, formulations of, 1600t
  efficacy by seizure type of, 1601t
  hepatic metabolism, enzyme induction/inhibition, pharmacokinetic interactions, and protein binding of, 1603t
  mechanism of action of, 1604t

F
F wave, 385, 385f
  in transcranial magnetic stimulation, 391–392
FA (fractional anisotropy), in dyslexia, 1315

Fabry disease, 1818.e7f, 1328.e1t, 1818.e7–1818.e8
  ischemic stroke due to, 943
  and stroke in children, 1001
Face-object recognition network, 94
Facet joint block, 729t
Facet joint disruption, structural imaging of, 454.e2, 454.e2f–454.e3f
Facet joint pain syndrome, 340–341
Facet joint rhizotomy, 729t
Facial angiofibromas, in tuberous sclerosis, 1539
Facial appearance, in myasthenia gravis, 1897f, 1898
Facial asymmetry, 534
Facial cutaneous angioma, in Sturge-Weber syndrome, 1546
Facial muscle weakness
  bedside examination of, 281
  clinical presentation of, 280
  differential diagnosis of, 289–290
Facial myokymia, 188–189, 1730
  in multiple sclerosis, 1165
Facial nerve, 1726f, 1728–1731
  anatomy of, 1728–1729, 1729f
  clinical lesions of, 1729–1731
    of facial nerve branches, 1731
    of facial nucleus and fascicle, 1730
    facial palsy as, appearance of, 1729–1730, 1729f
    of geniculate ganglion, 1730–1731
    intratemporal, 1730–1731
    of subarachnoid space, 1730
Facial nerve branch
  anatomy of, 1728
  clinical lesions of, 1731
Facial nerve fasciculus
  anatomy of, 1729
  clinical lesions of, 1730
Facial nerve involvement, neuropathies with, 1796, 1796b
Facial nerve root, clinical lesions of, 1730
Facial nerve schwannomas, intratemporal, 1730–1731
Facial neuralgia, 1716–1718
Facial nucleus
  anatomy of, 1729
  clinical lesions of, 1730
Facial pain, 197–204. *see also* Headache
  atypical, 1715
  dental causes of, 1695
  due to anesthesia dolorosa, 1716
  due to geniculate herpes zoster or Ramsay Hunt syndrome, 1715–1716
  due to glossopharyngeal neuralgia, 1717
  due to nervus intermedius neuralgia, 1717–1718
  due to occipital neuralgia, 1718
  due to postherpetic neuralgia, 1718
  due to temporomandibular joint disorders, 1695
  nasal causes of, 1694–1695
  persistent idiopathic, 1715
  sphenopalatine ganglion block for, 729–730, 729t
  types of, 1715–1718
Facial palsy, 1726.e1t
  appearance of, 1729–1730, 1729f
Facial paralysis, in newborn, 1969
Facial paresis, in multiple sclerosis, 1165
Facial recognition defect, 125
Facial sensation, impairment of, in multiple sclerosis, 1165
Facial spasm, functional, 1996, 1998f

Facilitatory I-wave interactions, in transcranial magnetic stimulation, 393
Faciobrachial dystonic seizures, in anti-LGI1 limbic encephalitis, 1199
Facioscapulohumeral dystrophy (FSHD), 1930–1932, 1931*f*
clinical features of
facial and bulbar weakness as, 289, 289*f*
scapular winging as, 289, 289*f*
diagnosis of, 1931, 1931*f*
hypotonic infant due to, 310
muscle biopsy of, 1931, 1931*f*
in pregnancy, 1977–1978
treatment of, 1931–1932
Factitious disorder, 1993
Factor V Leiden mutation, as risk factor for stroke, 924, 946
Factor VII, as risk factor for stroke, 924
Fahr disease, 1442
Failed back surgery syndrome (FBSS), 732, 1758
spinal cord stimulation for, 733–734
Faint, 11
Falls, 17–22
in aged, 20–22, 21*t*
causes and types of, 18*b*
collapsing, 252
cryptogenic, in middle-aged, 19–20
due to basal ganglia disorders, 20
due to cerebral/cerebellar disorders, 19
due to Duchenne muscular dystrophy, 1921–1922
due to myelopathy, 19
due to neuromuscular disorders, 19
due to other Parkinsonian syndromes, 20
due to Parkinson disease, 20
due to progressive supranuclear palsy, 20
due to stroke, 19
fear of, 260
and gait disorders, 252
intervention for, 21
medical history with, 17
neurological examination for, 17
toppling, 252
[¹⁸F]Fallypride, in chemical imaging of epilepsy, 509
FALS (familial amyotrophic lateral sclerosis), 1515–1516
False localizing signs, 6
Famciclovir, for viral infections, 1127*t*
FAME (familial adult myoclonic epilepsy), 1535
Familial adult myoclonic epilepsy (FAME), 1535
Familial amyloid polyneuropathy (FAP), 1818.*e*4–1818.*e*5, 1818.*e*4*t*
apolipoprotein A1 amyloidosis, 1818.*e*5
diagnosis of, 1818.*e*5
gelsolin amyloidosis, 1818.*e*5
transthyretin, 1818.*e*4–1818.*e*5
treatment of, 1818.*e*5
Familial amyotrophic lateral sclerosis (FALS), 1515–1516
Familial aneurysms, 983
Familial ataxia syndromes, vertigo due to, 587*t*, 594
treatment for, 603
Familial bilateral vestibulopathy (FBV), vertigo due to, 587*t*, 594
Familial cardiomyopathy with subsarcolemmal vermiform deposits, 1927
Familial Creutzfeldt-Jakob disease (fCJD), 1366*f*, 1374
Familial defective apolipoprotein B (APOB), 1326.*e*1*t*–1326.*e*2*t*

Familial desminopathy, 1927
Familial dysautonomia (FD), 1882–1883
Familial episodic ataxias, 1529–1530
clinical features of, 1530
diagnosis of, 1530, 1530*f*
genetic basis for, 1520*t*–1521*t*
pathophysiology of, 1530
treatment of, 1530
Familial erythromelalgia, 1531–1532
Familial hearing loss and vertigo, 594
Familial hemiplegic migraine (FHM), 942–943, 1528–1529, 1698
clinical features of, 1528, 1528*f*
diagnosis of, 1529
genetic basis for, 1520*t*–1521*t*
pathophysiology of, 1528–1529, 1529*f*
subtypes of, 1528
treatment of, 1529
Familial horizontal gaze palsy with scoliosis, 564
Familial hyperinsulinemic hypoglycemia of infancy (FPHHI), 1520*t*–1521*t*
Familial infantile myasthenia, 1911
Familial lateral temporal lobe epilepsy (FLTLE), 1533
Familial mesial temporal lobe epilepsy, 1578
Familial progressive vestibular-cochlear dysfunction, 594
Familial rectal pain syndrome, 1818.*e*3
Familial temporal lobe epilepsies, 1533
Family history, 4
for global developmental delay, 67
Family studies, of multiple sclerosis, 642–643
FAP. *see* Familial amyloid polyneuropathy (FAP)
Farber disease, 1333.*e*2*t*–1333.*e*3*t*
Farming, and brain tumors, 1022
FARR (Friedreich ataxia with retained reflexes), 1466
Fas ligand (FasL)
in apoptosis, 684, 685*f*
in CNS, 686
Fascicles, 904
Fascicular repair, for peripheral nerve trauma, 915
Fasciculation
in amyotrophic lateral sclerosis, 1508, 1513*t*
defined, 285
for lower motor neuron impairment, 1495
Fasciculation potentials
Lambert's criteria of, 383
in needle electromyography, 377*t*, 379
FasL. *see* Fas ligand (FasL)
Fast channel syndrome, 1911
Fast foot, 285–286
Fast (turbo) spin echo (FSE) techniques, 417.*e*1
Fast-foot maneuver, 285–286
Fastigial nuclei, in horizontal eye movements, 558
Fat embolism, ischemic stroke due to, 945
Fat saturation, for MRI, 417.*e*2, 417.*e*2*f*
Fatal familial insomnia (FFI), 1374, 1657
Fatigability, assessment of, in diplopia, 539
Fatigue
in amyotrophic lateral sclerosis, 1513*t*
defined, 1616
and functional disorders, 2002
in multiple sclerosis, 1166
treatment of, 1182
muscle weakness due to, 284
neuromedical problems during rehabilitation for, 797

Fatty acid oxidation defects, 1337
Fatty acids, in hepatic encephalopathy, 1214–1215
Fazio-Londe disease, 1501
FBI (Frontal Behavior Inventory), 76, 77*t*
FBV (familial bilateral vestibulopathy), vertigo due to, 587*t*, 594
Fc portion, of immunoglobulin, 678
Fc receptors, in adaptive immune response, 677
fCJD (familial Creutzfeldt-Jakob disease), 1366*f*
[¹⁸F]FCWAY , in chemical imaging of epilepsy, 509
FD (6-[¹⁸F]fluoro-L-dopa), in chemical imaging, 505
of epilepsy, 509
of Parkinson disease, 506–507, 507*f*
[¹⁸F]FDDNP, in chemical imaging, 506
of Alzheimer disease, 508–509
FDG-PET
of Alzheimer disease, 488*f*–489*f*, 489–490
in behavioral variant of frontotemporal dementia, 488*f*
for brain tumors, 495, 495*f*–496*f*
of corticobasal degeneration (CBD), 493, 494*f*
of dementia
frontotemporal, 489, 489*f*
with Lewy bodies, 490–491, 491*f*
Parkinson disease with, 491
vascular, 492–493
for epilepsy, 497, 497*f*–499*f*
of mild cognitive impairment, 490
of Parkinson disease, 493, 493*f*
for parkinsonism, 489–490, 495
in posterior cortical atrophy, 490*f*
for presurgical brain mapping, 499–500
of primary progressive aphasia, 489*f*
of progressive supranuclear palsy (PSP), 493, 494*f*
Febrile seizures, 1520*t*–1521*t*, 1580–1581
generalized epilepsy with, 1534, 1534*f*
neuroepidemiology of, 640–641
simple *versus* complex, 1580
Fecal incontinence, management of, 621, 621.*e*1
FEF (frontal eye field), in horizontal eye movements, 552, 557
Feigning, 2002–2003
Felbamate
for epilepsy
absorption, elimination half-life, formulations of, 1600*t*
efficacy by seizure type of, 1601*t*
hepatic metabolism, enzyme induction/inhibition, pharmacokinetic interactions, and protein binding of, 1603*t*
mechanism of action of, 1604*t*
psychotropic effects of, 89*t*
Female genitals, anatomy of, 624, 625*f*–626*f*
Female sexual dysfunction
due to spinal cord injury, 611
management of, 621
Female sexual function, primary impact of spinal cord lesions on, 629, 629*f*–630*f*
Female sexual response, 624–625
arousal and plateau phase, 624–625
dysfunction in, treatments for, 633
hormone and other (drug) therapy as, 633
natural potential and lubricants as, 633
phosphodiesterase inhibitors as, 633

Female sexual response *(Continued)*
  rehabilitation by Kegel exercises as, 633
  vacuum device, vibrostimulation, and
      sex toys as, 633
  neurological control of, 607
  orgasm and resolution, 625
Femoral nerve, 1809–1810
  applied anatomy of, 1809–1810
  motor and sensory function of, 334*t*
Femoral nerve entrapment, 1802*t*
Femoral nerve lesions, 1810
Femoral neuropathy, leg pain due to, 339
Fencing posture, with partial seizures of
    frontal lobe origin, 1568
Fenoprofen calcium (Nalfon), for chronic
    pain, 725*t*
Fentanyl
  half-life of, 1203*t*
  with induced hypothermia for
      cardiopulmonary arrest, 1204*b*
Fentanyl patch (Duragesic), for chronic pain,
    727*t*
Festinating speech, 225
Festination, 225–226
Fetal anticonvulsant syndrome, 1985
Fetal development, of nervous system,
    1279–1281
  mitotic proliferation of neuroblasts
      (neuronogenesis) in, 1282–1283
    disorders of, 1283, 1283*f*
  neurulation in, 1281–1282
    disorders of, 1282, 1293–1295
Fetal effects, of drug abuse, 1260
Fetal hydantoin syndrome, 1985
Fetal PCA, 432.*e*1–432.*e*2
Fetal watershed zones, 1292
α-fetoprotein, in ataxia-telangiectasia,
    1553
Fetor hepaticus, with coma, 39
Fetus, ischemic encephalopathy in, CNS
    malformations due to, 1292
Fever
  central, 757
  coma with, 38
  hypothalamus in, 700
  in neurointensive care, 756–757
F-fluorodeoxyglucose (FDG) positron
    emission tomography (PET), in
    disorders of consciousness, 56
Fiber degeneration, 1917
Fiber density, in single-fiber
    electromyography, 389
Fiber regeneration, 1917
Fiber splitting, 1916–1917
Fiber type grouping, for lower motor neuron
    impairment, 1495–1496
Fiber type predominance, 1918
Fiber-type disproportion, congenital, 1948,
    1948*f*
Fibric acids, necrotizing myopathy due to,
    1954
Fibrillary morphology, 1031
Fibrillation potentials
  Lambert's criteria of, 383
  in needle electromyography, 377–379,
      377*t*, 378*f*
Fibrillin-1 gene, in Marfan syndrome,
    1738–1739
Fibrinogen levels, as risk factor for stroke,
    924, 935, 946
Fibrinolysis, intraarterial, for acute ischemic
    stroke, 958
Fibrinolytic treatment, intracerebral
    hemorrhage due to, 969–971

Fibroblast growth factor receptor gene
    (FGFR3), in achondroplasia, 1738
Fibrocartilaginous emboli, spinal cord
    infarction due to, 1009, 1009*f*
Fibromas, ungual, in tuberous sclerosis,
    1539, 1541*t*
Fibromuscular dysplasia (FMD)
  CTA of, 460
  detection of patterns of, by MR
      angiography, 469
  ischemic stroke due to, 938, 939*f*
  and stroke in children, 1000
Fibromyalgia, 1764–1765
  arm and neck pain due to, 331
  muscle pain due to, 299, 304
  sleep disorders in, 1670–1671
  tender points in, 1764–1765, 1765*f*
Fibrosis, 1917
Fibular neck, common fibular neuropathy at,
    1808–1809
Fibular nerve, applied anatomy of, 1808
Fibular nerve entrapment, 1802*t*
Fibular neuropathy, monoplegia due to,
    270
"Fibular tunnel", 1808
Fifth-degree nerve injury, 371–373
Figure-of-4 posturing, 1567, 1567.*e*1*f*
Filamin-A (FLNA) gene, in neuroblast
    migration, 1286
Filopodia, in nerve regeneration, 907, 907*f*
Filoviruses, hemorrhagic fever due to,
    1145.*e*1
Final common integrator hypothesis, for
    horizontal eye movements, 555, 556*f*
Finger counting, 576
  in the quadrants, 576
  simultaneous, 576
Finger rub test, for hearing loss, 591
Fingolimod (Gilenya), for multiple sclerosis,
    690, 1179
Finkelnburg, Carl Maria, 115–116
First-degree nerve injury, 371–373
FISH. *see* Fluorescence in situ hybridization
    (FISH)
Fissures, development of, 1287–1288,
    1288*b*, 1288*f*
  disorders of, 1288
Fisting, in hypotonic infant, 306–307
Fistula testing, for dizziness, 591
Fitness training, in rehabilitation, 786
Fixation
  development of, 560
  spasm of, 564
  stability of, in diplopia, 535
Fixation subsystem, 552
Fixed battery approach, to
    neuropsychological evaluation, 512–513,
    513*b*
FKRP. *see* Fukutin-related protein (FKRP)
Flaccid dysarthria, 145, 146*t*
Flaccidity, due to lower motor neuron
    impairment, 1495
Flail leg presentation, of amyotrophic lateral
    sclerosis, 1508
FLAIR (fluid-attenuated inversion recovery),
    300
  for Creutzfeldt-Jakob disease, 1371–1372,
      1372*f*
Flavivirus
  dengue fever due to, 1145
  Japanese encephalitis virus as, 1138–1139
  Murray Valley encephalitis virus as,
      1139.*e*1
  Powassan virus as, 1137*t*, 1139

Flavivirus *(Continued)*
  St. Louis encephalitis virus as, 1137*t*, 1138
  tickborne encephalitis virus as, 1139.*e*1
  West Nile virus, 1136–1138
  yellow fever due to, 1145
Flexeril, for chronic pain, 726
Flexible battery approach, to
    neuropsychological evaluation, 513,
    514*f*
Flexion-compression injuries, 888–889
Flexion-distraction injuries, 888–889
FLNA (filamin-A) gene, in neuroblast
    migration, 1286
"Floating neurons," in dysembryoplastic
    neuroepithelial tumor, 1035
Flocculus, in horizontal eye movements, 558
Floppy infant. *see* Hypotonic infant
Flow gaps, in time-of-flight MR, 473–474
Flow velocity
  and cardiovascular reactivity, 483
  and carotid stenosis, 479
  changes in, 480
  and transcranial Doppler ultrasonography,
      480
  vasospasm and, 483
Flow-diversion devices, for cerebral
    aneurysms, 773–774
Flow-diversion stent, for intracranial
    aneurysm, 993
FLTLE (familial lateral temporal lobe
    epilepsy), 1533
Fludrocortisone (Florinef)
  for autonomic disorders, 1893
  for dystonia, 1452*t*
Fluent speech, 130
Fluid, in neurointensive care, 754–755, 755*t*,
    756*f*
Fluid overload, 1961
Fluid percussion (FP) injury model, 850
Fluid restriction, for SIADH, 709
Fluid-attenuated inversion recovery (FLAIR),
    170*f*, 1196
  for Creutzfeldt-Jakob disease, 1371–1372,
      1372*f*
  for stroke in children, 1004
Flumazenil, for hepatic encephalopathy,
    1214
[^{11}C]Flumazenil, in chemical imaging, 506
  of epilepsy, 509
Fluorescein angiography, 579
Fluorescence in situ hybridization (FISH),
    655, 1030
Fluorine-18 (^{18}F), for positron emission
    tomography, 504
6-[^{18}F]Fluoro-L-dopa (FD), in chemical
    imaging, 505
  of epilepsy, 509
  of Parkinson disease, 506–507, 507*f*
6-[^{18}F]Fluoro-meta-tyrosine (FMT), for
    chemical imaging, 505
[^{18}F] Fluorodeoxyglucose-positron emission
    tomography (FDG-PET)
  of Alzheimer disease, 1381, 1411*f*
  for paraneoplastic neurological syndromes,
      1188
[^{18}F]Fluorodopamine, in chemical imaging,
    505
5-Fluorouracil (5FU), ataxia due to,
    1461
Fluoxetine, for neuropathic pain,
    918*t*–919*t*
Fluphenazine, for dystonia, 1452*t*
Flurbiprofen (Ansaid), for chronic pain,
    725*t*

Flutter
  atrial, syncope due to, 10–11
  dysmetria, 542t, 549f, 550
  micro-, 546t, 550
  ocular, 549
    with coma, 44
    localization of, 542t
    oculographic diagram of waveforms in,
      549f
FMNS (fusion maldevelopment nystagmus
  syndrome), 543
FMT (6-[¹⁸F]fluoro-meta-tyrosine), for
  chemical imaging, 505
Focal lesions, 1156–1158
  diagnosis of, 1157, 1157t
  etiology and clinical presentation of,
    1156–1157
  prevention of, 1157–1158
Focal localizing signs, 6
Focal motor symptoms, of brain tumor,
  1045
Focal/multifocal hypoxic-ischemic brain
  injury, in newborn, 1962–1963
Focal nerve lesions
  blink reflex for, 386
  nerve conduction studies of,
    371–375
Focused neurological examination, 4
"Fogging" refraction, 581–582
"Fogging test", 2000
Foix-Chavany-Marie syndrome, 147,
  152–153
Folate deficiency, 1228–1229, 1362,
  1852–1853
  causes of, 1228–1229
  clinical features of, 1229
  cobalamin deficiency due to, 1227
  laboratory studies for, 1229
  treatment of, 1229
Folic acid, during pregnancy with epilepsy,
  1985–1986
Folic acid deficiency, psychiatric
  manifestations of, 103
Folinic acid, for inborn errors of
  metabolism, 1325–1326
Follicle-stimulating hormone (FSH),
  697t–698t
  hypothalamic peptides controlling release
    of, 702t
  in precocious puberty, 704
Follicle-stimulating hormone (FSH)-secreting
  tumors, 706
Food ingestion, for autonomic disorders,
  1892
FOOD Trial Collaboration, for dysphagia,
  795
Foot, striatal, 228, 229f
Foot deformities, in Charcot-Marie-Tooth
  disease type 1, 1812, 1814f
Foot drop, 254–255, 255b
  in amyotrophic lateral sclerosis, 1508
Foot dystonia, isolated, 1452–1453
Foot tremor, hypnagogic, 1668
Foramen magnum, in Chiari I malformation,
  1741, 1742f
Foramen magnum lesion, 275–276
Foramen magnum syndrome, 209
Foramen ovale, patent, cardiogenic
  embolism due to, 815, 935
Forced downgaze, 569
Forced ductions, for diplopia, 539b
Forced eyelid closure, 187f
Forced normalization, 526
Forced prolonged position, 590
Forced upgaze, 568
Forced-choice responding, 192

Forebrain, midline malformations of,
  1295–1299
"Foreign accent syndrome", 147
Forensic imaging, 503
Forestier disease, 1751
Fork stalling and template switching
  (FoSTeS), 667f
Forkhead box P2 (FOXP2) transcription
  factor, 653
Fornix, in memory, 62–63, 62f
Fortification spectra, 123
Fosamprenavir (Lexiva), for HIV infection,
  1108t–1109t
Foscarnet, for viral infections, 1127t
Fosphenytoin
  for neonatal seizures, 1958
  for trigeminal neuralgia, 1717
FoSTeS. see Fork stalling and template
  switching (FoSTeS)
Founder effect, 1328
Four-A Syndrome, 1517
Four-dimensional computed tomography
  angiography, 459, 462, 464
Four-dimensional time-resolved MRA (4D
  MRA), 466
FOUR score, 41
  for critically ill patients, 742, 743f
Fourier transform, in MRI, 413, 416–417
Fourth cranial nerve
  fundamental features of, 538–539
  palsy, 569
Fourth ventricle, rosette-forming
  glioneuronal tumor of, 1036
Fourth-degree nerve injury, 371–373
Fovea, 528–529, 573
Foveal displacement syndrome, 533
Foveation, 528–529
Foville syndrome, 214b, 1722t, 1728,
  1730
Fowler syndrome, 612, 618
FOX1 protein, 653
FOXP2. see Forkhead box P2 (FOXP2)
  transcription factor
FPHHI (familial hyperinsulinemic
  hypoglycemia of infancy), 1520t–1521t
Fractalkine, in CNS, 686
Fractional anisotropy (FA), in dyslexia,
  1315
Fractionated stereotactic radiotherapy, for
  brain metastases, 1090
Fractionation, of brain tumors, 1050
Fracture-dislocation injuries, 889
Fractures
  burst, 889
  cervical, with spinal cord injury, 887–889
    atlanto-occipital dissociation as, 887
    atlantoaxial injuries as, 887–888
    occipital condyle fractures as, 887
    subaxial, 888–889
  compression, 889
    vertebral, 889
      due to osteoporosis, 1749,
        1749f
      vertical, 888–889
  Hangman's, 888
  Jefferson, 887–888
  in newborn, 1968–1969
  ping-pong, 1968
  skull, 869
    basilar, 870f
    depressed, 869, 870f
    linear, 869
    in newborn, 1968–1969
  teardrop, 888–889
Fragile X permutation syndrome, structural
  imaging for, 444.e3

Fragile X syndrome
  in autism spectrum disorder, 1305
  cognitive and behavioral problems in,
    1309t
Fragile X tremor-ataxia syndrome (FXTAS),
  246–248, 653, 1479
Frameshift mutation, 651t, 654f
Francis grading system, 888
Francisella tularensis, meningitis due to,
  1147–1148
Frataxin, in Friedreich ataxia, 1466, 1467f
Frataxin gene, mutations in, 444.e3
Fraxiparine (nadroparin calcium), for acute
  ischemic stroke, 956
Free fragment, degenerative disc disease
  with, 455
Free radical injury, in amyotrophic lateral
  sclerosis, 1507–1508
Free radical production, 1344
Free radical reactions, in spinal cord injury,
  882
Free radical scavengers, for traumatic brain
  injury, 856
Free-running circadian rhythm disorder,
  1654
FreeHand, 803
Freezing, 251
  in Parkinson disease, 1428
  in parkinsonism, 225–226, 228
Fregoli syndrome, after stroke, 100–101
French Endarterectomy versus Stenting in
  Patients with Symptomatic Severe
  Carotid Stenosis (EVA-3S) trial, 765
Frenzel glasses, 587–588
Frequency encoding, in MRI, 413
Frequency encoding gradient, in MRI,
  416–417
Frequency-domain topographic maps, in
  EEG, 350, 351f
Freud, Sigmund, 122, 1623.e1
Friedreich, Nicholas, 1465
Friedreich ataxia (FA), 1465–1467, 1818.e3
  clinical features of, 1465, 1466f
  genetics and paradox of disease definition
    in, 671–672
  late-onset, 1466
  mutation in, 1466, 1466f
    point, 1466
  pathogenesis of, 1466, 1467f
  in pregnancy, 1980
  with retained reflexes, 1466
  structural imaging for, 444.e3
  transcranial magnetic stimulation for, 396
  treatment of, 1466–1467
Froment sign, 227–228
  in ulnar nerve entrapment at elbow, 1805
Frontal Behavior Inventory (FBI), 76, 77t
Frontal cortex
  in sense of self, 59
  in visual awareness, 58
Frontal encephalocele, 1295
Frontal eye field (FEF), in horizontal eye
  movements, 552, 557
Frontal lobe disturbances
  bladder dysfunction due to, 607–608
  bowel dysfunction due to, 608.e1
Frontal lobe epilepsy, 526
  nocturnal, autosomal dominant, 1520t–
    1521t, 1532–1533
Frontal lobe syndrome, 527
Frontal lobes
  as executive center of brain, 59
  in integration of functions, 59
Frontal nerve, 1721f, 1726f
Frontal subcortical circuits, general structures
  of, 96f

Hypoxic-ischemic brain injury, in term newborn, 1959–1962
  classification of, 1959
  clinical features of, 1959, 1960t
  control of brain swelling with, 1961
  diagnosis of, 1959–1960
  electroencephalography and cortical evoked responses in, 1960, 1962
  hypothermia for, 1961
  maintenance of adequate ventilation for, 1961
  management of, 1961
  metabolic biomarkers of, 1960
  neuroimaging of, 1960–1961, 1961f
  neuropathological patterns, 1960t
  prevention of metabolic derangements in, 1961
  prognosis of, 1961–1962, 1962b, 1962f
Hypoxic ischemic encephalopathy, cerebral palsy due to, 1311–1312
Hypoxic ventilatory responses, during sleep, 1630t
Hypsarrhythmia, 1573, 1573f
  in infantile spasms, 352, 353f
Hysterectomy, for menstrual migraine prophylaxis, 1705
Hysteria, 1993
Hysterical gait disorders, 260–261
Hytrin (terazosin hydrochloride), for bladder dysfunction, in multiple sclerosis, 1183

I

123I (iodine-123), for SPECT, 487
IAS (internal anal sphincter), in control of defecation, 606
Iatrogenic Creutzfeldt-Jakob disease (iCJD), 1375
Iatrogenic neuropathies, 1846
IBM. see Inclusion body myositis (IBM)
Ibotenic acid, in mushrooms, 1251t
Ibuprofen (Motrin)
  for chronic pain, 725t
  for migraine in children and adolescents, 1719
ICAM-1. see Intercellular adhesion molecule-1 (ICAM-1)
Ice cream headache, 1715
"Ice-pack" test, for myasthenia gravis, 1902
"Ice-pick pains", 198–199
Icepick headaches, 1712–1713
ICF (intracortical facilitation)
  short-interval, 393, 394t
  in transcranial magnetic stimulation, 393, 394t
iCJD (iatrogenic Creutzfeldt-Jakob disease), 1375
ICP. see Intracranial pressure (ICP)
ICSS (International Carotid Stenting Study), 963
Ictal nystagmus, 548
Ictal onset zone, 1595
Ictal phenomenology, 1564–1565
Ictal symptomatogenic zone, 1595
ICU (intensive care unit), sleep of, 1671
Ideational apraxia, 117
  testing, 120
Idebenone, for Friedreich ataxia, 1466–1467
Ideomotor apraxia
  disconnection variant of, 117
  parietal variant of, 117
  testing for, 119
IDH1, in diffuse gliomas, 1032–1033
IDH2, in diffuse gliomas, 1032–1033

Idiopathic brachial plexopathy, 1784–1786
  diagnosis of, 1785
  pathophysiology and etiology of, 1785
  treatment and prognosis of, 1785–1786
Idiopathic generalized epilepsy, 1533–1535, 1566
  benign familial neonatal seizures as, 1520t–1521t, 1533–1534, 1533f
  childhood absence epilepsy as, 1535
  EEG for, 352, 352f
  with febrile seizures plus, 1520t–1521t, 1534, 1534f
  juvenile myoclonic epilepsy, 1534–1535
  SCN2A mutation and other early childhood seizures as, 1534
  theoretical considerations for, 1535
Idiopathic hypersomnia, 1644
Idiopathic hypertrophic subaortic stenosis, cardiogenic embolism due to, 933–934
Idiopathic intracranial hypertension (IIH), 1272–1274
  brain edema in, 1274
  clinical features of, 1273
  drugs associated with, 1273, 1273b
  due to venous sinus occlusion, 1274
  fulminant, 1274
  headache due to, 1272–1273, 1688
  neurointerventional therapy for, 782–783, 783f
  papilledema due to, 172, 1272–1273
  during pregnancy, 1983–1984
  structural imaging of, 449.e1
  treatment of, 1273–1274
Idiopathic movement disorders, 223
Idiopathic neuroretinitis, 169f
Idiopathic Normal Pressure Hydrocephalus (iNPH), Japanese Diagnostic Criteria of, 1419t
Idiopathic Parkinson disease
  behavioral and personality disturbances in, 107, 104.e1b
  depression and, 107
  hallucination in, 107
  structural imaging for, 445.e1, 445.e1f
Idiopathic rapid eye movement sleep behavior disorder (iRBD), smell loss in, 194
Idiopathic reversible cerebral segmental vasoconstriction, ischemic stroke due to, 944–945
Idiopathic thrombocytopenic purpura, intracerebral hemorrhage due to, 969–971
Idiotopes, 684
IED. see Intermittent explosive disorder (IED)
IEP (Individualized Education Plan), 71
IFN-β-1a (Avonex, Rebif), for multiple sclerosis, 690
IFN-β-1b (Betaseron and Extavia), for multiple sclerosis, 690
Ifosfamide, for brain tumors, 1052t–1053t
IGF-1. see Insulin-like growth factor 1 (IGF-1)
IGF-2. see Insulin-like growth factor 2 (IGF-2)
IGLON5, antibodies to, encephalitis with, 1200
  with antibodies to IgLON5, 1200
Ignition hypothesis, for trigeminal neuralgia, 735
IHI (interhemispheric inhibition), in transcranial magnetic stimulation, 393–394, 394t

IIH. see Idiopathic intracranial hypertension (IIH)
Ilioinguinal entrapment, 1802t
Ilioinguinal nerve, 1810
Ilioinguinal neuropathy, 1810
Imagery, in rehabilitation, 802
Imatinib, for brain tumor, 1051–1053
Imbalance, 251–252
Imipramine (Tofranil)
  for bladder dysfunction, 796t
  for chronic pain, 725t
Imitrex, for migraine, 1701t
Immediate memory, 60
Immediately available store, in repetitive nerve stimulation, 386
Immittance measures, for hearing loss, 602
Immobilization, attempted for functional tremor, 1998
Immune privilege, in CNS, 10, 685–686
Immune reconstitution inflammatory syndrome (IRIS), 1107
Immune response
  in CNS, 685
  to infectious diseases, 693–694
  initiation of, 681–682
    accessory molecules for B-cell activation in, 682
    accessory molecules for T-cell activation in, 681–682
    antigen presentation in, 681
    CD3 in, 681
    CD4 and CD8 in, 681
    cell migration in, 681–682
    costimulatory molecules in, 681, 681f
  neuroglial cells and, 686
  organization of, 681–684
  regulation of, 682–683
    chemokines in, 682–683
    cytokines in, 682–683, 683t
  termination of, 683–684
    B-cell inhibition in, 684
    immunoglobulin in, 684
    T cells in, 684
  to tumors, 694
    paraneoplastic syndromes in, 694
Immune system, 676–679
  adaptive and innate, 676–677
  and CNS, 685–686
  genetics of, 679
    antigen receptor gene rearrangements in, 679
    major histocompatibility and human leukocyte antigens in, 679, 679f–680f
  neuropeptides and, 696–698, 699t
  normal functions and disorders of, 676, 677b
  principal components of, 677–679
    B lymphocytes as, 678
    immunoglobulins as, 678–679
    monocytes and macrophages as, 677
    natural killer cells as, 677
    T-cell receptors as, 678, 678f
    T lymphocytes as, 677
Immune-mediated disease, 686
  acute disseminated encephalomyelitis as, 690–691
  Alzheimer disease as, 693
  amyotrophic lateral sclerosis as, 693
  autoimmune myasthenia gravis as, 692
  immune-mediated neuropathies as, 691–692
  inflammatory muscle disease as, 692–693
  multiple sclerosis as, 688–690

Immune-mediated necrotizing myopathy, 1951
  prognosis and treatment of, 1951–1952
Immune-mediated neuropathies, 691–692
  neurogenic bladder dysfunction due to, 612
Immune-mediated strategies, for brain tumors, 1054–1055
Immunity
  adaptive and innate, 676–677
  and brain tumors, 1023–1024
  cell-mediated, 677, 682
Immunization, for congenital rubella, 1966
Immunoblot, of muscle histology, 1918–1919
Immunocompromised adults, cytomegalovirus in, 1130
Immunoglobulins (Igs)
  in adaptive immune response, 677
  classes of, 678
  in immune system, 678–679
  molecular and genetic organization of, 678f
  in multiple sclerosis, 1162
  in termination of immune response, 684
Immunohistochemistry, 1029–1030
  epithelial markers in, 1030
  glial markers in, 1029
  of muscle histology, 1918–1919
  neuronal markers in, 1029–1030
  s100 protein in, 1030
Immunological abnormalities, in amyotrophic lateral sclerosis, 1508
Immunologically privileged site, CNS as, 685
Immunology. *see also* Neuroimmunology
  adaptive and innate immunity in, 676–677
  antibody-associated neurological syndromes in, 694–695
  of central nervous system transplant, 695
  immune privilege in CNS in, 685–686
  neuroimmunological diseases in, 688–693
    acute disseminated encephalomyelitis as, 690–691
    Alzheimer disease as, 693
    amyotrophic lateral sclerosis as, 693
    autoimmune myasthenia gravis as, 692
    immune-mediated neuropathies as, 691–692
    inflammatory muscle disease as, 692–693
    multiple sclerosis as, 688–690
  putative mechanisms of human autoimmune disease, 686–688
    environmental factors as, 687–688
    genetic factors as, 687
  self-tolerance in, 684–685
    anergy due to failure of T-cell activation in, 684, 685f
    apoptosis in, 684, 685f
    central, 684
    peripheral, 684–685
    regulatory T cells in, 684–685
  tumor, 694
    paraneoplastic syndromes in, 694
Immunophilins, necrotizing myopathy due to, 1954
Immunoreceptor tyrosine-based activation motif (ITAM), in T-cell activation, 681
Immunoregulatory factors, in CNS, 686
Immunosuppressant drugs, for myasthenia gravis, 1906–1907
Immunosuppressives, for myasthenia gravis, 692

Immunotherapy
  for anti-AMPA receptor encephalitis, 1199
  for anti-GABA_B receptor encephalitis, 1198
  for anti-LGI1 limbic encephalitis, 1199
  for anti-NMDAR, 1200
  for viral infections, 1131t
Impaired pursuit, 557
Impaired sympathetic thoracolumbar outflow, bladder dysfunction and, 611
Impingement sign, 331
Imprinting, 662, 662f
Impulse control disorders (ICD), in Parkinson disease, 81
Impulsive behaviors, in autism spectrum disorder, 1307t
IMS (Interventional Management of Stroke) III trial, 958.e1
In vitro models, of traumatic brain injury, 851
Inattention, in autism spectrum disorder, 1307t
Inborn errors of metabolism (IEM), 1324–1341
  adolescent with, 1332–1333
  animal models of, 1333
  associated with abnormal brain development and encephaloclastic lesions, 1328, 1328.e1t
  associated with hearing abnormalities, 1328, 1328.e1t
  associated with thalamic lesions, 1328.e1t
  cerebrotendinous xanthomatosis, 1338
  clinical findings characteristic of, 1325.e3t–1325.e4t
  clinical manifestations, 1335
  commonly requested primary/secondary tests, 1326t
  congenital disorders of glycosylation, 1339
  creatine deficiency syndromes as, 1341
  developmental brain malformations associated with, 1329t
  diagnosis
    cardiomyopathy, 1326
    carnitine profile for, 1326t
    course in, 1324
    diet in, 1330
    imminent death prior to, 1330
    neuroimaging in, 1328–1330
    ophthalmologic findings, 1326.e1t–1326.e2t
    screening for, 1324
    tandem mass spectrometry, 1327
  diagnostic approach to, 1325–1328
  disorders associated with vitamin metabolism, 1338–1339
  disorders involving complex molecules, 1333–1335
    amino and organic acid metabolism, 1335–1336
    lysosomal storage disorders, 1333–1334
      classification of, 1333.e2t–1333.e3t
      clinical features of, 1334
      transmission of, 1334
  disorders involving small molecules, 1335–1337
  disorders of energy metabolism, 1336–1337
    disorders of gluconeogenesis as, 1337
    disorders of glycolysis as, 1337
    disorders of ketogenesis and ketolysis as, 1337
    fatty acid oxidation defects as, 1337
    glycogen storage diseases as, 1336–1337
    hyperammonemia-hyperornithinemia-homocitrullinemia syndrome as, 1336

Inborn errors of metabolism (IEM) (*Continued*)
    disorders of glycine and serine metabolism, 1340
    disorders of metals as, 1338
    disorders of polyol metabolism, 1338
    disorders of purine and pyrimidine metabolism, 1339
    dyslipidemias as, 1338
  genetic counseling in, 1324–1325
  genetic tests for, 1327–1328
  hepatosplenomegaly in, 1326
  histological examination for, 1327
  inheritance of, 1324
  management considerations following, 1330–1332
    enhancing excretion or detoxification of toxic metabolites in, 1331
    enzyme replacement therapy, 1332
    individualized approach to, 1330
    organ transplantation, 1332
    substrate reduction therapy in, 1331f
    symptomatic treatment in, 1332
  manifesting cerebellar lesions, 1328.e1t
  manifesting white matter abnormalities detected by DWI, 1328.e2t
  molybdenum cofactor and sulfite oxidase deficiency, 1339
  mutation analysis in, 1328
  special considerations in, 1328
  neuronal ceroid lipofuscinoses as, 1335
  neurotransmitter, 1340
  porphyrias as, 1339–1340, 1340.e1t
  during pregnancy, 1333
  psychiatric symptoms of, 1333
  strategies for, 1331
  subclassifications of, 1337–1341
INC (interstitial nucleus of Cajal), in vertical eye movements, 558–559, 559f
Inching technique, in nerve conduction studies, 369, 369f–370f
Incidence proportions (IPs), for brain metastases, 638
Incidence rate
  defined, 635–636
  for epilepsy, 640, 640f–641f
  for multiple sclerosis, 641–642
  for neurological disorders
    less common, 646t
    most common, 645t
  for Parkinson disease, 644
  of primary brain tumors, 638, 639f
  of stroke, 636–637
  for West Nile virus infection, 645.e1
Inclusion body myopathies, hereditary, 1920t–1921t, 1933–1934
  autosomal recessive, 1933–1934
  with early respiratory failure, 1927
Inclusion body myositis (IBM), 290, 1952–1953
  amyloid deposition in, 1952–1953, 1953f
  CD8+ cytotoxic cells in, 1953
  diagnosis of, 1952
  dysphagia in, 151
  immune mediation in, 692
  muscle biopsy for, 1952–1953, 1952f–1953f
  rimmed vacuoles in, 1952–1953, 1952f
Incontinentia pigmenti (IP), 1551–1552
  cutaneous features of, 1551–1552, 1552f
  genetics of, 1552
  neurological features of, 1552
Indinavir (Crixivan), for HIV infection, 1108t–1109t
Indirect wave, in transcranial magnetic stimulation, 391

Individualized Education Plan (IEP), 71
Individualized Family Service Plan, 71
Indoles, in mushrooms, 1251*t*
Indomethacin
for chronic pain, 725*t*
for exertional headache, 1714
for headache associated with sexual
activity, 1714
for hemicrania continua, 1712–1713
for paroxysmal hemicrania, 1711–1712
for primary cough headache, 1714
for primary stabbing headache, 1713
Indwelling catheters, for neurogenic bladder,
619
Inertial acceleration models, 851
Infancy
benign sleep myoclonus of, 1661
familial hyperinsulinemic hypoglycemia,
1520*t*–1521*t*
Infantile beriberi, 1231
Infantile botulism, 1914
Infantile facioscapulohumeral dystrophy,
hypotonic infant due to, 310
Infantile myotonic dystrophy, 1936,
1936*f*
Infantile neuroaxonal dystrophy, hypotonic
infant due to, 310
Infantile nystagmus syndrome (INS), 541,
542*t*, 543, 546*t*
Infantile spinal muscular atrophy with
respiratory distress type 1, hypotonic
infant due to, 311
Infants, primary nervous system tumors in,
1065–1083
Infarction
cerebral
headache due to, 1692
hyperhidrosis after, 1872*t*
myocardial
cardiogenic embolism due to,
933–934
and sleep, 1669
spinal cord, 1007–1010
causes of, 1009–1010, 1009*b*, 1009*f*
course of, 1008
examination findings in, 1007
investigations of, 1007–1008,
1008*f*
presentation and initial course of,
1007
prognosis of, 1008
treatment of, 1010
Infarcts of undetermined cause, ischemic
stroke due to, 949
Infection prophylaxis, for traumatic brain
injury, 875*t*–876*t*
Infections
associated with neuropathies,
1864
and brain tumors, 1023–1024
delirium due to, 30, 30*t*
headache due to, 1690–1691
hemiplegia due to, 265
monoplegia due to, 268
multiple sclerosis and, 1163
in neurointensive care, 756–757
neurological complications, of drug abuse,
1258
parasitic, seizures due to, 1582
and stroke, 939
in children, 1000
structural imaging of
of brain, 436
of spinal cord, 452

Infectious diseases
ataxia due to, 1462–1463
EEG in, 357–359
functional symptoms in, 1993*t*
immune response to, 693–694
of spine, 1759–1761
granulomatous vertebral osteomyelitis
as, 1760–1761, 1761*f*
pyogenic vertebral osteomyelitis and
epidural abscess as, 1759–1760,
1760*f*
versus viral nervous system disease,
1124*t*
Infectious radiculopathy, 1775–1777
herpes zoster as, 1776–1777
Lyme radiculoneuropathy as, 1776
polyradiculoneuropathy in human
immunodeficiency virus-infected
patients as, 1775–1776, 1776*f*
tabes dorsalis as, 1775
Infective endocarditis
cardiogenic embolism due to, 934
neurological complications of
in adults, 817*f*
in children, 836, 836*f*
Inferior altitudinal visual field defect, 577,
578*f*
Inferior alveolar nerve, 1726*f*
Inferior lateral pontine syndrome, 214*b*,
215*f*
Inferior medial pontine syndrome, 214*b*,
215*f*
Inferior oblique muscles, 528–529, 529*t*
anatomy of, 529*f*
Inferior parietal lobule (IPL), 557, 564
in praxis, 116
Inferior rectus muscle
actions of, 528–529, 529*t*
anatomy of, 529*f*
Inferior vena cava syndrome, due to
autonomic disorders, 1890
Inflammation, chemical imaging of, 505*t*,
506
Inflammatory abnormalities, in amyotrophic
lateral sclerosis, 1508
Inflammatory cells, in innate immune
system, 676
Inflammatory cytokines, in delirium, 27
Inflammatory demyelinating diseases,
1159–1186
acute disseminated encephalomyelitis as,
1183–1185, 1184*f*
acute hemorrhagic leukoencephalitis as,
1185
chronic relapsing inflammatory optic
neuropathy as, 1186
isolated optic neuritis as, 1186
neuromyelitis optica as, 1185–1186,
1185*f*
transverse myelitis as, 1186
Inflammatory demyelinating
polyradiculoneuropathies, 1818–1834
acute
HIV-associated, 1114*t*
immune mediation of, 686, 691
pathology of, 691
treatment of, 691–692
chronic, 1192
HIV-associated, 1114*t*
immune mediation of, 691
oral contraceptives and, 1974
in pregnancy, 1979
versus spinal muscular atrophy,
1502–1503

Inflammatory demyelinating
polyradiculoneuropathies (*Continued*)
chronic inflammatory demyelinating
polyradiculoneuropathy as,
1827–1832
clinical features of, 1827–1828
laboratory studies of, 1828–1830,
1829*b*, 1829*f*
prognosis of, 1832
treatment of, 1830–1832, 1831*f*
Guillain-Barré syndrome as, 1818–1827
HIV-associated, 1120
multifocal motor neuropathy as,
1832–1834
clinical features of, 1832
laboratory studies of, 1832–1833,
1832*f*, 1833*t*
treatment of, 1833–1834
needle electromyography of, 383
nerve conduction studies of, 375–376
in pregnancy, 1979
Inflammatory disorder
psychiatric manifestations of, 104
seizures due to, 1582–1583
Inflammatory joint disease, 1761–1763
rheumatoid arthritis as, 1761–1762
neurological manifestations of,
1761–1762, 1761.*e*1*f*
pathogenesis of, 1761
systemic presentation of, 1761
spondyloarthropathies as, 1762–1763
clinical presentation of, 1762, 1762.*e*1*f*
laboratory abnormalities in, 1763
neurological complications
nonspinal, 1762
spinal, 1762, 1762*t*,
1762.*e*1*f*–1762.*e*2*f*
pathogenesis of, 1762
Inflammatory myopathies, 1948–1953
dermatomyositis as, 1949–1950,
1949*f*–1950*f*
associated with neoplasia, 1951
associated with other collagen vascular
diseases, 1951
prognosis and treatment of, 1951–1952
dysphagia in, 150–151
immune-mediated necrotizing myopathy
as, 1951
prognosis and treatment of, 1951–1952
inclusion body myositis as, 1952–1953,
1952*f*–1953*f*
other, 1953
polymyalgia rheumatica as, 1953
polymyositis as, 1950–1951, 1951*f*
associated with neoplasia, 1951
associated with other collagen vascular
diseases, 1951
prognosis and treatment of, 1951–1952
in pregnancy, 1978
Inflammatory response, in spinal cord injury,
882
Inflammatory spondyloarthropathies,
1762–1763
clinical presentation of, 1762, 1762.*e*1*f*
laboratory abnormalities in, 1763
neurological complications
nonspinal, 1762
spinal, 1762, 1762*t*, 1762.*e*1*f*–1762.*e*2*f*
pathogenesis of, 1762
Inflammatory vasculitides, ischemic stroke
due to, 938–939
Influenza, vaccination of, with myasthenia
gravis, 1909
Influenza virus, 1144

Infraorbital nerve, 1721f, 1726f
Infratentorial tumor, 1027t
Inhalants, 1258t
drug dependence with, 1258
Inheritance
Mendelian, 657–659
autosomal dominant, 657–658, 658f
autosomal recessive, 658, 660f
gene identification by linkage analysis and chromosome mapping for, 659–660, 661f
pseudodominant, 658
sex-linked (X-linked), 658–659, 660f
non-Mendelian, 661–663
imprinting as, 662, 662f
mitochondrial disorders as, 661–662, 661f
uniparental disomy as, 662–663, 662f
Inhibitory cell-burst neurons, in horizontal eye movements, 554
Injection, peripheral nerve injury due to, 909
Innate immunity, 676–677
Innervation ratio, 376
Innominate artery syndrome, due to autonomic disorders, 1890
INO (internuclear ophthalmoplegia), in multiple sclerosis, 1165
In-office/outpatient diagnosis, sports and performance concussion and, 862
Inpatient rehabilitation unit, for rehabilitation, 791–792
Input-output curve, for motor evoked potentials, 392, 394t
INS (infantile nystagmus syndrome), 541, 542t, 543, 546t
Insect neurotoxins, 1247–1249
from scorpions, 1248–1249
from spiders, 1248
tick paralysis due to, 1249
Insertion, 654f
Insomnia
acute, 1638, 1638b
in amyotrophic lateral sclerosis, 1513t
behavioral, of childhood, 1671–1672
chronic, 1638, 1638b
classification of, 1637–1639
cognitive and behavioral therapy for, 1682t
fatal familial, 1374, 1657
hypnotic management for, 1681t
idiopathic and psychophysiological, 1638.e1
inadequate sleep hygiene, 1638.e1, 1638.e2b
medical disorders comorbid, 1638.e2b
neurological disorders comorbid, 1638.e2b
paradoxical, 1638.e1
physiological profiles of, 1638–1639
sporadic fatal, 1369–1370
treatment of, 1681–1682
Inspiratory gasp, 1645–1648
Instability, gait disorders due to perceptions of, 260
Instrumented biofeedback, in rehabilitation, 802
Insula, in speech and language disorders, 136–137
Insulin, 697t–698t
in appetite, 700, 701f
Insulin hypoglycemia test, 710t
Insulin levels, in inborn errors of metabolism, 1326t
Insulin-like growth factor 1 (IGF-1), 697t–698t, 703
Insulin-like growth factor 2 (IGF-2), 697t–698t, 703

Integrase inhibitors, for HIV infection, 1108t–1109t
Integrin, in immune response, 681–682
Integrin expression, agents targeting, 1054b
Integument examination, for coma, 39, 40t
Intelence (etravirine), for HIV infection, 1108t–1109t
Intellect, definition of, 57
Intellectual disability, 1307–1311
autism spectrum disorder and, 1302–1303
clinical features of, 1307
cognitive and behavioral problems in, 1309t
comorbidities in, 1307–1308
defined, 1307
diagnosis and etiology of, 1307–1308
environmental factors in, 1308
epidemiological studies on, 1307–1308
genetic defects in, 1308
management of, 1308–1311
metabolic disorders associated with, 1310t
mild, 1307
moderate, 1307
neuroimaging for, 1308
prevalence of, 1307
profound, 1307
prognosis for, 71
severe, 1307
Intellectual impairments, 57–65
Intelligence quotient (IQ)
in autism spectrum disorder, 1302–1303
in intellectual disability, 1307
Intensive care unit (ICU), sleep of, 1671
Intention tremor, 218, 230
Intercellular adhesion molecule-1 (ICAM-1)
in HIV disease, 1106
in T-cell activation, 681, 681f
Intercostobrachial nerve, 1807
Interference pattern, of motor unit action potentials, 381
Interferon alfa (IFN-α)
in immune response, 682
for viral infections, 1127t
Interferon alfa 2b (IFN-α-2b), myasthenia gravis due to, 1908
Interferon beta (IFN-β)
in immune response, 682
for multiple sclerosis, 690
Interferon beta-1a
for multiple sclerosis, 1177
during pregnancy, 1981–1982
Interferon beta-1b
for multiple sclerosis, 1177, 1181–1182
during pregnancy, 1981–1982
Interferon gamma (IFN-γ)
in immune response, 682, 683t
for low back pain, 732
Interferon-stimulated gene 15 (ISG15), in dermatomyositis, 1950
Interferons, 697t–698t
for multiple sclerosis
relapsing-remitting, 1177
side-effect of, 1177
Interhemispheric inhibition (IHI), in transcranial magnetic stimulation, 393–394, 394t
Interictal psychosis, 109
Interleukin-1 (IL-1), in immune response, 682, 683t
Interleukin-2 (IL-2)
in apoptosis, 684
in immune response, 682, 683t
Interleukin-3 (IL-3), in immune response, 682, 683t
Interleukin-4 (IL-4), in immune response, 682, 683t

Interleukin-5 (IL-5), in immune response, 682
Interleukin-6 (IL-6), in immune response, 682, 683t
Interleukin-9 (IL-9), in immune response, 682
Interleukin-10 (IL-10), in immune response, 682, 683t
Interleukin-12 (IL-12), in immune response, 682, 683t
Interleukin-13 (IL-13), in immune response, 682
Interleukin-17 (IL-17), in immune response, 682, 683t
Interleukin-23 (IL-23), in immune response, 682
Intermittent bladder drainage, for neurogenic bladder, 619
Intermittent claudication, neurogenic, 1758–1759
Intermittent explosive disorder (IED), in epilepsy, 89
Intermittent self-catheterization, for neurogenic bladder, 618
Intermyofibrillar network pattern, changes in, 1917–1918, 1918f
Internal anal sphincter (IAS), in control of defecation, 606
Internal capsule lesions, differential diagnosis of, 272.e1
Internal carotid artery, aneurysm at, imaging of, 989f
Internal carotid artery (ICA) dissection
CT angiography of, 460
MR angiography of, 470f
Internal carotid artery (ICA) stenosis, MR angiography of, 467f
time-of-flight, 467
International Carotid Stenting Study (ICSS), 765, 963
International Classification of Headache Disorders 3rd edition beta (ICHD-3 beta), 1686–1687, 1687b
International Classification of Sleep Disorders (ICSD-III), 1635
International Statistical Classification of Diseases, Injuries and Causes of Death (ICD), 635–636
International Stroke Trial, 956
International Study of Unruptured Intracranial Aneurysms (ISUIA), 472, 986
Interneurons, in horizontal eye movements, 554, 555f
Internodes, 903–904, 904f
Internuclear ophthalmoplegia (INO), 207, 567, 567b
in multiple sclerosis, 1165
Interpeduncular fossa
lesions in, 1721–1723
oculomotor nerve in, 1720
INTERPHONE study, 1021–1022
"Interstate illusions", 540
Interstimulus intervals (ISIs), in transcranial magnetic stimulation, 393
Interstitial fluid (ISF)
movement ventricles and around the spinal cord, 1264
production of, 1264–1265
Interstitial nucleus of Cajal (INC), in vertical eye movements, 558–559, 559f
Intertrial variability, in nerve conduction studies, 371
Interventional Management of Stroke (IMS) III trial, 958.e1

Interventional pain management, 729–734, 729t
  epidural corticosteroid injection for, 731–732, 732f
  Gasserian ganglion lesions for, 730–731, 731f
  greater occipital nerve block for, 729, 730f
  intrathecal drug delivery systems for, 734, 734f
  lumbar facet joint block for, 732
  motor cortex stimulation for, 734
  percutaneous disk decompression for, 732–733
  sphenopalatine ganglion block for, 729–730
  spinal cord stimulation for, 733–734, 733f
  stellate ganglion block for, 731, 731f
Intervertebral foramen, anatomy of, 1767, 1767f
Interview, neurological, 1–2
Interwave latencies, abnormal, 603
Intraarachnoid cyst, structural imaging of, 446.e8, 446.e9f
Intraarterial fibrinolysis, for acute ischemic stroke, 958
Intra-arterial thrombolysis, for ischemic stroke, 759
Intra-arterial vasodilators, for cerebral vasospasm, 774–775
Intraaxial primary brain tumors, 417, 418t–419t
  structural imaging of, 417–423
Intracavernous injections, for erectile dysfunction, 632
Intracellular adhesion molecules (ICAMs), 960.e1
Intracellular signal transduction pathways, small molecule inhibitors of, 1054b
Intracerebellar hemorrhage, in newborn, 1968t
Intracerebral hemorrhage, 968–982
  blood pressure management for, 753t, 754
  caudate, 977, 978t, 979f
  cerebellar, 978t, 979, 979.e1f
    surgical therapy for, 981, 982.e1f
  cerebral edema due to, 1270, 1272f
  clinical features of, 975–980, 976f–977f, 978t
  CT angiography of, 463
  versus hemorrhagic infarction, 975, 975f, 976f
  imaging of
    CTA, 976, 977f
    MRI, 976, 977t
  intraventricular, 978t, 980
    ventricular drainage for, 982
  lobar, 977–979, 978t, 981–982, 977.e1f
  mechanisms of, 968–975
    due to bleeding disorders, anticoagulants, and fibrinolytic treatment, 969–971, 972f–973f
    due to cerebral amyloid angiopathy, 971–972, 974f
    due to granulomatous angiitis of CNS and other vasculitides, 972–974
    due to head trauma, 975
    due to hypertension, 968
    due to intracranial tumors, 969, 970f
    due to sympathomimetic agents, 974–975, 975f
    due to vascular malformations, 968–969, 969f
    nonhypertensive, 969b
  medullary, 978t, 980, 980.e1f

Intracerebral hemorrhage (Continued)
  mesencephalic, 978t, 979, 979.e1f
  pontine, 978t, 979, 979f
  during pregnancy, 1987
  putaminal, 976–977, 978t, 976.e1f
  and stroke in children, 996
  thalamic, 977, 978t, 977.e1f
    ventricular drainage for, 982
  treatment of, 980–982
    general management for, 980–981
    hemostatic, 982
    for increased intracranial pressure, 981
    initial evaluation for, 980–981
    medical versus surgical, 981–982, 982.e1f
Intracortical facilitation (ICF)
  short-interval, 393, 394t
  in transcranial magnetic stimulation, 393, 394t
Intracortical inhibition, in transcranial magnetic stimulation
  long-interval, 392, 394t
  short-interval, 393, 394t
Intracranial aneurysms
  classification of, 984b
  conditions associated with, 983–984, 984b
  defined, 983
  diagnosis of, 987–990
  dissecting, 985, 986f–988f
  epidemiology of, 983–984
  familial, 983
  fusiform, 985, 986f
  headaches due to, 1691, 1713–1714
  imaging modalities for, 987–990
  incidental, treatment of, 990–993
  multiple, 983, 990
  natural history of, 985–987, 988t
  pathophysiology of, 984–985
  recurrence of, 992–993
  risk factors for, 984, 984b
  ruptured, treatment of, 993–994
  saccular, 984–985, 985f, 991f
  symptoms of, 990
  treatment of
    endovascular, 985f, 991–993, 992f
      flow-diversion stent in, 993
      recanalization and recurrence of, 992–993
      ruptured, 993–994
      stent-assisted coil embolization as, 991–992, 992f
    incidental, 990–993
    open surgical, 991, 991f–992f
Intracranial arteries, stenting of, 963.e1
Intracranial circulation
  CT angiography of, 461–464
  MR angiography of, 469–476, 471f
Intracranial cysts, versus viral nervous system disease, 1124t
Intracranial hemorrhage
  due to traumatic injuries, 1968, 1968t
  in newborn, drug- or toxin-induced, 1971
  and stroke in children, 996
  versus viral nervous system disease, 1124t
Intracranial hypertension, idiopathic
  headache due to, 1688
  papilledema due to, 172
  during pregnancy, 1983–1984
Intracranial injuries, 869–872
  contusions as, 869–870, 870f
  diffuse axonal injury as, 871–872, 872f
  epidural hematoma as, 870, 871f

Intracranial injuries (Continued)
  subdural hematoma as, 870, 871f
  traumatic subarachnoid hemorrhage as, 870–871, 871f
Intracranial pain-sensitive structures, 1686
Intracranial pressure (ICP)
  and cerebral perfusion pressure, 745
  increased
    with acute ischemic stroke, 964, 964b
    due to intracerebral hemorrhage
      clinical manifestations of, 975–976
      general measures for prevention of further, 981
      specific treatment of, 981
    from fungal infections, 1153
    with traumatic brain injury, 874
      escalating protocol for, 874, 876b
      guidelines for, 874–876, 875t–876t
      hemodynamic management in, 877
      high-dose barbiturates for, 875t–876t, 877
      hyperosmolar therapy in, 874, 875t–876t, 876b
      hyperventilation for, 875t–876t, 876–877, 876b
      hypothermia for, 875t–876t, 877
      monitoring of, 875t–876t
      multimodality monitoring in, 877
      paralysis for, 877
    normal, 745
    pressure-volume relationship for, 745, 745f
    waveforms of, 745, 745f
Intracranial pressure (ICP) monitoring
  for coma, 49
  devices for, 745–746
  in neurointensive care, 744t, 745–746
  purpose of, 745
  for traumatic brain injury, 875t–876t
  waveforms in, 745, 745f
Intracranial sinovenous occlusive disease, 964–966
  causes of, 967b
Intracranial stenosis
  CT angiography of, 462–463
  lesions of, ultrasound of, 482, 482f
Intracranial tumors
  intracerebral hemorrhage due to, 969, 970f
  versus viral nervous system disease, 1124t
Intradural vessels, enhancement of, 3D CE-MRA for, 476
Intramedullary lesions, arm and neck pain due to, 327
Intramedullary spinal cord tumor, structural imaging of, 450
Intramedullary spinal hemorrhage, 1013
Intramedullary spinal metastases, 1094
Intranuclear tubulofilaments, in oculopharyngeal muscular dystrophy, 1933
Intraoperative monitoring (IOM), 407–410
  and anesthesia, 410
  in clinical settings, 410, 410b
  electrocorticography (ECoG) for, 407
  electroencephalography (EEG) for, 407
    monitoring interpretation of, 409
  electromyography (EMG) for, 407
    neurotonic discharge in, 409
  evoked potentials for, 407
    brainstem auditory, 407, 408f, 409
    motor
      effect of anesthesia on, 410
      monitoring interpretation of, 409

Intraoperative monitoring (IOM)
  (*Continued*)
    for spinal cord monitoring, 407,
      410
    transcranial electrical, 407
    somatosensory, 407, 408*f*
      effect of anesthesia on, 410
      monitoring interpretation of, 409
      for spinal cord monitoring, 407
  interpretation of, 409
  with peripheral nerve trauma, 913–914
  and prediction of deficits, 409–410
  and response to change, 409
  spinal cord, 407–408
  for spinal surgery, 410
  techniques for, 407–408, 408*b*
Intraparenchymal abscess, headache and,
  1690
Intraparenchymal fiberoptic monitors, of
  intracranial pressure, 746
Intrasellar tumor, 1027*t*
Intraspinal canal lesions, nerve conduction
  studies of, 374–375
Intratemporal facial nerve schwannomas,
  1730–1731
Intrathecal chemotherapy, for
  leptomeningeal metastases, 1098–1099
Intrathecal drug delivery systems, for pain,
  734, 734*f*
Intrauterine growth retardation, due to drugs
  and toxins, 1971, 1971*f*
Intravascular malignant lymphomatosis,
  ischemic stroke due to, 944
Intravenous (IV) heparin, for acute ischemic
  stroke, 956
Intravenous immunoglobulin (IVIG)
  for acute inflammatory demyelinating
    polyneuropathy, 691–692
  for dermatomyositis, polymyositis, and
    immune-mediated necrotizing
    myopathy, 1951
  for Lambert-Eaton syndrome, 1913
  for multiple sclerosis, 1181
  for myasthenia gravis, 692, 1903*t*, 1905
  for postpolio syndrome, 1497–1498
  for viral infections, 1131*t*
Intravenous regional block, 729*t*
Intraventricular hemorrhage, 978*t*, 980
  in term newborn, 1964–1965, 1964*f*
    diagnosis of, 1965
    pathogenesis of, 1964–1965
    prognosis of, 1965
  ventricular drainage for, 982
Intraventricular meningiomas, headache due
  to, 1687
Intraventricular tumors, headache due to,
  1687
Intrinsic factor antibodies, in cobalamin
  deficiency, 1227
Introns, 649–650, 651*t*, 652*f*
Inverse Anton syndrome, 122
Inverse ocular bobbing, 44
Inversion, 654*f*
Inversion recovery sequences (FLAIR, STIR),
  in MRI, 300
Inversion time, 417.*e*2
  in MRI, 417.*e*2
Inverted isopters, 582
Invirase (saquinavir), for HIV infection,
  1108*t*–1109*t*
Involuntary movements, treatment of
  abnormal, 716
Involuntary muscle contraction syndromes
  diffuse, 303
    muscle cramps as, 302*b*, 303
    originating from muscle, 303

Inward deviation, of eyes, 44
Iodine-123 (^{123}I), for SPECT, 487
Ion channelopathies, 1936–1937
Ion channels, 1519–1522
  categorization of, 1519
  defined, 1519
  ligand-gated, 1519
    GABA$_A$ as, 1521–1522
    glycine receptors as, 1521–1522
    nicotinic acetylcholine receptors as,
      1521–1522, 1523*f*
  voltage-gated, 1519
    α-subunits of, 1519
    open, closed and inactivated, 1519
    phenotypic heterogeneity affecting, 1519
    potassium, 1519–1521, 1522*f*
    sodium and calcium, 1521, 1523*f*
Ionizing radiation
  effects of, 1245
    encephalopathy due to, 1245
    myelopathy due to, 1245
    plexopathy due to, 1245
  exposure, brain tumors and, 1021
  sensitization of tumor cells to, 1050
Iontophoresis, for hyperhidrosis, 1873*t*
Iowa-Benton method, for neuropsychological
  evaluation, 513, 514*f*
IPs. *see* Incidence proportions (IPs)
Ipsilateral gaze palsy, 565
IQ (intelligence quotient)
  in autism spectrum disorder, 1302–1303
  in intellectual disability, 1307
iRBD (idiopathic rapid eye movement sleep
  behavior disorder), smell loss in, 194
Ireton Child Development Inventory (CDI),
  66
Irinotecan, for brain tumors, 1052*t*–1053*t*
Iris ischemia, anisocoria due to, 183
Iris sphincter injury, anisocoria due to, 183
Iritis, anisocoria due to, 185–186
Irregular sleep/wake circadian rhythm
  disorder, 1654–1655, 1678*f*
Irritative zone, 1595
Isaacs syndrome, channelopathy in, 1536
Ischemia
  cerebral, headache due to, 1692
  spinal cord. *see* Spinal cord infarction
Ischemic arteriolar encephalopathy,
  structural imaging of, 433
Ischemic brain damage, posttraumatic, 855
Ischemic cerebrovascular disease, 920–967
  clinical syndromes of, 925–931
    anterior cerebral artery syndromes as,
      928, 928*f*
    anterior choroidal artery syndrome as,
      928
    carotid artery syndromes as, 927
    lacunar syndromes as, 928
    middle cerebral artery syndromes as,
      927–928
    posterior cerebral artery syndromes as,
      930–931, 931*f*
    thalamic infarction syndromes as, 931,
      931.*e*1*f*
    transient ischemic attacks as, 925–927,
      926*b*, 926*t*
    vertebrobasilar system syndromes as,
      929–931, 929*f*, 930.*e*1*f*
    watershed ischemic syndromes as, 931
  epidemiology and risk factors for,
    920–924
  pathology of, 925
  pathophysiology of, 924–925
Ischemic encephalopathy, in fetus, CNS
  malformations due to, 1292
Ischemic monomelic neuropathy, 1857

Ischemic optic neuropathy, anterior
  nonarteritic, 163–165
    visual field defects in, 577, 578*f*
    visual loss due to, 159–161
Ischemic stroke
  acute, 461–462, 461*f*
    Alberta Stroke Program Early CT Score
      (ASPECTS) on, 462*b*, 462*f*
    apparent diffusion coefficient map in,
      429–430
    blood pressure monitoring for, 963
    brain edema due to, 964
    cardiac monitoring for, 963
    Clot Burden Score (CBS) on, 461, 461*f*
    due to middle cerebral artery stenosis,
      461, 461*f*
    ischemic penumbra in, 431*f*
    pc-ASPECTS on, 462, 462*f*
    sensitivity and specificity of, 461
    source images in, 461
    structural imaging of, 428–429
    T2-weighted imaging of, 431
  apparent diffusion coefficient map of,
    429–430
  chronic, 432, 432.*e*1*f*
    with Wallerian degeneration, 432, 433*f*
  complications of, 964
    depression symptoms as, 964.*e*1
    falling as, 964.*e*1
    pressure sores as, 964.*e*1
    pulmonary, 963
    shoulder subluxation as, 964.*e*1
    urinary incontinence as, 964.*e*1
  diffusion-weighted imaging of, 429,
    430*f*–431*f*, 430.*e*1*f*
  drug abuse and, 939, 940*f*
  due to air embolism, 945
  due to amniotic fluid embolism, 945
  due to atheromatous embolization, 945
  due to cardiogenic embolism, 933–935,
    934*b*, 935*f*
  due to cerebral amyloid angiopathy, 945
  due to cerebral venous thrombosis,
    964–967, 966*f*, 967*b*, 966.*e*1*f*
  due to coarctation of aorta, 943
  due to coils and kinks of carotid artery,
    945
  due to coronary artery occlusions, 961
  due to dissections, 936–937, 937*f*,
    937.*e*1*f*, 936.*e*1*f*
  due to dolichoectasia, 945
  due to Eales disease, 944
  due to Ehlers-Danlos syndrome, 943
  due to Fabry disease, 943
  due to fat embolism, 945
  due to fibromuscular dysplasia, 938, 939*f*
  due to hereditary hemorrhagic
    telangiectasia, 944
  due to homocystinuria, 943
  due to hypercoagulable states
    primary, 945–947, 946*b*
    secondary, 946*b*, 947–949
  due to hypereosinophilic syndrome, 945
  due to idiopathic reversible cerebral
    segmental vasoconstriction, 944–945
  due to infarcts of undetermined cause,
    949
  due to inflammatory vasculitides,
    938–939
  due to inherited and miscellaneous
    disorders, 943–945, 943*b*
  due to large-artery atherothrombotic
    infarctions, 932–933, 932*f*–933*f*
  due to Marfan syndrome, 943
  due to microangiopathy of brain, retina,
    and inner ear, 944

Ischemic stroke (*Continued*)
due to moyamoya disease, 937–938, 938*f*
due to neoplastic angioendotheliomatosis, 944
due to nonatherosclerotic vasculopathies, 936–943, 936*b*
due to pseudoxanthoma elasticum, 943–944
due to radiation vasculopathy, 937
due to sickle cell disease, 949
due to small-vessel or penetrating artery disease, 933
due to Sneddon syndrome, 944
due to thrombotic thrombocytopenic purpura, 949
due to trauma, 937
emergency care for, 963
airway in, 963
blood studies in, 963–964
circulation assessment in, 963
neurological examination in, 963–964
epidemiology of, 920–924
diurnal and seasonal variation in, 924
essential investigations for, 949–953, 950*b*
cardiac evaluation as, 951–952
cerebral angiography as, 952–953, 952*f*
neuroimaging as, 950–951, 950*f*–951*f*
etiology of, 432
genetic causes of, 921
genome-wide association studies of, 664.*e1*
heritability of, 663*t*
increased intracranial pressure with, 964, 964*b*
infections and, 939
lacunar, 432.*e2*
late subacute, 432
migraine and, 942–943
neurointerventional therapy for, 758–767
acute treatment, 758–763
angioplasty and stenting, 762–763
endovascular revascularization therapy, 758–759, 759*b*
intra-arterial thrombolysis, 759
mechanical recanalization, 759–761
with MERCI device, 759, 760*f*, 762*f*
with Penumbra System, 760, 760*f*–761*f*
MR CLEAN, ESCAPE, EXTEND-IA, and SWIFT-PRIME trials, 761–762, 762*f*
sonothrombolysis, 758
nutritional status after, 964
pathology of, 925
perfusion-weighted imaging of, 431, 431*f*
during pregnancy, 1987–1988
preventing recurrence of, 953–955
oral anticoagulants for, 954–955
platelet antiaggregants for, 953–954
risk factors for, 921, 921*t*
age as, 921
alcohol consumption as, 923
aortic atherosclerosis as, 923–924
asymptomatic carotid artery disease as, 923
atrial fibrillation as, 923
cigarette smoking as, 923
diabetes mellitus as, 922
gender as, 921*t*
Heart Protection Study of, 922–923
hemostatic, 924
heredity as, 921
high cholesterol as, 922

Ischemic stroke (*Continued*)
hypertension as, 921–922
lifestyle, 920–921
modifiable, 921–924, 921*t*
non-lifestyle, 920–921
nonmodifiable, 920–921, 921*t*
obesity as, 923
obstructive sleep apnea as, 923
oral contraceptives as, 924, 947
race/ethnicity as, 921*t*
transient ischemic attacks as, 923
structural imaging of, 428–432
of anterior cerebral artery, 430.*e1f*
in left anterior watershed area, 431*f*
of middle cerebral artery, 430*f*
of posterior cerebral artery, 430.*e1f*
temporal evolution of, 429–432
subacute, 431
and systemic vasculitides, 940–942, 940*f*–942*f*
threatened, diagnosis and treatment of, 931–932
of thromboembolic origin, 432.*e1*–432.*e2*
treatment of, 956–963
defibrinogenating and hemorheological agents for, 960
general management in, 963–964
heparins and heparinoids for, 956–960, 957*t*
hypothermia for, 960.*e1*
neuroprotective agents for, 960
stenting for, 962–963, 962*f*, 963.*e1f*
surgical, 960–962
thrombolytic therapy for, 956–960
with Wallerian degeneration, 432, 433*f*
watershed, 432.*e1*
Isentres (raltegravir), for HIV infection, 1108*t*–1109*t*
Isolate sulfite oxidase deficiency, 1328.*e1t*–1328.*e2t*
Isolated central nervous system vasculitis, 1015–1017
approach to diagnosis of, 1016
clinical findings in, 1015
laboratory findings in, 1016
pathology of, 1015–1016
therapy for, 1016–1017
Isolated dystonia, 235–236
Isolated palatal tremor, 242
Isolation syndrome, 136*t*
Isometheptene mucate, for migraine, 1701
Isometrataxia, 218
Isoniazid
neuropathy due to, 1861
for tremor, in multiple sclerosis, 1182
Isopters
crossing, 582
inverted, 582
spiraling, 582, 582*f*
Isotropic diffusion, 417.*e4*
Isotype switching, 679
Isoxazoles, in mushrooms, 1251*t*
ISUIA (International Study of Unruptured Intracranial Aneurysms), 986
IT15 gene, 1446
ITAM. *see* Immunoreceptor tyrosine-based activation motif (ITAM)
ITPR1 receptor, in dominant ataxias, 1479
IV heparin, for acute ischemic stroke, 956
IVIg. *see* Intravenous immunoglobulin (IVIg)
I-wave interactions, facilitatory, in transcranial magnetic stimulation, 393

J
J (joining) gene segments, 679
Jabs and jolts, 1713
Jackson, John Hughlings, 115–116, 551–552
Jacksonian march, 1564
Jacobson nerve, 1731
Jactitation, 242
Jadassohn nevus phakomatosis, 1553
Jakob, Alfons, 1365–1366
Jamaican neuritis, 1236
Jamestown Canyon virus, 1139
Japanese encephalitis virus (JEV), 1138–1139
Jargon speech, 130
Jaw clenching, in amyotrophic lateral sclerosis, 1513*t*
JC virus (JCV), 1132–1133
progressive multifocal leukoencephalopathy due to, HIV-associated, 1114*t*, 1115
Jefferson fracture, 887–888
structural imaging for, 454.*e1*–454.*e2*, 454.*e2f*
Jerky (myoclonic) postural tremor, 227
Jerne, Niels, 684
Jet lag, 1653–1654
JEV (Japanese encephalitis virus), 1138–1139
Jimson weed, neurotoxins from, 1249
Jitter, in single-fiber electromyography, 389–390, 390*f*
Jitteriness, 1957
JMG. *see* Juvenile myasthenia gravis (JMG)
Joining (J) gene segments, 679
Joint disease, inflammatory, 1761–1763
rheumatoid arthritis as, 1761–1762
neurological manifestations of, 1761–1762, 1761.*e1f*
pathogenesis of, 1761
systemic presentation of, 1761
spondyloarthropathies as, 1762–1763
clinical presentation of, 1762, 1762.*e1f*
laboratory abnormalities in, 1763
nonspinal neurological complications of, 1762
pathogenesis of, 1762
spinal neurological complications of, 1762, 1762*t*, 1762.*e1f*–1762.*e2f*
Joint pains, in amyotrophic lateral sclerosis, 1513*t*
Joints, disorders of, 1736–1765
Jordan syndrome, 1884
Joubert syndrome, 570
Jugular bulb oximetry, in neurointensive care, 744*t*, 746–747
Jugular foramen
glossopharyngeal nerve at
anatomy of, 1731
clinical lesions of, 1731–1732
metastases to, 1095*t*
spinal accessory nerve at
anatomy of, 1733
clinical lesions of, 1733
vagus nerve at
anatomy of, 1732
clinical lesions of, 1732–1733
Jugular oximetry (SjvO$_2$), in neurointensive care, 744*t*, 746
Jumped facets, 888–889
Juvenile kyphosis, 1751
Juvenile/metameric arteriovenous malformation, neurointerventional therapy for, 780

Juvenile myasthenia gravis (JMG), 1909
  hypotonic infant due to, 312
Juvenile myoclonic epilepsy (JME), 352,
    352f, 1520t–1521t, 1534–1535, 1535f
  effect of sleep on, 1655
Juvenile pilocytic astrocytoma (JPA), 1034
  diffuse intrinsic pontine glioma *versus*,
    1075
  structural imaging of, 419
Juvenile rheumatoid arthritis (JRA),
    neurological complications of, 839
Juvenile segmental muscular atrophy, 1498

K

K complexes
  in NREM sleep, 1621–1622
  sleep staging, 1619f
KAL1 gene, 1298
Kaletra (lopinavir + ritonavir), for HIV
    infection, 1108t–1109t
Kallmann syndrome, 1298
Kaplan-Meier analysis, 1667f
Karnofsky Performance Score (KPS), 1086,
    1086t
Karyotype, 655, 657f
Kawasaki disease, neurological complications
    of, 838–839
Kayser-Fleischer (KF) ring, 103, 223–224,
    224f, 1454
KB (ketone bodies), with inborn errors of
    metabolism, 1337
KCNA1 gene, in familial episodic ataxia,
    1530
KCNJ2 gene, Andersen-Tawil syndrome,
    1527
KCNQ2 gene, in benign familial neonatal
    seizures, 1533–1534, 1533f
KCNQ3 gene, in benign familial neonatal
    seizures, 1533–1534, 1533f
Kearns-Sayre syndrome (KSS), 1358, 1945
  ataxia in, 1470
  myopathy in, 1945
  neuro-ophthalmological examination for,
    1355
  ocular weakness due to, 288
  threshold effect and mitotic segregation
    in, 1353
Kegel exercises, for sexual dysfunction in
    women, 633
Kennedy disease, 290, 1503–1505, 1503b,
    1504f
  clinical features of, 1504
  differential diagnosis of, 1504–1505
  laboratory studies of, 1504
  manifesting carrier of, 1505
  pathogenesis of, 1503–1504
  treatment of, 1505
Keratin, wet, in adamantinomatous
    craniopharyngioma, 1043
Kernicterus, neurological complications of,
    843
Ketoacidosis
  diabetic, hyperglycemia due to, 1220
    complications of treatment of, 1221,
      1221f
  due to inborn errors of metabolism,
    1337
Ketoconazole, for Cushing disease, 711
Ketogenesis, disorders of, 1337
Ketogenic diet, for epilepsy, 1609
Ketolysis, disorders of, 1337
Ketone bodies (KB), with inborn errors of
    metabolism, 1337
Ketoprofen (Orudis), for chronic pain,
    725t

Ketorolac
  for chronic pain, 725t
  for menstrual migraine, 1704
β-ketothiolase deficiency, 1337
KF (Kayser-Fleischer) rings, 103, 1454
Khat, 1256
Ki-67, 1030
  in anaplastic astrocytoma, 1031
Kilobase, 651t
Kinetic perimeter, 579
Kinetic tremor, 218, 230
Kinky hair syndrome, 1558–1560
  cutaneous features of, 1559
  diagnosis and treatment of, 1560
  genetic studies of, 1560
  neuroimaging of, 1559–1560
  neurological features of, 1559
  other clinical features of, 1559, 1559b
Kleine-Levin syndrome, 1644–1645, 1645f
Klinefelter syndrome (KS), 656
Klippel-Feil anomaly, 1740, 1740.e1f
Klüver-Bucy syndrome, 92, 125
Knee-buckling gait, 1999
Knife-edge atrophy, in frontotemporal lobar
    degeneration, 446, 446.e2f
Kocher-Cushing reflex, 38
Kohlmeier-Degos disease, ischemic stroke
    due to, 940
Kolmer cells, 686
Konzo, 1487t, 1494
Korsakoff syndrome, 1231–1233
KPS (Karnofsky Performance Score), 1086,
    1086t
Krabbe disease, 1329–1330, 1818.e8, 440.e1
  hypotonic infant due to, 310
Kratom, 1254
KS. *see* Klinefelter syndrome (KS)
K-space, in MRI, 415
KSS. *see* Kearns-Sayre Syndrome
Kugelberg-Welander disease, 1500t, 1501
  leg weakness in, 290–291
"Kuru", 1369–1370
Kuru plaques, 1374
Kussmaul breathing, 41
Kynurenin, in chemical imaging, 505t
Kyphosis, juvenile, 1751
Kytorphin, 697t–698t

L

L4 radiculopathy, 1771
L5 radiculopathy, 1770–1771
La belle indifference, 1995
La Crosse encephalitis, 1137t, 1139
Labetalol
  for acute ischemic stroke, 963
  for intracerebral hemorrhage, 981
Labia majora, 624
Laboratory investigations, 6
  abnormal test result in, 344
  biopsy as, 344
  blood tests as, 344
  for coma, 48, 49t
  decision analysis with, 347
  in diagnosis and management, of
    neurological disease, 343–347
  diagnostic yield of, 344
  genetic studies as, 343–344
  interpretation of results of, 344
  neuroimaging modalities of, 343
  normal range and standard deviations in,
    344
  patient confidentiality with, 347
  prioritization of tests in, 346–347
  purpose of, 343
  reliability of, 347

Laboratory investigations (*Continued*)
  in research investigations and teaching
    hospitals, 347
  risks and costs of, 345–346
    cost-to-benefit analysis of, 346
    risk-to-benefit analysis of, 345–346
      for brain biopsy, 345–346, 346f
      for cerebral arteriography, 345
      for lumbar puncture, 345
  role of, 347
Labyrinthine concussion, 592
Labyrinthitis, 595
Laceration, peripheral nerve injury due to,
    908
Lacosamide, for epilepsy
  absorption, elimination half-life,
    formulations of, 1600t
  efficacy by seizure type of, 1601t
  hepatic metabolism, enzyme induction/
    inhibition, pharmacokinetic
    interactions, and protein binding of,
    1603t
  mechanism of action of, 1604t
Lacrimal nerve, 1721f, 1726f
Lactate, 497
  with inborn errors of metabolism,
    1326t
Lactate dehydrogenase deficiency, myopathy
    due to, 1941
Lactate/pyruvate ratio, in mitochondrial
    diseases, 1355
Lactic acidosis, 1354
Lactulose, for hepatic encephalopathy,
    1215
Lacunae, EEG of, 356
Lacunar stroke, 1416
Lacunar syndromes, 928
Lafora body disease, 1579
Laing myopathy, 1934
Lambert-Eaton myasthenic syndrome
    (LEMS). *see* Lambert-Eaton syndrome
    (LES)
Lambert-Eaton syndrome (LES), 1912–1913
  channelopathy in, 1535–1536
  diagnostic procedures in, 1912
  fluctuating weakness due to, 292
  immune mediation of, 686–687
  immunopathology of, 1912–1913,
    1912f
  paraneoplastic, 1193
  repetitive nerve stimulation for, 388t
    rapid, 388, 389f
  treatment of, 1913
Lamellipodia, in nerve regeneration, 907,
    907f
Lamin A/C deficiency, 1924–1925
Lamina terminalis, 1295–1296
Laminar necrosis, after cardiac arrest, 1201
Laminectomy, decompressive, for spinal cord
    compression, 1094
Laminin-α2, 1919
Laminin-A₂ (merosin) deficiency, 1928
Lamivudine (3Tc, Epivir), for HIV infection,
    1108t–1109t
Lamotrigine
  for chronic pain, 726
  for epilepsy
    absorption, elimination half-life,
      formulations of, 1600t
    efficacy by seizure type of, 1601t
    hepatic metabolism, enzyme induction/
      inhibition, pharmacokinetic
      interactions, and protein binding
      of, 1603t
    mechanism of action of, 1604t
    during pregnancy, 1985

Luteinizing hormone (LH), 697t–698t
hypothalamic peptides controlling release
of, 702t
in precocious puberty, 704
Luteinizing hormone (LH)-secreting tumors,
706
Luteinizing hormone-releasing hormone,
697t–698t
lvPPA (logopenic variant primary progressive
aphasia), 489, 489f
Lyme borreliosis, peripheral nerve
manifestations of, 1864.e6
Lyme disease, 1776
structural imaging of, 436.e2
Lyme encephalitis, 436.e2
Lyme radiculoneuropathy, 1776
Lymph nodes, examination of, for coma, 39
Lymphadenopathy, in viral CNS disease,
1124t
Lymphocytic choriomeningitis virus (LCMV),
1145
Lymphocytosis, transient syndrome of
headache with neurological deficits and
CSF, 1690
Lymphoma, 1848
angiotropic, ischemic stroke due to, 944
central nervous system, pathology and
molecular genetics of, 1041–1042,
1042f
CNS vasculitis due to, 1017
Hodgkin, cerebellar ataxia associated with,
1200
neurological complications of, 826
peripheral neuropathy associated with,
1192–1193
primary central nervous system
HIV-associated, 1117, 1118f
management of, 1061f, 1062–1063
AIDS-related, 1063
for non-AIDS related disease,
1062–1063
pathology and molecular genetics of,
1041–1042, 1042f
structural imaging of, 418t–419t, 423,
424f
of spinal canal, structural imaging of, 449,
450f
subacute motor neuronopathy in,
1506
Lymphomatosis, intravascular malignant,
ischemic stroke due to, 944
Lymphoproliferative disorders, subacute
motor neuronopathy in, 1506
Lymphotoxin, in immune response, 683t
Lyonization, 651t, 658–659
in Kennedy disease, 1505
Lysinuric protein intolerance (LPI), 1333
Lysosomal disorders, hypotonic infant due
to, 310
Lysosomal storage disorders, 1333–1334
classification of, 1333.e2t–1333.e3t
clinical features of, 1334
transmission of, 1334
Lysosome, 1333–1334

M

M wave, in transcranial magnetic
stimulation, 391–392
Ma antibodies, 1190
MABC-2 (Movement Assessment Battery for
Children), 1316
MAC (mitral annular calcification),
cardiogenic embolism due to, 934

MACFIMS (Minimal Assessment of Cognitive
Function in Multiple Sclerosis), 1167
Machado-Joseph disease (MJD), 1471,
1474–1475, 1517
type 3
dystonia in, 1472f
MRI in, 1472f
type 6, 1473f, 1475
type 7, 1472f, 1475
MacLean, Paul, 58
Macrocephaly
in autism spectrum disorder, 1304
in neurofibromatosis type 1, 1544
Macroglobulinemia, Waldenström
neurological complications of, 825
peripheral neuropathy in, 1192
Macrophages
in immune system, 677
in multiple sclerosis, 1161
in spinal cord injury, 882
Macropsia, 123
Macrosquare wave jerks, 219, 566f, 567
Macular cherry-red spot, with global
developmental delay, 69t
Macular degeneration, with global
developmental delay, 69t
Macular rash, confluent, in viral CNS
disease, 1123t
Macule, 585
Maculopapular eruption, in viral CNS
disease, 1123t
Maculopathy, in spinocerebellar atrophy type
7, 1472f
Mad cow disease, 1375
MADD. see Multiple acyl-coenzyme A
dehydrogenation deficiency (MADD)
Maddox rod test, for diplopia, 536, 537f
Magnesium, for migraine prophylaxis, 1703
menstrual, 1705
Magnesium disturbances, neurological
complications of, 831
Magnesium metabolism, encephalopathy,
due to disorders of, 1224–1225
Magnesium sulfate
for migraine, 1702
for preeclampsia and eclampsia, 1991
Magnetic coil, in transcranial magnetic
stimulation, 391
Magnetic coil stimulation, 365.e7–365.e9
Magnetic feet, 254
Magnetic field, in transcranial magnetic
stimulation, 391
"Magnetic" gait, 219
Magnetic grasp and grope reflexes, 121
Magnetic resonance angiography (MRA),
459–460, 464–476
3T or greater, 466
4D time-resolved, 466
7T scanners, 466
applications of, 467–476
for acute ischemic stroke, 472
for cerebral aneurysms, 472–473,
472f–473f
in extracranial carotid and vertebral
circulation, 467–469, 467f
in intracranial circulation, 469–476,
471f
in spine disorders, 476, 477f
for subclavian steal syndrome, 471–472
for vascular malformations, 474–476,
475f, 475t
for venous disorders, 473–474
digital subtraction, 466
headache and, 201–202

Magnetic resonance angiography (MRA)
(Continued)
for intracranial aneurysms, 987–988
limitations of, 466–467
metal implant contraindications as, 467
nephrogenic systemic fibrosis as,
466–467
maximum intensity projection in, 466,
468f
methods of, 464–466, 466f
phase-contrast, 464–466, 471–472
of spinal vascular malformations,
1011–1012, 1012f
for stroke in children, 1004, 1004f
three-dimensional contrast-enhanced,
468–469, 468f–471f
of carotid and vertebral circulation, 466
after stent placement, 469, 471f
with basilar artery stenosis, 469, 469f
with carotid artery dissection, 469,
470f–471f
with carotid stenosis, 468f
with fibromuscular dysplasia, 469
with vertebral artery dissection, 469,
470f
fast, dynamic, or time-resolved, 466
time-of-flight, 467–468, 467f
of extracranial carotid and vertebral
circulation, 467–469, 467f
Magnetic resonance imaging (MRI),
412–417, 486
of anoxic-ischemic encephalopathy,
1206–1208, 1207f–1208f
basic principles, 412–413, 413f
of brain metastases, 1085, 1085f
for chronic infectious meningitis, 1149
for coma, 48
for Creutzfeldt-Jakob disease, 1372f
versus CT, 458.e1
defined, 412
in diagnosis of multiple sclerosis,
1168–1170, 1169f
brain atrophy in, 1169–1170, 1171f
high-field strength, 1169
lesion differentiation based on,
1168–1169, 1169f–1170f
of spinal cord, 1170, 1172f
diffusion tensor imaging in, 417.e4,
417.e4f
diffusion-weighted, 417.e3
for dizziness, 598
echoplanar imaging in, 417.e2–417.e3
fat saturation in, 417.e2, 417.e2f
flipping net magnetization vector in, 413,
413f
Fourier transform in, 413, 416–417
frequency encoding gradient in, 416–417
frequency encoding in, 413
functional, 486
in disorders of consciousness, 55–56
for presurgical brain mapping, 499
prior to epilepsy surgery, 1598
for global developmental delay, 69
gradient-recalled echo sequences and
partial flip angle for, 417.e1
gyromagnetic ratio in, 416
headache and, 201–202
of hepatic encephalopathy, 1211, 1211f
for HIV-associated dementia, 1111, 1112f
image reconstruction in, 416–417, 417f
indications for, 457–458
inversion recovery sequences (FLAIR,
STIR), 300
Larmor frequency in, 416

Magnetic resonance imaging (MRI)
  (Continued)
  of leptomeningeal metastases, 1097–1098
  for lower back and leg pain, 335, 336*t*
  magnetic field in, 412–413, 413*f*
  magnetization in, 413, 413*f*
  magnetization transfer contrast imaging
    in, 417.*e*4–417.*e*5
  for movement disorder, 246–248
  for neonatal hypoxic-ischemic brain
    injury, 1960, 1961*f*
  for paraneoplastic neurological syndromes,
    1188
  perfusion -weighted, 417.*e*3
  phase encoding gradient in, 416–417
  precession in, 413, 413*f*
  during pregnancy, 1975
  receiver coils in, 413
  repetition time in, 414–415, 414*f*
  resonance in, 413
  signal intensity in, 413, 416*t*
  slice selection gradient, 416, 417*f*
  spin echo and fast (turbo) spin echo
    techniques for, 417.*e*1
  of spinal cord compression, 1093,
    1093*f*
  of spinal cord ischemia, 1007–1008,
    1008*f*
  for spinal epidural abscess, 1152, 1152*f*
  of spinal vascular malformations,
    1011–1012, 1012*f*
  for stroke in children, 1004
  of subarachnoid hemorrhage, 987, 989*f*
  T1 and T2 relaxation times, 413–414,
    414*f*
  T1 contrast in, 415
  T1 weighting in, 415, 415*f*–416*f*, 416*t*
  T2 contrast in, 415
  T2 weighting in, 415, 415*f*–416*f*, 416*t*
  temporal evolution of ischemic stroke on,
    429–432
  for threatened stroke, 950, 951*f*
  time to echo in, 414–415
    effective, 417.*e*1
  tissue contrast (T1, T2, and proton density
    weighting) in, 415, 415*f*–416*f*, 416*t*
  transverse magnetization, 413
  water molecules as basis for, 1265
Magnetic resonance spectroscopy (MRS),
    497, 444.*e*2
  of hepatic encephalopathy, 1211
  with inborn errors of metabolism, 1341
  for movement disorder, 248–249
  prior to epilepsy surgery, 1597
  sports and performance concussion in,
    862
  for stroke in children, 1004
Magnetic resonance venography (MRV), 434,
    463
Magnetization transfer contrast imaging,
    417.*e*4–417.*e*5
Magnetization transfer ratio (MTR),
    417.*e*5
Magnetoencephalography, 365.*e*1
  prior to epilepsy surgery, 1597–1598
Magnocellular layers, in visual pathways,
    573, 574*f*
Ma-huang, ischemic stroke due to, 939
Maintenance of wakefulness test (MWT),
    1675
Major depressive disorder (MDD)
  electroconvulsive therapy for, 113
  repetitive transcranial magnetic
    stimulation, 113
Major histocompatibility complex (MHC),
    in multiple sclerosis, 1163

Major histocompatibility complex (MHC)
    antigens
  in CNS, 685
  in immune response, 677, 679, 679*f*–680*f*
Major histocompatibility complex (MHC)
    class I restricted T cells, 679, 680*f*
Major histocompatibility complex (MHC)
    class II restricted T cells, 679, 680*f*
Major histocompatibility complex (MHC)
    restriction, 679*f*
Mal de débarquement syndrome, 540
Malabsorption syndromes, neuropathy
    associated with, 1854–1855
Male genital and reproductive system,
    innervation of, 626*f*
Male sexual dysfunction
  due to spinal cord injury, 610–611
  management of
    for ejaculation dysfunction, 621
    for erectile dysfunction, 620–621, 621*t*
Male sexual function, primary impact of
    spinal cord lesions on, 628–629
Male sexual response, 622–624
  ejaculation, 622, 624*f*
  erection, 622, 623*f*–624*f*
  neurological control of, 607
  orgasm, 622–624
Malignancies, peripheral neuropathy in,
    1845–1848
Malignant atrophic papulosis, ischemic
    stroke due to, 940
Malignant hypertension, optic disc swelling
    due to, 172
Malignant hyperthermia, 700, 1520*t*–1521*t*,
    1527–1528
  ryanodine receptor in, 1937
Malignant inflammatory sensory
    polyganglionopathy (paraneoplastic
    sensory neuronopathy), 1847–1848
  clinical features of, 1847
  differential diagnosis of, 1847
  laboratory features of, 1847
  prognosis of, 1847–1848
Malignant parkinsonism, 227
Malignant peripheral nerve sheath tumor
    (MPNST), 1041
  management of, 1061
Malingering, 1993, 2002–2003
Mallampati classification, in central sleep
    apnea syndrome, 1650*f*
Mallory body myopathy, 1927
Malnutrition, protein-calorie, 1236
Mammillary bodies, in memory, 62–63, 62*f*
Mammillothalamic tract, in memory, 62*f*
"Man-in-the-barrel" syndrome, 1202, 1203*t*
Management, of neurological disorders, 7
Management of Atherothrombosis with
    Clopidogrel in High-Risk Patients
    (MATCH) trial, 953–954
Mandibular nerve
  anatomy of, 1721*f*, 1725, 1726*f*
  clinical lesions of, 1727
Manganese
  in hepatic encephalopathy, 1215
  occupational exposure to, 1243–1244
Manganese metabolism, encephalopathy due
    to disorders of, 1225
Manganese toxicity, parkinsonism due to,
    1442
Mania, after stroke, 99–100
Manifest latent nystagmus (MLN), 543
Manipulative automatisms, 1564–1565
Mannitol, for cerebral edema, 1272
MAOI (monoamine oxidase inhibitor),
    111–112
  for migraine, 1703

MAP. *see* Mean arterial pressure (MAP)
Maple syrup urine disease (MSUD), 1330
  disorders of neurotransmitter synthesis in,
    1290
MAPT mutations, 1409–1410, 1409*f*
MAR (melanoma-associated retinopathy),
    1194
Maraviroc (Selzentry), for HIV infection,
    1108*t*–1109*t*
Marburg variant, of multiple sclerosis,
    1174–1175, 1175*f*
Marburg virus, 1145.*e*1
Marchiafava-Bignami disease, 1234–1235,
    440.*e*1
Marcus Gunn pupil, 179–180, 575–576,
    576*b*, 576*f*
Marfan syndrome, 1738–1739
  dural ectasia in, 1739
  ischemic stroke due to, 943
  and stroke in children, 998
Marginal glioneuronal heterotopia, 1287
Marie, Pierre, 1465
Marie ataxia, 1471
Marijuana
  acute effects of, 1257*b*
  drug dependence with, 1257
  use, and seizures, 1583
Marine neurotoxins, 1251–1253, 1914
  from ciguatera fish, 1251–1252
  from puffer fish, 1252
  from shellfish, 1252–1253
Marinesco-Sjögren syndrome, 1469
Marker, 651*t*, 659–660, 661*f*
Markesbery-Griggs myopathy, 1920*t*–1921*t*,
    1927, 1933
Maroteaux-Lamy disease, 1333.*e*4*t*
Martin-Gruber anastomosis, nerve
    conduction studies with, 370–371
Mass lesions
  headache attributed to, 1687
  hemiplegia due to, 264
  psychiatric manifestations of, 105
MASS syndrome. *see* Mitral valve, aorta,
    skeletal, and skin involvement (MASS
    syndrome)
Mastitis, in viral CNS disease, 1124*t*
Mastoiditis, headache and, 1690
MATCH (Management of Atherothrombosis
    with Clopidogrel in High-Risk Patients)
    trial, 953–954
Maternal brachial plexus neuropathy, 1979
Maternal inheritance, 661*f*
  of mtDNA, 1350
Maternal obstetric palsy, 1979–1980, 1979*f*
Maternally inherited diabetes and deafness
    (MIDD), 1360, 1326.*e*1*t*–1326.*e*2*t*
Maternally inherited Leigh syndrome
    (MILS), 1360
Matrix metalloproteinases (MMPs), in
    immune response, 681–682
Maturation, defined, 1279
Maxillary nerve
  anatomy of, 1721*f*, 1725, 1726*f*
  clinical lesions of, 1727
Maxillary nerve block, 729*t*
Maxillary sinusitis, headache and facial pain
    due to, 1694–1695
Maximum intensity projection (MIP), 459
  algorithm for, 466
Mayo Asymptomatic Carotid Endarterectomy
    Trial, 961–962
MBP (myelin basic protein), in multiple
    sclerosis, 1163
McArdle disease, 1336–1337, 1940
McCarley-Hobson reciprocal interaction
    model, of REM sleep, 1624.*e*1

McDonald criteria, for multiple sclerosis, 1167, 1168*t*

M-CHAT-R (Modified Checklist for Autism in Toddlers-Revised), 1304

McKittrick-Wheelock syndrome, due to autonomic disorders, 1890

McLeod syndrome, 1448

MCMD (minor cognitive motor disorder), 101

MD (myoclonus dystonia), 1454

MDAS (Memorial Delirium Assessment Scale), 28–29

MDCTA (multidetector CTA), of cerebral venous thrombosis, 463

MDDS (mitochondrial DNA depletion syndrome), 1360

[¹¹C]MDL 100,907, in chemical imaging, 506

MDS-UPDRS (Movement Disorder Society Unified Parkinson's Disease Rating Scale), 1428

Mean arterial pressure (MAP), and cerebral perfusion pressure, 745

Measles, 1141–1143
  acute encephalitis due to, 1141
  inclusion body encephalitis due to, 1142
  postviral encephalomyelitis due to, 1141
  subacute sclerosing panencephalitis due to, 1142–1143, 1142*f*

Measles hyperimmunoglobulin, 1131*t*

Measles inclusion body encephalitis, 1142

MEB. *see* Muscle-eye-brain (MEB) disease

Mechanical assistive devices, 802–803
  for mobility, 802–803
  for upper extremities, 802

Mechanical circulatory support, and stroke in children, 997

Mechanical dysphagia, 149, 149*b*

Mechanical pain, lower back pain due to, 334*t*, 340

Mechanical recanalization, for ischemic stroke, 759–761
  with MERCI device, 759, 760*f*, 762*f*
  with Penumbra System, 760, 760*f*–761*f*

Mechanical Retrieval and Recanalization of Stroke Clots Using Embolectomy (MR RESCUE) study, 958.*e1*

Mechanical thrombectomy, for acute ischemic stroke, 958, 960*t*

Meckel-Grüber syndrome, 1295*f*

Meclofenamate sodium (Meclomen), for chronic pain, 725*t*

MECP2. *see* Methyl-CpG-binding protein 2 (MECP2)

Medial branch block, 729*t*

Medial inferior pontine syndrome, 930

Medial longitudinal fasciculus (MLF), in eye movements
  horizontal, 554, 555*f*
  rostral interstitial nucleus of, 560
  vertical, 558–559, 559*f*

Medial medullary (Dejerine) syndrome, 930, 1722*t*, 1734
  sensory deficit due to, 319

Medial preoptic area (MPOA), 625

Medial rectus muscle
  actions of, 528–529, 529*t*
  anatomy of, 529*f*
  weakness of, 533–534, 536–537

Median nerve
  applied anatomy of, 1802
  neuropathy of, monoplegia due to, 269–270
    differential diagnosis of, 272.*e2*

Median nerve entrapment, 324, 1801*t*
  at elbow, 1804
  at ligament of Struthers, 1804
  at wrist (carpal tunnel syndrome), 1802–1803, 1803*f*, 1803*t*

Median nerve pain, 324

Median nerve stimulator, 919*f*

Median spinal vein, 1007.*e1*–1007.*e2*

Medical Research Council Muscle Grading System, 883, 883*t*

Medically unexplained, 1993

Medicated urethral system for erection (MUSE), 621

Medication overuse headache (MOH), 1706–1708
  pathogenesis of, 1707
  treatment of, 1707–1708
    pharmacological, 1708

Medicinal herbs, neurotoxins from, 1250

Medium-chain acyl-CoA dehydrogenase (MCAD) deficiency, 1337
  DNA testing for, 1328

Medroxyprogesterone, anticonvulsants and, 1974

Medullary hemorrhage, 978*t*, 980, 980.*e1f*

Medullary radicular artery, 1007.*e1f*

Medullary stroke syndromes, 212–216, 216*b*

Medulloblastoma
  anaplastic/large-cell variant of, 1038
  desmoplastic/nodular variant of, 1038
  familial forms of, 1038–1039
  management of, 1059–1060
  with melanotic differentiation, 1038
  with myogenic differentiation, 1038
  pathology and molecular genetics of, 1038–1039, 1038*f*
  pediatric, 1065–1069
    classification of, 1065
    clinical presentation of, 1067
    desmoplastic, 1066
    diagnosis of, 1067, 1068*f*
    etiology of, 1065–1067
    management of, 1067–1069
    prognosis of, 1069
    risk stratification for, 1067–1068
    staging of, 1067–1068
    structural imaging of, of brain, 418*t*–419*t*, 424, 426*f*

Medulloepithelioma, pediatric, 1066

Medullomyoblastoma, 1038

Medulloradicular arteries, 1007.*e1f*

Mees lines, in arsenic neuropathy, 1242, 1242*f*

Megabase, 651*t*

Megalencephaly, in epidermal nevus syndrome, 1554

Megaloblastic anemia, neurological complications of, 824

Meiosis, 651*t*

Melanocyte-stimulating hormone, 697*t*–698*t*

α-Melanocyte-stimulating hormone
  in appetite, 701
  immunoregulatory effects of, 699*t*

Melanoma-associated retinopathy (MAR), 1194

Melanomas, structural imaging of, 449.*e1*

Melanosis
  leptomeningeal, 1555, 1555*f*
  neurocutaneous, 1554–1555
    cutaneous features of, 1554–1555
    laboratory findings of, 1555
    neuroimaging of, 1555, 1556*f*
    neurological features of, 1555

MELAS (mitochondrial encephalomyopathy with lactic acidosis and stroke-like episodes), 444.*e2*
  ataxia in, 1470

Melatonin
  in circadian rhythm, 1625–1626
  in menstrual migraine, 1704
  during sleep, 1631, 1631*f*

MELD. *see* Model for End-stage Liver Disease (MELD)

Melkersson-Rosenthal syndrome, 1722*t*, 1731

Melodic intonation therapy (MIT), 806

Meloxicam (Mobic), for chronic pain, 725*t*

Memantine (Namenda XR), 1398
  for dystonia, 1452*t*

Membrane polarity, 1289
  disorders of, 1289

Memorial Delirium Assessment Scale (MDAS), 28–29

Memory
  bedside tests of, 64–65, 64*b*, 65*f*
  classical conditioning as, 63–64
  declarative (explicit), 63, 63*t*
  defined, 57, 60
  immediate (working), 60, 61*t*
  long-term (remote), 60, 61*t*
  motor, 61–62, 61*t*
  nondeclarative (implicit), 63–64, 63*t*
  priming, 63–64
  probabilistic classification learning and, 63–64
  procedural, 61*t*, 63
    in Alzheimer disease, 1387
  semantic, 60, 61*t*
    in Alzheimer disease, 1387
  short-term (recent), 60, 61*t*
  stages of, 60–61, 61*t*
  testing, in Alzheimer disease, 1389–1391

Memory consolidation, during sleep, 1628

Memory disturbances, during rehabilitation, 807–808
  frequency of, 807
  outcomes of, 808
  pharmacological adjuncts in, 807–808, 808*b*
  treatments in, 807, 808*b*

Memory impairment, 57–65
  in Alzheimer disease, 521, 1387
  in delirium, 26
  in epilepsy, 526
  in Huntington disease, 524–525
  treatment of, 717
  in vascular dementia, 521–522

Memory loss
  in amnestic syndrome, 61–63, 62*b*
  partial, syndromes of, 63

Memory network, 94

Memory symptoms, functional, 2001–2002

Mendelian inheritance, 657–659
  autosomal dominant, 657–658, 658*f*
  autosomal recessive, 658, 660*f*
  defined, 651*t*
  gene identification by linkage analysis and chromosome mapping for, 659–660, 661*f*
  pseudodominant, 658
  sex-linked (X-linked), 658–659, 660*f*

Meniere, Prosper, 583

Meniere disease
  drop attacks due to, 19
  hearing loss due to, 596
  tinnitus in, 596–598

Meniere disease *(Continued)*
    treatment of, 603
    vertigo due to, 587*t*, 591–592, 595
    vestibular, 583–584, 591–592
Meningeal carcinomatosis, headache due to,
        1687–1688
Meningeal/extra-axial tumors, pathology and
        molecular genetics of, 1039–1041
Meningeal sarcomas, headache due to,
        1687–1688
Meningeal tumor
    management of, 1061–1062
    pathology and molecular genetics of,
        1039–1041
Meninges, disorders of, 1736–1765
Meningioma
    anaplastic, 1040
    atypical, 1039–1040
    en plaque, 1039
    fibroblastic, 1039
    headache due to, 1687–1688
    malignant progression of, 1040
    management of, 1061–1062, 1061*f*
    meningothelial, 1039, 1040*f*
    molecular features of, 1040
    optic nerve sheath, structural imaging of,
        449.*e*1
    optic neuritis due to, 165*f*
    pathology and molecular genetics of,
        1039, 1040*f*
    of planum sphenoidale, 174*f*
    structural imaging of
        of brain, 418*t*–419*t*, 423–424, 425*f*
        of spine, 450, 451*f*
Meningismus, coma with, 37, 39
Meningitic hydrocephalus, 1965
Meningitis
    bacterial, 1147–1150
        acute, 1147
            headache due to, 1690
        in children, 1147
        clinical presentation of, 1148
        diagnosis of, 1148–1149
        EEG in, 359
        etiology of, 1147–1148
        management of, 1149–1150,
            1149*t*–1150*t*
        pathogens of, 1148*t*
        recurrent, 1763–1764
        and stroke in children, 1000
        structural imaging of, 436.*e*1
        subacute or chronic, 1147–1148
        versus viral, 1149
    carcinomatous, 1687–1688
    chronic, 1147–1148, 1763–1764
        diagnosis of, 1149
        due to chronic adhesive arachnoiditis,
            1763, 1763.*e*1*b*
        due to superficial hemosiderosis, 1764,
            1765*f*
        due to uveomeningitis syndromes,
            1764, 1764.*e*1*b*
        pachymeningitis as, 1764, 1764*f*,
            1764.*e*1*b*
        presentation of, 1148
        recurrent, 1763–1764
    from *Cryptococcus neoformans*, HIV-
        associated, 1114*t*
    defined, 1265–1266, 1265*t*
    fungal, 1153
        clinical presentation of, 1153
        diagnosis of, 1153
        etiology of, 1153
        headache due to, 1690
        management of, 1153, 1154*t*
    mastoiditis-associated, 1147

Meningitis *(Continued)*
    Mollaret
        headache due to, 1690
        recurrent, 1763–1764
    neonatal, 1965
        management of, 1965
        prognosis of, 1965, 1966*f*
    neoplastic, 1149
    pachy, 1764, 1764*f*, 1764.*e*1*b*
    parasitic
        acute, 1155
            diagnosis of, 1155, 1156*t*
            etiology and clinical presentation of,
                1155
            management of, 1155
        chronic, 1155–1156
            diagnosis of, 1156
            etiology and clinical presentation of,
                1155–1156
            management of, 1156
    recurrent, 1763–1764
    S. pneumoniae, 1149–1150
    tuberculous, headache due to, 1690
    viral. *see* Viral meningitis
Meningocele, 1744, 1745*f*
Meningococcal glycoconjugate vaccine,
        tetravalent, 1147
Meningoencephalitis
    defined, 1265–1266, 1265*t*
    due to non-polio enterovirus, 1136
    neonatal herpes simplex virus, 1126–1128
Meningoencephalitis syndromes, HIV-
        associated, 1115
Meningomyelocele, 1282, 1295
Menkes disease, 1338, 1558–1560, 1328.*e*1*t*
    cutaneous features of, 1559
    diagnosis and treatment of, 1560
    genetic studies of, 1560
    neuroimaging of, 1559–1560
    neurological features of, 1559
    other clinical features of, 1559, 1559*b*
Menkes kinky hair syndrome
        (trichopolydystrophy, X-linked copper
        deficiency), 1888
Menopause, migraine in, 1706
Menstrual migraine, 1704
    management of, 1704–1705
        acute, 1704
        prophylactic, 1704–1705, 1704*b*
Mental retardation, genetic basis for,
        1520*t*–1521*t*
Mental status
    changes in, due to brain tumor, 1047
    in screening neurological examination, 5*t*
Mental status examination, for delirium, 28
Meperidine (Demerol), for chronic pain,
        727, 727*t*
Meralgia paresthetica, 1810
    leg pain due to, 336*t*, 339
    in pregnancy, 1979
Mercaptans, in hepatic encephalopathy, 1215
MERCI coil retriever catheter, 958.*e*1
MERCI study, 958.*e*1
Mercury, occupational exposure to, 1244
Mercury poisoning, ataxia due to,
        1461–1462
Merlin, in neurofibromatosis type 2, 1546
Merosin, 1919
Merosin deficiency, 1928
Merosin-deficient congenital muscular
        dystrophy, hypotonic infant due to, 313
MERRF (myoclonic epilepsy with ragged-red
        fibers)
    ataxia in, 1470
    seizures and, 1360
    sensorineural hearing loss in, 1360

MES (microembolic signals), 476–477
    of transient ischemic attacks, 481
MESCC (metastatic epidural spinal cord
        compression), 1091
Mesencephalic hemorrhage, 978*t*, 979,
        979.*e*1*f*
Mesial temporal lobe epilepsy (MTLE)
    familial, 1578
    with hippocampal sclerosis, 1578–1579,
        1578*f*–1579*f*
Mesoneurium, 904
Messenger RNA (mRNA), 649–650,
        650*f*
Mestinon Bromide (Pyridostigmine
        bromide), for myasthenia gravis, 1904,
        1904*t*
Mestinon Timespan, for myasthenia gravis,
        1904*t*
Metabolic biomarkers, for neonatal
        hypoxic-ischemic brain injury, 1960
Metabolic bone disease, spinal deformities
        with, 1749–1751
    diffuse idiopathic skeletal hyperostosis as,
        1751, 1751.*e*1*f*
    juvenile kyphosis as, 1751
    ossification of posterior longitudinal
        ligament or ligamentum flavum as,
        1751, 1752*f*
    osteomalacia and rickets as, 1749
    osteopetrosis as, 1749–1750,
        1749.*e*1*f*
    osteoporosis as, 1749, 1749*f*
    Paget disease as, 1750, 1750*f*
        cranial neurological complications of,
            1750
        diagnosis of, 1750
        spinal neurological complications of,
            1750
        treatment of, 1750
    scoliosis as, 1751
"Metabolic depression", 861
Metabolic derangements
    in neurointensive care, 755–756
    prevention of, with neonatal hypoxic-
        ischemic brain injury, 1961
Metabolic disorders
    childhood and young adult- onset, ataxia
        due to, 1470, 1470*t*
    psychiatric manifestations of, 102.*e*1*t*
    structural imaging of, 444
    syncope due to, 12
Metabolic disturbances, 1218–1225
    delirium due to, 29–30, 30*t*
    due to disorders of glucose metabolism,
        1218–1221
        clinical aspects of
            with hyperglycemia, 1220–1221
            with hypoglycemia, 1218–1220,
                1219*b*
        complications of treatment for, 1221,
            1221*f*
        physiology of, 1218
            cerebral glucose metabolism in,
                1218
            glucose homeostasis in, 1218
    due to disorders of water and electrolyte
        metabolism, 1221–1225
        with disordered osmolality, 1221–1224
            clinical features of, 1222–1223
            hyperosmolality as, 1224
            hypo-osmolality and hyponatremia
                as, 1222, 1222*b*
            osmotic homeostasis and, 1221–
                1222, 1222*f*
        disorders of calcium metabolism as,
            1224

Metabolic disturbances (*Continued*)
  disorders of magnesium metabolism as, 1224–1225
  disorders of manganese metabolism as, 1225
Metabolic encephalopathies
  clinical manifestations of, 1209–1210
  EEG of, 357, 357f
    continuous, 747
  falls due to, 19
Metabolic myelopathies, structural imaging of, 454
Metabolic myopathies, 1940–1943
  defined, 1915
  due to abnormal nucleotide metabolism, 1943
    myoadenylate deaminase deficiency as, 1943
  due to disorders of carbohydrate metabolism, 1940–1942
    β-enolase deficiency as, 1941
    α-glucosidase deficiency (acid maltase deficiency), 1941–1942
    lactate dehydrogenase deficiency as, 1941
    myophosphorylase deficiency as, 1940–1941
    phosphofructokinase deficiency as, 1941
    phosphoglycerate kinase deficiency as, 1941
    phosphoglycerate mutase deficiency as, 1941
    treatment of, 1942
  due to disorders of lipid metabolism, 1942–1943
    carnitine deficiency myopathy as, 1942–1943, 1943f
    carnitine palmitoyl transferase deficiency as, 1942
    other, 1943
Metabolic pathways, 1325f
Metabolic studies, for hypotonic infant, 308
Metabolic syndromes, stroke in children due to, 998, 1001
  treatment of, 1005
Metachromatic leukodystrophy (MLD), 1329–1330, 1818.e8, 440.e1
  hypotonic infant due to, 310
Metal artifacts, with CT angiography, 459–460
Metal implant
  as contraindications to MR angiography, 467
  CT angiography with, 459–460
Metals
  disorders of, 1338
  occupational exposure to, 1242–1245
    aluminum as, 1242
    arsenic as, 1242
    lead as, 1243
    manganese as, 1243–1244
    mercury as, 1244
    tellurium as, 1244
    thallium as, 1244
    tin as, 1244–1245
Metamorphopsia, 123, 158
Metastases
  brain. *see* Brain metastases
  of brain tumors, structural imaging of, 428, 428f–429f
  dural, 1094–1095
  leptomeningeal, 1095–1100
    clinical features of, 1096
    diagnosis of, 1098

Metastases (*Continued*)
  diagnostic tests for, 1096–1097, 1097t
    cerebrospinal fluid examination as, 1096–1097, 1097t
  differential diagnosis of, 1092b
  epidemiology of, 1095–1096
  neuroimaging of, 1097–1098
  pathogenesis of, 1096, 1096f
  prognosis of, 1099–1100
  treatment of, 1098–1100, 1098b
    chemotherapy for, 1098–1099
    hormonal, 1099
    radiation therapy for, 1098
    surgery for, 1098
    systemic, 1099
  peripheral nerve, 1101
    in peripheral neuropathy, 1846
  plexus, 1100–1101
    brachial plexopathy, 1100–1101
    lumbosacral plexopathy, 1101
  skull, 1094–1095, 1095t
  spinal, intramedullary, 1094
  vertebral, structural imaging of, 449, 450f
    intermedullary, 451
    leptomeningeal, 450
Metastatic and radiation-induced brachial plexopathy, with cancer, 1783–1784
  metastatic plexopathy, 1783
  radiation-induced plexopathy, 1784
Metastatic brain tumors, neuroepidemiology of, survival in, 637–638
Metastatic epidural spinal cord compression (MESCC), 1091
Metastatic plexopathy, 1783
Methadone (Dolophine), for chronic pain, 727t
Methamphetamine, 1255
  acute effects of, 1256b
  CNS vasculitis due to, 1017
Methanol poisoning, structural imaging for, 444.e1
[^{11}C] methionine, 487
Methotrexate (MTX)
  for brain tumors, 1051, 1052t–1053t
    complications of, 1048
  for dermatomyositis, polymyositis, and immune-mediated necrotizing myopathy, 1952
  for leptomeningeal metastases, 1099
  during pregnancy, 1982
Methsuximide, for epilepsy
  absorption, elimination half-life, formulations of, 1600t
  efficacy by seizure type of, 1601t
  hepatic metabolism, enzyme induction/inhibition, pharmacokinetic interactions, and protein binding of, 1603t
  mechanism of action of, 1604t
1-Methyl-4-phenyl-1,2,3,6-tetrahydropyridine (MPTP), parkinsonism due to, 1422–1423
Methyl bromide, occupational exposure to, 1239–1240
Methyl-CpG-binding protein 2 (MECP2), 653
α-[^{11}C] Methyl-L-tryptophan (AMT), in chemical imaging, 506
  of epilepsy, 509
3,4-Methylenedioxymethamphetamie (MDMA), 1256
Methylenetetrahydrofolate reductase deficiency (MTHFR), 1328.e1t

Methylmalonic acid, in cobalamin deficiency, 1227, 1227b
Methylphenidate (Ritalin), for fatigue, in multiple sclerosis, 1182
Methylprednisolone
  for cluster headaches, 1710
  for migraine, during pregnancy, 1706
  for multiple sclerosis, chronic, 1181
Methylprednisolone acetate (MPA), 1153–1154
Methysergide, for cluster headache maintenance prophylaxis, 1710
Metoclopramide, 1702
  for migraine in children and adolescents, 1719
Metronidazole, neuropathy due to, 1862
Metyrapone, for Cushing disease, 711
Metyrapone test, 710t
Mevalonic aciduria (MVA), 1337
Mexiletine, for neuropathic pain, 918t–919t
Meyer loop, in visual pathways, 573, 574f
MFM. *see* Myofibrillar myopathy (MFM)
MFN2. *see* Mitofusin 2 (MFN2) gene
MG. *see* Myasthenia gravis (MG)
mGluR5 receptors, in chemical imaging, 505t, 506
MGMT gene, methylation of, in glioblastoma, 1033
MHC (major histocompatibility complex), in multiple sclerosis, 1163
MI (myocardial infarction)
  cardiogenic embolism due to, 933–934
  and sleep, 1669
MIB-1, 1030
  in anaplastic astrocytoma, 1031
Microangiopathy, of brain, retina, and inner ear, ischemic stroke due to, 944
Microarray, 651t
Microarray technology, 655–656, 664.e1
Microdialysis, in neurointensive care, 744t, 748–749
Microembolic signals (MES), 476–477
  of transient ischemic attacks, 481
Microflutter, ocular, 546t, 550
Microgemistocytes, in oligodendroglioma, 1031–1032
Microglia
  in amyotrophic lateral sclerosis, 693
  and immune response, 686
  in immune surveillance, 685–686
  in multiple sclerosis, 1162
  in spinal cord injury, 882
Microinfarcts, 1416
Micropsia, 123, 540
Micro-RNAs (miRNAs), 650f, 652
Microsaccadic ocular flutter, 550
"Microsleep" episodes, 1631.e1
Microtubule-Associated Protein Tau, 1413
Microtubule dysfunction, in amyotrophic lateral sclerosis, 1508
Microvascular decompression (MVD)
  of posterior fossa, 1717
  for trigeminal neuralgia, 736, 1717
Microvascular ischemic changes, structural imaging of, 432
Microvascular ischemic white matter lesions, 432–434, 434f
  clinical significance, 433
Microvascular proliferation, 1028, 1029f
Microwave equipment, and brain tumors, 1021–1022
Micturition, neurological control of, 605, 606f
Micturition syncope, 12–13

MID (multi-infarct dementia), 1414
Midazolam
    half-life of, 1203t
    with induced hypothermia for
        cardiopulmonary arrest, 1204b
Midbrain hemorrhage, 979.e1f
Midbrain reticular formation (MRF), in eye
        movements
    horizontal, 555
    vertical, 558–559, 559f
Midbrain stroke syndromes, 211–212, 212b
Midbrain syndrome of Foville, 929–930
MIDD (maternally inherited diabetes and
        deafness), 1360
Middle cerebral artery (MCA)
    dense, 950, 950f
    hyperdense, 429, 429f
    infarction of, hemiplegia due to, 263–264
Middle cerebral artery (MCA) aneurysms
    endovascular treatment of, 991–992
    imaging of, 989f
Middle cerebral artery (MCA) stenosis
    CT angiography of, 461, 461f
    MRA of, 471f
Middle cerebral artery (MCA) stroke
    ASPECTS for, 461–462, 462b, 462f
Middle cerebral artery syndromes, 927–928
Middle column, 889
Middle cranial fossa, metastases to, 1095t
Middle ear testing, for hearing loss, 602
Middle lateral pontine syndrome, 214b, 215f
Middle medial pontine syndrome, 214b, 215f
Middle superior alveolar nerve, 1726f
Middle-aged, cryptogenic falls in, 19–20
Midfacial hypoplasia, and
        holoprosencephaly, 1297
Midget cells, 163
Midline malformations, of forebrain,
        1295–1299
Midodrine
    for autonomic disorders, 1893–1894
    for dystonia, 1452t
Midposition pupils, 42
Mifepristone (RU-486), for Cushing disease,
        711
Miglusta, for inborn errors of metabolism,
        1331
Migraine, 1695–1706
    abdominal, 1719
    acephalgic, 1696
    atrial, syncope due to, 12
    attack, 1696–1697
        frequency of, 1696
        headache phase of, 1697
        migraine aura, 1696–1697
        migraine postdrome, 1697
        migraine prodrome, 1696
        triggers of, 1696
    with aura, 1696–1697
        with brainstem aura, 1697
        language, 1697
        sensory, 1696–1697
        visual, 159, 1692, 1696
        without headache, 1697
    basilar, 265, 1697
    with brainstem aura, 1697
    breastfeeding and, 1976
    as cause of dizziness, 584
    in children and adolescents, 1718–1719
    chronic, 1696, 1707
    classic, 265
    common, 265
    complicated, 265
    cutaneous allodynia in, 1697
    definition and classification, 1695–1696,
        1696b

Migraine (Continued)
    diagnostic testing for, 1698
    differential diagnosis of, 272.e1, 272.e1t
        versus epilepsies, 1591–1592
    EEG of, 356
    epidemiology, 1696
    epilepsy and, 1585
    episodic, 1696
    episodic syndromes associated with, 1719
    familial hemiplegic, 942–943
    genetic predisposition to, 1696
    genetics of, 1698
    hemiplegia due to, 265
    hemiplegic, 265, 1002, 1697
        familial, 1528–1529, 1698
            clinical features of, 1528, 1528f
            diagnosis of, 1529
            genetic basis for, 1520t–1521t
            pathophysiology of, 1528–1529,
                1529f
            subtypes of, 1528
            treatment of, 1529
    and hormone replacement therapy, 1706
    and hormones, 1703–1704
    in menopause, 1706
    menstrual migraine, 1704
        management, 1704–1705
            acute, 1704
            prophylactic, 1704–1705, 1704b
        pathogenesis of, 1704
    monoplegia due to, 268
    neurogenic inflammation in, 1699
    oligemia in, 1698
    oral contraception in female migraineurs,
        1705–1706
    oral contraceptives and, 1973–1974
    pathophysiology of, 1698–1699
        cortical spreading depression in, 1699
        hyperexcitable migraine brain in,
            1699
        migraine generator, 1698–1699
        and trigeminocervical system in, 1699
        vascular versus neuronal, 1698
    physical findings, 1697
    and pregnancy, 1706, 1975–1976
        before, 1975–1976
        during, 1976
        postpartum, 1976
    with referred pain to occipital and nuchal
        regions, 1695
    remission of, during pregnancy, 1706
    retinal, 158
    rTMS for, 399
    stress and, 1700
    and stroke, 942–943
        in children, 1000
    treatment and management of, 603,
        1699–1700
        dietary factors in, 1700
        in emergency room, 1702
        pharmacotherapy in, 1700
        prophylactic, 1702–1703
            anticonvulsants for, 1703
            antidepressants as, 1702–1703
            β-adrenergic blockers, 1702
            calcium channel blockers as,
                1702
            riboflavin for, 1703
            selective serotonin reuptake inhibitors
                for, 1703
            serotonergic agents, 1703
        symptomatic, 1700–1702
            ergots in, 1701–1702, 1701t
            triptans in, 1700–1701, 1700.e1t
    trigeminal nucleus caudalis in, 1699
    vertigo due to, 587t, 593–595

Migraine auras, 1696–1697
    with brainstem aura, 1697
    language, 1697
    sensory, 1696–1697
    visual, 159, 1692, 1696
    without headache, 1697
Migraine Disability Assessment Scale
        (MIDAS), 200
Migraine equivalent, 265, 1591, 1697
Migraine hangover, 1697
Migraine headaches, 197, 1695, 1697
Migraine-triggered epilepsy, 1591–1592
Migraine-triggered seizures, 1591–1592
Migrainous infarction, 265, 942
Migrainous syndrome with CSF pleocytosis,
        1690
"Migralepsy", 1591–1592
Migrant sensory neuritis of Wartenberg, 1811
Migrating motor complex, during sleep,
        1630t, 1631
Migration, in multiple sclerosis, 643.e1
Mild cognitive impairment, 490
    and Alzheimer disease, 490
    chemical imaging of, 508–509
    in chronic renal disease, 1218
    and dementia, 488–493
    dementia and, 1381–1382, 1381t, 1382f
    functional neuroimaging for, 490
    neuropsychological characteristics of,
        518–521
    prognostic value of, 519–521
    psychiatric manifestations of, 106
    subtypes of, 518–519
Military models, of traumatic brain injury,
        851
Milkmaid's grip, 239
Millard-Gubler syndrome, 1722t, 1728, 1730
Miller-Dieker syndrome, 1286, 1300.e1,
        1300.e1f
    clinical features of, 1294t
    copy number variation in, 668t
Miller Fisher syndrome (MFS), 1819
Millikan-Siekert syndrome, due to
        autonomic disorders, 1890
MILS (maternally inherited Leigh syndrome),
        1360
Mineralocorticoid secretion, neurological
        complications in children of excess, 847
Mini-Mental State Examination (MMSE), 64,
        515–518, 519f
    advantages and disadvantages of, 64
    Modified, 518
    normative data for, 520t
        drawbacks of, 517–518
        normative data for, 517
Miniature end plate potential, 386
Minigemistocytes, in oligodendroglioma,
        1031–1032
Minimal Assessment of Cognitive Function
        in Multiple Sclerosis (MACFIMS), 1167
Minimally conscious state, 34–35, 54–55
    consciousness in, 59
    decision-making and bioethics for, 56
    interventions for, 55b
Minimally invasive techniques, for complex
        regional pain syndrome, 739
Minipolymyoclonus, in spinal muscular
        atrophy, 1500
Minor cognitive motor disorder (MCMD),
        101
Minor neurocognitive disorder (MND),
        HIV-associated, 1110–1111
    clinical features of, 1111
    neuropsychological tests for, 1111
MIP (maximum intensity projection), 459
    algorithm for, 466

MIRACL (Myocardial Ischemia Reduction with Aggressive Cholesterol Lowering) trial, 922
miRNAs. *see* Micro-RNAs (miRNAs)
Mirror movements, 1740
Mirror neuron system, 95
Mirror therapy, in rehabilitation, 802
Miscellaneous movement disorders, 1459–1460
   hemifacial spasm, 1459
   painful legs-moving toes syndrome, 1459
   psychogenic, 1460
   stiff person syndrome, 1459–1460
Misidentification phenomena, in Alzheimer disease, 79
MISME (multiple inherited schwannomas, meningiomas, and ependymomas) syndrome, 1546
Misonidazole, neuropathy due to, 1862
Missense mutation, 651*t*, 654, 654*f*
Missing heritability, 665
MIT-MANUS, 802
Mitgehen, 121
Mitmachen, 121
Mitochondria, 661–662
   bacterial hypothesis of origin of, 1349
   in cellular homeostasis, 1353–1354
Mitochondria dynamics, mitiphagy and abnormalities of, 1344–1345
Mitochondrial cytopathies and polyneuropathy, 1818.*e*9–1818.*e*10
Mitochondrial disorders, 1349–1364
   approach to diagnosis of, 1354–1358
   and ataxia, 1360, 1470–1471
   clinical features in, 1355*b*
   clinical syndromes in, 1358–1360
   diagnosis
      DNA-based, 1357–1358
      laboratory findings in, 1355
      neuro-ophthalmology, 1355
   due to inborn errors of metabolism, 1336
   dysfunction, 1363
      Alzheimer disease, 1363
      Huntington disease, 1363–1364
      Parkinson disease, 1363
   dysphagia in, 151
   enzyme and metabolite replacement, 1362
   gene therapy, 1362–1363
   genetics of, 1350–1353
      heteroplasmy and mitotic segregation of mtDNA in, 1350–1353
      human mtDNA map, 1350, 1351*f*
      major gene mutations in, 1352*t*–1353*t*
      maternal inheritance of mtDNA in, 1350
      threshold effects of mtDNA mutations in, 1353
   historical background, 1349–1350
   Kearns-Sayre syndrome as, 1358
   Leber hereditary optic neuropathy as, 1360
   management of, 1360–1363
      genetic counseling, prenatal diagnosis, and reproductive options as, 1361
      treatment of associated complications, 1360–1361
         diabetes, 1361
         gastrointestinal, 1361
         hearing and vision, 1360
         heart, 1361
         movement disorders, 1360–1361
         respiratory, 1361
         seizures, 1360

Mitochondrial disorders *(Continued)*
   mitochondrial DNA depletion syndrome and, 1360
   mitochondrial encephalomyopathy, lactic acidosis, and stroke-like episodes (MELAS) as, 1358
   mitochondrial myopathies without progressive external ophthalmoplegia, 1358
   mitochondrial neurogastrointestinal encephalomyopathy (MNGIE) as, 1358–1360
   mitochondrial peripheral neuropathy as, 1358
   muscle biopsy in, 1356–1358
      biochemistry of, 1357
      blue native polyacrylamide gel electrophoresis of, 1357
      electron microscopy of, 1357
      histochemistry of, 1356–1357
      prenatal, 1361
   myoclonic epilepsy with ragged-red fiber myopathy as, 1358
   neurodegenerative diseases, 1364
   neuropathy, ataxia, retinitis pigmentosa syndrome as, 1360
   neuroradiology, 1355–1356, 1356*f*
   nuclear DNA-related, 1350
   Parkinson disease, 1363
   pathophysiology of, 1353–1354
   patterns of inheritance in, 661–662, 661*f*
   pharmacological approaches in, 1361–1362
   progressive external ophthalmoplegia as, 1358
   removal or neutralization of toxic metabolites, 1362
   sensorineural deafness as, 1360
   and stroke in children, 1001, 1002*f*
   subacute necrotizing encephalomyelopathy (Leigh Syndrome) as, 1360
Mitochondrial DNA
   coenzyme Q10 (CoQ10), 1350
   gene therapy approaches for, 1362–1363
   heteroplasmy and mitotic segregation of, 1350–1353
   map of, 1351*f*
   maternal inheritance of, 1350
   nuclear DNA-related, 1350
   resistance exercise training to shift, 1362
   respiratory chain, 1350
   threshold effect of, 1353
Mitochondrial DNA depletion syndrome, 1946
Mitochondrial dysfunction
   in amyotrophic lateral sclerosis, 1508
   leading to oxidative stress, 1344
Mitochondrial Encephalomyopathy, Lactic Acidosis, and Stroke-like Episodes (MELAS), 1356*f*, 1358, 1945, 1818.*e*10
   myopathy in, 1945
   seizures and, 1360
   sensorineural hearing loss in, 1360
   threshold effect and mitotic segregation in, 1353
Mitochondrial metabolic test battery, 1355
Mitochondrial myopathies, 1354*f*, 1358, 1943–1946, 1944*f*
   Kearns-Sayre syndrome as, 1945
   mitochondrial DNA depletion syndrome as, 1946
   mitochondrial encephalopathy, lactic acidosis, and stroke-like episodes as, 1945

Mitochondrial myopathies *(Continued)*
   myoclonic epilepsy with ragged-red fibers as, 1945
   noninvasive techniques to monitor muscle metabolism in, 1944
   with progressive external ophthalmoplegia, 1945–1946
   with recurrent myoglobinuria, 1945
   treatment of, 1944
   without progressive external ophthalmoplegia, 1358
Mitochondrial neurogastrointestinal encephalopathy (MNGIE), 1358–1360, 1818.*e*10
   imaging, 1356*f*
Mitochondrial peripheral neuropathy, 1358
Mitochondrial recessive ataxia syndrome, 1467
Mitochondrial respiratory chain, 1350, 1351*f*
Mitochondrial trifunctional protein (MTP) deficiency, 1337
Mitofusin 2 (MFN2) gene, in Charcot-Marie-Tooth disease type 1, 1815–1816
MitoMap database, 1357
Mitosis, 651*t*
Mitotic index, 1030
Mitotic proliferation, of neuroblasts, 1282–1283
   disorders of, 1283, 1283*f*
Mitotic segregation, of mtDNA, 1350–1353
Mitoxantrone (Novantrone)
   for multiple sclerosis, 1181
   during pregnancy, 1982
Mitral annular calcification (MAC), cardiogenic embolism due to, 934
Mitral stenosis, cardiogenic embolism due to, 934
Mitral valve, aorta, skeletal, and skin involvement (MASS syndrome), 1739
Mitral valve prolapse, cardiogenic embolism with, 815
Mixed dysarthria, 146
Mixed ependymoma/subependymoma, 1037
Mixed germ cell tumors, management of, 1063
Mixed malignant germ cell tumors (MMGCT), pediatric, 1079
   background of, 1079–1080
   clinical presentation of, 1080
   diagnosis and management of, 1080–1081, 1080*f*
   prognosis for, 1081
Mixed nerve action potential (MNAP), 366
Mixed nerve conduction studies, 369
Mixed neuronal-glial tumors
   management of, 1059
   pediatric, 1076–1077
Mixed spinal nerve, 1766–1767, 1767*f*
Mixed transcortical aphasia, 136
Mixed vascular malformation, 447.*e*1
Miyoshi myopathy, 1933
MLF (medial longitudinal fasciculus), in eye movements
   horizontal, 554, 555*f*
   rostral interstitial nucleus of, 560
   vertical, 558–559, 559*f*
MLN (manifest latent nystagmus), 543
MM (mononeuritis multiplex), HIV-associated, 1120
MMF. *see* Mycophenolate mofetil (MMF)
MMNCB (multifocal motor neuropathy with conduction block), 1498
MMPs. *see* Matrix metalloproteinases (MMPs)

MMSE. *see* Mini-Mental State Examination (MMSE)

MNAP (mixed nerve action potential), 366

MND (minor neurocognitive disorder), HIV-associated, 1110–1111
clinical features of, 1111
neuropsychological tests for, 1111

MNK gene, in kinky hair syndrome, 1560

Mobile health devices, in rehabilitation, 804

Mobilization, in primary neurorrhaphy, 915

Mobilization store, in repetitive nerve stimulation, 386

Möbius syndrome, 1292

Modafinil (Provigil), for fatigue, in multiple sclerosis, 1182

Mode of onset, 2

Model for End-stage Liver Disease (MELD), for hepatic encephalopathy, 1216

Moderate head injury, defined, 1581

Modified Checklist for Autism in Toddlers-Revised (M-CHAT-R), 1304

Modified Effendi system, 888

Modified Mini-Mental State Examination (3MS), 518

Modified Telephone Interview for Cognitive Status (mTICS), 517, 518*f*

Modifier genes, 664

Modulation, 722

Modules, 57

MOH (medication overuse headache), 1706–1708

Molar tooth sign, 563–564, 570

Molecular biology, defined, 1279

Molecular cascade, in brain edema, 1267, 1267*f*

Molecular chaperones, in protein folding, 1426

Molecular development, defined, 1279

Molecular diagnostic testing, for inherited ataxias, 1480–1482

Molecular diagnostics, 1030

Molecular genetics, pathology and, 1026–1044

Molecular imaging techniques, 486

Molecular mimicry
in autoimmune disease, 687
in multiple sclerosis, 1162

Mollaret meningitis
headache due to, 1690
recurrent, 1763–1764

Molybdenum cofactor deficiency, 1326.*e*1*t*–1326.*e*2*t*

Monitoring, in neurointensive care
brain. *see* Brain monitoring
systemic, 743–744

Monkeypox, 1135.*e*1

Monoamine oxidase inhibitor (MAOI), 111–112
for migraine, 1703

Monoamines, in chemical imaging, 505–506, 505*f*, 505*t*

Monoballism, 240

Monoclonal antibody, for multiple sclerosis, 1178

Monoclonal gammopathy of undetermined significance (MGUS), 1834–1836, 1834*t*
clinical features of, 1835–1836, 1835*f*
neurological complications of, 825
treatment of, 1836, 1836*f*

Monocular bobbing, 44

Monocular elevator deficiency, 540, 568
acquired, 568

Monocular elevator palsy, 540, 568
acquired, 568

Monocular nystagmus, 545, 545*b*

Monocular temporal crescent, 573

Monocular temporal crescent syndrome, 578

Monocytes, in immune system, 677

Monomelic amyotrophy
arm weakness in, 290
monoplegia due to, 272

Monomelic presentation, of amyotrophic lateral sclerosis, 1508

Monomethylhydrazines, in mushrooms, 1251*t*

Mononeuritis multiplex (MM), HIV-associated, 1120

Mononeuropathies, 1800–1812, 1864.*e*2
axon-loss
needle electromyography of, 383
nerve conduction studies of, 374, 374*f*
axonotmesis as, 1801
classification of, 1800–1801
defined, 1795, 1800–1801
diagnostic clues in, 1795
fifth-degree, 1801
first-degree, 1800
fourth-degree, 1801
localized perineurial hypertrophic, 1811–1812, 1811*f*
of lower extremities, 1802*t*, 1808–1812
of femoral nerve, 1802*t*, 1809–1810
of fibular (peroneal) nerve, 1802*t*, 1808–1809
of ilioinguinal nerve, 1802*t*, 1810
of lateral femoral cutaneous nerve, 1802*t*, 1810
of obturator nerve, 1802*t*, 1811
of saphenous nerve, 1810
of sciatic nerve, 1802*t*, 1808
of sural nerve, 1809
of tibial nerve, 1802*t*, 1809
migrant sensory neuritis of Wartenberg, 1811
monoplegia due to, 269–270, 269*t*
multiple (multiplex), 1795
causes of, 1796*b*
diagnostic clues in, 1795–1796
needle electromyography of, 382–383, 382*f*
neurapraxia as, 1800
neurotmesis as, 1801
second-degree as, 1801
sensory abnormalities due to, 321
third-degree, 1801
of upper extremities, 1801–1808, 1801*t*
of dorsal scapular nerve, 1801*t*
in double crush syndrome, 1807–1808
of intercostobrachial nerve, 1807
of lower trunk of brachial plexus or C8/T1 roots, 1801*t*
of median nerve, 1801*t*, 1802–1804
of musculocutaneous nerve, 1807
of radial nerve, 1801*t*, 1806–1807
of suprascapular nerve, 1801*t*, 1807
of ulnar nerve, 1801*t*, 1804–1806

Mononeuropathy multiplex
causes of, 1796*b*
defined, 1795
diagnostic clues in, 1795–1796
hemiplegia due to, 267

Mononucleosis, in viral CNS disease, 1124*t*

Monoplegia, 262–272
anatomy and physiology of, 262–263
due to brainstem lesions, 268
due to cerebral lesions, 268
from infarction, 268
from infections, 268
from migraine, 268
from multiple sclerosis, 268

Monoplegia (*Continued*)
from seizure, 268
from transient ischemic attack, 268
from tumors, 268
due to peripheral lesions, 268–272
from mononeuropathies, 269–270, 269*t*
femoral neuropathy, 270
median nerve, 269–270
peroneal (fibular) neuropathy, 270
radial nerve palsy, 270
sciatic neuropathy, 270
ulnar nerve, 270
neuronopathies as, 272
monomelic amyotrophy as, 272
multifocal motor neuropathy as, 272
poliomyelitis as, 272
from plexopathies, 271–272
brachial and lumbar, 271
diabetic amyotrophy as, 272
due to neoplastic plexus infiltration, 271
due to trauma, 271
from hematomas, 271
radiation, 271
thoracic outlet syndrome as, 271–272
from pressure palsies, 268–269
hereditary neuropathy with predisposition of, 269
in polyneuropathy, 269
from radiculopathies, 270–271, 270*t*
due to spinal lesions, 268
pitfalls in differential diagnosis of, 272.*e*1–272.*e*2
with focal weakness of apparently central origin, 272.*e*1
with leg weakness, 272.*e*2
with weakness of hand and wrist, 272.*e*2

Monopolar needle electrodes, 376

Monoradiculopathy, 1757–1758
clinical presentation of, 1757
diagnostic studies of, 1757–1758, 1757*f*, 1757.*e*1*f*
treatment of, 1758

Monosomy, 656

Monosomy X, 656

Monro-Kellie doctrine, 745, 1262

Montages, in EEG, 350

Montreal Cognitive Assessment (MoCA), 515–517, 516*f*, 517*t*
normative data for, 517

Mood disorders, *versus* delirium, 32

Morbidity, excessive daytime sleepiness and, 1632

Morbidity rates
for cerebrovascular disease, 636–637
defined, 635–636
for epilepsy, 640, 640*f*–641*f*
for movement disorders, 644
for multiple sclerosis, 641–642, 642*f*–643*f*
for primary neoplasms, 638, 639*f*

Morning glory, neurotoxins from, 1250

Morning glory disc, 176

Morning types, 1622

Moro reflex, in hypotonic infant, 306–307

Morphine
for chronic pain, 727, 727*t*
half-life of, 1203*t*

Morphine SR (MS Contin), for chronic pain, 727*t*

Morphology, 128

Mortality, excessive daytime sleepiness and, 1632

Mortality rates
  for cerebrovascular disease, 636, 636f
  defined, 635–636
  for epilepsy, 638–640, 640f
  for HIV infection, 644
  for movement disorders, 644
  for multiple sclerosis, 641
  for primary neoplasms, 637–638
Mortality ratio, standardized, 635–636
Morvan syndrome, 1199, 1536
Mosaic, 658–659
Mosaic pattern, with denervation, 1916,
  1917f
Motor aprosodia, 139–140
Motor block, in Parkinson disease, 1428
Motor conduction velocity, 368
Motor cortex, upper motor neurons in,
  1484–1485
Motor cortex stimulation, 729t
  for pain, 734
  in rehabilitation, 803–804
Motor dysfunctions, in complex regional
  pain syndrome, 738
Motor evoked potential (MEP), 365.e7–
  365.e9, 365.e9f
  for intraoperative monitoring, 407
    effect of anesthesia on, 410
    monitoring interpretation of, 409
    for spinal cord monitoring, 407, 410
    transcranial electrical, 407
  recruitment curve for, 392, 394t
  in transcranial magnetic stimulation,
    391
Motor examination, for dizziness, 586
Motor excitability measurements, in
  transcranial magnetic stimulation,
  392–394, 394t
Motor fluctuations, drug-related, in
  Parkinson disease, 1435
  delayed on, 1435
  dose failure, 1435
  dyskinesias, 1435
  management of, 1437b
  off-period dystonia, 1435
  on/off as, 1435
  protein-related, 1435
  wearing off, 1435
Motor impatience, 244
Motor impersistence, 121
Motor learning approaches, in rehabilitation,
  787
Motor manifestations
  polyneuropathies with predominantly,
    1796, 1796b
  of seizures, 1564
Motor nerve conduction studies, 367–368,
  367f
Motor nerve conduction velocity, 368
Motor neuron disorders, 5
  acute, 1136
  defined, 1484
  lower, 1494–1506
    acute poliomyelitis as, 1496–1497
    benign focal amyotrophy as, 1498–1499
      differential diagnosis of, 1499
      treatment of, 1499
    clinical features of, 1495, 1495b
    due to West Nile Virus, 1498
    Kennedy disease (X-linked recessive
      bulbospinal neuronopathy) as,
      1503–1505, 1503b, 1504f
      clinical features of, 1504
      differential diagnosis of, 1504–1505
      laboratory studies of, 1504

Motor neuron disorders (Continued)
      manifesting carrier of, 1505
      pathogenesis of, 1503–1504
      treatment of, 1505
    laboratory evidence of, 1495–1496
    multifocal motor neuropathy as, 1498
    neuroanatomy of lower motor neurons
      and, 1494–1495
    postirradiation lower motor neuron
      syndrome, 1506
    postpolio syndrome/progressive
      postpoliomyelitis muscular atrophy
      as, 1497–1498, 1497b
    progressive muscular atrophy as,
      1505–1506
      clinical features of, 1505
      differential diagnosis of, 1505–1506
      etiology of, 1505
      laboratory studies of, 1505
      treatment of, 1506
    spinal muscular atrophy as, 1499–1503
      clinical features of, 1500–1502
      differential diagnosis of, 1502–1503
      genetic counseling and prenatal
        diagnosis of, 1503
      laboratory studies of, 1502
      treatment of, 1503
      type 0 (prenatal), 1500t
      type 1 (infantile, Werdnig-Hoffmann
        disease), 1500, 1500t, 1501f
      type 2 (intermediate, chronic),
        1500–1501, 1500t
      type 3 (juvenile, Kugelberg-Welander
        disease), 1500t, 1501
      type 4 (adult-onset,
        pseudomyopathic), 1500t,
        1501–1502, 1502f
    subacute motor neuronopathy, in
      lymphoproliferative disorders,
      1506
  upper, 1484–1494
    adrenomyeloneuropathy, 1487t,
      1493–1494
    due to plant excitotoxins, 1494
      Konzo as, 1487t, 1494
      lathyrism as, 1487t, 1494
    hereditary spastic paraplegia as,
      1487–1488, 1487t, 1489t–1493t
      diagnosis of, 1488
      treatment of, 1488
    HTLV-1-associated myelopathy (tropical
      spastic paraparesis) as, 1487t,
      1488–1493
    HTLV-2-associated myelopathy (tropical
      spastic paraparesis) as, 1487t,
      1493
    key characteristics of, 1487t
    laboratory evidence of, 1486
      MRS imaging in, 1486
      neuroimaging in, 1486
      transcranial magnetic stimulation in,
        1486
    and lower, 1484–1518
    neuroanatomy of upper motor neurons,
      1484–1485, 1485b
      brainstem control in, 1485
      corticospinal and corticobulbar tracts
        in, 1484–1485
      limbic motor control in, 1485
      motor cortex, 1484–1485
    primary lateral sclerosis, 1486–1487
      diagnosis of, 1487
      key characteristics, 1487t
      treatment of, 1487

Motor neuron disorders (Continued)
  signs and symptoms of, 1485–1486,
    1485b
    loss of dexterity as, 1485
    loss of muscle strength (weakness),
      1485
    pathological hyper-reflexia and
      pathological reflexes as, 1486
    pseudobulbar (spastic bulbar) palsy
      as, 1486
    spasticity as, 1485–1486
Motor neuronopathy, subacute, in
  lymphoproliferative disorders, 1506
Motor neuropathy, multifocal, 1498
  with conduction block, 1498
Motor pathways, impairment of, in multiple
  sclerosis, 1166
Motor perseveration, 121
Motor signs
  for arm and neck pain, 326–327, 326t
  of Parkinson disease with dementia,
    523
Motor speech disorders, 145–147
  acquired stuttering as, 147
  aphasia *versus*, 130
  aphemia as, 147
  apraxia of speech as, 146–147
  dysarthrias as, 145–146
  foreign accent syndrome as, 147
  opercular syndrome as, 147
  oral or buccolingual apraxia as, 147
Motor system, examination of, for coma,
  45–46
Motor threshold (MT), in transcranial
  magnetic stimulation, 392, 394t
Motor tics, 240
Motor unit, 279, 306, 309–310, 376
Motor unit action potentials, voluntary,
  380–381
  amplitude of, 380
  duration of, 380, 380f
  firing patterns of, 381
  morphology of, 380–381, 380f
  phases of, 380–381
  stability of, 381, 381f
Motor unit discharge, 381
Motor unit diseases, neuromuscular
  transmission disorder in, 1914
Motor unit number estimation (MUNE),
  for lower motor neuron impairment,
  1495
Motor unit potential (MUP), with disk
  herniation, 1771–1772
Motor unit size, 376
Motorcycle potentials, in myotonic
  dystrophy, 1935–1936
Motoric difficulties, in developmental
  coordination disorders, 1315, 1316b
Movement
  gait disorders due to illusions of, 260
  slowness of, 716
Movement Assessment Battery for Children
  (MABC-2), 1316
Movement Disorder Society Unified
  Parkinson's Disease Rating Scale
  (MDS-UPDRS), 227, 1428
Movement disorders
  and basal ganglia, 1422–1426
    anatomy, 1423
    biochemistry of, 1425–1426, 1426t
    functional organization of, 1423–1425,
      1423f
  description of, 223
  diagnosis and assessment of, 223–249

Movement disorders *(Continued)*
  functional, 1996–1999
    dystonia as, 1999, 1999*f*
    of gait, 1999
    myoclonus as, 1999
    parkinsonism as, 1998–1999
    tremor as, 1997–1998
  genetic and degenerative disorders
      primarily causing, 445
  investigation of, 245–249, 246*b*,
      247*t*–248*t*
  mechanisms of neurodegeneration,
      1426–1427, 1426*t*, 1427*b*, 1427*f*
  miscellaneous, 244–245, 1459–1460
  in mitochondrial disorders, 1360–1361
  neuroepidemiology of, 644
    morbidity rates in, 644
    mortality rates in, 644
  paroxysmal, 1455–1456
  peripherally induced, posttraumatic
      dystonia, 1455
  in pregnancy, 1980–1981
  structural imaging for, 458.*e5*
  tardive dyskinesia, 1450
  transcranial magnetic stimulation for,
      394–396, 395*t*
Moyamoya disease
  disorders associated with, 1001*t*
  ischemic stroke due to, 937–938, 938*f*
  oral contraceptives and, 1974
  and stroke in children, 1000
[¹¹C]MP4A, in chemical imaging, 506
MPNST (malignant peripheral nerve sheath
      tumor), 1041
  management of, 1061
[¹⁸F]MPPF, in chemical imaging of epilepsy,
      509
MPTP (1-methyl-4-phenyl-1,2,3,6-
      tetrahydropyridine), parkinsonism due to,
      1422–1423
MPZ. *see* Myelin protein zero (MPZ)
MR CLEAN trial, for ischemic stroke,
      761–762, 762*f*
MR RESCUE (Mechanical Retrieval and
      Recanalization of Stroke Clots Using
      Embolectomy) study, 958.*e1*
M-region, in neurological control of bladder,
      605
MRF (midbrain reticular formation), in eye
      movements
  horizontal, 555
  vertical, 558–559, 559*f*
MRI. *see* Magnetic resonance imaging (MRI)
mRNA. *see* Messenger RNA (mRNA)
MRS. *see* Magnetic resonance spectroscopy
      (MRS)
MS. *see* Multiple sclerosis (MS)
3MS (Modified Mini-Mental State
      Examination), 518
MSLT (Multiple Sleep Latency Test),
      1635–1637
MT (motor threshold), in transcranial
      magnetic stimulation, 392, 394*t*
MTA (Multimodal Treatment Study of
      ADHD), 1320–1321, 1321*f*
mTICS (Modified Telephone Interview for
      Cognitive Status), 517, 518*f*
MTP (mitochondrial trifunctional protein)
      deficiency, 1337, 1326.*e1t*–1326.*e2t*
Mucocele, optic neuropathy due to, 169
Mucolipidosis II, 1333.*e2t*–1333.*e3t*
Mucopolysaccharidoses, 1333.*e4t*,
      1328.*e1t*
Mucous membrane findings, suggestive of
      viral central nervous system diseases,
      1123*t*

Mulberry lesions, in tuberous sclerosis,
      1541–1542, 1543*f*
Mulberry-shaped eosinophilic granular
      bodies, in pilocytic astrocytoma, 1034,
      1034*f*
Müller muscle, 184
Multicystic encephalomalacia, 1292
Multidetector CTA (MDCTA), of cerebral
      venous thrombosis, 463
Multifocal motor neuropathy (MMN), 1498,
      1832–1834
  clinical features of, 1832
  laboratory studies of, 1832–1833, 1832*f*,
      1833*t*
  monoplegia due to, 272
  treatment of, 1833–1834
Multifocal motor neuropathy with
      conduction block (MMNCB), 1498
  muscle weakness in, 293
Multi-infarct dementia (MID), 1414
Multimodal Treatment Study of ADHD
      (MTA), 1320–1321, 1321*f*
Multimodality monitoring, in neurointensive
      care, 744, 748, 749*f*
Multinucleated giant cells, in HIV
      encephalitis, 1106*f*
Multiple acyl-coenzyme A dehydrogenation
      deficiency (MADD), myopathy due to,
      1943
Multiple mononeuropathies, 1843, 1848,
      1864.*e2*
  causes of, 1796*b*
  defined, 1795
  diagnostic clues in, 1795–1796
Multiple myeloma, 1837
  peripheral neuropathy in, 1192
  spinal, 449
Multiple sclerosis (MS), 689*t*, 1159–1186,
      1347
  animal models for, 689
  behavior and personality disturbances in,
      83–84
    anxiety as, 84, 84*b*
    depression as, 83–84
    euphoria as, 84
    pseudobulbar affect as, 84, 85*t*
  benign, 1172
  and bowel dysfunction, 610.*e1*
  clinical course of, 1171–1174, 1173*f*
    clinically isolated syndrome as,
        1172
    exogenous factors on, 1173
    measures of disability in, 1173
    predictive value of MRI in conversion to
        clinically definite multiple sclerosis
        in, 1172–1173
    pregnancy in, 1173–1174
    radiographically isolated syndrome as,
        1173
  clinical symptoms and physical findings
      in, 1165–1167, 1167*t*
    affective disorders as, 1167
    cognitive impairment as, 1166–1167
    cranial nerve dysfunction as, 1165
      impairment of ocular motor pathways
          due to, 1165
      impairment of visual pathways due
          to, 1165
      other impairments due to, 1165
    fatigue as, 1166
    impairment of bladder, bowel and
        sexual functions as, 1166
    impairment of cerebellar pathways as,
        1166
    impairment of motor pathways as,
        1166

Multiple sclerosis (MS) *(Continued)*
    impairment of sensory pathways as,
        1165–1166
    vertigo as, 1165
  clinically isolated syndrome of, 1166
  cognitive impairment in, 105, 525
  cytokines in, 688–689
  diagnostic criteria for, 1167
  diagnostic studies for, 1167–1171
    cerebrospinal fluid analysis in, 1170,
        1172*t*
    evoked potentials in, 1171, 1172*t*
    magnetic resonance imaging in,
        1168–1170, 1169*f*
    optic coherence tomography in, 1170
  differential diagnosis in, 1176, 1176*b*
  dysphagia as, 153–154
  environmental contributions to, 671
  environmental risk factor for, 688
  epidemiology of, 1163–1165
    age of onset in, 1163–1164, 1164*f*
    geographical distribution in, 1164–1165,
        1164*f*
    mortality in, 1165
    racial distribution in, 1164–1165
    sex distribution in, 1164
  epitope spreading in, 689
  Epstein-Barr virus and, 687
  erectile dysfunction in, 610–611
  etiology of, 1162–1163
    autoimmunity in, 1162–1163
    genetics in, 1163
    infection in, 1163
    smoking in, 1163
    vitamin D in, 1163
  functional outcomes with, 812–813
  genetic factors in, 688
  genetic studies in, 642–643
  genome-wide association studies of,
      663.*e1t*–663.*e2t*
  hemiplegia due to, 264
  heritability of, 663*t*
  human leukocyte antigen in, 687,
      1163
  immune mediation of, 686
  immunopathogenesis of, 688–689
  impact of, on sexual function, 630–631
    primary, 630–631
    secondary, 631
    tertiary, 631
  malignant, 1172
  monoplegia due to, 268
  myelin antigens in, 688
  neuroepidemiology of, 641–644
    epidemics in, 644.*e1*, 644.*e1f*–644.*e2f*
    genetic studies in, 642–643
    migration in, 643.*e1*
    morbidity rates in, 641–642,
        642*f*–643*f*
    mortality rates and survival in, 641
  neuropsychological characteristics of,
      525
  oligoclonal bands in, 688
  with optic neuritis, 166, 1165
  pain after, 740
  pathologic subtypes of, 1161–1162, 1161*t*
  pathological laughing and crying as,
      104–105
  pathology of, 688, 1160–1162
    B cells and Ig in, 1162
    blood-brain barrier in, 1160–1161
    gray matter in, 1162
    macrophages in, 1161
    microglia in, 1162
    molecular mimicry in, 1162
    oligodendroglia in, 1161

Multiple sclerosis (MS) (Continued)
plaques in
chronic inactive, 1162, 1162f
gross examination of, 1160–1161,
1160f–1161f
histological examination of, 1161
remyelination in, 1161
T cells in, 1162
pathophysiology of, 1159–1160, 1160f
in pregnancy, 1981–1982
primary progressive, 688
clinical course of, 1172
prognosis of, 1174
progressive
pathology of, 1162
treatment of, 1180–1182
progressive relapsing, 688
clinical course of, 1172
psychiatric manifestations of, 104–105
relapsing-remitting, 688
clinical course of, 1171
cognitive impairment in, 1166
sacral neuromodulation for, 618
secondary progressive, 688
clinical course of, 1171
seizures in, 1582–1583
and sexual dysfunction, 610–611
female, 611
male, 610–611
sleep and, 1660, 1660f, 1661b
structural imaging of, 437–440, 439f
Dawson fingers in, 438, 439f
diffusion-weighted imaging, 440
FLAIR of, 440
of spinal cord, 452, 453f
T cells in, 688
therapeutic strategies
immune response, 690
nonspecific, 690
transcranial magnetic stimulation for,
397
treatment and management of,
1176–1183
for acute attacks, 1176–1177
disease modifying, 1177–1180, 1181f
alemtuzumab for, 1178–1179
dimethyl fumarate for, 1179–1180
fingolimod for, 1179
glatiramer acetate for, 1177–1178
infusion therapies for, 1178–1179
injectable agents for, 1177–1178
interferons for, 1177
natalizumab for, 1178
oral therapies for, 1179–1180
teriflunomide for, 1179
strategies and goals in, 1180
symptomatic, 1182
for bladder dysfunction, 1182–1183
for cognitive impairment, 1183
for depression, 1183
for fatigue, 1182
for gait and ambulatory dysfunction,
1182
for paroxysmal symptoms, 1183
for sexual dysfunction, 1183
for spasticity, 1182
for tremor, 1182
types of, 688
urinary incontinence in, 610
variants of, 1174–1176
Balo concentric sclerosis as, 1175, 1175f
Marburg, 1174–1175, 1175f
tumefactive multiple sclerosis, 1174,
1174f

Multiple sclerosis (MS) (Continued)
vertigo due to, 587t, 593, 595
vitamin D in, 688
weighted genetic risk score for, 1163
Multiple Sleep Latency Test (MSLT),
1635–1637, 1675
Multiple subpial transection, for epilepsy,
1607–1608
Multiple system atrophy (MSA), 394–395,
1403–1404, 1437–1439, 1660–1661,
1888–1889
bladder dysfunction and, 609
sphincter EMG for, 615, 615f
clinical manifestations of, salient,
1661b
dysphagia in, 154
erectile dysfunction and, 609
functional neuroimaging of, 493, 494f
nonautonomic, 1873
treatment of, 1438–1439
Mumps, 1143
Munchausen syndrome, 1993
MUNE (motor unit number estimation),
for lower motor neuron impairment,
1495
MUP. see Motor unit potential (MUP)
Murray Valley encephalitis virus, 1139.e1
Muscarine, in mushrooms, 1251t
Muscarinic receptors
in basal ganglia, 1426
in chemical imaging, 505t, 506
Muscimol, in mushrooms, 1251t
Muscle
balance of, in diplopia, 536–537
histology of, 1915–1919
with changes of denervation, 1916
angulated fibers in, 1916, 1916f
checkerboard or mosaic pattern due
to, 1916, 1917f
group atrophy due to, 1916, 1917f
reinnervation after, 1916, 1917f
target fiber in, 1916, 1917f
immunohistochemistry and
immunoblot, 1918–1919
with myopathic changes, 1916–1918,
1918f
normal, 1915, 1916f
with perifascicular atrophy, 1918
with type 1 fiber atrophy, 1918
with type 2 fiber atrophy (cachectic
atrophy), 1918, 1918f
Muscle atonia, during REM sleep, 1625
Muscle atrophy, due to lower motor neuron
impairment, 1495
Muscle biopsy, 1915
with changes of denervation, 1916
angulated fibers in, 1916, 1916f
checkerboard or mosaic pattern due to,
1916, 1917f
group atrophy due to, 1916, 1917f
reinnervation after, 1916, 1917f
target fiber in, 1916, 1917f
for Duchenne muscular dystrophy, 1922,
1922f–1923f
for hypotonic infant, 308
immunohistochemistry and immunoblot
for, 1918–1919
for lower motor neuron impairment,
1495–1496
of mitochondrial disorders, 1356–1358
for muscle weakness, 287
with myopathic changes, 1916–1918,
1918f
normal, 1915, 1916f

Muscle biopsy (Continued)
with perifascicular atrophy, 1918
with type 1 fiber atrophy, 1918
with type 2 fiber atrophy (cachectic
atrophy), 1918, 1918f
Muscle bulk, bedside examination of,
282–283
Muscle contraction syndromes, involuntary
diffuse, 303
muscle cramps as, 302b, 303
originating from muscle, 303
Muscle contractures, muscle pain due to,
303
Muscle cramps, 296–304. see also Muscle
pain
in amyotrophic lateral sclerosis, 1508
due to lower motor neuron impairment,
1495
Muscle disorders
myotonic, in pregnancy, 1977
in pregnancy, 1977–1978
Muscle exercise test, for mitochondrial
disease, 1355
Muscle-eye-brain (MEB) disease, 1920t–
1921t, 1929–1930
hypotonic infant due to, 310
Muscle fibers, 376
degeneration and regeneration of, 1917
with denervation, 1916
angulated fibers in, 1916, 1916f
checkerboard or mosaic pattern due to,
1916, 1917f
group atrophy due to, 1916, 1917f
reinnervation after, 1916, 1917f
target fiber in, 1916, 1917f
necrosis of, 1916–1917
normal, 1915, 1916f
splitting of, 1916–1917
type 1, 1916, 1916f
atrophy of, 1918
type 2, 1916, 1916f
atrophy of, 1918, 1918f
Muscle hypotonia, during REM sleep,
1625
Muscle hypotonicity, due to lower motor
neuron impairment, 1495
Muscle pain, 296–304
basic concepts of, 296–299
clinical features of, 299–300
evaluation of, 299–300
general features of, 299
nociceptive axons in, 297–299
nociceptor terminal stimulation and
sensitization in, 296–297
specific causes of, 300–304
drugs and toxins as, 301b
muscle cramps as, 302b, 303
myalgia syndromes without chronic
myopathy, 302b, 303–304
myopathies with, 300–303, 300b
other involuntary muscle contraction
syndromes, 302b, 303
diffuse, 303
originating from muscle, 303
Muscle relaxants, for chronic pain, 726
Muscle spasm, arm and neck pain due to,
324
Muscle specific tyrosine kinase (MuSK),
immunopathology and, 1899
Muscle strength, 283–284, 284t
abnormalities of, 218
loss of, 1485
due to lower motor neuron impairment,
1495

Muscle tone, 283
  abnormalities of, 218
  in coma, 46
Muscle weakness, 279–295
  acquired disorders causing, 293
  in amyotrophic lateral sclerosis, 1508
  of axial muscles, 280
  bedside examination for, 281–285
    of fasciculations, cramps, and other
      abnormal muscle movements, 285
    of fatigue, 284
    of muscle bulk and deformities,
      282–283
    muscle palpation, percussion, and range
      of motion in, 283
    of muscle strength, 283–284, 284t
    of muscle tone, 283
    observation in, 281–282, 282f
    of peripheral nerve enlargement,
      284–285
    of reflexes, 284
    of sensory disturbances, 284
  clinical investigations for, 286–288
    electromyography in, 286
    exercise testing in, 287–288
    genetic testing in, 287
    muscle biopsy in, 287
    serum creatine kinase in, 286
  constant, 292–293
  of diaphragm, 280
  differential diagnosis of, 288–295, 288f
  due to lower motor neuron impairment,
    1495
  exacerbated by exercise, 292
  of facial and bulbar muscles
    clinical presentation of, 280
    differential diagnosis of, 289–290
  fluctuating, 291–292
  functional evaluation for, 285–286
    arising from floor in, 285
    psychogenic weakness in, 286
    stepping onto stool in, 285–286
    walking in, 285
  general considerations with, 279–280
  of legs, 251
  lifelong, 294–295
    nonprogressive, 294, 294f
    progressive, 294–295
  of lower extremity, clinical presentation of
    distal, 281
    proximal, 281
  myopathic, 255
  of neck muscles, 280
  neurogenic, 255
  of ocular muscles
    clinical presentation of, 280
    differential diagnosis of, 288–289
  other conditions causing, 295
  progressive, 458.e5
  of respiratory muscles, differential
    diagnosis of, 290
  of upper extremity, clinical presentation of
    distal, 281
    proximal, 280
Muscle-contraction headache, 1713
Muscular channelopathies, 1520t–1521t,
  1522–1528
  Andersen-Tawil syndrome as, 1527
    clinical features of, 1527
    diagnosis of, 1527
    genetic basis for, 1520t–1521t
    pathophysiology of, 1527
    treatment of, 1527
  central core disease as, 1520t–1521t
  congenital myasthenic syndromes as,
    1520t–1521t, 1528

Muscular channelopathies (Continued)
  hyperkalemic periodic paralysis as, 1525
    clinical features of, 1524t, 1525
    diagnosis of, 1525
    genetic basis for, 1520t–1521t, 1523f
    pathophysiology of, 1525
    treatment of, 1525
  hypokalemic periodic paralysis as,
    1522–1524
    clinical features of, 1522–1523,
      1524t
    diagnosis of, 1524
    genetic basis for, 1520t–1521t
    pathophysiology of, 1523
    treatment of, 1524, 1524t
  malignant hyperthermia as, 1520t–1521t,
    1527–1528
  myotonia congenita as, 1526
    clinical features of, 1524t, 1526
    diagnosis of, 1526
    genetic basis for, 1520t–1521t
    pathophysiology of, 1526
    treatment of, 1526
  paramyotonia congenita as, 1525–1526
    clinical features of, 1524t, 1525
    diagnosis of, 1525–1526
    genetic basis for, 1520t–1521t
    pathophysiology of, 1525
    treatment of, 1526
  potassium-aggravated myotonia as,
    1526–1527
    clinical features of, 1524t, 1526
    diagnosis of, 1527
    genetic basis for, 1520t–1521t
    pathophysiology of, 1526–1527
    treatment of, 1527
Muscular dystrophies, 1919–1936,
  1920t–1921t
  Becker, 1923–1924
    clinical characteristics of, 1923
    copy number variation in, 668t
    diagnosis of, 1923–1924
    molecular defects of, 1919–1924,
      1920t–1921t
    treatment of, 1924
  congenital, 1920t–1921t, 1927–1930
    classical, 1928, 1928f
    due to laminin-A2 (merosin) deficiency,
      1928
    Fukuyama-type, 1928–1929, 1929f
      biopsy of, 1929, 1929f
      computed tomography scan of, 1929,
        1929f
      molecular defects of, 1920t–1921t
    with rigid spine syndrome, 1920t–1921t,
      1930
    Ullrich, 1920t–1921t, 1930
    Walker-Warburg syndrome and
      muscle-eye-brain disease,
      1929–1930
  defined, 1915
  distal, 1920t–1921t, 1933–1934
    Laing myopathy as, 1934
    Markesbery-Griggs, 1920t–1921t, 1927,
      1933
    Miyoshi myopathy as, 1933
    Nonaka myopathy as, 1933–1934
    Udd myopathy as, 1933
    Welander myopathy as, 1933
    William myopathy as, 1934
  Duchenne, 1921–1923
    copy number variation in, 668t
    creatine kinase in, 1922, 1922f
    genetic counseling for, 1924
    molecular defects of, 1919–1924,
      1920t–1921t

Muscular dystrophies (Continued)
    muscle biopsy for, 1922, 1922f–1923f
    treatment of, 1922–1923
      bracing for, 1923
      pharmacological, 1923
      physical therapy for, 1922–1923
      surgery, 1923
  dysphagia of, 150
  Emery-Dreifuss, 1920t–1921t, 1930
    autosomal dominant, 1924–1925,
      1930
  facioscapulohumeral, 1930–1932, 1931f
    diagnosis of, 1931, 1931f
    molecular defects in, 1920t–1921t
    muscle biopsy of, 1931, 1931f
    treatment of, 1931–1932
  Fukuyama, clinical features of, 1294t
  hereditary inclusion body myopathies as,
    1920t–1921t, 1933–1934
    autosomal recessive, 1933–1934
    with early respiratory failure, 1927
  limb-girdle, 1920t–1921t, 1924–1927
  molecular defects of, 1920t–1921t
  myofibrillar myopathy as, 1920t–1921t,
    1927
  myotonic, 1920t–1921t, 1934–1936
    congenital, 1936, 1936f
    type 1, 1934–1936, 1934f–1935f
      cardiac disease in, 1935
      diagnosis of, 1936
      excessive daytime somnolence in,
        1935
      molecular defects of, 1920t–1921t
      treatment of, 1936
    type 2, 1920t–1921t, 1936
  oculopharyngeal, 150, 1932–1933, 1932f
    molecular defects of, 1920t–1921t
    muscle biopsy of, 1932–1933, 1932f
    myotonic dystrophy, 150
    ptosis due to, 188
    treatment of, 1933
  reducing body myopathy as, 1920t–1921t,
    1927
  scapuloperoneal, 1920t–1921t, 1932
  X-linked, 1920t–1921t
Musculocutaneous nerve, 1807
Musculoskeletal disorders, gait disorders due
  to, 261
MUSE (medicated urethral system for
  erection), 621
MuSK. see Muscle specific tyrosine kinase
  (MuSK)
MuSK-antibody myasthenia gravis (MuSK-
  MG), 1900, 1900f, 1900t
  antibody testing for, 1902
Mutation
  frameshift, 651t, 654f
  missense, 651t, 654, 654f
  nonsense, 651t, 654, 654f
  point, 654–655, 654f
  silent, 651t, 654, 654f
  types of, 653–655
Muteness, 130
Mutism
  akinetic, 59
  cerebellar, 1083.e1
Myasthenia, familial infantile, 1911
Myasthenia gravis (MG), 1193–1194,
  1896–1910
  anesthetic management with, 1909
  autoantibodies in, 1901–1902
    AChR-abs, 1901–1902
    anti-MuSK, 1902
    anti-striational, 1902
  autoimmune, 692
  channelopathy in, 1535

Neural integrator (NI), in eye movements
horizontal, 554, 555*f*–556*f*
vertical, 560
Neural prostheses, in rehabilitation, 804
Neural stem cells (NSCs), 695
Neuralgia
cranial, 1716–1718
facial, 1716–1718
geniculate, 1717–1718
Hunt, 1717–1718
nevus intermedius, 1717–1718
occipital, 1718
occipital, greater occipital nerve block for, 729, 729*t*
postherpetic, 1129, 1718
trigeminal, Gasserian ganglion lesions for, 730–731, 731*f*
Neuralgic amyotrophy, 328
hereditary, 1818
Neuraminidase inhibitors, for viral infections, 1127*t*
Neurapraxia, 371–373, 905, 1800
Neuraxis tumors, derived from hematopoietic system, 1062–1063
Neurectomy, for neuropathic pain, 917
Neurilemoma, pathology and molecular genetics of, 1041
Neurite growth, disorders of, 1288–1289
Neuritic plaques (NP), in Alzheimer disease, 1397
Neuritis
Jamaican, 1236
migrant sensory, of Wartenberg, 1811
optic, structural imaging for, 449.*e1*–449.*e3*, 449.*e3f*
paraneoplastic, 1194
vestibular, 585, 587*t*, 591, 595
treatment of, 603
Neuroacanthocytosis, 237–238, 1448
Neurobehavioral Rating Scale-Revised (NRS-R), 76, 77*t*
Neurobehavioral symptoms and disorders, classification of, 76
Neuroblast migration, 1284–1287
disorders of, 1286–1287, 1286*f*
early, 1299–1300
late, 1300.*e2*
lissencephaly as, 1286, 1299–1300
in Miller-Dieker syndrome, 1286, 1294*t*, 1300.*e1*, 1300.*e1f*
in Walker-Warburg syndrome, 1294*t*, 1300.*e1*–1300.*e2*
X-linked recessive, with abnormal genitalia, 1300.*e2*
pachygyria as, 1286–1287, 1294*t*
periventricular nodular heterotopia as, 1286, 1300.*e2*
polymicrogyria as, 1286–1287
schizencephaly as, 1300.*e2*
subcortical laminar heterotopia as, 1286, 1300.*e2*
in formation of gyri and sulci, 1284, 1285*f*
major mechanisms of, 1284–1286, 1285*f*
subependymal germinal matrix in, 1284, 1284*f*
synaptogenesis and, 1289
Neuroblastic rosette, 1028
Neuroblastic tumors, peripheral, management of, 1059
Neuroblastoma
central or cerebellar, 1028, 1038
limbic and brainstem encephalitis and, 1191

Neuroblasts, mitotic proliferation of, 1282–1283
disorders of, 1283, 1283*f*
Neurochemical tracers, for chemical imaging, 505*t*
Neurocognitive disorders
classification of, 76
HIV-associated, 1110–1112
cerebrospinal fluid analysis of, 1111
clinical features of, 1111
management of, 1111–1112
neuroimaging of, 1111, 1112*f*
neuropsychological tests for, 1111
Neurocognitive impairment
from radiation therapy, 1087
from WBRT, 1089
Neurocutaneous melanosis, 1554–1555
cutaneous features of, 1554–1555
laboratory findings of, 1555
neuroimaging of, 1555, 1556*f*
neurological features of, 1555
Neurocutaneous syndromes, 1538–1562
ataxia-telangiectasia as, 1552–1553
cutaneous features of, 1552–1553
immunodeficiency and cancer risk of, 1553
laboratory diagnosis of, 1553
neurological features of, 1553
cerebrotendinous xanthomatosis as, 1557–1558
clinical features of, 1557*b*
neurological features of, 1557
treatment of, 1557–1558
xanthomas in, 1557
cortical tubers, structural imaging of, 446.*e2*
Ehlers-Danlos syndrome as, 1555–1557, 1556*f*
neurovascular features of, 1556–1557
epidermal nevus syndrome as, 1553–1554
cutaneous features of, 1554
neuroimaging of, 1554
neurological features of, 1554
other features of, 1554
hamartoma , structural imaging of, 446.*e2*
hereditary hemorrhagic telangiectasia as, 1550–1551
neurological features of, 1550–1551
treatment of, 1551
hypomelanosis of Ito, 1551
cutaneous features of, 1551
neurological features of, 1551
systemic features of, 1551
incontinentia pigmenti as, 1551–1552
cutaneous features of, 1551–1552, 1552*f*
genetics of, 1552
neurological features of, 1552
kinky hair syndrome (Menkes disease), 1558–1560
cutaneous features of, 1559, 1559*f*
diagnosis and treatment of, 1560
genetic studies of, 1560
neuroimaging of, 1559–1560
neurological features of, 1559
other clinical features of, 1559, 1559*b*
neurocutaneous melanosis as, 1554–1555
cutaneous features of, 1554–1555
laboratory findings of, 1555
neuroimaging of, 1555, 1556*f*
neurological features of, 1555
neurofibroma, structural imaging of, 446.*e2*

Neurocutaneous syndromes *(Continued)*
neurofibromatosis, structural imaging of, 446.*e2*
type 1, 446.*e2*, 446.*e3f*
type 2, 446.*e2*, 446.*e3f*
neurofibromatosis as, 1543–1546
type 1
cutaneous features of, 1544, 1545*f*
diagnostic criteria of, 1544*b*
neurological features of, 1544–1546, 1545*f*–1546*f*
type 2
clinical features of, 1546, 1546*f*
diagnostic criteria of, 1544*b*
other cutaneous manifestations of, 1562
progressive facial hemiatrophy as, 1558
clinical features of, 1558, 1558*f*
structural imaging of, 446
Sturge-Weber syndrome, 1546–1548, 1547*f*
cutaneous features of, 1546–1547
diagnostic studies of, 1547–1548, 1548*f*
neurological features of, 1547
ocular features of, 1547
structural imaging of, 446.*e2*–446.*e4*
treatment of, 1548
subependymal nodules, structural imaging of, 446.*e2*
tuberous sclerosis as, 1538–1543
cutaneous features of, 1539
confetti lesions as, 1539
facial angiofibromas (adenoma sebaceum) as, 1539, 1540*f*, 1541*t*
hypomelanotic macules (ash leaf spots) as, 1539, 1540*f*, 1541*t*
poliosis as, 1539
shagreen patch as, 1539, 1541*t*
ungual fibromas, 1539
diagnostic criteria of, 1539*b*
neurological features of, 1540–1541, 1541*f*–1542*f*
retinal features of, 1541–1542
structural imaging of, 446.*e2*, 446.*e4f*
systemic features of, 1542–1543
cardiac, 1542
pulmonary, 1543
renal, 1542–1543
Von Hippel-Lindau disease, structural imaging of, 446.*e2*
von Hippel-Lindau syndrome as, 1548–1550
Cambridge screening protocol for, 1550*b*
molecular genetics of, 1550
neurological features of, 1549, 1549*f*
ocular features of, 1549
systemic features of, 1549
treatment of, 1550
white matter lesions, structural imaging of, 446.*e2*
xeroderma pigmentosum as, 1560–1562
complementation groups of, 1560
cutaneous and ocular features of, 1561, 1561*b*
related syndromes of, 1560
treatment of, 1561–1562
Neurocysticercosis (NCC)
diagnostic criteria for, 1157*t*
neuroepidemiology of, 645.*e1*–645.*e2*, 645.*e1t*
seizures due to, 1582
suggested treatment for, 1158*t*
Neurocytic rosettes, 1036

Neurocytoma
  atypical, 1036
  central
    management of, 1059
    pathology and molecular genetics of,
      1036
    pediatric, 1077.e1–1077.e2, 1077.e2f
    structural imaging of, 418t–419t, 426.e1
  extraventricular, 1036
Neurodegeneration
  with brain iron accumulation, 1455
  falls due to, 20–22
  mechanisms of, 1426–1427, 1427b
  mechanisms of cell loss in, 1344–1348
  protein spread and prion hypothesis of,
    1347
Neurodegenerative disorders
  beginning, 1343–1344
  brain in, 1345f–1346f
  of central nervous system, 1342, 1343t
  processes, 1342–1348
  regression due to, 72
  transcranial magnetic stimulation for,
    395t, 396
  vertigo due to, 587t, 593
Neuroectodermal tumors, primitive,
  pathology and molecular genetics of,
    1038–1039
Neuroendocrine tumors, 712
  carcinoid tumors as, 712
  pheochromocytomas as, 712
Neuroendocrinology, 696–712
  anterior pituitary, 703–707
    hyperfunction of, 704–706
      Cushing disease and Nelson
        syndrome due to, 705–706, 706b,
        711
      due to gonadotropin-secreting
        tumors, 706, 711
      excessive secretion of thyroid-
        stimulating hormone due to,
        706, 711
      gigantism and acromegaly due to,
        705, 705b, 711
      hyperprolactinemia due to, 704–705,
        710–711
      precocious puberty due to, 704
    hypofunction of, 703–704, 704b, 704t
    hypothalamic control of, 702t, 703
    tumors and hyperplasia of, 707, 707t
      medical management of, 710–711
      radiotherapy for, 711
      surgery for, 711
  approach to hypothalamic-pituitary
    dysfunction in, 710–712
    endocrinological investigation in, 710,
      710t
    history and physical examination in, 710
    imaging studies in, 710
  hypophysitis of, 707
  hypothalamus
    endocrine, 702–703
      blood supply to, 703, 703f
      functional anatomy of, 702–703,
        702t, 703f
    nonendocrine, 698–702
      in appetite, 700–701, 701f
      in biological rhythms, 702
      in emotion and libido, 701–702
      in temperature regulation, 698–700,
        699f
  neuroendocrine tumors in, 712
    carcinoid tumors as, 712
    pheochromocytomas as, 712
  neurohormones in, 696
    and immune system, 696–698, 699t

Neuroendocrinology (Continued)
    neuropeptides in, 696, 697t–698t
      and immune system, 696–698, 699t
    neurotransmitters in, 696
  other tumors, 707
  posterior pituitary in, 707–710
    in cerebral salt wasting, 709–710
    in diabetes insipidus, 708
      etiology of, 708
      management of, 708
    physiology of, 707–708
      atrial natriuretic peptide in, 708
      oxytocin in, 708
      in sodium homeostasis, 708
      in thirst and drinking, 708
      vasopressin in, 707–708
    in syndrome of inappropriate
      antidiuretic hormone secretion,
      708–709
      clinical features of, 709
      etiology and pathophysiology of,
        708–709, 709b
      treatment of, 709
Neuroenteric cysts, pathology and molecular
  genetics of, 1043–1044
Neuroepidemiology, 635–647
  of cerebrovascular disease, 636–637
    morbidity rates in, 636–637
    mortality rates in, 636, 636f
    transient ischemic attacks in, 637
  of convulsive disorders, 638–641
    febrile seizures in, 640–641
    morbidity rates in, 640, 640f–641f
    mortality rates in, 638–640, 640f
  of HIV infection, 644–645, 645b
  of movement disorders, 644
    morbidity rates in, 644
    mortality rates in, 644
  of multiple sclerosis, 641–644
    epidemics in, 644.e1, 644.e1f–644.e2f
    genetic studies in, 642–643
    migration in, 643.e1
    morbidity rates in, 641–642, 642f–643f
    mortality rates and survival in, 641
  of neurocysticercosis, 645.e1–645.e2,
    645.e1t
  of neurological disorders, 645–647
    less common
      incidence of, 646t
      prevalence of, 647t
    most common
      incidence of, 645t
      prevalence of, 646t
  population-based rates in, 635–636
  of primary neoplasms, 637–638
    morbidity rates in, 638, 639f
    mortality rates and survival in, 637–638
  of West Nile virus infection, 645.e1
Neuroepithelial cyst, 1043–1044
Neuroepithelial tumors, 1030–1039
  astrocytoma as
    anaplastic, 1031
    diffuse, 1031
  central neurocytoma as, 1036
  choroid plexus tumors as, 1037, 1037f
  circumscribed ("favorable prognosis"),
    1033–1036
    pilocytic astrocytoma as, 1034, 1034f
    pleomorphic xanthoastrocytoma as,
      1034
    subependymal giant cell astrocytoma as,
      1034–1035
  dysembryoplastic, 1035, 1077.e1, 1077.e1f
  embryonal tumors/primitive
    neuroectodermal tumors as, 1038–
    1039, 1038f

Neuroepithelial tumors (Continued)
    ependymoma as, 1036
    ganglioglioma/gangliocytoma, 1035,
      1035f
    glioblastoma as, 1032, 1032f
    glioneuronal tumors as, 1035–1036
    management of, 1055–1060
    oligoastrocytoma as, 1032
    oligodendroglioma as, 1031–1032, 1031f
    pathology and molecular genetics of,
      1029f
    subependymoma as, 1037
    of unknown origin, management of, 1056
Neurofibrillary tangles (NFTs), in Alzheimer
  disease, 693, 1396–1397
Neurofibroma
  management of, 1060–1061
  in neurofibromatosis type 1
    plexiform, 1544
    subcutaneous, 1544, 1545f
  pathology and molecular genetics of, 1041
  structural imaging of, of brain, 418t–419t,
    446.e2
Neurofibromatosis, 1543–1546
  central, 1546
  structural imaging of, 446.e2
    type 1, 446.e2, 446.e3f
    type 2, 446.e2, 446.e3f
Neurofibromatosis type 1
  and brain tumors, 1024, 1025t
  copy number variation in, 668t
  cutaneous features of, 1544, 1545f
  diagnostic criteria for, 1544b
  intracranial aneurysm in, 983–984
  neurological features of, 1544–1546,
    1545f–1546f
  optic pathway glioma in, 1071, 1072f
  and stroke in children, 998
  systemic features of, 1544
Neurofibromatosis type 2
  and brain tumors, 1024, 1025t
  clinical features of, 1546, 1546f
  diagnostic criteria for, 1544b
Neurofilament dysfunction, in amyotrophic
  lateral sclerosis, 1507
Neurofilament light (NEFL) subunit, in
  Charcot-Marie-Tooth disease,
  1815–1816
Neurofilament protein, 1029
Neurogenetic disease
  clinical approach to patient with
    suspected, 672–675
    evaluation and diagnosis in, 672–674,
      672t–673t
    genetic counseling in, 674
    prognosis and treatment in, 674–675
  environmental contributions to, 671
  future role of systems biology in, 669–671,
    670f
Neurogenetics resources, 659t
Neurogenic bladder, 896–897, 896.e1f
Neurogenic bladder dysfunction, 607–612
  causes of, 608t
    due to basal ganglia, 608–609
    due to brainstem lesions, 609–610
    due to conus and cauda equina lesions,
      611
    due to cortical lesions, 607–608
    due to disturbances of peripheral
      innervation, 611–612
      in amyloid neuropathy, 611–612
      in autoimmune autonomic
        ganglionopathy, 612
      in diabetic nephropathy, 611
      in immune-mediated neuropathies,
        612

Neurogenic bladder dysfunction (*Continued*)
  due to impaired sympathetic
    thoracolumbar outflow, 611
  due to multiple sclerosis, 610–611
  due to multiple system atrophy, 609
  due to pure autonomic failure, 609
  due to spinal cord injury, 610
  due to spinal cord lesions, 610
  due to urinary retention in young
    women, 612
  complications of, 616
  diagnostic evaluation of, 612–616
    bladder scan in, 613, 613*f*
    electromyography in, 615–616
      for cauda equina lesions, 615
      for multiple system atrophy, 615, 615*f*
      for penilo-cavernosus reflex, 616
      for urinary retention in young
        women, 615–616
    history in, 612
      bladder diary for, 612, 612*f*
    investigations in, 613–616
    physical examination in, 612–613
    pudendal nerve terminal motor latency
      (PNMTL), 616
    pudendal somatosensory evoked
      potentials, 616
    screening for urinary tract infections in,
      613
    ultrasound scan in, 613
    urodynamic studies, 613–615
      noninvasive, 613, 614*f*
      requiring catheterization, 613–615,
        614*f*
    uroneurophysiology in, 615
  management of, 616–620
    algorithm for, 617*f*
    external devices, 619
    general measures, 616
    nerve root stimulators in, 619
    other options, 619
      beta-3-receptor agonists, 619
      vanilloids, 619
    permanent indwelling catheters in, 619
    referral for specialist urology service,
      620*b*
    sacral neuromodulation in, 618
    stepwise approach to, 619, 620*f*
    storage dysfunction, 617–619
      botulinum toxin in, 618
      percutaneous tibial nerve stimulation
        in, 618
      peripheral nerve stimulation in, 618
      surgery in, 618, 619*t*
    for storage dysfunction
      anti-muscarinic medications in, 617,
        617*t*
      cannabinoids, 619
      desmopressin in, 617–618
Neurogenic bowel dysfunction, causes of
  due to amyloid neuropathy, 612.*e*1
  due to basal ganglia lesions, 608–609
  due to conus and cauda equina lesions,
    611
  due to cortical lesions, 607–608
  due to multiple sclerosis, 610
  due to spinal cord injury, 610.*e*1
Neurogenic dysphagia, 151–156, 152*b*
  in amyotrophic lateral sclerosis, 155
  due to brainstem processes, 155
  due to cervical spinal cord injury,
    155–156
  due to cranial neuropathies, 155
  due to other processes, 156

Neurogenic dysphagia (*Continued*)
  due to stroke, 152–153
  in multiple sclerosis, 153–154
  in other basal ganglia disorders, 154–155
  in Parkinson disease, 154
Neurogenic gait, 255
Neurogenic inflammation, in migraine, 1699
Neurogenic intermittent claudication,
  1758–1759
Neurogenic muscle weakness, ataxia, and
  retinitis pigmentosa (NARP),
  1818.*e*9–1818.*e*10
Neurogenic myocardial stunning,
  1881–1882
Neurogenic pain, central, due to spinal
  lesions, 277–278
Neurogenic sexual dysfunction
  causes of
    due to amyloid neuropathy, 611–612
    due to autoimmune autonomic
      ganglionopathy, 612
    due to basal ganglia lesions, 609
    due to conus and cauda equina lesions,
      611
    due to cortical lesions, 608
    due to diabetic neuropathy, 611
    due to epilepsy, 608
    due to impaired sympathetic
      thoracolumbar outflow, 611
    due to spinal cord injury, 610–611
      female, 611
      male, 610–611
  female
    due to spinal cord injury, 611
    management of, 621
  male
    due to spinal cord injury, 610–611
    management of
      for ejaculation dysfunction, 621
      for erectile dysfunction, 620–621,
        621*t*
  management of, 620–621
    in men
      for ejaculation dysfunction, 621
      for erectile dysfunction, 620–621,
        621*t*
    in women, 621
Neurogenic thoracic outlet syndrome,
  1782–1783, 1783*f*
Neurogenic weakness, 255
Neuroglial cells, and immune response, 686
Neuroglial cyst, 446.*e*9, 446.*e*12*f*
Neurohormones, 696
  and immune system, 696–698, 699*t*
Neuroimaging
  of ADHD, 1320
  of anoxic-ischemic encephalopathy,
    1206–1208, 1207*f*–1208*f*
  of brain metastases, 1085–1086
  of cerebral palsy, 1312
  of dizziness and vertigo, 583
  of epidermal nevus syndrome, 1554
  of global developmental delay, 69
  of hepatic encephalopathy, 1211, 1211*f*
  of HIV-associated dementia, 1111, 1112*f*
  of hypotonic infant, 307
  of hypoxic-ischemic brain injury, in
    newborns, 1960–1961, 1961*f*
  of inborn errors of metabolism,
    1328–1330
  of intellectual disability, 1308
  of kinky hair syndrome, 1559–1560
  of leptomeningeal metastases, 1097–1098
  of neurocutaneous melanosis, 1555, 1556*f*

Neuroimaging (*Continued*)
  of Parkinson disease, 1429
  of spinal cord compression, 1093, 1093*f*
  sports and performance concussion and,
    862
  of threatened stroke, 950–951, 950*f*–951*f*
  of TIA, 950
Neuroimaging biomarkers, 1391–1393
Neuroimaging studies, in sleep disorders,
  1676–1678
Neuroimmunological diseases, 688–693
  acute disseminated encephalomyelitis as,
    690–691
  Alzheimer disease as, 693
  amyotrophic lateral sclerosis as, 693
  autoimmune myasthenia gravis as, 692
  immune-mediated neuropathies as,
    691–692
  inflammatory muscle disease as, 692–693
  multiple sclerosis as, 688–690
Neuroimmunology, 676–695
Neuroinflammation
  chemical imaging for, 505*t*
  vasogenic edema and, 1268
Neurointensive care
  brain monitoring in, 744–745, 744*t*
    cerebral blood flow monitoring for,
      744*t*, 747–748
      laser Doppler flowmetry for, 744*t*,
        748
      thermal diffusion flowmetry for, 744*t*,
        748
      xenon-133, 744*t*, 747
    electroencephalogram for, 744*t*, 747
    global techniques for, 745–747
    intracranial pressure monitoring in,
      744*t*, 745–746, 745*f*
    jugular oximetry for, 744*t*, 746–747
    local cerebral oxygenation monitoring
      for, 748
      brain tissue PO$_2$ for, 744*t*, 748
      near-infrared spectroscopy for, 744*t*,
        748
    microdialysis for, 744*t*, 748–749
    multimodality monitoring for, 744,
      748, 749*f*
    somatosensory evoked potentials for,
      744*t*, 748
    transcranial Doppler for, 744*t*, 748
  clinical assessment in, 742–743, 743*f*
  fluid and electrolytes in, 754–755, 755*t*,
    756*f*
  principles of, 742–757
  principles of management in, 749–757
    airway and ventilatory assistance in,
      750–752
    analgesia and sedation in, 749–750,
      751*t*
    blood pressure management in,
      753–754, 753*t*
      for acute ischemic stroke, 753*t*, 754
      for intracerebral hemorrhage, 753*t*,
        754
      for subarachnoid hemorrhage, 753*t*,
        754
      for traumatic brain injury, 753*t*, 754
    cardiovascular care in, 752–754
      for acute coronary syndrome,
        752–753, 753*f*
      for cardiac arrhythmias, 753
      for congestive heart failure, 753
    for fever and infections, 756–757
    for hematological complications,
      757

Neurointensive care *(Continued)*
  for nutrition and metabolic
    derangements, 755–756
  for pulmonary complications, 752
  regional/focal techniques for, 747–749
  systemic monitoring in, 743–744
Neurointerventional therapy
  for carotid artery disease, 763–765
    angioplasty and stenting, 763–765
      clinical trials for, 763–765, 764*b*
      procedure for, 763, 763*f*–764*f*
  for cerebral aneurysms, 768–774
    alternative treatments for, 773–774,
      773*f*
    endovascular treatment modalities for,
      769–771
      balloon remodeling as, 770,
        770*f*–771*f*
      coil embolization as, 769–770, 770*f*
        stent-assisted, 770–771, 771*f*–772*f*
    ruptured, 768–769
    unruptured, 769
  for cerebral arteriovenous fistulas,
    777–779
    carotid-cavernous, 778–779, 778*f*–779*f*,
      779*b*
    cranial dural, 777–778, 777*b*
  for cerebral arteriovenous malformations,
    775–777
    embolization procedure for, 775–777,
      776*f*
      with ethylene vinyl alcohol
        copolymer, 776–777
      with *n*-butyl cyanoacrylate, 776
      with polyvinyl alcohol, 775–776
    stereotactic radiosurgery for, 777
  for cerebral vasospasm, management of,
    774–775
    balloon angioplasty for, 774, 774*f*
    intra-arterial vasodilators for, 774–775
  for idiopathic intracranial hypertension,
    782–783, 783*f*
  for intracranial arteriosclerotic disease,
    765–767
    angioplasty and stenting as, 765–767,
      766*f*
      clinical trials of, 766–767
      procedure for, 766, 767*f*
    angioplasty as, 765
  for ischemic stroke, 758–767
    acute treatment, 758–763
    angioplasty and stenting, 762–763
    endovascular revascularization therapy,
      758–759, 759*b*
    intra-arterial thrombolysis, 759
    mechanical recanalization, 759–761
      with MERCI device, 759, 760*f*, 762*f*
      with Penumbra System, 760,
        760*f*–761*f*
    MR CLEAN, ESCAPE, EXTEND-IA, and
      SWIFT-PRIME trials, 761–762, 762*f*
    sonothrombolysis, 758
  principles of, 758–783
  for spinal vascular malformations,
    779–780, 780*f*
    arteriovenous fistula as
      glomus, 780
      juvenile/metameric, 780
      perimedullary, 780
      spinal dural, 780
  for tumor embolization, 780–782
    clinical evidence on, 782
    materials for, 781–782
    procedure for, 781–782, 781*f*–782*f*
    vessel selection for, 782
  for vertebral artery disease, 767, 768*f*

Neuroleptic malignant syndrome (NMS),
  700
Neuroleptics, 244
Neuroleukins, 697*t*–698*t*
Neurological deficit, sudden, 458.*e*4
Neurological disease
  diagnosis of, 1–7
  management of, 713–719
Neurological examination, 4–5
  for acute ischemic stroke, 963–964
  for Alzheimer disease, 1384–1385
  for coma, 40–46
    eye deviation in, 44
    motor system in, 45–46
    ocular motility in, 43–45, 47
    pupil reactivity in, 42–43, 43*f*–44*f*, 47
    pupil size in, 42–43, 43*f*–44*f*, 47
    reflex ocular movements in, 44–45,
      45*t*–46*t*, 47
    respiration in, 41–42, 42*f*, 47
    resting position abnormalities in, 44
    spontaneous eye movements in, 44, 47
    state of consciousness in, 40–41, 41*t*,
      47
  for dizziness, 586
  focused, 4
  prior to epilepsy surgery, 1596
  screening, 4, 5*t*
Neurological history
  for global developmental delay, 66–67
  prior to epilepsy surgery, 1595–1596
Neurological illnesses, 1646*f*
Neurological impairment, defined, 714
Neurological interview, 1–2
Neurological management
  evidence-based medicine in, 713–714
  explanation of prognosis in, 717–718
  genetic counseling in, 718
  goals of, 714–715
    arresting an attack as, 714
    circumventing functional disability as,
      715
    relieving symptoms as, 714
    slowing disease progression as, 714
  implications for clinical practice in, 719
  legal issues in, 718–719
  palliation and care of terminally ill patient
    in, 718
  principles of, 713, 714*b*
  for secondary effects, 717
  symptom management in, 715–717
    for aphasia and dysarthria, 716
    for ataxia, 716
    for memory impairment and dementia,
      717
    for pain, 715
    for respiratory failure, 716–717, 716*b*
    for sensory loss, paresthesias, and
      burning pain, 715
    slowness of movement or abnormal
      involuntary movements, 716
    for weakness, 715–716
Neurological practice, 92–114, 92.*e*1*b*
Neurological rehabilitation. *see*
  Rehabilitation
Neurolymphomatosis, 1848
Neurolysis
  for nerve root avulsion, 1768–1769
  for peripheral nerve trauma, 914
Neurometabolic cascade, 860–861
Neuromodulation
  applications of
    for dystonia, 404
    for epilepsy, 406
      closed-loop stimulation in, 406
      vagal-nerve stimulation (VNS), 406

Neuromodulation *(Continued)*
    for neuropsychiatric disorders,
      404–406
      depression as, 405
      drug addiction as, 405–406
      obsessive-compulsive disorder as,
        405
      Tourette syndrome as, 404–405
    for pain, 406
    for Parkinson disease, 401–404
      long-term efficacy of, 404
    for tremor, 404
  for neuropathic pain, 917
  techniques of, deep brain stimulation as,
    401–406
    clinical benefits of, 401
    clinical evidence for, randomized
      controlled trials, 402–404, 403*t*
    conclusions and the future of, 406
    lead placement for, 401
    mechanism of action of, 401
    patient selection for, 401
    technology of, 401, 402*f*
Neuromodulators, in rehabilitation, 804
Neuromuscular disorders
  falls due to, 19
  HIV-associated, 1118–1120
  sleep disorders associated with, 1658
Neuromuscular dysphagia, 149–151, 150*b*
  in inflammatory myopathies, 150–151
  in mitochondrial disorders, 151
  in muscular dystrophy
    myotonic, 150
    oculopharyngeal, 150
    other, 150
  in myasthenia gravis, 151
Neuromuscular junction (NMJ), 1896. *see
  also* Neuromuscular transmission (NMT)
  disorders
Neuromuscular junctional disorders, 1658
Neuromuscular respiratory weakness, in
  critically ill patients, 742–743
Neuromuscular transmission (NMT)
  disorders, 1896–1914
  botulism as, 1913–1914
    clinical features of, 1913–1914
    electromyographic findings in, 1914
    forms of, 1913
    infantile, 1914
    treatment of, 1914
  congenital myasthenic syndromes as,
    1910–1912
    due to AChR deficiency, 1911
    due to choline acetyl transferase (ChAT)
      deficiency, 1911
    due to congenital acetylcholinesterase
      (AChE) deficiency, 1911
    due to DOK-7 mutations, 1911–1912
    due to GFPT1 and DPAGT1 mutations,
      1912
    due to rapsyn mutations, 1911
    with episodic apnea, 1911
    fast channel, 1911
    slow-channel, 1911
  in critically ill patients, 1914
    due to animal toxin envenomation, 1914
    due to heavy metal intoxication, 1914
    due to marine neurotoxins, 1914
    due to motor unit diseases, 1914
    due to organophosphates, 1914
    due to snakebite envenomation, 1914
  Lambert-Eaton syndrome as, 1912–1913
    diagnostic procedures in, 1912
    immunopathology of, 1912–1913,
      1912*f*
    treatment of, 1913

Ocular motor apraxia *(Continued)*
  disorders associated with, 563*b*
  early-onset, with ataxia, 564
  type 1, with ataxia, 564
  type 2, with ataxia, 564
Ocular motor examination, for dizziness, 586–588
Ocular motor nuclei syndromes, 208
  sixth cranial nerve nucleus, 208
  third cranial nerve nucleus, 208
Ocular motor pathway impairment, in multiple sclerosis, 1165
Ocular motor syndromes, 205–208
  combined vertical gaze ophthalmoplegia as, 205–206, 206*b*
  downgaze paresis as, 206
  global paralysis of gaze as, 207–208, 208*b*
  horizontal gaze paresis as, 207
  internuclear ophthalmoplegia as, 207
  one-and-a-half syndrome as, 208
  upgaze paresis (dorsal midbrain or Parinaud syndrome) as, 206, 206*b*
Ocular motor system, 528–572
  development of, 560
  extraocular muscles in, 553
    actions of, 528–529, 529*f*, 529*t*
    anatomy of, 528–529, 529*f*–530*f*
    yoked pairs of, 528–529, 529*t*
  eye movements in
    generation and control of, 551–560, 553*f*
    horizontal, 553–558, 555*f*–556*f*
    recording techniques for, 571–572
    types of, 554*b*
    vergence, 553*f*, 558
    vertical, 558–560, 559*f*–560*f*
  fibromuscular connective tissues in, 528–529, 530*f*
  sensory fusion and stereopsis in, 529, 531*f*
  subsystems of, 552–553, 554*f*
  yoked muscle pairs in, 528–529, 529*t*
Ocular motor system disorders, eye movement recording techniques for, 571–572
Ocular muscle overaction, in diplopia, 535, 535*f*
Ocular muscle weakness
  clinical presentation of, 280
  differential diagnosis of, 288–289
Ocular muscles
  actions of, 528–529, 529*f*, 529*t*
  anatomy of, 528–529, 529*f*–530*f*
  in myasthenia gravis, 1897, 1897*b*, 1897*f*–1898*f*
  yoked pairs of, 528–529, 529*t*
Ocular myasthenia gravis (OMG), 1899, 1900*t*, 1909
Ocular myoclonus, 542*t*, 546*t*, 551
Ocular neuromyotonia, 546*t*, 571
Ocular oscillations, 542*t*, 549–551
  flutter dysmetria as, 542*t*, 549*f*, 550
  ocular bobbing as, 550–551
    causes of, 550, 551*t*
    inverse, 550–551, 551*t*
    localization of, 542*t*
    reverse, 550–551, 551*t*
    reverse dipping, 550–551, 551*t*
    V-pattern pretectal pseudobobbing as, 551, 551*t*
  ocular dysmetria as, 549*f*, 550
  ocular flutter as, 542*t*, 549, 549*f*
  ocular microflutter as, 546*t*, 550
  ocular myoclonus (oculopalatal tremor) as, 542*t*, 546*t*, 551

Ocular oscillations *(Continued)*
  ocular neuromyotonia as, 546*t*
  opsoclonus as, 549–550
    age-related causes of, 550*t*
    causes of, 549–550, 550*b*
    localization of, 542*t*
    treatment of, 546*t*, 549–550
  overshoot dysmetria as, 549*f*
  saccadic, 551, 552*b*
  square-wave jerks as, 542*t*, 546*t*
  square-wave oscillations as, 546*t*
  square-wave pulses as, 542*t*
  superior oblique myokymia as, 541, 551
    detection of, 551
    versus monocular nystagmus, 545
    treatment of, 546*t*, 551
  undershoot dysmetria as, 549*f*
Ocular tilt reaction (OTR), 563, 569–570, 569*f*
Ocular-palatal myoclonus, 44
Oculoauricular phenomenon, 571
Oculocephalic reflex, 563
  with coma, 44–45, 45*t*
Oculo-facial-skeletal myorhythmia, 1463
Oculography, 571–572
Oculogyric crises, 570
Oculomasticatory myorhythmia (OMM), 544, 546*t*, 1463
Oculomotor apraxia, 1468
  ataxia with
    type 1, 1469
    type 2, 1469
    type 2, copy number variation in, 668*t*
  type 1, ataxia with, 1469
  type 2, ataxia with, 1469
Oculomotor circuit, 96
Oculomotor disturbances, in cerebellar ataxia, 218–219
Oculomotor nerve, 1720–1724
  anatomy of, 1720, 1721*f*, 1720.*e*1*f*
  clinical lesions of, 1720–1724
    of brainstem fascicle, 1721
    of cavernous sinus, 1723
    of interpeduncular fossa and subarachnoid space, 1721–1723
    of oculomotor nucleus, 1720
    oculomotor palsy as
      appearance of, 1721, 1723*f*
      isolated, 1724
    of orbital apex, 1723–1724
  oculomotor palsy, cyclical, 186, 571
Oculomotor nerve fascicle, 1720
Oculomotor nucleus
  anatomy of, 1720
  lesions of, 1720
Oculomotor palsy, 182–183
  appearance of, 1721, 1723*f*
  cyclical, 186, 571
  isolated, 1724
Oculopalatal myoclonus, 542*t*, 546*t*, 551
Oculopalatal syndrome, 551
Oculopalatal tremor, 542*t*, 546*t*, 551
Oculopharyngeal muscular dystrophy (OPMD), 1932–1933, 1932*f*
  clinical features of, ocular weakness as, 288
  dysphagia in, 150, 1932
  molecular defects of, 1920*t*–1921*t*
  ptosis as, 188, 1932, 1932*f*
  treatment of, 1933
  weakness as, 1932
Oculovestibular reflexes, brain death and, 52
Odds ratio (OR), for brain tumors, 1020–1021

Odontoid fracture, structural imaging for, 454.*e*1, 454.*e*1*f*
Odor detection threshold test, 192–193
OFC (orbitofrontal cortex), 94
Off-period dystonia, in Parkinson disease, 1435
Ohtahara syndrome, 1572
OKN (optokinetic nystagmus), 549, 560, 588, 599, 599*f*
Olecranon bursitis, of elbow, 331
Olfaction, 190–191, 191*f*
  anatomy and physiology, 190–192, 191*f*
  disorders of, 193–194
  treatment and management of, 195–196
Olfactory agenesis, in holoprosencephaly, 1296
Olfactory agnosia, 193
Olfactory bulb, 190, 191*f*
Olfactory epithelium, 191*f*
Olfactory function, disorders and conditions associated with, 193*t*
Olfactory hallucinations, 1565
Olfactory neuroblastoma, 424.*e*1
Olfactory receptor cells, 190
Oligemia, in migraine, 1698
Oligoastrocytoma
  anaplastic, 1058
  biphasic, 421.*e*1
  management of, 1056*f*, 1058
  pathology and molecular genetics of, 1032
  structural imaging of, 418*t*–419*t*, 421.*e*1
Oligoclonal bands, in multiple sclerosis, 688
Oligodendrocytes, gliofibrillary, in oligodendroglioma, 1031–1032
Oligodendroglia, in multiple sclerosis, 1161
Oligodendroglial tumors, management of, 1058
Oligodendroglioma, 1077–1078
  anaplastic, 1058
  management of, 1058
  pathology and molecular genetics of, 1031–1032, 1031*f*
  structural imaging of, 418*t*–419*t*, 421, 421*f*
Oligometastases, WBRT in, 1090–1091
Olivo-ponto-cerebellar atrophy (OPCA), 246–248, 1660, 444.*e*2
Omer, George E., 903
OMG. *see* Ocular myasthenia gravis (OMG)
OMM (oculomasticatory myorhythmia), 544, 546*t*, 1463
Omnipause neurons in, in horizontal eye movements, 554
On/off, in Parkinson disease, 1435
Onabotulinum toxin A, 618
  for migraine, 1703
    chronic, 1707
Oncolytic viruses, for brain tumors, 1055
One-and-a-half syndrome, 208, 567, 1727
  vertical, 568
1-year rule, dementia with Lewy bodies *versus* Parkinson disease, 491
Onion bulb, 1792–1794
Onset latency, 368
ONYX-015, for brain tumors, 1055
Oophorectomy, for menstrual migraine prophylaxis, 1705
Oophoritis, in viral CNS disease, 1124*t*
Opalski syndrome, 1722*t*, 1732
Open-loop stimulation, for epilepsy, 1611
Opercular syndrome, 147
Ophelia syndrome, 1200
Ophthalmic artery, 163, 164*f*
  transcranial Doppler ultrasonography of, 480

Ophthalmic Graves disease, 832
Ophthalmic nerve
    anatomy of, 1721*f*, 1725, 1726*f*
    clinical lesions of, 1727
Ophthalmodynia periodica, 1713
Ophthalmologic findings, with inborn errors
        of metabolism, 1326.*e*1*t*–1326.*e*2*t*
Ophthalmoplegia
    bilateral
        acute, 539, 540*b*
        chronic, 539, 540*b*
    cause of, 561*t*–562*t*
    chronic progressive external, 187
    combined vertical gaze, 205–206, 206*b*
    with global developmental delay, 69*t*
    internuclear, 207, 540, 567, 567*b*
        in multiple sclerosis, 1165
    progressive external, 1358, 1945–1946
        ataxia with, 1470
        mitochondrial myopathies without,
            1358
        myopathy in, 1945–1946
        neuro-ophthalmological examination
            for, 1358
    total, 207, 208*b*
Ophthalmoscope, 587–588
Opioid
    for chronic pain, 727–729, 727*t*
    classification of, 727
    physical dependence of, 728
    route of administration of, 727
        intrathecal, 728
        transdermal, 728
    tolerance to, 728
Opioid abstinence syndrome, 728
Opioid antagonists, in chemical imaging of
        epilepsy, 509
Opioid family, 697*t*–698*t*
Opioid-induced hyperalgesia (OIH),
        728–729
Opioid receptors
    in chemical imaging, 505*t*, 506
    classes of, 721
    in pain pathway, 721–722
Opioids
    agonists, 1254, 1255*b*
    commonly used, 1255*b*
    drug dependence with, 1254–1255
    and medication overuse headache,
        1707
    overdose from, treatment of, 1255*b*
    and pain perception, 1686
    withdrawal from, symptoms and signs of,
        1255*b*
OPMD. *see* Oculopharyngeal muscular
        dystrophy (OPMD)
Oppenheim dystonia, 1451
Opsin, 1235
Opsoclonus, 219, 549–550
    age-related causes of, 550*t*
    causes of, 549–550, 550*b*
    in children, 1187–1188
    with dizziness, 588
    localization of, 542*t*
    in newborns, 560
    treatment of, 546*t*, 549–550
Opsoclonus-myoclonus, 1190–1191
Optic anomia, 124–125
Optic aphasia, 124–125
Optic ataxia, 123
Optic atrophy
    dominant, 161–162
    with global developmental delay, 69*t*
    optic neuropathies with, 174–175,
        174*f*–175*f*
Optic chiasm, 703*f*

Optic chiasmal disease, visual field defects
        due to, 578, 578*f*
Optic coherence tomography (OCT),
        in multiple sclerosis diagnosis,
        1170
Optic disc
    congenital anomalies, 175–176
        optic nerve dysplasia, 175–176
    optic neuropathies with
        bilateral, 174
        normal-appearing, 174
        unilateral, 174
    pallor, 168*f*
    swollen, 163–174
        bilateral, 170–173
            diabetic papillopathy, 172, 172*f*
            due to malignant hypertension, 172,
                172*f*
            due to optic disc drusen, 173–174,
                174*f*
            due to papilledema, 170–172
            due to pseudopapilledema, 173–174,
                173*f*
            other causes, 172–173
        unilateral, 163–170
            due to optic neuritis, 165–166,
                165*f*–166*f*
    tilted, 175, 175*f*
Optic disc coloboma, 176, 176*f*
Optic disc drusen, 173–174, 174*f*
Optic nerve
    abnormalities of, 163–178
    anatomy and physiology, 163, 164*f*
    anatomy of, 1721*f*
    blood supply to, 163, 164*f*
Optic nerve dysplasia, 175–176
Optic nerve glioma
    in neurofibromatosis type 1, 1544–1545,
        1545*f*
    structural imaging of, 449.*e*1
Optic nerve head, drusen of, 162
Optic nerve hypoplasia, 175*f*
Optic nerve infarction, retrobulbar,
        159–161
Optic nerve ischemia, visual loss due to,
        161
Optic nerve sheath meningioma, structural
        imaging of, 449.*e*1
Optic neuritis
    fundus examination of, 165–166
    isolated, 1186
    multiple sclerosis with, 1165
    optical coherence tomography, 166
    paraneoplastic, 1194
    structural imaging for, 449.*e*1–449.*e*3,
        449.*e*3*f*
    sudden visual loss due to, 161, 165–166,
        165*f*–166*f*
    visual field defects due to, 577, 578*f*
Optic neuropathies
    anterior ischemic
        arteritic, 166
        nonarteritic, 167
            acute, 168*f*
            visual loss due to, 159–161
        arteritic posterior, 167
    compressive, visual field defects due to,
        577, 578*f*
    ischemic, 166–167, 167*f*
    Leber hereditary, 170, 170*f*
        historical background, 1349
        visual loss due to, 161
    nonarteritic anterior ischemic, visual field
        defects due to, 577, 578*f*
    with normal-appearing optic discs, 174
    with optic atrophy, 174–175, 175*f*

Optic neuropathies (*Continued*)
    with optic disc
        bilateral, 174
        normal-appearing, 174
        unilateral, 174
    other causes, 167–170, 169*f*, 171*f*
    paraneoplastic, 170
    posterior ischemic, 159–161
    progressive, 162
    radiation therapy, 170
    swollen optic disc, bilateral
        diabetic papillopathy, 172, 172*f*
        due to malignant hypertension, 172,
            172*f*
        due to papilledema, 170–172
        due to pseudopapilledema, 173–174,
            173*f*
        other causes, 172–173
    toxic and nutritional, 162
    traumatic, 161
    visual field defects, 165*f*
Optic pathway glioma (OPG)
    in neurofibromatosis type 1, 1544–1545
    pediatric, 1071–1072, 1072*f*
Optic pathway tumor, 1027*t*
Optic pit, 176
Optic tract, 703*f*
Optical coherence tomography (OCT), 579,
        581*f*
    of optic neuritis, 166, 166*f*
Optokinetic nystagmus (OKN), 549, 560,
        588, 599, 599*f*
Optokinetic system, 552
OR (odds ratio), for brain tumors,
        1020–1021
Oral anticoagulants, for preventing stroke
        recurrence, 954–955
Oral apraxia, 147
Oral contraceptives
    and migraine, 1705–1706, 1973–1974
    neurological complications of, 1973–1974
    as risk factor for stroke, 924, 947
        in adolescents, 1006
Oral examination, for coma, 39
Orbicularis oculi myokymia, 571
Orbital apex
    abducens nerve in, lesions of, 1728
    oculomotor nerve in, lesions of,
        1723–1724
    trochlear nerve in, lesions of, 1725
Orbital connective tissues, 530*f*
Orbital lesions, structural imaging of, 449
Orbital metastases, 1095*t*
Orbital myectomy, for blepharospasm, 1453
Orbital pseudomotor, structural imaging for,
        449.*e*3
Orbitofrontal cortex (OFC), 94
    in visual awareness, 58
Orchitis, in viral CNS disease, 1124*t*
Orexin A
    in narcolepsy, 194
    in wakefulness, 1624
Orexin B, in wakefulness, 1624
Orexins, 697*t*–698*t*
    in appetite, 701
Organ transplantation, management of,
        1332
Organic acid analysis, in inborn errors of
        metabolism, 1326*t*
Organic acidemias, 1335
Organic chemicals, occupational, 1238–1242
    acrylamide as, 1238
    allyl chloride as, 1238
    carbon disulfide as, 1238–1239
    carbon monoxide as, 1239
    ethylene oxide as, 1239

Organic chemicals, occupational *(Continued)*
hexacarbon solvents as, 1239
methyl bromide as, 1239–1240
organocholine pesticides as, 1240
organophosphates as, 1240–1241
pyrethroids as, 1241
pyriminil as, 1241
solvent mixtures as, 1241
styrene as, 1241
toluene as, 1241
trichloroethylene as, 1241–1242
Organizational effects, of neurohormones
and neuropeptides, 696
Organocholine pesticides, occupational
exposure to, 1240
Organoid nevus syndrome, 1553
Organophosphates, 1914
occupational exposure to, 1240–1241
Orgasm
dysfunction in, from multiple sclerosis,
630–631
in female sexual response, 607
in females, 625
effect of spinal cord lesions on, 629
in male sexual response, 607
in males, 622–624
effect of spinal cord lesions on,
628–629
of sexual response, 607
ORL (otorhinolaryngological) examination,
for taste disorders, 195
Ornithine aminotransferase (OAT)
deficiency, 1326.*e1t*–1326.*e2t*
Ornithine transcarbamylase (OTC)
deficiency, 1324, 1326.*e1t*–1326.*e2t*
Oromandibular dystonia, 235,
1452–1453
Oropharyngeal dysfunction, with acute
ischemic stroke, 963
Oropharyngeal muscles, in myasthenia
gravis, 1897–1898
Orphenedine (Norflex), for chronic pain,
726
Orthopoxviruses, 1135.*e1*
Orthosis, 789
ankle-foot, 789, 790*f*
dynamic, 789
knee-ankle-foot, 789–790
mechanical and robotic-assistive devices
as, 802–803
for mobility, 802–803
for upper extremities, 802
reciprocal gait, 789–790
static, 789
upper limb, 790, 790*f*
Orthostatic hypotension (OH), 586
acute, 1870
chronic, 1870
defined, 1870
differential diagnosis of, 1885*b*
history of, 1873
hyperadrenergic, 1887
hypoadrenergic, 1887
nonpharmacological interventions for,
1891, 1892*f*
symptoms of, 1870
Orthostatic intolerance, 1870, 1873
Orthostatic syncope, 11–12
Orthostatic test, 1874–1875
Orthostatic tremor, 1444
Orthotists, in rehabilitation, 789–790
Oscillopsia, 541, 543, 592
in multiple sclerosis, 1165
Oseltamivir, for viral infections, 1127*t*

Osmolality
changes of, on brain edema, 1269–1270,
1270*f*
encephalopathy due to disordered,
1221–1224
clinical features of, 1222–1223
hyperosmolality as, 1224
hypo-osmolality and hyponatremia as,
1222, 1222*b*
osmotic homeostasis and, 1221–1222,
1222*f*
Osmolar gap, 48
Osmotic homeostasis, 1221–1222,
1222*f*
Ossicles, 585
Ossification, of posterior longitudinal
ligament or ligamentum flavum, 1751,
1752*f*
Osteoarthritis
spinal, 1751
cervical, 1752
vertebral artery stroke caused by,
1754–1755
spinal cord compression *versus*,
1092–1093
Osteogenesis
circumscripta, 1750
imperfecta, 1737
Osteomalacia, 1749
Osteomyelitis
structural imaging of, 452, 452*f*
vertebral
granulomatous, 1760–1761, 1761*f*
pyogenic, 1759–1760, 1760*f*
Osteopetrosis, 1749–1750, 1749.*e1f*
Osteoporosis, 1749, 1749*f*
Osteosclerotic myeloma, 1837–1838, 1837*f*
peripheral neuropathy in, 1192–1193
Otalgia, reflex, 1732
OTC (ornithine transcarbamylase) deficiency,
1324
Otitis media, hearing loss due to, 596
Otolith crisis, drop attacks due to, 19
Otolithic catastrophes of Tumarkin, 592
Otolithic (gravireceptive) pathways,
569–570
Otoliths, 552
Otorhinolaryngological (ORL) examination,
for taste disorders, 195
Otorrhea, CSF, 1689–1690
Otosclerosis, hearing loss due to,
596–597
Otoscopic examination, for coma, 39
Otoscopy, 591
Ototoxicity, vestibular, hearing loss due to,
592
OTR (ocular tilt reaction), 563, 569–570,
569*f*
Oval window, 585
Ovarian hyperstimulation syndrome,
ischemic stroke due to, 948
Overactive bladder (OAB), in Parkinson
disease, 609
Overactive bladder syndrome, 612
Overlap syndromes, with dermatomyositis
and polymyositis, 1951
Overshoot dysmetria, 549*f*
"Owls", 1622
Oxcarbazepine
for chronic pain, 726
for epilepsy
absorption, elimination half-life,
formulations of, 1600*t*
efficacy by seizure type of, 1601*t*

Oxcarbazepine *(Continued)*
hepatic metabolism, enzyme induction/
inhibition, pharmacokinetic
interactions, and protein binding
of, 1603*t*
mechanism of action of, 1604*t*
Oxcarbazepine, for neuropathic pain,
918*t*–919*t*
OXPHOS defects, 1326.*e1t*–1326.*e2t*
OXPHOS enzymes, in mitochondrial
disorders, 1357
Oxybutynin (Ditropan)
for bladder dysfunction, 796*t*
for bladder dysfunction, in multiple
sclerosis, 1182–1183
Oxycodone (OxyContin, Percocet), for
chronic pain, 727*t*
Oxygen inhalation, for cluster headaches,
1710
Oxytocin, 697*t*–698*t*, 708
immunoregulatory effects of, 699*t*

P
P/Q type voltage-gated calcium channels, in
Lambert-Eaton syndrome, 1912–1913
P13K/Akt (phosphoinositide-3-kinase/
protein kinase B), inhibition of, for
brain tumors, 1053, 1054*b*
p16/CDK4/RB pathway, in diffuse gliomas,
1033
Pacemaker placement, for autonomic
disorders, 1894
Pacemaker zone, 1595
Pachygyria, 1286–1287, 1299–1300
clinical features of, 1294*t*
structural imaging for, 446.*e5*, 446.*e6f*
Pachymeningitis, 1764, 1764*f*, 1764.*e1b*
idiopathic hypertrophic, 1764
Paclitaxel, for brain tumors, 1051,
1052*t*–1053*t*
PAF (pure autonomic failure), neurogenic
bladder dysfunction due to, 609
PAGD (periodic alternating gaze deviation),
565
Paget disease, 1750, 1750*f*
cranial neurological complications of,
1750
defined, 1750
diagnosis of, 1750, 1750*f*
spinal neurological complications of,
1750
treatment of, 1750
Pain, 715
acute, defined, 720
burning, 715
chronic, defined, 720
cranial and facial, 197–204
deep brain stimulation for, 406
defined, 296, 720
and functional disorders, 2002
with gait disorders, 252
general features of, 296
mechanical, of lower back and leg, 334*t*
neuropathic, 315
of lower back and leg, 334*t*
in peripheral nerve disorders, 1795,
1864–1866, 1865*b*
management of, 1865–1866
with peripheral nerve trauma
interventional strategies for, 917
management of, 917
pharmacological options for, 917,
918*t*–919*t*

Pain (*Continued*)
  non-neurologic, of lower back and leg, 334*t*
  rTMS for, 399
Pain management
  chronic
    psychological therapy, 734–735, 735*t*
    rehabilitation in, 735, 735*t*
  for common pain syndromes, 735–741
    cervicogenic headache as, 737, 737*f*
    complex regional pain syndrome as, 737–739, 738*f*
    low back pain as, 736–737
    pain in multiple sclerosis as, 740
    phantom limb pain and stump pain as, 740–741
    post-stroke pain syndrome as, 739
    spinal cord injury and pain as, 739–740
    trigeminal neuralgia as, 735–736, 736*b*
  definition and challenge of, 720
  interventional, 729–734, 729*t*
    epidural corticosteroid injection for, 731–732, 732*f*
    Gasserian ganglion lesions for, 730–731, 731*f*
    greater occipital nerve block for, 729, 730*f*
    intrathecal drug delivery systems for, 734, 734*f*
    lumbar facet joint block for, 732
    motor cortex stimulation for, 734
    percutaneous disk decompression for, 732–733
    sphenopalatine ganglion block for, 729–730
    spinal cord stimulation for, 733–734, 733*f*
    stellate ganglion block for, 731, 731*f*
  multidisciplinary approach to, 722–723, 723*t*, 724*f*
  pharmacological, 723–729
    anticonvulsants for, 725–726
    antidepressants for, 723–726
    muscle relaxants for, 726
    N-methyl-D-aspartate receptor blockers for, 726–727
    nonsteroidal anti-inflammatory drugs for, 723, 725*t*
    opioid analgesics for, 727–729, 727*t*
    systemic local anesthetic therapies for, 726
    topical analgesics for, 726
  principles of, 720–741
Pain modulation, as related to headache, 1686
Pain pathways
  anatomy and physiology of, 720–722
  central modulation of nociception in, 721
  central nervous system, 299*f*
  opioid receptors in, 721–722
Pain sensation, 1770*f*
Pain syndrome, 277, 735–741
  cervicogenic headache as, 737, 737*f*
  complex regional pain syndrome as, 737–739, 738*f*
  low back pain as, 736–737
  pain in multiple sclerosis as, 740
  phantom limb pain and stump pain as, 740–741
  post-stroke pain syndrome as, 739
  spinal cord injury and pain as, 739–740
  trigeminal neuralgia as, 735–736
Pain transmission, as related to headache, 1686
Painful legs-moving toes syndrome, 1459

Painful post-traumatic trigeminal neuropathy, 1716
Pain-sensitive intracranial structures, 1686
Paired-associative stimulation (PAS), 394, 397–398
Palatal myoclonus, 242, 1424–1425, 1458
Palatal tremor, 232–234, 242, 1424–1425
  with coma, 44
Palilalia, 225
Palinacusis, 541*f*
Palinopia, 540–541
  cerebral, 541*f*
Palinopsia, 123, 540–541, 541*f*
Palisading, 1028, 1028*f*
Palliation, 718
Palliative care, 714, 718
Pallid breath-holding spells, 15–16
Palpebral fissures
  pathologically narrowed, 188
  pathologically widened, 187–188
PAMPs. *see* Pathogen-associated molecular patterns (PAMPs)
PAN (periodic alternating nystagmus), 542*t*, 545–547
  and albinism, 547
  and PAGD, 565
  treatment of, 546*t*, 547
Panayiotopoulos syndrome, 1574
Pancreatic cholera, due to autonomic disorders, 1890
Pancreatic cysts, in von Hippel- Lindau syndrome, 1549
Pancreatic encephalopathy, 828
Pancreatic polypeptide, 697*t*–698*t*
Pancreatic tumors, in von Hippel- Lindau syndrome, 1549
Pancuronium bromide, 1964
PANDAS. *see* Pediatric autoimmune neuropsychiatric disorders associated with streptococcal infection (PANDAS)
Panencephalitis
  progressive rubella, 1143–1144
  subacute sclerosing, 1142–1143, 1142*f*
Panhypopituitarism, 703
  neurologic complications in, children of, 847
Panic attacks, functional symptoms of, 1994
Pannus, 1761
Papez circuit, in memory, 62–63
Papillary glioneuronal tumor, pathology and molecular genetics of, 1035
Papilledema, 170–172
  acute, 171*f*
  atrophic, 171
  chronic, 172*f*
    progressive visual loss due to, 162
  defined, 163
  due to brain tumor, 1046
  due to idiopathic intracranial hypertension, 1272–1273
  pseudo-, 173–174, 173*t*
Papillopathy, diabetic, 172, 172*f*
Paraballism, 240
Paradoxical breathing, 1645
  in critically ill patients, 742–743
Paradoxical photophobia, 158
Paraganglioma, 1036–1037
Paragrammatism, 132
Parahippocampal gyrus, in memory, 62*f*
Parainfectious encephalomyelitis, 264
"Parakinesia", 115–116
Parakinesis, 239
Paralimbic regions, 94
Paralysis
  agitans, 1427
  functional, 1996

Paralytic shellfish poisoning (PSP), 1252–1253
Paramedian cerebral cortical lesion, differential diagnosis of, 272.*e*2
Paramedian pontine reticular formation (PPRF), in eye movements
  horizontal, 553, 555*f*
  vertical, 558–559, 559*f*
Paramedian thalamus, and vergence, 558
Paramnesia, reduplicative
  after stroke, 100–101
  in delirium, 26
Paramyotonia congenita, 1525–1526, 1938–1939
  clinical features of, 1524*t*, 1525
  diagnosis of, 1525–1526
  genetic basis for, 1520*t*–1521*t*
  muscle hypertrophy due to, 282–283
  pathophysiology of, 1525
  treatment of, 1526
Paraneoplastic autonomic neuropathy, 1848
Paraneoplastic brainstem encephalitis,, horizontal gaze palsies due to, 565
Paraneoplastic cerebellar degeneration (PCD), 1188–1189, 1463–1464
  ataxia due to, 1463–1464
  channelopathy in, 1536
  clinical findings in, 1188–1189
  immune responses in, 1189, 1189*f*
  treatment of, 1189
  tumor association of, 1189
Paraneoplastic encephalomyelitis, 1189–1190
Paraneoplastic gaze palsies, 565
Paraneoplastic motor neuron disease, 1518
Paraneoplastic myelopathy, spinal cord compression *versus*, 1092
Paraneoplastic necrotizing myopathy, acute, 1194
Paraneoplastic neurological syndromes (PNSs), 1187, 1188*b*
  affecting CNS, 1188*b*
  affecting peripheral nervous system, 1188*b*
  cerebellar degeneration as, 1188–1189
  general diagnostic approach, 1187–1188
  pathogenesis of, 1187, 1188*t*
  specific, 1188–1195
    acute necrotizing myopathy as, 1194
    dermatomyositis as, 1194
    Lambert-Eaton myasthenic syndrome as, 1193
    limbic and brainstem encephalitis as, 1190
    myasthenia gravis as, 1193–1194
    paraneoplastic encephalomyelitis as, 1190
    paraneoplastic opsoclonus-myoclonus as, 1190–1191
    paraneoplastic sensory neuropathy as, 1191–1192
    peripheral neuropathy associated with plasma cell dyscrasias and B-cell lymphoma as, 1192–1193
    Stiff-man syndrome as, 1191
    subacute and chronic peripheral neuropathies as, 1192
    vasculitis of the nerve as, 1192
    visual syndromes as, 1194–1195
Paraneoplastic neuropathy, 1846–1847, 1846*t*
  sensory, 1191–1192
    clinical findings in, 1191–1192
    immune responses, 1192
    treatment of, 1192
    tumor association, 1192

Peroneal nerve graft, 916*f*
Peroneal nerve stimulation, in rehabilitation, 801, 801*f*
Peroneal neuropathy
   leg pain due to, 336*t*, 339
   monoplegia due to, 270
      differential diagnosis of, 272.*e*2
Peroxisomal disorders, 1335, 1328.*e*1*t*, 1333.*e*1*t*
Peroxisome, 1335
Perseveration, 130
Perseverative automatisms, 1564
Persistent idiopathic facial pain, 1715
Persistent vegetative state (PVS), 34, 35*t*, 54
   consciousness in, 59
   interventions for, 55*b*
   prognosis for, 50
Persistently poor readers, 1315
Personality change
   after traumatic brain injury, 91
   in amyotrophic lateral sclerosis, 85–86
Personalized medicine, 665*b*
Pervasive developmental disorder-not otherwise specified (PDD-NOS), 1301
Perverted nystagmus, 548
Pes cavus
   in Charcot-Marie-Tooth disease type 1, 1812, 1814*f*
   due to muscle weakness, 283, 283*f*
Pesticide exposure, and brain tumors, 1022
PET. *see* Positron emission tomography (PET)
Petit mal epilepsy, 352, 353*f*
   impulsive, 1577
Petrosal ganglion
   anatomy of, 1731
   clinical lesions of, 1731–1732
Petrous apex, abducens nerve in, clinical lesions of, 1728
Peyote, neurotoxins from, 1250
PFC (prefrontal cortex), in horizontal eye movements, 556
PFO (patent foramen ovale), cardiogenic embolism due to, 935
PFS (posterior fossa syndrome), 1083.*e*1
PGE$_1$ (prostaglandin E$_{1)}$, for erectile dysfunction, 621
PGE$_2$. *see* Prostaglandin E$_2$ (PGE$_2$)
PGK (phosphoglycerate kinase) deficiency, 1337
P-glycoprotein , in chemical imaging, 505*t*
PH (paroxysmal hemicrania), 1711–1712
Phagocytes, in innate immune system, 676
Phakomatosis, 178, 1538
   pigmentokeratotica, 1553
Phalen maneuver, 1802
   reversed, 1802
Phantom limb pain, 740–741
Phantosmia, 193
Pharmacogenetics, 665*b*
Pharmacological adjuncts
   for memory disturbances, 807–808, 808*b*
   in rehabilitation, 804
Pharyngeal manometry, for dysphagia, 157
Pharyngitis, in viral CNS disease, 1123*t*
Phase cancellation, in nerve conduction studies, 371, 372*f*
   of demyelinative conduction block, 373–374
Phase encoding, in MRI, 413
Phase encoding gradient, in MRI, 416–417
Phase-contrast MRA (PC-MRA), 464–466
   for subclavian steal syndrome, 471–472
Phencyclidine, drug dependence with, 1258

Phenelzine, for migraine, 1703
Phenobarbital
   for epilepsy
      absorption, elimination half-life, formulations of, 1600*t*
      efficacy by seizure type of, 1601*t*
      hepatic metabolism, enzyme induction/ inhibition, pharmacokinetic interactions, and protein binding of, 1603*t*
      mechanism of action of, 1604*t*
   for neonatal seizures, 1958, 1959*t*
   for passive addiction and withdrawal syndrome, 1972
   during pregnancy, and vitamin K deficiency, 1986
   for spasticity, 799*t*
Phenomenology, 1
Phenothiazine, for vertigo, 603–604, 603*t*
Phenotype, 651*t*, 652–653
   in neurogenetic evaluation, 672*t*
Phenotypic heterogeneity, 1519, 664.*e*1
Phenylbutazone (Butazolidin), for chronic pain, 725*t*
Phenylketonuria (PKU)
   disorders of neurotransmitter synthesis in, 1290
   management of, 1330
Phenylpropanolamine, 1256
   intracerebral hemorrhage due to, 974–975
Phenytoin
   ataxia due to, 1462
   for epilepsy
      absorption, elimination half-life, formulations of, 1600*t*
      efficacy by seizure type of, 1601*t*
      hepatic metabolism, enzyme induction/ inhibition, pharmacokinetic interactions, and protein binding of, 1603*t*
      mechanism of action of, 1604*t*
   for glossopharyngeal neuralgia, 1717
   and levonorgestrel, 1974
   for neonatal seizures, 1958, 1959*t*
   for neuropathic pain, 918*t*–919*t*
   neuropathy due to, 1862
   during pregnancy, and vitamin K deficiency, 1986
   psychotropic effects of, 89*t*
   for spasticity, 799*t*
Pheochromocytoma, 712
   headache due to, 1694
   neurological complications of, in adults, 833
   in von Hippel- Lindau syndrome, 1549
Phlebovirus
   Rift Valley fever virus as, 1139.*e*1
   Toscana virus as, 1139–1140
Phlegmon, paravertebral, structural imaging of, 452, 453*f*
PHM (posthypoxic myoclonus), 1457–1458
Phonagnosia, 126
Phoneme-based treatment, for aphasia, 805–806
Phonemes, 128
Phonic tics, 240–241
Phonologic variant, of frontotemporal dementia, 522–523
Phonological agraphia, 139
Phonological dyslexia, 139
Phosphodiesterase inhibitors
   for erectile dysfunction, 632
   for sexual dysfunction in women, 633

Phosphodiesterase type 5 inhibitors, for erectile dysfunction, 620–621, 621*t*
Phosphoenolpyruvate carboxykinase (PEPCK) deficiency, 1337
Phosphofructokinase deficiency, myopathy due to, 1941
Phosphoglycerate kinase deficiency, myopathy due to, 1941
Phosphoglycerate mutase deficiency, myopathy due to, 1941
Phosphoinositide-3-kinase/protein kinase B (P13K/Akt), inhibition of, for brain tumors, 1053, 1054*b*
Photic stimulation, for EEG, 350, 351*f*
Photoelectric capture, 411–412
Photoelectric effect, in CT, 411
Photophobia
   with global developmental delay, 69*t*
   paradoxical, 158
Photopsias, 158
Photo-stress test, 574
PHQ-9 (Patient Health Questionnaire), 76, 76*t*
Phrenitis, 23
Physical activity, return to, concussion and, 863–864, 864*t*
Physical aids and appliances, for functional motor symptoms, 2007
Physical dependence, 1254
   on opioids, 728
Physical examination, 5
Physical therapists, in rehabilitation, 786–787, 786*b*
Physical therapy, for Duchenne muscular dystrophy, 1922–1923
Physicians, in rehabilitation, 785
Physiological nystagmus, 544–545
Physiotherapy, for functional symptoms, 2006
Phytanic acid storage disease, 1818.*e*9
Pial surfaces, gap junctions on, 1266
PiB (Pittsburgh Compound B), in chemical imaging, 506
   of Alzheimer disease, 508–509
   in healthy aging, 508–509
PiB-PET (Pittsburgh Compound B positron emission tomography), of Alzheimer disease, 1393*f*
PICA (posterior inferior cerebellar artery) aneurysm, 987*f*
PICA (posterior inferior cerebellar artery) infarctions, 929
Pick, Arnold, 1405
Pick bodies, 1412
   pathology, 1412*f*
"Pick complex", 489–490
Pick disease, structural imaging of, 446, 446.*e*2*f*
Pigmentary retinopathy, in mitochondrial disease, 1355
Pili torti, in kinky hair syndrome, 1559
Pill rolling tremor, 230
Pilocytic astrocytoma
   juvenile, 1034
      diffuse intrinsic pontine glioma *versus*, 1075
   management of, 1055
   pathology and molecular genetics of, 1034, 1034*f*
   pediatric, 1070–1071, 1071*f*
   structural imaging of, 418*t*–419*t*, 419
Pilomyxoid astrocytoma, 1034
PIN. *see* Posterior interosseous nerve (PIN) lesions

Pinch sign, 1804
Pineal parenchymal tumors, management of, 1059
Pineal region tumors, structural imaging of, 418t–419t, 425–426
Pineal tumor, 1027t
Pineoblastoma
    management of, 1059
    pediatric, 1066–1067
    structural imaging of, 418t–419t, 424–425
Pineocytoma
    management of, 1059
    structural imaging of, 418t–419t, 425–426
Ping-pong fractures, 1968
Ping-pong gaze, 565
Pinhole test, for monocular diplopia, 533
Pinpoint pupils, 42
PION (posterior ischemic optic neuropathy), 159–161
PIP (postictal psychosis), 108
Pipeline Embolization Device (PED), for cerebral aneurysms, 773–774, 773f
Piribedil, for Parkinson disease, 1432–1435
Piriformis syndrome, 1808
    leg pain due to, 336t, 339
Piroxicam (Feldene), for chronic pain, 725t
Pisohamate hiatus, 1806
Pittsburgh Compound B (PiB), in chemical imaging, 506
    of Alzheimer disease, 508–509
    in healthy aging, 508–509
Pittsburgh Compound B positron emission tomography (PiB-PET), of Alzheimer disease, 1393f
Pituitary adenoma, 707, 707t
    management of, 1061f, 1064
        radiotherapy for, 711
        surgical, 711
    neurological complications of, in adults, 831, 831f
    structural imaging of, 418t–419t, 426–427, 427f, 427.e1f
Pituitary apoplexy, 161, 704
Pituitary diseases, neurological complications of, 831–832, 831f
Pituitary dysfunction, approach to patient with, 710–712
    endocrinological investigation in, 710, 710t
    history and physical examination in, 710
    imaging studies in, 710
Pituitary fossa, and cavernous sinus, 703f
Pituitary function, modulation by hypothalamic peptides of, 697t–698t
Pituitary gland, 702–703
    anterior, 703–707
        hyperfunction of, 704–706
            Cushing disease and Nelson syndrome due to, 705–706, 706b, 711
            due to gonadotropin-secreting tumors, 706, 711
            excessive secretion of thyroid-stimulating hormone due to, 706, 711
            gigantism and acromegaly due to, 705, 705b, 711
            hyperprolactinemia due to, 704–705, 710–711
            precocious puberty due to, 704
        hypofunction of, 703–704, 704b, 704t
        hypophysitis of, 707
        hypothalamic control of, 702t, 703
        other tumors of, 707

Pituitary gland (Continued)
        tumors and hyperplasia of, 707, 707t
            medical management of, 710–711
            radiotherapy for, 711
            surgery for, 711
    blood supply to, 703, 703f
    functional anatomy of, 702–703, 702t, 703f
    posterior, 707–710
        in cerebral salt wasting, 709–710
        in diabetes insipidus, 708
            etiology of, 708
            management of, 708
        physiology of, 707–708
            atrial natriuretic peptide in, 708
            oxytocin in, 708
            in sodium homeostasis, 708
            in thirst and drinking, 708
            vasopressin in, 707–708
        in syndrome of inappropriate antidiuretic hormone secretion, 708–709
            clinical features of, 709
            etiology and pathophysiology of, 708–709, 709b
            treatment of, 709
Pituitary hyperplasia, 707
Pituitary insufficiency, 703, 704b, 704t
Pituitary peptides, 697t–698t
Pituitary tumors, 707, 707t
    headache due to, 1687–1688
    medical management of, 710–711
    during pregnancy, 1983
    radiotherapy for, 711
    surgery for, 711
Pixel, in CT, 411
[¹¹C]PK 11195, in chemical imaging, 506
    of Alzheimer disease, 509
    of Parkinson disease, 508
PKC (protein kinase C), inhibition of, for brain tumors, 1053, 1054b
Plagiocephaly, 1739t
Plain radiographs, headache and, 202
Plantar reflex, in coma, 46
Plants neurotoxins, 1249–1251
    excitatory amino acids as, 1250
    of Jimson weed, 1249
    of medicinal herbs, 1250
    of morning glory, 1250
    of peyote, 1250
    of poison hemlock, 1249
    of water hemlock, 1249–1250
Plaques
    in multiple sclerosis
        chronic inactive, 1162, 1162f
        gross examination of, 1160–1161, 1160f–1161f
        histological examination of, 1161
        neuritic, in Alzheimer disease, 1397
        thickness of, measurement of, 478
Plasma cell dyscrasias
    neurological complications of, 824–826
    peripheral neuropathy associated with, 1192–1193
Plasma exchange (PLEX)
    for Lambert-Eaton syndrome, 1913
    for myasthenia gravis, 1903t, 1904–1905
Plasma viscosity, as risk factor for stroke, 935
Plasmacytoid dendritic cells (PDCs), in dermatomyositis, 1950
Plasmapheresis
    for acute inflammatory demyelinating polyneuropathy, 691–692
    for myasthenia gravis, 692

Plasminogen activator inhibitor-1 excess, as risk factor for stroke, 924
Plasmodium falciparum, 1155, 1156t
Plateau phase, 607
    of sexual response, 624–625
Plateau waves
    due to brain tumor, 1047
    in intracranial pressure monitoring, 745, 745f
Platelet antiaggregants, for preventing stroke recurrence, 953–954
Platelet-derived growth factor receptor (PDGFR) inhibitors, for brain tumors, 1053, 1054b
Platinum compounds, for brain tumors, 1051, 1052t–1053t
Platybasia, 1740
Play, abnormalities of, in autism spectrum disorder, 1303
Plectin-1 deficiency, 1927
Pleocytosis, migrainous syndrome with CSF, 1690
Pleomorphic xanthoastrocytoma, 1075
    management of, 1055–1056, 1056f
    pathology and molecular genetics of, 1034
    structural imaging of, 418t–419t, 419.e1
PLEX. see Plasma exchange (PLEX)
Plexiform neurofibromas, in neurofibromatosis type 1, 1544
Plexopathy
    brachial, 1100–1101
    idiopathic brachial, 1784–1786
        diagnosis of, 1785
        pathophysiology and etiology of, 1785
        treatment and prognosis of, 1785–1786
    isolated leg pain due to, 336t, 340
    lower back pain and leg pain due to, 335t, 338
    lumbosacral, 1101
    metastatic, 1783
    monoplegia due to, 271–272
    needle electromyography of, 382, 382f
    neoplastic, lumbosacral, 338
    radiation, 1245
    radiation-induced, 1784
    traumatic, 1782
        early management of, 1782
        long-term management of, 1782
Plexus injury
    from retroperitoneal abscess, 338
    from retroperitoneal hematoma, 338
Plexus metastases, 1100–1101
    brachial plexopathy, 1100–1101
    lumbosacral plexopathy, 1101
Plexus pain, arm and neck pain due to, 324–325, 325f
Plexuses, disorders of, 1766–1790
PLP1 (proteolipid protein 1), in hereditary spastic paraplegia, 1487–1488
Plumboporphyria, psychiatric manifestations of, 103–104
PM (palatal myoclonus), 1424–1425
PMC (pontine micturition center), neurological control of, 605
PMCA (protein misfolding cyclic amplification), 1372–1373
PMD-TCD (power motion-mode Doppler), of acute ischemic stroke, 480
[¹¹C]PMP, in chemical imaging, 506
PMR. see Proportionate mortality (PMR)
PNES (psychogenic nonepileptic seizures), 15
PNET (primitive neuroectodermal tumors), supratentorial, management of, 1060
Pneumatoscopy, 591

Pneumonia
 with acute ischemic stroke, 963
 in viral CNS disease, 1124t
PNKD (paroxysmal nonkinesiogenic
 dyskinesia), 1520t–1521t, 1532
PNTML (pudendal nerve terminal motor
 latency), 616
PO₂. *see* Partial pressure of oxygen (PO₂)
POEMS syndrome, 1192–1193, 1837–1838,
 1837f
Point mutations, 654–655, 654f
Poison hemlock, neurotoxins from,
 1249
POLG (polymerase γ) gene, in mitochondrial
 recessive ataxia syndrome, 1467
Polio wall, 1497
Poliomyelitis, 1135, 1496–1497
 clinical features of, 1496
 differential diagnosis of, 1496
 laboratory features of, 1496
 monoplegia due to, 272
 sleep disturbances in, 1658
 treatment of, 1496
 vaccination of, 1496–1497
Poliomyelitis-like illness, enterovirus-68
 associated, 1136
Poliosis, in tuberous sclerosis, 1539
Poliovirus, 1135
Polyangiitis, granulomatosis with,
 820–821
Polyarteritis nodosa (PAN)
 intracerebral hemorrhage due to,
 972–974
 neurological complications of
 in adults, 819–820, 820f
 in children, 838
Polychondritis, relapsing, 822
Polycythemia, neurological complications of,
 in adults, 826
Polycythemia vera, 1848
 ischemic stroke due to, 948
Polyethylene glycol, for constipation,
 621.e1
Polyganglionopathy, dorsal, 1792, 1793f
Polyglutamine tract, in neurodegenerative
 movement disorders, 1426t
Polymerase chain reaction (PCR), 1030
 of viral nervous system disease, 1125t
Polymerase chain reaction (PCR) assays, for
 meningitis, 1148–1149
Polymerase γ (POLG) gene, in mitochondrial
 recessive ataxia syndrome, 1467
Polymicrogyria, 1286–1287, 1292
 structural imaging for, 446.e5, 446.e6f
Polymorphism, 651t, 654–655
 single nucleotide, 651t, 654
 genome-wide association studies for,
 663–664, 664f
Polymorphonuclear cells, in innate immune
 system, 676
Polymyalgia rheumatica, 1953
 arm and neck pain due to, 331
 due to giant-cell arteritis, 1692
 muscle pain due to, 304
Polymyositis, 1194, 1950–1951, 1951f
 associated with neoplasia, 1951
 associated with other collagen vascular
 diseases, 1951
 diagnostic studies for, 1950
 dysphagia in, 150
 HIV-associated, 1114t
 immune mediation in, 686, 692
 immune system activation in,
 1950–1951

Polymyositis *(Continued)*
 needle electromyography of, 384
 neuromuscular examination in, 1950
 prognosis for, 1951–1952
 treatment of, 693, 1951–1952
Polyneuropathy
 axonal
 needle electromyography of, 383
 nerve conduction studies of, 375f
 defined, 1795
 demyelinating
 needle electromyography of, 383
 nerve conduction studies of, 375–376
 diabetic, in adults, 833
 diagnostic clues in, 1796
 distal sensory, HIV-associated, 1119
 dying-back or length-dependent, 1792
 generalized, nerve conduction studies of,
 375–376
 gestational, 1979
 leg pain due to, 339–340
 peripheral, needle electromyography of,
 382f
 with predominant sensory involvement,
 1796–1797, 1797f
 with predominantly motor manifestations,
 1796, 1796b
Polyol metabolism, disorders of, 1338
Polyomaviruses, 1132–1133
Polyopia, 123, 540
Polyphenotypical tumor, 1039
PolyQ disorders, neurodegenerative
 movement disorders due to, 1427
Polyradiculomyelitis, lumbosacral, HIV-
 associated, 1120
Polyradiculoneuropathy
 acute paraneoplastic, 1193
 diabetic, in adults, 833
 inflammatory demyelinating, HIV-
 associated, 1114t, 1120
Polyradiculopathy, defined, 1766
Polyvinyl alcohol, for embolization
 procedure, of cerebral arteriovenous
 malformations, 775–776
POMGnT1. *see* Protein O-mannose-β-1,2-N-
 acetylglucosaminyl transferase
 (POMGnT1)
Pompe disease, 1336–1337
 myopathy due to, 1941
POMT1. *see* Protein O-mannosyltransferase
 1 (POMT1)
POMT2. *see* Protein O-mannosyltransferase 2
 (POMT2)
Pontine hemorrhage, 978t, 979, 979f
Pontine micturition center (PMC),
 neurological control of, 605
Pontine reticular formation (PRF), in REM
 sleep, 1624.e1
Pontine stroke syndromes, 212, 214b
Pontine syndromes, 930
Pontocerebellar hypoplasia, disorders of
 programmed cell death in, 1284
Population-based rates, 635–636
Porencephaly, structural imaging for, 446.e5,
 446.e6f
Porphyrias, 1339–1340, 1340.e1t
 acute intermittent, psychiatric
 manifestations of, 103–104
 psychiatric manifestations of, 103–104
 variegated, psychiatric manifestations of,
 103–104
Porphyric attack, acute
 clinical features of, 1818.e6
 management of, 1818.e7f

Porphyric neuropathy, 1818.e5–1818.e7,
 1818.e6t
 clinical features of, 1818.e6
 laboratory studies of, 1818.e6–1818.e7
 pathogenesis of, 1818.e7
 treatment and management of, 1818.e7,
 1818.e7f
Porphyrins, 1339–1340
Portal systemic encephalopathy, 827, 828f,
 1210t
Port-wine nevus, in Sturge-Weber syndrome,
 1546, 1547f
Positional plagiocephaly, hypotonic infant
 due to, 305–306
Positional testing, for dizziness, 589–591,
 590f
Positive motor manifestations, of seizures,
 1564
Positive myoclonus, 242
Positive predictive values, in
 neuropsychological evaluation, 514
Positive sensory symptoms, in peripheral
 nerve disorders, 1795
Positive sharp wave, in needle
 electromyography, 377–378, 377t, 378f
Positron emission tomography (PET),
 486–487, 487t
 for chemical imaging
 principles of, 504
 versus single-photon emission computed
 tomography, 504
 FDG
 in behavioral variant of frontotemporal
 dementia, 488f
 for brain tumors, 495, 495f–496f
 of corticobasal degeneration (CBD), 493
 of dementia, 488
 and Alzheimer disease, 488f
 with Lewy bodies, 490–491, 491f
 Parkinson disease with, 491
 vascular, 492–493
 for epilepsy, 497–498, 497f–498f
 of Parkinson disease, 493, 493f
 for Parkinsonism, 489–490, 493–495,
 493f–494f
 in multiple system atrophy, 493, 494f
 in Parkinson disease, 493, 493f
 in progressive supranuclear palsy,
 493, 494f
 in posterior cortical atrophy, 490f
 for presurgical brain mapping, 499–500
 of primary progressive aphasia, 489f
 of progressive supranuclear palsy (PSP),
 493, 494f
 fluorodeoxyglucose (FDG), of Alzheimer
 disease, 1388f–1389f, 1392f,
 1409f–1410f, 1412f
 of hepatic encephalopathy, 1212, 1213f
 of Parkinson disease, 1429, 1429f
 prior to epilepsy surgery, 1596
 radionuclides used in, 487
 sports and performance concussion in,
 862
Postactivation depression, 899–900
Postanoxic vegetative state, 54
Postconcussion syndrome (PCS), 527,
 864–865, 869, 879, 1690
Posterior branch, 1007.e1f
Posterior cerebral artery (PCA), infarction of,
 hemiplegia due to, 264
Posterior cerebral artery infarctions, of
 penetrating branches, 929–930
Posterior cerebral artery syndromes,
 930–931, 931f

Posterior ciliary arteries, 163
Posterior circulation Alberta Stroke Program Early CT score (pc-ASPECTS), 462, 462f
Posterior column, 889
Posterior column syndrome, 884, 884f
Posterior commissure (PC), in vertical eye movements, 558–559, 559f
Posterior communicating artery (PCOM), oculomotor nerve and, 1720
Posterior communicating artery (PCOM) aneurysm, 1721–1723
Posterior cortical atrophy (PCA), 1387–1388, 1388f
Posterior cranial fossa, in Chiari I malformation, 1741, 1742t
Posterior elements, degenerative changes of, 457, 457f
Posterior fossa, microvascular decompression of, 1717
Posterior fossa abnormalities, drop attacks due to, 18
Posterior fossa headache, in Chiari I malformation, 1743
Posterior fossa mass lesion, headache due to, 1688
Posterior fossa structural abnormalities, vertigo due to, 587t, 593
    treatment for, 603
Posterior fossa syndrome (PFS), 1083.e1
Posterior fossa tumors, structural imaging of, 418t–419t
Posterior inferior cerebellar artery (PICA) aneurysm, 987f
Posterior inferior cerebellar artery (PICA) infarctions, 929
Posterior interosseous nerve (PIN) lesions, 1806–1807
Posterior interosseous neuropathy, 1806–1807
Posterior ischemic optic neuropathy (PION), 159–161
Posterior longitudinal ligament, ossification of, 1751, 1752f
Posterior midline regions, in memory, 61
Posterior parietal cortex (PPC), in horizontal eye movements, 556
Posterior pituitary, 707–710
    in cerebral salt wasting, 709–710
    in diabetes insipidus, 708
        etiology of, 708
        management of, 708
        physiology of, 707–708
        atrial natriuretic peptide in, 708
        oxytocin in, 708
        in sodium homeostasis, 708
        in thirst and drinking, 708
        vasopressin in, 707–708
    in syndrome of inappropriate antidiuretic hormone secretion, 708–709
        clinical features of, 709
        etiology and pathophysiology of, 708–709, 709b
        treatment of, 709
Posterior radicular veins, 1007.e1–1007.e2
Posterior reversible encephalopathy syndrome (PRES), 1218
    structural imaging of, 440.e1–440.e2, 440.e2f
Posterior spinal arteries (PSA), 1007.e1, 1007.e1f
Posterior-circulation cerebrovascular disease, evaluation of
    with 3D CE-MRA, 469, 469f
    with TOF-MRA, 467–468
Postexercise exhaustion, in myasthenia gravis, 387

Postganglionic parasympathetic dysfunction, anisocoria due to, 180–182, 183f
Postherpetic neuralgia, 1129, 1718
Posthypoxic myoclonus, 1457–1458
Postictal depression, 108
Postictal psychosis (PIP), 108
Postirradiation, lower motor neuron syndrome, 1506
Postmyelographic computed tomography, for lower back and leg pain, 335
Postoperative causes, of delirium, 31
Postpartum migraine, 1976
Postpartum myasthenia gravis, 1977
Postpartum stroke, 947, 1988–1989
Postpolio syndrome, 1135, 1497–1498, 1497b, 1658
Poststroke depression (PSD), 99–100
Post-stroke pain syndrome (PSP), 739
Postsynaptic neuromuscular junction disorder, repetitive nerve stimulation for rapid, 388t
    slow, 387, 387f, 388t
Posttetanic facilitation, in myasthenia gravis, 387
Posttetanic pseudofacilitation, 388
Post-transplant acute limbic encephalitis (PTALE), 1132
Posttraumatic fusion deficiency, 571
Posttraumatic headache, 1690
Postural instability, 508
    in parkinsonian disorders, 228
"Postural instability gait difficulty" (PIGD), 227
Postural manifestation, of seizures, 1564
Postural orthostatic hypotension (POTS), 1737
Postural responses, 254
Postural tachycardia syndrome (POTS)
    gastrointestinal dysfunction in, 1871, 1878–1880, 1879b, 1879f
    syncope due to, 11–12
Postural tremor, 231, 231b
    definition of, 230
Posture
    examination of, 252–254, 253b
    trunk, 253–254
Posturing
    decerebrate, 45
    decorticate, 45–46
Posturography, in vestibular testing, 601
Postvaccinal encephalomyelitis (PVEM), 1135.e1
Postvaccination encephalomyelitis, acute disseminated, 1184
Postvoid residual urine, 613f
Potassium channel, 1937
    voltage-gated, 1519–1521, 1522f
Potassium channelopathy, 1939
Potassium disturbances, neurological complications of, 830
Potassium-aggravated myotonia, 1526–1527, 1939
    clinical features of, 1524t, 1526
    diagnosis of, 1527
    genetic basis for, 1520t–1521t
    pathophysiology of, 1526–1527
    treatment of, 1527
Potassium-sensitive periodic paralysis, 1938
Potocki-Lupski syndrome, copy number variation in, 668t
POTS. see Postural orthostatic hypotension (POTS)
Pott disease, 1760, 1761f
Pott paraplegia, 1760–1761
Powassan virus, 1137t, 1139

Power Doppler imaging (PDI), 477
    for high-grade stenosis, 479
    of transient ischemic attack, 480–481
Power motion-mode Doppler (PMD-TCD), of acute ischemic stroke, 480
Powers ratio, 890–891
PPC (posterior parietal cortex), in horizontal eye movements, 556
PPN (pedunculopontine nucleus), 1423
PPRF (paramedian pontine reticular formation), in eye movements horizontal, 553, 555f
PPT (pedunculopontine tegmental) nucleus, in REM sleep, 1624
Prader-Willi syndrome, 662, 662f
    cognitive and behavioral problems in, 1309t
    copy number variation in, 668t
    hypotonic infant due to, 309
Pragmatics, 128
Pramipexole, for Parkinson disease, 1433t–1434t
Pramipexole on Underlying Disease (PROUD) study, 1432
Pravastatin, for ischemic stroke, 922
Praxis, model for, 116, 116f
Praxis testing, memory and, 64
Prazosin, for bladder dysfunction, 796t
Precoeruleus (PC), in NREM sleep, 1625.e1
Precession, 413, 413f
Precocious puberty, 704
Precursor peptides, 697t–698t
Prednisolone, for migraine, 1702
Prednisone
    for cluster headache maintenance prophylaxis, 1710
    for dermatomyositis, polymyositis, and immune-mediated necrotizing myopathy, 1951
    for Duchenne muscular dystrophy, 1923
    for giant-cell arteritis, 1694
    for medication overuse headache, 1708
    for myasthenia gravis, 1903t, 1905
Preeclampsia
    defined, 1990
    headache due to, 1694
    and ischemic stroke, 1988
    severe, 1990
Prefrontal cortex (PFC)
    in horizontal eye movements, 556
    in memory, 61, 62f
Pregabalin
    for chronic pain, 726
    for epilepsy
        absorption, elimination half-life, formulations of, 1600t
        efficacy by seizure type of, 1601t
        hepatic metabolism, enzyme induction/inhibition, pharmacokinetic interactions, and protein binding of, 1603t
        mechanism of action of, 1604t
    for neuropathic pain, 918t–919t
    for trigeminal neuralgia, 736
Preganglionic (intraspinal canal) lesions, nerve conduction studies of, 374–375
Preganglionic parasympathetic dysfunction, anisocoria due to, 182–183
Pregnancy
    in adolescence, after stroke, 1006
    cerebrovascular disease in, 1987–1990
        antiphospholipid antibody syndrome as, 1988
        arteriovenous malformations as, 1987
        cerebral venous thrombosis as, 1989–1990

Pregnancy (*Continued*)
intracranial hemorrhage as, 1987
ischemic stroke as, 1987–1988
postpartum stroke as, 1988–1989
eclamptic encephalopathy in, 1990–1991
effect of drugs and toxins during, 1970–1972, 1970*t*
passive addiction and withdrawal syndrome as, 1971–1972
risk for intracranial hemorrhage as, 1971
teratogenic effects and intrauterine growth retardation as, 1971, 1971*f*
epilepsy in, 1984–1987
common advice and management strategy for, 1985–1987, 1986*f*
fetal considerations with, 1984–1985, 1985*f*
maternal considerations with, 1984
ethical considerations in, 1974–1975
headache in, 1975–1976
migraine, 1975–1976
before, 1975–1976
during, 1976
postpartum, 1976
tension, 1975
imaging in, 1975
inborn errors of metabolism during, 1333
leg muscle cramps in, 1976
lumbosacral plexopathy and, 1789
migraine in, 1706
movement disorders in, 1980–1981
chorea gravidarum as, 1980
dystonia as, 1980
Friedreich ataxia as, 1980
Huntington disease as, 1980
Parkinson disease as, 1980–1981
restless legs as, 1980
Tourette syndrome as, 1981
Wilson disease as, 1981
with multiple sclerosis, 1173–1174, 1981–1982
muscle disorders in, 1977–1978
facioscapulohumeral dystrophy as, 1977–1978
inflammatory myopathy as, 1978
limb-girdle muscular dystrophy as, 1978
myotonic dystrophy as, 1977
myasthenia gravis and, 1910, 1976–1977
before, 1976–1977
during, 1977
outcome with, 1977
postpartum, 1977
neurological problems of, 1973–1991
neuromyelitis optica-Devic syndrome, 1982
neuropathy in, 1978–1980
acute polyradiculoneuropathy (Guillain-Barré syndrome) as, 1979
Bell palsy as, 1978
carpal tunnel syndrome as, 1978
Charcot-Marie-Tooth disease type 1 as, 1979
chronic inflammatory demyelinating polyneuropathy as, 1979
gestational polyneuropathy as, 1979
low back pain as, 1978–1979
maternal brachial plexus neuropathy as, 1979
maternal obstetric palsy as, 1979–1980, 1979*f*
meralgia paresthetica, 1979

Pregnancy (*Continued*)
tumors in, 1982–1984
choriocarcinoma as, 1983
idiopathic intracranial hypertension (pseudotumor cerebri) as, 1983–1984
pituitary, 1983
primary brain, 1982–1983
Wernicke encephalopathy in, 1981
Pregnancy in Multiple Sclerosis (PRIMS), 1173–1174
Prehypertension, as risk factor, for stroke, 921–922
Premature ejaculation, 633
Premature infants, hypoxic-ischemic brain injury in, 1963
Premotor area, upper motor neurons in, 1484
Premotor cortex, upper motor neurons in, 1484
Premotor region, in praxis, 116
Prenatal diagnosis, of spinal muscular atrophy, 1503
Prenatal testing, for Huntington disease, 1446
Prenuclear gaze disturbances, 563
Preoccipital cortex, in vergence, 558
Preorgasmic headache, 1714
PRES. *see* Posterior reversible encephalopathy syndrome (PRES)
Presbycusis, 597
Presenilin 1 (PSEN1) Chromosome 14, in Alzheimer disease, 1394
Presenilin 2 (PSEN2) Chromosome 1, in Alzheimer disease, 1394
Present illness, history of, 2–3
Pressure palsies
hereditary neuropathy with liability to, 269, 1818, 1819*f*
hereditary neuropathy with liability to, copy number variation in, 668*t*
monoplegia due to, 268–269
in polyneuropathy, 269
Prestriate cortex, 557
Presurgical brain mapping, functional neuroimaging of, 499–500
Presynaptic neuromuscular junction disorders, repetitive nerve stimulation for
rapid, 388, 388*t*
slow, 387, 388*t*
Pretectum, and vergence, 558
PREVAIL (Prevention of VTE after Acute Ischemic Stroke with LMWH) study, 964
Prevalence rate
defined, 635–636
for epilepsy, 640, 640*f*–641*f*
lifetime, 635–636
for multiple sclerosis, 641, 642*f*
for neurological disorders
less common, 647*t*
most common, 646*t*
for Parkinson disease, 644
point, 635–636
of stroke, 637
Prevention of VTE after Acute Ischemic Stroke with LMWH (PREVAIL) study, 964
Previous illness, history of, 3
Prezista (darunavir), for HIV infection, 1108*t*–1109*t*
PRF (pontine reticular formation), in REM sleep, 1624.*e*1

Primary α-dystroglycanopathy deficiency, 1927
Primary angiitis of CNS, and stroke in children, 1000
Primary aphasia, neuropsychological characteristics of, 522–523
Primary central nervous system lymphoma, management of
AIDS-related, 1063
for non-AIDS related disease, 1062–1063
Primary CNS lymphoma (PCNSL), 495, 496*f*
HIV-associated, 1117, 1118*f*
pathology and molecular genetics of, 1041–1042, 1042*f*
structural imaging of, 418*t*–419*t*, 423, 424*f*
Primary deviation, 530, 532*f*
Primary erythermalgia, 1520*t*–1521*t*
Primary generalized seizure, 1566
Primary headache, 197, 198*b*
Primary lateral sclerosis, 1486–1487
diagnosis of, 1487
key characteristics, 1487*t*
treatment of, 1487
Primary progressive aphasia (PPA), 1407–1408
functional neuroimaging of
logopenic variant, 489, 489*f*
nonfluent variant, 489–490
semantic variant, 489–490
language and speech disorders in, 140–141, 142*f*
semantic variant, 1407–1408
Primary progressive multiple sclerosis (PPMS), 688
age of onset of, 1163–1164
clinical course of, 1172
Primary sensory areas, 94
Primary sensory cortex, 57
Primary stabbing headaches, 198–199
Primary store, in repetitive nerve stimulation, 386
Primary systemic amyloidosis, 1838–1839
clinical features of, 1838–1839, 1839*f*
Primary thunderclap headache, 1715
Primary vestibular afferent nerve fibers, 585, 585*f*
Primary visual cortex, 58
Primary writing tremor, 231
Primidone (Mysoline)
for epilepsy
absorption, elimination half-life, formulations of, 1600*t*
efficacy by seizure type of, 1601*t*
hepatic metabolism, enzyme induction/inhibition, pharmacokinetic interactions, and protein binding of, 1603*t*
mechanism of action of, 1604*t*
for Parkinson disease, 1433*t*–1434*t*
during pregnancy, and vitamin K deficiency, 1986
for tremor
essential, 1444
in multiple sclerosis, 1182
Priming, 63–64
for memory disturbances, 807
Primitive neuroectodermal tumor (PNET)
pediatric, 1065–1069
background of, 1065
classification of, 1065
clinical presentation of, 1067
diagnosis of, 1067
etiology of, 1065–1067
management of, 1067–1069

Primitive neuroectodermal tumor (PNET)
(Continued)
prognosis of, 1069
risk stratification for, 1067–1068
staging of, 1067–1068
supratentorial, 1067
structural imaging of, 424
Primitive neuroectodermal tumors (PNET)
cerebellar, 1038
pathology and molecular genetics of, 1038–1039
peripheral nervous system, 1038
supratentorial, management of, 1060
Primitive reflexes, in vegetative state, 54
PRIMS (Pregnancy in Multiple Sclerosis), 1173–1174
Principle of parsimony, 6
Prion, defined, 1365
Prion decontamination, 1377
Prion diseases, 1365–1379
animal, 1377–1378
defined, 1365
fatal familial insomnia, 1374
molecular classification, 1369–1370
genetic, 1373–1374, 1373*f*
Gerstmann-Sträussler-Scheinker Disease as, 1366*f*, 1374
human, 1365–1367
clinical aspects of, 1367–1370
differential diagnosis of, 1378–1379
epidemiology, 1365
treatments of, 1378
kuru as, 1369–1370
neuropathology of, 1369*f*
prion decontamination of, 1377
sporadic, 1367–1370
Prion protein, 1367*f*, 1379*f*
Prion protein gene (PRNP), 1367*f*, 1369*t*
human prion protein gene, 1373*f*
Prion-related protein (PrP), 1365
Prion-specific diagnostic test, development of, 1372–1373
Prisms, 536–537, 537*f*, 539
PRNP (prion protein gene), 1367*f*, 1369*t*
Probabilistic classification learning, 63–64
Probe, 651*t*
Probst bundles, 446.*e*5
Procarbazine, for brain tumors, 1052*t*–1053*t*
complications of, 1048
Procedural memory, 61*t*, 63
in Alzheimer disease, 1387
Procedural skills, 63*t*
"Procerus sign", 227
Process-oriented therapies, for developmental coordination disorders, 1317
Prochlorperazine
for migraine, 1701
menstrual, 1704
during pregnancy, 1706
for migraine in children and adolescents, 1719
Procyclidine, for dystonia, 1452*t*
Prodrome
with dissociative (nonepileptic) attack, 1995, 1996*f*
with simple partial seizures, 1567
Productivity, excessive daytime sleepiness and, 1632
Proenkephalins, 697*t*–698*t*
Progestins, for migraine, in menopause, 1706
Proglucagon, 697*t*–698*t*
Prognosis, explanation of, 717–718
Programmed cell death, 1283–1284
disorders of, 1283–1284

Progranulin (PGRN) mutations, 1410
Progranulin protein, 1413
Progressive agrammatic/(nonfluent) aphasia, 1407
Progressive damage, after traumatic brain injury, 852–853, 853*f*
Progressive dialysis dementia, in children, 848
Progressive encephalomyelitis with rigidity and myoclonus (PERM), 1191, 1200
horizontal gaze palsies due to, 565
Progressive external ophthalmoplegia (PEO), 1358, 1945–1946
ataxia in, 1470
mitochondrial myopathies without, 1358
myopathy in, 1945–1946
for neuro-ophthalmological examination, 1355
Progressive facial hemiatrophy, 1558
clinical features of, 1558, 1558*f*
Progressive multifocal leukoencephalopathy (PML), 1132–1133, 1134*f*
hemiplegia due to, 264–265
HIV-associated, 1114*t*, 1115–1117, 1116*f*
structural imaging of, 436.*e*5
Progressive multiple sclerosis, pathology of, 1162
Progressive muscular atrophy, 1505–1506
clinical features of, 1505
differential diagnosis of, 1505–1506
etiology of, 1505
laboratory studies of, 1505
treatment of, 1506
Progressive myoclonus epilepsies (PME), 1579–1580
Progressive postpoliomyelitis muscular atrophy (PPMA), 1497–1498, 1497*b*
Progressive relapsing multiple sclerosis, 688, 1172
Progressive rubella panencephalitis, 1143–1144
Progressive supranuclear palsy (PSP), 1404–1405, 1439–1440, 1439*f*
clinical features of, 1439–1440
diagnosis of, 1439
dysphagia in, 154
falls due to, 20
functional neuroimaging for, 493, 494*f*
neurodegenerative disorders, 1342
pathology, 1406*f*
pseudo-, 559*f*, 560–563
structural imaging for, 445.*e*1–445.*e*2, 445.*e*1*f*
transcranial magnetic stimulation for, 394–395
Progressive systemic sclerosis, neurological complications of, 822
Proinsulin, 697*t*–698*t*
Projected pain, due to spinal lesions, 277
Prolactin, 697*t*–698*t*
hypothalamic peptides controlling release of, 702*t*
immunoregulatory effects of, 699*t*
during sleep, 1631
Prolactin-releasing peptide, 697*t*–698*t*
Prolactinoma
medical management of, 710–711
during pregnancy, 1983
Promethazine, for migraine in children and adolescents, 1719
PROMM. *see* Proximal myotonic myopathy (PROMM)
Promoters, 649, 651*t*
Pronator teres syndrome, 270, 1804
Pro-opiomelanocortin, 697*t*–698*t*
Prophylactic cranial irradiation (PCI), 1087

Prophylactic hypothermia, for traumatic brain injury, 875*t*–876*t*
Propofol
half-life of, 1203*t*
with induced hypothermia for cardiopulmonary arrest, 1204*b*
Proportionate mortality (PMR), for epilepsy, 638
Propranolol (Inderal)
for essential tremor, 1444
for migraine prophylaxis, 1702
in children and adolescents, 1719
for Parkinson disease, 1433*t*–1434*t*
for tremor, in multiple sclerosis, 1182
Propriospinal myoclonus, at sleep onset, 1661
Proptosis, 186–187
in diplopia, 534
Propulsion, 254
Prosaposin, 1334
Prosopagnosia, 125
Prostaglandin E$_1$, for erectile dysfunction, 621
Prostaglandin E$_2$ (PGE$_2$), in fever, 700
Prostaglandins, in menstrual migraine, 1704
Prostheses, neural, 804
Prosthetic heart valves, cardiogenic embolism with, 934
Prostigmin Bromide (Neostigmine bromide), for myasthenia gravis, 1904, 1904*t*
Prostigmin Methylsulfate (Neostigmine methylsulfate), for myasthenia gravis, 1904*t*
Protamine sulfate, for intracerebral hemorrhage, 980
Protease inhibitors (PIs), for HIV infection, 1108*t*–1109*t*
Proteasome inhibitors, for brain tumors, 1053, 1054*b*
Protein
defined, 651*t*
toxic, and neurodegenerative movement disorders, 1426*t*
translation into, 650–652, 650*f*
Protein aggregation
in amyotrophic lateral sclerosis, 1507
neurodegenerative movement disorders due to, 1426–1427
Protein C deficiency
ischemic stroke due to, 946
and stroke in children, 1005
Protein deposition, abnormal, chemical imaging of, 505*t*, 506
Protein kinase C (PKC), inhibition of, for brain tumors, 1053, 1054*b*
Protein misfolding cyclic amplification (PMCA), 1372–1373
Protein O- mannosyltransferase 1 (POMT1), 1926, 1930
Protein O-mannose-β-1,2-N-acetylglucosaminyl transferase (POMGnT1), 1927, 1930
Protein O-mannosyltransferase 2 (POMT2), 1927, 1930
Protein S deficiency
ischemic stroke due to, 946
and stroke in children, 1005–1006
Proteinaceous infectious particle, 1365
Protein-calorie malnutrition, 1236
Protein-related offs, in Parkinson disease, 1435
Proteolipid protein, in multiple sclerosis, 1163
Proteolipid protein 1 (PLP1), in hereditary spastic paraplegia, 1487–1488
Proteus syndrome, 1553

Proton density weighting, 415
Proton MR spectroscopic techniques, of hepatic encephalopathy, 1211–1212
Proton radiosurgery, for brain tumors, 1050
Protriptyline, for migraine, 1702–1703
PROUD (Pramipexole on Underlying Disease) study, 1432
Prourokinase, intracerebral hemorrhage due to, 971, 972f
Prourokinase in Acute Cerebral Thromboembolism (PROACT) II trial, 958
Proust, Marcel, 60
Proximal diabetic neuropathy, 1842
Proximal great vessels, ultrasonography of, 477–478
Proximal latency, of compound muscle action potential, 367–368, 367f
Proximal myotonic myopathy (PROMM), 1936
Proximal segment changes, in wallerian degeneration, 906
Proximal sensory loss, 320
PrP (prion-related protein), 1365
PRRs. *see* Pattern recognition receptors (PRRs)
Prusiner, Stanley, 1365
PS1 (presenilin-1) Chromosome 14, in Alzheimer disease, 1394
PS2 (presenilin-2) Chromosome 1, in Alzheimer disease, 1394
PSA (posterior spinal arteries), 1007.e1, 1007.e1f
Psammoma bodies, 1039, 1040f
PSD (poststroke depression), 99–100
Pseudallescheria boydii, brain abscess due to, 1154
Pseudo-Cushing syndrome, 706
Pseudo-Foster Kennedy syndrome, 167
Pseudo-progressive supranuclear palsy (pseudo-PSP) syndrome, 559f, 560–563
Pseudoachondroplasia, 1738
Pseudoaneurysm
    subarachnoid hemorrhage with, 992f
    traumatic, 867
Pseudoathetosis, in peripheral nerve disorders, 1796–1797
Pseudobobbing, v-pattern pretectal, 551, 551t
Pseudobulbar affect
    in amyotrophic lateral sclerosis, 85
    in multiple sclerosis, 84, 85t, 104–105, 1167
    in stroke, 90
Pseudobulbar laughing or crying, in amyotrophic lateral sclerosis, 1513t
Pseudobulbar palsy
    in amyotrophic lateral sclerosis, 1508
    due to upper motor neuron impairment, 1486
Pseudochereria boydii, meningitis due to, 1153
Pseudocoma, 34–35, 35t
    versus metabolic or structural coma, 47–48
Pseudodominant pattern of inheritance, 658
Pseudoepileptic seizures, 1590
Pseudohypertrophy, 282–283
    in Duchenne muscular dystrophy, 1921, 1922f
Pseudomigraine with temporary neurological symptoms, lymphocytic pleocytosis and, 1690
Pseudomonas aeruginosa, neonatal meningitis due to, 1965

Pseudoneuritic presentation (flail leg), in amyotrophic lateral sclerosis, 1510
Pseudopalisades, 1028, 1028f
Pseudopapilledema, 173–174, 173f, 173t
Pseudopseudoseizures, 15
Pseudoptosis, 188, 568
Pseudorosette, perivascular, 1028f
Pseudoseizures, 15, 1590
Pseudo-status epilepticus, 1591
Pseudotumor cerebri, 1688
Pseudoxanthoma elasticum
    ischemic stroke due to, 943–944
    and stroke in children, 998
Psilocin, in mushrooms, 1251t
Psilocybin, in mushrooms, 1251t
Psychiatric conditions, *versus* delirium, 32
Psychiatric illness, sleep disturbances in, 1671
Psychiatric manifestations
    catatonia as, 111
    delirium as, 110–111
    depression-related cognitive impairment as, 110
    due to degenerative, 105–109
        Alzheimer disease as, 106
        epilepsy as, 107–109
        frontotemporal dementia as, 106–107
        Huntington disease as, 107
        idiopathic Parkinson disease, 107
        Lewy body dementia as, 107
    infectious, 101–102
        Creutzfeldt-Jakob disease, 101–102
        Human Immunodeficiency Virus, 101
        neurosyphilis, 102
    metabolic and toxic, 102–105, 102.e1t
        drug abuse as, 104
        multiple sclerosis as, 104–105
        porphyrias as, 103–104
        systemic lupus erythematosus as, 104
        thyroid disease as, 102–103
        vitamin B$_{12}$ and folic acid deficiency as, 103
        Wilson disease as, 103
    neoplastic, 105
    neurological abnormalities in, 99.e1t
    of neurological disease, 99–111
    traumatic brain injury, 109–110
    vascular, stroke and cerebral vascular disease, 99–101, 100b
Psychiatric neurosurgery, 113–114
Psychiatry, functional symptoms in, 1993t
Psychic dependence, 1254
Psychodynamic psychotherapies, for functional symptoms, 2006–2007
Psychogenic convergence paralysis, 570
Psychogenic disorder, 2
Psychogenic gait disorders, 260–261
Psychogenic movement disorders, 1460
Psychogenic nonepileptic events, 1590
Psychogenic nonepileptic seizure (PNES), 15, 16t, 526, 1590–1591
Psychogenic weakness, 286
Psychological treatment, for functional symptoms, 2006–2007, 2007t
Psychologists, in rehabilitation, 789
Psychomotor activity, altered, in delirium, 25–26
Psychophysical tests, of chemosensory function, 192
Psychosis, 92–114, 92.e1b
    in Alzheimer disease, 78–79, 79f, 79t
    in autism spectrum disorder, 1307t
    biology of, 97–98

Psychosis (*Continued*)
    clinical symptoms and signs suggesting neurological disease, 99
    degenerative, 105–109
        Alzheimer disease as, 106
        epilepsy as, 107–109
        frontotemporal dementia as, 106–107
        Huntington disease as, 107
        idiopathic Parkinson disease, 107
        Lewy body dementia as, 107
    in dementia with Lewy bodies, 82
    in epilepsy, 88–89
    in Huntington disease, 83
    infectious, 101–102
        with Creutzfeldt-Jakob disease, 101–102
        with human immunodeficiency virus, 101
        with neurosyphilis, 102
    metabolic and toxic
        drug abuse as, 104
        multiple sclerosis as, 104–105
        porphyrias as, 103–104
        systemic lupus erythematosus as, 104
        vitamin B$_{12}$ and folic acid deficiency as, 103
        Wilson disease as, 103
    neuroanatomy corresponding, 93t
        cortical networks, 94–97
    in Parkinson disease, 80t–81t, 81
    principles
        of differential diagnosis, 92–93, 93t
        of neuropsychiatric evaluation, 93–94, 95f
    in stroke, 90
    in traumatic brain injury, 109–110
    treatment modalities, 111–114
        electroconvulsive therapy as, 113
        psychiatric neurosurgery (psychosurgery) as, 113–114
        repetitive transcranial magnetic stimulation as, 113
        vagus nerve stimulation as, 113
    treatment principles of, 114
Psychosomatic disorder, 1993
Psychostimulants, 1255b
    drug dependence with, 1255–1256
    overdose, treatment of, 1256, 1256b
    withdrawal from, 1256
Psychosurgery, 113–114
PTALE (post-transplant acute limbic encephalitis), 1132
PTEN gene, in diffuse gliomas, 1033
Pterygopalatine ganglion, 1726f
PTO (parietotemporo-occipital junction), in control of eye movements, 552
Ptosis, 187f
    acquired, 188
    cerebral, 188
    congenital, 188
    in diplopia, 534
    enhanced, 187
    in myasthenia gravis, 1897, 1897f, 1899
    in oculopharyngeal muscular dystrophy, 188, 1932–1933, 1932f
    pseudo-, 188
PTU (paroxysmal tonic upward) gaze, "benign", 568–569
Puberty
    delayed or absent, 703–704
    precocious, 704
Puborectalis muscle, in control of defecation, 606
Pudendal nerve terminal motor latency (PNTML), 616

Pudendal somatosensory evoked potentials, 616
"Pull test", 254
Pulmonary arteriovenous fistula, in hereditary hemorrhagic telangiectasia, 1550
Pulmonary arteriovenous malformations, in hereditary hemorrhagic telangiectasia, 1550
Pulmonary complications
 of acute ischemic stroke, 963
 in neurointensive care, 752
Pulmonary features, of autonomic disorders, 1870
Pulmonary function tests, in sleep disorders, 1678
Pulpitis, headache due to, 1695
Pulsed-wave Doppler, 476–477
Pulseless disease, neurological complications of, in children, 839
Pulvinar sign, in Creutzfeldt-Jakob disease, 1372f
Pupil
 anatomy of, 179, 180f–181f
 Argyll-Robertson, 186
 diencephalic, 42
 examination of, 574–576, 575t, 576b, 576f
 Marcus Gunn, 179–180, 575–576, 576b, 576f
 midposition, 42
 neural control of, 179, 180f–181f
 normal phenomena, 179
 tadpole, 186
 tonic, 180, 183f
Pupil reactivity
 in coma, 42–43, 43f–44f, 47
 measurement of, 574, 575t
Pupil size
 in coma, 42–43, 43f–44f, 47
 measurement of, 574, 575t
 neural control of, 179
Pupillary abnormalities, 179–186
 afferent, 179–180
 anisocoria
  episodic, 186
  greater in dark, 184–186
   due to Horner syndrome, 184–185, 184f–185f
   due to iritis, 185–186
   due to pupillary light-near dissociation, 186
  episodic, 186
  greater in light, 180–184
   due to iris sphincter injury and ischemia, 183
   due to pharmacological mydriasis, 183–184
   due to postganglionic parasympathetic dysfunction, 180–182, 183f
   due to preganglionic parasympathetic dysfunction, 182–183
 efferent, 180–186
Pupillary defect, relative afferent, 179–180
Pupillary dilation, wide, 42
Pupillary eyedrop testing, 181t
Pupillary light reflex, 179
 in toxic and metabolic encephalopathies, 1209
Pupillary light-near dissociation, 186
Pupillary near response, 180
Pupillary unrest, 179
Pupilloconstrictor pathway, parasympathetic, 43f

Pure agraphia, 139
Pure autonomic failure (PAF), 1885–1886, 1886t
 neurogenic bladder dysfunction due to, 609
Pure menstrual migraine (PMM), 1704
Pure word deafness, 126, 126f
Pure-tone testing, 601, 602f
Purine bases, 649
Purine metabolism, disorders of, 1339
Purkinje cells
 after cardiac arrest, 1201, 1202f
 in dominant ataxias, 1473
Purple toe syndrome, ischemic stroke due to, 945
Purpura
 Henoch-Schönlein, neurological complications of, 839
 idiopathic thrombocytopenic, intracerebral hemorrhage due to, 969–971
 thrombotic thrombocytopenic, ischemic stroke due to, 949
 in viral CNS disease, 1123t
Pursuit, disorders of, 219
Pursuit movements
 bidirectionally defective, 552
 control of, 557, 558f
 development of, 560
 in diplopia, 535, 535f
Pursuit pathways, 557, 558f
Pursuit system, 552
Purulent maxillary sinus, 1686
Putaminal hemorrhage, 976–977, 978t, 981–982, 976.e1f
Putaminal slit sign, 445.e2
PVEM (postvaccinal encephalomyelitis), 1135.e1
PVN. see Paraventricular nucleus (PVN)
PWI (perfusion-weighted imaging) of ischemic stroke, 431, 431f
Pyknolepsy, 1576–1577
Pyogenic vertebral osteomyelitis, 1759–1760, 1760f
Pyomyositis, 1953
 HIV-associated, 1120
Pyramidal tract, motor system anatomy of, 262
Pyramidal tract syndrome, 274
Pyrethroids, occupational exposure to, 1241
Pyrexia
 coma with, 38
 in multiple sclerosis, 610
Pyridostigmine, for autonomic disorders, 1894
Pyridostigmine bromide (Mestinon Bromide), for myasthenia gravis, 1904, 1904t
Pyridoxal, 1230
Pyridoxamine, 1230
Pyridoxine
 neuropathy due to, 1862
 for tremor, in multiple sclerosis, 1182
Pyridoxine (vitamin B_6) deficiency, 1230–1231, 1852
Pyridoxine-dependent seizure, 1958
Pyrimidine bases, 649
Pyrimidine metabolism, disorders of, 1339
Pyriminil, occupational exposure to, 1241
Pyrophosphate analog, for viral infections, 1127t
Pyrroline-5′-carboxylic acid synthetase deficiency, 1326.e1t–1326.e2t
Pyruvate carboxylase (PC) deficiency, 1337, 1328.e1t

Q

QSART. see Quantitative sudomotor axon reflex test (QSART)
QT interval, prolonged, in Andersen-Tawil syndrome, 1527
Quadriplegic myopathy, acute, 1955
Quality of life, excessive daytime sleepiness and, 1632
Quantitative sudomotor axon reflex test (QSART), 1875
 for peripheral nerve disorders, 1798
Quantum, in repetitive nerve stimulation, 386
Queen Square mitochondrial disease investigation pathway, 1359f
Quetiapine (Seroquel), for dystonia, 1452t

R

RA. see Rheumatoid arthritis (RA)
RAB7 gene, in Charcot-Marie-Tooth disease, 1815–1816
Rabbit syndrome, 232–234
Rabies, 1140–1141
 diagnosis of, 1140
 differential diagnosis of, 1140
 dysphagia due to, 156
 neuropathological characteristic of, 1140, 1140f
 postexposure prophylaxis for, 1141
 preexposure prophylaxis for, 1141
 treatment for, 1141
Rabies immunoglobulin (RIG), 1131t
Raccoon eyes, with coma, 39
Race, and stroke, 921t
Rachischisis, 1282
[^{11}C]Raclopride, in chemical imaging
 of epilepsy, 509
 of Parkinson disease, 507–508
Radar equipment, and brain tumors, 1021–1022
Radial glial fiber, in neuroblast migration, 1284–1286, 1285f
Radial nerve, applied anatomy of, 1806
Radial nerve compression, 1806
Radial nerve entrapment, 1801t
Radial nerve palsy, monoplegia due to, 270
Radial neuropathy, sensory abnormalities due to, 321
Radial sensory neuropathy, superficial, 1807
"Radial tunnel", 1806
Radial tunnel syndrome, 1807
Radial veins, 1007.e1–1007.e2
Radiation
 for brain tumor, complications of, 1048
 detection of, 504
Radiation damage, visual loss from, 162
Radiation exposure, brain tumors and, 1021–1022
Radiation leukoencephalopathy, structural imaging of, 440.e1, 440.e2f
Radiation myelopathy
 spinal cord compression versus, 1092
 spinal cord infarction due to, 1009
Radiation necrosis, 1083.e1
Radiation plexopathy
 lumbosacral plexopathy and, 1790
 monoplegia due to, 271
Radiation somnolence syndrome (RSS), 1083.e1
Radiation therapy
 for brain metastases, 1086–1087
  after surgical resection, 1087–1088
  prophylactic, 1087
  with stereotactic radiosurgery, 1089–1090

Radiation therapy (Continued)
    toxicity of, 1087
    whole-brain, 1089
    for brain tumors, 1050–1051
        brachytherapy as, 1050
        conventional fractionated, 1050
        sensitization of tumor cells to ionizing
            radiation in, 1050
        stereotactic radiosurgery techniques in,
            1050–1051
    complications from, in pediatric nervous
        system tumors, 1083.e1–1083.e2
    effects of
        ionizing, 1245
            encephalopathy due to, 1245
            myelopathy due to, 1245
            plexopathy due to, 1245
        nonionizing, 1245–1246
    for leptomeningeal metastases, 1098
    peripheral nerve injury due to, 908
    for spinal cord compression, 1093–1094
        with surgery, 1094
Radiation Therapy Oncology Group (RTOG),
    1086
Radiation vasculopathy, ischemic stroke due
    to, 937
Radiation-induced plexopathy, 1784
Radicular arteries, 1007.e1
Radiculitis, arm and neck pain due to, 328
Radiculomedullary veins, 1007.e1–1007.e2
Radiculopathies
    cervical, 1752–1753
        clinical presentation of, 1752–1753
        imaging of, 1752–1753, 1753f
        treatment of, 1753
    infectious, 1775–1777
        herpes zoster as, 1776–1777
        Lyme radiculoneuropathy as, 1776
        polyradiculoneuropathy in human
            immunodeficiency virus-infected
            patients as, 1775–1776, 1776f
        tabes dorsalis as, 1775
    leg pain due to, 336t
    lower back pain and leg pain due to, 335t
    monoplegia due to, 270–271, 270t
    needle electromyography of, 382, 382f
    sensory abnormalities due to, 321, 321t
    simulating motor neuron disease, 1779
    traumatic, 1768–1772
        due to disk herniation, 1769–1772,
            1769f
            clinical features of, 1770–1771, 1770f
            diagnosis of, 1771–1772, 1772f
            treatment of, 1772
        due to nerve root avulsion, 1768–1769
            clinical features and diagnosis of,
                1768
            treatment of, 1768–1769
Radiofrequency lesioning, 729t
Radiofrequency (RF) radiation, and brain
    tumors, 1021–1022
Radiographically isolated syndrome (RIS), of
    multiple sclerosis, 1173
Radioisotope, for positron emission
    tomography, 504
Radioisotope studies, for cerebrospinal fluid
    leaks, 202
Radioligands, 509
Radionecrosis, 1083.e1
Radionuclides
    for PET, 487
    for SPECT, 487
Radiosurgery, for epilepsy, 1611
Radiotherapy, for pituitary tumors, 711

Radiotracer, positron-emitting, 486–487
Raf/MEK/ERK pathway, inhibition of, for
    brain tumors, 1053, 1054b
Ragged-red fiber (RRF), 1356–1358
Ragged-red fiber myopathy, myoclonic
    epilepsy with, 1358
Raltegravir (Isentres), for HIV infection,
    1108t–1109t
Ramsay Hunt syndrome, 243, 1715–1716,
    1722t, 1730, 1776–1777
RAPD (relative afferent pupillary defect),
    179–180, 574, 576b, 576f
Rapid eye movement sleep, 1615, 1668f
    dreams during, 1623.e1
    muscle hypotonia or atonia during, 1625
    neuroanatomical substrates for,
        1623–1625
    sleep staging, 1619f
Rapid eye movement sleep behavior disorder
    in anti-LGI1 limbic encephalitis, 1199
    features of, 1665b
    parasomnias, 1663–1666, 1666f–1667f
Rapid initial examination, for coma, 35–37
Rapid plasma reagin (RPR), 1149
Rapid repetitive nerve stimulation, 388,
    388t, 389f
Rapidly progressive dementias, 1420, 1421b
Rapid-onset dystonia parkinsonism (RDP),
    1454
Rapsyn mutations, 1911
Rare variants
    and candidate gene resequencing,
        665–666, 665f
    common disease with, 665f, 666
    common versus, 653–654
    defined, 665
Ras signaling pathway, inhibition of, for
    brain tumors, 1054b
Rasagiline, for Parkinson disease,
    1433t–1434t
Rashes, in coma, 40t
Rasmussen encephalitis, 695
Rasmussen syndrome, 1579, 1579f
Rathke cleft cysts, pathology and molecular
    genetics of, 1043–1044
Rathke pouch, 702
Ravel, Maurice, 127
Raw test scores, in neuropsychological
    evaluation, 513
Raymond syndrome, 1722t, 1728
RB1 gene, in diffuse gliomas, 1033
RCDP (rhizomelic chondrodysplasia
    punctata), 1335, 1326.e1t–1326.e2t,
    1333.e1t
RDP (rapid-onset dystonia parkinsonism),
    1454
Reactive arthritis
    clinical presentation of, 1762
    neurological complications of, 1763b
    pathogenesis of, 1762
Reactive gliosis, in chronic ischemic stroke,
    432, 432.e1f
Reactive postural responses, 254
Readers
    compensated, 1315
    persistently poor, 1315
Reading
    assessment of, 131
    neurolinguistic model of, 139f
Re-bleeding, after subarachnoid hemorrhage,
    993
Rebound headache, 199, 1704–1705
Rebound nystagmus, 542t, 547
    in ataxia, 219

Recall bias, in studies of brain tumors,
    1021–1022
Recanalization, after endovascular treatment
    of intracranial aneurysm, 992–993
Receiver coils, in MRI, 413
"Recent onset" headache, 197
Recent-onset seizures, 1592–1594
    electroencephalography in, 1593–1594,
        1593f
    history in, 1592–1593
    neuroimaging in, 1594
    other testing in, 1594
    physical and neurological examination in,
        1593
Recessive, defined, 651t
Recessive X-linked transmission, 659, 660f
Reciprocal gait orthoses, 789–790
Reciprocal inhibition, Sherrington law of,
    528–529
Reckless gait patterns, 260
Recombinant activated factor VII (rFVIIa),
    for intracerebral hemorrhage, 982
Recombinant prourokinase (r-pro-UK), for
    acute ischemic stroke, 958
Recombinant tissue plasminogen activator
    (rtPA), for acute ischemic stroke,
    956–957
Recording electrodes, for nerve conduction
    studies, 367
Recording procedure, for nerve conduction
    studies, 367
Recreational therapists, 789
Recruitment curve, for motor evoked
    potentials, 392, 394t
Recruitment frequency, of motor unit action
    potentials, 381
    early or rapid, 381
Recruitment ratio, of motor unit action
    potentials, 381
Rectal stimulation, 606
    processing of, 606
Rectum, 606
Recumbency, 1688–1689
Red desaturation, 574
Red glass test, for diplopia, 536, 536f
Redirection, for Alzheimer disease, 77–78,
    78t
Redox state, 1354
Reducing body myopathy, 1920t–1921t,
    1927
Reducing substances (urine), in inborn
    errors of metabolism, 1326t
Reduplicative paramnesia
    after stroke, 100–101
    in delirium, 26
Reelin (RLN) gene, in neuroblast migration,
    1286
Re-emergent tremor, 227, 231
Reflex(es), pathological, due to upper motor
    neuron impairment, 1486
Reflex blepharospasm, 188
Reflex cardiac arrhythmias, syncope due to,
    11
Reflex ocular movements, 44–45, 45t–46t,
    47
Reflex otalgia, 1732
Reflex sympathetic dystrophy (RSD), 235
    dystonia with, 1444
Reflex syncope, 1877–1878
Reflex voiding, 616–617
Reflexes
    "altered", 1996
    muscle weakness due to, 284
    primitive, in hypotonic infant, 306–307

Reflexogenic erection, 622
Reflux esophagitis, sleep disturbances with, 1670
Refractory seizures, in anti-GABA_A receptor encephalitis, 1199
Refsum disease, 1818.e9
Regional cerebral blood flow (CBF)
    monitoring, in neurointensive care, 744t, 747–748
    laser Doppler flowmetry for, 744t, 748
    thermal diffusion flowmetry for, 744t, 748
    xenon-133, 744t, 747
Regression, 72
Regulatory factors, in immune response, 682
Regulatory T cells (T_reg), in self-tolerance, 684–685
Rehabilitation, 784–813
    aims of, 784–785
    biological bases for, 792–793
        network and neuronal plasticity as, 793b
    for cognitive and behavioral disabilities, 804–810, 805b
        affective disorders as, 810
            incidence of, 810
            treatment of, 810
        aphasia as, 805–806
            outcomes of, 806
            pharmacological adjuncts in, 806
            treatments in, 805–806
        apraxia as, 806
        attentional disorders as, 806–807
        behavioral disorders as, 809–810
            treatments in, 809–810, 809b–810b
        hemineglect as, 808–809
            frequency of, 808–809
            treatments in, 809, 809b
        memory disturbances as, 807–808
            frequency of, 807
            outcomes of, 808
            pharmacological adjuncts in, 807–808, 808b
            treatments in, 807, 808b
    frequency of complications in, 793–794
        with spinal cord injury, 793–794, 794t
        with stroke, 793, 794t
        with traumatic brain injury, 794
    functional outcomes with, 810–813
        and aging with neurological disabilities, 813
        for multiple sclerosis, 812–813
        for other diseases, 813
        for Parkinson disease, 812
        for spinal cord injury, 811–812
        for stroke, 810–811, 810t
            ambulation as, 811
            self-care skills as, 811
        for traumatic brain injury, 810t, 812
    future directions for, 813
    as goal of treatment, 715
    goals and structure of, 784–792
    for impairments and disabilities, 799–804
        acupuncture as, 802
        bimanual upper extremity therapy as, 801
        brain-computer interfaces as, 804
        brain stimulation as, 803–804
        constraint-induced upper extremity therapy as, 801
        functional neuromuscular stimulation as, 803, 803f
        gait training as, 799–801, 800f–801f
        instrumented biofeedback as, 802

Rehabilitation (Continued)
        mechanical and robotic-assistive devices as, 802–803
            for mobility, 802–803
            for upper extremities, 802
        mirror therapy and imagery as, 802
        mobile health and wireless sensing devices as, 804
        neural prostheses as, 804
        pharmacological adjuncts as, 804
        virtual reality training as, 801–802
        visual field deficits as, 802
    measurement tools for, 790–791, 791b
    neuromedical problems during, 793–799
        bowel and bladder dysfunction as, 796–797, 796t
        central pain as, 797
        contractures as, 795
        dysautonomia as, 795–796
        dysphagia as, 794–795
        fatigue as, 797
        heterotopic ossification as, 795
        management of, 794–799
        skin ulcers as, 795
        sleep disorders as, 797
        spasticity and upper motor neuron syndrome as, 797–799
            assessments for, 797–798, 798t
            chemical injections for, 799
            mechanisms of, 797
            pharmacotherapy for, 798–799, 799t
            physical modalities for, 798
            surgical interventions for, 799
            treatment for, 798
    organization of services for, 791–792
    personnel for, 785–790
        nursing as, 785
        occupational therapists as, 787–788
        orthotists as, 789–790
        physical therapists as, 786–787, 786b
        physicians as, 785
        psychologists as, 789
        recreational therapists as, 789
        social workers as, 789
        speech and cognitive therapists as, 788–789
    service provision in, 791–792
        community-based services in, 792
        in inpatient rehabilitation unit, 791–792
    stimulation-facilitation approaches for aphasia, 788–789, 789b
    by stimulation of bulbocavernous reflex, 632
    strategies for, 785–790
        adaptive aids as, 787–788, 788b, 788f
        assistive equipment as, 787
        bracing as, 789–790
        conditioning and strengthening as, 786
        exercise and compensatory functional training as, 786
        motor learning approaches as, 787
        neurophysiological schools as, 786–787
        task-oriented practice as, 787
Reinnervation, after denervation, 1916, 1917f
Re-irradiation, for brain metastases, 1091
Reiter syndrome
    clinical presentation of, 1762
    neurological complications of, 1763b
    pathogenesis of, 1762
Relapsing polychondritis, neurological complications of, 822
Relapsing-remitting multiple sclerosis (RRMS), 688, 1171
    cognitive impairment in, 1166

Relative afferent pupillary defect (RAPD), 179–180, 574, 576b, 576f
Relative risk, 651t
Reliability, of laboratory investigations, 347
Relpax, for migraine, 1701t
REM sleep latency, 1673
Remacemide, for Huntington disease, 1447
Remote memory, test for, 64
Remyelination, in multiple sclerosis, 1161
Renal angiomyolipoma, in tuberous sclerosis, 1539, 1541t
Renal cysts
    in tuberous sclerosis, 1541t
    in von Hippel-Lindau syndrome, 1549
Renal failure
    chronic, sleep disturbances in, 1670
    neurological complications of, 829–830. see also Uremic encephalopathy
Renal transplantation, neurological complications of
    in adults, 830
    in children, 848–849
Renin, during sleep, 1631
Reparative strategies, for traumatic brain injury, 858–859
Repeat expansion disorders, 654f, 655, 656t
Repeat expansion testing, 673t
Repetition, in language examination, 131
Repetition time, in MRI, 414–415, 414f
Repetitive damage, after traumatic brain injury, 853, 854f
Repetitive nerve stimulation (RNS), 386–388
    for myasthenia gravis, 1902
    principles of, 386–387
    rapid, 388, 388t, 389f
    slow, 387–388, 387f, 388t
Repetitive nucleotide expansions, in dominant ataxias, 1473f
Repetitive transcranial magnetic stimulation (rTMS), 113
    basic principles of, 397–398
    for epilepsy, 1610–1611
    rationale for, 397
    therapeutic application of, current concepts of, 398–400
        for amyotrophic lateral sclerosis, 399–400
        for auditory hallucinations and negative symptoms in schizophrenia, 398
        for depression, 398
        for dystonia, 399
        for epilepsy, 400
        for pain and migraine, 399
        for Parkinson disease, 398–399
        for stroke with motor deficits, aphasia, and hemispatial neglect, 399
        for tinnitus, 399
Replacement phenomena, 1147
RER. see Respiratory exchange ratio (RER)
Rescriptor (delavirdine), for HIV infection, 1108t–1109t
Resequencing, 651t
Reserpine, for dystonia, 1452t
Reserve store, in repetitive nerve stimulation, 386
Resolution, 607
Resolution phase, of sexual response, 625
Resonance, in MRI, 413
Respiration
    Cheyne-Stokes, 41
    with coma, 38, 41–42, 47
Respiratory care, for amyotrophic lateral sclerosis, 1514
Respiratory chain, mitochondrial, 1350, 1351f

Respiratory changes, during sleep, 1629–1630
Respiratory complications, in neurointensive care, 752
Respiratory diseases
  neurological complications of, in adults, 822
  in sleep disorders, 1670
Respiratory drive, brain death and, 52–54
Respiratory exchange ratio (RER), 287–288
  for carnitine palmitoyl transferase deficiency, 1942
Respiratory failure
  in amyotrophic lateral sclerosis, 1513t
  with spinal cord injury, 893
  treatment of, 716–717
    ethical considerations in, 716–717
    terminal, 717
Respiratory muscle weakness, differential diagnosis of, 290
Respiratory muscles, electrodiagnosis of, 1678
Respiratory patterns, abnormal, 41, 42f
Respiratory rate
  with coma, 38
  during sleep, 1630t
Respiratory system, functional symptoms in, 1993t
Respiratory weakness, in critically ill patients, 742–743
Responsive neurostimulator (RNS), for epilepsy, 406
Rest tremor
  definition of, 230
  in parkinsonism, 230, 231b
Resting motor threshold (RMT), in transcranial magnetic stimulation, 392
Resting position, of eyes, in coma, 44
Restless leg syndrome (RLS), 1217, 1650–1653, 1650b–1651b
  clinical manifestations of, 1650–1651
  comorbidities with, 1653b
  conditions that mimic, 1652b
  differentiate it from, 1653b
  genome-wide association studies of, 663.e1t–663.e2t
  heritability of, 663t
  pathophysiology of, 1651–1652, 1653f
  periodic limb movements in sleep in, 1654b
  pharmacological treatment of, 1683t
  pharmacotherapy in, 1684b
  upper airway resistance syndrome, 1649.e1, 1649.e1f
Restless legs, in pregnancy, 1980
Restorative theory, of sleep, 1628
Restricted diffusion, 417.e3
Reticular activating system, in consciousness, 59
Reticular passive hypothesis, of NREM sleep, 1625.e1
Reticulospinal tracts, in control of, upper motor neurons, 1485
Retina, in vision, 552
Retinal angiomas, in von Hippel-Lindau disease, 178
Retinal arterial disease, 176–177
  branch retinal artery occlusions and encephalopathy (Susac syndrome) as, 177, 177f
  central retinal artery occlusion, 176f–177f
  ocular ischemic syndrome as, 177
Retinal arterioles, microemboli in, with TIAs, 927

Retinal artery occlusion, 161
  branch, 177
  central, 176f
Retinal artery vasospasm, visual loss due to, 158
Retinal astrocytomas, in tuberous sclerosis, 1543f
Retinal degenerations, 177–178, 177f
Retinal detachment, in incontinentia pigmenti, 1552
Retinal disorders, 176–178
  branch retinal artery occlusions and encephalopathy (Susac syndrome), 177, 177f
  central retinal artery occlusion as, 176f–177f
  retinal arterial disease of, 176–177
    ocular ischemic syndrome, 177
    retinal degenerations, 177–178, 177f
  retinal vein occlusion as, 177, 177f
Retinal ganglion cells, 163
Retinal hamartomas, in tuberous sclerosis, 1541–1542
Retinal hemangioblastomas, in von Hippel-Lindau syndrome, 1549
Retinal ischemia, visual loss due to, 159–161
Retinal migraine, 158
Retinal slip, 560
Retinal vein occlusion, 159
  due to antiphospholipid antibody syndrome, 947.e1f
Retinitis, in viral CNS disease, 1124t
Retinitis pigmentosa (RP), 177, 177f
  with global developmental delay, 69t
  in mitochondrial syndromes, 1360
Retinoblastoma
  structural imaging of, 449.e1, 449.e2f
  trilateral, 1066–1067
Retinocochleocerebral vasculopathy, ischemic stroke due to, 944
Retinol, 1235
Retinopathy
  cancer-associated, 177–178
  idiopathic central serous, 161
  melanoma-associated, 1194
  pigmentary, in mitochondrial disease, 1355
Retinotopic defects, 557
Retrobulbar optic nerve infarction, 159–161
Retrochiasmal visual loss, in mitochondrial disease, 1355
Retrograde/psychogenic amnesia, functional, 2002
Retropulsion, 254
Retrovir (zidovudine), for HIV infection, 1108t–1109t
Rett syndrome
  cognitive and behavioral problems in, 1309t
  copy number variation in, 668t
Reverse bobbing, 550–551
Reverse dipping, 550–551, 551t
Reverse ocular bobbing, 44
Reverse Shapiro syndrome, 698
Reversed Phalen maneuver, 1802
Reversible cerebral segmental vasoconstriction, ischemic stroke due to, 944–945
Reversible posterior leukoencephalopathy syndrome (RPLS), 1269
  postpartum, 1988–1989
Reversible segmental cerebral vasoconstriction (RSCV), 1016
  postpartum, 1988–1989

Review
  of patient-specific information, 3–4
  of systems, 3
Reyataz (atazanavir), for HIV infection, 1108t–1109t
RF (radiofrequency) radiation, and brain tumors, 1021–1022
rFVIIa (recombinant activated factor VII), for intracerebral hemorrhage, 982
Rhabdoid cell, 1039
Rhabdoid tumor
  pathology and molecular genetics of, 1039
  pediatric, 1069–1070
Rhabdomyolysis, 1955
  with muscle pain, 300–302, 300b
Rhabdomyoma, cardiac, in tuberous sclerosis, 1542, 1543f
Rheumatic heart disease, cardiogenic embolism with, 815
Rheumatoid arthritis (RA), 1761–1762
  neurological complications of
    in adults, 821, 821f
  neurological manifestations of, 1761–1762, 1761.e1f
  neuropathy in, 1852.e1
  pathogenesis of, 1761
  of spine, neck pain due to, 330
  systemic presentation of, 1761
Rheumatology, functional symptoms in, 1993t
Rhinorrhea, CSF, 1689–1690
Rhinosinusitis, headache and facial pain due to, 1694–1695
Rhizomelic chondrodysplasia punctata (RCDP), 1335, 1326.e1t–1326.e2t, 1333.e1t
Rhizopus spp., brain abscess due to, 1154
Rhizotomy, for trigeminal neuralgia, 1717
Rhodococcus equi, brain abscess from, 1150
Rhodopsin, 1235
Rhombencephalosynapsis, 1298
Rhombomeric deletions, 1298
Rhythmic movement disorder, 1661
Rhythmic myoclonus, with coma, 46
Ribavirin, for viral infections, 1127t
Riboflavin
  for inborn errors of metabolism, 1338–1339
  for migraine, 1703
Ribonucleic acid (RNA), 649, 650f, 651t
  messenger, 649–650, 650f
Ribonucleic acid viruses, encephalitis and meningitis due to, 1135–1146
Ribosome, 650–652, 650f
Richardson syndrome, 1439–1440
Riche-Cannieu anastomosis, nerve conduction studies with, 371
Rickets, 1749
Rickettsial infections, versus viral nervous system disease, 1124t
Riddoch phenomenon, 576
Rifaximin, for hepatic encephalopathy, 1216
Rift Valley fever virus, 1139.e1
RIG (rabies immunoglobulin), 1131t
Right hemisphere disorders, language in, 139–140
Right hemisphere syndrome, 1315.e1
Rigid spine syndrome, congenital muscular dystrophies with, 1920t–1921t, 1930
Rigidity, 227–228
Riley-Day syndrome, 1882–1883, 1818.e2–1818.e3
Rilpivirine (Edurant), for HIV infection, 1108t–1109t

Riluzole (Rilutek), for amyotrophic lateral sclerosis, 1512

riMLF (rostral interstitial nucleus of medial longitudinal fasciculus), in vertical eye movements, 560, 560f

Rimmed vacuoles, in inclusion body myositis, 1952-1953, 1952f

Rinne test, 591

RIS (radiographically isolated syndrome), of multiple sclerosis, 1173

Risk-to-benefit analysis, of laboratory investigations, 345-346
  for brain biopsy, 345-346, 346f
  for cerebral arteriography, 345
  for lumbar puncture, 345

Ritonavir (Norvir), for HIV infection, 1108t-1109t

Rituximab
  for multiple sclerosis, 690
  for myasthenia gravis, 1903t, 1907

Rivastigmine, 1397-1398

Rivastigmine (Exelon) patch, for dystonia, 1452t

Rizatriptan, for migraine, 1701t, 1700.e1t
  in children and adolescents, 1719

RLN (reelin) gene, in neuroblast migration, 1286

RMT (resting motor threshold), in transcranial magnetic stimulation, 392

RNA. see Ribonucleic acid (RNA)

RNA inclusions, 653

RNA metabolism, in amyotrophic lateral sclerosis, 1508

RNA processing, in amyotrophic lateral sclerosis, 1508

RNA splicing, 649-650, 650f, 651t, 652f

RNS (responsive neurostimulator), for epilepsy, 406

Robinul (glycopyrrolate), for hyperhidrosis, 1873t

Robotic-assistive devices, in rehabilitation, 802-803
  for mobility, 802-803
  for upper extremities, 802

Robotic frameless stereotactic radiosurgery, for brain tumors, 1050-1051

Rolandic epilepsy, benign, 352, 354f, 1574

Rolandic spikes, benign focal epilepsy of childhood with, 1655

Romberg position, for dizziness, 591

Romberg sign, in peripheral nerve disorders, 1796-1797

Romberg test, in screening neurological examination, 5t

Roos test, 324-325

Root abscess, 1695

Root pain, 1770, 1770f

Ropinirole, for Parkinson disease, 1433t-1434t

Rosenthal fibers, 1034, 1034f

Rosette-forming glioneuronal tumor, of fourth ventricle, 1036

Rosettes, 1028, 1028f
  in central neurocytoma, 1036

Rostral interstitial nucleus of medial longitudinal fasciculus (riMLF), in vertical eye movements, 560, 560f

Rostral medulla, in horizontal eye movements, 554

Rostral ventromedial medulla (RVM), in medication overuse headache, 1707

Rotational testing, in vestibular testing, 600, 600f

Rotational vertebral artery syndrome, vertigo due to, 595

Rotigotine patch, for Parkinson disease, 1433t-1434t

Roussy-Lévy syndrome, 1812

Routine electrophysiological testing, for movement disorder, 249

Roving eye movements, 44

RP (retinitis pigmentosa), 177, 177f
  in mitochondrial syndromes, 1360

RPLS. see Reversible posterior leukoencephalopathy syndrome (RPLS)

r-pro-UK (recombinant prourokinase), for acute ischemic stroke, 958

RRF (ragged-red fibers), 1356-1357
  myoclonic epilepsy with, 1358

RSCV (reversible segmental cerebral vasoconstriction), 1016

RSD (reflex sympathetic dystrophy), dystonia with, 1444

RSS (radiation somnolence syndrome), 1083.e1

rTMS (repetitive transcranial magnetic stimulation), 113

RTOG (Radiation Therapy Oncology Group), 1086

rtPA (recombinant tissue plasminogen activator), for acute ischemic stroke, 956-957

RU-486 (mifepristone), for Cushing disease, 711

Rubella, congenital, 1966, 1966f

Rubella virus, 1143-1144

Rubinstein-Taybi syndrome, copy number variation in, 668t

Rubra tremor, 218

Rubral tremor, 1444-1445

Rufinamide, for epilepsy
  absorption, elimination half-life, formulations of, 1600t
  efficacy by seizure type of, 1601t
  hepatic metabolism, enzyme induction/ inhibition, pharmacokinetic interactions, and protein binding of, 1603t
  mechanism of action of, 1604t

Russell syndrome, 208-209

RVM (rostral ventromedial medulla), in medication overuse headache, 1707

Ryanodine receptor, 1937

Ryanodine receptor gene (RYR1), in central core disease, 1946

RYR1. see Ryanodine receptor gene (RYR1)

S

4S (Scandinavian Simvastatin Survival Study), 922

S1 radiculopathy, 1770

S100 protein, 1030
  in anoxic-ischemic encephalopathy, 1206

SA (sinoatrial block), syncope due to, 10

Sabin trivalent oral poliovirus vaccine, 1496-1497

Saccades
  in cerebellar ataxia, 218-219
  defined, 556-557
  development of, 560
  in diplopia, 535, 535f
  disorders of, 219
  with dizziness, 588
  electronystagmographic recordings of, 599f
  externally triggered, 556
  generation and control of, 552, 556-557
    abducens nucleus in, 554, 555f
    cerebellum in, 555
    cerebral cortex in, 556

Saccades (Continued)
    cerebrum in, 554
    electrophysiological events during, 556f
    excitatory burst neurons in, 553, 555f
    final common integrator hypothesis for, 555, 556f
    frontal eye field in, 552, 557
    gain of, 555
    hippocampus in, 556
    inhibitory cell-burst neurons in, 554
    interneurons in, 554, 555f
    latch neurons in, 554
    lateral intraparietal area in, 556
    medial longitudinal fasciculus in, 554, 555f
    midbrain reticular formation in, 555
    neural integrator in, 554, 555f-556f
    ocular motor events in, 556f
    oculomotor neurons in, 556f
    omnipause neurons in, 554
    paramedian pontine reticular formation in, 553, 555, 555f
    parietal eye field in, 556-557
    pause cells in, 555f
    posterior parietal cortex in, 556
    prefrontal cortex in, 556
    rostral medulla in, 554
    spontaneous, 556
    superior colliculus in, 554
    supplementary eye field in, 556-557
    vestibular cortex, 556
    vestibular nuclei in, 555f
    vestibular system in, 555-556
  intentional, 554b
  internally triggered, 556
  reflexive, 554b
  simulated eye movement recordings of, 554f
  slow, 566, 566b
  spontaneous, 554b
  torsional, 565
  vertical, 558-560, 559f, 565
    paralysis of, 567-568
  in vestibular testing, 588, 598-599, 599f

Saccadic dysmetria, 558

Saccadic failure, 563-564

Saccadic intrusions, 219, 546t, 549-551
  with dizziness, 588
  and oscillations, 551, 552b

Saccadic latency, prolonged, 566

Saccadic lateropulsion, 565

Saccadic oscillations
  with dizziness, 588
  macro-. see Macrosquare wave jerks

Saccadic palsy, congenital, 563

Saccadic pulses, 551, 566f

Saccadic pursuit, 535
  with dizziness, 588

Saccadic system, 552, 560

Saccular aneurysm, 984-985, 985f, 991f

Saccule, 584f, 585

Sacks, Oliver, 122

Sacral fractures, lumbosacral plexopathy due to, 1789

Sacral plexopathy. see Lumbosacral plexopathy

Sacral plexus, 1786-1787

Sacral roots, anatomy of, 1767f

Sacral sparing, 318

Sacroiliac joint inflammation, lower back pain due to, 340

Sacroiliac joint injection, for pain, 729t

Sacroiliac joint separation, lumbosacral plexopathy due to, 1789

Sacroiliitis, 1762
  lower back pain due to, 340

Safety factor, in repetitive nerve stimulation for, 386–387
Sagging eye syndrome, 537–538, 568
Sagittal sinus occlusion, 1271f
SAH. see Subarachnoid hemorrhage (SAH)
SAHA (suberoylanilide hydroxamic acid), for brain tumors, 1053
SAI (short-latency afferent inhibition), in transcranial magnetic stimulation, 393
Salaam attacks, 1570
Salivary cortisol determination, for Cushing disease, 706
Salivary flow, during sleep, 1630t
Salk inactivated poliovirus vaccine, 1135
Salsalate (Disalcid), for chronic pain, 725t
Salt wasting, cerebral, 709–710
in neurointensive care, 755, 755t
Saltatory conduction, 904f, 1792
SAMMPRIS (Stenting vs Aggressive Medical Management for Preventing Recurrent Stroke in Intracranial Stenosis) trial, 963.e1
Samuels, Martin, 1881
Sandhoff disease, 1333.e2t–1333.e3t
SANDO (sensory ataxic neuropathy, dysarthria, and ophthalmoplegia), 1818.e9–1818.e10
Sanfilippo syndrome, 1332
intellectual disability associated with, 1310t
Sanger sequencing, in disease gene discovery, 666–667, 669t
Saphenous nerve, motor and sensory function of, 334t
Saphenous nerve lesions, 1810
Saposin, 1334
SAPPHIRE (Stenting and Angioplasty with Protection in Patients at High Risk for Endarterectomy) study, 962–963
Saquinavir (Invirase), for HIV infection, 1108t–1109t
Sarcoglycan, 1919
immunohistochemistry of, 1918–1919
Sarcoglycan deficiencies, 1925–1926
Sarcoglycanopathies, 291
Sarcoidosis
myopathy in, 1953
neurological complications of
in adults, 823, 823f
in children, 842
neuropathy in, 1852.e2–1852.e3
polyradiculopathy associated with, 1775
Sarcoma, meningeal, 1687–1688
SAS. see Sleep apnea syndrome (SAS)
Satellite potential, 380–381
Saturday-night palsy, 1806
Sawtooth waves, in REM sleep, 1620f
Saxitoxin (STX), 1252
SC (superior colliculus), in horizontal eye movements, 554
SCA (superior cerebellar artery) infarction, 929
Scandinavian Simvastatin Survival Study (4S), 922
"Scanning speech", 145
Scaphocephaly, 1739t
Scapular winging, in facioscapulohumeral muscular dystrophy, 281–282, 282f
Scapuloperoneal spinal muscular atrophy, 1520t–1521t, 1532
Scapuloperoneal syndromes, 1920t–1921t, 1932
SCCMS. see Slow-channel congenital myasthenic syndrome (SCCMS)

SCD (subacute combined degeneration), 103
SCD (superior canal dehiscence)
hearing loss due to, 592, 597
vertigo due to, 583
Scharrer, Berta, 702
Scharrer, Ernst, 702
Scheuermann disease, 1751
Schiff-Sherrington phenomenon, 886–887
Schiller-Duval bodies, 1042
Schimmelpenning syndrome, 1553
Schindler disease, 1334
Schistosoma spp., parasitic meningitis or encephalitis due to, 1155–1156
Schizencephaly, 1300.e2
structural imaging for, 446.e5
Schizophrenia
versus Alzheimer disease, 79t
biology of, 97
copy number variants, 97
copy number variation in, 668t
versus delirium, 32, 32t
functional imaging studies, 99
negative symptoms in, rTMS for, 398
susceptibility genes of, 97
School, return to, concussion and, 863
School performance, excessive daytime sleepiness and, 1632
Schwann cell, 1792
Schwannomas
intratemporal facial nerve, 1730–1731
management of, 1060–1061
pathology and molecular genetics of, 1041
spinal, 1041
structural imaging of, 418t–419t, 424.e1
Sciatic nerve, 1808
applied anatomy of, 1808
motor and sensory function of, 334t
Sciatic nerve entrapment, 1802t
Sciatic nerve lesions, at sciatic notch, 1808
Sciatic neuropathy, 1808
leg pain due to, 339
monoplegia due to, 270
Sciatic notch, sciatic neuropathy at, 1808
Sciatica, 1757, 1770
treatment of, 1758
Scintillating scotomas, 123, 1696
Scissors gait, 256
Sclerotome, 1770
SCN (suprachiasmatic nucleus), in NREM sleep, 1626f, 1625.e2f
SCN1A gene
in familial hemiplegic migraine, 1529
in generalized epilepsy with febrile seizures plus, 1534, 1534f
SCN1B gene, in generalized epilepsy with febrile seizures plus, 1534, 1534f
SCN2A gene
and early childhood seizures, 1534
in generalized epilepsy with febrile seizures plus, 1534, 1534f
SCN4A gene
in hyperkalemic periodic paralysis, 1525
in hypokalemic periodic paralysis, 1523
in paramyotonia congenita, 1525
in potassium-aggravated myotonia, 1526–1527
SCN9A gene, in primary erythermalgia, 1531–1532
SCNA4A gene, in potassium-sensitive periodic paralysis, 1938

Scoliosis, 1751
due to spinal muscular atrophy, 1503
with familial horizontal gaze palsy, 564
Scotomas, 576
cecocentral, 577–578, 578f
central and cecocentral, 158
junctional, 158, 578
negative, 1696
positive, 158
scintillating, 123, 1696
Scrapie, 1366
Scrapie prion protein (PrPSc), 1366f
Screening neurological examination, 4, 5t
SDH (succinate dehydrogenase), in mitochondrial disorders, 1356–1357
Seadornavirus, Banna virus as, 1139
Seasonal variation, of ischemic events, 924
Seat belt injuries, 889
Second-degree nerve injury, 371–373
Second European-Australasian Acute Stroke Study, 958
Second impact syndrome (SIS), 864
Second-wind phenomenon, in McArdle disease, 1940
Secondarily generalized seizure, 1566, 1566t
Secondary damage, after traumatic brain injury, 853
Secondary deviation, 530, 532f
Secondary effects, of neurological disease, 717
Secondary headache, 197, 198b
Secondary impact syndrome, 853
Secondary insults, posttraumatic, 855
Secondary malignancies, pediatric, 1083.e1
Secondary motor cortex, upper motor neurons and, 1484
"Secondary narcolepsy", 1643
Secondary progressive multiple sclerosis, 688, 1171
Secondary store, in repetitive nerve stimulation, 386
Secretin, 697t–698t
Sedation
for functional motor symptoms, 2007
in neurointensive care, 749–750, 751t
Sedatives
delirium due to, 30
drug dependence with, 1256–1257
excessive daytime sleepiness due, 1634
half-life of, 1203t
miscellaneous, 1257b
for traumatic brain injury, 875t–876t, 876b
Seddon, Herbert, 903
SEER (Surveillance, Epidemiology, and End Results) Program, 1018
Seesaw nystagmus (SSN), 542t, 546t, 547–548
SEF (supplementary eye field), in horizontal eye movements, 556–557
Segmental artery, 1007.e1f
Segmental demyelination, 905, 1792–1794, 1794f
Segmental muscle atrophy, juvenile, 1498
Segmental stimulation, in nerve conduction studies, 369, 369f–370f
Segregation, in linkage analysis, 659–660, 661f
SEH (spinal epidural hemorrhage), 1013–1014
Seipin gene, in hereditary spastic paraplegia, 1487–1488
Seizure onset zone, 1595

Seizures, 13–15, 525–526
  absence, 14, 14t
    EEG of, 1569
    generalized, 1569, 1570f
    simple *versus* complex, 1569
  alcohol-withdrawal, 1233
  antiepileptic drugs for
    absorption, elimination half-life,
      formulations of, 1600t
    adverse effects of, 1605
    based on age and gender, 1602
    breakthrough seizures with, 1583–1584
    discontinuation of, 1606
    efficacy by seizure type of, 1601t
    hepatic metabolism, enzyme induction/
      inhibition, pharmacokinetic
      interactions, and protein binding
      in, 1603t
    initiation of, 1599–1602
    mechanism of action of, 1604t
    pharmacoresistance, tolerance, and
      seizure aggravation with,
      1602–1605
    therapeutic drug monitoring in,
      1605–1606
  astatic, 1564
  atonic, 1565–1566
    generalized, 1571
  in autism spectrum disorder, 1305, 1307t
  autonomic phenomena with, 1565
  benign familial
    infantile, 1520t–1521t
    neonatal, 1520t–1521t
    neonatal-infantile, 1520t–1521t
  causes and risk factors for, 1581–1583
    brain tumors as, 1582
    head trauma as, 1581–1582
    inflammatory and autoimmune
      disorders as, 1582–1583
    other, 1583
    parasitic infections as, 1582
    stroke as, 1582
    vascular malformations as, 1582, 1582f
  cephalic sensation with, 1565
  childhood, due to SCN2A mutation, 1534
  classification of, 1563–1566, 1565b, 1566t
  clinical features of, 9t
  clonic, 1565–1566
    generalized, 1570
  clonic-tonic-clonic, 1570–1571
  complex, 1565–1566
  complex partial, 14, 14t
  definitions of, 1563–1564
  drop attacks due to, 18
  due to brain tumor, 1046
  dyscognitive phenomena with, 1565
  EEG for
    for focal-onset (partial), 352, 353f
    for generalized seizure, 352, 352f
  elementary motor of, 1564
  epidemiology of, 1584
    comorbidity and, 1584–1585
    descriptive, 1584
    first unprovoked, 1584
  epileptic spasms as, 1570
  evaluation of, 1592–1598
    for drug-resistant seizures, 1594–1595
    for recent-onset seizures, 1592–1594
  experiential phenomena with, 1565
  faciobrachial, in anti-LGI1 limbic
    encephalitis, 1199
  febrile, 1520t–1521t, 1580–1581
    generalized epilepsy with, 1534, 1534f
    neuroepidemiology of, 640–641
    simple *versus* complex, 1580
  focal-onset (partial), EEG for, 352, 353f

Seizures (*Continued*)
  gelastic, with hypothalamic hamartoma,
    1580, 1580f
  generalized (idiopathic), 1565–1566,
    1569–1571
    EEG for, 352, 352f
    with focal evolution, 1571
    histopathology of, 1587
    molecular pathology of, 1587–1588,
      1587t
    physiology of, 1586
    primary, 1566
    secondarily, 1566
    symptomatic, 1566
  hemiplegia due to, 265
  history and physical examination for, 13
  ictal phenomenology of, 1564–1565
  with intracerebral hemorrhage, 981
  investigations of, 14–15
  monoplegia due to, 268
    differential diagnosis of, 272.e1, 272.e1t
  motor manifestations of, 1564
  myoclonic, 1565–1566
    generalized, 1569–1570
    myoclonic-astatic, 1569–1570
    myoclonic-tonic, 1569–1570
  neocortical focal, 1589–1590
    molecular pathophysiology of,
      1589–1590
    physiological abnormalities of, 1589
  neonatal, 1956–1959
    determination of underlying cause of,
      1957, 1958t
    diagnosis of, 1957
    differentiation of, from nonconvulsive
      movements, 1957
    duration of treatment and outcome of,
      1958–1959, 1959t
    electroencephalography for, 1957
    management of, 1958
    types of, 1957t
  neurological complications, of drug abuse,
    1258
  partial (focal, local), 1565–1569
    complex, 14, 14t, 1566–1567
    evolving to generalized tonic-clonic
      activity, 1567
    of femoral lobe origin, 1568
    originating in insular cortex, 1569
    originating in occipital lobe, 1569
    originating in parietal lobe, 1568–1569
    semiology in relation to localization,
      1567–1569
    simple, 1566–1567
    of temporal lobe origin, 1567–1568
  positive motor manifestations of, 1564
  post-traumatic, 879
  postural manifestation of, 1564
  precipitants of, 1583–1584
  psychogenic nonepileptic, 15, 16t
  for recent-onset seizures, 1592–1594
    electroencephalography in, 1593–1594,
      1593f
    history in, 1592–1593
    neuroimaging in, 1594
    other testing in, 1594
    physical and neurological examination
      in, 1593
  refractory, in anti-GABA_A receptor
    encephalitis, 1199
  from rTMS, 398
  sensory phenomena with, 1565
  simple partial, 1565–1566
  sleep, differential diagnosis, 1656
  special electroencephalographic studies in
    nocturnal, 1676

Seizures (*Continued*)
  and stroke in children, 998–999, 1002
  in Sturge-Weber syndrome, 1547
  symptomatic, acute, causes of, 1583
  versus syncope, 9t
  temporal lobe
    mesial, 1588–1589
      histopathology of, 1588–1589
      molecular pathology of, 1589
      physiology of, 1588
  terminology for, 1566
  tonic, 1565–1566
    generalized, 1570
  tonic-clonic (grand mal), 14, 1565–1566
    generalized, 1570–1571
  in toxic and metabolic encephalopathies,
    1209–1210
  types of, 1566–1571
  versive manifestation of, 1564, 1564.e1f
Select exon sequencing, 673t
Select exon testing, 673, 673t
Selectins, in immune response, 681–682
Selection bias, in studies of brain tumors,
  1021–1022
Selective amygdalohippocampectomy, for
  epilepsy, 1607
Selective neuronal vulnerability, after
  traumatic brain injury, 852
Selective serotonin reuptake inhibitors
  (SSRIs), 78, 99
  in Alzheimer disease, 1398
  for depression, in multiple sclerosis, 1183
  for fatigue, in multiple sclerosis, 1182
  for migraine prophylaxis, 1703
  for neuropathic pain, 918t–919t
  for premature ejaculation, 633
Selegiline (Deprenyl, Eldepryl), for
  Parkinson disease, 1432, 1433t–1434t
Selegiline transdermal patch, for depression,
  112t
Self-care skills
  after spinal cord injury, 811–812
  after stroke, 811
Self-catheterization, in management of
  voiding dysfunction, 616
Self-mutilation, in autism spectrum disorder,
  1307t
Self-tolerance, 684–685
  anergy due to failure of T-cell activation
    in, 684, 685f
  apoptosis in, 684, 685f
  central, 684
  defined, 676, 684
  peripheral, 684–685
  regulatory T cells in, 684–685
Sella turcica, 703f
  tumors in region of, 707
Sellar region tumors
  management of, 1063–1064
  structural imaging of, 418t–419t, 426–427
Selzentry (maraviroc), for HIV infection,
  1108t–1109t
Semantic dementia, behavior and personality
  disturbances in, 80
Semantic memory, 60, 61t
  in Alzheimer disease, 1387
Semantic variant, of frontotemporal
  dementia, 522–523
Semantic variant primary progressive aphasia
  (svPPA), functional neuroimaging of,
  489–490
Semantics, 128
Semicircular canals, in auditory system, 584f,
  585
SEN(s) (subependymal nodules), in
  tuberous sclerosis, 1540

Senataxin (SETX) gene, in ataxia with oculomotor apraxia type 2, 1469
Senile chorea, 1450
Sense strand, 649, 650f, 651t
Sensitivity data, in neuropsychological evaluation, 514
Sensitization
    central, 722
    of nociceptor terminals, 296–297
    peripheral, 722
    of tumor cells to ionizing radiation, 1050
Sensorimotor polyneuropathy, 1848
Sensorimotor striatum, 1423
Sensorineural hearing loss (SNHL), 596
    asymmetrical, 597
    in mitochondrial disorders, 1360
    sudden, 597
Sensory abnormalities, 315
    diagnosis of, 316t
    functional, 1999–2000, 2000f
    of limbs, trunk, and face, 314–323
    localization of, 315–319, 316t
    pattern of symptoms of
        dysesthesia and paresthesia as, 315
        hyperesthesia as, 315
        hyperpathia as, 315
        neuropathic pain as, 315
        sensory ataxia as, 315
Sensory afferents, 314.e1t
Sensory ataxia, 221b, 315
    gait disorders in, 255
    neurological signs in, 219
    symptoms in, 217
Sensory ataxic neuropathies, 1796–1797, 1798b
Sensory ataxic neuropathy, dysarthria, and ophthalmoplegia (SANDO), 1818.e9–1818.e10
Sensory aura, 1696–1697
Sensory axons, 368
Sensory conduction velocity, 368–369, 368f
Sensory disturbances, muscle weakness due to, 284
Sensory examination, for gait disorders, 254–255
Sensory fusion, 529, 531f
Sensory innervation, of skin and muscle, 298f
Sensory involvement, polyneuropathies with predominantly, 1796–1797, 1797f
Sensory lesions
    brainstem, 318–319
    cerebral, 319
        cortical, 319
        thalamic, 319
    peripheral, 316, 317f–318f
    spinal, 317–318
        dissociated sensory loss in, 318
        sacral sparing in, 318
        sensory level in, 317–318
        suspended sensory loss in, 318
Sensory level, 317–318
Sensory loss, treatment of, 715
Sensory nerve action potentials (SNAPs), 366
    amplitude of, 368, 368f
        aging and, 370
    conduction velocity of, 368–369, 368f
        with disk herniation, 1771
    latencies of, 368, 368f
    observation of, 368–369, 368f
    and physiological temporal dispersion, 371, 372f

Sensory nerve conduction studies, 368–369, 368f
    for motor neuron disease, 383
Sensory neuronopathy, 1792, 1793f
Sensory neuropathy, 319t
    ataxic, 1796–1797, 1798b
    paraneoplastic, 1191–1192
        clinical findings in, 1191–1192
        immune responses, 1192
        treatment of, 1192
        tumor association, 1192
Sensory pathways, impairment of, in multiple sclerosis, 1165–1166
Sensory polyneuropathy, 319–320
Sensory receptors, 314.e1t
Sensory signs, for arm and neck pain, 326–327, 326f
Sensory symptoms
    dysesthesia and paresthesia as, 315
    with gait disorders, 252
    hyperesthesia as, 315
    hyperpathia as, 315
    neuropathic pain as, 315
    sensory ataxia as, 315
Sensory syndromes, 319–323, 319t
    brain, 322–323
        cortical infarction as, 322
        deficits of higher sensory perception as, 322–323
        mental neuropathy (numb chin syndrome) as, 322
        thalamic infarction and hemorrhage as, 322
        thalamic pain syndrome (central post-stroke pain) as, 322
        trigeminal neuralgia as, 322
    functional (psychogenic), 323
    peripheral, 319–321
        acquired immunodeficiency syndrome-associated neuropathies as, 320
        acute inflammatory demyelinating polyradiculoneuropathy as, 320–321
        amyloid neuropathy as, 320
        carpal tunnel syndrome as, 321
        diabetic neuropathies as, 320
        mononeuropathy as, 321
        proximal sensory loss as, 320
        radial neuropathy as, 321
        radiculopathy as, 321, 321t
        sensory polyneuropathy as, 319–320
        small fiber neuropathy as, 320
        temperature-dependent sensory loss as, 320
        toxic neuropathies as, 320
        ulnar neuropathy as, 321
    spinal, 321–322
        myelopathy as, 321–322
        spinal hemisection as, 322
        syringomyelia as, 322
        tabes dorsalis and related disorders as, 322
Sensory system
    anatomy and physiology and, 314–315
    brain pathways in, 314
        brainstem in, 314
        cerebral cortex in, 314
        thalamus in, 314
    peripheral pathways in, 314
    sensory afferents in, 314.e1t
    sensory input processing in, 314–315
    sensory receptors in, 314.e1t
    spinal cord pathways in, 314, 315f
Sensory visual function, in diplopia, 535

Sentence Level Auditory Comprehension Program, 806
Sentinel headache, in subarachnoid hemorrhage, 990
Sentinel headaches, in subarachnoid hemorrhage, 1691
Sepiapterin reductase deficiency, 1326.e1t–1326.e2t
Septo-optic dysplasia, structural imaging for, 446.e5
Septo-optic-pituitary dysplasia, 1294t, 1298
Sequestrated fragment, degenerative disc disease with, 455
Serial recitation tasks, for delirium, 28
Serial reversal test, for delirium, 28
Serine metabolism, disorders of, 1340
Serology, of hypotonic infant, 308–309
Seronegative myasthenia gravis, 1899–1900, 1900t
Serotonergic neurons, in nociception, 721
Serotonin
    in appetite, 701f
    in basal ganglia, 1425–1426
    in chemical imaging, 505t, 506
    of epilepsy, 509
Serotonin and norepinephrine reuptake inhibitors (SNRIs), 111–112
Serotonin syndrome, 700
Serous otitis, 596
Serum creatine kinase, for muscle weakness, 286
[^{18}F]Setoperone, in chemical imaging, 506
Setting sun sign, 569
SETX (senataxin) gene, in ataxia with oculomotor apraxia type 2, 1469
Severe head injury, defined, 1581
Severity profile, 2
Sex chromosomes, 658–659
Sex distribution, in multiple sclerosis, 1164
Sex-linked (X-linked) disorders, 658–659, 660f
Sex toys, for sexual dysfunction in women, 633
Sexual activity, headache associated with, 1714
Sexual arousal, 624
Sexual compulsive behavior, hypersexuality due to, 609
Sexual dysfunction
    due to basal ganglia lesions, 609
    due to cortical lesions, 608
    due to epilepsy, 608
    due to spinal cord injury, 610–611
        in females, 611
        in males, 610–611
    female
        due to spinal cord injury, 611
        management of, 621
    male
        due to spinal cord injury, 610–611
        management of
            for ejaculation dysfunction, 621
            for erectile dysfunction, 620–621, 621t
    management of
        in men
            for ejaculation dysfunction, 621
            for erectile dysfunction, 620–621, 621t
        in women, 621
    in neurological disorders, 622–634
    potential factors predisposing to, in neurological disease, 620b

Sexual function, impact of neurological conditions on, 627–632
  multiple sclerosis, 630–631
  Parkinson disease, 632
  spinal cord lesions, 627–630, 627f–628f
    primary
      on female sexual function, 629, 629f–630f
      on male sexual function, 628–629
    secondary, 630
    tertiary, 630
  stroke, 631
  traumatic brain injury, 631–632
  treatment options
    for primary impacts, 632–633
      for ejaculation disorders, 633
      for erectile dysfunction, 632–633
      for sexual dysfunction in women, 633
    for secondary impacts, 633–634
    for tertiary consequences, 634
Sexual function changes, during sleep, 1631
Sexual functions, neurological control of, 607
  female, 607
  male, 607
SFT (solitary fibrous tumor), pathology and molecular genetics of, 1040–1041
SH3TC2 gene, in Charcot-Marie-Tooth disease, 1816–1817
Shagreen patch, in tuberous sclerosis, 1539, 1541t
Shapiro syndrome, 698
  reverse, 698
Sheehan syndrome, 703
Shellfish poisoning, 1252–1253
  amnestic, 1253
  neurotoxic, 1253
  paralytic, 1252–1253
Sherrington law of reciprocal inhibition, 528–529
SHH (sonic hedgehog) gene, in holoprosencephaly, 1296
Shift-worker sleep disorder, 1654
Shift workers, sleep deprivation in, 1632
Shingles, 1776–1777
Shock, spinal, 273
Short ciliary nerves, 1721f
Short-cycle periodic breathing, 41
Short-interval intracortical facilitation (SICF), in transcranial magnetic stimulation, 393, 394t
Short-interval intracortical inhibition, in transcranial magnetic stimulation, 393, 394t
Short-lasting unilateral neuralgiform headache, 1712
  with conjunctival injection and tearing (SUNCT), 198–199
Short-latency afferent inhibition (SAI), in transcranial magnetic stimulation, 393, 394t
Short QT syndrome, syncope due to, 10–11
Short syndrome, due to autonomic disorders, 1890
Short-term (recent) memory, 60
Shoulder-girdle weakness, differential diagnosis of, 290
Shoulder pain, due to tendonitis, bursitis, and arthritis, 331
Shprintzen-Goldberg syndrome, 1739
Shy-Drager syndrome, 1888
SI (surround inhibition), in transcranial magnetic stimulation, 393, 394t
SIADH. see Syndrome of inappropriate antidiuretic hormone secretion (SIADH)

Sialorrhea, in amyotrophic lateral sclerosis, 1508, 1513t
SICF (short-interval intracortical facilitation), in transcranial magnetic stimulation, 393, 394t
SICI (short-interval intracortical inhibition), in transcranial magnetic stimulation, 393, 394t
Sick sinus syndrome
  cardiogenic embolism due to, 934–935
  drop attacks due to, 17–18
  due to autonomic disorders, 1890
Sickle cell anemia, and stroke in children, 996–997, 997f
  treatment of, 1005
Sickle cell disease
  ischemic stroke due to, 949
  neurological complications, in children, 843–844, 844f
  neurological complications of, in adults, 824
  ultrasound of, 483
Siderosis, superficial
  ataxia in, 1464, 1464f
  structural imaging of, 441, 436.e1f
Signal intensity, in MRI, 413, 416t
Signal-to-noise ratio, 367
Sildenafil (Viagra)
  for erectile dysfunction, 620–621, 621t
  for sexual dysfunction, in multiple sclerosis, 1183
  for sexual dysfunction in women, 621
Silent brain infarcts, 521
Silent mutation, 651t, 654, 654f
Silent period (SP), in transcranial magnetic stimulation, 392, 392f, 394t
Silver-Russell syndrome, copy number variation in, 668t
Silver syndrome, 1487–1488
Simian hand, 282
Simian virus 40 (SV40), and brain tumors, 1022
Simmonds disease, 703
Simultanagnosia, 123
Simvastatin, for ischemic stroke, 922
Single-fiber electromyography (SFEMG), 388–390
  fiber density in, 389
  jitter in, 389–390, 390f
  for myasthenia gravis, 1902
  stimulation, 388–389
  voluntary, 388–389
Single-nucleotide polymorphisms (SNPs), 651t, 654
  and brain tumors, 1025
  genome-wide association studies for, 663–664, 664f
Single-photon emission computed tomography (SPECT), 486–488, 487t, 504, 1392
  for coma, 48
  ictal, for epilepsy, 497–498, 497f
    and seizure focus, 498
  versus positron emission tomography, 504
  prior to epilepsy surgery, 1597, 1597f
  for stroke in children, 1004
Single TMS pulses (sTMS), 399
Sinoatrial block, syncope due to, 10
Sinus headaches, 1695
Sinuses
  imaging of, headache and, 202
Sinusitis
  headache and facial pain due to, 1694–1695
  optic neuropathy due to, 169
Sitting, arising from, 252

Situational syncope, 12
Sixth cranial nerve nucleus, lesions of, 208
Sjögren syndrome
  dementia in, 1419–1420
  neurological complications of
    in adults, 821–822
    in children, 841
  neuropathy in, 1852.e1–1852.e2, 1852.e2f
Skeletal deformity, gait disorders due to, 261
Skeletal dysplasias, 1738
Skeletal muscle disorders, 1915–1955
  channelopathies as, 1936–1940
    of calcium channel
      familial hypokalemic periodic paralysis type 1 as, 1937
      secondary hypokalemic paralysis as, 1937–1938
    of chloride channel, 1939–1940
      myotonia congenita as, 1939–1940
    ion, 1936–1937
    of potassium channel, 1939
      Andersen-Tawil syndrome as, 1939
    of sodium channel, 1938–1939
      hyperkalemic periodic paralysis as, 1938
      hypokalemic periodic paralysis type 2 as, 1939
      paramyotonia congenita as, 1938–1939
      potassium-aggravated myotonias as, 1939
      potassium-sensitive periodic paralysis as, 1938
      secondary hyperkalemic periodic paralysis as, 1939
  congenital myopathies as, 1946–1948
    central core disease as, 1946, 1947f
    centronuclear myopathy as, 1947–1948
    congenital fiber-type disproportion as, 1948, 1948f
    nemaline myopathy as, 1946–1947, 1947f
  inflammatory myopathies as, 1948–1953
    dermatomyositis as, 1949–1950, 1949f–1950f
      associated with neoplasia, 1951
      associated with other collagen vascular diseases, 1951
      prognosis and treatment of, 1951–1952
    immune-mediated necrotizing myopathy as, 1951
      prognosis and treatment of, 1951–1952
    inclusion body myositis as, 1952–1953, 1952f–1953f
    other, 1953
    polymyalgia rheumatica as, 1953
    polymyositis as, 1950–1951, 1951f
      associated with neoplasia, 1951
      associated with other collagen vascular diseases, 1951
      prognosis and treatment of, 1951–1952
  metabolic myopathies as, 1940–1943
    due to abnormal nucleotide metabolism, 1943
      myoadenylate deaminase deficiency as, 1943
    due to disorders of carbohydrate metabolism, 1940–1942
      β-enolase deficiency as, 1941
      α-glucosidase deficiency (acid maltase deficiency), 1941–1942
      lactate dehydrogenase deficiency as, 1941

Spinal deformities, with metabolic bone disease *(Continued)*
  osteomalacia and rickets as, 1749
  osteopetrosis as, 1749–1750, 1749.e1f
  osteoporosis as, 1749, 1749f
  Paget disease as, 1750, 1750f
    cranial neurological complications of, 1750
    diagnosis of, 1750
    spinal neurological complications of, 1750
    treatment of, 1750
  scoliosis as, 1751
Spinal diseases, structural imaging of, 449–457
Spinal dysraphism, 1282, 1295, 1744–1746
  Dandy-Walker syndrome as, 1745
  defined, 1744
  myelomeningocele and encephalocele as, 1744–1745, 1744f–1745f, 1744.e1f
  spina bifida occulta as, 1744, 1744b, 1744.e1f
  tethered cord syndromes as, 1745–1746, 1745b
Spinal epidural abscess, 1151–1152, 1759–1760
  clinical presentation of, 1151
  diagnosis of, 1151–1152, 1152f
  etiology of, 1151
  lower back pain due to, 341
  management of, 1149t, 1152
  risk factors for, 1151
Spinal epidural hematoma, structural imaging of, 454.e2, 454.e3f
Spinal epidural hemorrhage (SEH), 1013–1014
Spinal generator of ejaculation, 622
Spinal hemisection, 266
  sensory abnormalities due to, 322
Spinal hemorrhage, 1013–1014
  epidural and subdural, 1013–1014
  hematomyelia as, 1013
  subarachnoid, 1013
Spinal infections, structural imaging of, 452
Spinal locomotor centers, 250–251
Spinal metastases, intramedullary, 1094
Spinal muscular atrophy, 1499–1503
  clinical features of, 1500–1502
  copy number variation in, 668t
  differential diagnosis of, 1502–1503
  disorders of programmed cell death in, 1283–1284
  distal, congenital, 1520t–1521t, 1532
  distal, hereditary, 1812
  genetic counseling and prenatal diagnosis of, 1503
  hypotonic infant due to, 311
  laboratory studies of, 1502
  scapuloperoneal, 1520t–1521t, 1532
  treatment of, 1503
  type 0 (prenatal), 1500t
  type 1 (infantile, Werdnig-Hoffmann disease), 1500, 1500t, 1501f
  type 2 (intermediate, chronic), 1500–1501, 1500t
  type 3 (juvenile, Kugelberg-Welander disease), 1500t, 1501
  type 4 (adult-onset, pseudomyopathic), 1500t, 1501–1502, 1502f
Spinal muscular atrophy with respiratory distress (SMARD), 1500
Spinal myoclonus, 1458

Spinal nerves, 1767–1768, 1767f
  anatomy of, 903–905, 904f
  axon in, 903–904
  peripheral nerve trunks in, 904–905
Spinal osteoarthritis, 1751
  cervical, 1752
  vertebral artery stroke caused by, 1754–1755
Spinal reflexes, in coma, 46
Spinal roots, magnetic stimulation of, 391–392
Spinal sensory lesions, 317–318
  dissociated sensory loss in, 318
  sacral sparing in, 318
  sensory level in, 317–318
  suspended sensory loss in, 318
Spinal shock, 273, 886–887, 887t
Spinal stability, 895
Spinal subarachnoid hemorrhage, 454.e3, 454.e3f
Spinal subdural hematoma, 454.e2–454.e3
Spinal subdural hemorrhage (SSH), 1013–1014
Spinal subluxations, due to rheumatoid arthritis, 1762
Spinal surgery, intraoperative monitoring for, 410
Spinal tumors, structural imaging of, 449–451
Spinal vascular malformations, 1010–1013
  arteriovenous fistula as
    glomus, 780
    juvenile/metameric, 780
    perimedullary, 780
    spinal dural, 780
  classification of, 1010b
  clinical presentation and course of, 1010–1011
  distribution and prevalence of, 1010, 1011f
  investigations of, 1011–1012, 1012f
  neurointerventional therapy for, 779–780, 780f
  treatment of, 1012–1013
Spinal vasculature, anatomy of, 1007.e1–1007.e2, 1007.e1f
Spine disorders, MR angiography of, 476, 477f
Spine trauma, structural imaging for, 454
  in absence of neurologic deficit, 458.e5
Spinocerebellar Ataxia Type 3 (Machado-Joseph disease), 1517
Spinocerebellar ataxias, 1520t–1521t, 1818.e3
  classification of, 1471
  clinical features of, 1471–1472, 1471t
  dentatorubral pallidoluysian atrophy as, 1477
  gene mutations and phenotype-genotype correlations in, 1473–1477
  imaging and other laboratory studies in, 1472, 1472f
  neuropathology of, 1472–1473
  pathogenesis of, 1478–1479
  structural imaging for, 444.e2–444.e3, 444.e2f
  transcranial magnetic stimulation for, 396
  type 1, 1474
  type 2, 1474
  type 3 (Machado-Joseph disease), 1474–1475
    dystonia in, 1472f
    MRI in, 1472f

Spinocerebellar ataxias *(Continued)*
  type 4, 1475
  type 5, 1475
  type 6, 1475
  type 7, 1475
  type 8, 1475
  type 10, 1475
  type 11, 1475
  type 12, 1475–1476
  type 13, 1476
  type 14, 1476
  type 15, 1476
  type 16, 1476
  type 17, 1476
  type 18, 1476
  type 19, 1476
  type 20, 1476
  type 21, 1476
  type 22, 1476
  type 23, 1476
  type 25, 1476
  type 26, 1476
  type 27, 1476
  type 28, 1476–1477
  type 29, 1477
  type 30, 1477
  type 31, 1477
  type 32, 1477
  type 34, 1477
  type 35, 1477
  type 36, 1477
Spiral CT, 412, 459, 463
Spiraling isopters, 582, 582f
SPIRIT (Stroke Prevention in Reversible Ischemia Trial), 971
Spirometra genus, CNS lesions due to, 1157
Spliceosome, 649–650
Splint, for Duchenne muscular dystrophy, 1922–1923
Split-brain patients, 59–60
Spondylitis, ankylosing
  clinical presentation of, 1762
  pathogenesis of, 1762
  spinal neurological complications of, 1762, 1762t, 1762.e1f–1762.e2f
Spondyloarthropathies, inflammatory, 1762–1763
  clinical presentation of, 1762, 1762.e1f
  laboratory abnormalities in, 1763
  nonspinal neurological complications of, 1762
  pathogenesis of, 1762
  spinal neurological complications of, 1762, 1762t, 1762.e1f–1762.e2f
Spondylolisthesis, 1755–1757
  structural imaging of, 457, 458f, 454.e2, 454.e2f–454.e3f
Spondylolysis, 1755–1757
  structural imaging of, 457, 458f
Spondylosis, 1751
  cervical, 1752, 1752.e1f
  and disk herniation, 1769–1770
  lumbar, 1755–1757
  thoracic, 1755, 1755f–1756f
Spondylotic myelopathy, cervical, 1753–1754, 1754f
Spontaneous eye movements, 44, 47
Spontaneous intracranial hypotension, 1689
Spontaneous speech, 130
Sporadic ataxia, with added non-cerebellar deficits, 1480
Sporadic cortical cerebellar atrophy, 1480

Sporadic Creutzfeldt-Jakob disease (sCJD)
  clinical aspects of, 1367
  diagnosis of, 1370
  diagnostic tests for, 1370–1373
    development of prion-specific,
      1372–1373
    electroencephalogram in, 1371f
  molecular classification of, 1369–1370
  neuropathological features of, 1369
Sporadic fatal insomnia (sFI), 1369–1370
Sporotrichosis, 1154t
Sports concussion, 860–866
  acute and subacute management of,
    862–864
  definition in, 860
  diagnosis of, 861–862, 861t
  epidemiology of, 860
  long-term effects of, 864–865
  pathophysiology of, 860–861
  prevention of, 866
  risk involved with premature return to
    participation, 864
Spot sign
  on CT angiography, 463
  in intracerebral hemorrhage, 976, 977f
Spurling sign, 1752
Squamous epithelial cyst, structural imaging
  of, 446.e7, 446.e7f
Square-wave jerks (SWJs), 219, 566–567,
  566f
  causes of, 566b
  definition of, 566–567
  with dizziness, 588
  localization of, 542t
  macro-, 542t, 546t, 567
  treatment of, 546t
Square-wave oscillations, 546t
Square-wave pulses (SWPs), 542t, 567
  localization of, 542t
  treatment of, 546t
SRT (stereotactic radiation therapy), for
  brain tumors, 1050
SSADH deficiency, 1328.e2t
SSEP. see Somatosensory evoked potentials
  (SEPs, SSEPs)
SSH (spinal subdural hemorrhage),
  1013–1014
SSN (seesaw nystagmus), 542t, 546t,
  547–548
SSPE (subacute sclerosing panencephalitis),
  1142–1143, 1142f
SSR. see Sympathetic skin response (SSR)
SSRIs. see Selective serotonin reuptake
  inhibitors (SSRIs)
SSYLVIA (Stenting of Symptomatic
  Atherosclerotic Lesions in the Vertebral
  or Intracranial Arteries) study, 963.e1
St. Jude Medical DBS Study Group, 404
St. Louis encephalitis (SLE) virus, 1137t,
  1138
Stabbing headaches, 1713
Stable headache, 197
Stage shifts, 1673
Staging, tumor, 1028
"Staircase procedure", 192–193
Stalevo (carbidopa, levodopa, and
  entacapone), for Parkinson disease,
  1435
Stance, 252–253, 253t
  of ataxia, 218
Standard deviations (SDs), 344
Standardization sample, in
  neuropsychological evaluation, 513
Standardized mortality ratio (SMR),
  635–636
  for epilepsy, 638

Stanford Sleepiness Scale (SSS), 1635, 1637b
Stapedius muscle, 602
Stapes, 585
Start codon, 650–652
Start hesitation, 251, 254
Startle response, in vegetative state, 54
Startle syndrome, 245, 1458
State shifts, 1673
Static perimeters, in visual field testing, 579
Statin, necrotizing myopathy due to, 1954
Status epilepticus, 1611–1614
  classification of, 1612
  convulsive, 1612–1613
    generalized, 1612
      treatment of, 1613
    during pregnancy, 1986–1987
    subtle, 1613
  defined, 1612
  EEG of, 1613
  etiology of, 1613
  incidence of, 1613
  myoclonus, in anoxic-ischemic
    encephalopathy, 1202–1203
  nonconvulsive, 1612–1613
    continuous EEG monitoring for, 747
  outcome of, 1614
  treatment of, 1613–1614, 1614t
Status migrainosus, 1702, 1706
Stavudine (d₄T, Zerit), for HIV infection,
  1108t–1109t
Steinthal, Heymann, 116
Stellate ganglion block, for pain, 729t, 731,
  731f
Stem cell transplantation
  autologous peripheral blood, for brain
    tumors, 1051
  hematopoietic, for inborn errors of
    metabolism, 1332
Stem cells, neural, 695
Stenosis, duplex ultrasonography of, 478,
  478f
Stent-assisted coil embolization
  for cerebral aneurysms, 770–771,
    771f–772f
  for intracranial aneurysm, 991–992, 992f
Stent placement, three-dimensional
  contrast-enhanced magnetic resonance
  angiography after, 469, 471f
Stent-Supported Percutaneous Angioplasty of
  the Carotid Artery versus Endarterectomy
  (SPACE), 963
Stenting and Angioplasty with Protection in
  Patients at High Risk for Endarterectomy
  (SAPPHIRE) study, 962–963
Stenting of Symptomatic Atherosclerotic
  Lesions in the Vertebral or Intracranial
  Arteries (SSYLVIA) study, 963.e1
Stenting vs Aggressive Medical Management
  for Preventing Recurrent Stroke in
  Intracranial Stenosis (SAMMPRIS) trial,
  963.e1
Steppage gait, 255
Stepping, 254
Stereopsis, 529, 531f
Stereotactic radiation therapy (SRT), for
  brain tumors, 1050
Stereotactic radiosurgery (SRS)
  for brain metastases, 1089–1090
  for brain tumors, 1050–1051
  for trigeminal neuralgia, 736
Stereotypies, 237
  in autism spectrum disorder, 1306, 1307t
Steroids, with traumatic brain injury,
  875t–876t
STICH (Surgical Trial of Intracerebral
  Haemorrhage), 981

Stickler syndrome, 1738
Stiff leg syndrome (SLS), 1200
Stiff-man syndrome, paraneoplastic, 1191
Stiff-person spectrum disorder, and
  antibodies to glycine receptors, 1200
Stiff person syndrome, 246, 1459–1460
  supranuclear gaze disturbances due to,
    560
Stimulants, for ADHD, 1321, 1322f–1323f
Stimulation parameters, for transcranial
  magnetic stimulation, 391–394,
  394t
Stimulators, for nerve conduction studies,
  366–367
Stimulus response curve, for motor evoked
  potentials, 392, 394t
Stokes-Adams attack
  drop attacks due to, 17–18
  syncope due to, 10
Stop codons, 650–652
Strabismus
  comitant, 529–530
  nonconcomitant (incomitant, paralytic,
    restrictive), 529–530
StrAbs. see Anti-striational muscle antibodies
  (StrAbs)
Strachan syndrome, 1236
Straight leg-raising test, 1757
Strategic infarcts, 1414
Strengthening, in rehabilitation, 786
Streptococcal infections, and antibody-
  associated neurological syndromes,
  695
Streptococcus, group B, neonatal meningitis
  due to, 1965
Streptococcus aureus, spinal epidural abscess
  due to, 1151
Streptococcus pneumoniae, meningitis due to,
  1147
Streptococcus pyogenes, and Sydenham chorea,
  695
Streptokinase, intracerebral hemorrhage due
  to, 971
Stress, and migraines, 1700
Stress-induced cardiomyopathy, 1881–1882
Stretch, peripheral nerve injury due to,
  907–908
Striatal toe, in dystonic gait, 257
Striate cortex, in smooth-pursuit eye
  movements, 557
Striatonigral degeneration, 1437, 1660
Striatopallidodentate calcification, bilateral,
  1442
Striatum
  in basal ganglia, 1423
  divisions of, 1424t
Stribild, for HIV infection, 1108t–1109t
Stroke
  acute, temporal evolution of, 429–431
  behavior and personality disturbances
    after, 89–90
    aggression as, 90
    depression as, 89–90
    pseudobulbar affect as, 90
    psychosis as, 90
  brainstem syndromes of, 210–216, 210f
    medullary, 212–216, 215f, 216b
    midbrain, 211–212, 212b
      territories involved in, 212, 213f
    pontine, 212, 214b
      territories involved in, 212, 215f
    thalamic, 210–211, 211b
      arterial territories and, 210–211,
        211f
      blood supply of thalamus and,
        210–211, 210f

Stroke *(Continued)*
  as cause of vertigo, 583, 587*t*, 592–593
  in children, 996–1006
    with arteriovenous malformation, 996, 997*f*
    with bleeding disorders, 996, 999
    with cancer, 997–998, 998*f*
    cardiac causes of, 999
    with complex congenital heart disease, 997, 998*f*
    with connective tissue disorders, 998
    and developing cerebrovascular system, 996
    differential diagnosis of, 1002
    with Down syndrome, 998
    due to drugs/toxins, 1000–1001
    due to infection, 1000
    due to metabolic syndromes, 998
      treatment of, 1005
    due to trauma, 999–1000
    due to vascular compression, 999–1000
    epidemiology of, 996–998
      in full-term and near-term neonates, 996
      in general population, 996
      in high-risk subgroups, 996–998
    ethnicity in, 1001
    etiology of, 999–1002
    evaluation of, 1002–1005
      cardiac, 1004–1005
      coagulation workup in, 1004
      history and physical examination in, 1002, 1003*t*
      imaging studies in, 1004
      other studies in, 1005
    gender in, 1001
    genetic risk factors of, 1001–1002
    and HIV infection, 1000
    with mechanical circulatory support, 997
    with neurofibromatosis type 1, 998
    outcome of, 1006
    presentations of, 998–999
    seizures due to, 998–999, 1002
    with sickle cell anemia, 996–997, 997*f*
    treatment of, 1005–1006
      in acute period, 1005
      additional issues in chronic therapy for, 1005–1006
      initiating chronic therapy in, 1005
    with vascular malformations/vasculopathy/migraine, 996, 1000
  with congenital heart disease, 836
  dysphagia due to, 152–153
  falls due to, 19
  functional outcomes with, 810–811, 810*t*
    ambulation as, 811
    self-care skills as, 811
  genome-wide association studies of, 663.*e*1*t*–663.*e*2*t*, 664.*e*1
  HIV-associated, 1117
  impact of, on sexual function, 631
    primary, 631
    secondary, 631
    tertiary, 631
  with motor deficits, rTMS for, 399
  neuroepidemiology of, 636–637
    morbidity rates in, 636–637
    mortality rates in, 636, 636*f*
    transient ischemic attacks in, 637
  neurological complications, of drug abuse, 1259

Stroke *(Continued)*
  postpartum, 1988–1989
  psychiatric manifestations and, 99–101, 100*b*
  rehabilitation for, 793, 794*t*
  seizures due to, 1582
  and sleep/wake disturbance, 1659
  transcranial magnetic stimulation for, 396–397
  ultrasonography of, 480–481
  urinary incontinence after, 608
Stroke Prevention by Aggressive Reduction in Cholesterol Levels (SPARCL) study, 922–923
Stroke Prevention in Reversible Ischemia Trial (SPIRIT), 971
Stroke Prevention Trial in Sickle Cell Anemia, 949
Stroke Treatment with Ancrod Trial, 960
Strokes, delirium due to, 30–31
Strongyloides stercoralis, parasitic meningitis or encephalitis due to, 1155–1156
Structural imaging, 411–458
  advanced neuroimaging, for planning of brain tumor surgery, 428.*e*1, 428.*e*1*f*
  of brain tumors, 417, 418*t*–419*t*
    astrocytoma as
      anaplastic, 418*t*–419*t*, 420–421
      low-grade, 418*t*–419*t*, 419–420, 420*f*
      pilocytic, 418*t*–419*t*, 419
      subependymal giant cell, 418*t*–419*t*, 426
    central neurocytoma as, 418*t*–419*t*, 426.*e*1
    choroid plexus papilloma as, 418*t*–419*t*, 426
    craniopharyngioma as, 418*t*–419*t*, 427, 427*f*
    ependymoma as, 418*t*–419*t*, 423
    esthesioneuroblastoma as, 418*t*–419*t*, 424.*e*1, 424.*e*1*f*
    extraaxial, 418*t*–419*t*, 423–426
    ganglioma and gangliocytoma as, 417–419, 418*t*–419*t*
    germinoma as, 418*t*–419*t*, 426
    glioblastoma multiforme as, 418*t*–419*t*, 422, 423*f*
    gliomatosis cerebri as, 418*t*–419*t*, 422
    hemangioblastoma as, 418*t*–419*t*, 423.*e*1
    intraaxial, 417–423, 418*t*–419*t*
    medulloblastoma as, 418*t*–419*t*, 424, 426*f*
    meningioma as, 418*t*–419*t*, 423–424, 425*f*
    metastatic, 428, 428*f*–429*f*
    neurofibroma as, 418*t*–419*t*
    oligoastrocytoma as, 418*t*–419*t*, 421.*e*1
    oligodendroglioma, 418*t*–419*t*, 421, 421*f*
    of parasellar region, 426–427
    of pineal region, 418*t*–419*t*
    pineoblastoma as, 418*t*–419*t*, 424–425
    pineocytoma as, 418*t*–419*t*, 425–426
    pituitary adenoma as, 418*t*–419*t*, 426–427, 427*f*, 427.*e*1*f*
    pleomorphic xanthoastrocytoma as, 418*t*–419*t*, 419.*e*1
    of posterior fossa, 418*t*–419*t*
    primary CNS lymphoma as, 418*t*–419*t*, 423, 424*f*
    primitive neuroectodermal tumor as, 424
    schwannoma as, 418*t*–419*t*, 424.*e*1

Structural imaging *(Continued)*
    of sellar and pineal regions, 418*t*–419*t*
    subependymoma as, 418*t*–419*t*, 426.*e*1
    of ventricular region, 418*t*–419*t*
  of cerebral amyloid angiopathy, 436.*e*1, 436.*e*1*f*
  of cerebral infection, 436
    bacterial meningitis as, 436.*e*1
    cerebral toxoplasmosis as, 436.*e*5
    cerebritis, abscess as, 436.*e*1, 436.*e*2*f*
    CNS tuberculosis as, 436.*e*2, 436.*e*3*f*
    Creutzfeldt-Jakob disease as, 436.*e*5, 436.*e*6*f*
    cysticercosis as, 436.*e*2–436.*e*3, 436.*e*3*f*
    cytomegalovirus as, 436.*e*5
    herpes simplex encephalitis as, 436.*e*3–436.*e*4, 436.*e*4*f*
    human immunodeficiency virus encephalitis as, 436.*e*4–436.*e*5, 436.*e*5*f*
    limbic encephalitis as, 436.*e*5, 436.*e*6*f*
    Lyme disease as, 436.*e*2
    progressive multifocal leukoencephalopathy as, 436.*e*5
  of cerebrospinal fluid circulation disorders, 447–449
    Chiari malformation as, 448–449
      type 1, 448–449, 449*f*
      type 2, 449
    hydrocephalus
      normal-pressure, 447–448, 448*f*
      obstructive, noncommunicating, 447, 447*f*
    idiopathic intracranial hypertension (pseudomotor cerebri) as, 449.*e*1
    intracranial hypotension as, 449.*e*1, 449.*e*1*f*
  in clinical practice of neurology, 417–457
  computed tomography for, 411–412, 412*f*
    indications for, 457–458
    versus MRI, 458.*e*1
  of congenital anomalies of the brain, 446
    agenesis of corpus callosum, 446.*e*5, 446.*e*5*f*
    Dandy-Walker malformation as, 446.*e*5
    gray matter heterotopia as, 446.*e*5, 446.*e*6*f*
    holoprosencephaly as, 446.*e*5
    hydranencephaly as, 446.*e*5–446.*e*6
    lipomas as, 446.*e*6–446.*e*7, 446.*e*7*f*
    pachygyria, polymicrogyria, lissencephaly, 446.*e*5, 446.*e*6*f*
    porencephaly as, 446.*e*5, 446.*e*6*f*
    schizencephaly as, 446.*e*5
    septo-optic dysplasia, 446.*e*5
  of degenerative disorders causing dementia, 445–446
    age-related involutional changes as, 445–446, 446*f*
    Alzheimer disease as, 446, 446.*e*1*f*
    frontotemporal lobar degeneration, including Pick disease as, 446, 446.*e*2*f*
  of degenerative spine disease, 454–457
    degenerative end plate changes, 456, 457*f*
    of disc, 454–456
      with disc bulge, 455, 455*f*
      with disc extrusion, 455, 456*f*
      with disc herniation, 455*f*–456*f*
      with disc migration, 455, 456*f*
      with disc protrusion, 455, 455*f*
      versus normal intervertebral discs, 455*f*

Structural imaging (*Continued*)
  with sequestrated or free fragment, 455
  with spinal cord compression, 455–456, 456*f*
  of posterior elements, 457, 457*f*
  of spondylolysis and spondylolisthesis, 457, 458*f*
  of vertebral bodies, 456–457
echoplanar imaging in, 417.*e*2–417.*e*3
of genetic and degenerative disorders
  primarily causing ataxia (cerebellar disorders), 444
    ataxia-telangiectasia as, 444.*e*3
    fragile X permutation syndrome as, 444.*e*3
    Friedreich ataxia as, 444.*e*3
    multiple system atrophy, cerebellar subtype, 444.*e*2
    spinocerebellar ataxias as, 444.*e*2–444.*e*3, 444.*e*2*f*
  primarily causing Parkinsonism or other movement disorders, 445
    Huntington disease, 445.*e*2, 445.*e*2*f*
    idiopathic Parkinson disease as, 445.*e*1, 445.*e*1*f*
    multiple system atrophy, Parkinsonian variant (striatonigral degeneration), 445.*e*2
    progressive supranuclear palsy as, 445.*e*1–445.*e*2, 445.*e*1*f*
of hemorrhagic cerebrovascular disease, 435–436
  acute, 435–436, 437*f*
  chronic, 436, 438*f*
  early subacute, 436
  hyperacute, 436
  late subacute, 436, 438*f*
indications for, 457–458, 458.*e*4
  cognitive or behavioral impairment as, 458.*e*5
  epilepsy as, 458.*e*5
  headache as, 458.*e*4
  low back pain as, 458.*e*5
  movement disorders as, 458.*e*5
  progressive ataxia, gait disorder as, 458.*e*5
  progressive weakness or numbness of central or peripheral origin as, 458.*e*5
  sudden neurological deficit as, 458.*e*4
  vertigo and hearing loss as, 458.*e*4–458.*e*5
  visual impairment as, 458.*e*4
of inflammatory or white matter disease of brain, 436
  acute disseminated encephalomyelitis as, 440
  central pontine myelinolysis as, 440.*e*2
  lesions of corpus callosum as, 440.*e*1
  leukodystrophy as, 440.*e*1
    adreno-, 440.*e*1, 440.*e*1*f*
    Krabbe disease, 440.*e*1
    metachromatic, 440.*e*1
  multiple sclerosis as, 436–440, 439*f*
  neurosarcoidosis as, 440, 441*f*
  posterior reversible encephalopathy syndrome as, 440.*e*1–440.*e*2, 440.*e*2*f*
  radiation leukoencephalopathy as, 440.*e*1, 440.*e*2*f*
of ischemic stroke, 428–432
  acute, 428–429
    of anterior cerebral artery, 430.*e*1*f*
    diffusion-weighted imaging of, 429, 430*f*–431*f*, 430.*e*1*f*

Structural imaging (*Continued*)
    of middle cerebral artery, 430*f*
    of posterior cerebral artery, 430.*e*1*f*
    temporal evolution of, 429–432
  chronic, 432, 432.*e*1*f*
  for etiology, 432
  lacunar, 432.*e*1*f*, 432.*e*2
  late subacute, 432
  perfusion-weighted imaging in, 431, 431*f*
  subacute, 431
  of thromboembolic origin, 432.*e*1–432.*e*2
  watershed, 432.*e*1
of metabolic and hereditary myelopathies, 454
  adrenomyeloneuropathy as, 454.*e*4
  amyotrophic lateral sclerosis, hereditary spastic paraplegia as, 454.*e*4
  Friedreich ataxia as, 454.*e*4
  spinocerebellar ataxias as, 454.*e*4
  subacute combined degeneration as, 454.*e*4, 454.*e*5*f*
of metabolic and toxic disorders, 444
  carbon monoxide poisoning as, 444.*e*1
  due to ethanol, 444.*e*1
  methanol poisoning as, 444.*e*1
  mitochondrial disease, 444.*e*2
  Wilson disease as, 444.*e*1
MRI for, 412–417
  basic principles, 412–413, 413*f*
  versus CT, 458.*e*1
  diffusion tensor imaging in, 417.*e*4, 417.*e*4*f*
  diffusion-weighted, 417.*e*3
  fat saturation for, 417.*e*2, 417.*e*2*f*
  gradient-recalled echo sequences and partial flip angle for, 417.*e*1
  image reconstruction in, 416–417, 417*f*
  inversion recovery sequences (FLAIR, STIR), 300
  magnetization transfer contrast imaging in, 417.*e*4–417.*e*5
  perfusion -weighted, 417.*e*3
  repetition time and time to echo in, 414–415, 414*f*
  spin echo and fast (turbo) spin echo techniques for, 417.*e*1
  T1 and T2 relaxation times, 413–414, 414*f*
  tissue contrast (T1, T2, and proton density weighting) in, 415, 415*f*–416*f*, 416*t*
of neurocutaneous syndromes, 446
  cortical tubers as, 446.*e*2
  hamartoma , as, 446.*e*2
  neurofibroma as, 418*t*–419*t*, 446.*e*2
  neurofibromatosis as, 446.*e*2
    type 1, 446.*e*2, 446.*e*3*f*
    type 2, 446.*e*2, 446.*e*3*f*
  Sturge-Weber syndrome as, 446.*e*2–446.*e*4
  subependymal nodules as, 446.*e*2
  tuberous sclerosis (Bourneville disease) as, 446.*e*2, 446.*e*4*f*
  Von Hippel-Lindau disease as, 446.*e*2
  white matter lesions as, 446.*e*2
of noninfectious encephalitis, 436
of noninfectious inflammatory disorders, 452–454
  acute disseminated encephalomyelitis as, 452, 454*f*
  multiple sclerosis as, 452, 453*f*
  sarcoidosis as, 454.*e*1
  transverse myelitis as, 452–454, 454*f*
  vacuolar myelopathy as, 454.*e*1

Structural imaging (*Continued*)
  of nonneoplastic congenital cystic lesions, 446
    arachnoid cyst as, 446.*e*8, 446.*e*9*f*
    choroid fissure cyst, 446.*e*9, 446.*e*11*f*
    choroid plexus cyst as, 446.*e*9, 446.*e*11*f*
    colloid cyst as, 446.*e*8, 446.*e*8*f*
    dermoid as, 446.*e*8
    dilated Virchow-Robin spaces as, 446.*e*8, 446.*e*10*f*
    ependymal cyst as, 446.*e*9, 446.*e*11*f*
    epidermoid as, 446.*e*7, 446.*e*7*f*
    neuroglial cyst as, 446.*e*9, 446.*e*12*f*
  of orbital lesions, 449
    ocular tumors as, 449.*e*1
    optic nerve tumors, 449.*e*1
    optic neuritis as, 449.*e*1–449.*e*3, 449.*e*3*f*
    orbital pseudomotor as, 449.*e*3
    thyroid ophthalmopathy as, 449.*e*1, 449.*e*2*f*
  of other cerebrovascular occlusive diseases, 432–435
    CADASIL as, 434.*e*1, 434.*e*1*f*
    cerebral venous sinus thrombosis as, 434–435, 435*f*
    hippocampal sclerosis as, 434, 434.*e*2*f*
    microvascular ischemic white matter lesions, "White matter disease," Binswanger disease as, 432–434, 434*f*
    venous stroke as, 434.*e*2, 434.*e*3*f*
  of spinal infections, 452
    discitis and osteomyelitis as, 452, 452*f*
    epidural abscess, paravertebral phlegmon as, 452, 453*f*
  of spinal tumors, 449–451
    astrocytoma as, 450–451, 451*f*
    embryonal, 450.*e*1
    ependymoma as, 450
    extramedullary intradural, 450
    intermedullary metastases, 451
    intramedullary, 450
    leptomeningeal metastases as, 450
    meningiomas as, 450, 451*f*
    nerve sheath tumors as, 450.*e*1, 450.*e*1*f*
    vertebral metastases, extradural tumors as, 449, 450*f*
  of spine trauma, 454
    burst fracture as, 454.*e*1, 454.*e*1*f*
    facet joint disruption, traumatic spondylolisthesis as, 454.*e*2, 454.*e*2*f*–454.*e*3*f*
    Hangman's fracture as, 454.*e*1
    Jefferson fracture as, 454.*e*1–454.*e*2, 454.*e*2*f*
    odontoid fracture as, 454.*e*1, 454.*e*1*f*
    spinal cord injury without radiologic abnormality, 454.*e*4
    spinal cord trauma as, 454.*e*3–454.*e*4, 454.*e*4*f*
    spinal epidural hematoma as, 454.*e*2, 454.*e*3*f*
    spinal subarachnoid hemorrhage as, 454.*e*3, 454.*e*3*f*
    spinal subdural hematoma as, 454.*e*2–454.*e*3
  of superficial siderosis, 441, 436.*e*1, 436.*e*1*f*
  of trauma, cerebral, 440–444, 442*f*
    with cerebral parenchymal hematoma, 444
    with cortical contusion, 443–444, 445*f*
    with diffuse axonal injury, 444, 445*f*
    with epidural hemorrhage, 442
    with subarachnoid hemorrhage, 440–441, 442*f*

Structural imaging (*Continued*)
  with subdural hemorrhage, 441–442
    acute, 441–442, 443*f*
    chronic, 442, 444*f*
    subacute, 441–442, 443*f*
  in various clinical situations, 458,
    458.*e*1t–458.*e*4t
  of vascular disease, 451
    arteriovenous malformation as, 451.*e*1,
      451.*e*1f
    cavernous malformation as, 451.*e*1
    dural arteriovenous fistula as, 451.*e*1
    spinal cord infarction as, 451.*e*1
  of vascular malformations, 447
    arteriovenous malformations as, 447.*e*1
    capillary telangiectasia as, 447.*e*1
    cavernous malformation as, 447.*e*1
    developmental venous anomaly as,
      447.*e*1
Stump pain, 740–741
Stupor, 23, 34–50
Sturge-Weber syndrome, 1546–1548, 1547*f*
  and brain tumors, 1025*t*
  cutaneous features of, 1546–1547
  diagnostic studies of, 1547–1548, 1548*f*
  neurological features of, 1547
  ocular features of, 1547
  structural imaging of, 446.*e*2–446.*e*4
  treatment of, 1548
Stuttering, acquired, 147
Styrene, occupational exposure to, 1241
Subacute and chronic peripheral
    neuropathies, 1192
Subacute combined degeneration (SCD),
    103, 1853–1854
  due to vitamin B$_{12}$ deficiency, 1228,
    1228*f*
  structural imaging for, 454.*e*4, 454.*e*5f
Subacute motor neuronopathy, 1779
  in lymphoproliferative disorders, 1506
Subacute necrotizing encephalomyelopathy,
    1360
Subacute sclerosing panencephalitis (SSPE),
    1142–1143, 1142*f*
Subaortic stenosis, idiopathic hypertrophic,
    cardiogenic embolism due to, 933–934
Subarachnoid hemorrhage (SAH)
  acute coronary syndrome due to, 752,
    753*f*
  aneurysmal, ultrasound of, 482–483,
    483*f*
  benign perimesencephalic, 990
  blood pressure management for, 753*t*,
    754
  with cerebral vasospasm, 994–995, 994*f*
  continuous EEG monitoring for, 747
  with delayed cerebral ischemia, 994–995
  diagnosis of, 987–990
  due to saccular aneurysm, 985*f*, 991*f*
  grading of, 990, 990*t*
  headache due to, 990, 1691
  imaging of, 987–990
    CT for, 987, 988*b*, 988*f*
  management of, 993–995
  misdiagnosis of, 990
  natural history of, 986
  during pregnancy, 1987
  with pseudoaneurysm, 992*f*
  re-bleeding after, 993
  SIADH with, 1222
  spinal, 1013
  structural imaging of
    of brain, 440–441, 442*f*
    spinal, 454.*e*3, 454.*e*3f

Subarachnoid hemorrhage (SAH)
    (*Continued*)
  symptoms of, 990
  transcranial Doppler ultrasonography for,
    748
  traumatic, 870–871, 871*f*
Subarachnoid space
  abducens nerve in
    anatomy of, 1727
    clinical lesions of, 1728
  facial nerve in, clinical lesions of, 1730
  oculomotor nerve in, 1720
    lesions in, 1721–1723
  trigeminal nerve in, clinical lesions of,
    1725–1726
  trochlear nerve in
    anatomy of, 1724
    clinical lesions of, 1725
Subaxial cervical spine injuries, 888–889
Subaxial subluxations, due to rheumatoid
    arthritis, 1762
Subclavian steal syndrome (SSS), 926
  due to autonomic disorders, 1890
  MR angiography of, 471–472
  neurological complications of, 819
Subcortical aphasia, 136–137, 137*f*
Subcortical arcuate fibers, 434.*e*1
Subcortical dementia, neuropsychological
    characteristics of, 511, 512*t*
Subcortical laminar heterotopia, 1286,
    1300.*e*2
Subcortical lesions, hemiplegia due to,
    264–265
Subcortical profile, 522
Subcutaneous neurofibromas, in
    neurofibromatosis type 1, 1544
Subdural empyema
  defined, 1265–1266, 1265*t*
  HIV-associated, 1115
Subdural hematoma
  headache due to, 1691
  structural imaging of, 441–442
    acute, 441–442, 443*f*
    chronic, 442, 444*f*
    spinal, 454.*e*2–454.*e*3
    subacute, 441–442, 443*f*
Subdural hemorrhage
  spinal, 1013–1014
  structural imaging of, 441–442
    acute, 441–442, 443*f*
    chronic, 442, 444*f*
    subacute, 441–442, 443*f*
Subdural monitors, of intracranial pressure,
    746
Subependymal germinal matrix, 1284, 1284*f*
Subependymal giant cell astrocytoma
    (SEGA)
  management of, 1056
  pathology and molecular genetics of,
    1034–1035
  pediatric, 1072–1073
  structural imaging of, 418*t*–419*t*, 426
  in tuberous sclerosis, 1035, 1541
Subependymal giant cell tumor, 1035
Subependymal nodules
  structural imaging of, 446.*e*2
  in tuberous sclerosis, 1540
Subependymoma
  management of, 1058
  pathology and molecular genetics of, 1037
  structural imaging of, 418*t*–419*t*, 426.*e*1
Suberoylanilide hydroxamic acid (SAHA),
    for brain tumors, 1053
Subgaleal hemorrhage, in newborn, 1969*t*

Subjective cognitive impairment,
    1382–1383, 1385*t*
  DSM-V, 1385
  laboratory evaluation, 1385
  neuroimaging, 1385
Sublaterodorsal (SLD) nucleus, in NREM
    sleep, 1625.*e*1
Subliminal fringe, 392
Submandibular ganglion, 1726*f*
Suboccipital decompressive craniectomy,
    965*f*
Subplate neurons, of fetal brain, 1291
Subretinal neovascular membrane, 533
Subsarcolemmal vermiform deposits,
    familial cardiomyopathy with, 1927
Substance P, 697*t*–698*t*
  immunoregulatory effects of, 699*t*
Substantia nigra, 1396
  in basal ganglia, 1422–1423
Substantia nigra pars reticulata (SNr), 557
Substrate reduction therapy, for inborn
    errors of metabolism, 1331*f*
Subthalamic nucleus (STN)
  in basal ganglia, 1422–1423
  in Huntington disease, 1422–1423
Subthalamic nucleus (STN) deep brain
    stimulation
  for dopamine dysregulation syndrome,
    405–406
  for Parkinson disease, 402
α-subunits, of voltage-gated ion channels,
    1519
Succinate dehydrogenase (SDH), in
    mitochondrial disorders, 1356–1357
Sudden give-way, 284
Sudden neurological deficit, structural
    imaging for, 458.*e*4
Sudden unexplained death in epilepsy
    (SUDEP), 640, 1585
Sudden unexplained nocturnal death
    syndrome (SUNDS), 1669–1670
Suicide
  after traumatic brain injury, 91
  in epilepsy, 88
  in Huntington disease, 82*t*, 83
  in multiple sclerosis, 84
Suicide headache, 1708
Sulci, development of, 1287–1288
  disorders of, 1288
  neuroblast migration in, 1284, 1285*f*
Sulfite oxidase deficiency, 1325–1326
Sulindac (Clinoril), for chronic pain, 725*t*
Sumatriptan
  for cluster headache, 1710
  for migraine, 1700, 1700.*e*1t
    menstrual, 1704
    oral, intranasal, subcutaneous, 1700,
      1700.*e*1t
Summating potential, 603
Sunderland, Sydney, 903
Sunderland plexus, 904
Sundowning syndrome
  in delirium, 25
  in dementia, 1656–1657
SUNDS (sudden unexplained nocturnal
    death syndrome), 1669–1670
Sunitinib, for brain tumors, 1053–1054
Superantigens, in autoimmune disease, 687
Superficial cervical plexus block, 729*t*
Superficial hemosiderosis, 1764, 1765*f*
Superficial peroneal nerve, motor and
    sensory function of, 334*t*
Superficial radial sensory neuropathy, 1807
Superficial sensory division, 557

Superficial siderosis
  ataxia in, 1464, 1464f
  structural imaging of, 441, 436.e1f
Superficial vein thrombosis, 966
Superior canal dehiscence (SCD)
  hearing loss due to, 592, 597
  vertigo due to, 583
Superior cerebellar artery (SCA) aneurysm,
    symptoms of, 990
Superior cerebellar artery (SCA) infarction,
    929
Superior colliculus, in horizontal eye
    movements, 554
Superior lateral pontine syndrome, 214b,
    215f
Superior medial pontine syndrome, 214b,
    215f
Superior oblique muscle
  actions of, 528–529, 529t
  anatomy of, 529f
  palsy, 532–533, 535f
  weakness of, 533–534
Superior oblique myokymia, 551
  defined, 541
  detection of, 551
  versus monocular nystagmus, 545
  treatment of, 546t, 551
Superior rectus muscle
  actions of, 528–529, 529t
  anatomy of, 529f
Superior sagittal sinus thrombosis, 966f
Supine hypertension, treatment of,
    1894–1895
Supine hypotensive syndrome, due to
    autonomic disorders, 1890
Supplementary eye field (SEF), in horizontal
    eye movements, 556–557
Supplementary motor area (SMA)
  in praxis, 116
  upper motor neurons and, 1484
Supplements, for viral infections, 1127t
Suppressor T cells, in self-tolerance,
    684–685
Suppurative otitis, 596
Suprachiasmatic nucleus (SCN), in NREM
    sleep, 1625.e2f
Supramaximal stimulation, for nerve
    conduction studies, 366–367
Supramodal cortex, 58
Supranormal fusional amplitudes, 536–537
Supranuclear bulbar palsy, 210
Supranuclear gaze disturbances, 560–571
  cause of, 561t–562t
  disorders of convergence as, 570–571,
      570b
  disorders of divergence as, 571, 572b
  disorders of vertical gaze as, 567–570,
      569f
  evaluation of, 563
  horizontal gaze palsy as
    acquired, 564–565
    familial, 564
  internuclear ophthalmoplegia as, 567,
      567b
  ocular motor apraxia as, 563–564, 563b
    autosomal recessive, 564
    early-onset, with ataxia, 564
    type 1 syndrome, 564
    type 2, 564
  one-and-a-half syndrome as, 567
  periodic alternating gaze deviation as,
      565
  ping-pong gaze as, 565
  prolonged saccadic latency as, 566
  saccadic lateropulsion as, 565
  slow saccades as, 566, 566b

Supranuclear gaze disturbances (Continued)
    spasm of fixation as, 564
    square-wave jerks as, 542t, 546t, 566–567,
      566b, 566f
    torsional saccades as, 565
    wrong-way eyes as, 565
Supranuclear gaze palsy, 560
Supraorbital nerve, 1726f
Suprapubic catheter, for neurogenic bladder
    dysfunction, 619
Suprascapular nerve, 1807
Suprascapular nerve block, 729t
Suprascapular nerve entrapment, 1801t
    arm and neck pain due to, 328
Suprasellar tumor, 1027t
Supratentorial primitive neuroectodermal
    tumor
    management of, 1060
    pediatric, 1067
Supratentorial tumor, 1027t
Suprathreshold static perimetry, in visual
    field testing, 579
Supratrochlear nerve, 1726f
Supraventricular tachycardias, syncope due
    to, 10–11
Sural nerve, motor and sensory function of,
    334t
Sural nerve lesions, 1809
Suramin, neuropathy due to, 1862–1863
Surface dysgraphia, 139
Surface dyslexia, 139
Surgery
    for brain metastases, 1087–1088
    for brain tumor, 1049–1050
      complications of, 1047
    complications from, in pediatric nervous
      system tumors, 1083.e1
    for Duchenne muscular dystrophy,
      1923
    with inborn errors of metabolism, 1332
    for leptomeningeal metastases, 1098
    for neurogenic bladder dysfunction, 618,
      619t
    for pituitary tumors, 711
    for spinal cord compression, 1094
      with radiation therapy, 1094
Surgical clipping, of intracranial aneurysm,
    991, 991f
Surgical therapy
    for acute ischemic stroke, 960–962
    for carotid artery stenosis
      asymptomatic, 961–962
      symptomatic, 960–961
    for cerebellar hemorrhage, 981, 982.e1f
    for cluster headache, 1711
    of intracranial aneurysm, 991, 991f–992f
Surgical Trial of Intracerebral Haemorrhage
    (STICH), 981
Surround inhibition (SI), in transcranial
    magnetic stimulation, 393, 394t
Surveillance, Epidemiology, and End Results
    (SEER) Program, 1018
Survival rate
    for multiple sclerosis, 641
    with primary neoplasms, 637–638
Susac syndrome, 161, 440.e1
    ischemic stroke due to, 944, 944f
Susceptibility-weighted imaging, 417.e3–
    417.e4, 417.e4f
Suspected non-Alzheimer pathway (sNAP),
    1394
Suspended sensory loss, 318
Sustiva (efavirenz), for HIV infection,
    1108t–1109t
SV40 (simian virus 40), and brain tumors,
    1022

svPPA (Semantic variant primary progressive
    aphasia), functional neuroimaging of,
    489–490
Swallowing
    central control of, 148–149
    esophageal phase of, 148
    horizontal and vertical subsystems of, 148
    neurophysiology of, 148–149
    normal, 148
    oral (swallowing-preparatory) phase of,
      148
    pharyngeal phase of, 148
    reflex, 148
    during sleep, 1630t, 1631
    stages of, 148
    volitional, 148
Swallowing symptoms, functional,
    2000–2001
Sweat testing, for autonomic disorders, 1875
Sweating
    abnormalities, in autonomic disorders,
      1872, 1872t
    gustatory, 1872t
SWIFT-PRIME trial, for ischemic stroke,
    761–762
Swine influenza vaccination, and Guillain-
    Barré syndrome, 1144
Swinging flashlight test, 575–576, 576b,
    576f
Sydenham chorea, and Streptococcus pyogenes,
    695
Sylvian fissure, development of, 1287–1288,
    1288f
    disorders of, 1288
Symmetrically impaired pursuit, 557
Symmetry, disorders of, 1293
Sympathetic activity, during sleep, 1629,
    1630t
Sympathetic division, 1867–1868
Sympathetic skin response (SSR), 1875
Sympathomimetic agents, intracerebral
    hemorrhage due to, 974–975, 975f
Symptom management, 715–717
    for aphasia and dysarthria, 716
    for ataxia, 716
    for memory impairment and dementia,
      717
    for pain, 715
    for respiratory failure, 716–717, 716b
      ethical considerations in, 716–717
      terminal, 717
    for sensory loss, paresthesias, and burning
      pain, 715
    slowness of movement or abnormal
      involuntary movements, 716
    treatment of common neurological
      symptoms, 715–717
    for weakness, 715–716
Symptomatic cyclical oculomotor palsy, 571
Symptomatic generalized epilepsy, 1566
"Symptomatic narcolepsy", 1643
Symptoms, functional, 1993t
Synapsins, 697t–698t
Synaptic plasticity, sports and performance
    concussion and, 861
Synaptic trafficking abnormalities,
    1346–1347
Synaptogenesis, 1289–1290
    disorders of, 1289–1290
Synaptophysin, 1029–1030
Syncopal migraine, 1878
Syncope, 8–13
    in adults, 815–816
    causes of, 10–13
      atrioventricular block as, 10
      cardiac arrhythmias as, 10

Syncope (Continued)
  cerebrovascular ischemia as, 12
  decreased cardiac output as, 11
  hyperventilation as, 12
  hypotension as, 11–12
  hypovolemia as, 11
  metabolic disorders as, 12
  miscellaneous, 12–13
  paroxysmal tachycardia as, 10–11
  reflex cardiac arrhythmias as, 11
  sinoatrial block as, 10
  classification and etiology of, 9b
  clinical features of, 9t
  convulsive, 12–13
  cough (tussive), 12
  defecation, 12–13
  defined, 8
  drop attacks due to, 17–18
  due to brain tumor, 1047
  versus epilepsy, 1591
  glossopharyngeal neuralgia with, 11, 1732
  history and physical examination for, 8–10
  investigations of patients with, 13
  micturition, 12–13
  orthostatic, 11–12
  versus seizures, 9t
  situational, 12
  temporal lobe, 14
  vasovagal or vasodepressor, 11
Syndrome of inappropriate antidiuretic hormone secretion (SIADH), 708–709, 1222
  causes of, 1223b
  clinical features of, 709
  etiology and pathophysiology of, 708–709, 709b
  in neurointensive care, 755, 755t
  with subarachnoid hemorrhage, 1222
  treatment of, 709
SYNE1 gene, in autosomal recessive cerebellar ataxia type 1, 1469–1470
Synergies, in neurophysiological schools, for rehabilitation, 786
Synovial cyst, 457, 457f
Syntax, 128
α-Synuclein, 1401
  neurodegenerative movement disorders due to, 1426–1427, 1438f
Synucleinopathy
  dementia due to, 1399–1404
  neurodegenerative movement disorders due to, 1430
  in sleep disorder, 1656–1657, 1656f
Syphilis
  ischemic stroke due to, 939
  neuro-, psychiatric manifestations and, 102
Syringobulbia, 209–210, 1746–1749
  defined, 1746
Syringomyelia, 1746–1749
  clinical correlations with, 1748–1749, 1748f
  clinical presentation of, 1746
  communicating and noncommunicating, 1747
  defined, 1746
  diagrammatic representation of, 1746f
  MRI of, 1746, 1747f
  post-traumatic, 898
  sensory abnormalities due to, 319t, 322
  treatment of, 1748

Syrinx
  associated with other focal spinal cord pathologies, 1748–1749
  associated with spinal cord trauma, 1748
  associated with spinal cord tumors, 1747, 1747.e1f
  clinical presentation of, 1746
  communicating and noncommunicating, 1747
  defined, 1746
  due to abnormalities of cervicomedullary junction, 1747
  treatment of, 1748
System disorder, 5
Systemic diseases, neurologic complications in children of, 835–849
  of adrenal gland dysfunction, 847
    in Addison disease, 847
    in Cushing syndrome, 847
    with excess mineralocorticoid secretion, 847
  of cardiac disorders and the nervous system, 835–838
    acquired, 838
    congenital heart disease as, 835–836
    due to cardiac transplantation, 837
    due to intervention and cardiac surgery, 837, 837f
  of connective tissue diseases and vasculitides, 838–841
    Behçet disease as, 841
    Churg-Strauss syndrome as, 839
    granulomatosis with polyangiitis (Wegener) as, 840–841
    Henoch-Schönlein purpura as, 839
    juvenile rheumatoid arthritis as, 839
    Kawasaki disease as, 838–839
    primary angiitis of CNS as, 841
    Sjögren syndrome as, 841
    systemic lupus erythematosus as, 839–840, 840f
    Takayasu arteritis as, 839
  of diabetes mellitus, 847–848
  of gastrointestinal disorders, 845–846
    hepatic encephalopathy as, 845
    with liver transplantation, 845–846
  of hematological disorders, 843–845
    hemolytic disease of newborn and kernicterus as, 843
    hemolytic-uremic syndrome as, 845
    hemophilia as, 844
    hemorrhagic disease of newborn, 843
    neonatal polycythemia as, 843
    sickle cell disease as, 843–844, 844f
    thrombotic thrombocytopenic purpura as, 844–845
  of parathyroid disorders, 846–847
    hyperparathyroidism as, 847
    hypoparathyroidism as, 846–847
  of pituitary disorders, 847
  of renal disorders, 848–849
    complications of dialysis as, 848
    due to renal transplantation, 848–849
    renal failure as, 848
  of respiratory disorders, 841–842
    bronchopulmonary dysplasia as, 841–842
    cystic fibrosis as, 842
    of hypertension, 842–843, 843f
    periodic breathing and apnea as, 841
    sarcoidosis as, 842
  of thyroid disorders, 846
    hyperthyroidism as, 846
    hypothyroidism as, 846

Systemic diseases, neurological complications in adults, 814–834
  of adrenal glands, 833
    Addison disease as, 833
    pheochromocytoma as, 833
  of antiphospholipid antibody syndromes, 827, 827f
  of cardiac disorders and the nervous system, 815–818
    cardiac arrest as, 816
    cardiogenic embolism as, 815
    due to complications of cardiac catheterization and surgery, 816–817, 817f
    infective endocarditis as, 817–818, 817f
    medication and, 817
    syncope as, 815–816
  of connective tissue diseases and vasculitides, 819–822
    Behçet disease as, 822
    giant cell arteritis as, 820
    granulomatosis with polyangiitis, 820–821
    isolated angiitis of nervous system as, 821
    polyarteritis nodosa, Churg-Strauss syndrome, and overlap syndrome as, 819–820, 820f
    progressive systemic sclerosis as, 822
    relapsing polychondritis as, 822
    rheumatoid arthritis as, 821, 821f
    Sjögren syndrome as, 821–822
    systemic lupus erythematosus as, 821
  of diabetes insipidus, 832
  of diabetes mellitus, 833–834
    in central nervous system, 833–834
    due to hypoglycemia, 834
    in peripheral nervous system, 833
  diseases of aorta and, 818–819
    aortic aneurysms as, 818
    aortitis as, 818–819
    coarctation of aorta as, 819
    complications of aortic surgery as, 819
    subclavian steal syndrome as, 819
  of electrolyte disturbances, 830–831
    of calcium, 830–831
    of magnesium, 831
    of potassium, 830
    of sodium, 830
  of gastrointestinal diseases, 828
    celiac disease as, 828
    gastric surgery and, 828
    small-bowel disease as, 828
    Whipple disease as, 828, 829f
  of hematological disorders with anemia, 824
    acanthocytic syndromes as, 824
    megaloblastic anemia as, 824
    sickle cell disease as, 824
    thalassemias as, 824
  of hemorrhagic diseases, 826–827
    disseminated intravascular coagulation as, 826
    hemophilia as, 826
    iatrogenic, 826–827
    thrombocytopenia as, 826
    thrombotic thrombocytopenic purpura as, 826
  of liver disease, 827–828, 827f
    chronic non-Wilsonian hepatocerebral degeneration as, 827–828
    liver transplantation as, 828

Systemic diseases, neurological
complications in adults *(Continued)*
portal-systemic encephalopathy as, 827,
828*f*
pancreatic encephalopathy as, 828
of parathyroid disease, 833
hyperparathyroidism as, 833
hypoparathyroidism as, 833
of pituitary diseases, 831–832, 831*f*
Cushing disease and syndrome as,
831–832
hypopituitarism as, 832
pituitary adenomas as, 831, 831*f*
of proliferative hematological disorders,
824–826
amyloidosis as, 825
cryoglobulinemia as, 825–826
leukemias as, 824
lymphoma as, 826
monoclonal gammopathy of
undetermined significance as,
825
myelomatosis as, 824–825
plasma cell dyscrasias as, 824–826
polycythemia as, 826
Waldenström macroglobulinemia as,
825
of renal failure, 829–830
complications of dialysis as,
829–830
complications of renal transplantation
as, 830
overview of, 829
of respiratory diseases, 822
hypercapnia as, 822
hypocapnia as, 822
hypoxia as, 822
of sarcoidosis, 823, 823*f*
of systemic inflammatory response
syndrome, 822–823
of thyroid disease, 832–833
Hashimoto thyroiditis as, 832–833
hyperthyroidism as, 832
hypothyroidism as, 832
Systemic inflammatory response syndrome,
neurological complications of, 822–823
Systemic lupus erythematosus (SLE)
dementia in, 1419–1420
ischemic stroke due to, 940, 940*f*
neurological complications of, in children,
839–840, 840*f*
neuropathy in, 1852.*e*1
optic neuropathy due to, 167–168
oral contraceptives and, 1974
psychiatric manifestations of, 104
seizures due to, 1582–1583
sex and, 687
Systemic sclerosis, neuropathy in, 1852.*e*1
Systemic therapy, for leptomeningeal
metastases, 1099
Systemic vasculitides, stroke and, 940–942,
940*f*–942*f*
Systems, review of, 3
Systems biology, future role in neurogenetic
disease, 669–671, 670*f*
Systolic acceleration slope, 476–477

T

T cell(s)
in central tolerance, 684
cytotoxic
in immune response, 677
antigenic recognition in, 680*f*
cytotoxic, in paraneoplastic neurological
syndromes, 1187

T cell(s) *(Continued)*
helper
B cells and, 682
cytokine secretion by, 682
in immune response, 677
antigenic recognition in, 680*f*
helper, in HIV disease, 1103
in immune system, 677
immunoglobulin, and mucin-domain
containing molecules (Tim), in
immune response, 683
MHC class I and class I restricted, 679,
680*f*
in multiple sclerosis, 1162
in myasthenia gravis, 1899
regulatory, 684–685
termination of immune response of,
684
for viral infections, 1131*t*
T-cell activation
accessory molecules for, 681–682
CD3 as, 681
CD4 and CD8, 681
and cell migration, 681–682
costimulatory molecules as, 681, 681*f*
anergy due to failure of, 684, 685*f*
two-signal model of, 685*f*
T-cell-mediated autoimmune disease,
686–687
T-cell receptors (TCRs)
in immune system, 678, 678*f*
and superantigens, 687
T-cytotoxic (T$_C$) cells, in immune response,
677
antigenic recognition in, 680*f*
T dependent. *see* Thymus-dependent
(T-dependent)
T-helper (T$_H$) cells
B cells and, 682
cytokine secretion by, 682
in immune response, 677
antigenic recognition in, 680*f*
T1 contrast, in MRI, 415
T1 relaxation time, 413–414, 414*f*
T1 weighting, 415, 415*f*–416*f*, 416*t*
T2 contrast, in MRI, 415
T2 relaxation time, 413–414, 414*f*
T2-shine-through, in diffusion-weighted
imaging, 415
T2 weighting, 415, 415*f*–416*f*, 416*t*
T2* weighting, in MRI, 417.*e*1
T$_3$ (triiodothyronine), 112
T$_4$ (levothyroxine), 112
[^{18}F] T807, in chemical imaging, 509
Tabes dorsalis, 1775
Tachycardias, in neurointensive care,
753
Tachykinins, 697*t*–698*t*
Tachyphemia, 225
Tacrine, 1397
Tacrolimus
for myasthenia gravis, 1903*t*, 1906
necrotizing myopathies due to,
1954
neuropathy due to, 1863
TACs (trigeminal-autonomic cephalalgias),
1709, 1711–1713
Tactile agnosias, 127
Tactile aphasia, 127
Tadalafil, for erectile dysfunction, 621, 621*t*,
632
Tadpole pupil, 186
Taenia genus, CNS lesions due to,
1157
Taenia solium, 1156–1157, 1156*t*
Tailored resection, for epilepsy, 1607

Takayasu arteritis
ischemic stroke due to, 940, 940*f*
neurological complications of, in children,
839
syncope due to, 12
Takotsubo "broken heart" syndrome,
1881–1882, 1881*f*–1882*f*
Takotsubo cardiomyopathy, 1881
in neurointensive care, 753
Tamsulosin, for bladder dysfunction, 796*t*
Tandem gait, 4, 254
Tandem mass spectrometry (TMS), for
inborn errors of metabolism, 1327,
1327.*e*1*t*
Tangential migration, along axons,
1284–1286
Tangier disease, 1338, 1818.*e*9
Tapentadol, for chronic pain, 728
Tapia syndrome, 1722*t*, 1732–1733
Tardive dyskinesia, 237, 239–240, 239*t*,
1450–1451
Tardive dystonia, 1450–1451
Target fiber, with denervation, 1916, 1917*f*
Targeted mutation analysis, 673*t*
Targeted sequence analysis, 673, 673*t*
Targeted therapies, for brain tumors, 1054*b*
Tarsal tunnel syndrome, 1809
Task-Free Functional MRI, 1392–1393
Task-oriented practice, in rehabilitation, 787
Task-oriented therapies, for developmental
coordination disorders, 1317
Task-specific dystonia, 235, 1452–1453
Taste, 190–196
anatomy and physiology of, 190–192
chemosensory testing of, 192–193, 192*f*
clinical evaluation of, 195
disorders of, 194–195
treatment and management of, 195–196
Taste buds, 191
Taste papillae, 192*f*
Tau imaging, in Alzheimer disease, 1393
Tau-opathy, in sleep disorder, 1656–1657,
1656*f*
Tau protein
in Alzheimer disease, 1413
in chemical imaging, 505*t*, 506
in neurodegenerative movement disorders,
1439
Tauopathy, in neurodegenerative movement
disorders, 1441
Taxanes
for brain tumors, 1051, 1052*t*–1053*t*
neuropathy due to, 1863
Tay-Sachs disease, 1333.*e*2*t*–1333.*e*3*t*
Tay syndrome, 1560
TBE (tickborne encephalitis) virus, 1139.*e*1
T$_C$ (T-cytotoxic) cells, in immune response,
677
antigenic recognition in, 680*f*
TCCD (transcranial color-coded duplex)
ultrasonography, 480
TD (tardive dyskinesia), 1450–1451
TDP-43 (TAR DNA-binding protein 43),
1413
in Alzheimer disease, 1397
TDP-43-opathy, in sleep disorder, 1656*f*
TDP1 (tyrosyl-DNA phosphodiesterase 1)
mutation, ataxia due to, 1469
TE (time to echo), in MRI, 414–415
effective, 417.*e*1
TE (toxoplasmic encephalitis), HIV-
associated, 1114*t*
Tea, and brain tumors, 1023
TEACCH (Treatment and Education of
Autistic and Related Communication-
Handicapped Children), 1306

Teardrop fractures, 888–889
Techenetium-99m (^{99m}Tc), for SPECT, 487
^{99m}Tc (technetium-99m), for SPECT, 487
Tectal deafness, 209
Tectospinal tract, in control of upper motor neurons, 1485
TEE (transesophageal echocardiography), for threatened stroke, 952
Teichopsia, 123
Telangiectasia
  in ataxia-telangiectasia, 1552–1553
  conjunctival, 1468f
  hereditary hemorrhagic, 1550–1551
    neurological features of, 1550–1551
    treatment of, 1551
  hereditary hemorrhagic, ischemic stroke due to, 944
Telegraphic speech, 131
Telencephalic flexure, 1287–1288, 1288f
  disorders of, 1288
Telephone Interview for Cognitive Status-Modified (mTICS), 517, 518f
Telethonin deficiency, 1926
Tellurium, occupational exposure to, 1244
Temazepam (Restoril), for dystonia, 1452t
Temozolomide
  for brain tumor, complications of, 1048
  for brain tumors, 1052t–1053t
Temperature
  with coma, 38
  and nerve conduction studies, 370
Temperature-dependent sensory loss, 320
Temperature regulation, hypothalamus in, 698–700, 699f
Temporal arteritis, ischemic optic neuropathy due to, 166, 167f
Temporal arteritis, ischemic stroke due to, 941–942
Temporal cortex, in memory, 61
Temporal dispersion, in nerve conduction studies, 371, 372f
Temporal isthmus, 136
Temporal lobe epilepsy (TLE)
  familial, 1533
    lateral, 1533
    mesial, 1578
  mesial
    familial, 1578
    with hippocampal sclerosis, 1578–1579, 1578f–1579f
Temporal lobe syncope, 14
Temporal lobectomy
  and amnestic syndrome, 62
  for epilepsy, 1607
Temporal patterns, of neuronal damage after traumatic brain injury, 851–852, 852f
Temporal-severity profile, 2
Temporomandibular joint, imaging of, headache and, 202
Temporomandibular joint disorders (TMJ), headache and facial pain due to, 1695
Temporoparietal cortex (TPC), 399
Tender points, in fibromyalgia, 1764–1765, 1765f
Tendon reflexes, for arm and neck pain, 327
Tendonitis, arm and neck pain due to, 331
Tenecteplase (TNK), for acute ischemic stroke, 958
"Tennis elbow", 331
Tenosynovitis, de Quervain, 1807
Tensilon (edrophonium) test, for diplopia, 539
Tension headache, in pregnancy, 1975

Tension-type headache, 1713
  in children and adolescents, 1719
  pathophysiology of, 1713
  physical examination in, 1713
  prevalence of, 1713
Teratogenic effects
  of antiepileptic drugs, 1985
  of drugs and toxins, 1971, 1971f
Teratoid tumor, atypical
  pathology and molecular genetics of, 1039
  pediatric, 1069–1070
Teratoma
  immature, management of, 1063
  immature, pathology and molecular genetics of, 1042
  mature, management of, 1063
  mature, pathology and molecular genetics of, 1042
Terazosin hydrochloride (Hytrin), for bladder dysfunction, in multiple sclerosis, 1183
Terbinafine, taste disorders due to, 195
Teriflunomide (Aubagio), for multiple sclerosis, 1179
Terminal tremor, 230, 234
Terminally ill patient, care of, 718
Tertiary store, in repetitive nerve stimulation, 386
Test administration, for neuropsychological evaluation, 512–513
  fixed battery approach to, 512–513, 513b
  flexible battery approach to, 513, 514f
Test interpretation, for neuropsychological evaluation, 513–515
  current *versus* past performance in, 515
  cut scores, 514
Test stimulation (TS), in transcranial magnetic stimulation, 392, 392f
Test validation studies, in neuropsychological evaluation, 514
Testosterone, during sleep, 1631
Tetany, muscle pain due to, 303
Tethered cord syndromes, 1745–1746, 1745b
Tetrabenazine
  for dystonia, 1452t
  for Huntington disease, 1448
Tetrahydrobiopterin (BH4), in inborn errors of metabolism, 1331–1332
TETRAS (The Essential Tremor Rating Assessment Scale), 1443
TGA (transient global amnesia), 926
TGF-β. *see* Transforming growth factor beta (TGF-β)
Thalamic aphasia, 136
Thalamic damage, after traumatic brain injury, 852
Thalamic hemorrhage, 322, 977, 978t, 977.e1f
  ventricular drainage for, 982
Thalamic infarction, 319t, 322
  syndromes of, 931, 931.e1f
Thalamic nuclei, in delirium, 26
Thalamic pain syndrome, 319t, 322
Thalamic stroke syndromes, 210–211, 211b
  arterial territories and, 210–211, 211f
  blood supply of thalamus and, 210–211, 210f
Thalamic syndrome, 209
Thalamocingulate tract, in memory, 62f
Thalamoperforate arteries, infarction of, hemiplegia due to, 264

Thalamus
  arterial territories of, 210–211, 211f
  blood supply of, 210–211, 210f
  in memory, 62f
  in sensory system, 314
  tumor of, 1027t
Thalassemias, neurological complications of, 824
Thalidomide, neuropathy due to, 1863
Thallium, occupational exposure to, 1244
THAN (transitory hyperammonemia of newborn), 1336
The Essential Tremor Rating Assessment Scale (TETRAS), 1443
Theiler murine encephalomyelitis virus-induced disease (TMEV-IDD), 689–690
Thenar atrophy, in carpal tunnel syndrome, 1802, 1803f
Theory of Mind, 59
"Theory of mind" deficits, 96
Therapy Wilmington Robotic Exoskeleton (T-WREX), 802
Thermal diffusion flowmetry, in neurointensive care, 744t, 748
Thermoregulation, during sleep, 1630t, 1631
Thermoregulatory function theory, of sleep, 1628–1629
Thermoregulatory sweat test (TST), 1875
Theta activity
  on EEG, 349–350
  sleep staging, 1619f
Thiamine
  for coma, 35–37
  defined, 1231
  and inborn errors of metabolism, 1338–1339
  metabolism of, 1231
  requirement of, 1231
Thiamine deficiency, 1231
Thiamine deficiency neuropathy, 1231
Thick filament, myopathy associated with, 1955
Thick phlegm, in amyotrophic lateral sclerosis, 1513t
Thiotepa
  for brain tumors, 1052t–1053t
  for leptomeningeal metastases, 1099
Third cranial nerve nucleus, lesions of, 208
Third cranial nerve palsy, due to intracranial aneurysms, 990
Third-degree nerve injury, 371–373
Third ventricle tumor, 1027t
Third ventricular abnormalities, drop attacks due to, 18
Thirst, posterior pituitary in, 708
Thomsen disease, 1526
Thoracic disk herniation, 1755, 1755f
Thoracic outlet syndrome
  arm and neck pain due to, 328
  monoplegia due to, 271–272
Thoracic roots, anatomy of, 1767f
Thoracic segmental artery, 1007.e1f
Thoracic spinal cord, herniation through dura of, 1755, 1756f
Thoracic spondylosis, 1755, 1755f–1756f
Thoracolumbar injuries, 889, 889f
Thoracolumbar outflow, neurogenic bladder dysfunction due to impaired sympathetic, 611
Three-dimensional carotid ultrasound, 479

Three-dimensional contrast-enhanced MRA (3D CE-MRA), 466, 470–471
  of carotid and vertebral circulation, 466
    after stent placement, 469, 471*f*
    with basilar artery stenosis, 469, 469*f*
    with carotid artery dissection, 469, 470*f*–471*f*
    with carotid stenosis, 468*f*
    with fibromuscular dysplasia, 469
    with vertebral artery dissection, 469, 470*f*
  fast, dynamic, or time-resolved, 466
Three-step test, for vertical diplopia, 538–539, 538*f*, 539*b*
3-ounce water swallow test, for dysphagia, 157
3Tc (lamivudine), for HIV infection, 1108*t*–1109*t*
Threshold, 192–193
Threshold effect, of mtDNA mutations, 1353
Threshold for electrical failure, in cerebral ischemia, 925
Threshold of membrane failure, in cerebral ischemia, 925
Threshold static perimetry, in visual field testing, 579
Thrombectomy, mechanical, for acute ischemic stroke, 958, 960*t*
Thromboangiitis obliterans, ischemic stroke due to, 941–942
Thrombocythemia, ischemic stroke due to, 948
Thrombocytopenia
  heparin-induced, ischemic stroke due to, 948–949
  immune-mediated, intracerebral hemorrhage due to, 969–971
  in neurointensive care, 757
  neurological complications of, 826
Thromboembolic complications, in neurointensive care, 757
Thromboembolic origin, ischemic stroke of, 432.*e*1–432.*e*2
Thromboembolism
  spinal cord infarction due to, 1009
  with spinal cord injury, 901
Thrombolysis, intra-arterial, for ischemic stroke, 759
Thrombolytic therapy
  for acute ischemic stroke, 956–960, 959*f*
  for stroke, in children, 1005
Thrombophilia, specialized laboratory tests for, 950*b*
Thrombotic thrombocytopenic purpura (TTP)
  ischemic stroke due to, 949
  neurological complications of
    in adults, 826
    in children, 844–845
Thunderclap headache, 198, 1691
Thymectomy, for myasthenia gravis, 1907–1908
Thymidine phosphorylase deficiency, removal or neutralization of toxic metabolites for, 1362
Thymidine phosphorylase replacement therapy, 1362
Thymocytes, in central tolerance, 684
Thymomatous myasthenia gravis, 1899, 1900*t*
Thymopentin, 697*t*–698*t*
Thymosin, 697*t*–698*t*
Thymus, in myasthenia gravis, 1899
Thymus-dependent (T-dependent), 682

Thyroid disease
  neurological complications of, in adults, 832–833
  psychiatric manifestations of, 102–103
Thyroid hormone, 112
Thyroid ophthalmopathy, structural imaging for, 449.*e*1, 449.*e*2*f*
Thyroid-stimulating hormone (TSH), excessive secretion of, 706, 711
Thyroid-stimulating hormone deficiency, treatment of, 711
Thyroid storm, psychiatric manifestations of, 102
Thyroiditis, Hashimoto, neurological complications of, 832–833
Thyrotoxic periodic paralysis, 832, 1524, 1937
Thyrotropin, during sleep, 1627–1628
Thyrotropin (TSH)
  hypothalamic peptides controlling release of, 702*t*
  immunoregulatory effects of, 699*t*
Thyrotropin-releasing hormone (TRH), 697*t*–698*t*
Thyrotropin-releasing hormone (TRH) test, 710*t*
TI (inversion time), in MRI, 417.*e*2
Tiagabine
  for chronic pain, 726
  for epilepsy
    absorption, elimination half-life, formulations of, 1600*t*
    efficacy by seizure type of, 1601*t*
    hepatic metabolism, enzyme induction/inhibition, pharmacokinetic interactions, and protein binding of, 1603*t*
    mechanism of action of, 1604*t*
  psychotropic effects of, 89*t*
Tibial nerve, 1809
  applied anatomy of, 1809
  motor and sensory function of, 334*t*
Tibial nerve entrapment, 1802*t*, 1809
Tic douloureux. *see* Trigeminal neuralgia
Tick paralysis, 1249
Tickborne encephalitis (TBE) virus, 1139.*e*1
Ticlopidine, for preventing stroke recurrence, 953
Tics, 240–242, 240*b*, 1456–1457
  in autism spectrum disorder, 1307*t*
  common symptoms of, 241
  etiological classification of, 241*b*
  examination of, 242
  in Tourette syndrome, 1456–1457
    clinical features of, 1456–1457
    pathogenesis of, 1457
    treatment of, 1457
Tidal wave, in intracranial pressure monitoring, 745
Tightrope walker's gait, 1999
Tilt-table testing, 1875
Tilted optic disc, 175, 175*f*
Time-locked digitally recorded video image, in EEG, 351
Time-of-flight MRA (TOF-MRA), 464–466
  accuracy of, 469
  for arteriovenous malformations, 474–475
  of carotid stenosis, 467
  for cerebral aneurysms, 472
  of coiled intracranial aneurysms, 467
  of extracranial carotid and vertebral circulation, 467–469, 467*f*
  sensitivity and specificity of, 467
Time-resolved imaging of contrast kinetics (TRICKS) MRA (trMRA) technique, 475–476

Time to echo
  effective, 417.*e*1
  in MRI, 414–415
Timed swallowing tests, for dysphagia, 156–157
Tin, occupational exposure to, 1244–1245
Tincture of opium, for passive addiction and withdrawal syndrome, 1972
Tinel sign, 1802
Tinnitus, 596–598
  gaze-evoked, 571
  laboratory testing for, 601–603
    acoustic reflex testing, 602
    auditory testing, 601–603
      pure-tone testing for, 601, 602*f*
      speech testing for, 601–602
    evoked potentials, 602–603
    middle ear testing for, 602
    other tests, 603
  management of, 604
  rTMS for, 399
Tinofovir (Viread), for HIV infection, 1108*t*–1109*t*
Tipranavir (Aptivus), for HIV infection, 1108*t*–1109*t*
TIPSS. *see* Transjugular intrahepatic portosystemic shunt (TIPSS)
Tissue contrast, in MRI, 415, 415*f*–416*f*, 416*t*
Tissue magnetization, in MRI, 412
Tissue plasminogen activator (tPA), 603
  for acute ischemic stroke, 959*f*
  intracerebral hemorrhage due to, 971
Titin, 1926
Titubation, 227, 230
Tivicay (dolutegravir), for HIV infection, 1108*t*–1109*t*
Tizanidine
  for chronic pain, 726
  for spasticity, 799*t*
  for spasticity, in multiple sclerosis, 1182
TLRs. *see* Toll-like receptors (TLRs)
TMEM106B, 1413
TMEV-IDD. *see* Theiler murine encephalomyelitis virus-induced disease (TMEV-IDD)
TMJ (temporomandibular joint disorders), headache and facial pain due to, 1695
TMS (tandem mass spectrometry), for inborn errors of metabolism, 1327
TN (torsional (rotary) nystagmus), 542*t*, 546*t*, 548, 569
TNC (trigeminal nucleus caudalis), in migraine, 1699
TNF-α blockers, neuropathy due to, 1863
TNK (tenecteplase), for acute ischemic stroke, 958
TNMG. *see* Transient neonatal myasthenia gravis (TNMG)
Tobacco
  and brain tumors, 1023
  as risk factor for stroke, 923
Tobacco-alcohol amblyopia, 1234
α-Tocopherol transfer protein (TTPA)
  mutations in, 1229–1230
    ataxia with isolated vitamin E deficiency, 1467–1468
Todd paresis, stroke *versus*, 1002
TOF-MRA (time-of-flight MRA), 464–466
  accuracy of, 469
  for arteriovenous malformations, 474–475
  of carotid stenosis, 467
  for cerebral aneurysms, 472
  of coiled intracranial aneurysms, 467
  of extracranial carotid and vertebral circulation, 467–469, 467*f*
  sensitivity and specificity of, 467

Tolcapone, for Parkinson disease, 1435
Toll-like receptors (TLRs)
  in innate immune system, 676
  microglia and, 686
Tolmetin (Tolectin), for chronic pain, 725*t*
Tolosa-Hunt syndrome, 1722*t*, 1723
Tolterodine, for bladder dysfunction, 796*t*
Toluene
  ataxia due to, 1462
  occupational exposure to, 1241
Tolvaptan, for SIADH, 709
TOM (theory of mind) deficits, 96
Tomography, defined, 411
Tongue atrophy, in amyotrophic lateral
  sclerosis, 290, 290*f*, 1509*f*
Tonic activity, 1564
Tonic-clonic seizures, 14
  generalized, epilepsy with, 1578
Tonic downward deviation of gaze, 569
Tonic neck reflex, in hypotonic infant,
  306–307
Tonic neurons, in vertical eye movement,
  560, 560*f*
Tonic pupil, 180, 183*f*
Tonic seizures, 1565–1566
  generalized, 1570
Tonic tics, 240
Tonic upward gaze
  benign paroxysmal, 568–569
  deviation of, 568
Tooth grinding, 1661
Top of the Basilar Syndrome, 560
Topical analgesics, for chronic pain, 726
Topiramate, 526
  for chronic pain, 726
  for epilepsy
    absorption, elimination half-life,
      formulations of, 1600*t*
    efficacy by seizure type of, 1601*t*
    hepatic metabolism, enzyme induction/
      inhibition, pharmacokinetic
      interactions, and protein binding
      of, 1603*t*
    mechanism of action of, 1604*t*
  for migraine, 1703
    chronic, 1707
    prophylaxis, 1703
  for neuropathic pain, 918*t*–919*t*
  psychotropic effects of, 89*t*
  for tremor, in multiple sclerosis, 1182
Topographic maps, in EEG, 350, 351*f*
Topoisomerase inhibitors, for brain tumors,
  1051, 1052*t*–1053*t*
Topotecan, for brain tumors, 1052*t*–1053*t*
TORCH, 1966
Torsional (rotary) nystagmus (TN), 542*t*,
  546*t*, 548, 569
Torsional saccades, 565
Torticollis, benign paroxysmal, 1719
Tortopia, 541
Toscana virus, 1139–1140
Total ophthalmoplegia, 207, 208*b*
Total unilateral inferior pontine syndrome,
  930
Total unilateral medullary syndrome (of
  Babinski-Nageotte), 930
Touch imprints, 1028–1029
Touch sensation, 1770, 1770*f*
Tourette syndrome, 1456–1457
  behavior and personality disturbances in,
    83
  clinical features of, 1456–1457
  deep brain stimulation for, 404–405
  pathogenesis of, 1457

Tourette syndrome (*Continued*)
  in pregnancy, 1981
  streptococcal infections and, 695
  TICS and, 1456–1457
  treatment of, 1457
Tourette Syndrome Association, 404–405
Toxic disorders
  ataxia due to, 1461–1462
  psychiatric manifestations of, 102–105,
    102.*e*1*t*
  structural imaging of, 444
Toxic encephalopathies, 1210–1218
  clinical manifestations of, 1209–1210
  due to acute liver failure, 1210*t*,
    1216–1217
  hepatic. *see* Hepatic encephalopathy (HE)
  uremic, 1217
    calcium and parathyroid hormone in,
      1217
Toxic gain of function, 657
Toxic myopathies, 1953–1955
  acute quadriplegic myopathy/critical
    illness myopathy as, 1955
  amphiphilic, 1954
    due to amiodarone, 1954
    due to chloroquine, 1954
  antimicrotubular, 1954
    due to colchicine, 1954
  corticosteroid myopathy as, 1954–1955
  necrotizing, 1953–1954
    cholesterol-lowering drugs, 1953–1954
    due to immunophilins (cyclosporine
      and tacrolimus), 1954
Toxic neuropathies, 1858–1864
  nucleoside analog-associated, 1119–1120
  sensory abnormalities due to, 320
Toxic proteins, and neurodegenerative
  movement disorders, 1426*t*
Toxin- and drug-induced myoclonus,
  1458–1459
Toxin hypersensitivity, 1210
Toxin-induced parkinsonism, 1442
Toxin-related hypersomnolence, 1634–1635
Toxins
  effects on newborns of, 1970–1972, 1970*t*
    passive addiction and withdrawal
      syndrome as, 1971–1972
    risk for intracranial hemorrhage as,
      1971
    teratogenic effects and intrauterine
      growth retardation as, 1971, 1971*f*
  and stroke in children, 1000–1001
Toxins and physical agents
  animals and insects neurotoxins,
    1247–1249
    from scorpions, 1248–1249
    from snakes, 1248
    from spiders, 1248
    tick paralysis due to, 1249
  burns as, 1247
  effects on nervous system, 1237–1253
  electric current and lightning as, 1246
  hyperthermia as, 1246–1247
  hypothermia as, 1247
  marine neurotoxins as, 1251–1253
    from ciguatera fish, 1251–1252
    from puffer fish, 1252
    from shellfish, 1252–1253
  metals as, 1242–1245
    aluminum as, 1242
    arsenic as, 1242
    lead as, 1243
    manganese as, 1243–1244
    mercury as, 1244

Toxins and physical agents (*Continued*)
    tellurium as, 1244
    thallium as, 1244
    tin as, 1244–1245
  organic chemicals as, 1238–1242
    acrylamide as, 1238
    allyl chloride as, 1238
    carbon disulfide as, 1238–1239
    carbon monoxide as, 1239
    ethylene oxide as, 1239
    hexacarbon solvents as, 1239
    methyl bromide as, 1239–1240
    organocholine pesticides as, 1240
    organophosphates as, 1240–1241
    pyrethroids as, 1241
    pyriminil as, 1241
    solvent mixtures as, 1241
    styrene as, 1241
    toluene as, 1241
    trichloroethylene as, 1241–1242
  plants and fungi as, 1249–1251
    excitatory amino acids as, 1250
    from Jimson weed, 1249
    from medicinal herbs, 1250
    from morning glory, 1250
    from mushroom poisoning, 1250–1251,
      1251*t*
    from peyote, 1250
    from poison hemlock, 1249
    from water hemlock, 1249–1250
  radiation as
    ionizing, 1245
      encephalopathy due to, 1245
      myelopathy due to, 1245
      plexopathy due to, 1245
    nonionizing, 1245–1246
  vibration as, 1246
Toxocara genus, parasitic meningitis or
  encephalitis due to, 1155–1156
Toxoplasma gondii, 1156*t*, 1157
Toxoplasmic encephalitis (TE), 1157
  HIV-associated, 1114*t*, 1115
Toxoplasmosis
  cerebral
    HIV-associated, 1115, 1116*f*
    structural imaging of, 436.*e*5
  neonatal, 1967
TP53 mutations, in diffuse gliomas, 1033
tPA (tissue plasminogen activator)
  for acute ischemic stroke, 959*f*
  intracerebral hemorrhage due to, 971
TPM, for dystonia, 1452*t*
TR (repetition time), in MRI, 414–415, 414*f*
Tr antibodies, 1189
Traction, peripheral nerve injury due to,
  907–908
Traction response, in hypotonic infant,
  305–306
Tragus, 591
Trans-acting factors, 651*t*, 653
Transcortical aphasia, 135–136, 136*t*
Transcortical motor aphasia, 136, 136*t*
Transcortical sensory aphasia, 136, 136*t*
Transcranial color-coded duplex
  ultrasonography (TCCD), 480
Transcranial Doppler (TCD)
  of acute ischemic stroke, 480
  and brain death, 484
  of cervical carotid stenosis, 481
  and increased ICP, 483–484, 484*f*
  of intracranial atherosclerotic plaque, 482,
    482*f*
  in neurointensive care, 744*t*, 748
  of periprocedural monitoring, 484

Transcranial Doppler (TCD) (*Continued*)
  for threatened stroke, 951
  and thrombolytic agents, monitoring the
      effect of, 480
  for vasospasm, 994
  of vasospasms, 483
Transcranial magnetic stimulation (TMS),
      391–400
  acute effects of neurological drugs on,
      395t
  clinical applications for diagnostic use of,
      394–397
    for cervical myelopathy and other spinal
        cord lesions, 397
    for epilepsy and antiepileptic drugs,
        396
    for migraine, 397
    for movement disorders, 394–396,
        395t
      dystonia, 395–396
      Huntington disease, 396
      Parkinson disease and Parkinson plus
          syndromes, 394–395
    for multiple sclerosis, 397
    for other neurodegenerative disorders,
        395t, 396
      amyotrophic lateral sclerosis,
          396
      cerebellar disorders, 396
      dementia and mild cognitive
          impairment, 396
    for stroke, 396–397
  historical background of, 391
  methods and their neurophysiological
      background for, 391
    central motor conduction measurements
        in, 391–392, 394t
    cerebellar inhibition in, 394, 394t
    interhemispheric inhibition (IHI),
        393–394, 394t
    intracortical facilitation in, 393, 394t
      short-interval, 393, 394t
    intracortical inhibition in
      long-interval, 392, 394t
      short-interval, 393, 394t
    MEP recruitment curve in, 392, 394t
    motor excitability measurements in,
        392–394, 394t
    motor thresholds in, 392, 394t
    other inhibitory phenomena of the
        motor cortex, 393–394, 394t
    short-latency and long latency afferent
        inhibition in, 393, 394t
    silent period in, 392, 392f, 394t
    stimulation parameters for diagnostic
        use of, 391–394, 394t
    surround inhibition in, 393, 394t
  for migraine, 1702
  motor cortical plasticity measurements in,
      394
  paired-pulse, 393f
  repetitive
    basic principles of, 397–398
    rationale for, 397
    therapeutic application of, current
        concepts of, 398–400
      for amyotrophic lateral sclerosis,
          399–400
      for auditory hallucinations and
          negative symptoms in
          schizophrenia, 398
      for depression, 398
      for dystonia, 399
      for epilepsy, 400
      for pain and migraine, 399
      for Parkinson disease, 398–399

Transcranial magnetic stimulation (TMS)
      (*Continued*)
      for stroke with motor deficits,
          aphasia, and hemispatial neglect,
          399
      for tinnitus, 399
    therapeutic applications of, 397–400
    for upper motor neuron disorders, 1486
Transcription, 649, 650f, 651t
Transcriptional dysregulation, 1344
Transcriptome, 651t
Transesophageal echocardiography (TEE), for
      threatened stroke, 952
Transformed migraine, 1707
Transforming growth factor beta (TGF-β)
    in CNS, 686
    in immune response, 682, 683t
Transient amnesia, 63
Transient cortical blindness, 159
Transient global amnesia (TGA), 926
    versus epilepsy, 1590
Transient ischemic attacks (TIAs), 925–927
    ABCD2 score for, 925, 926t
    from atherothromboembolism, 927
    carotid, 925–926, 926b
    defined, 925
    differential diagnosis of, 927
    differential diagnosis of, *versus* epilepsy,
        1590
    drop attacks due to, 18–19, 926–927
    EEG of, 356
    essential investigations for, 949–953, 950b
      cardiac evaluation as, 951–952
      cerebral angiography for, 952–953, 952f
      neuroimaging as, 950
    microemboli in retinal arterioles in, 927
    monoplegia due to, 268
      differential diagnosis of, 272.e1, 272.e1t
    neuroepidemiology of, 637
    as risk factor for stroke, 923, 925
    with subclavian steal syndrome, 926
    transient global amnesia due to, 926
    treatment of, 927
    vertebrobasilar, 925–926, 926b
    vertigo due to, 595
Transient monocular visual loss (TMVL),
      158–159, 159b
    in bright light, 159
    due to amaurosis fugax, 158
    due to angle-closure glaucoma, 158
    due to retinal artery vasospasm, 158
    due to Uhthoff phenomenon, 159
    other causes of, 159
    transient visual obscurations as, 159
Transient neonatal myasthenia gravis
      (TNMG), 1910
Transient receptor potential vanilloid 4
      (TRPV4) channel, of nociceptor
      terminals, 296
Transient syndrome of headache with
      neurological deficits and CSF
      lymphocytosis, 1690
Transient visual obscurations, 159
Transitory hyperammonemia of newborn
      (THAN), 1336
Transjugular intrahepatic portosystemic
      shunt (TIPSS), encephalopathy related
      to, 1210
Translation, 650–652, 650f, 651t
Translocation, 654f
Translocator Protein (TSPO) ligand, in
      chemical imaging, 506
Transmissible diseases, ataxia due to,
      1462–1463
Transmissible spongiform encephalopathies
      (TSEs), 1365–1366

Transmodal areas, 94
Transmodal cortical areas, lesions of, 94
Transplantation strategies, for traumatic
      brain injury, 858–859
Transportin 3 deficiency, 1925
Transposition, in primary neurorrhaphy, 915
Transsexuals, hormone treatment in,
      ischemic stroke due to, 948
Transthoracic echocardiogram (TTE), for
      threatened stroke, 951–952, 952f
Transthyretin familial amyloid
      polyneuropathy, 1818.e4–1818.e5
Transverse magnetization, in MRI, 413,
      417.e1
Transverse myelitis, 1186
    hemiplegia due to, 266
    structural imaging of, 452–454, 454f
Trapezoid body, 585
TRAPPC11 deficiency, 1927
Trauma
    ischemic stroke due to, 937
    lumbosacral plexopathy and, 1789
    neurological complications, of drug abuse,
        1258
    plexus, monoplegia due to, 271
    and stroke in children, 999–1000
Traumatic aneurysms, 867
Traumatic brain hemorrhages, 975
Traumatic brain injury (TBI), 867–880
    basic mechanisms of, 855
      primary, 855
      secondary, 855
    basic neuroscience of, 850
    behavior and personality disturbances
        after, 90–91, 90t–91t
      anosognosia as, 90
      anxiety as, 91
      apathy as, 91
      depression as, 90–91
      personality change as, 91
    blood pressure management in, 753t,
        754
    cerebral perfusion pressure after, 872
    cerebrovascular dysregulation after, 872
    classification of, 867–872, 868t
      by injury severity, 868–869, 869b
      by mechanism, 867–868
      by morphology, 869–872
        contusions as, 869–870
        diffuse axonal injury as, 871–872,
            872f
        epidural hematoma as, 870, 871f
        intracranial injuries as, 869–872
        skull fractures as, 869
        subdural hematoma as, 870, 871f
        traumatic subarachnoid hemorrhage
            as, 870–871, 871f
    concussion as
      defined, 869
      postconcussion syndrome after, 869
    diffuse cerebral swelling after, 872
    due to blast injury, 867
    due to blunt injury, 867
    due to gunshot wounds, 867, 868f
    epidemiology of, 867
    evaluation of, 873
    experimental models of, 850–851
      acceleration concussion as, 851
      military, 851
      percussion concussion as, 850–851
      in vitro, 851
    functional outcomes with, 810t, 812
    future directions of, 859
    future of, 880
    Glasgow Coma Scale for, 868
    headache after, 1690

Traumatic brain injury (TBI) (*Continued*)
impact of, on sexual function, 631–632
primary, 631
secondary, 631
tertiary, 631–632
inflammation after, 872–873
late complications of, 879
mild, 527
diagnosis of, 869
epidemiology of, 868–869
mild, seizures due to, 1581
moderate, 526–527, 873
neuronal damage after, 851–855
axonal and dendritic, 853–854, 854*f*
gender in, 854–855
progressive, 852–853, 853*f*
secondary and repetitive, 853, 854*f*
selective neuronal vulnerability to, 852
temporal patterns of, 851–852, 852*f*
neuropsychological characteristics of,
526–527, 527*t*
in olfactory impairment, 193–194
outcome of, 879–880
pathophysiology of, 872–873
psychiatric manifestations of, 109–110
recovery of function after, 858–859
environmental enrichment for, 858
reparative and transplantation strategies
for, 858–859
rehabilitation for, 794
and sleep disturbances, 1659–1660
therapeutic interventions directed against
pathophysiological processes for,
856–857, 856*f*
antiapoptotic agents as, 857, 858*f*
free radical scavengers as, 856
glutamate antagonists as, 856
inflammation and, 857–858
neurotrophic factors as, 856
nitric oxide-related species as,
856–857
therapeutic hypothermia as, 857–858
treatment of, 873–879
for concussions, 873–874, 873*t*–874*t*
for diffuse injuries, 873–878
for focal injuries, 878–879
for increased intracranial pressure,
874
antiseizure prophylaxis in, 875*t*–876*t*
cerebral oxygenation in, 875*t*–876*t*
deep vein thrombosis prophylaxis in,
875*t*–876*t*
escalating protocol for, 874, 876*b*
guidelines for, 874–876, 875*t*–876*t*
hemodynamic management in,
877
high-dose barbiturates for, 877
hyperosmolar therapy in, 874, 876*b*
hyperventilation for, 876–877, 876*b*
hypothermia for, 877
monitoring, 875*t*–876*t*
multimodality monitoring in, 877
paralysis for, 877
infection prophylaxis in, 875*t*–876*t*
nutrition in, 875*t*–876*t*
steroids in, 875*t*–876*t*
vascular injury with, 867
Traumatic coma, prognosis for, 50
Traumatic injuries, in newborns
mechanical, 1968–1969
extracranial hemorrhage, 1968, 1969*t*
intracranial hemorrhage, 1968, 1968*t*
skull fractures due to, 1968–1969
spinal cord injury as, 1969

Traumatic injuries, in newborns (*Continued*)
of the peripheral nervous system,
1969–1970
brachial plexus injury as, 1969–1970,
1969*f*
facial paralysis as, 1969
Traumatic optic neuropathy, 161
Traumatic plexopathy, 1782
early management of, 1782
long-term management of, 1782
Traumatic radiculopathies, 1768–1772
disk herniation as, 1769–1772, 1769*f*
clinical features of, 1770–1771, 1770*f*
diagnosis of, 1771–1772, 1772*f*
treatment of, 1772
nerve root avulsion as, 1768–1769
clinical features and diagnosis of, 1768
treatment of, 1768–1769
Trazodone, for dystonia, 1452*t*
Treatment and Education of Autistic and
Related Communication-Handicapped
Children (TEACCH), 1306
Treatment-refractory depression (TRD), 113
T$_{reg}$. *see* Regulatory T cells (T$_{reg}$)
Tremblement affirmatif, 232–234
Tremblement negatif, 232–234
Tremor, 230–235, 1442–1445
cerebellar outflow (rubral, wing-beating,
midbrain, Holmes), 1444–1445
chin (hereditary geniospasm), 1445
classification and differential diagnosis of,
231*b*
clues in history, 232
common symptoms of, 230–232
deep brain stimulation for, 404
definition of, 404
due to fragile X premutation, 1445
essential, 1442–1444
diagnostic criteria for, 1443, 1443*b*
epidemiology and clinical features of,
1442–1443, 1443*f*
etiology of, 1443–1444
treatment of, 1444
examination of, 232–235, 232*b*–233*b*,
234*f*
functional, 1997–1998
in multiple sclerosis, treatment of,
1182
neuropathic, 1444
orthostatic, 1444
palatal, 1424–1425
with coma, 44
physiological, 1442
classification of, 1443*b*
types of, 218, 227, 231–232
in viral CNS disease, 1124*t*
writing, 1444
Tremor Research Group (TRG) Essential
Tremor Rating Scale (TETRAS), 1443
"Trench foot", 908–909
Treponema pallidum, meningitis due to,
1147–1148, 1148*t*
TRG Essential Tremor Rating Scale (TETRAS),
232–234, 232*b*–233*b*
TRG (Tremor Research Group) Essential
Tremor Rating Scale (TETRAS), 1443
TRH. *see* Thyrotropin-releasing hormone
(TRH)
Triamcinolone, for cluster headache
maintenance prophylaxis, 1710
Trichinella spiralis, 1155
CNS lesions due to, 1157
Trichinosis, 1155
myopathy due to, 1953

Trichloroethylene, occupational exposure to,
1241–1242
Trichopolydystrophy, 1888
Trichorrhexis nodosa, in kinky hair
syndrome, 1559
Trichothiodystrophy, 1560
Tricyclic antidepressants (TCAs), 111–112
for chronic pain, 723–725, 725*t*
for migraine prophylaxis, 1702–1703
in children and adolescents, 1719
menstrual, 1704
Trifluridine, for viral infections, 1127*t*
Trigeminal-autonomic cephalalgias (TACs),
1709, 1711–1713
Trigeminal ganglion
anatomy of, 1725, 1726*f*
clinical lesions of, 1727
Trigeminal motor root, anatomy of, 1725,
1726*f*
Trigeminal nerve, 1725–1727
anatomy of, 1721*f*, 1725, 1726*f*
clinical lesions of, 1725–1727
of subarachnoid space, 1725–1726
of trigeminal ganglion, 1727
of trigeminal nerve branches, 1727
of trigeminal nucleus, 1725
microvascular decompression of, for
short-lasting unilateral neuralgiform
headache attack, 1712
Trigeminal nerve branches
anatomy of, 1725
clinical lesions of, 1727
Trigeminal nerve stimulation, for epilepsy,
1610
Trigeminal neuralgia, 319*t*, 322, 735–736,
1716–1717, 1725–1726, 1726.e1*t*
cause of, 735
classic, 735–736, 1726
clinical symptoms, 1716
course and prognosis of, 1716
diagnosis of, 735–736
epidemiology of, 1716
Gasserian ganglion lesions for, 730–731,
731*f*
laboratory and radiological findings, 1716
pain in, 198–199
pathogenesis and etiology of, 1716
pathology of, 1716
physical findings in, 1716
symptomatic, 735–736
treatment of, 1716–1717
microvascular decompression for,
736
stereotactic radiosurgery for, 736
trigeminal radiofrequency rhizotomy
for, 736
trigger zone in, 1716
White and Sweet criteria for, 735–736,
736*b*
Trigeminal neuropathy, 1716
Trigeminal nucleus
anatomy of, 1725
clinical lesions of, 1725
modulation of afferent pain impulses into,
1686
Trigeminal nucleus caudalis (TNC), in
migraine, 1699
Trigeminal radiofrequency rhizotomy, 736
Trigeminal sensory neuropathy, in
connective tissue disorders, 1852.*e*2
Trigeminal sensory nucleus, anatomy of,
1725
Trigeminal sensory root, anatomy of, 1725,
1726*f*

Trigger areas, for trigeminal neuralgia, 735
Trigger factors, for trigeminal neuralgia, 735
Trigonocephaly, 1739t
Trihexiphenidyl
    for Parkinson disease, 1433t–1434t
Trihexyphenidyl
    for Parkinson disease, 1452t, 1454
Triiodothyronine (T₃), 112
TRIM32 mutations, 1926
Trimethobenzamide
    for migraine in children and adolescents,
        1719
    for Parkinson disease, 1433t–1434t
Triple flexion response, in coma, 46
Triplopia, 540
Triptans
    for headache associated with sexual
        activity, 1714
    and medication overuse headache, 1707
    for migraine, 1700–1701, 1700.e1t
Trisomy, 656
Trisomy 21, 656
    cognitive and behavioral problems in,
        1309t
Triterpene, in plants, 1250t
Trizivir (zidovudine + lamivudine +
    abacavir), for HIV infection, 1108t–1109t
Trochlear nerve, 1724–1725
    anatomy of, 1721f, 1724
    clinical lesions of, 1724–1725
        of cavernous sinus, 1725
        of orbital apex, 1725
        of subarachnoid space, 1725, 1725.e1f
        of trochlear nucleus and fascicle, 1724
        trochlear palsy as, 1724–1725, 1724f
Trochlear nerve fascicle, 1724
Trochlear nucleus, 1724
Trochlear palsy
    appearance of, 1724–1725, 1724f
    isolated, 1725
Trochleitis, headache due to, 1694
Trombone tongue, 237–238
Tropane (belladonna) alkaloids, in plants,
    1250t
Tropical ataxic neuropathy, 1864.e4
Tropical spastic paraparesis (TSP), 1487t,
    1488–1493
TRPV4 gene, in hereditary peripheral nerve
    disorders, 1532
Trudeau, Edward, 713
True kinetic (intention) tremor, 227
Truncal ataxia, 217
    gait disorders due to, 256
Truncal dystonia, pure, 1452–1453
Truncal neuropathy, 1842–1843, 1843f
Trunk posture, 253–254
Truvada (tenofovir + emtricitabine), for HIV
    infection, 1108t–1109t
Trypanosoma brucei, 1155
Trypanosomiasis, 1634
    sleep disorders in, 1671
Trypanosomiasis, African, 1155
Tryptophan hydroxylase, in chemical
    imaging, 505t
TS (test stimulation), in transcranial
    magnetic stimulation, 392, 392f
TSC1, in tuberous sclerosis, 1539
TSC2, in tuberous sclerosis, 1539
TSP (tropical spastic paraparesis), 1487t,
    1488–1493
TST. see Thermoregulatory sweat test
    (TST)
TTE (transthoracic echocardiogram), for
    threatened stroke, 952f
TTPA. see α-Tocopherol transfer protein
    (TTPA)

TTPA (α-tocopherol transfer protein) gene
    mutations, in ataxia with isolated
    vitamin E deficiency, 1467–1468
Tuberculosis (TB)
    of CNS, structural imaging for, 436.e2,
        436.e3f
    myopathy in, 1953
    of spine, 1760, 1761f
Tuberculous meningitis, 1148t, 1149
    headache due to, 1690
Tuberous sclerosis, 509, 1538–1543
    astrocytic hamartoma in, 178f
    in autism spectrum disorder, 1305
    and brain tumors, 1025t
    clinical features of, 1294t
    copy number variation in, 668t
    cutaneous features of, 1539
        confetti lesions as, 1539
        facial angiofibromas (adenoma
            sebaceum) as, 1539, 1540f, 1541t
        hypomelanotic macules (ash leaf spots)
            as, 1539, 1540f, 1541t
        poliosis as, 1539
        shagreen patch as, 1539, 1541t
    diagnostic criteria of, 1539b
    neurological features of, 1540–1541,
        1541f–1542f
        cortical dysplasia/tubers as, 1541t
        subependymal giant cell astrocytoma as,
            1541, 1542f
        subependymal nodules as, 1541t
    retinal features of, 1541–1542
    structural imaging of, 446.e2, 446.e4f
    subependymal giant cell astrocytoma with,
        1072
    systemic features of, 1542–1543
        cardiac, 1542
        pulmonary, 1543
        renal, 1542–1543
Tubular constriction, 582
Tufted cells, 190
Tullio phenomenon, 569–570, 592
Tumefactive multiple sclerosis, 1174, 1174f
Tumescence, 622
Tumor embolization, 780–782
    clinical evidence on, 782
    materials for, 781–782
    procedure for, 781–782, 781f–782f
    vessel selection for, 782
Tumor grading, 1028
Tumor immunology, 694
    paraneoplastic syndromes in, 694
Tumor immunosurveillance, 694
Tumor necrosis factor alpha (TNF-α), in
    immune response, 682, 683t
Tumor necrosis factor beta (TNF-β), in
    immune response, 683t
Tumor-reactive antibodies, 694
Tumor staging, 1028
Tumor vaccination, for brain tumors,
    1054–1055
Tumors
    hemiplegia due to, 265
    monoplegia due to, 268
    during pregnancy, 1982–1984
Tuning fork tests, for hearing loss, 591
Tunnels, in visual field, 576, 577f
Turbo spin echo techniques, 417.e1
Turcot syndrome, and brain tumors, 1024,
    1025t
Turner syndrome, 656
Turning, 254
Turning en bloc, 225–226
Tussive syncope, 12
Twin studies, of multiple sclerosis, 642
Twining line, in Chiari I malformation, 1741

Twitch convulsive syndrome, 1217
Tympanic membrane, examination of,
    591
Tympanosclerosis, 591
Typical ocular bobbing, 44
Tyrosinemia type I, 1331
Tyrosyl-DNA phosphodiesterase 1 (TDP1)
    mutation, ataxia due to, 1469
Tysabri (natalizumab), for multiple sclerosis,
    690, 1178

U
Ubiquitin-dependent proteasome
    proteolysis, 1427f
Ubiquitin-proteasomal dysfunction, 1345
UBOs (unidentified bright objects), in
    neurofibromatosis type 1, 1545–1546
Udd myopathy, 1933
UES (upper esophageal sphincter), in
    swallowing, 148
UFH. see Unfractionated heparin (UFH)
UFH (unfractionated heparin), for acute
    ischemic stroke, 956, 964
Uhthoff phenomenon, 1159–1160
    in multiple sclerosis, 1167
    visual loss due to, 159
Ulegyria, 1292
Ullrich congenital muscular dystrophy,
    1920t–1921t, 1930
    hypotonic infant due to, 313
Ulnar clawing, 1805
Ulnar groove syndrome, 1804–1805
Ulnar nerve
    applied anatomy of, 1804
    neuropathy of, monoplegia due to,
        270
    differential diagnosis of, 272.e2
Ulnar nerve entrapment, 1801t
    at elbow, 329, 1804–1806
    at wrist, 1806
Ulnar nerve pain, arm and neck pain due to,
    324
Ulnar neuropathy, sensory abnormalities due
    to, 319t, 321
Ultrasound, 476–485
    applications of, 480–485
        for acute ischemic stroke, 480
        for aneurysmal subarachnoid
            hemorrhage, 482–483, 483f
        for brain death, 483–484, 484f
        for cerebrovascular reactivity, 483
        for external stenotic lesions, 481–482
        for intracranial stenotic lesions, 482,
            482f
        for periprocedural monitoring,
            484–485, 484f
        for recent transient ischemic attack or
            stroke, 480–481
        for sickle cell disease, 483
    B-mode imaging, 477
        high-resolution, 478
            of atherosclerotic plaques, 478–479,
                478f
            of intima-media thickening,
                481–482
            of transient ischemic attack, 480–481
        carotid, 477–479, 478f–479f
    Doppler
        continuous-wave, 476–477
            microembolic signals in, 476–477
            of transient ischemic attacks, 481
        power, 477
            for high-grade stenosis, 479
            of transient ischemic attack, 480–481
        power motion-mode, 480

Ultrasound (*Continued*)
 pulsed-wave, 476–477
 transcranial, 480
  of acute ischemic stroke, 480
  and brain death, 484
  of cervical carotid stenosis, 481
  and increased ICP, 483–484, 484*f*
  of intracranial atherosclerotic plaque,
   482, 482*f*
  microembolic signals detected by, 481
  neurointensive care, 744*t*, 748
  of periprocedural monitoring, 484
  and thrombolytic agents, monitoring
   the effect of, 480
  of vasospasms, 483
 duplex, 477–478, 477*f*
  color flow, 477, 478*f*
  sensitivity of, 479
  transcranial color-coded, 480
  of transient ischemic attack, 480–481
 methods of, 476–477, 477*f*–478*f*
 for stroke in children, 1004
 techniques for, 477–480
 transcranial color-coded duplex, 480
 vertebral, 479–480
Ultrasound scan, for neurogenic bladder
  dysfunction, 613
Ultrastructural pathology, 1029
"Unconscious" mental processing, 58
Unconscious process, functional
  neuroimaging of, 503
Undershoot dysmetria, 549*f*
Unfolded protein response, 1346
Unfractionated heparin (UFH)
 for acute ischemic stroke, 956, 964
 during pregnancy, 1988
Ungual fibromas, in tuberous sclerosis,
  1539
Unidentified bright objects (UBOs), in
  neurofibromatosis type 1,
  1545–1546
Unified Parkinson's Disease Rating Scale
  (UPDRS), 1428
Unified Parkinson's Disease Rating Scale
  motor score (UPDRS-III), 402
Unilateral transverse lesion, 273–274
"Unilateral upper motor neuron" (UUMN)
  dysarthria, 145
Unimodal association areas, 94
Unimodal association cortex, 57
Uniparental disomy, 662–663, 662*f*
University of Pennsylvania Smell
  Identification Test (UPSIT), 192, 192*f*,
  194*f*
"Unresponsiveness wakefulness syndrome",
  54
Unverricht-Lundborg disease, 1579
Upbeat nystagmus, 545, 546*t*
UPDRS (Unified Parkinson's Disease Rating
  Scale), 1428
Upgaze, forced, 568
Upgaze paralysis, 568
Upgaze paresis, 206, 206*b*
Upper airway muscle tone, during sleep,
  1630*t*
Upper airway resistance, during sleep,
  1630*t*
Upper airway resistance syndrome, 1649,
  1649.*e*1, 1649.*e*1*f*
Upper and lower motor neuron disorders,
  1506–1518
Upper cervical spine lesion, 275–276
Upper esophageal sphincter (UES), in
  swallowing, 148

Upper extremities
 entrapment neuropathy of, 1801*t*
 mechanical and robotic-assistive devices
  for, 802
 mononeuropathies of, 1801–1808, 1801*t*
Upper extremity weakness, clinical
  presentation of
 distal, 281
 proximal, 280
Upper-limb motor involvement,
  polyneuropathies with predominantly,
  1796*b*
Upper limb orthoses, 790, 790*f*
Upper motor neuron (UMN) disorder, 381
Upper motor neuron lesions, needle
  electromyography of, 382*f*, 384
Upper motor neuron syndrome,
  neuromedical problems during
  rehabilitation for, 797–799
Upper motor neurons disorders, 1484–1494
 adrenomyeloneuropathy, 1487*t*,
  1493–1494
 due to plant excitotoxins, 1494
  Konzo as, 1487*t*, 1494
  lathyrism as, 1487*t*, 1494
 hereditary spastic paraplegia as, 1487–
  1488, 1487*t*, 1489*t*–1493*t*
  diagnosis of, 1488
  treatment of, 1488
 HTLV-1-associated myelopathy (tropical
  spastic paraparesis) as, 1487*t*,
  1488–1493
 HTLV-2-associated myelopathy (tropical
  spastic paraparesis) as, 1487*t*, 1493
 key characteristics of, 1487*t*
 laboratory evidence of, 1486
  MRS imaging in, 1486
  neuroimaging in, 1486
  transcranial magnetic stimulation in,
   1486
 neuroanatomy of, 1484–1494, 1485*b*
  brainstem control in, 1485
  corticospinal and corticobulbar tracts in,
   1484–1485
  limbic motor control in, 1485
  motor cortex, 1484–1485
 primary lateral sclerosis, 1486–1487
  diagnosis of, 1487
  key characteristics, 1487*t*
  treatment of, 1487
 signs and symptoms of, 1485–1486,
  1485*b*
  loss of dexterity as, 1485
  loss of muscle strength (weakness),
   1485
  pathological hyper-reflexia and
   pathological reflexes as, 1486
  pseudobulbar (spastic bulbar) palsy as,
   1486
  spasticity as, 1485–1486
 upper motor neurons, neuroanatomy of,
  1484–1485, 1485*b*
  brainstem control in, 1485
  corticospinal and corticobulbar tracts in,
   1484–1485
  limbic motor control in, 1485
  motor cortex, 1484–1485
Upper respiratory infections, 195
UPSIT (University of Pennsylvania Smell
  Identification Test), 192*f*, 194*f*
Uremic encephalopathy, 1217
 calcium and parathyroid hormone in,
  1217
Uremic encephalopathy, in children, 848

Uremic neuropathy, 1855–1856
 treatment of, 1856
Uremic optic neuropathy, 829
Urethral pressure profile, 614–615
Urethral sphincter muscles, neurological
  control of, 605, 606*f*
Urge syndrome, 612
Urgency-frequency syndrome, 612
Uric acid, in inborn errors of metabolism,
  1326*t*
Urinary flow meter, 613, 614*f*
Urinary incontinence
 after stroke, 608
 in amyloid neuropathy, 611–612
 in dementia, 608
 in hydrocephalus, 608
 in multiple sclerosis, 610
Urinary ketones, in inborn errors of
  metabolism, 1326*t*
Urinary problems, in viral CNS disease,
  1124*t*
Urinary retention, in young women, 612
 sphincter EMG for, 615–616
Urinary tract
 of autonomic disorders, 1871
 neurological control of, lower, 605–606,
  606*f*
Urinary tract infections (UTIs)
 in multiple sclerosis, 610
 screening for, 613
Urine, postvoid residual, 613*f*
Urodynamic studies, 613–615
 noninvasive, 613, 614*f*
 requiring catheterization, 613–615,
  614*f*
Uroflowmetry, 613, 614*f*
Uroneurophysiology, 615
UTIs (urinary tract infections)
 in multiple sclerosis, 610
 screening for, 613
Utricle, 584*f*, 585
UUMN (unilateral upper motor neuron)
  dysarthria, 145
Uveitis, with meningitis, 1764, 1764.*e*1*b*
Uveomeningitis syndromes, 1764
 versus viral nervous system disease, 1124*t*

V

V. *see* Variable (V) gene segment
V-pattern pretectal pseudobobbing, 551,
  551*t*
VABS-2 (Vineland Adaptive Behavior
  Scale-II), 1307
Vacuolar myelopathy (VM), HIV-associated,
  1117–1118
Vacuolation, 1365–1366
Vacuum constriction devices, for erectile
  dysfunction, 621
Vacuum device
 for erectile dysfunction, 633
 for sexual dysfunction in women, 633
Vagal nerve stimulation (VNS), for epilepsy,
  406
Vaginal lubrication, 624
Vagus nerve, 1732–1733
 anatomy of, 1732
 branches, clinical lesions of, 1733
 clinical lesions of, 1732–1733
  of nodose ganglion and jugular
   foramen, 1732–1733
  of vagus nerve branches, 1733
  of vagus nucleus, 1732
  vagus palsy due to, 1732

Vagus nerve stimulation
  for epilepsy, 1610
  treatment-refractory depression, 113
Vagus nucleus, clinical lesions of, 1732
Vagus palsy, 1732
Valacyclovir, for viral infections, 1127t
Valganciclovir, for viral infections, 1127t
Valosin-containing protein, 1441
Valproate
  for epilepsy
    absorption, elimination half-life,
      formulations of, 1600t
    efficacy by seizure type of, 1601t
    hepatic metabolism, enzyme induction/
      inhibition, pharmacokinetic
      interactions, and protein binding
      of, 1603t
    mechanism of action of, 1604t
  psychotropic effects of, 89t
Valproic acid
  for chronic pain, 725
  for migraine, 1703
  during pregnancy, 1985
Valsalva maneuver, 896–897
Vancomycin
  for brain abscess, 1151
  for meningitis, 1149–1150
Vanilloids, for neurogenic bladder, 619
Vardenafil, for erectile dysfunction, 621,
  621t, 632
Variable (V) gene segment, 679
Variably protease-sensitive proteinopathy
  (vPSPr), 1373
Variant Creutzfeldt-Jakob disease (vCJD),
  1376f
  current diagnostic criteria for, 1376t
  definitive diagnosis of, 1375
Variants
  common
    common disease with, 665f, 666
    and genome-wide association studies,
      663–665, 664f, 665b, 663.e1t–
      663.e2t, 664.e1b
  rare
    and candidate gene resequencing,
      665–666, 665f
    common disease with, 665f, 666
    defined, 665
Variation, common versus rare, 653–654
Varicella vaccine, 1129
Varicella-zoster immunoglobulin (VZIG),
  1131t
Varicella zoster virus (VZV)
  and brain tumors, 1023–1024
Varicella-zoster virus (VZV), 1128–1129
  Bell's palsy due to, 1730
  herpes zoster due to, 1128–1129
  primary infection with, 1128
  Ramsay Hunt syndrome due to, 1730
  and stroke in children, 1000
Varicella-zoster virus encephalitis, 1128
Varicella-zoster virus meningitis, 1128
Varicella-zoster virus vasculopathy, 1128
Variegate porphyria (VP), 1339–1340
  psychiatric manifestations of,
    103–104
Variola major, 1135.e1
Variola minor, 1135.e1
Vascular adhesion molecule-1 (VCAM-1), in
  HIV disease, 1106
Vascular cell adhesion molecule 1 (VCAM-
  1), in T-cell activation, 681
Vascular cognitive impairment, 521,
  1413–1417, 1415t
Vascular compression, and stroke in
  children, 999–1000

Vascular dementia, 492–493, 1413–1417,
  434.e1f
  behavior and personality disturbances in,
    80
    additional disorders in, 80
    depression as, 80
  behavioral and personality disturbances
    in, 101, 104.e1b
  clinical presentation of, 1414
  diagnostic criteria for, 1414
  epidemiology of, 1414
  functional neuroimaging of, 492–493
  large vessel stroke and, 1414
  mixed pathology of, 1416
  neuropsychological characteristics of,
    521–522
    clinical presentation of, 521–522
    memory problems in, 521–522
  neuropsychological testing and,
    1416–1417
  risk factors of, 1414
  subtypes of, 1414
  treatment of, 1417
Vascular endothelial growth factor (VEGF),
  inhibition of, for brain tumors,
  1053–1054, 1054b
Vascular endothelial growth factor (VEGF)
  receptor antagonists, for brain tumors,
  1054b
Vascular imaging, 459–485
  computed tomography angiography for,
    459–464
    accuracy of, 463
    applications of, 460–464
      for acute ischemic stroke, 461–462,
        461f–462f, 462b
      for brain death, 464
      for carotid and vertebral dissection,
        460
      for carotid artery stenosis, 460, 460f
      for cerebral aneurysms, 463–464,
        464f–465f
      for cerebral vascular malformations,
        464
      for cerebral venous thrombosis, 463
      in extracranial circulation, 460
      for intracerebral hemorrhage, 463
      in intracranial circulation, 461–464
      for intracranial stenosis, 462–463
    disadvantages of, 463
    limitations of, 459–460
      contrast-induced nephropathy as, 459
      metal artifacts as, 459–460
    methods of, 459
  magnetic resonance angiography for,
    464–476
    3T or greater, 466
    4D time-resolved, 466
    after stent placement, 469, 471f
    applications of, 467–476
      for acute ischemic stroke, 472
      for cerebral aneurysms, 472–473,
        472f–473f
      in extracranial carotid and vertebral
        circulation, 467–469, 467f
      in intracranial circulation, 469–476,
        471f
      in spine disorders, 476, 477f
      for subclavian steal syndrome,
        471–472
      for vascular malformations, 474–476,
        475f, 475t
      for venous disorders, 473–474
    of basilar artery stenosis, 469, 469f
    digital subtraction, 466
    of fibromuscular dysplasia, 469

Vascular imaging (Continued)
  limitations of, 466–467
    metal implant contraindications as,
      467
    nephrogenic systemic fibrosis as,
      466–467
    maximum intensity projection in, 466,
      468f
    methods of, 464–466, 466f
    phase-contrast, 464–466, 471–472
    three-dimensional contrast-enhanced,
      466, 468–471, 468f–471f
      of carotid artery dissection, 469,
        470f–471f
      of carotid stenosis, 468f
      fast, dynamic, or time-resolved, 466
      of vertebral artery dissection, 469,
        470f
    time-of-flight, 467–468, 467f
      of extracranial carotid and vertebral
        circulation, 467–469, 467f
  ultrasound for, 476–485
    applications of, 480–485
      for acute ischemic stroke, 480
      of aneurysmal subarachnoid
        hemorrhage, 482–483, 483f
      for brain death, 483–484, 484f
      for cerebrovascular reactivity, 483
      for external stenotic lesions,
        481–482
      for intracranial stenotic lesions, 482,
        482f
      for periprocedural monitoring,
        484–485, 484f
      for recent transient ischemic attack or
        stroke, 480–481
      for sickle cell disease, 483
    methods of, 476–477, 477f–478f
    techniques for, 477–480
      carotid, 477–479, 478f–479f
      transcranial color-coded duplex,
        480
      transcranial Doppler, 480
      vertebral, 479–480
Vascular injury, with traumatic brain injury,
  867
Vascular leakage, brain edema due to, 1267
Vascular malformations
  intracerebral hemorrhage due to,
    968–969, 969f
  MR angiography of, 474–476, 475f,
    475t
  seizures due to, 1582, 1582f
  spinal, 1010–1013
    classification of, 1010b
    clinical presentation and course of,
      1010–1011
    distribution and prevalence of, 1010,
      1011f
    investigations of, 1011–1012, 1012f
    treatment of, 1012–1013
  and stroke in children, 996, 1000
  structural imaging of, 447
Vascular parkinsonism, 1441
Vasculitides
  intracerebral hemorrhage due to,
    972–974
  neurological complications of, in adults,
    819–822
Vasculitis
  central nervous system, 1015–1017
    due to amyloid, 1017
    due to cutaneous herpes zoster
      infection, 1017
    due to drug abuse, 1017
    due to lymphoma, 1017

Vasculitis *(Continued)*
    isolated, 1015–1017
        approach to diagnosis of, 1016
        clinical findings in, 1015
        laboratory findings in, 1016
        pathology of, 1015–1016
        therapy for, 1016–1017
        types of, 1015
    lumbosacral plexopathy and, 1790
    of the nerve, 1192
Vasculopathy
    and stroke in children, 1000
    varicella-zoster virus, 1128
Vasoactive intestinal peptide,
    immunoregulatory effects of, 699*t*
Vasoactive intestinal polypeptide gene
    product, 697*t*–698*t*
Vasoconstriction
    reversible segmental cerebral, 1016
    reversible segmental cerebral, postpartum,
        1988–1989
Vasoconstriction, reversible cerebral
    segmental, ischemic stroke due to,
        944–945
Vasodepressor syncope, 11
Vasodilators
    for cerebral vasospasm, 994–995
    intra-arterial, for cerebral vasospasm,
        774–775
Vasopressin, 697*t*–698*t*, 707–708
    for diabetes insipidus, in neurointensive
        care, 755
    immunoregulatory effects of, 699*t*
Vasovagal syncope, 11
VCAM-1 (vascular adhesion molecule-1), in
    HIV disease, 1106
vCJD (variant Creutzfeldt-Jakob disease),
    1376*f*
    current diagnostic criteria for, 1376*t*
    definitive diagnosis of, 1375
Vecuronium, with induced hypothermia for
    cardiopulmonary arrest, 1204*b*
VEE (Venezuelan equine encephalitis), 1137*t*,
    1139
Vegetative state, 54
    decision-making and bioethics in, 56
VEGF (vascular endothelial growth factor),
    inhibition of, for brain tumors,
        1053–1054, 1054*b*
VEGF (vascular endothelial growth factor)
    receptor antagonists, for brain tumors,
        1054*b*
Velocardiofacial syndrome
    cognitive and behavioral problems in,
        1309*t*
    copy number variation in, 668*t*
Velocity storage, 552
VEMP (vestibular evoked myogenic
    potentials), 601
Venezuelan equine encephalitis (VEE), 1137*t*,
    1139
Venlafaxine, for neuropathic pain, 918*t*–919*t*
Venous angiomas, 447.*e*1
Venous disorders, MR angiography of,
    473–474
Venous infarction, spinal cord infarction due
    to, 1009–1010
Venous occlusion, cerebral edema due to,
    1270, 1271*f*
Venous sinus thrombosis, 434–435, 435*f*
Venous stroke, structural imaging for, 434.*e*2,
    434.*e*3*f*
Ventilation, adequate, for neonatal hypoxic-
    ischemic brain injury, 1961

Ventilatory assistance, in neurointensive care,
    750–752
Ventral posterolateral (VPL) nucleus, in pain
    pathway, 721
Ventral root, 1767, 1767*f*
Ventral stream, 552
    in visual system, 58
Ventralis intermedius (VIM) nucleus, 404
    deep brain stimulation, for tremor, 403*t*,
        404
Ventricular drainage, for intracerebral
    hemorrhage, 982
Ventricular fibrillation, syncope due to,
    10–11
Ventricular monitoring, of intracranial
    pressure, 745–746
Ventricular region tumors, structural imaging
    of, 418*t*–419*t*
Ventricular system, tumors in, headache due
    to, 1687
Ventricular tachycardia, syncope due to,
    10–11
Ventriculitis
    cytomegalovirus, 1129*f*
    due to neonatal meningitis, 1965, 1966*f*
Ventriculoencephalitis, cytomegalovirus,
    1114–1115
Ventriculomegaly
    in Alzheimer disease, 1417–1418
    from radiation therapy, 1087
Ventriculoperitoneal shunt, for normal-
    pressure hydrocephalus, 1277–1278
Ventriculostomy, for intracerebral
    hemorrhage, 982
Ventrolateral pattern generator, in
    swallowing, 149
Ventrolateral periaqueductal gray matter
    (vlPAG), 1624.*e*1
Ventrolateral preoptic (VLPO)
    in NREM sleep, 1625
    in wakefulness, 1625
Ventromedial nucleus, in appetite, 700, 701*f*
Verapamil
    for cluster headache maintenance
        prophylaxis, 1710
    for migraine prophylaxis, 1702
Verbal auditory agnosia, in autism spectrum
    disorder, 1302–1303
Verbal fluency, in Alzheimer disease, 1388
Verbal memory tests, 513
Vergence system, 553
Vermal aplasia, selective, 1300.*e*2
Verner-Morrison syndrome, due to
    autonomic disorders, 1890
Vernet syndrome, 1722*t*, 1731–1733
Verocay bodies, 1028, 1041
Versions, 571
    in diplopia, 535, 535*f*
Versive manifestation, of seizures, 1564,
    1564.*e*1*f*
Vertebral artery, 479–480, 1007.*e*1*f*
    aneurysm, imaging of, 986*f*
    CTA of, 459
Vertebral artery disease, neurointerventional
    therapy for, 767, 768*f*
Vertebral artery dissection
    CE-MRA of, 469, 470*f*
    CT angiography of, 460
    headache due to, 1692, 1692.*e*1*f*
    MR angiography of, 469, 470*f*
Vertebral artery occlusion, headache due to,
    1692, 1692.*e*1*f*
Vertebral artery stenosis, MR angiography of,
    467–468

Vertebral artery stroke, caused by cervical
    osteoarthritis, 1754–1755
Vertebral bodies, degenerative changes of,
    456–457
Vertebral compression fractures, due to
    osteoporosis, 1749, 1749*f*
Vertebral corpectomies, for spinal cord
    compression, 1094
Vertebral metastases, structural imaging of,
    449, 450*f*
Vertebral osteomyelitis
    granulomatous, 1760–1761, 1761*f*
    pyogenic, 1759–1760, 1760*f*
Vertebral ultrasonography, 479–480
Vertebral venous plexus, 1007.*e*2
Vertebrobasilar insufficiency, drop attacks
    due to, 18
Vertebrobasilar system syndromes, 929–931,
    929*f*, 930.*e*1*f*
Vertebroplasty, 729*t*
    in spinal cord injury, 895
Vertex sharp waves, sleep staging, 1619*f*
Vertical compression fractures, 888–889
Vertical diplopia, 532–533, 534*b*
    three-step test for, 538–539, 538*f*, 539*b*
Vertical gaze
    disorders of, 567–570, 569*f*
    impaired, 568
Vertical gaze ophthalmoplegia, combined,
    205–206, 206*b*
Vertical nystagmus, with coma, 44
Vertical pendular nystagmus, 544
Vertical suspension, in hypotonic infant,
    305–306, 306*f*
Vertigo
    benign paroxysmal, 1719
    causes, 591–594
        central nervous system disorders, 587*t*,
            592–593
            brainstem or cerebellar ischemia/
                infarction as, 587*t*, 592–593
            epilepsy as, 587*t*, 593
            multiple sclerosis as, 587*t*, 593
            neurodegenerative disorders as, 587*t*,
                593
            posterior fossa structural
                abnormalities as, 587*t*, 593
        inherited, 587*t*, 593–594
            familial bilateral vestibulopathy, 587*t*,
                594
            familial hearing loss and vertigo as,
                594
            migraine as, 587*t*, 593–595
        peripheral vestibular disorders, 587*t*,
            591–592
            benign paroxysmal positional vertigo
                as, 587*t*, 591
            Meniere disease as, 587*t*, 591–592
            other, 592
            vestibular fistulae as, 587*t*, 592
            vestibular neuritis as, 587*t*, 591
            vestibular paroxysmia as, 587*t*,
                592
    common presentations of, 595–596
        acute severe, 595
        recurrent attacks of, 595
        recurrent positional, 595–596
    definition, 583
    due to multiple sclerosis, 1165
    epidemiology of, 584
    and gait, 255–256
    historical background of, 583–584,
        587*t*
    history of present illness with, 586

Vertigo (*Continued*)
  laboratory investigations in diagnosis and
      management, 598–603
    general tests, 598
    imaging in, 598
    vestibular testing, 598–601
      bithermal caloric testing, 599
      eye movement recording for, 598
      eye movement subtests for, 598
      posturography for, 601
      quantitative head-thrust testing for,
          601
      recording pathological spontaneous
          eye movements for, 598
      rotational testing, 600, 600*f*
      vestibular evoked myogenic potentials
          for, 601
      visual ocular motor control for,
          598–599, 599*f*
  management of, 603–604
    symptomatic treatment of, 603–604,
        603*t*
    treatments of specific disorders, 603
  physical examination of, 586–591
    general medical examination, 586
    general motor examination, 586
    general neurological examination, 586
    neuro-otological examination, 587–591
      auditory examination, 591
      fistula testing, 591
      of gait, 591
      gaze testing, 588
      ocular motor, 587–588
        optokinetic nystagmus and fixation
            suppression of the vestibulo-
            ocular reflex, 588
        positional testing, 589–591, 590*f*
        saccades, 588
        smooth pursuit, 588
        vestibular nerve examination,
            588–589, 589*f*
  positional
    benign paroxysmal, 583, 589–590
      treatment of, 589–590
    recurrent, 584, 595–596
  recurrent, 584
    positional, 595–596
  structural imaging for, 458.e4–458.e5
Very long-chain fatty acids (VLCFAs)
  in adrenomyeloneuropathy, 1493–1494
  for inborn errors of metabolism, 1335
Vesicular cholinergic transporter, in chemical
    imaging, 505*t*, 506
Vesicular eruption, in viral CNS disease,
    1123*t*
Vesicular monoamine transporter type 2
    (VMAT2), in chemical imaging, 505,
    505*t*
  of Parkinson disease, 506–507, 507*f*
Vestibular aqueduct, enlarged, vertigo due to,
    594
Vestibular bulbs, 624
Vestibular cortex, in horizontal eye
    movements, 556
"Vestibular drop attacks", 19
Vestibular evoked myogenic potentials,
    601
Vestibular eye movement subsystem, 552
Vestibular fistulae, dizziness due to, 587*t*,
    592
Vestibular imbalance, and gait, 255–256
Vestibular nerve examination, 588–589,
    589*f*
Vestibular neuritis, 585, 587*t*, 591, 595
  treatment of, 603
Vestibular nystagmus, 544

Vestibular-ocular reflex (VOR), 219
Vestibular ototoxicity, 592
Vestibular paresis formula, 599
Vestibular paroxysmia, 585, 587*t*, 592
  treatment of, 603
Vestibular responses, in toxic and metabolic
    encephalopathies, 1209
Vestibular schwannomas, 592, 596–597
Vestibular system
  at birth, 560
  in horizontal eye movements, 555–556
Vestibular testing, 598–601
  bithermal caloric testing, 599
  eye movement recording for, 598
  eye movement subtests for, 598
  posturography for, 601
  quantitative head-thrust testing for, 601
  recording pathological spontaneous eye
      movements for, 598
  rotational testing, 600, 600*f*
  vestibular evoked myogenic potentials for,
      601
  visual ocular motor control for, 598–599,
      599*f*
Vestibule, 584–585, 584*f*
Vestibulo-ocular reflex (VOR), 583
  fixation suppression of, 588
Vestibulocerebellum, 558
Vestibulopathy, bilateral, familial, 587*t*,
    594
Veteran's Administration CSP 468 Study
    Group, 402
Veterans Administration (VAH) Trial of
    Carotid Endarterectomy in Symptomatic
    Carotid Stenosis, 961
Veterans Affairs Asymptomatic Carotid
    Endarterectomy Trial, 961–962
VGCCs (voltage-gated calcium channels),
    1521
  in repetitive nerve stimulation, 387
VGKC (voltage-gated potassium channels),
    1519–1521, 1522*f*
VHL gene
  in hemangioblastoma, 1043
  in von Hippel-Lindau syndrome, 1550
Viagra (sildenafil)
  for erectile dysfunction, 620–621, 621*t*
  for sexual dysfunction, in multiple
      sclerosis, 1183
  for sexual dysfunction in women, 621
Vibration, effects of, 1246
Vibratory phase, of generalized tonic-clonic
    seizures, 1570–1571
Vibrostimulation
  for ejaculation disorders, 633
  for sexual dysfunction in women, 633
"Victory sign", 228–230
Video-EEG monitoring, for seizures, 1595
Video image, time-locked digitally recorded,
    in EEG, 351
Video-nystagmography (VNG), 598
Video polysomnographic study, 1675,
    1676*f*
Video polysomnography, for encephalitis
    with antibodies to IgLON5, 1200
Videocystometry, 614
Videoendoscopy, for dysphagia, 157
Videomanofluorometry, for dysphagia, 157
Videx (didanosine), for HIV infection,
    1108*t*–1109*t*
Vietnam Head Injury Study (VHIS), 1581
Vigabatrin
  for epilepsy
    absorption, elimination half-life,
        formulations of, 1600*t*
    efficacy by seizure type of, 1601*t*

Vigabatrin (*Continued*)
    hepatic metabolism, enzyme induction/
        inhibition, pharmacokinetic
        interactions, and protein binding
        of, 1603*t*
    mechanism of action of, 1604*t*
  psychotropic effects of, 89*t*
Villaret syndrome, 1722*t*, 1731–1733
Villous adenoma, due to autonomic
    disorders, 1890
VIM (ventralis intermedius) nucleus deep
    brain stimulation, for tremor, 403*t*, 404
Vinblastine, for brain tumors, 1052*t*–1053*t*
Vinca alkaloids
  for brain tumors, 1051, 1052*t*–1053*t*
  neuropathy due to, 1863–1864
Vincristine
  for brain tumor, 1052*t*–1053*t*
  complications of, 1048
Vineland Adaptive Behavior Scale-II
    (VABS-2), 1307
Viracept (nelfinavir), for HIV infection,
    1108*t*–1109*t*
Viral encephalitis, 1121–1146
  additional causes of, 1123*t*
  diseases that can mimic, 1121, 1124*t*
  due to adenovirus, 1133–1135
  due to arboviruses, 1136–1140, 1137*t*
    Banna virus as, 1139
    California serogroup of viruses as,
        1137*t*, 1139
    causing hemorrhagic fevers, 1145
      dengue as, 1145
      filoviruses (Ebola and Marburg
          viruses) as, 1145.*e1*
      yellow fever as, 1145
    Colorado tick fever virus as, 1137*t*, 1139
    equine encephalitis viruses as, 1137*t*,
        1139
    Japanese encephalitis virus as,
        1138–1139
    Murray Valley encephalitis virus as,
        1139.*e1*
    Powassan virus as, 1137*t*, 1139
    Rift Valley fever virus as, 1139.*e1*
    St. Louis encephalitis virus as, 1137*t*,
        1138
    tickborne encephalitis virus as, 1139.*e1*
    Toscana virus as, 1139–1140
    West Nile virus as, 1136–1138, 1137*t*
  due to arenaviruses, 1144–1145
  due to Australian bat lyssavirus, 1141.*e1*
  due to Chandipura virus, 1141.*e1*
  due to deoxyribonucleic acid viruses,
      1121–1135
  due to henipaviruses, 1144
    Hendra virus as, 1144.*e1*
    Nipah virus as, 1144
  due to hepatitis viruses, 1145–1146
  due to herpes simplex, structural imaging
      of, 436.*e3*–436.*e4*, 436.*e4f*
  due to herpesviruses, 1121–1132
    cytomegalovirus as, 1129–1130,
        1129*f*–1130*f*
    Epstein-Barr virus as, 1130–1132
    herpes B virus (cercopithecine
        herpesvirus 1) as, 1132.*e1*
    herpes simplex viruses type 1 and 2 as,
        1121–1128
      brain biopsy for, 1125, 1126*f*
      clinical presentations of, 1121
      CSF examination for, 1122–1125
      diagnosis of, 1122
      MRI for, 1125, 1126*f*
      PCR for, 1125, 1125*t*
      treatment of, 1125–1126

Viral encephalitis *(Continued)*
human herpesvirus type 6 as, 1132,
1132*f*
varicella-zoster virus as, 1128–1129
due to influenza, 1144
due to measles, 1141–1143, 1142*f*
due to mumps, 1143
due to non-polio enteroviruses,
1135–1136
due to orthopoxviruses, 1135.*e1*
monkeypox as, 1135.*e1*
smallpox as, 1135.*e1*
due to parvovirus, 1135
due to poliovirus, 1135
due to polyomaviruses (JC), 1132–1133
due to rabies, 1140–1141, 1140*f*
due to ribonucleic acid viruses, 1135–1146
due to rubella, 1143–1144
EEG of, 357–359
immunotherapy for, 1131*t*
other specific findings associated with,
1124*t*
primary causes of, 1122*t*
progressive multifocal
leukoencephalopathy and, 1132–
1133, 1134*f*
skin/mucous membrane findings
suggesting, 1123*t*
treatment and prophylaxis of, 1127*t*
Viral infections
and brain tumors, 1023–1024
immunotherapy of, 1131*t*
neonatal, 1966–1968
congenital rubella as, 1966, 1966*f*
cytomegalovirus as, 1967
herpes simplex as, 1967
human immunodeficiency virus as,
1967–1968
toxoplasmosis as, 1967
and neuropathy, 1864.*e1*–1864.*e4*
Viral meningitis, 1121–1146
additional causes of, 1123*t*
diseases that can mimic, 1121, 1124*t*
due to adenovirus, 1133–1135
due to arboviruses, 1136–1140, 1137*t*
Banna virus as, 1139
California serogroup of viruses as,
1137*t*, 1139
causing hemorrhagic fevers, 1145
Colorado tick fever virus as, 1137*t*, 1139
equine encephalitis viruses as, 1137*t*,
1139
Japanese encephalitis virus as,
1138–1139
Murray Valley encephalitis virus as,
1139.*e1*
Powassan virus as, 1137*t*, 1139
Rift Valley fever virus as, 1139.*e1*
St. Louis encephalitis virus as, 1137*t*,
1138
tickborne encephalitis virus as, 1139.*e1*
Toscana virus as, 1139–1140
West Nile virus as, 1136–1138, 1137*t*
due to arenaviruses, 1144–1145
due to Australian bat lyssavirus, 1141.*e1*
due to Chandipura virus, 1141.*e1*
due to coxsackievirus, 1136
due to deoxyribonucleic acid viruses,
1121–1135
due to Epstein-Barr virus, 1131
due to henipaviruses, 1144
due to hepatitis viruses, 1145–1146
due to herpes simplex virus, 1128
due to herpesviruses, 1121–1132

Viral meningitis *(Continued)*
cytomegalovirus as, 1129–1130,
1129*f*–1130*f*
Epstein-Barr virus as, 1130–1132
herpes B virus (cercopithecine
herpesvirus 1) as, 1132.*e1*
herpes simplex viruses type 1 and 2 as,
1121–1128
human herpesvirus type 6 as, 1132,
1132*f*
varicella-zoster virus as, 1128–1129
due to influenza, 1144
due to measles, 1141–1143, 1142*f*
due to mumps, 1143
due to non-polio enteroviruses,
1135–1136
due to orthopoxviruses, 1135.*e1*
due to parvovirus, 1135
due to poliovirus, 1135
due to polyomaviruses (JC), 1132–1133
due to rabies, 1140–1141, 1140*f*
due to ribonucleic acid viruses,
1135–1146
due to rubella, 1143–1144
immunotherapy for, 1131*t*
other specific findings associated with,
1124*t*
primary causes of, 1122*t*
progressive multifocal
leukoencephalopathy and, 1132–
1133, 1134*f*
skin/mucous membrane findings
suggesting, 1123*t*
treatment and prophylaxis of, 1127*t*
Viramune (nevirapine), for HIV infection,
1108*t*–1109*t*
Virchow-Robin spaces, 1266
dilated, structural imaging for, 446.*e8*,
446.*e10f*
Viread (tinofovir), for HIV infection,
1108*t*–1109*t*
Virtual reality training, in rehabilitation,
801–802
Vision
of autonomic disorders, 1868–1870
double, 2000
Visual acuity
best-corrected, 573–574
definition of, 573–574
examination of, 573–574, 575*f*
with homonymous hemianopia, 579
near, 574, 575*f*
Visual agnosia, 122–125
Balint syndrome and simultanagnosia as,
123
cortical visual distortions as, 123
cortical visual disturbances as, 122–123
Klüver-Bucy syndrome as, 125
optic aphasia as, 124–125
prosopagnosia as, 125
visual object, 123–124
apperceptive, 123–124, 124*f*
associative, 124
Visual allesthesia, 123
Visual attention, impaired, 123
Visual auras, 1696
Visual awareness, 58
Visual axis misalignment, 529–530,
531*f*
amblyopia due to, 529
clinical assessment of, 533–539
convergence in, 535–536
cover-uncover test in, 536–537, 537*f*
cross-cover test in, 537

Visual axis misalignment *(Continued)*
of ductions, 535*f*, 536
forced, 539, 539*b*
edrophonium (Tensilon) test, 539
fatigability in, 539
general inspection in, 534
of head posture, 534–535, 535*f*
Hess screen test in, 536
Hirschberg test in, 536, 537*f*
history in, 533–534
Lancaster red-green test in, 536
Maddox rod test in, 536, 537*f*
of ocular alignment and muscle balance,
536–537
pinhole test in, 533
red glass test in, 536, 536*f*
sagging eye syndrome in, 537–538
of sensory visual function, 535
of stability of fixation, 535
three-step test for vertical diplopia in,
538–539, 538*f*, 539*b*
versions (pursuit, saccades, and ocular
muscle overaction), 535, 535*f*
convergent eyes due to, 529–530
diplopia due to, 529, 531*f*, 532–533
in anisoiconia, 533
crossed, 529, 531*f*
uncrossed, 529, 531*f*
vertical, 532–533, 534*b*
three-step test for, 538–539, 538*f*,
539*b*
visual confusion with, 532, 533*f*
dissociated vertical deviation (divergence)
due to, 537
esotropia due to
causes of, 531*b*
defined, 529–530
uncrossed diplopia due to, 529, 531*f*
exotropia due to, 529, 531*f*
heterophorias due to, 529–541
heterotropias due to, 529–541
hypertropia due to, 529–530
hypotonia due to, 529–530
latent hypotonia due to, 530
physiological hyperdeviation due to,
529–530
related disorders to, 540–541
asthenopia as, 540
"interstate illusions" (highway
hallucinosis) as, 540
mal de débarquement as, 540
micropsia as, 540
monocular elevator deficiency (double
elevator palsy) as, 540
acquired, 568
oscillopsia as, 540
palinopsia as, 540–541, 541*f*
polyopia as, 540
superior oblique myokymia as, 541, 551
detection of, 551
versus monocular nystagmus, 545
treatment of, 546*t*, 551
tortopia as, 541
triplopia as, 540
strabismus
comitant, 529–530
nonconcomitant (incomitant, paralytic,
restrictive), 529–530
vertical, 529–530, 531*f*
Visual confusion, 532, 533*f*
Visual cortex, in visual pathways, 573,
574*f*
Visual distortions, cortical, 123
Visual disturbances, cortical, 122–123

Visual evoked potentials (VEPs), 579–581, 365.*e1*–365.*e3*, 365.*e1f*
  in neurological disease, 365.*e2*–365.*e3*, 365.*e3b*, 365.*e3f*
  for nonorganic visual field defects, 582
  normal, 365.*e1*–365.*e2*, 365.*e2f*
Visual field defects, 160*f*
  interpretation of, 577–579, 577*b*
    binasal hemianopia as, 578, 578*f*
    bitemporal hemianopia as, 578
    from chiasmal disease, 578, 578*f*
    from compressive optic neuropathy, 577, 578*f*
    homonymous hemianopia as
      congruous, 578–579, 579*f*
      cortical blindness, 579
      incongruous, 578*f*
      visual acuity with, 579
    inferior altitudinal, 577, 578*f*
    monocular temporal crescent syndrome, 578
    from nonarteritic anterior ischemic optic neuropathy, 577, 578*f*
    from optic neuritis, 577, 578*f*
    pseudobitemporal hemianopia, 578, 578*f*
    scotoma
      cecocentral, 577–578, 578*f*
      junctional, 578
  nonorganic (functional), 581–582, 581*b*
    diagnostic techniques, 581–582
    prognosis, 582
    visual field testing in, 582, 582*f*
Visual field deficits, in rehabilitation, 802
Visual field loss, in IIH, 1688
Visual field testing, 576–577, 577*f*
  Amsler grid in, 577, 577*f*
  confrontation testing for, 576
  funnels and tunnels in, 576, 577*f*
Visual hallucinations, in PDD, 523
Visual impairment, structural imaging for, 458.*e4*
Visual loss, 158–162
  monocular/partial, 2000, 2001*f*
  pattern of, 158
    central, 158, 159*f*
    peripheral, 158, 160*f*
    progressive, 161–162, 162*b*
  sudden
    with progression, 161, 162*b*
    without progression
      binocular, 161, 161*b*
      monocular, 159–161, 160*b*
  temporal profile of, 158–162
    sudden-onset, 158–161
  total, 2000
  transient
    binocular, 159, 160*b*
    monocular, 158–159, 159*b*
      in bright light, 159
      due to amaurosis fugax, 158
      due to angle-closure glaucoma, 158
      due to retinal artery vasospasm, 158
      due to Uhthoff phenomenon, 159
      transient visual obscurations as, 159
Visual migraine aura, 159
Visual object agnosia, 123–124
Visual obscurations, transient, 159
Visual ocular motor control, in vestibular testing, 598–599, 599*f*
Visual pathways, impairment of, in multiple sclerosis, 1165
Visual problems, due to brain tumor, 1046
Visual processing, in cortex, 552, 553*f*
Visual radiations, 574*f*

Visual-spatial-constructional tasks, 64
Visual symptoms
  ataxia and, 217
  functional, 2000, 2001*f*
Visual syndromes, 1194–1195
  clinical findings, 1194
  immune responses, 1195
  treatment of, 1195
  tumor association of, 1195
Visuospatial disturbances, in delirium, 26
Visuospatial learning disability
  in developmental coordination disorders, 1317*b*
  in nonverbal learning disability, 1315.*e1*
Vital signs, for headache, 200–201
Vitamin A, for viral infections, 1127*t*
Vitamin A deficiency, 1235
Vitamin A overdose, 1235
Vitamin A toxicity, 1235
Vitamin B$_6$, for inborn errors of metabolism, 1331.*e1t*
Vitamin B$_6$ deficiency, 1230–1231, 1852
Vitamin B$_{12}$
  biochemical reactions dependent on, 1226
  for inborn errors of metabolism, 1339
Vitamin B$_{12}$ deficiency, 1226–1228, 1853–1854
  causes of, 1226–1227
  clinical features of, 1227
  laboratory studies for, 1227–1228, 1227*b*, 1228*f*
  pathology of, 1228, 1228*f*
  psychiatric manifestations and, 103
  treatment of, 1228
Vitamin B$_{12}$ deficiency myelopathy, 1228, 1228*f*
Vitamin C, and brain tumors, 1023
Vitamin D, in multiple sclerosis, 688, 1163
Vitamin D deficiency, 1235
Vitamin E
  for Alzheimer disease, 1398
  and brain tumors, 1023
  defined, 1229
Vitamin E deficiency, 1229–1230, 1854
  ataxia with isolated, 1467–1468
  causes of, 1229*b*
  clinical features of, 1230
  laboratory studies of, 1230
  treatment of, 1230
Vitamin K deficiency, 1986
  and stroke in children, 999
Vitamin metabolism, disorders associated with, 1338–1339
Vitamins, and brain tumors, 1023
VLCFAs (very long-chain fatty acids)
  in adrenomyeloneuropathy, 1493–1494
  for inborn errors of metabolism, 1335
vlPAG (ventrolateral periaqueductal gray matter), in NREM sleep, 1624.*e1*
VLPO (ventrolateral preoptic) nucleus
  in NREM sleep, 1625
  in wakefulness, 1625
VM (vacuolar myelopathy), HIV-associated, 1117–1118
VMAT2 (vesicular monoamine transporter type 2), in chemical imaging, 505, 505*t*
  of Parkinson disease, 506–507, 507*f*
Voiding, neurological control of, 605, 606*f*
Voiding dysfunction, management of, 616–617
Volition, and movement, 262
Volitional movements, foot tapping leg rocking, 1652*b*
Voltage attenuation, on EEG, 350

Voltage-gated calcium channels (VGCCs), 1521
  in Lambert-Eaton syndrome, 1912–1913
  in repetitive nerve stimulation, 387
Voltage-gated ion channels, 1519
  α-subunits of, 1519
  open, closed and inactivated, 1519
  phenotypic heterogeneity affecting, 1519
  potassium, 1519–1521, 1522*f*
  sodium and calcium, 1521, 1523*f*
Voltage-gated potassium channels (VGKC), 1519–1521, 1522*f*
Volume depletion, in neurointensive care, 755
Volume expansion, in neurointensive care, 755
Volume flow rate
  of CCA, 479, 479*f*
  and transient ischemic attack, 480–481
Voluntary Control of Involuntary Utterance Program, 806
Voluntary nystagmus, 582
Vomiting
  cyclical, 1719
  due to brain tumor, 1047
von Gierke disease, 1332, 1337
von Graefe sign, 188
von Hippel-Lindau disease
  and brain tumors, 1025*t*
  hemangioblastoma in, 1043
  retinal angiomas in, 178
  structural imaging of, 446.*e2*
von Hippel-Lindau syndrome, 1548–1550
  Cambridge screening protocol for, 1550*b*
  molecular genetics of, 1550
  neurological features of, 1549, 1549*f*
  ocular features of, 1549
  systemic features of, 1549
  treatment of, 1550
von Willebrand factor, elevated, as risk factor for stroke, 924
VOR (vestibulo-ocular reflex), 583
  fixation suppression of, 588
Voriconazole, 1155
VP (variegate porphyria), 1339–1340
  psychiatric manifestations of, 103–104
VPS13A gene, in neuroacanthocytosis, 1448
vPSPr (variably protease-sensitive proteinopathy), 1373
VR (virtual reality) training, in rehabilitation, 801–802
VZV. *see* Varicella-zoster virus (VZV)

W
Waardenburg syndrome, vertigo due to, 594
Wada test, 526
  prior to epilepsy surgery, 1598
WAGR syndrome, copy number variation in, 668*t*
Wake after sleep onset, 1673
Wakefulness, 23, 1615
  neuroanatomical substrates for, 1623
Waldenström macroglobulinemia (WM), 1836–1837
  neurological complications of, 825
  peripheral neuropathy in, 1192
Walker-Warburg syndrome, 1929–1930
  clinical features of, 1294*t*
  hypotonic infant due to, 310
  lissencephaly in, 1286*f*, 1300.*e1*–1300.*e2*
Walkers, in rehabilitation, 787
Walking
  associated and synergistic limb movements while, 254
  slowness of, 251

Wallenberg syndrome, 930, 1722*t*, 1725, 1732
 vertigo due to, 592–593
Wallerian degeneration, 906, 906*f*, 1792
 ischemic stroke with, 432, 433*f*
Wall-eyed bilateral internuclear ophthalmoplegia (WEBINO) syndrome, 567
Warfarin
 for antiphospholipid antibody syndrome, 947
 with atrial fibrillation, 815
 intracerebral hemorrhage due to, 971, 980
 during pregnancy, 1989–1990
 for preventing stroke recurrence, 954–955
 for stroke, in children, 1005–1006
Warfarin-Aspirin Recurrent Stroke Study trial, 947
Warm-up phenomenon, in myotonia congenita, 1526
Wartenberg sign, 1805
Warts, brain, 1287
Water balance, 1222*f*
Water drinking, for autonomic disorders, 1892
Water hemlock, neurotoxins from, 1249–1250
Water metabolism, encephalopathy due to disorders of, 1221–1225
Water molecules, as basis for magnetic resonance imaging, 1265
Watershed ischemic stroke, structural imaging for, 432.*e*1
Watershed ischemic syndromes, 931
Watershed zones, fetal, 1292
Watson, James, 57
Weakness, treatment of, 715–716
Wearing off, in Parkinson disease, 1435
Weber syndrome, 929–930, 1721, 1722*t*
Weber test, for hearing loss, 591
WEBINO (wall-eyed bilateral internuclear ophthalmoplegia) syndrome, 567
Wegener's granulomatosis, neurological complications of, in children, 840–841
Weighted gene coexpression network analysis (WGCNA), 670*f*
Weighted genetic risk score (wGRS), for multiple sclerosis, 1163
Weir Mitchell, Silas, 903
Weir Mitchell disease, 1531–1532
Weisenberg syndrome, due to autonomic disorders, 1890
Welander myopathy, 1933
 arm weakness in, 290
Werdnig-Hoffmann disease, 1500, 1501*f*
 clinical features of, 1500–1502
 leg weakness in, 290–291
Wernicke, Carl, 1231–1232
Wernicke aphasia, 59, 129*f*, 132–133, 133*t*, 134*f*–135*f*
 versus delirium, 32, 32*t*
Wernicke area, 129*f*
Wernicke encephalopathy, 1218, 1232, 1232*b*
 laboratory studies for, 1232
 in pregnancy, 1981
 structural imaging of, 444.*e*1, 444.*e*1*f*
 treatment of, 1233
Wernicke-Korsakoff syndrome, 1231–1233
 amnestic syndrome and, 62–63
 associated conditions in nonalcoholic patients with, 1232*b*

Wernicke-Korsakoff syndrome (*Continued*)
 laboratory studies for, 1232
 pathology of, 1232, 1232*f*
 treatment of, 1233
West Haven Scale, for hepatic encephalopathy, 1210
West Nile fever (WNF), 1137, 1498
West Nile virus (WNV), 1136–1138, 1137*t*, 1498
 neuroepidemiology of, 645.*e*1
West Nile virus motor neuronopathy, 1864.*e*4
West syndrome, 1573
 EEG for, 352, 353*f*
Western blot, of muscle biopsy, 1919
Western equine encephalitis, 1137*t*
Western Pacific Amyotrophic Lateral Sclerosis, 1516–1517
Wet keratin, in adamantinomatous craniopharyngioma, 1043
WGCNA. *see* Weighted gene coexpression network analysis (WGCNA)
wGRS (weighted genetic risk score), for multiple sclerosis, 1163
Wheelchairs, in rehabilitation, 787, 787*b*
Whiplash injury, neck pain due to, 330
Whipple disease (WD)
 ataxia due to, 1463
 excessive sleepiness due to, 1633–1634
 neurological complications of, 828, 829*f*
 oculomasticatory myorhythmia in, 544
Whisper test, for hearing loss, 591
White epidermoid, 446.*e*7
White matter disease
 inflammatory, 436
 microvascular, 432–434, 434*f*
 clinical significance, 433
White matter hyperintensity, in vascular dementia, 1416
White matter lesions, structural imaging of, 446.*e*2
WHO (World Health Organization), tumor classification system of, 1027, 1027*t*
Whole-brain dynamic time-resolved CTA, 462
Whole-brain radiotherapy (WBRT), for brain metastases, 1086, 1089
 after surgical resection, 1088
 following radiosurgery, 1090
 recurrent, 1091
 with stereotactic radiosurgery, 1090
 toxicity of, 1087
Wilhelmsen-Lynch disease, 1441
Williams-Beuren syndrome, copy number variation in, 668*t*
Williams myopathy, 1934
Williams syndrome
 cognitive and behavioral problems in, 1309*t*
 visuospatial difficulties in, 1315.*e*2
Wilms tumor, and brain tumors, 1024
Wilson disease, 1326, 1454–1455, 1328.*e*1*t*–1328.*e*2*t*
 clinical features, 1454–1455
 clinical features of, 1454–1455
 dysphagia in, 154–155
 Kayser-Fleischer rings in, 103, 1454
 pathogenesis, 1455
 pathology, 1455
 in pregnancy, 1981
 psychiatric manifestations of, 103
 structural imaging of, 444.*e*1
 treatment, 1455
Wind-up phenomenon, 722

Windowing, 411, 412*f*
Wine, port-wine, in Sturge-Weber syndrome, 1546, 1547*f*
"Wing-beating position", 227
Wing-beating tremor, 218
Wingspan stent, for intracranial arterial stenosis, 766, 766*f*
WINGSPAN study, 963.*e*1
Wireless sensing devices, in rehabilitation, 804
WM (Waldenström macroglobulinemia), peripheral neuropathy in, 1192
WNF (West Nile fever), 1137, 1498
WNT1 gene, 1298
WNV. *see* West Nile virus (WNV)
Wolff-Parkinson-White syndrome, syncope due to, 10–11
Wolman disease, 1333.*e*2*t*–1333.*e*3*t*
Women's Estrogen for Stroke Treatment study, 924
Woodhall, Barnes, 903
Word-finding difficulty, 2002
"Word salad", 130
Work, return to, concussion and, 863
Working memory, 60, 61*t*
 in Alzheimer disease, 1380
Working memory network, 94
World Health Organization (WHO), tumor classification system of, 1027, 1027*t*
"Worst ever" headache, 197
Wrist
 pain in, 331
 tendonitis of, 331
Writer's cramp, 1452–1453
Writing
 assessment of, 131
 neurolinguistic model of, 140*f*
Writing disturbance, in delirium, 26, 26*f*
Writing tremor, 1444
Wrong-way eyes, 565
Wyburn-Mason disease, retinal findings, 178, 178*f*

X

X chromosome, 658–659
X chromosome inactivation, skewed, in Kennedy disease, 1505
X-linked adrenoleukodystrophy, genetics and paradox of disease definition, 671–672
X-linked ataxias, 1479
X-linked Charcot-Marie-Tooth disease (CMTX), 1816
X-linked copper deficiency, 1888
X-linked cutis laxa, 1559
X-linked disorders, 658–659, 660*f*
X-linked dystonia-parkinsonism, 1453–1454
X-linked dystrophies, 1920*t*–1921*t*
X-linked intellectual disability (XLID), 1307
X-linked recessive lissencephaly, with abnormal genitalia, 1300.*e*2
X-linked spinal muscular atrophy, hypotonic infant due to, 311
X-ray exposure, and brain tumors, 1021
X-rays, hard, 411
Xanthoastrocytoma, pleomorphic, 1075
 management of, 1055–1056, 1056*f*
 pathology and molecular genetics of, 1034
 structural imaging of, 418*t*–419*t*, 419.*e*1
Xanthoma, in cerebrotendinous xanthomatosis, 1557

Xanthomatosis, cerebrotendinous, 1338,
    1557–1558
  clinical features of, 1557b
  neurological features of, 1557
  treatment of, 1557–1558
  xanthomas in, 1557
Xenon-133, in neurointensive care, 744t, 747
Xeroderma pigmentosum (XP), 1560–1562
  ataxia in, 1469
  complementation groups of, 1560
  cutaneous and ocular features of, 1561,
    1561b
  related syndromes of, 1560
  treatment of, 1561–1562
XLID (X-linked intellectual disability), 1307
XPCC gene, in xeroderma pigmentosum,
    1560

Y

Y chromosomes, 658–659
Yellow fever, 1145

Yohimbine, for ejaculation dysfunction, 621
Yolk sac tumor, 1042
Young adult-onset ataxia, due to metabolic
    disorder, 1470, 1470t

Z

Zalcitabin (ddC, Hivid), for HIV infection,
    1108t–1109t
Zaleplon, 1681
Zanaflex. see Tizanidine
Zanamivir, for viral infections, 1127t
Z-disc-derived bodies, in myofibrillar
    myopathy, 1927
ZDS (Zung Depression Scale), 76t
Zeitgeber, 1625–1626
Zellweger syndrome, 1326.e1t–1326.e2t
Zerit (stavudine), for HIV infection,
    1108t–1109t
Ziagen (abacavir), for HIV infection,
    1108t–1109t
Ziconotide, for pain, 734

Zidovudine
  for HIV infection, 1108t–1109t
  myopathy due to, 1120
Zolmitriptan
  for cluster headaches, 1710
  for migraine, 1701t, 1700.e1t
    menstrual, 1704
Zomig, for migraine, 1701t
Zonisamide
  for chronic pain, 726
  for epilepsy
    absorption, elimination half-life,
        formulations of, 1600t
    efficacy by seizure type of, 1601t
    hepatic metabolism, enzyme induction/
        inhibition, pharmacokinetic
        interactions, and protein binding
        of, 1603t
  mechanism of action of, 1604t
Zung Depression Scale (ZDS), 76t
Zygomatic nerve, 1726f
Zygomycosis, 1154t